$\mathcal{P}$ATHOLOGY *of the* HUMAN PLACENTA

Third Edition

$\mathcal{P}$ATHOLOGY
of the HUMAN
PLACENTA
Third Edition

Kurt Benirschke

Peter Kaufmann

With 642 Illustrations

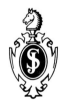

Springer-Verlag
New York Berlin Heidelberg London Paris
Tokyo Hong Kong Barcelona Budapest

Kurt Benirschke, MD
Professor of Pathology and Reproductive Medicine
University of California, San Diego
University Medical Center
San Diego, California 92103-8321, USA

Professor Dr. med. Peter Kaufmann
Institut für Anatomie der Medizinischen Fakultät
Rheinisch-Westfälische Technische Hochschule Aachen
52057 Aachen, Germany

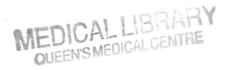
Library of Congress Cataloging-in-Publication Data
Benirschke, Kurt.
    Pathology of the human placenta / Kurt Benirschke, Peter Kaufmann.
    3rd ed.
      p.   cm.
    Includes bibliographical references and index.
    ISBN 0-387-94335-8. — ISBN 3-540-94335-8
    1. Placenta—Diseases. I. Kaufmann, Peter, 1942– . II. Title.
    [DNLM: 1. Placenta—pathology. WQ 212 B467p 1995]
RG591.B38   1995
618.3′4—dc20
DNLM/DLC
for Library of Congress   94-25783

Printed on acid-free paper.

Production coordinated by Chernow Editorial Services, Inc. and managed by Laura Carlson; manu-
facturing supervised by Jacqui Ashri.
Typeset by Best-set Typesetter Ltd, Hong Kong.
Printed and bound by Edwards Brothers, Ann Arbor, MI.
Printed in the United States of America.

9 8 7 6 5 4 3 2 1

ISBN 0-387-94335-8 Springer-Verlag New York Berlin Heidelberg
ISBN 3-540-94335-8 Springer-Verlag Berlin Heidelberg New York

Preface

Most obstetricians and pediatricians would agree that examination of the placenta often helps to explain abnormal neonatal outcome. As early as in 1892 Ballantyne wrote that:

A diseased foetus without its placenta is an imperfect specimen, and a description of a foetal malady, unless accompanied by a notice of the placental condition, is incomplete. Deductions drawn from such a case cannot be considered as conclusive, for in the missing placenta or cord may have existed the cause of the disease and death. During intrauterine life the foetus, the membranes, the cord and the placenta form an organic whole, and disease of any part must react upon and affect the others.

Similar thoughts were succinctly detailed in Price's 1950 discussion of his concept of "prenatal biases" as they affected twins. His contribution admonished us that placental study is a sine qua non for a more perfect understanding of fetal development. Despite this understanding of our past, there is still great resistance to performing the task of placental examination routinely. For many pathologists, therefore, the placenta has remained a mysterious organ.

In 1967 Shirley G. Driscoll and I (K.B.) wrote the chapter on placental pathology for the *German Handbook of Pathology*, the *Henke-Lubarsch*. Because there seemed to be a need for wider dissemination of the text, it was reprinted by Springer-Verlag New York; it soon became unavailable. Since then several books on placental pathology have been written in French, English, and German (Fox, 1978; Perrin, 1984; Philippe, 1986; Baldwin & Lavery, 1987; Becker & Röckelein, 1989; Naeye, 1992; Vogel, 1992; Baldwin, 1994), and much more interest has been accorded this so readily available but poorly studied organ. A journal (*Placenta*) has appeared. Regular "Trophoblast Conferences" have been held in Rochester, N.Y.; and European and international meetings have been organized. Much other new information has been obtained, and the enigma of placental nonrejection has been tackled by numerous investigators. In addition, the availability of the placenta for biochemical study has stimulated many cell biologists and molecular biologists to use this organ as a convenient source of human tissue. Genetic information is currently being gathered.

The decision to rewrite the original text to create the second edition was made in 1989 because of the large amount of newly created knowledge, the fact that the placenta had become a focal point of litigation in regard to cerebral palsy and fetal death, and because the anatomic pathologist performing surgical pathological diagnosis still had problems when faced with the task of having to undertake a decisive examination of this organ. Moreover, I (K.B.) had continued to collect material and had the good fortune to be associated with many inquiring minds. Pathologist Marjorie Grafe, dysmorphologists Drs. Kenneth L. Jones and his wife

Marilyn Jones, and ultrasonographers/radiologists Drs. George R. Leopold, Dolores Pretorius, and David K. Edwards continue to challenge me and require that I provide explanations for perinatal deaths and abnormalities. Having examined all placentas of all deliveries in the institutions with which I was affiliated for over two decades, I had gathered a large amount of new material. Professor Peter Kaufmann agreed to write about the normal anatomical and histological aspects of placental structure and development.

This third edition has been written because of the many new findings and the ever-growing need to have documentation for legal purposes; moreover, organization of the second edition left some aspects uncovered. Many changes have been made in the book. Not only was the text updated, a better index was created, the order of chapters is presented more logically, new chapters have been added, and others were combined. Much new information has been incorporated to bring the text to the current state of knowledge.

Now that many more pathologists are required to examine placentas, the need to make some introductory chapters was apparent. To make it easier for the novice of placental morphology, we have added new chapters that serve as guides to normal histology (Chapter 4) and to the principal histopathological aspects of the placenta (Chapter 15).

The text was written with WordPerfect 6.0. A complete set of diskettes containing the references is available from the authors, if desired.

I (K.B.) am indebted to many people, foremost to my wife for her understanding and patience with me and this task; the publisher with its many people has been gracious and patient; my colleagues at the university, secretaries, computer consultants, and other persons who have all helped gather data, are gratefully acknowledged. Many students and colleagues have graciously read most chapters, and they have made many helpful suggestions and corrections, for which I am grateful. Most of all, however, I am grateful to Dr. Geoffrey Altshuler, Oklahoma City, for many stimulating discussions and for his willingness to read and correct much of this manuscript. He undertook this task with endless patience and friendship.

I (P.K.) gratefully acknowledge the scientific cooperation of many former and present coworkers: Mario Castellucci, Caterina Crescimanno, Hans-Georg Frank, Berthold Huppertz, Sonya Kertschanska, Gaby Kohnen, Georg Kosanke, Vladimir Mironov, Azizbek Nanaev, Iris Scheffen, and the late Gertfried Schweikhart. Many of my data are based on their material, their findings, and their ideas.

Many colleagues and friends from other laboratories have contributed by discussion and by offering technical help. In this respect I am particularly grateful to Graham Burton, Anthony Carter, Ramazan Demir, Gernot Desoye, Gottfried Dohr, Jean-Michel Foidart, Renate Graf, Michaele Hartmann, John Kingdom, Hubert Korr, Rudolf Leiser, Lena Macara, Hobe Schröder, Tullia Todros, Carla Verkeste, and the late Elizabeth Ramsey. In many cases it is virtually impossible to differentiate between their and my ideas.

These chapters have required not only scientific inspiration but also much artistic, technical, and secretarial work. The artistic help of Wolfgang Graulich and the photographic assistance of Gaby Bock and Ute Kaufmann are gratefully acknowledged. The histological and electron microscopic pictures are based on material processed by Marianne von Bentheim, Christine Eherer, Michaela Nicolau, Linda Philippens, Barbara Witte, and Uta Zahn. Perfect secretarial assistance was provided by Jutta Jacobs and Michael Kaufmann.

The collaboration of these coworkers and friends was the basis for my contribution. Last but not least, I am very much indebted to my wife for her support and understanding.

KURT BENIRSCHKE
La Jolla, California

PETER KAUFMANN
Aachen, Germany

1994

References

Baldwin, V.J.: Pathology of Multiple Pregnancy. Springer-Verlag, New York, 1994.

Ballantyne, J.W.: The Diseases and Deformities of the Foetus. Vol. 1. Oliver & Boyd, Edinburgh, 1892.

Becker, V., and Röckelein G.: Pathologie der weiblichen Genitalorgane. I. Pathologie der Plazenta und des Abortes. Springer-Verlag, Heidelberg, 1989.

Benirschke, K., and Driscoll, S.G.: The Pathology of the Human Placenta. Springer-Verlag, New York, 1967.

Benirschke, K., and Kaufmann, P.: Pathology of the Human Placenta. 2nd ed. Springer-Verlag, New York, 1990.

Fox, H.: Pathology of the Placenta. Saunders, Philadelphia, 1978.

Lavery, J.P., ed.: The Human Placenta. Clinical Perspectives. Aspen Publishers, Rockville, MD, 1987.

Naeye, R.L.: Disorders of the Placenta, Fetus, and Neonate. Mosby Year Book, St. Louis, 1992.

Perrin, V.D.K., ed.: Pathology of the Placenta. Churchill Livingstone, New York, 1984.

Philippe, E.: Pathologie Foeto-Placentaire. Masson, Paris, 1986.

Price, B.: Primary biases in twin studies: review of prenatal and natal differences-producing factors in monozygotic pairs. Am. J. Hum. Genet. 2:293–352, 1950.

Vogel, M.: Atlas der morphologischen Plazentadiagnostik. Springer-Verlag, Heidelberg, 1992.

Contents

1
Placental Types

Throughout pregnancy the viviparous vertebrates develop a system of membranes that surround the fetus. The apposition or fusion of these fetal membranes with the uterine mucosa, for purposes of maternofetal physiological exchange, initiates the formation of the placenta. To put it differently, the fetus is surrounded by the fetal membranes, to which it is connected by the umbilical cord (Figure 1). The sac of membranes lies in the uterine cavity and has contact with the endometrium over almost its entire surface. The maternofetal contact zone, provided by membranes and endometrium, is the placenta.

This nonspecific definition points to the great structural and functional variability of the organ. There is probably no other organ that exhibits such an extent of species differences as the placenta. When comparing species, the outer shape and inner structure can vary to such a degree that nonplacentologists, who are familiar with the structure of only the human placenta, probably cannot identify any other type as a placenta at all. There is only one structural component that all placental types have in common (i.e., the existence of two separate circulatory systems: the maternal system and the fetal system). Under normal conditions the vessels of the two systems remain separated by several tissue layers throughout pregnancy. Even the origin of these separating tissue layers, making up the so-called placental barrier or interhemal membrane, varies. They may be derived from such fetal tissues as (1) the blastocyst wall (trophoblast), which after fusion with the fetal mesenchyme is called chorion; (2) the allantois, which is the extracorporeal embryonic urinary bladder; or (3) the yolk sac, an extracorporeal vesicular extension of the gut (Figure 2). Each of these membranes is completed by the amnion, which forms a second fetally derived membranous sac surrounding the em-

bryo. In some cases these fetal constituents are completed by maternal tissues (i.e., remainder of the endometrium).

The placenta is unique among all other organs in that it conducts the functional activities of most fetal organs (except the locomotor apparatus and the central nervous system) from its early beginning onward throughout its development. The following fetal functions are partially or completely taken over by the placenta during pregnancy as a substitute for still immature embryonic and fetal organs.

1. Gas transfer (later done by the lung)
2. Excretory functions, water balance, and pH regulation later done by the kidney
3. Catabolic and resorptive functions later done by the gut
4. Synthetic and secretory functions of most endocrine glands
5. Numerous metabolic and secretory functions of the liver
6. Hematopoiesis of the bone marrow (during early stages of pregnancy)
7. Heat transfer of the skin
8. Immunological functions (to a largely unknown degree)

It is highly unlikely that these functional requirements can be fulfilled by phylogenetic development of an identical structural solution for all the species, as species exhibit large variations in size, pregnancy length, litter size, and living conditions. The logical result of this situation has been the development of numerous placental types, differing from each other with respect to outer shape, type of maternofetal interdigitation, structure of the maternofetal barrier, and maternofetal blood flow interrelations. As a basis for better under-

1

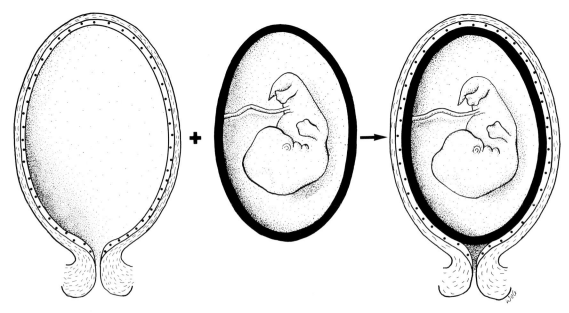

FIGURE 1. A placenta is formed when the fetal membrane (black, central figure) comes into close contact by apposition or fusion with the endometrial lining (point shading, left figure) of the uterus. This theoretically most simple type of a placenta (i.e., a placenta diffusa with a smooth contact area, as shown on the right figure) is not known to exist. (Modified after Kaufmann, 1981, with permission.)

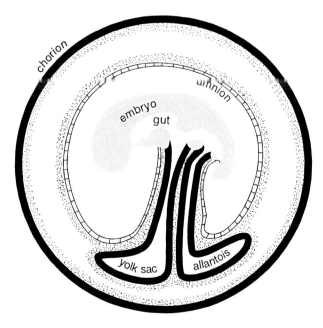

FIGURE 2. Synoptic representation of the fetal membranes that may contribute to the formation of a placenta. The trophoblast, as derivative of the blastocyst wall, together with the fetal mesenchyme forms the chorion, which is the main exchange membrane of most mammals. The chorion does not develop its own vessels but, rather, becomes vascularized by either the allantois (chorioallantoic placenta) or the yolk sac (choriovitelline placenta). In some species the chorion is replaced locally by the yolk sac, thus forming a yolk sac placenta. The amnion is not vascularized and never replaces the chorion; rather, it serves as an additional, inner membrane that separates the chorion or yolk sac from the amnionic fluid.

standing the human placenta, we present a brief overview of the so-called allantochorial placentas only. This group comprises all the placentas that develop from the blastocyst wall and that become fetally vascularized from the allantois (i.e., the embryonic bladder) (Figure 2). This placental type is the most common among mammals and is also represented in the human. For more detailed information we refer to the fundamental monographs on comparative placentology by Björkman (1970), Steven (1975), Ramsey (1982), and Mossman (1987) and to the reviews by Wimsatt (1962), Enders (1965), Kaufmann (1981), and Leiser and Kaufmann (1994).

Among the numerous possibilities for classifying the allantochorial placentas (Amoroso, 1952; Wimsatt, 1962; Steven, 1975; Kaufmann, 1981; Ludwig, 1981; King, 1982; Ramsey, 1982; Mossman, 1987; Dantzer et al., 1988) the following proved to be the most successful for characterizing the organ structurally and, to a limited degree, functionally: (1) outer shape and surface extension around the chorionic sac; (2) kind and intensity of interdigitation of maternal and fetal tissues; (3) number, kind, and structure of tissue layers separating maternal and fetal blood; and (4) spatial arrangement of maternal and fetal vessels or of blood flow directions.

It is impossible to cite the vast comparative placentological literature dealing with the various placental types. Rather, for each placental type or for each group of animals we refer to one or two detailed publications that may provide characteristic representations.

Placental Shapes

The extent of maternofetal and fetomaternal transfer depends largely on the size of the maternofetal contact area available for exchange (Kaufmann, 1981; Ludwig, 1981; Schröder, 1982). The smooth contact area of the chorion (derivative of the blastocyst wall, outer layer of the fetal membranes) with the endometrium seems to be insufficient to meet fetal demands, even if the contact is established over the entire surface of the chorionic sac, as depicted in Figure 1. This placental type does not exist in mammals. Rather, mammals increase the placental exchange area by interdigitation of the opposing maternal and fetal tissue surfaces. In most cases the surface enlargement by interdigitation is so intense that enough exchange surface can be provided even if interdigitation takes place only on a limited surface area of the chorionic sac. This interdigitating part is called the placenta, whereas those parts of the chorionic sac that maintain a more or less plane apposition to the uterine surface are called smooth chorion, chorion laeve, paraplacenta, or simply outer fetal membrane. Each animal order or suborder has a typical shape and surface extension of its placenta. In the light of phylogeny it is interesting to note that most of these typical placental shapes have been observed as more or less rare malformations in humans as well. However, it is still a matter of discussion whether placental shapes of certain animal orders and the respective human malformations are comparable results of placental development rather than merely products of external similarity in shape.

Maternofetal interdigitation extending over the entire surface of the chorionic sac is called *placenta diffusa* (placenta membranacea) (Figure 3). This type is seen in perissodactyla (Amoroso, 1952), cetacea (Wislocki & Enders, 1941), suiforma (MacDonald & Bosma, 1985), tylopoda (Ramsey, 1982), and some lower primates (Ramsey, 1982). According to Torpin (1969), it occurs rarely in the human as well (see Chapter 14).

In all other cases, maternofetal interdigitations are locally restricted and highly concentrated. Many such spot-like regions of intense maternofetal interdigitations, such as those in ruminants (Björkman, 1969), are called *placenta cotyledonaria* or placenta multiplex (Figure 3). To our knowledge, a corresponding malformation has not been described so far for the human.

In carnivores (Bjrökman, 1970), sirenia (Wislocki, 1935), hyracoidea (Mossman, 1937), and proboscidea (Mossman, 1937), the placenta forms a ring-like zone in the chorionic sac surrounding the fetus like a girdle, the *placenta zonaria*, placenta annularis, or girdle-like placenta (Figure 3). The incidence of this kind of maldevelopment in the human is far less than 0.1%. It

has been interpreted as a result of implantation in the uterine cervix, where the fetal membranes establish intense contact with the uterine wall in a ring-like fashion (Torpin, 1969).

Several lower and higher primates (Luckett, 1970; Ramsey, 1982), as well as the tupaia (Kaufmann et al., 1985; Luckhardt et al., 1985), as a phylogenetic link between insectivores and lower primates, develop two disk-like areas of intimate contact, the *placenta bidiscoidalis* (Figure 3). In the human it is represented by the placenta duplex (0.1%). Incomplete subdivision of the placental disk in the human is described as placenta bilobata or placenta bipartita (2–8%). The placenta succenturiata in the human (0.5–1.0%) shows an asymmetrical complete or incomplete subdivision into a large and a small disk. All three types of placental malformation in the human have been discussed to be a result of lateral implantation in the corner between the anterior and posterior walls of the uterus (Torpin, 1969).

The highest degree of concentration of maternofetal interdigitation is realized in the *discoidal placenta* (Figure 3), which provides only a single disk-like zone of intimate maternofetal contact. This most common type of placenta exists in rodents (Enders, 1965; Kaufmann & Davidoff, 1977; Ramsey, 1982), great apes (Ludwig & Baur, 1971), and humans (Boyd & Hamilton, 1970).

Types of Maternofetal Interdigitation

If that part of the surface area of the chorionic sac in which maternofetal interdigitation takes place is reduced, it must be compensated for by an increased intensity of the interdigitations. The simplest form of interdigitation, consequently, is combined with the large-surfaced diffuse placenta: It is called the *folded* type of placenta (Figure 4a) and is characterized by poorly branching, ridge-like folds of the chorion that fit into corresponding grooves of the uterine mucosa. Examples are seen in the pig (MacDonald & Bosma, 1985) and some lower primates (Ramsey, 1982), which have a diffuse placenta.

A generally similar but more complex construction is typical for the *lamellar* placenta (Figure 4b). This type is represented in carnivores (Leiser & Kohler, 1984). In this case, the ridges branch into complicated systems of slender chorionic lamellae, oriented in parallel to each other and separated by correspondingly branching endometrial folds.

Even more exchange surface per placental volume is provided by a tree-like branching pattern of the chorion, resulting in the placental villous tree. The villi fit into

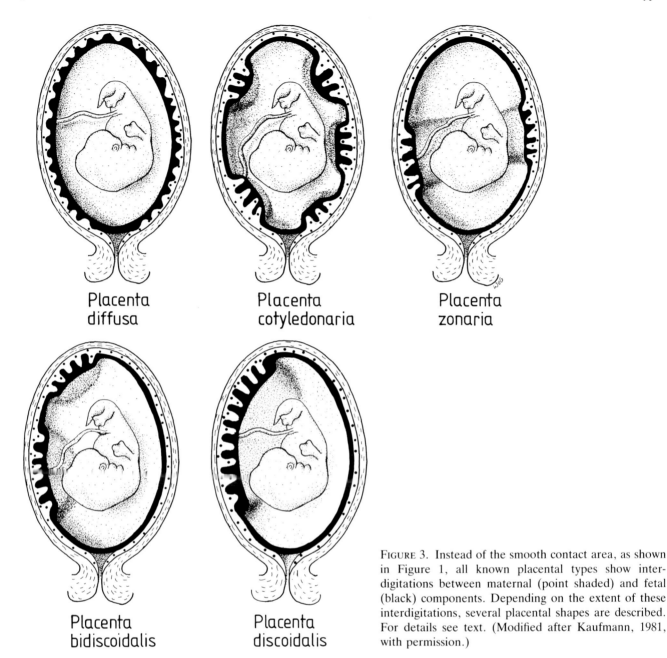

Placenta
diffusa

Placenta
cotyledonaria

Placenta
zonaria

Placenta
bidiscoidalis

Placenta
discoidalis

FIGURE 3. Instead of the smooth contact area, as shown in Figure 1, all known placental types show interdigitations between maternal (point shaded) and fetal (black) components. Depending on the extent of these interdigitations, several placental shapes are described. For details see text. (Modified after Kaufmann, 1981, with permission.)

corresponding endometrial crypts or are directly surrounded by maternal blood. This *villous* type of placenta (Figure 4d) exists in ruminants (Steven, 1975; Kaufmann, 1981) and most higher primates (Boyd & Hamilton, 1970; King & Mais, 1982).

An intermediate stage between the lamellar and the villous condition is represented by the *trabecular* type of placenta (Figure 4c). It has been described for some higher monkeys, such as *Callithrix* (Luckett, 1974; Merker et al., 1987). This placental type is characterized by branching folds from which leaf-like and finally finger-like villi branch off.

The most common and most effective kind of interdigitation can be found in the *labyrinthine* type of placenta (Figure 4e). It has been described so far only in placentas that have a discoidal or bidiscoidal shape. It is the typical type of interdigitation for the placentas of rodents (Kaufmann & Davidoff, 1977), lagomorphs (Mossman, 1937), insectivores (Malassine & Leiser, 1984), bats (Wimsatt & Enders, 1980), and some lower monkeys (Ramsey, 1982; Kaufmann et al., 1985; Mossman, 1987). As the characteristic feature, a tissue bloc of trophoblast is penetrated by web-like channels that are filled with maternal blood or fetal capillaries.

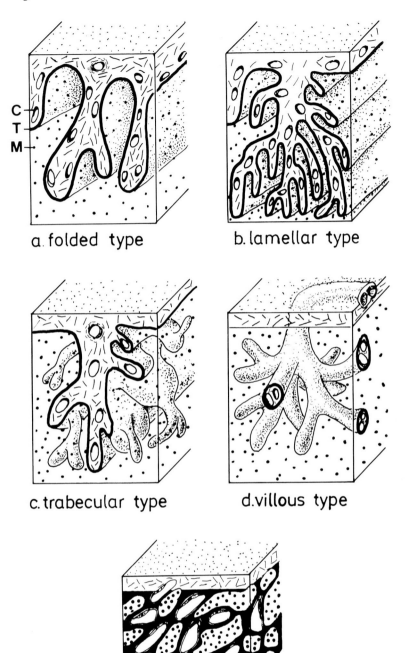

a. folded type

b. lamellar type

c. trabecular type

d. villous type

e. labyrinthine type

FIGURE 4. Types of interdigitation between maternal and fetal tissues. M = maternal tissue or maternal blood (fat dots); T = fetal trophoblast (black); C = fetal capillaries and fetal connective tissue. For details see text. (Modified and extended after Kaufmann, 1981, with permission.)

Maternofetal Barrier

The two preceding systems of classification are just structurally descriptive. Grosser (1909, 1927) initiated a more functional system of classification, describing structure and composition of the so-called placental barrier. This system was later extended by Enders (1965). Though criticized often because it fails to consider structural variation within the same placenta, this system still has its merits, "if for no other reason than that it serves as a ready reminder of the different components that need to be analyzed before drawing functional conclusions" (King, 1982). Maternofetal and fetomaternal diffusional transfer depends on the thickness of the separating layers, whereas facilitated transport, active transport, and vesicular transfer are influenced by the number and kind of layers of the barrier. The terms maternofetal barrier and placental barrier are traditional descriptions of the tissue layers separating maternal and fetal circulations in the placenta. These terms are still in use despite the fact that they are somewhat misleading (King, 1982): Increasing knowledge of placental physiology has taught us that synthetic, secretory, and transport functions of the placenta are as important aspects of this organ as the barrier role, separating the maternal and the fetal circulations. As an alternative, the term interhemal membrane is in use because it avoids any functional connotation for the separating layers. However, the use of the term membrane for a complex layer composed of several cells, rather than for the unit membrane of a cell, is misleading.

In the most complete cases of a placental barrier—in the artiodactyla (Wooding et al., 1980), the perissodactyla (Amoroso, 1952; Ramsey, 1982), and some prosimians (Mossman, 1987)—the fetal chorion directly faces the intact endometrial epithelium. The blastocyst did not invade the endometrium but simply remained attached to it. This condition is called the *epitheliochorial placenta*. Maternal and fetal blood are separated by six tissue layers (Figure 5): maternal capillary endothelium, maternal endometrial connective tissue, maternal endometrial epithelium, and three layers of fetal origin (trophoblast, chorionic connective tissue, and fetal endothelium). From the six layers, the trophoblast or the maternal epithelium may fuse syncytially. Sometimes even hybrid syncytia are formed by fusion of trophoblastic (fetal) and uterine epithelial (maternal) cells (e.g., in ruminants) (Wooding, 1992).

This maximum six-layer barrier can be reduced during invasion by the blastocyst by stepwise removal of maternal tissue layers. If invasion stops after destruction

of the uterine epithelium, the
(Figure 5) results. Originally, ʲ
to belong to this type. More ʲ
this five-layer barrier has been ʲ
Ramsey, 1982). Sheep and ʲ
an epitheliochorial or synepiʲ
(Wooding et al., 1980; Wooding
artiodactyla.

Deeper invasion with subsequʲ
metrial connective tissue, establishi
of trophoblast and maternal end
the development of the *endothʲ
(Figure 5). This placental barrier is ʲ
carnivores (Björkman, 1970), and iʲ
some insectivores (Malassine & Leʲ ʲ, ʲower
primates (Kaufmann et al., 1985), and bats (Ramsey, 1982).

As the next and final step of invasion, the maternal vessels are eroded and finally completely destroyed by the invasive trophoblast. The trophoblastic surfaces now directly face the maternal blood. This respective placental type is called *hemochorial placenta* (Figure 5). It has been described, for instance, for all rodents and lagomorphs, some insectivores, bats, and sirenia, and for the higher primates including the human (Enders, 1965; Ramsey, 1982). Depending on the number of trophoblastic epithelial layers, Enders (1965) has proposed a more detailed subdivision into *hemotrichorial* (rat; Enders, 1965; mouse: Björkman, 1970; hamster: Carpenter, 1972), *hemodichorial* (rabbit: Enders, 1965; human in the first trimester: Boyd & Hamilton, 1970; beaver: Fischer, 1971), and *hemomonochorial* (human placenta at term: Boyd & Hamilton, 1970; caviomorph rodents, e.g., guinea pig: Kaufmann & Davidoff, 1977).

Some authors (Wimsatt, 1962) have described less common types of placenta in insectivores and bats, in which even fetal tissue components are subjected to destruction, resulting in endothelioendothelial and even hemoendothelial conditions. In most cases, these descriptions have not been based on ultrastructural studies and thus need to be corroborated.

When stating that the placental barrier is made up of three to six tissue layers, it does not necessarily imply that a corresponding number of cells must be passed transcellularly by each transported molecule. This situation is mandatory only for the trophoblast, which in most species with invasive implantation is a syncytium that can be passed only transcellularly by transport mechanisms such as diffusion, facilitated transfer, active transport, and vesicular transfer. In both connective tissue layers, however, transport may easily take place paracellularly by diffusion. In terms of smaller mole-

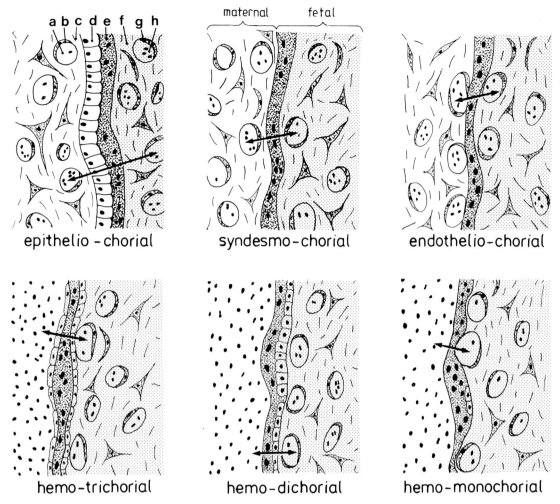

FIGURE 5. Tissue layers of the maternofetal barrier according to the Grosser classification. a = maternal blood; b = maternal endothelium; c = endometrial connective tissue; d = endometrial epithelium; e = trophoblast; f = fetal connective tissue; g = fetal endothelium; h = fetal blood. The fetal components of the placental barrier (e, f, g) come together under the name chorion. The maternal components are reduced step by step until the chorion comes into direct contact with the maternal blood (a, black dots). The tropho-

blast, normally consisting of a syncytium (e), may be covered on one side (hemodichorial) or on both sides (hemotrichorial) by cytotrophoblast. In most species the trophoblast fuses syncytially. In some species, mostly those with epitheliochorial placentation, either the maternal epithelium fuses syncytially instead of the trophoblast or both epithelia remain cellular. For further details see text. (Modified and extended after Kaufmann, 1981, with permission.)

cules, the same is valid for the uterine epithelium (so far as it is cellular in nature) and for both endothelia. These epithelial and endothelial linings offer limited paracellular transfer to small molecules along the lateral intercellular clefts. As a consequence, the syncytiotrophoblast in most placentas, including that of the human, is the decisive barrier limiting or supporting transplacental transfer processes.

According to Fick's law of diffusion, the net amount of substance crossing the membrane depends (inter alia) on the concentration difference of the substance across the membrane, as well as on the area and the thickness

of the membrane. Thus reduction of the distance between maternal and fetal blood is of decisive importance for the maternofetal diffusional exchange. It makes the Grosser classification valuable for determining diffusional efficiency of the organ. However, it is important to note that it is valid only for passive diffusion (oxygen, carbon dioxide, water) (Schröder, 1982; Faber & Thornburg, 1983). For most transport mechanisms, the product of exchange surface available and the activity of the uptake mechanisms (carrier molecules, enzymes, and receptors for active and vesicular transport) are the limiting factors, not the barrier thickness. The latter situation is comparable to being on an escalator, the capacity of which is limited by its width and speed rather than by its length. It is valid for transplacental transport processes, such as facilitated diffusion (e.g., glucose), active transport (e.g., ions and many amino acids), and vesicular transport (peptides, proteins, lipids). As a consequence, we must conclude that the applicability of the Grosser classification is limited to the interpretation of the capacity of the placenta for passive diffusion. The findings by Dantzer et al. (1988) make it likely that it is primarily the fetal demands during transplacental oxygen diffusion that determine placental size.

Maternofetal Blood Flow Interrelations

Similar advantages and similar limitations, as discussed for the Grosser classification, are valid for a more physiological attempt to classify the placentas, that is, according to the geometric arrangement of maternal and fetal capillaries or blood flows in the exchange area (Bartels & Moll, 1964; Faber, 1969; Moll, 1972, 1981; Martin, 1981; Schröder, 1982; Faber & Thornburg, 1983; Dantzer et al., 1988). The relative efficiencies of various types of the following theoretical exchanges for the diffusion of, for example, oxygen have been calculated. Physiologists have defined several theoretical

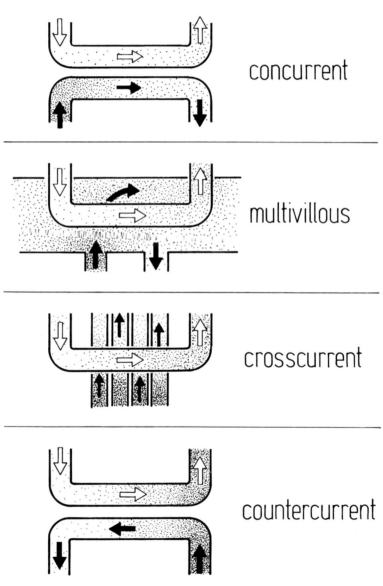

FIGURE 6. Idealized arrangement of the fetal (white arrows) and maternal (black arrows) bloodstreams of different placental exchange types, according to Faber (1969), Moll (1972), and Martin (1981). The density of dots in the venous limbs of the fetal vessel loops (upper right vessel of each single drawing) illustrates the efficiency of the various exchangers in diffusional exchange (e.g., oxygen). For further details see text. (From Dantzer et al., 1988, with permission.)

models of diffusional exchangers and calculated their efficiency for diffusional transfer. The results have been compared with real structural and functional findings in various mammals.

The *concurrent flow exchanger* (Figure 6) is the most inefficient system. Its fetal and maternal capillaries are thought to be arranged in parallel, having identical blood flow directions. Obviously it is not represented in placentas of mammals (Martin, 1981). Also, with the *countercurrent flow exchanger*, maternal and fetal capillaries are arranged in parallel but with blood flow in opposite directions (Figure 6). This vascular arrangement is the most effective one for passive diffusion. It is nearly perfectly realized in the placentas of all rodents (Kaufmann & Davidoff, 1977; Dantzer et al., 1988) and lagomorphs (Mossmann, 1926). Accordingly, these animals exhibit small placentas compared to their fetal weight (fetoplacental weight ratios of up to 20:1). The remaining theoretical and real exchange systems have an intermediate position between concurrent and countercurrent exchangers regarding efficiency. Among them, for placentology the most important ones are *simple cross-current flow* (Figure 6) (carnivores: Leiser & Kohler, 1984; Dantzer et al., 1988), *double cross-current flow* (Figure 6) (lower primates: Luckhardt et al., 1985; pig: Dantzer et al., 1988), and *multivillous flow* (Figure 6) (higher primates and human: Moll, 1981; ruminants: Dantzer et al., 1988). The importance of this classification system for the fetal oxygen supply is stressed by the fact that the animals showing a less efficient vessel arrangement have a worse fetoplacental weight relation at term (pig 9:1, cat 8:1, human 6:1) compared to the highly effective, small rodent placentas (up to 20:1) (Dantzer et al., 1988).

Placental Types and Phylogeny

The above systems of placental classification have been accused of being merely structurally descriptive but of being functionally more or less irrelevant. This reproach is supported by several facts. The pig seems to have one of the most primitive placentas possible: a diffuse, epitheliochorial, folded, cross-current placenta (Dantzer et al., 1988). This seemingly primitive placenta, however, guarantees embryonic development in the pig as satisfactorily as does the highly sophisticated guinea pig placenta for its embryos. Moreover, the latter placenta is thought to be one of the most effective ones, being of the discoidal, labyrinthine, hemomonochorial, countercurrent type (Kaufmann & Davidoff, 1977). Probably no one would state that the reproductive qualities of the guinea pig are superior to that of the pig. One must therefore be careful when describing a placenta as "primitive" or "highly developed." Independent from

the simplicity or complexity of their structure, all placentas fulfill their biological tasks—when necessary, compensating for missing complexity simply by having an increased mass.

Schröder (1993) has stressed another interesting view explaining the phylogenetic variabilities of placental sizes and efficiencies. Animals with a rather short gestational period relative to their neonatal weight have a relatively large daily fetal growth rate. If such species want to produce their large fetuses within a short time with a small placenta (e.g., rodents), their choice of placental type is restricted to the high efficiency type, such as labyrinthine and hemochorial with countercurrent flow. With low daily fetal growth rates, however, it does not really matter which placental type and efficiency is available to the species; all grades of efficiencies are possible, ranging from the villous, synepitheliochorial, multivillous sheep placenta, to the villous, hemomonochorial, multivillous human placenta, to the labyrinthine, hemomonochorial, countercurrent capybara placenta.

Unquestioned is the importance of the classification systems when characterizing certain placentas in comparison to the human one. The delivered human term placenta has been easily available for any kind of research. Animal experiments are required for nearly all in situ studies. The only placentas that are directly comparable to the human placenta are those of the great apes. For several reasons (expense and protection of rare species), however, they are not a real alternative for placental research. Thus one must work with laboratory animals with placentas that are largely different from the human placenta. The classification systems described above provide a certain orientation regarding differences and similarities between the various animal models and the human placenta. Moreover, as stated by King (1982), they remind us that we must take into consideration the differences before drawing functional conclusions.

When inspecting Table 1, one realizes that there is no evident relation between placental classification and taxonomy. Some orders, such as the carnivores, lagomorphs, and rodents, seem to be homogeneous regarding placental structure. Others, such as insectivores and primates, may even give us the impression that several animals have acquired their respective placental types by chance. Perhaps it is due to the special situation of the placenta, which has been developed for single use over a limited life-span. Most placentas show considerable excess capacity, which makes a significant difference when evaluating efficiency. It is an important factor in pathology: The human placenta, which compared to the fetus is rather large, can compensate for 50% tissue degeneration, perhaps even more, without severe disturbance of

TABLE 1. Placental classification at term in various animal orders.

Order/species	Placental shape	Fetomaternal interdigitation	Placental barrier	Fetomaternal blood flow interrelations	Neonatal/placental weight ratio
Marsupialia				—	—
Opossum	Discoidal	Folded	Epitheliochorial		
Insectivora					
Sorex	Discoidal	Labyrinthine	Endotheliochorial	—	—
European mole	Discoidal	Labyrinthine	Endotheliochorial	—	—
Pacific mole	Diffuse	Labyrinthine	Hemochorial	—	—
Primates					
Tupaia	Bidiscoidal	Labyrinthine	Endotheliochorial	Double cross-current	18:1
Galago	Diffuse	Folded	Epitheliochorial	—	—
Marmoset	Bidiscoidal	Trabecular	Hemomonochorial	Multivillous	—
Rhesus monkey	Bidiscoidal	Villous	Hemomonochorial	Multivillous	—
Great apes	Discoidal	Villous	Hemomonochorial	Multivillous	—
Human	Discoidal	Villous	Hemomonochorial	Multivillous	6:1
Chiroptera					
Microchiroptera	Discoidal	Labyrinthine	Endotheliochorial	—	—
Molossidae	Discoidal	Labyrinthine	Hemodichorial	—	—
Lagomorpha					
Rabbit	Discoidal	Labyrinthine	Hemodichorial	Countercurrent	6:1
Hare	Discoidal	Labyrinthine	Hemodichorial	—	—
Rodentia					
Guinea pig	Discoidal	Labyrinthine	Hemomonochorial	Countercurrent	20:1
Chinchilla	Discoidal	Labyrinthine	Hemomonochorial	Countercurrent	30:1
Hamster	Discoidal	Labyrinthine	Hemodichorial	Countercurrent	—
Beaver	Discoidal	Labyrinthine	Hemodichorial	—	—
Mouse	Discoidal	Labyrinthine	Hemodichorial	Countercurrent	—
Rat	Discoidal	Labyrinthine	Hemodichorial	Countercurrent	10:1
Cetacea					
Dolphin	Diffuse	Villous	Epitheliochorial	—	—
Carnivora					
Dog	Zonary	Lamellar	Endotheliochorial	—	—
Cat	Zonary	Lamellar	Endotheliochorial	Simple cross-current	8:1
Bear	Zonary	Lamellar	Endotheliochorial	—	—
Hyena	Zonary	Villous/labyr.	Hemomonochorial	—	—
Sirenia					
Manatee	Zonary	Labyrinthine	Hemochorial	—	—
Pholidota					
Pangolin	Diffuse	Villous	Epitheliochorial	—	—
Proboscidea					
Elephant	Zonary	Villous	Endotheliochorial	—	—
Hyracoidea					
Hyrax	Zonary	Labyrinthine	Hemochorial	—	—
Edentata					
Sloth	Discoidal	Labyrinthine	Endotheliochorial	—	—
Armadillo	Discoidal	Villous	Hemochorial	—	—
Perissodactyla					
Horse	Diffuse	Villous	Epitheliochorial	—	—
Rhinoceros	Diffuse	Villous	Epitheliochorial	—	—
Artiodactyla					
Pig	Diffuse	Folded	Epitheliochorial	Double cross-current	9:1
Alpaca	Diffuse	Folded/villous	Epitheliochorial	—	—
Sheep	Cotyledonary	Villous	Epitheliochorial	Multivillous	10:1
Goat	Cotyledonary	Villous	Epitheliochorial	Multivillous	10:1
Cow	Cotyledonary	Villous	Epitheliochorial	Multivillous	—

The data were assembled from the following publications: Wimsatt (1962), Enders (1965), Björkman (1970), Starck (1975), Ramsey (1982), Mossman (1987), Dantzer et al. (1988).

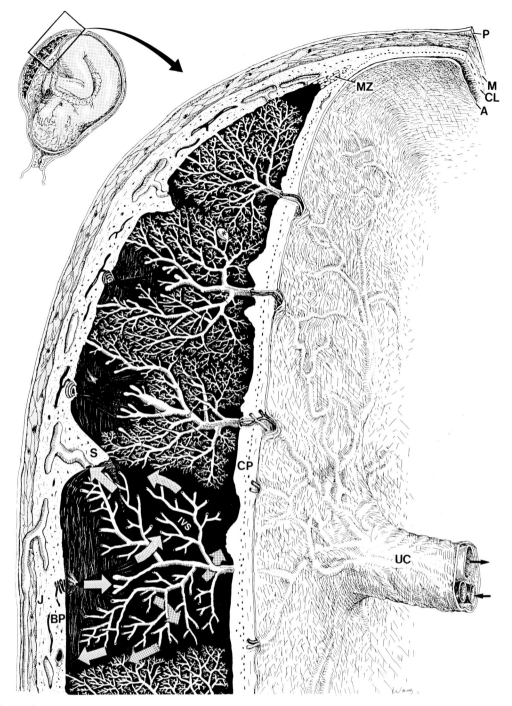

FIGURE 7. Mature human placenta in situ. It is composed of the chorionic plate (CP) and the basal plate (BP) surrounding the intervillous space (IVS) as cover and as bottom. The fetally vascularized villous trees project from the chorionic plate into the intervillous space and are directly surrounded by the maternal blood that circulates through the intervillous space. The loose centers of villous trees, arranged around the maternal arterial inflow area, are frequent features. P = perimetrium; M = myometrium; CL = chorion leave; A = amnion; MZ = marginal zone between placenta and fetal membranes, with obliterated intervillous space and ghost villi; * = cell island, connected to a villous tree; S = placental septum; J = junctional zone; UC = umbilical cord. (From Kaufmann & Scheffen, 1992, with permission.)

pregnancy. In animals with relatively small placentas compared to the fetus (e.g., guinea pig or tupaia), fetal death is the normal result as soon as only a small amount of placental parenchyma is destroyed (Van der Heijden, 1981).

Human Placenta

According to the classification systems described herein, the human placenta is discoidal, villous, and hemochorial in structure. The arrangement of its maternal and fetal blood flows corresponds to the multivillous type of exchange system.

These basic structural characteristics are realized by the following design: The human placenta at term is a local, disk-like thickening of the membranous sac (Figure 7, inset) that is formed by splitting of the membranes into two separate sheets, the chorionic plate and the basal plate (Figure 7). These two plates confine the intervillous space, serving as cover and bottom. The intervillous space is perfused with maternal blood, which circulates directly around the trophoblastic surfaces of the placental villi. The villi are complex tree-like structures of the chorionic plate that project into the intervillous space. Inside the villi are fetal vessels that are connected to the fetal circulatory system via the chorionic plate and the umbilical cord. At the placental margin the intervillous space is obliterated so the chorionic plate and the basal plate fuse with each other and thus form the chorion leave.

References

Amoroso, E.C.: Placentation. In, Marshall's Physiology of Reproduction. 3rd Ed., A.S. Parkes, ed., pp. 127–316. Longmans Green, London, 1952.

Bartels, H., and Moll, W.: Passage of inert substances and oxygen in the human placenta. Pflügers Arch. Ges. Physiol. 280:165, 1964.

Björkman, N.: Light and electron microscopic studies on cellular alterations in the normal bovine placentome. Anat. Rec. 163:17–30, 1969.

Björkman, N.: An Atlas of Placental Fine Structure. Baillière, London; Williams & Wilkins, Baltimore, 1970.

Boyd, J.D., and Hamilton, W.J.: The Human Placenta. Heffer & Sons, Cambridge, 1970.

Carpenter, S.J.: Light and electron microscopic observations on the morphogenesis of the chorioallantoic placenta of the golden hamster (Cricetus auratus): days seven through nine of gestation. Am. J. Anat. 135:445–476, 1972.

Dantzer, V., Leiser, R., Kaufmann, P., and Luckhardt, M.: Comparative morphological aspects of placental vascularization. Trophoblast Res. 3:235–260, 1988.

Enders, A.C.: A comparative study of the fine structure in several hemochorial placentas. Am. J. Anat. 116:29–67, 1965.

Faber, J.J.: Application of the theory of heat exchangers to the transfer of inert materials in placentas. Circ. Res. 24:221–234, 1969.

Faber, J.J., and Thornburg, K.L.: Placental Physiology. Structure and Function of Fetomaternal Exchange. Raven Press, New York, 1983.

Fischer, T.V.: Placentation in the American beaver (Castor canadensis). Am. J. Anat. 131:159–184, 1971.

Grosser, O.: Vergleichende Anatomie und Entwicklungsgeschichte der Eihäute und der Placenta mit besonderer Berücksichtigung des Menschen. Braumüller, Vienna, 1909.

Grosser, O.: Frühentwicklung, Eihautbildung und Placentation des Menschen und der Säugetiere. Deutsche Frauenheilkunde, Geburtshilfe, Gynäkologie und Nachbargebiete in Einzeldarstellungen. Vol. 5. R.T. Jaschke, ed. Bergmann, Munich, 1927.

Kaufmann, P.: Functional anatomy of the non-primate placenta. Placenta Suppl. 1:13–28, 1981.

Kaufmann, P., and Davidoff, M.: The guinea pig placenta. Adv. Anat. Embryol. Cell Biol. 53:1–90, 1977.

Kaufmann, P., and Scheffen, I.: Placental development. In, Neonatal and Fetal Medicine—Physiology and Pathophysiology, Vol. 1. R. Polin and W. Fox, eds., pp. 47–55. Saunders, Orlando, FL, 1992.

Kaufmann, P., Luckhardt, M., and Elger, W.: The structure of the tupaia placenta. II. Ultrastructure. Anat. Embryol. (Berl.) 171:211–221, 1985.

King, B.F.: Comparative anatomy of the placental barrier. Bibl. Anat. 22:13–28, 1982.

King, B.F., and Mais, J.J.: Developmental changes in rhesus monkey placental villi and cell columns. Anat. Embryol. (Berl.) 165:361–376, 1982.

Leiser, R., and Kohler, T.: The blood vessels of the cat girdle placenta: observations on corrosion casts, scanning electron microscopical and histological studies. II. Fetal vasculature. Anat. Embryol. (Berl.) 170:209–216, 1984.

Leiser, R., and Kaufmann, P.: Placental structure: in a comparative aspect. Exp. Clin. Endocrinol. 102:122–134, 1994.

Luckett, W.P.: The fine structure of the placental villi of the rhesus monkey (Macaca mulatta). Anat. Rec. 167:141–164, 1970.

Luckett, W.P.: Comparative development and evolution of the placenta in primates. Contrib. Primatol. 3:142–223, 1974.

Luckhardt, M., Kaufmann, P., and Elger, W.: The structure of the tupaia placenta. I. Histology and vascularisation. Anat. Embryol. (Berl.) 171:201–210, 1985.

Ludwig, K.S.: Vergleichende Anatomie der Plazenta. In, Die Plazenta des Menschen. V. Becker, Th.H. Schiebler, and F. Kubli, eds. Thieme, Stuttgart, 1981.

Ludwig, K.S., and Baur, R.: The chimpanzee placenta. In, The Chimpanzee, Vol. 4. G.H. Bourne, ed., pp. 349–372. University Park Press, Baltimore, 1971.

Macdonald, A.A., and Bosma, A.A.: Notes on placentation in Suina. Placenta 6:83–92, 1985.

Malassine, A., and Leiser, R.: Morphogenesis and fine structure of the near-term placenta of Talpa europaea. I. Endotheliochorial labyrinth. Placenta 5:145–158, 1984.

Martin, C.B.: Models of placental blood flow. Placenta Suppl. 1:65–80, 1981.

Merker, H.-J., Bremer, D., Barrach, H.-J., and Gossrau, R.: The basement membrane of the persisting maternal blood vessels in the placenta of Callithrix jacchus. Anat. Embryol. (Berl.) 176:87–97, 1987.

Moll, W.: Gas exchange in concurrent, countercurrent and crosscurrent flow systems: the concept of the fetoplacental unit. In, Respiratory Gas Exchange and Blood Flow in the Placenta. L.D. Longo and H. Bartèls, eds., pp. 281–294. DHEW Publ. No. (NIH) 73–361. Department of Health, Education and Welfare, Bethesda, 1972.

Moll, W.: Theorie des plazentaren Transfers durch Diffusion. In, Die Plazenta des Menschen. V. Becker, Th.H. Schiebler, and F. Kubli, eds., pp. 129–139. Thieme, Stuttgart, 1981.

Mossman, H.W.: The rabbit placenta and the problem of placental transmission. Am. J. Anat. 37:433–497, 1926.

Mossman, H.W.: Comparative morphogenesis of the fetal membranes and accessory uterine structures. Carnegie Contrib. Embryol. 26:129–246, 1937.

Mossman, H.W.: Vertebrate Fetal Membranes: Comparative Ontogeny and Morphology; Evolution; Phylogenetic Significance; Basic Functions; Research Opportunities. Macmillan, London, 1987.

Ramsey, E.M.: The Placenta. Human and Animal. Praeger, New York, 1982.

Schröder, H.: Structural and functional organization of the placenta from the physiological point of view. Bibl. Anat. 22:4–12, 1982.

Schröder, H.: Placental diversity: transport physiology diversity. Keynote Lecture, 5th Meeting of the European Placenta Group, Manchester, UK, 1993.

Starck, D.: Embryologie. Thieme, Stuttgart, 1975.

Steven, D.H., ed.: Comparative Placentation. Academic Press, Orlando, FL, 1975.

Torpin, R.: The Human Placenta. Charles C Thomas, Springfield, IL, 1969.

Van der Heijden, F.L.: Compensation mechanisms for experimental reduction of the functional capacity in the guinea pig placenta. I. Changes in the maternal and fetal placenta vascularization. Acta Anat. (Basel) 111:352–358, 1981.

Wimsatt, W.A.: Some aspects of the comparative anatomy of the mammalian placenta. Am. J. Obstet. Gynecol. 84:1568–1594, 1962.

Wimsatt, W.A., and Enders, A.C.: Structure and morphogenesis of the uterus placenta, and paraplacental organs of the neotropical disc-winged bat Thyroptera tricolor spix (Microchiroptera: Thyropteridae). Am. J. Anat. 159:209–243, 1980.

Wislocki, G.B.: The placentation of the manatee (Trichechus latirostris). Mem. Museum Comp. Zool. Harvard 54:159–178, 1935.

Wislocki, G.B., and Enders, R.K.: The placentation of the bottle-nosed porpoise (Tursiops truncatus). Am. J. Anat. 68:97–125, 1941.

Wooding, F.B.F.: The synepitheliochorial placenta of ruminants: binucleate cell fusion and hormone production. Placenta 13:101–113, 1992.

Wooding, F.B.P., Chamber, S.G., Perry, J.S., George, M., and Heap, R.B.: Migration of binucleate cells in the sheep placenta during normal pregnancy. Anat. Embryol. (Berl.) 158:361–370, 1980.

2
Examination of the Placenta

Macroscopic Examination

Storage

Most placentas are normal, as are most neonates. Therefore an examination of all placentas is not warranted even though it has been advocated repeatedly. Salafia and Vintzileos (1991) made a strong plea for the study of all placentas by pathologists. We concur with this view, as the sporadic examination does not provide sufficient training for young pathologists, and it does not allow the routine pathologist to obtain sufficient background knowledge as to what constitutes a truly normal placenta. Another reason is the litigious climate of today (see Chapter 27). It has been shown repeatedly that a placental examination is needed in order to assess the cause of a perinatal death. Most recently this point was demonstrated especially for stillbirths by Las Heras et al. (1994). The most important lesions were found in the cord (18%), with inflammatory lesions second most common. Because placentas differ widely in shape, size, and appearance, the novice must become familiar with this spectrum of placental shapes. To do so, a large number of placentas must be examined routinely. It is therefore prudent in hospitals with large numbers of deliveries to select placentas for examination. To facilitate this practice, storage is required. The American College of Obstetricians and Gynecologists, on the other hand, has suggested that routine study of the placenta is not warranted (ACOG, 1991), a decision with which we strongly disagree.

Placentas should *not* be frozen prior to examination, as it obliterates the most useful histological characteristics and even makes the macroscopic examination more difficult. We believe that formalin fixation has similar effects. It is best to store the delivered placentas in containers, such as plastic jars. We have found ice cream cartons, made from styrofoam, the most convenient and least expensive. Cardboard containers absorb the fluids, and the placentas tend to stick to them. Styrofoam containers can also be readily labeled and stored in a refrigerator at 4°C. In this state, the placenta is preserved for a meaningful examination for many days. Autolysis is minimal. We cannot agree with Naeye (1987) that such storage causes significant artifacts that render a subsequent examination difficult. Indeed the immediate fixation of the organ in formalin, recommended by others (Bartholomew et al., 1961) as a good means to evaluate the extent of infarction, makes the placenta more difficult to evaluate critically, aside from the storage problems, expense, and odor. For maximal convenience, it is a good idea to have a refrigerator with seven shelves, labeled Monday through Sunday, and to discard the normal placentas on one shelf when the next identical weekday arrives. In this way, all placentas from problem births are available for study.

During storage the placenta loses some weight. In part, the loss is due to evaporation, but most weight is lost by leakage of blood and serum occasioned by the weight of placental tissue resting on other portions. The quantity of weight loss depends on the length of storage and the degree of edema but is not great in the normal placenta. It is most significant in the edematous placentas of hydrops. (We observed a 180 g fluid extravasation within 1 day from a 740 g hydropic placenta.) The freshly examined placenta is thus softer, bloodier, and thicker than one that has been stored. On the other hand, it must be noted that the placenta gains weight when it is stored in formalin, particularly during the first day of fixation. Not all organs increase in weight uniformly after such fixation, as the detailed report by Schremmer (1967) specified. The placenta, according to Schremmer, gains between 0.7% and 23.0%, with an average of +9.9%. It is among the organs with the largest deviations in weight gain after fixation. Our findings are summarized in Figure 8.

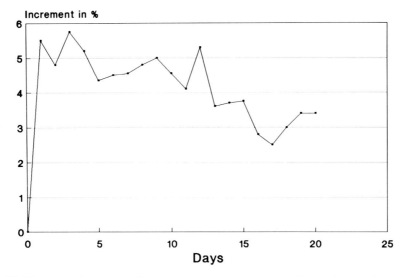

FIGURE 8. Weight gain of placentas (trimmed, without cord or membranes) after formalin fixation.

Selection

Placentas from all premature infants and all twins should be examined routinely, at least macroscopically, and many of them require histological study as well. In addition, many circumstances arise during the first few days of life of an infant where the neonatologist is interested in placental findings. They often help to clarify whether a particular disease had a prenatal onset. Furthermore, there are some maternal conditions that warrant placental examination (e.g., preeclampsia, the condition known as lupus anticoagulant, diabetes, fever, and many more). In our routine study of placentas, the obstetricians and neonatologists alert us as to which placentas they believe warrant more scrutiny; and so perhaps 5% to 10% of all placentas undergo histological examination.

Photography

A photographic record is often desirable and is useful for many purposes. Most pathology laboratories are equipped with cameras that can take Kodachrome color pictures, which are valuable for teaching purposes. It has been our experience, however, that the color tends to disappear; and certainly these photographs cannot generally be retrieved years later when they may be of interest in litigation or for review of material. For this reason it is good practice to make a black and white photograph of the entire pathological placenta that exhibits special features or of its salient portions. We employ Kodak Plus-X film for this purpose, and the print is attached permanently to the protocol. It has been most convenient to mount two cameras side by side on a sliding platform, one for color and the other for black and white film. The photographic task is thus quickly accomplished. Others may use Polaroid photography, which serves the same purpose. Some are amused by this recommendation, but they agree that a good picture is worth many words.

Examination

Detailed protocols for the placental examination have been reported in the past (Snoeck, 1958; Benirschke, 1961a,b; Gruenwald, 1964; Fox, 1978). Some were designed to allow an unbiased examination of the placenta and its recording by the many medical centers of the "Collaborative Study" so ultimately correlations could be made regarding fetal outcome. Our routine procedure now is to examine all placentas and to select for histological study those that appear abnormal or whose perinatal circumstances demand such an examination. The selection process just outlined has been helpful, and we have rarely missed a placenta that was of importance. Other recommendations for a triage of placental study and other ramifications come from a joint conference held in 1990 (Travers & Schmidt, 1991). This volume provides useful information on many aspects of placental pathology.

The tools for the examination are simple (Figure 9). They consist of a ruler, a long, sharp knife, a toothed forceps, a pair of scissors, and a scale. Our ruler is permanently mounted over the cutting board, thus enabling rapid measurement of the length of the umbilical cord and the placenta's diameter. A butcher's scale with removable bucket that weighs items up to 2 kg is

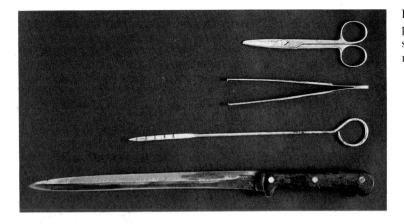

FIGURE 9. Instruments most practical for the placental examination. From top to bottom: scissors; forceps; "dipstick" to measure the thickness of placental tissue; long, stiff knife.

also available. The long knife, best obtained from a butcher supply house, is sharpened just before examination.

The placenta is removed from its container. At this time one often perceives rather characteristic odors. For instance, when a mother has recently eaten garlic, the intense smell of its diallyl sulfides is readily apparent. Also, in infected placentas the fetid smell due to *Escherichia coli* and the rather sweeter smell due to *Listeria monocytogenes* can be distinguished by an experienced pathologist. Storage in the refrigerator enhances the growth and hence the recognition of these organisms.

The shape of the placenta is then ascertained by stretching it flat on the cutting board. Is it round or oval, or are there accessory (succenturiate) lobes? One finds that during the delivery the membranes have generally inverted over the maternal surface (Schultze procedure) and rarely are they found in the position they held in utero (Duncan) (Pritchard et al., 1985). They are then inverted by the examiner so they assume the in utero configuration, and one ascertains the completeness of the membranes. It is also noted at this time if the tear that allowed the infant to escape from its membranous enclosure extends to the edge of the placenta or if free membranes extend beyond the edge. If there is *any* margin of intact membranes, this placenta could not have been a placenta previa, provided it was from a vaginal delivery. If the edge of the membranous tear is far from the placental border (often the case with circumvallate placentas), a fundal position can be deduced. Torpin and Hart (1941) made the point that when the minimally disturbed sac is immersed in a bucket of water the sac assumes the configuration of the uterus, and that its position before birth can be reasonably accurately determined by this study. At this time it is prudent to inspect the color and appearance of the fetal surface of the placenta. Normally it is shiny, and the

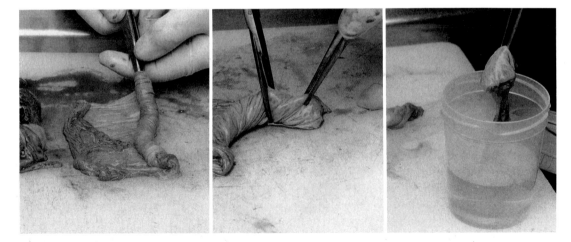

FIGURE 10. Rolling of membranes for fixation and later sectioning. It is best to prepare them in a standardized fashion (e.g., amnion inside) starting at the site of rupture and proceeding toward the edge of the placenta, as shown at left. A segment is then taken from a well rolled portion (center) and is fixed for a day (right).

FIGURE 11. Edge of the placenta (right) with an intrauterine device embedded in degenerating decidua (partly removed) and old blood clot.

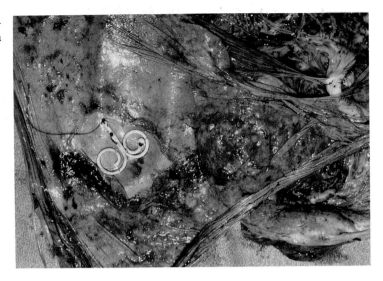

subjacent blood is seen as a clear blue hue, particularly in the immature organ. When chorioamnionitis is present, the membranes become opaque by the interposition of leukocytes, and the surface usually loses its sheen.

Next the membranes are cut off the edge of the placenta with the knife. If one anticipates making sections of the placenta for histological study, it is wise to follow a routine protocol for doing it, as it enhances subsequent interpretation. Therefore it is recommended that one become accustomed to doing it the same way each time. It is preferable to cut the membranes off in such a manner that one knows the point of rupture; then when sections are made, the membrane roll is prepared in such a fashion that the point of rupture is in the center of the roll with the amnion inward (Figure 10). This method of preparing a roll of membranes (the "jelly roll") in order to obtain a maximum amount of membranes with decidua capsularis was first described by Zeek and Assali (1950). In immature placentas there

may be a large amount of decidua, and it is often ragged. In more mature organs the decidua atrophies and often degenerates. Occasionally, one finds an intrauterine device in this decidua capsularis, usually at the edge of the placenta and associated with old clot and debris (Figures 11, 12). Frequently, there are areas of brown to green discoloration in the membranes that are from former hemorrhages, or they may have been induced by amniocentesis.

In many placentas that come from patients after labor, in contrast to those after cesarean section, the amnion is disrupted or sheared off the underlying chorion. In fact, the amnion may be totally detached. Often, though, there is milky, white vernix caseosa that has dissected underneath the amnion; it is readily moved about by pressure. It has no significance. Moreover, the membranes near the edge of the placenta frequently contain the remnant of the yolk sac, a small, white to yellow, oval disk that is located underneath the amnion.

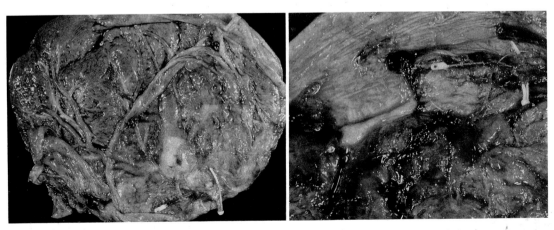

FIGURE 12. Intrauterine devices at the placental margin at term (left) and in a slightly immature (right) pregnancy. Note the attending hemorrhagic degeneration of the adjacent tissues.

The yolk sac can now be visualized ultrasonographically. Measurements have shown that the size of the yolk sac is variable, and that it is not a useful prognosticator for fetal well-being (Reece et al., 1988). Occasionally, one sees remnants of tiny vessels traversing from it to the insertion of the cord.

The color of the membranes is noted, as are the surface characteristics. A slimy feeling is often the result of meconium discharge, as is of course a green color. The duration of meconium discharge can be estimated by the presence of green discoloration in different layers. When it is only in the amnion, a short time interval is suggested; when meconium is found also in the chorion after the amnion is stripped off, a longer interval has passed since discharge (Miller et al., 1985). We found that at 1 hour the meconium macrophages are visible within the amnion; after 3 hours they may be seen in the chorionic membrane. Greenish or brownish discolorations in immature placentas are more often due to blood breakdown products (hematoidin, hemosiderin) following hemolysis than to meconium. Hemosiderin, of course, can be stained with the Prussian blue method for iron, and the bilirubin of meconium stains with bile stains. The immature fetus cannot discharge meconium, lacking the hormonal maturation for intestinal propulsion (Lucas et al., 1979). The surface of the membranes, the amnion, is normally shiny. Around the insertion of the cord one may find squamous metaplasia in the form of concentric nodules that are hydrophobic (Figure 13). They are a normal feature. Amnion nodosum, usually represented by a finely granular, dull appearance of the amnionic surface, correlates with oligohydramnios. One must, of course, be cognizant of whether the amnion is present at all and, if not, whether amnionic bands exist. Often some blood has dissected underneath the amnion during delivery or, especially, when fetal blood has been aspirated for diagnostic tests from the fetal surface blood vessels.

The placenta is next measured, and then the cord is examined. Is it central, eccentric, marginal, or membranous (velamentous) in its insertion? What is its length, and is it spiraled? We now understand that the length of the umbilical cord is determined primarily by fetal movements, and that excessive spiraling implies unusual fetal motions (Moessinger et al., 1982). There may be a genetic component to the spiraling and the length, as the umbilical cords of some animals have different and consistent lengths; but this characteristic is so far unknown for human umbilical cords. Are there knots, thrombi, or discolorations? Can any other unusual features be detected?

The cord is then severed from the bulk of the placenta, and its cut surface is studied at several locations. The most important observation to be made here is whether there are three vessels and if other unusual features are present. Single umbilical artery (SUA) is the commonest abnormality. One must also appreciate that there is almost always an anastomosis between the two umbilical arteries, and that it is usually found near the point of insertion on the placental surface (Priman, 1959). Thus counting the number of vessels is best done farther away from the insertion. When a velamentous insertion of the cord is found, the examiner must pursue the ramifications of the fetal vessels after they leave the site of cord insertion, at times finding thrombi, particularly in membranous vessels. These vessels may be disrupted, as in vasa previa, and acute exsanguination of the fetus is common in such circumstances.

The weight of the remaining disk is ascertained. It is generally useless to know the weight of the entire organ, including cord and membranes. Correlations with fetal

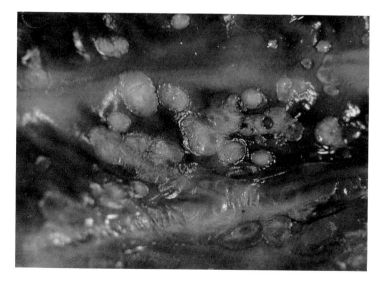

Figure 13. Squamous metaplasia of amnion in concentric patches, usually found near the insertion of the umbilical cord. The plaques are water-repellent.

weight and development can be made only by knowing the "net" weight of the placental tissue (Walker, 1954; Gruenwald & Minh, 1961). Excessive amounts of maternal, retroplacental clots must, of course, also have been removed before weighing. Note again that the weight of formalin-fixed placentas is greater than that of fresh organs (Figure 8) (Schremmer, 1967).

When studying the fetal surface of the placenta, one notes its color and the possible presence of granular excrescences. Most importantly, however, one must inspect the fetal vessels, which are carried in the chorion; the amnion has no blood vessels. In nearly all placentas, one can recognize the fetal arteries as those vessels that cross *over* the veins (Hyrtl, 1870; Bacsich & Smout, 1938; Boe, 1953; Crawford, 1962). It can be observed that the terminal branches of arteries dip singly into a cotyledon; and next to it a vein emerges to return the blood to the cord (Figure 14). One often finds thrombi in these vessels in placentas of abnormal newborns. They appear as white-yellow streaks on the vessel's surface and are usually not completely occlusive. When they are, an area of hemolysis is often seen adjacent to the thrombosis. Thrombi may also calcify. They must be sampled for histologic study.

The fetal surface of the mature placenta is often described as "bosselated" or "tesselated," meaning that tiny white elevations are present underneath the chorion, giving the surface a mosaic, irregular pattern. These protrusions represent accumulations of fibrin in the intervillous space, and they increase in number with advancing maturity. Larger patches of fibrin also exist; at times they have a liquefied center, but they are of little significance (Geller, 1959). Cysts from the subchorionic "X cells" (nonvillous cytotrophoblast) may bulge on the surface and contain a clear, slightly viscid mucoid substance. At times this substance is discolored

with blood. Finally, the insertion of the membranes is observed. Was the insertion at the edge, or was there a ring of "circumvallation"?

When the placenta is turned over then, exposing the maternal surface, the first step is to identify possible areas of abruptio. When an abruptio placentae is fresh, one may not be able to differentiate it from the normally present postpartum maternal blood clot that adheres. Within a few hours, though, the blood dries, becomes firmer and stringy, and then changes color to brown and eventually greenish. In such cases the placenta underneath is usually infarcted or is at least compressed. Abruptios are common, and most are clinically silent. Most are located at the margin of the placenta; and on occasion one finds old clot behind the membranes. Calcification on the maternal surface is then sought; it appears as small yellow-white granules in the decidua basalis and septa. Calcifications vary a good deal in quantity; they are usually found only in mature organs. The quantity has no clinically important correlations (Fujikura, 1963a,b; Jeacock et al., 1963), but clinicians have paid much attention to the recognition of calcification. It may be detected by sonography and has served as a method to "grade" (age) the placenta (Fisher et al., 1976). This step is rarely done now, as it has not been found to be helpful. At this point one also observes the cotyledons, the major subdivisions of the placental tissue. They increase in size and differentiation with advancing gestation, being absent early. One needs to ascertain now whether all of the placental "floor" is present or there are missing cotyledons. If no cotyledonary subdivisions exist in the mature placenta, the floor is often too thick and it may be infiltrated with an excess amount of fibrin. This condition is known as "maternal floor infarction" and is best noted at this time (Naeye, 1985).

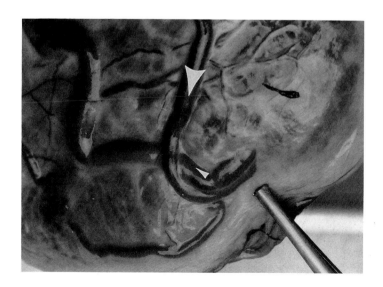

FIGURE 14. Entrance of fetal vessels of the chorionic plate into the cotyledon. One artery (large arrowhead) brings the fetal blood; the vein (small arrowhead) next to it returns it to the fetus.

Long, parallel cuts are now made with the long knife, and, most importantly, the color of the villous tissue is observed. The color of the villous tissue is almost wholly determined by its content of *fetal* blood. Thus a congested placenta (as in maternal diabetes, for instance) is dark. That of an anemic, hydropic, exsanguinated, or erythroblastotic fetus is pale, and it is usually much more friable. Such a placenta is also commonly thicker, 3 to 5 cm, in contrast to the normal placenta, which averages 2.0 to 2.5 cm at term.

It is normal to find "holes" in the center of many placentas (Fritschek, 1927). Such holes were filled in vivo with maternal blood and represent the areas of first blood distribution into the intervillous space from the maternal injection jet. Intervillous thrombi, often located in these spaces, may be dark when fresh; alternatively, they are composed of layered white fibrin when older. The intervillous thrombi differ from infarcts in that they displace villous tissue. Furthermore, infarcts are granular, in contrast, because they are composed of dead villous tissue. Fresh infarcts are red, and older ones are yellow to white. When sectioning the placenta, one also finds that the intercotyledonary septa contain some calcium and often some cystic spaces filled with clear mucoid material. They too arise from X cells. Occasionally one encounters round tumors of a solid nature, chorioangiomas. *Gitterinfarcts* or *netzinfarcts* (because they appear to form a network of fibrin) accompany maternal floor infarction. They may be prominent and appear as dense fibrin patches throughout the organ. It is good practice to estimate the total amount of infarction and record it; in fact, it is ultimately of some importance and may have medicolegal implications for infants with growth retardation. Single marginal infarcts are common and do not correlate with either fetal or maternal conditions. Other lesions are seen occasionally. Thus some lesions that appear grossly as "infarcts" may turn out to be choriocarcinoma on histological study (Driscoll, 1963).

Placentas of Multiple Births

Placentas of multiple births are important records for the infants, and they are routinely examined. A recording of the membrane relation between the twins, triplets, and so on is mandatory. Of course, for meaningful analysis it is necessary that the umbilical cords be labeled with sutures or clamps by the obstetrician, in the order of the births. The most important decisions to be made when examining placentas of multiple births are (1) the number of membranous sacs (one, two, or four) and (2) the types of vascular anastomoses present only in monochorionic twin placentas (Schatz, 1886). Fraternal (dizygotic) twins always have diamnionic/dichorionic (DiDi) placentas. Fused pla-

centas may be DiDi; they may be diamnionic/monochorionic (DiMo); or there may be no "dividing membranes" between the fetuses, as in the monoamnionic/monochorionic twin placenta (MoMo). All monochorionic placentas belong to monozygotic (MZ, or "identical") twins. The time at which MZ twins separated one from another during the early embryonic stages determines the type of placentation that develops, and the time can be estimated from an examination of the membrane relation. It is easiest, but not necessarily best, to separate the "dividing" membranes from each other. If there are four distinctive leaves it is a DiDi placenta, whereas if only two membranes are apposed it is a DiMo placenta. Equally readily, the diagnosis of a DiDi twin placenta is made by ascertaining that the dividing membranes are opaque, containing remnants of old vessels or other debris (old decidua, degenerated villi). The dividing membranes of DiMo placentas are transparent. Also, in DiDi placentas one usually finds a ridge at the site where the membranes meet over the placenta. It is caused by the buckling of tissues from the collision of the two expanding placental tissue masses. The diagnosis is, of course, easiest and most permanently established by a histological section of a membrane roll of this tissue or by a "T section" that includes this area (Figure 15).

The location of the cord insertion is especially important in twin placentas, as it is much more frequently marginal or membranous than in singletons; this positioning may reflect some problems during early placental development. Moreover, the presence of only a single umbilical artery is more common in multiple births (Heifetz, 1984).

After the membrane relation is established, the "vascular equator" (i.e., the area where the two chorionic vascular districts meet) is examined. In DiDi placentas there is never confluence of fetal blood vessels; if one were found, it would be exceptional and would be the basis for blood chimerism in fraternal twins. It must be cautioned here that ascertainment of a DiDi relation does not make the diagnosis of fraternal twins. Approximately one-third of identical twins have this placentation (discussed in greater detail in Chapter 25). In monochorionic placentas (DiMo, MoMo) there are almost always some anastomoses, particularly in the prematurely delivered placentas. These anastomoses have a great influence on the well-being of the developing fetus (Benirschke, 1961b; Bejar et al., 1988). They take three forms: artery to artery (AA), vein to vein (VV), and artery to vein (AV). The latter is doubtless the most important and is the basis for the "transfusion syndrome." It must here be remembered that arteries lie on top of veins, and that they are thus readily identified macroscopically. An AV anastomosis carries the blood of one twin, through a cotyledon in a one-way

FIGURE 15. Preparation of a "T section" of the meeting point of the dividing membranes in twin placentas.

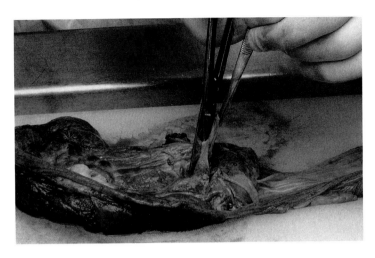

direction, to the other twin. Often various types of anastomosis coexist, and the consequences for fetal development may be different depending on the arrangements that are present. When in doubt, one injects the vessels in question with colored water or milk, all being readily available in obstetrical suites. Only the most sophisticated studies require injection with plastics (Panigel, 1962). Injection of vessels has presented some problems for novices. First it must be remembered that most placentas have suffered some disruption during delivery, especially the immature twin placentas. Therefore only small, selected areas should be injected, and it should be done only after the cords have been cut off, to reduce resistance. One should seek to identify the areas most "profitable" for injection by careful inspection. Large interarterial anastomoses (common) may be identified by one's ability to push blood back and forth from one side to the other. When one attempts to demonstrate the areas that reflect shared cotyledons, as in the transfusion syndrome, it is best to use a 20 ml syringe and a large (15 gauge) blunt needle. The needle is inserted into an arterial branch a little away from the prospective site, after which one gradually fills the area with water or milk. The cotyledon first rises and, when completely filled, empties into the vein that drains it. It is also advisable to make a drawing or photograph of the anastomotic arrangements among multiple placental vascular areas—just to have it available for the record.

Examination of the maternal surface and other parameters of the placentas of twins follows that of the regular protocol. It must be borne in mind that when the blood content of twins differs considerably it may be reflected in the macroscopic placental examination as well. One portion of such a twin placenta may be severely congested and large, with the other portion pale and small. This condition is present when only one AV anastomosis exists. Here, with the classical mechanism of the transfusion syndrome, one twin constantly loses blood through this one-way AV shunt, whereas the other becomes plethoric. Usually it leads to hydramnios, premature birth, and disparate birth weights of these "identical twins." It must be recognized, however, that differences in neonatal hemoglobin content of monochorionic twins may also occur acutely, when large AA and VV anastomoses exist. Thus after the delivery of one twin, the other twin may bleed through anastomoses if the cord of the delivered twin is not promptly clamped. Likewise, when one of such twins dies in utero, significant shifts of blood may occur from the live twin through such large anastomoses into the relaxed vascular bed of the deceased twin.

Finally, it is our practice to dissect the two halves of the twin placenta at the site of the vascular equator in order to determine the placental weight of each twin. Multiple births are handled the same way.

Fixation

The pathologist is accustomed to fixing tissues for histological study in 10% formalin (a 1:10 dilution of the commercial 40% formaldehyde), and there is no need to make an exception with the placenta. For *routine histopathology* we prefer Bouin's solution, however, because it makes embryonic and placental tissue considerably harder and allows one to trim the tissue more readily before embedding. After a membrane roll is made with the help of the forceps, it is also much easier to trim this "jelly-roll" when Bouin's solution (rather than formalin) has been used. Bouin's solution is made by preparing a saturated solution (1.2%) of picric acid in water and adding 40% formaldehyde solution and glacial acetic acid in proportions of 15:5:1. After overnight fixation, the tissue is ready to be trimmed.

Carnoy solution is a useful alternative if immediate fixation is required directly after delivery and if obstetricians refuse to use formaldehyde in the vicinity of the delivery room. This fixative is composed of 60 ml absolute ethanol, 30 ml chloroform, and 10 ml glacial acetic acid. It guarantees good structural preservation, provided the thickness of the tissue blocks does not exceed 3 to 4 mm.

Many other fixatives have been used. Jiricka and Preslickova (1974) made a detailed study of seven solutions and evaluated the effect for the staining characteristics with different dyes. They found that none is ideal for all purposes, so the fixative must be chosen that gives the best results for a specific reason. The authors presented this information in tabular form, and their paper must be consulted if optimal results are to be obtained.

Ideally, the sectioned slices, when Bouin-fixed, are immersed in a saturated lithium carbonate solution before embedding. This step is not absolutely required, but it helps to remove extraneous pigments. Moreover, some intervillous blood is lysed, and pigments derived from blood ("formalin pigment," acid hematin) are more frequently present when lithium carbonate is omitted. Note, however, that occasionally the use of Bouin's fixation is disadvantageous. For instance, Altshuler and Hyde (1985) reported that infection with fusobacteria was less readily appreciated after Bouin's fixation than when formalin was used.

Furthermore, as Gleich pointed out, Bouin's solution is not useful for fixation when the purpose is to conduct an immunofluorescence study of major basic protein (MBP), produced by X cells, and for in situ hybridization studies (Gleich, personal communication, 1989). Today many *immunohistochemical studies* can be carried out on paraffin sections, such as the demonstration of most cytoskeletal proteins, extracellular matrix molecules, and several proliferation markers (Frank et al., 1994). For all these purposes we suggest that fixation be done in 4% neutral buffered formaldehyde solution for a maximum of 24 hours followed by paraffin embedding not exceeding 60°C.

Another important issue is the manner of tissue handling prior to fixation. The time and mode of cord clamping (Bouw et al., 1976), the ischemic period before onset of fixation (Voigt et al., 1978; Kaufmann, 1985), and the composition of the fixative (Kaufmann, 1980) may well influence the distension of the fetal vascular bed and the width of the intervillous space (Tables 15, 17–19). We recommend, particularly for all studies concerning the pathology of the fetoplacental vessels (e.g., in cases with a Doppler high resistance index), that a strictly standardized sampling and fixation protocol be used.

Other techniques, of course, may also require special handling, as for instance in the studies by Becker and Bleyl (1961) on toxemia. They employed fluorescence microscopy of villi to understand the various compositions of these structures in this disease.

It is the recommended practice to save at least one section of umbilical cord, a membrane roll, and three pieces of placental tissue for histological examination. Of course, having more sections of umbilical cord available for histological study is ideal, as an inflammatory response, thrombi, and other features are not always uniformly distributed throughout the length of the umbilical cord. Preparing more than one piece of placental tissue for histological study is also desirable because so many areas of the placenta show histological variations. Thus one can much better determine the existence of inflammatory lesions and is less apt to overlook changes that are not ascertained macroscopically. Moreover, it is wise to obtain sections from the more normal portions of the placenta as well. Although the pathologist is used to sampling abnormal areas for histological study, it is not desirable to take only abnormal areas of the placenta. Indeed, almost all infarcts are histologically alike; and because they also have a typical macroscopic appearance, they are rarely worth the trouble of histological study, except that the sections provide verifiable evidence of the existence of infarcts. It is much more important to save normal-appearing placental tissue for microscopy. One must sample both the fetal and maternal surfaces in order to include some fetal surface blood vessels. Because it is generally impossible to anticipate from macroscopic inspection whether chronic villitis and many other lesions exist, it is better to preserve too much than too little in the fixative. It goes without saying that unusual-appearing areas must also be sampled.

For histological examination, we prefer the hematoxylin and eosin stain. On many occasions, however, it is useful to employ special stains, such as elastica preparations, bacterial and spirochete stains, periodic acid-Schiff preparations, and specific immunohistochemical stains that disclose the presence of viruses (e.g., cytomegalovirus and herpes antigens) and specific proteins (e.g., human chorionic gonadotropin, placental lactogen, MBP, cytokeratin, vimentin, fibrin, and proliferation markers) (see Chapter 4). These tests have given much insight into the sites of hormone production and the involvement by organisms as well as other pathological processes. The report form used by us during placental examination is reproduced on the following page for the benefit of the reader.

Special Procedures

The placenta can serve as a good source of tissue for *chromosome analysis*. It is especially useful when the fetus is macerated. One proceeds best by disinfecting the amnion with some alcohol and then stripping the amnion off a portion of the placental surface. For the

REPORT OF PLACENTAL EXAMINATION

NAME of PATIENT:_____   Path. #_____
                                                                 Unit #_____

HISTORY:_____

_____

_____

INFANT:_____

_____

Macroscopic:

WEIGHT (disk only)_____g   Formalin-fixed_____ Fresh_____

SIZE___ x___ x___cm

CORD: INSERTION: Central___ Eccentric:_____cm from margin

                 Marginal__Velamentous__Vasa previa_____

        Vessels: 3__ 2__ Thrombosis: Yes__ No__ Knots:_____

MEMBRANES: Marginal___ Circumvallate___ Color: Green___ Opaque___ Normal___

       Point of rupture from margin:_____cm

       Amnion nodosum_____

SURFACE VESSELS:_____

TWINS: Yes___ No_____   HIGHER MULTIPLES:_____

       DiDi___ DiMo___ MoMo___

Describe twin placenta_____ Anastomoses_____

MATERNAL SURFACE: Intact: Yes___ No___ Calcification: Marked___ normal___ no__

       Color:_____ (Normal?)_____ (Pale?)_____

       Abruptio: Yes___ No___ Size_____cm Old___ Recent___

CUT SURFACE: Infarct___ % of total placenta___ Old___ Recent___

TUMORS_____

OTHER_____

Microscopic:_____

_____

_____

DIAGNOSIS:

_____

Pathologist

purpose of obtaining a biopsy specimen from chorion, sterile instruments are recommended. A small piece of chorion, ideally with a bit of fetal surface vessel, is the best choice for the purpose of establishing a tissue culture. The specimens are placed in tissue culture medium with antibiotics and transferred to the laboratory. Touch preparations of amnionic surface or from the undersurface of the amnion may be useful for the *identification of bacteria or leukocytes*. It is of parenthetical interest that Jauniaux and Campbell (1990) showed that many structural abnormalities of the placenta can be anticipated using *sonography*.

References

ACOG: Placental Pathology. Committee Opinion. Vol. 102, pp. 1–2, 1991.

Altshuler, G., and Hyde, S.: Fusobacteria: an important cause of chorioamnionitis. Arch. Pathol. Lab. Med. 109:739–743, 1985.

Bacsich, P., and Smout, C.F.V.: Some observations on the foetal vessels of the human placenta with an account of the corrosion technique. J. Anat. 72:358–364, 1938.

Bartholomew, R.A., Colvin, E.D., Grimes, W.H., Fish, J.S., Lester, W.M., and Galloway, W.H.: Criteria by which toxemia of pregnancy may be diagnosed from unlabeled formalin-fixed placentas. Am. J. Obstet. Gynecol. 82:277–290, 1961.

Becker, V., and Bleyl, U.: Placentarzotte bei Schwangerschaftstoxicose und fetaler Erythroblastose im fluorescenzmikroskopischen Bilde. Virchows Arch. Pathol. Anat. 334:516–527, 1961.

Bejar, R., Wozniak, P., Allard, M., Benirschke, K., Vaucher, Y., Coen, R., Berry, C., Schragg, P., Villegas, I., and Resnik, R.: Antenatal origin of neurologic damage in newborn infants. I. Preterm infants. Am. J. Obstet. Gynecol. 159:357–363, 1988.

Benirschke, K.: Examination of the placenta. Obstet. Gynecol. 18:309–333, 1961a.

Benirschke, K.: Twin placenta and perinatal mortality. N.Y. State J. Med. 61:1499–1508, 1961b.

Boe, F.: Studies on vascularization of the human placenta. Acta Obstet. Gynecol. Scand. Suppl. 5 32:1–92, 1953.

Bouw, G.M., Stolte, L.A.M., Baak, J.P.A., and Oort, J.: Quantitative morphology of the placenta. 1. Standardization of sampling. Eur. J. Obstet. Gynecol. Reprod. Biol. 6:325–331, 1976.

Crawford, J.M.: Vascular anatomy of the human placenta. Am. J. Obstet. Gynecol. 84:1543–1567, 1962.

Driscoll, S.G.: Choriocarcinoma: an "incidental finding" within a term placenta. Obstet. Gynecol. 21:96–101, 1963.

Fisher, C.C., Garrett, W., and Kossoff, G.: Placental aging monitored by gray scale echography. Am. J. Obstet. Gynecol. 124:483–488, 1976.

Fox, H.: Pathology of the Placenta. Saunders, London, 1978.

Frank, H.G., Malekzadeh, F., Kertschanska, S., Crescimanno, C., Castellucci, M., Lang, I., Desoye, G., and Kaufmann, P.: Immunohistochemistry of two different types of placental fibrinoid. Acta Anat. (Basel) 150:55–68, 1994.

Fritschek, F.: Über "leere" Placentarhohlräume. Anat. Anz. 64:65–73, 1927.

Fujikura, T.: Placental calcification and maternal age. Am. J. Obstet. Gynecol. 87:41–45, 1963a.

Fujikura, T.: Placental calcification and seasonal difference. Am. J. Obstet. Gynecol. 87:46–47, 1963b.

Geller, H.F.: Über die Bedeutung des subchorialen Fibrinstreifens in der menschlichen Placenta. Arch. Gynecol. 192:1–6, 1959.

Gruenwald, P.: Examination of the placenta by the pathologist. Arch. Pathol. 77:41–46, 1964.

Gruenwald, P., and Minh, H.N.: Evaluation of body and organ weights in perinatal pathology. II. Weight of body and placenta of surviving and of autopsied infants. Am. J. Obstet. Gynecol. 82:312–319, 1961.

Heifetz, S.A.: Single umbilical artery: a statistical analysis of 237 autopsy cases and review of the literature. Perspect. Pediatr. Pathol. 8:345–378, 1984.

Hyrtl, J.: Die Blutgefässe der Menschlichen Nachgeburt Unter Normalen und Abnormen Verhältnissen. Braumüller, Vienna, 1870.

Jauniaux, E., and Campbell, S.: Ultrasonographic assessment of placental abnormalities. Am. J. Obstet. Gynecol. 163:1650–1658, 1990.

Jeacock, M.K., Scott, J., and Plester, J.A.: Calcium content of the human placenta. Am. J. Obstet. Gynecol. 87:34–40, 1963.

Jiricka, Z., and Preslickova, M.: The effect of fixation on staining of placental tissue. Z. Versuchstierkd. 16:127–130, 1974.

Kaufmann, P.: Der osmotische Effekt der Fixation auf die Placentastruktur. Verh. Anat. Ges. 74:351–352, 1980.

Kaufmann, P.: Influence of ischemia and artificial perfusion on placental ultrastructure and morphometry. Contrib. Gynecol. Obstet. 13:18–26, 1985.

Las Heras, J., Micheli, V., and Kakarieka, E.: Placental pathology in perinatal deaths [abstract 26]. Mod. Pathol. 7(1):5P, 1994.

Lucas, A., Christofides, N.D., Adran, T.E., Bloom, S.R., and Aynsley-Green, A.: Fetal distress, meconium, and motilin. Lancet i:718, 1979.

Miller, P.W., Coen, R.W., and Benirschke, K.: Dating the time interval from meconium passage to birth. Obstet. Gynecol. 66:459–462, 1985.

Moessinger, A.C., Blanc, W.A., Marone, P.A., and Polsen, D.C.: Umbilical cord length as an index of fetal activity: experimental study and clinical implications. Pediatr. Res. 16:109–112, 1982.

Naeye, R.L.: Maternal floor infarction. Hum. Pathol. 16:823–828, 1985.

Naeye, R.L.: Functionally important disorders of the placenta, umbilical cord, and fetal membranes. Hum. Pathol. 18:680–691, 1987.

Panigel, M.: Placental perfusion experiments. Am. J. Obstet. Gynecol. 84:1664–1683, 1962.

Priman, J.: A note on the anastomosis of the umbilical arteries. Anat. Rec. 134:1–5, 1959.

Pritchard, J.A., MacDonald, P.C., and Gant, N.F.: Williams Obstetrics. 17th ed. Appleton-Century-Crofts, Norwalk, CN, 1985.

Reece, E.A., Scioscia, A.L., Pinter, E., Hobbins, J.C., Green, J., Mahoney, M.J., and Naftolin, F.: Prognostic significance of the human yolk sac assessed by ultrasonography. Am. J. Obstet. Gynecol. 159:1191–1194, 1988.

Salafia, C.M., and Vintzileos, A.M.: Why all placentas should be examined by a pathologist in 1990. Am. J. Obstet. Gynecol. 163:1282–1293, 1990. See also discussion Am. J. Obstet. Gynecol. 165:783–784, 1991.

Schatz, F.: Die Gefässverbindungen der Placentakreisläufe eineiiger Zwillinge, ihre Entwicklung und ihre Folgen. Arch. Gynecol. 27:1–72, 1886.

Schremmer, B.-N.: Gewichtsveränderungen verschiedener Gewebe nach Formalinfixierung. Frankfurt Z. Pathol. 77:299–304, 1967.

Snoeck, J.: Le Placenta Humain. Masson & Cie, Paris, 1958.

Torpin, R., and Hart, B.F.: Placenta bilobata. Am. J. Obstet. Gynecol. 42:38–49, 1941.

Travers, H., and Schmidt, W.A.: College of American Pathologists Conference XIX on the Examination of the Placenta. Arch. Pathol. Lab. Med. 115:660–731, 1991. [a composite of many articles by numerous authors].

Voigt, S., Kaufmann, P., and Schweikhart, G.: Zur Abgrenzung normaler, artefizieller und pathologischer Strukturen in reifen menschlichen Plazentazotten. II. Morphometrische Untersuchungen zum Einfluss des Fixationsmodus. Arch. Gynecol. 226:347–362, 1978.

Walker, J.: Weight of the human fetus and of its placenta. Cold Spring Harbor Symp. Quant. Biol. 19:39–40, 1954.

Zeek, P.M., and Assali, N.S.: Vascular changes in the decidua associated with eclamptogenic toxemia of pregnancy. Am. J. Clin. Pathol. 20:1099–1109, 1950.

3
Macroscopic Features of the Delivered Placenta

The full-term, delivered placenta in more than 90% of the cases is a disk-like, flat, round to oval organ. In nearly 10% it has an abnormal shape, such as placenta bilobata, placenta duplex, placenta succenturiata, placenta zonaria, or placenta membranacea (Torpin, 1969). The average diameter is 22 cm, the average thickness in the center of the delivered organ is 2.5 cm, and the average weight is 470 g (Table 2, p. 42). The respective measurements show considerable interindividual variation and strongly depend on such factors as mode of birth, time of cord clamping (Table 9, p. 46), and time elapsed between delivery and fixation.

The fetal (chorionic or amnionic) surface, facing the amnionic cavity, has a glossy appearance due to the intact epithelial surface of the amnion. This membrane covers the chorionic plate, including the chorionic vessels. The latter branch in a star-like pattern centrifugally from the cord insertion over the fetal surface (Figure 34, left). Where arteries and veins cross, the arterial branches are usually closer to the amnion; they cross the veins on their amnionic aspect. Wentworth (1965) reported that only about 3% show the opposite condition. According to Boyd and Hamilton (1970), the superficial position of one or few venous branches at points of arteriovenous crossing is not unusual.

In the vicinity of the larger chorionic vessels, the chorionic plate normally has an opaque appearance due to the increased number of collagen fibers that accompany the vessels. Those areas of the chorionic plate located between the chorionic vessels are mostly transparent and are dark lilac to black owing to maternal blood in the intervillous space shining through. Opaque spots (bosselations) or large opaque areas independent of chorionic vessels usually point to large subchorionic deposits of Langhans' fibrinoid.

Near the placental margin, where the most peripheral branches of the chorionic vessels bend vertically toward the marginal villous trees, the transparency of the chorionic plate decreases, resulting in a largely incomplete, opaque subchorial closing ring that is a result of increased amounts of cytotrophoblast and collagen fibers (see Chapter 11). It connects the placenta with the membranes. In the case of a particularly broad, prominent subchorial closing ring, the specimen is called a placenta marginata. A placenta circumvallata is formed as soon as the closing ring is peripherally undergrown by villous trees. In such cases it does not represent the outermost margin of the placenta; rather, the membranes insert superficially from the fetal surface of the placenta.

The uterine (maternal) surface of the placenta is opaque, as it is an artificial surface originating from laminar degenerative processes within the junctional zone that led to the separation of the organ. This surface could not be identified prior to placental separation in in situ specimens that were fixed before the onset of labor (Figure 7). It is composed of a heterogeneous mixture of trophoblastic and decidual cells embedded in prevailing amounts of extracellular debris, fibrinoid, and blood clot.

An incomplete system of grooves subdivides the basal surface of the placenta into 10 to 40 slightly elevated areas called lobes (lobules or maternal cotyledons) (Figure 16, right; Figure 17). Internally, the grooves correspond to the septa (Figures 7, 236). In histological sections, the septa often can be seen indented at their basal surfaces (Figure 236). It is likely that these grooves and the respective basal indentations of the septa are the postpartal results of tearing at sites of minor mechanical resistance, as the basal central parts of the septa are often characterized by necrotic zones, clefts (Figure 236), and (locally) pseudocysts. Despite their possibly artifactual genesis, the grooves delineate the lobes and mark the position of the septa. As described in Chapter 11, the septa must not be misunderstood to be separating structures that subdivide the intervillous space into chambers; rather, they are

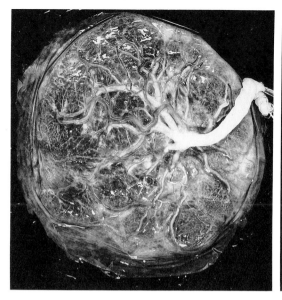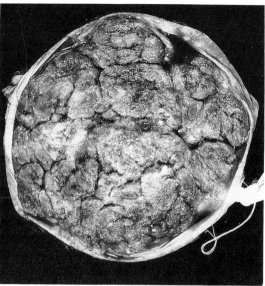

FIGURE 16. Apical (left) and basal (right) views of a freshly delivered, mature human placenta. Note the slightly eccentric insertion of the cord, which is the usual situation. The chorionic arteries (dark vessels) cross over the corresponding veins (light vessels). The basal surface is subdivided into placental lobules of varying size by an interrupted net of grooves. ×0.30.

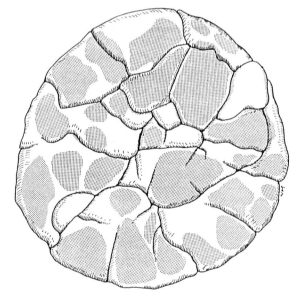

FIGURE 17. Basal view of the placenta, drawn in combination with a radiograph of the same placenta after injection of a radiopaque medium into the fetal vessels. The borderlines of the placental lobules (maternal cotyledons) as seen in Figure 16 are marked by lines. The radiographic projections of 29 villous trees are represented by stippled areas. This combination demonstrates a fairly good harmony of villous trees and maternal lobes. One to three villous trees are projected on one lobe. (From Kaufmann & Scheffen, 1992, with permission; based on photographs by Boyd & Hamilton, 1970.)

irregular pillars or short sails that only trace the lobular borders.

The lobes show fairly good harmony with the position of the villous trees. From the chorionic plate at term, 60 to 70 villous stems arise, each branching into one villous tree (or fetal cotyledon) (Figures 7, 81). According to Boyd and Hamilton (1970) and Kaufmann (1985), each lobe is occupied by one or several villous trees. When projecting a radioangiogram of the villous trees on the basal view of the same placenta (Figure 17), the borderlines of the lobes usually coincide with the borderlines of single villous trees or small groups of trees. Small marginal lobes are likely to be occupied by only a single villous tree and so correspond to what Schuhmann (1981) and his group described as representing a placentone.

When describing human placentation, terms such as fetal placenta and maternal placenta must be avoided because they are misleading and often cause misinterpretation. This point may become important as soon as morphologically inexperienced biochemists or endocrinologists isolate respective parts of the organ, trust in their putative and designated origin, and draw functional conclusions. A typical example is the questionable interpretation that decidua may produce human placental lactogen (hPL). The basal plate, often referred to as maternal placenta, represents a colorful mixture of trophoblastic and endometrium-derived cells. The term fetal placenta is also inappropriate. With the possible exception of central parts of the chorionic plate, there are no placental structures of which the mere fetal composition can be ensured. The marginal zone of the chorionic plate contains decidua. The same is true for parts of the cell islands and septa. Because the latter may be attached to the villous trees, one is never sure that villous preparations are devoid of maternal tissues, even if we disregard maternal blood and fibrinoid deposits that partly are maternal blood clot products. A corresponding warning is necessary regarding the placental bed. It is often thought to represent only the maternal remains of the placental site after separation of the placenta. Trophoblastic streamers deeply invade the endometrium, however, and even penetrate the myometrium. They remain in utero after delivery and can be found as fetal admixtures in the placental bed.

Placental shape and cord insertion are sometimes regarded as structurally impressive but functionally unimportant parameters. Becker (1989) stressed that both are influenced by the intrauterine position of the placenta. According to Schultze (1887), the location of the cord insertion represents the epicenter of implantation. Eccentric or marginal cord insertion thus points to an eccentric implantation on the anterior or posterior uterine wall, which causes asymmetrical development of the organ for mechanical and nutritional reasons.

References

Becker, V.: Plazenta. In, Pathologie der Plazenta und des Abortes. V. Becker and G. Röckelein, eds., pp. 1–155. Springer-Verlag, Berlin, 1989.

Boyd, J.D., and Hamilton, W.J.: The Human Placenta. Heffer & Sons, Cambridge, 1970.

Kaufmann, P.: Basic morphology of the fetal and maternal circuits in the human placenta. Contrib. Gynecol. Obstet. 13:5–17, 1985.

Kaufmann, P., and Scheffen, I.: Placental development. In, Neonatal and Fetal Medicine—Physiology and Pathophysiology, Vol. 1. R. Polin and W. Fox, eds., pp. 47–55. Saunders, Orlando, FL, 1992.

Schuhmann, R.: Plazenton: Begriff, Entstehung, funktionelle Anatomie. In, Die Plazenta des Menschen. V. Becker, T.H. Schiebler, and F. Kubli, eds., pp. 199–207. Thieme Verlag, Stuttgart, 1981.

Schultze, B.S.: Über velamentöse und placentale Insertion der Nabelschnur. Arch. Gynecol. 30:47–56, 1887.

Torpin, R.: The Human Placenta. Charles C Thomas, Springfield, IL, 1969.

Wentworth, P.: Some anomalies of the foetal vessels of the human placenta. J. Anat. 99:273–282, 1965.

4
Microscopic Survey

For the beginner in placental histology and histopathology, paraffin sections of the organ are confusing as they contain not only a broad variety of differently structured villi but many nonvillous structures as well. It is the intention of this chapter to provide an introduction to those basic histologic features that leap into eyesight during inspection of a paraffin section and thus provide a quick orientation for the inexperienced. For this purpose we have selected a collection of conventional photographs from routine histologic sections and of routine quality. For further reading concerning the various structures, we refer to later chapters.

Ideally, routine histological examination of the human placenta requires vertically oriented sections that cover all placental structures from the chorionic plate, to the intervillous space, to the basal plate (Figures 18A, 19A). Such sections are easily obtained from most second and third trimester placentas, as well as from the rare in situ specimens obtained by hysterectomy during the first trimester (Figure 18A). Tissue biopsies from legal interruptions of pregnancy are in most cases less ideal for good survey pictures; usually the basal plate and its neighboring tissues, such as septa, anchoring villi, and cell columns, are either absent or at least difficult to identify because they are destroyed and mixed up among the villi.

Typical Histological Features of the First Trimester Placenta

Figure 18A: Complete and well preserved survey sections of the first trimester placenta, such as the vertical section of an in situ specimen from the 6th week postmenstruation (p.m.) shown in Figure 18A, cover the following structures: chorionic plate, intervillous space surrounding the placental villi, cell islands, and the basal plate, from which in Figure 18A a septum

protrudes into the intervillous space; some anchoring villi may be connected via cell columns to the septum or to the basal plate.

The *intervillous space* (see pp. 139ff) is the diffuse space surrounded by the chorionic plate on one side and the basal plate on the other. From the 13th week on it contains maternal blood, the volume of which increases to about 100 to 200 ml at term. Up to the 12th week p.m. only plasma has been found in the intervillous space; it is filtered out of the uteroplacental vessels (see p. 231). The maternal plasma, and in later stages maternal blood, flows around the villous trees, cell islands, septa, and fibrinoid deposits. During early pregnancy the mean width of the intervillous space (between neighboring villi) usually amounts to several hundred micrometers.

Figure 18B: Histological specimens of the first trimester *chorionic plate* (see pp. 213ff) usually are devoid of amnion, as amnion is only superficially attached to the chorionic plate and is usually removed during preparation. Occasionally, pieces of amnion can be found curled up or upside down somewhere at the section's margin. As it is a regular constituent of most third trimester survey sections, it is dealt with on p. 34 (Figures 19A,B).

If the amnion is missing, as it is in this case, the surface of the chorionic plate toward the fetus is covered by an inconspicuous, incomplete layer of mesothelium. It follows a thick layer of chorionic mesoderm in which the chorionic branches of the umbilical vessels are embedded. Toward the intervillous space, the surface is covered in the early stages by a layer of syncytiotrophoblast, which with progressing pregnancy is replaced by fibrinoid (Figure 19C).

Figure 18C: The tree-like placental villi arise from the chorionic plate and protrude into the intervillous space, the villous trophoblastic surface being bathed directly in maternal plasma or blood. The trophoblastic surface of the villi is composed of an outer continuous layer of *villous syncytiotrophoblast*, underneath which is a discontinuous layer of *villous cytotrophoblast* (Langhans' cells) (see pp. 71ff). The villous cytotrophoblast represents the proliferating stem cells for the syncytiotrophoblast, which forms the decisive maternofetal transport barrier. The relative number of Langhans' cells decreases toward term.

The stroma of the villi is composed of the *fetal vessels*, which are embedded in a mixture of fixed connective tissue cells, macrophages, and connective tissue fibers. Throughout the first 2 months of pregnancy, *nucleated red blood cells* inside the fetal villous vessels are a regular finding (see p. 345).

Figure 18D: Early in gestation the *central stems* of the villous trees show signs of fibrosis (Figure 18D) around larger central vessels that gradually achieve the structural characteristics of arteries and veins. The superficial stromal layer has an unfibrosed, reticular appearance (see p. 121, Figures 67, 84–87). Arrows indicate the syncytial sprouts (Figure 18D). Before the 8th week p.m. even the largest villi show a homogeneous mesenchymal stroma that is mostly not fibrosed and is devoid of the reticular structure; arteries and veins are absent as well (Figures 82, 83).

Figure 18E: Most of the large, bulbous villi of the first and second trimester are *immature intermediate villi* with reticular stroma and without stromal fibrosis. The fixed connective tissue cells surround channel-like spaces within the reticular stroma (Figure 18E) (see p. 121). These channels contain stromal macrophages (Hofbauer cells) that are easily identifiable by their rounded shape and their vacuolated or granular cytoplasm (see p. 84).

Figure 18F: The peripheral branches of the immature intermediate villi are the *mesenchymal villi* (see p. 124). They usually have diameters of 60 to 200 µm and are characterized by a dense cellular stroma; they possess few fetal vessels or collagen fibers. Peripherally, the mesenchymal villi extend into *syncytial sprouts* (see p. 128), mere syncytiotrophoblastic, multinucleated structures. Often the sprouts appear as dark cross sections (Figure 18D) that seemingly do not have contact with villous surfaces.

Syncytial or trophoblastic sprouts are the first steps in the formation of new villi. They are invaded by mesenchymal stroma and fetal capillary sprouts and thus transform into mesenchymal villi. Later, the mesenchymal villi grow in size and achieve the typical structure of immature intermediate villi (see p. 130). For a description of the structural aspects of trophoblastic knotting and sprouting, see Chapter 10; for the pathohistological significance see p. 142 and p. 411.

Figure 18G: *Cell islands* are globular accumulations of extravillous trophoblast cells that adhere to one or several villi (see pp. 237ff). They are directly continuous with villous cytotrophoblast in places were the villous syncytiotrophoblast is interrupted. Parts of the surfaces of these islands may be covered with plaques of syncytiotrophoblast. The extravillous trophoblast cells are usually embedded in matrix-type fibrinoid (see below and p. 204). Cell islands are the still proliferating remainders of the free-floating primary villi from early pregnancy stages that were never excavated by villous stroma.

Figure 18H: *Placental septa* are veil-like or pillar-shaped extensions of the basal plate that protrude into the intervillous space. They are rudimentary walls that are unable to completely subdivide the intervillous space into separate chambers. Structurally, they have the same composition as the basal plate, as they contain mostly extravillous trophoblast cells and sometimes also decidual cells (Figure 140). Often anchoring villi can be seen attached to the septa. In this stage of pregnancy they belong to the mesenchymal or immature intermediate type of villi. Cross sections of tips of septa resemble cell islands and can be confused with the latter. For further information see p. 234.

Figure 18I: *Anchoring villi* are peripheral villi that are connected to the basal plate or the placental septa (Figure 18H) via cell columns. They stabilize the position of the villous trees in the maternal intervillous bloodstream. For their development see p. 53.

Cell columns are the trophoblastic feet of the anchoring villi. During early stages of pregnancy they consist of several layers of proliferating extravillous cytotrophoblast serving as a proliferative source of villous and basal plate cytotrophoblast (see pp. 184ff, p. 240).

Figure 18J: The *basal plate* is the bottom of the intervillous space and is that part of the maternofetal junctional zone that adheres to the delivered placenta (see pp. 219ff). The basal portion of the maternofetal junctional zone—that which adheres to the myometrium and remains in utero after delivery—is called the placental bed. The basal plate is composed of an admixture of extravillous trophoblast cells, various endometrial stromal cells, decidual cells, uteroplacental vessels, and endometrial glands, all embedded in ample fibrinoid, which makes up the glossy to fibrillar ground substance.

Extravillous trophoblast cells is the summarizing term for all trophoblast cells located outside the villi: in the chorionic plate, cell islands, septa, basal plate, cell columns, and membranes. Apparent inhomogeneities within the population are mostly due to different stages of proliferation and differentiation: Those cells resting on the basal lamina facing the chorionic mesoderm (chorionic plate, membranes) or the villous stroma (cell columns, cell islands) seem to be the proliferating stem cells (Langhans' cells), whereas the nonproliferating extravillous trophoblast cells represent higher differentiated, invasive daughter cells of the former

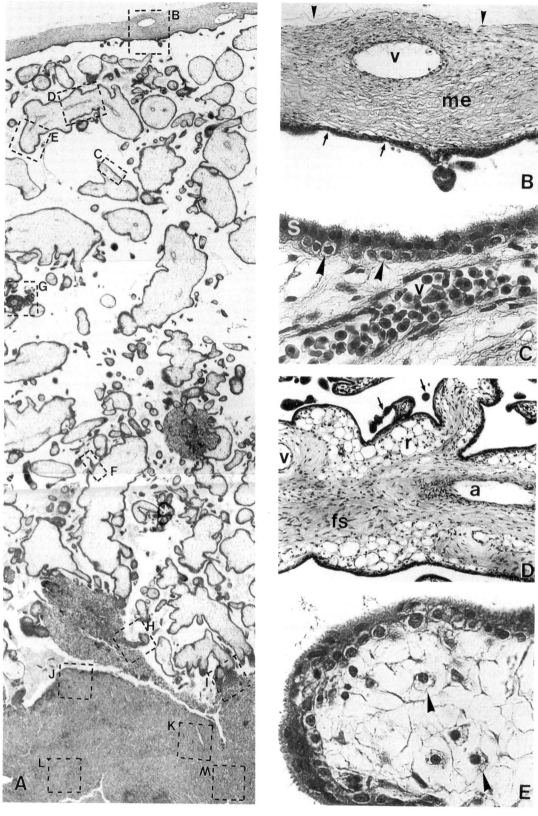

FIGURE 18. Typical features of the first trimester placenta as seen in paraffin sections after H&E staining. All specimens are from the 6th week p.m., except when otherwise stated. For details see the text. (A) Vertical survey section of an in situ specimen, 6th week p.m. The marked frames refer to the following detailed pictures. ×20. (B) Chorionic plate. v = vein; arrowheads = mesothelium; me = chorionic mesoderm; arrows = incomplete layer of syncytiotrophoblast. ×100. (C) Surface of an immature intermediate villus with trophoblast and a fetal vessel (v) containing nucleated red blood cells. s = syncytiotrophoblast; arrowheads = cytotrophoblast. ×400. (D) Transitional form of an immature intermediate villus to become a stem villus (18th week p.m.). a = artery; v = vein; r = reticular stroma; fs = fibrous stroma; arrows = sprouts. ×100. (E) Immature intermediate villus showing characteristic reticular stroma with macrophages (arrowheads). ×400. (F) Mesenchymal villus (m) arising from an immature intermediate villus (i) and extending into syncytial sprouts

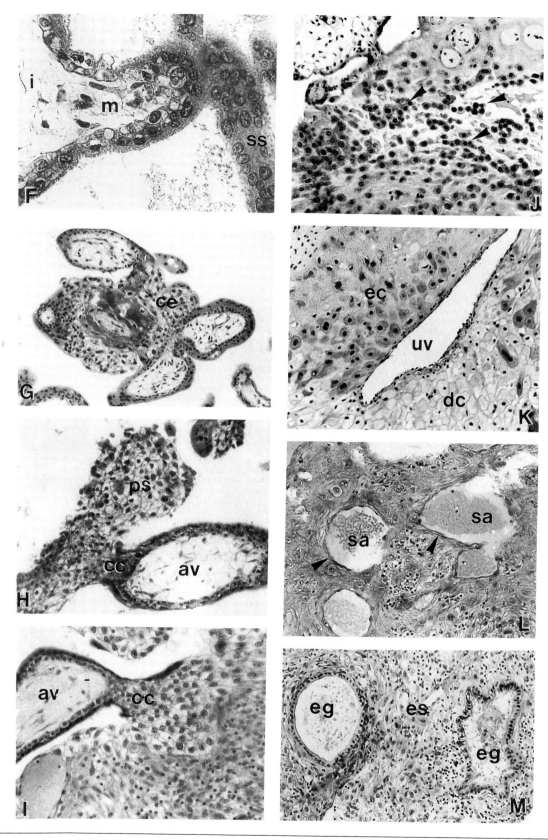

(ss). ×400. (G) Cell island (ce) attached to some villi. ×100. (H) Placental septum (ps) connected to a villus (av) by a cell column (cc). ×200. (I) Anchoring villus (av) connected to the basal plate by a cell column (cc). ×200. (J) Surface of the basal plate showing extravillous trophoblast cells (arrowheads) embedded in fibrinoid (10th week p.m.). ×100. (K) Deep part of the basal plate showing a uteroplacental vein (uv) sur-

rounded by extravillous cytotrophoblast (ec) and decidua (dc) (37th week p.m., similar to the first trimester situation). ×140. (L) Multiple cross sections across a spiral artery (sa), the wall of which is replaced by fibrinoid (arrowheads). ×100. (M) Endometrial glands (eg) of the junctional zone embedded in endometrial stroma (es). ×200. For further details see the text.

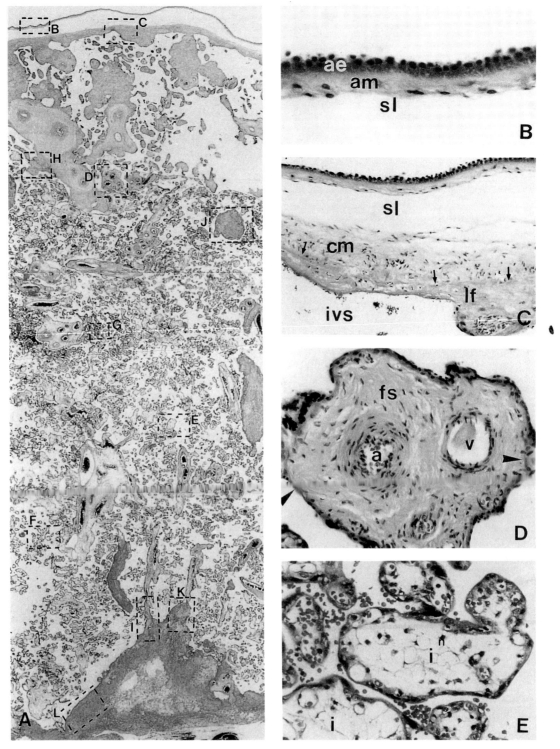

FIGURE 19. Typical features of the third trimester placenta as seen in paraffin sections after H&E staining. All specimens are from the 40th week p.m. For details see the text. (A) Vertical survey section. The marked frames refer to the following detailed pictures. ×10. (B) Amnion. ae = amnionic epithelium; am = amnionic mesoderm; sl = spongy layer. ×120. (C) Chorionic plate, covered by the amnion. lf = Langhans fibrinoid stria; arrows = basement membrane; cm = chorionic mesoderm. ×60. (D) Peripheral stem villus. fs = fibrous stroma; a = artery; v = vein; arrowheads = syncytiotrophoblast. ×180. (E) Two immature intermediate villi (i) surrounded by some mature intermediate and terminal villi. ×180. (F) Longitudinally sectioned mature intermediate villus (mv) together with some terminal villi and villous fibrinoid necrosis (if). ×180. (G) Group of terminal villi (t) showing considerable knotting (k). ×360. (H) Small stem villus, the trophoblastic cover of which is partly replaced by a thick plug of perivillous fibrinoid (f). ×180. (I) Anchoring villus (av), connected to the basal plate by fibrinoid (rf) as the originally connecting cell column has vanished. ×180. (J) Cell island. mf = matrix-type fibrinoid. ×90. (K) Tip of a placental septum with ample matrix. ×90. (L) Basal plate with obvious layering. rf = Rohr fibrinoid; nf = Nitabuch fibrinoid; dc = decidual cells; ec = extravillous cytotrophoblast; v = vein. ×90. For further details see text.

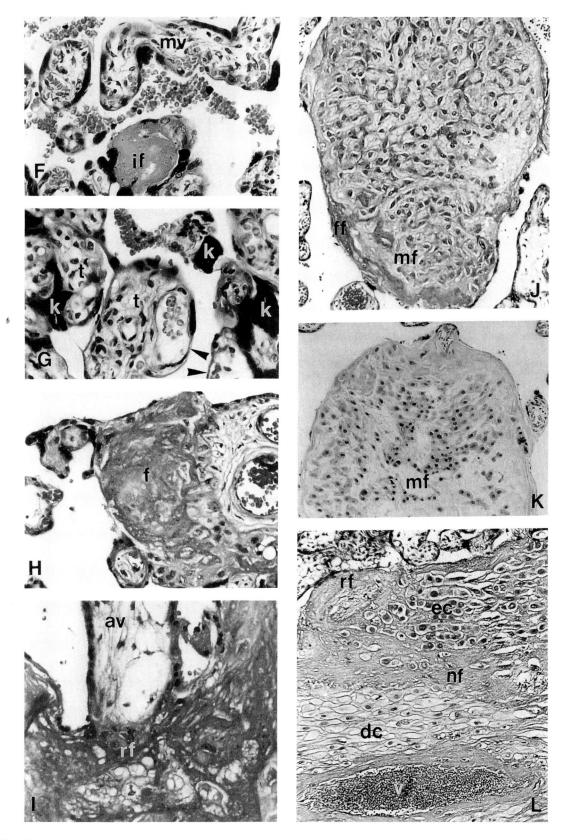

Figure 19. Continued

(see pp. 182ff). Histologically, extravillous trophoblast cells appear as rounded to polygonal cells that may be isolated or grouped in strings. They differ from decidual cells in that, in paraffin sections, most of the cell bodies show nuclear cross sections (Figures 18K, 19L).

Figure 18K: *Decidual cells* are enlarged endometrial stromal cells that have elongated, partly branched bodies (Figure 118). Neighboring decidual cells are usually arranged in parallel, resulting in a peculiar histological appearance: All of the cellular sections in one area have the same shape (round, ellipsoid, or longitudinal) (Figure 19L), depending on the sectional angle. Due to the elongated cell body, cross sections of the ovoid nuclei are rarely found (see pp. 196ff).

Uteroplacental veins are endothelial tubes surrounded by few regressive medial and adventitial cells and embedded in decidua and extravillous trophoblast cells (Figure 18K); the latter rarely invade the venous walls and never the venous lumens (see pp. 231ff).

Figure 18L: *Uteroplacental arteries (spiral arteries)* traverse the basal plate in spiral turns and connect the maternal uterine arteries to the intervillous space. Because of their shape, usually several cross sections are found close together (see pp. 228ff). Different from the uteroplacental veins, the endothelial lining is largely replaced by intravascular trophoblast, a special form of extravillous trophoblast (see p. 231). These cells may form large plugs that narrow or even occlude the arterial lumen (not shown). Arterial media and adventitia are replaced by trophoblast cells and fibrinoid, the latter substance also forming the immediate surrounding of most arteries (intramural fibrinoid, see p. 204, p. 233).

Figure 18M: In the depth of the basal plate, the remains of *endometrial glands* can be found. They are regular findings throughout the first 2 months of pregnancy, forming round to star-shaped lumens lined by cuboidal epithelium. They are surrounded by endometrial stroma or decidualized endometrial stromal cells. During subsequent stages of pregnancy, the glands disintegrate and only degenerative epithelial remainders may be found (see p. 201).

Typical Histological Features of the Third Trimester Placenta

Third trimester sections of the placenta, such as the vertical survey section of a mature placenta in Figure 19A, are more difficult to examine as the villi are smaller and often stick so close together it is difficult to find the intervillous space in between. Figure 19A covers the chorionic plate including the amnion, different types of villi, fibrinoid deposits in various locations, anchoring villi with rudimentary cell columns, cell islands, septa, and the basal plate.

Figure 19A: Different from the first trimester situation, the width of the *intervillous space* is highly variable, with large "subchorionic lakes" below the chorionic plate and narrow intervillous clefts between the terminal villi. In the term placenta, the mean width of the clefts including the subchorionic lakes is between 16 and 32 µm (see p. 140).

Figure 19B: The *amnion* covers the chorionic plate toward the amnionic cavity. It consists of a single layer of cuboidal to columnar cells that participate in the turnover of the amnionic fluid (see p. 277). Seemingly multilayered segments of the amnionic epithelium represent oblique or tangential sections across the surface in most cases. In addition, nearly 50% of mature placentas also possess foci of real squamous metaplasia of the amnionic epithelium that may become up to 15 cellular layers in thickness (see pp. 273ff). Underneath the amnionic epithelium there exists a thin layer of amnionic mesoderm (about 15–30 µm in thickness) (see p. 279). It is only loosely connected with the next layer, the chorionic mesoderm via the spongy or intermediate layer, a reticular zone showing larger clefts (Figure 19C) (see p. 282). Because of this unstable connection, the amnion may start gliding, or it may even become lost during preparation.

Figure 19C: The third trimester *chorionic plate* is a multilayered structure. It consists of the spongy layer with numerous clefts, followed by the compact layer of chorionic mesoderm that is separated from the Langhans fibrinoid stria by a rudimentary basement membrane. On the lower side of this basement membrane, highly variable amounts of extravillous cytotrophoblast can be found. During early pregnancy they form a complete and usually multilayered stratum. During later pregnancy this layer becomes rarified. Some of the cells deeply invade the fibrinoid (see pp. 213ff). Attached to or embedded into the fibrinoid one finds numerous stem villi, representing the first branches of villous trunci branching from the chorionic plate nearby (upper third of Figure 19A). The chorionic plate represents the cover of the intervillous space, which follows directly below.

Figure 19D: The villous trees measure 1 to 4 cm in diameter. Their central branches are made up of *stem villi* (Figure 81), which are the large caliber villi that range from 80 to several thousand micrometers in diameter (see pp. 116ff). The highest concentration of stem villi and those with the largest calibers are found near the chorionic plate. Histologically, they are characterized by one or several arteries and veins, or arterioles and venules, with clearly visible muscular walls and surrounded by a fibrous stroma that contains few paravascular capillaries (see p. 131). Near term the trophoblastic cover is focally or largely replaced by fibrinoid (see Chapter 7). This process is more pronounced in large stem villi.

Figure 19E: The immature forerunners of the stem villi are the *immature intermediate villi*. They are easily identifiable by their large caliber and pale staining. Large arteries and veins are usually absent, as are large amounts of collagen fibers. The prevailing structure within the stroma is a reticularly arranged loose connective tissue with few fetal vessels. It is composed of fixed connective tissue cells in a net-like arrangement that surround round spaces, the so-called stromal channels (see pp. 119ff), which contain the Hofbauer cells (macrophages) (see pp. 84ff). The latter are characterized by their rounded cell body and their numerous vacuoles or lysosomes.

Immature intermediate villi are the dominating villous type during early pregnancy (Figures 18D,E). At term they usually persist in small groups (<10% of the total villous volume) in the centers of the villous trees. They are absent in hypermature placentas, and their number increases with persisting immaturity of the placenta (see p. 171).

Figure 19F: *Mature intermediate villi* are slender, multiply curved branches of stem villi that exhibit diameters ranging from 60 to about 100 µm. They differ from stem villi by the absence of both stromal fibrosis and fetal stem vessels (arterioles and venules) with a light-microscopically identifiable media. Their stroma is composed of slender fetal capillaries embedded in a loose connective tissue that is rich in cells but poor in fibers (see p. 122). Longitudinal sections of mature intermediate villi are easily identifiable, whereas cross sections can easily be confused with terminal villi (see below).

Figure 19G: *Terminal villi* are the grape-like terminal side branches of the mature intermediate villi (Figure 70; see also p. 124). Their diameters range from 40 µm to about 80 µm. The dominating structures within the loose stroma are sinusoidally dilated and highly coiled fetal capillaries (see Chapter 8). Typically, they bulge against the trophoblastic surface and transform it into thin vasculosyncytial membranes that are devoid of nuclei.

The terminal villi, together with mature intermediate villi, comprise the main exchange area of the third trimester placenta. Mature intermediate villi with slender capillaries and terminal villi with dilated sinusoids are easily discernible in placentas after early cord clamping and immediate fixation. Placentas that were fixed late after delivery and that have lost large amounts of fetal blood have collapsed sinusoids, so the terminal villi can no longer be discriminated from mature intermediate villi, which have slender capillaries.

A typical feature of terminal villi and, to a certain degree also of other villous types, is the *trophoblastic knotting*. This term is usually applied to an increased appearance of seemingly polypoid trophoblastic outgrowths at the villous surfaces and to the trophoblastic bridges connecting neighboring villi. Only a small percentage of both structures represents real trophoblast protrusions and real bridges during the third trimester (see p. 167). Rather, almost all are flat sections across trophoblastic surfaces of irregularly shaped and branched villi. Toward term, as well as under hypoxic conditions (see pp. 176ff), the outer shape of terminal villi becomes more irregular, thereby increasing the chance of trophoblastic flat sectioning (knotting).

Figure 19H: *Fibrinoid* is an acellular, intensely staining, eosinophilic material that is mostly related to the intervillous space (Figures 19C,D,F). When it replaces the trophoblastic cover of villi, as shown in Figure 19D,H, it is called perivillous fibrinoid. In other villi, it may replace the stroma underneath a largely intact trophoblastic surface (intravillous fibrinoid, villous fibrinoid necrosis) (Figure 19F). Other sites of fibrinoid deposition are a prominent fibrinoid layer below the chorionic plate (Langhans' fibrinoid, Figure 19C), a corresponding layer at the surface of the basal plate (Rohr fibrinoid, Figures 19I,L), the Nitabuch fibrinoid in the depth of the maternofetal junctional zone (Figure 19L), and the extracellular matrix of cell islands (Figure 19J) and septa (Figure 19K).

Despite the fact that fibrinoid appears to be homogeneous histologically, it is composed of two completely different materials: (1) *fibrin-type fibrinoid* (Figure 21C), a blood clotting product that is free of extravillous trophoblast cells and usually in contact with the intervillous space; and (2) *matrix-type fibrinoid* (Figure 20D), in which are embedded varying numbers of extravillous trophoblast cells and which itself is a secretory product of these cells. Both substances may be deposited close together or separately (see p. 204).

Figure 19I: With the increasing development of free-floating villi that takes place during the course of the last trimester, *anchoring villi* become less prominent. They are still connected to the basal plate or to septa by *cell columns* (Figures 18H,I). As the proliferative activity of the columnar cytotrophoblast slows, the cells are rarified to one layer that is sometimes even incomplete. In some cases, extravillous trophoblast may be completely replaced by matrix-type fibrinoid so the stroma of the anchoring villus directly borders Rohr's fibrinoid of the basal plate. Some cell columns maintain their proliferative activity and thus act as growth zones for the anchoring villi as well as for the basal plate, even near term (see pp. 184ff).

Figure 19J: *Cell islands* increase in size throughout pregnancy owing to continuous proliferation of their extravillous trophoblast cells. The amount of fibrinoid embedding these cells increases steadily by apposition of fibrin-type fibrinoid from the intervillous space and by secretion of matrix-type fibrinoid from the trophoblast cells. Large cell islands may contain central cavities, or "cysts" (Figure 148). They must be con-

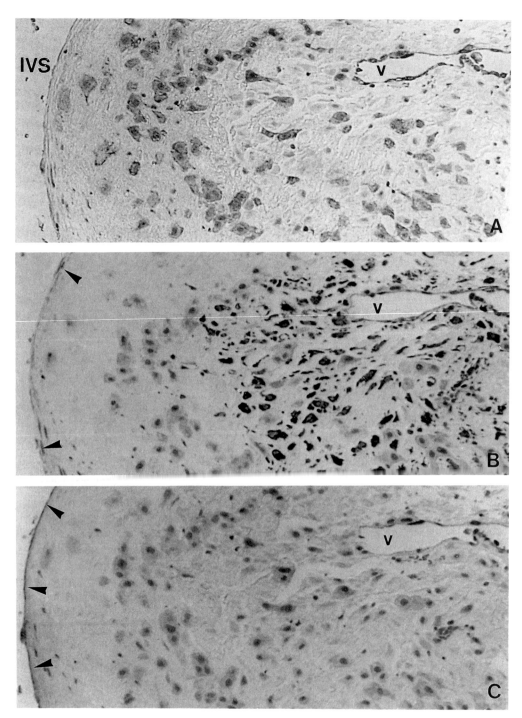

FIGURE 20. Serial sections of a superficial part of the mature basal plate bordering the intervillous space (IVS) and showing a colorful mixture of extravillous trophoblast cells with decidual cells as well as a uteroplacental vein (v). Owing to the hematoxylin counterstain, all nuclei are black. (A) Anticytokeratin, an epithelial marker, binds to evenly spread extravillous trophoblast cells. The surface of the basal plate and the luminal lining of the vessel remain unstained. (B) Anti-vimentin, a mesenchymal marker, stains the decidual cells as well as the lining of the vessel (v) and partly that of the basal plate surface (arrowheads). (C) Staining with antibodies to factor VIII-related antigen, a specific endothelial marker, reveals that the surface of this part of the basal plate is covered by (maternal) endothelium (arrowheads). The same is true for the uteroplacental vein (v). ×200. (Courtesy Dr. Sonya Kertschanska, Aachen.)

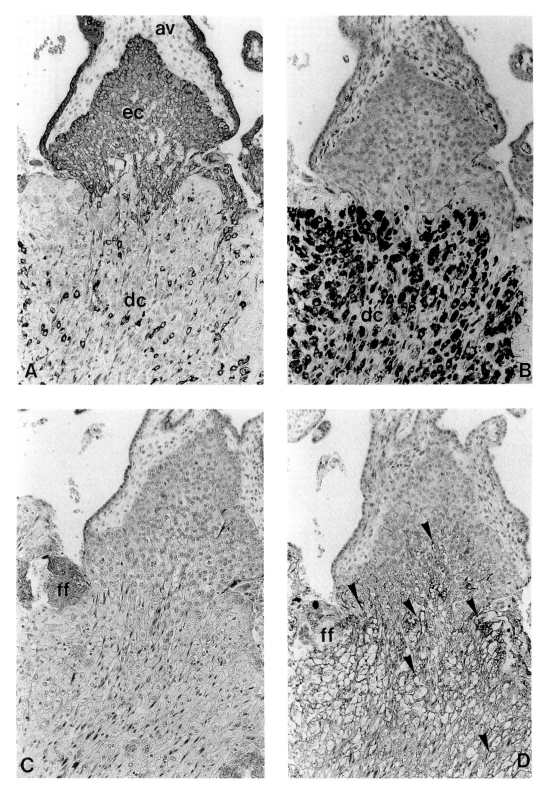

FIGURE 21. Serial sections of a cell column of a first trimester placenta. (A) Anti-cytokeratin stains the villous trophoblastic surface as well as extravillous trophoblast (ec) that forms a compact layer at the border to the anchoring villus (av) and invades the basal plate (below). dc = decidual cells. (B) Anti-vimentin staining reveals that most of the basal plate cells are of mesenchymal origin (decidual cells, dc). The trophoblast cells (largely unstained) invade the decidual layer. (C) Anti-fibrin binds to a deposit of fibrinoid (ff) that is closely related to the intervillous space and devoid of extravillous trophoblast cells (fibrin-type fibrinoid). (D) In contrast, anti-oncofetal fibronectin binds to the reticular fibrinoid deposits (matrix-type fibrinoid) (arrowheads) around the invading extravillous trophoblast cells and decidua cells rather than to the fibrin-type fibrinoid (ff). ×80. (Courtesy Dr. Hans-Georg Frank, Aachen.)

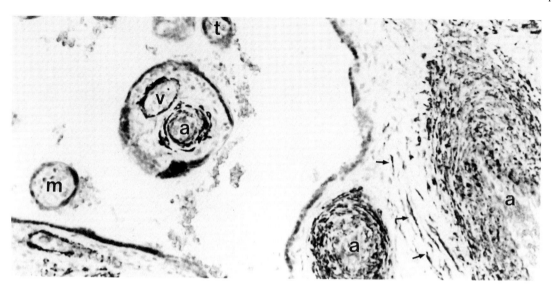

FIGURE 22. Anti-γ-enteric actin specifically stains smooth muscle cells of arteries/arterioles (a) and veins/venules (v) of stem villi as well as highly differentiated myofibroblasts (arrows), which are characteristic for the extravascular stroma of only the largest stem villi (>300 μm caliber). The stroma of mature intermediate (m) and terminal (t) villi remains unstained. The trophoblastic cover of the villi appears black owing to nuclear counterstaining with hematoxylin. ×200. (Courtesy Dr. Gaby Kohnen, Aachen.)

sidered the result of degeneration of trophoblast cells and subsequent liquefaction. Occasionally, structures looking like cell islands contain some decidual cells in addition to extravillous trophoblast cells. Such islands can be interpreted either as cross sections of placental septa or as disrupted parts of such. For an understanding of their development and structure see pp. 237ff.

Figure 19K: *Placental septa* are the result of folding of the basal plate, probably supported by the tension of anchoring villi (see pp. 234ff). They are rudimentary pillarshaped structures, insufficient to subdivide the intervillous space into separate chambers. They are attached to the basal plate at their base (Figure 19A) and are usually composed of extravillous trophoblast and decidual cells, both embedded in ample fibrinoid. Sometimes large cysts similar to those of the cell islands can be found (Figure 143) (see pp. 241ff). These sites of minor mechanical resistance during delivery usually give rise to deep basal tears of the placenta, the grooves delineating the placental lobes (Figures 16, 17). The septal tips (Figure 19K) are composed mostly of extravillous trophoblast and matrix-type fibrinoid, and they are surrounded by fibrin-type fibrinoid. Their cross sections are hardly distinguishable from cell islands.

Figure 19L: Only in a few exceptional places is the *basal plate* of the term placenta as clearly layered as depicted here. There is a superficial stria of Rohr fibrinoid, followed by extravillous cytotrophoblast, a layer of Nitabuch fibrinoid, and a compact decidual layer. A uteroplacental vein is embedded in the latter. In most cases, however, there is no clearly defined fetomaternal border; rather, extravillous cytotropho-

blast, decidual cells, uteroplacental vessels, and glandular residues are intermingled with ample fibrinoid, in no identifiable order (Figure 135) (see p. 222). In such cases immunohistochemical markers may facilitate orientation (see below). For a consideration of the uteroplacental vessels and intraarterial trophoblast see the description of the first trimester placenta.

IMMUNOHISTOCHEMICAL MARKERS

Structural orientation in histological sections can be considerably facilitated by immunohistochemical markers. Some of those may even be applied to paraffin sections, provided the tissue has been fixed with formalin only. We prefer fixation in a 4% neutrally buffered formaldehyde solution (10% formalin solution) for a maximum of 24 hours and at temperatures below 60°C during the paraffin embedding. Correspondingly prepared paraffin blocks may be used even years later for many immunohistochemical reactions (e.g., intermediate filaments, extracellular matrix proteins, proliferation markers).

The following immunohistochemical reactions may be useful for routine histological examination of placental paraffin sections. All of them work with human material, some even cross-react with the respective molecules in several animal placentas.

Anti-cytokeratin stains epithelial structures such as amnionic epithelium, villous syncytio- and cytotrophoblast, and extravillous cytotrophoblast. It is a useful marker in particular for the discrimination between extravillous cytotrophoblast (Figures 20A, 21A) and decidual cells (Figures 20B, 21B) or intraarterial trophoblast (Figure 20A) and maternal endothelium (Figure 20C). We prefer an antibody directed against cytokeratins 10, 17, and 18, which stains all cellular epithelial elements. Syncytiotrophoblast is only partly stained. Sometimes some cross reaction occurs with vascular smooth muscle cells and contractile perivascular stromal cells in the larger stem villi.

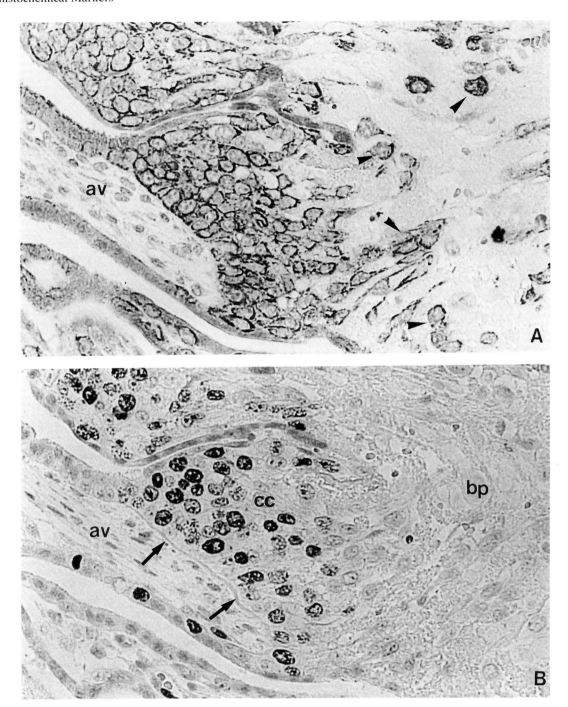

FIGURE 23. Serial paraffin sections of a cell column (cc) connecting an anchoring villus (av) to the basal plate (bp). The comparison of anti-cytokeratin staining (A) of the extravillous cytotrophoblast with MIB 1 staining (B) of proliferating trophoblast cells reveals that only those extravillous trophoblast cells close to the basal lamina (arrows) of the anchoring villus undergo mitosis. In contrast, those invasive daughter cells (arrowheads) that have left the cell column and deeply invaded the basal plate are no longer proliferative. In conclusion, those cells resting on the basal lamina are the proliferating stem cells of all extravillous trophoblast cells. ×200. (Courtesy Dr. Gaby Kohnen, Aachen.)

Anti-vimentin stains all mesenchyme-derived cells, such as connective tissue cells, macrophages, decidual cells, smooth muscle cells, and endothelial cells. We use it as control on paraffin sections used in parallel to those stained for cytokeratin: Placental cells and syncytia should be positive either for cytokeratin (epithelial) or vimentin (mesenchymal). It is a useful tool for identifying decidual cells (Figures 20B, 21B) as opposed to extravillous trophoblast cells (Figures 20A, 21A) or for discriminating maternal endothelium from intraarterial trophoblast.

Anti-factor VIII-related antigen (the former anti-von Willebrand factor) is a marker that is largely specific for most endothelial cells. Application of this antibody provided proof that the intervillous space adjacent to venous openings is lined by maternal endothelium (Figure 20C). It does not always work on paraffin sections. In those cases, the less problematical anti-vimentin may be helpful.

Anti-fibrin can be used as a specific marker for fibrin-type fibrinoid as a blood clotting product (Figure 21D), only if an antibody is available (e.g., Immunotech, clone E8) that does not cross-react with the nearly universally present fibrinogen.

Anti-oncofetal fibronectin (directed against the ED-B sequence of cellular fibronectin) is a specific marker for matrix-type fibrinoid (Figure 20D). Different from other fibronectin isoforms, it cross-reacts with neither fibrin-type fibrinoid nor connective tissue.

Anti-γ-enteric actin is largely specific for vascular smooth muscle cells and myofibroblasts. It is a useful tool for identifying the vessel walls of fetal villous arteries and arterioles and of veins and venules. It may be used as a marker for stem villi (Figure 22) and their immature forerunners, the immature intermediate villi, as both villous types are the only villi having these stem vessels.

The more easily available *anti-α-smooth muscle actin* (not shown) has a staining pattern that is largely comparable. It also covers, however, earlier stages of myofibroblast differentiation and vascular pericytes. Because the latter are also present in mature intermediate and terminal villi, this antibody is less useful for the discrimination of different villous types.

Anti-collagen IV and *anti-laminin* (not shown) bind to basal laminas and partly also to placental connective tissue. They also bind to matrix-type fibrinoid.

Anti-leu-M3 (not shown) is the most consistent immunohistochemical marker of macrophages, the Hofbauer cells. It detects the CD14 monocyte differentiation antigen. Its application to placental villi demonstrates that a much larger share of villous stromal cells than had been expected from ultrastructural and enzyme histochemical studies are in fact macrophages. Like most antibodies directed against cell surface receptors, this antibody works only on unfixed cryostat sections. Other macrophage specific antibodies are available, however, that also work on paraffin sections.

The antibodies *Ki-67, MIB-1*, and *anti-PCNA* (clones PC10, 19A2, 19F4) bind to nuclear proteins that are expressed in proliferating cells. Ki-67 is applicable only to cryostat sections. MIB-1 is its analogue for carefully fixed paraffin sections; it can be applied also on cryostat sections. Anti-PCNA can be used only for paraffin material. Whereas Ki-67/MIB-1 binds only to cells in the mitotic cycle, because of its longer biological half-life PCNA can also be detected in cells that have already left the cell cycle up to 24 hours earlier. These antibodies are useful markers for distinguishing proliferating stem cell populations from differentiated ones and identifying growth zones (Figures 23A,B).

5
Normative Values and Tables

Quantitative structural and biochemical data concerning pregnancy, placental development, and composition of the term placenta are given in Tables 2 to 11. When examining the tables on placental morphometry and comparing the results from various authors, it is important to note that quantitative structural data are heavily influenced by the mode of sampling and by the preparation of the material. Because of the high degree of maternal and fetal vascularization, the placenta reacts immediately to changes in intravascular pressure. Thus, the mode of birth, the time elapsing from cessation of maternal and fetal blood flows to tissue fixation (Tables 7, 10), and the nature of cord clamping (Table 9) directly influence the volumetric relations of villi and intervillous space. In particular, parameters such as the width of fetal vessels, degree of fetal vascularization, maternofetal diffusion distance, and trophoblastic thickness are easily affected. Moreover, the composition of the fixative and its osmolarity (Table 11) as well as the mode of fixation (immersion versus perfusion fixation) are of importance. Normally, immersion fixation of the entire placenta or of small pieces is used. The more advanced methods, such as perfusion fixation (Burton et al., 1987) or puncture biopsy of the still maternally perfused placenta during cesarean section (Schweikhart & Kaufmann, 1977; Voigt et al., 1978; Sen et al., 1979), are time-consuming. When studying immersion-fixed material, however, one should keep in mind that this material differs quantitatively and qualitatively from the in vivo conditions (Tables 7, 10). It is impossible to include the results of numerous other valuable contributions to placental morphometry into these table. For further information on special issues, we refer to the following publications: placental growth development in relation to birth weight (Bouw et al., 1978); relation of placental weight to body size at 7 years of age and to abnormalities in children (Naeye, 1987); fetal and placental weights in relation to maternal weight (Auinger & Bauer, 1974); ultrasonographic measurements of volumetric growth of the placenta (Bleker et al., 1977); weight development of placenta and membranes during early pregnancy (Abramovich, 1969); ratio of gestational sac volume to crown-rump length during early pregnancy (Goldstein et al., 1986); villous surface area and villous volume densities in various placental regions and along different levels of the chorial basal axis (Teasdale, 1978; Boyd et al., 1980; Cabezon et al., 1985; Bacon et al., 1986); local variations of villous surface, fetal vascularization, and amount of vasculosyncytial membranes in the placentone (maternofetal circulatory unit) (Schuhmann et al., 1988); total villous surface in relation to fetal weight in normal and various pathological conditions (Clavero-Nunez & Botella-Llusia, 1961, 1963); morphometric data affecting placental oxygen diffusion (Mayhew et al., 1984, 1986); computer measurement of the mass of syncytiotrophoblast (Boyd et al., 1983); ultrastructural morphometric analysis of the villous syncytiotrophoblast (Sala et al., 1983); microvillous surface enlargement of the villous surface (Teasdale & Jean-Jacques, 1985); comparison of villous structure after immersion and perfusion fixation (Burton et al., 1987).

TABLE 2. Length and weight data for placenta and fetus. (1) extrapolated data from Boyd & Hamilton (1970) and O'Rahilly (1973); (2) data from Johannigmann et al. (1972); (3) data from Winckel (1893).

Pregnancy week (post conception)	Pregnancy week (post menstruation)	Pregnancy month (post menstruation)	crown rump length (mm) [1]	embryonic/fetal weight (gm) [1]	diameter of the chorionic sac (mm) [1]	placental diameter (mm) [1]	placental weight (gm) [1]	placental thickness post partum (mm) [1]	placental thickness incl. uterine wall measured by ultrasound in vivo (mm) [2]	length of the umbilical cord (mm) [3]
	1	1								
	2									
1	3									
2	4									
3	5		2.5		5–12					
4	6	2	5		13–21					5
5	7		9		22–28					
6	8		14	1.1	29–34		6			
7	9		20	2	35–42					
8	10	3	26	5	43–58		14			
9	11		33	11	59–64					
10	12		40	17	65–68		26			
11	13		48	23	68	50				160
12	14	4	56	30			42	10		
13	15		65	40	—	—				—
14	16		75	60	90	75	65	12		180
15	17		88	90		75				220
16	18	5	99	130			90			
17	19		112	180		—				—
18	20		125	250		100	115	15	28	300
19	21		137	320		100				330
20	22	6	150	400			150			
21	23		163	480		—				—
22	24		176	560		125	185	18	34	350
23	25		188	650		125				370
24	26	7	200	750			210			
25	27		213	870		—				—
26	28		226	1,000		150	250	20	38	400
27	29		236	1,130		150				420
28	30	8	250	1,260			285			
29	31		263	1,400		—				—
30	32		276	1,550		170	315	22	43	450
31	33		289	1,700		170				460
32	34	9	302	1,900			355			
33	35		315	2,100		—				—
34	36		328	2,300		200	390	24	45	490
35	37		341	2,500		200				500
36	38	10	354	2,750			425			
37	39		367	3,000		—				—
38	40		380	3,400		220	470	25	45	520

TABLE 3. Quantitative data of various placental tissues as related to fetal weight and stage of pregnancy. (1) data from Knopp (1960); (2) data from Kloos & Vogel (1974); (3) data from Kaufmann (1981).

Pregnancy week (post conception)	Pregnancy week (post menstruation)	Pregnancy month (post menstruation)	fetal weight (gm) per 1 gm of placental weight [1]	placental weight index–placental weight (gm) per 1 gm of fetal weight [2]	villous volume (gm) per placenta [1] (percentage of total placental weight)	villous surface (cm²) per placenta [1]	fetal weight (gm) per 10,000 cm² villous surface [1]	villous surface (cm²) per 1 gm of placental villi [1]	number of villous cross sections per mm² of paraffin sections [3]	number of villous cross sections per mm² of paraffin sections [1]	villous diameter (mean of all villous types) (µm) [3]
	1										
	2	1									
1	3										
2	4										
3	5										
4	6	2									
5	7										
6	8		0.18	10.0–9.3	5 (83%)	830		166	15	47	204
7	9										
8	10	3	0.36								
9	11										
10	12		0.65	3.9–3.3	18 (69%)	3,020	29.8	168	20		
11	13										
12	14	4	0.71								
13	15										
14	16		0.92	2.5–1.0	28 (43%)	5,440	64.3	194	25	104	158
15	17										
16	18	5	1.44								
17	19										
18	20		2.17	0.97–0.57	63 (55%)	14,800	104.7	235	30	131	108
19	21										
20	22	6	2.67								
21	23										
22	24		3.03	0.49–0.38	102 (55%)	28,100	156.6	275	40	202	61
23	25										
24	26	7	3.57								
25	27										
26	28		4.00	0.31–0.26	135 (54%)	42,200	191.9	313	60		
27	29			0.26						205	53
28	30	8	4.42	0.242							
29	31			0.208							
30	32		4.92	0.203	191 (61%)	72,000	184.5	377	90		
31	33			0.180							
32	34	9	5.35	0.168							
33	35			0.163							
34	36		5.90	0.157	234 (60%)	101,000	198.0	432	140		
35	37			0.145						264	52
36	38	10	6.47	0.138							
37	39			0.132							
38	40		7.23	0.130	273 (58%)	125,000	230.0	458	150	321	48

TABLE 4. Histomorphometrical evaluation of placental villi. The data presented here are mean data for the complete villous tree including all villous types. (1) data from Glöde (1984); (2) data from Kaufmann (1972); (3) calculated from data from Kaufmann (1981); (4) data from Kaufmann & Scheffen (1992).

Pregnancy week (post conception)	Pregnancy week (post menstruation)	Pregnancy month (post menstruation)	trophoblastic volume as a percentage of the villous volume (%) [1]	mean trophoblastic thickness (μm) [1]	villous cytotrophoblast volume as a percentage of villous trophoblast (%) [2]	villous stromal volume as a percentage of villous volume (%) [1]	villous connective tissue volume as a percentage of villous volume (%) [3]	volume of fetal vessel lumina as a percentage of villous volume (%) [3]	percentage of the villous surface which is characterized by a double layered trophoblast (syncytium and Langhans cells) (%) [2]	materno fetal diffusion distance (μm) [4]
	1									
	2	1								
1	3									
2	4									
3	5									
4	6	2								
5	7		31.7	18.9		68.3	65.6	2.7		55.9
6	8				30					
7	9		33.5	19.1		66.5	63.5	3.0	85	
8	10	3								
9	11		34.5	21.6		65.8	61.8	4.0		
10	12				35				80	
11	13									
12	14	4								
13	15									
14	16				43			6.0	80	40.2
15	17									
16	18	5	24.8	11.6		75.2	68.9	6.3		
17	19									
18	20				35			6.6	60	22.4
19	21									
20	22	6								
21	23									
22	24				30				55	21.6
23	25									
24	26	7								
25	27									
26	28		30.1	9.7	25	69.9	60.8	9.1	45	
27	29									
28	30	8								
29	31									
30	32				20				35	20.6
31	33									
32	34	9								
33	35									
34	36		30.8	5.2	15	69.2	47.9	21.3	25	11.7
35	37									
36	38	10								
37	39									
38	40		32.9	4.1	14	67.1	38.7	28.4	23	4.8

TABLE 5. Fetal and placental weight as related to the number of pregnancies.

	Male neonates				Female neonates			
Pregnancy no.	Mat. age (years)	Neo. length (cm)	Neo. wt. (g)	Plac. wt. (g)	Mat. age (years)	Neo. length (cm)	Neo. wt. (g)	Plac. wt. (g)
First ($n = 101$)	22.37	51.04	3,141.3	548.7	22.42	50.96	2,974.0	560.7
Second ($n = 71$)	25.24	51.95	3,442.8	607.9	25.15	51.29	3,133.6	565.5
Third ($n = 27$)	30.21	50.29	3,495.0	603.2	26.69	50.29	3,228.1	553.9
Fourth ($n = 18$)	30.00	53.83	3,677.5	599.6	29.00	50.83	3,095.0	568.3

From Lips (1891).
Mat. = maternal; Neo. = neonatal; Plac. = placental.
All results are given as the mean value.

TABLE 6. Quantitative data for the human placenta at term. The data were taken or calculated from (1) Knopp 1960; (2) Aherne & Dunnill (1966); (3) Baur (1970); (4) Wördehoff (1971); (5) Laga et al. (1973); (6) Ehrhardt & Gerl (1970); (7) Bacon et al. (1986); (8) Mayhew et al. (1986); (9) Bouw et al. (1976); (10) Feneley & Burton (1991); (11) Voigt et al. (1978).

Mean placental volume (cm^3) (without cord and membranes)	448 (2)	448 (5)	540 (9)	408 (10)
Percentage of villous volume per placenta (%)	57.5 (1)	57.9 ± 5.7 (2)	45.6 (5)	62.9 ± 2.1 (7)
Mean villous volume per placenta (gm)	273 (1)	214 (5)	224 (2)	239 (9)
Percentage of intervillous space per placenta (post partum) (%)	35.8 ± 3.2 (2)	23.29 (5)	29.3 ± 2.0 (7)	37.9 (8)
Volume of intervillous space (cm^3)	144 (2)	110 (5)	210 (9)	173 (8)
Percentage of intervillous fibrinoid per placenta (%)	4.3 ± 2.1 (2)	2.58 (5)		
Villous surface covered with fibrinoid (%)	0.364 (6)			
Percentage of villous tissues per placenta (chorionic plate, basal plate, septa, cell islands, infarctions) (%)	27.6 (5)			
Villous surface per placenta (m^2)	13.3 ± 0.47 (4)	12.0 (3)	11.8 (6)	11.0 ± 1.3 (2)
Villous surface per 1 cm^3 of villous volume (cm^2)	330 (1)	248 (3)	301.2 (4)	
Inner fetal capillary surface per placenta (m^2)	12.2 ± 1.5 (2)	12.0 (5)		
Total length of all villi per placenta (kms)	90 (1)			
Arithmetic mean thickness of villous membrane (mean maternofetal diffusion distance) (μm)	3.5 (2)	4.5 (10)	5.0 (11)	
Harmonic mean thickness of villous membrane (μm)	10.0 (5)	4.9 (8)		

TABLE 7. Quantitative composition of peripheral villous types (diameter <80 μm) after resin embedding.

Parameter	All villous types after spon. del.	After in situ puncture of placenta					
		All villous types	SV	IIV	MIV	TV, neck	TV, no neck
Villous surface showing cytotrophoblast below the syncytium (%)	27.5	22.8	21.4	23.4	24.6	20.0	23.5
Cytotrophoblastic volume as a percentage of total villous trophoblast (%)	13.3	14.0	11.7	14.3	13.8	11.6	15.7
Percent of total villous volume { Trophoblast	41.7	37.7	30.0	33.8	38.0	46.2	29.6
Villous stroma	58.3	62.3	70.0	66.2	62.0	53.8	70.4
Fetal vessel lumens	20.0	28.4	26.0	15.7	21.0	20.2	45.2
Connective tissue including vessel walls	38.4	33.9	44.0	50.5	41.0	33.6	25.2
Mean trophoblastic thickness	4.7	4.1	4.7	5.2	4.4	4.0	3.3
Distribution of maternofetal diffusion distances in % of villous surface { 0–2 μm	10.4	21.0	9.2	10.9	13.1	21.8	37.1
2.1–5 μm	29.9	40.2	27.3	27.3	37.5	41.4	36.5
5.1–10 μm	40.3	32.4	50.5	37.7	37.8	32.6	25.1
10.1–∞ μm	19.5	6.4	13.0	24.1	11.6	4.4	1.3
Mean maternofetal diffusion distance (μm)	7.1	5.0	6.8	7.5	6.0	4.8	3.7
Macrophages (no.)/mm^2 of histological section		24	730	241	83	192	
Mast cells (no.)/mm^2 of histological section		18	10	5	<1	<1	

The data obtained from spontaneous deliveries (fixation about 10 minutes after cord clamping, ischemic period far longer than 10 minutes) (Voigt et al., 1978) are compared with data obtained by puncture aspiration from the still maternally perfused in situ placenta (ischemic period: 0 minutes) (Voigt et al., 1978). In addition, data have been separately measured and calculated for various villous types (Sen et al., 1979). Spon. del. = spontaneous delivery; SV = stem villi; IIV = immature intermediate villi; MIV = mature intermediate villi; TV, neck = neck regions of terminal villi; TV, no neck = terminal villi, excluding neck regions.

TABLE 8. Villous cross sections, surface, and volume in various groups of villi.

Parameter	Villous cross sections (% of total no.)	Surface of villi (% of total)	Volume of villi (% of total)	Type of villus	Mean caliber (μm)	Mean length of cross sections (μm)
Diameter of villi (μm)						
>1,500	0.003	0.1	1.2	Trunci chorii		
1,201–1,500	0.002	0.1	0.8			
901–1,200	0.007	0.1	1.4	Rami chorii		
601–900	0.02	0.5	2.4			
301–600	0.2	1.9	9.0			
226–300	0.3	1.7	6.4	Ramuli chorii, mature and immature intermediate villi, terminal villi[a]		
151–225	0.6	3.2	7.7			
76–150	7.1	15.1	20.8			
0–75	91.8	77.2	50.4			
Type of villus						
Ramuli	5.1	12.4	22.7		120.5	340.1
Immature intermediate	5.1	8.4	10.1		76.6	233.5
Mature intermediate	29.1	31.0	27.8		60.6	153.5
Terminal	55.1	46.3	38.7		50.8	118.4
Neck regions	5.5	2.0	0.8		34.3	46.4

Modified from Sen et al. (1979).
[a] The villi are classified according to diameter (using data from Hansen and König, personal communication, 1978) and compared according to structure.

TABLE 9. Influence of cord clamping on placental structure.

Parameter	Early clamped ($n = 9$)	Late clamped ($n = 7$)
Placental weight (g)	567.4 ± 114.5	407.1 ± 74.0
Birth weight (g)	$3,593.5 \pm 380.0$	$3,404.3 \pm 313.5$
Placental weight index	0.156 ± 0.021	0.116 ± 0.088
Villous volume (cm^3)	239.1 ± 51.9	185.3 ± 39.5
Villous vessel volume (cm^3)	74.9 ± 28.2	33.4 ± 18.3
Villous vessel volume (%)	30.4 ± 5.8	17.4 ± 6.9
Villous vessel surface (mm^2) per mm^3 of villous volume	66.9 ± 10.0	46.3 ± 10.5
Total villous surface (m^2)	13.3 ± 2.6	9.3 ± 2.1
Volume of intervillous space (cm^3)	210.3 ± 50.0	116.0 ± 21.7

Data from Bouw et al. (1976).
A group of spontaneously delivered placentas of which the cord was clamped as early as possible compared with a group in which the cord was clamped after cessation of the arterial pulsation.
Results are given as the mean $\pm$ SD.

TABLE 10. Influence of total ischemia of varying duration on the structure of terminal villi.

Parameter	0 min	2 min	5 min	10 min	20 min
Fetal capillary volume (%)	45	32	19	13	17
Connective tissue volume (%)	25	42	49	54	47
Trophoblastic volume (%)	23	26	32	33	36
Mean maternofetal diffusion distance (μm)	3.2	3.7	5.2	7.1	7.4
Epithelial plates (percentage of villous surface) (%)	40.4	—	—	—	14.7
Mean mitochondrial diameter (syncytiotrophoblast) (μm)	0.30	0.34	0.51	0.63	0.61

(column header: Ischemic period)

Data from Kaufmann (1985).

TABLE 11. Influence of total osmolarity of the fixative on guinea pig placenta.

Parameter	235	290	340	390	600
Trophoblastic volume (%)	39.5	39.3	33.3	32.7	24.6
Fetal capillary volume (%)	12.1	14.7	25.5	16.9	19.3
Extracellular space (%)	<1.0	<1.0	<1.0	2.3	11.7
Mean mitochondrial diameter (syncytiotrophoblast) (μm)	0.68	0.56	0.30	0.26	0.25

(column header: Osmolarity of the fixative)

Data from Kaufmann (1980).
[a] The fixative was 2.2% phosphate-buffered glutaraldehyde.

References

Abramovich, D.R.: The weight of placenta and membranes in early pregnancy. Obstet. Gynaecol. Br. Commonw. 76: 523–526, 1969.

Aherne, W., and Dunnill, M.S.: Morphometry of the human placenta. Br. Med. Bull. 22:5–8, 1966.

Auinger, W., and Bauer, P.: Zum Zusammenhang zwischen Kindsgewicht, Placentagewicht, Muttergewicht und Muttergröße. Arch. Gynecol. 217:69–83, 1974.

Bacon, B.J., Gilbert, R.D., and Longo, L.D.: Regional anatomy of the term human placenta. Placenta 7:233–241, 1986.

Baur, R.: Über die Relation zwischen Zottenoberfläche der Geburtsplacenta und Gewicht des Neugeborenen bei verschiedenen Säugetieren. Z. Anat. Entwicklungsgesch. 131:31–38, 1970.

Bleker, O.P., Kloosterman, G.J., Breur, W., and Mieras, D.J.: The volumetric growth of the human placenta: a longitudinal ultrasonic study. Am. J. Obstet. Gynecol. 127: 657–661, 1977.

Bouw, G.M., Stolte, L.A.M., Baak, J.P.A., and Oort, J.: Quantitative morphology of the placenta. 1. Standardization of sampling. Eur. J. Obstet. Gynecol. Reprod. Biol. 6: 325–331, 1976.

Bouw, G.M., Stolte, L.A.M., Baak, J.P.A., and Oort, J.: Quantitative morphology of the placenta. 3. The growth of the placenta and its relationship to birth weight. Eur. J. Obstet. Gynecol. Reprod. Biol. 8:73–76, 1978.

Boyd, J.D., and Hamilton, W.J.: The Human Placenta. Heffer & Sons, Cambridge, 1970.

Boyd, P.A., Brown, R.A., and Stewart, W.J.: Quantitative structural differences within the normal term human placenta: a pilot study. Placenta 1:337–344, 1980.

Boyd, P.A., Brown, R.A., Coghill, G.R., Slidders, W., and Stewart, W.J.: Measurement of the mass of syncytiotrophoblast in a range of human placentae using an image analysing computer. Placenta 4:255–262, 1983.

Burton, G.J., Ingram, S.C., and Palmer, M.E.: The influence of mode of fixation on morphometrical data derived from terminal villi in the human placenta at term: a comparison of immersion and perfusion fixation. Placenta 8:37–51, 1987.

Cabezon, C., De la Fuente, F., Jurado, M., and Lopez, G.: Histometry of the placental structures involved in the respiratory interchange. Acta Obstet. Gynecol. Scand. 64: 411–416, 1985.

Clavero-Nunez, J.A., and Botella-Llusia, J.: Measurement of the villus surface in normal and pathologic placentas. Am. J. Obstet. Gynecol. 86:234–240, 1961.

Clavero-Nunez, J.A., and Botella-Llusia, J.: Ergebnisse von Messungen der Gesamtoberfläche normaler und krankhafter Placenten. Arch. Gynecol. 198:56–60, 1963.

Ehrhardt, G., and Gerl, D.: Eine einfache Methode zur Bestimmung der Zottenoberfläche von Placenten mit Hilfe der Flächenintegration nach der "Nadelmethode." Zentralbl. Gynakol. 92:728–731, 1970.

Feneley, M.R., and Burton, G.J.: Villous composition and membrane thickness in the human placenta at term: A stereological study using unbiased estimators and optimal fixation techniques. Placenta 12:131–142, 1991.

Glöde, B.: Morphometrische Untersuchungen zur Reifung menschlicher Placentazotten. Medical thesis, University of Hamburg, 1984.

Goldstein, S.R., Subramanyam, B.R., and Snyder, J.R.: Ratio of gestational sac volume to crown-rump length in early pregnancy. Hum. Pathol. 31:320–321, 1986.

Johannigmann, J., Zahn, V., and Thieme, V.: Einführung in die Ultraschalluntersuchung mit dem Vidoson. Elektromedica 2:1–11, 1972.

Kaufmann, P.: Untersuchungen über die Langhanszellen in der menschlichen Placenta. Z. Zellforsch. 128:283–302, 1972.

Kaufmann, P.: Der osmotische Effekt der Fixation auf die Placentastruktur. Verh. Anat. Ges. 74:351–352, 1980.

Kaufmann, P.: Entwicklung der Plazenta. In, Die Plazenta des Menschen. V. Becker, Th.H. Schiebler, and F. Kubli, eds. Thieme Verlag, Stuttgart, 1981.

Kaufmann, P.: Influence of ischemia and artificial perfusion on placental ultrastructure and morphometry. Contrib. Gynecol. Obstet. 13:18–26, 1985.

Kaufmann, P., and Scheffen, I.: Placental development. In, Neonatal and Fetal Medicine—Physiology and Pathophysiology. R. Polin and W. Fox, eds., pp. 47–55. Saunders, Orlando, FL, 1992.

Kloos, K., and Vogel, M.: Pathologie der Perinatalperiode. Grundlage, Methodik und erste Ergebnisse einer Kyematopathologie, pp. 1–361. Thieme, Stuttgart, 1974.

Knopp, J.: Das Wachstum der Chorionzotten vom 2. bis 10. Monat. Z. Anat. Entwicklungsgesch. 122:42–59, 1960.

Laga, E.M., Driscoll, S.G., and Munro, H.N.: Quantitative studies of human placenta. 1. Morphometry. Biol. Neonate 23:224–231, 1973.

Lips, F.: Über die Gewichtsverhaeltnisse der neugeborenen Kinder zu ihren Placenten. Medical thesis, University of Erlangen, 1891.

Mayhew, T.M., Joy, C.F., and Haas, J.D.: Structure-function correlation in the human placenta: the morphometric diffusing capacity for oxygen at full term. J. Anat. 139:691–708, 1984.

Mayhew, T.M., Jackson, M.R., and Haas, J.D.: Microscopical morphology of the human placenta and its effects on oxygen diffusion: a morphometric model. Placenta 7:121–131, 1986.

Naeye, R.L.: Do placental weights have clinical significance? Hum. Pathol. 18:387–391, 1987.

O'Rahilly, R.: Developmental stages in human embryos. Part A, Publication 631. Carnegie Institute, Washington, DC, 1973.

Sala, M.A., Valeri, V., and Matheus, M.: Stereological analysis of syncytiotrophoblast from human mature placenta. Arch. Anat. Microsc. 72:99–106, 1983.

Schuhmann, R., Stoz, F., and Maier, M.: Histometric investigations in placentones (materno-fetal circulation units) of human placentae. Trophoblast Res. 3:3–16, 1988.

Schweikhart, G., and Kaufmann, P.: Zur Abgrenzung normaler, artefizieller und pathologischer Strukturen in reifen menschlichen Plazentazotten. I. Ultrastruktur des Syncytiotrophoblasten. Arch. Gynecol. 222:213–230, 1977.

Sen, D.K., Kaufmann, P., and Schweikhart, G.: Classification of human placental villi. II. Morphometry. Cell Tissue Res. 200:425–434, 1979.

Teasdale, F.: Functional significance of the zonal morphologic differences in the normal human placenta. Am. J. Obstet. Gynecol. 130:773–778, 1978.

Teasdale, F., and Jean-Jacques, G.: Morphometric evaluation of the microvillous surface enlargement factor in the human placenta from mid-gestation to term. Placenta 6:375–381, 1985.

Voigt, S., Kaufmann, P., and Schweikhart, G.: Zur Abgrenzung normaler, artefizieller und pathologischer Strukturen in reifen menschlichen Plazentazotten. II. Morphometrische Untersuchungen zum Einfluss des Fixationsmodus. Arch. Gynecol. 226:347–362, 1978.

Winckel, F.K.L.W.: Lehrbuch der Geburtshilfe. 2nd Ed. Veit, Leipzig, 1893.

Wördehoff, B.: Zur Bestimmung der Zottenoberfläche der menschlichen Plazenta. Medical thesis, University of Würzburg, 1971.

6
Early Development of the Human Placenta

For many years understanding placental pathology was thought to demand only limited knowledge of implantation and early placental development, as disturbances of these early steps of placentation seemed to cause abortion, rather than affect placental structure and function. Increasing experience with assisted fertilization, however, has taught us that a high percentage of these cases have impaired fetal and neonatal outcome, such as an increased incidence of intrauterine growth retardation and retroplacental hematoma, as well as increased perinatal mortality (Beck & Heywinkel, 1990). The causal connections are still unknown, although there are some arguments that placental causes must be discussed. It is speculated that improper conditions during implantation handicap early development and finally result in inappropriate functioning of the fetoplacental unit.

Basic information concerning the early development may achieve increasing importance and so is presented in this chapter. The pathologically interesting interactions between implantation site and the shape of the placenta are dealt with in Chapter 14.

Prelacunar Stage

According to the general definition of the placenta, its development begins as soon as the fetal membranes establish close, stable contacts with the uterine mucosa (i.e., as soon as the blastocyst implants). The first step of implantation is called apposition. In the human it takes place around day 6 to 7 postcoitus (p.c.) (day 1 p.c. = the first 24 hours after conception). During this stage the implanting blastocyst is composed of 107 to 256 cells (Hertig, 1960; Boyd & Hamilton, 1970). It is a flattened vesicle measuring about $0.1 \times 0.3 \times 0.3$ mm in diameter. Most of the cells make up the outer wall (*trophoblast*) surrounding the blastocystic cavity (Figure 24a). Generally speaking, the trophoblast is the fore-runner of the fetal membranes, including the placenta. The inner cell mass, a small group of larger cells that form the *embryoblast*, is apposed to the inner surface of the trophoblastic vesicle. The embryo, cord, and amnion are derived from these cells. Moreover, both embryoblast-derived mesenchyme and embryoblast-derived vessels contribute to the formation of the placenta.

In most cases the blastocyst is oriented in such a way that the embryonic pole (that part of the blastocyst bearing the embryoblast at its inner surface) is attached to the endometrium first (Boyd & Hamilton, 1970). Accordingly, this part of the circumference is also called the implantation pole. Rotation of the blastocyst in such a way that the embryonic pole and the implantation pole are not identical results in abnormal cord insertion. In moderate cases we find an eccentric or marginal insertion of the cord; in severe cases a velamentous cord insertion may be the consequence (see Chapter 13). The usual implantation site is the upper part of the posterior wall of the uterine body, near the midsagittal plane. According to Mossman (1937, 1987), this region is homologous with the antimesometrial wall of a bicornuate uterus, where primary attachment takes place in most mammals.

In all species, implantation is introduced by attachment of the apical plasma membranes of the blastocystic trophoblast to the apical plasma membranes of the uterine epithelium. This phenomenon has been described as a cell biological paradox by Denker (1990), as apical plasma membranes of epithelia are normally known to be nonadhesive. Adhesiveness is a normal quality of basolateral epithelial plasma membranes, which are attached to each other and to their basal laminas as well.

The blastocyst and the endometrium demonstrate this usual epithelial behavior throughout the entire preimplantation phase so long as the blastocyst moves in the fallopian tube and uterine cavity. Apical adhesive-

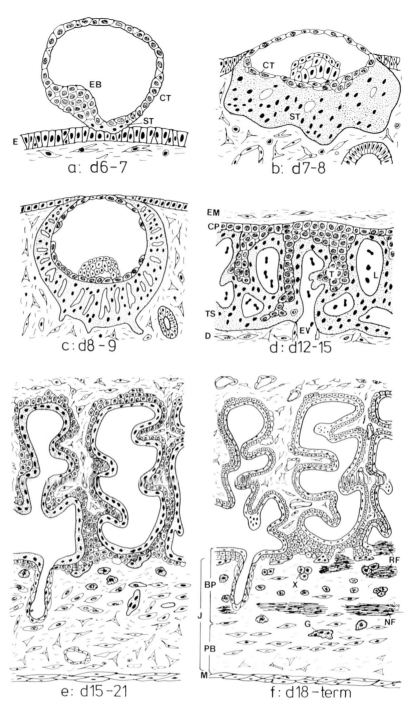

FIGURE 24. Typical stages of early placental development. (a, b) Prelacunar stages. (c) Lacunar stage. (d) Transition from lacunar to primary villous stage. (e) Secondary villous stage. (f) Tertiary villous stage. Note that the basal segments of the anchoring villi (e, f) remain merely trophoblast-forming cell columns. E = endometrial epithelium; EB = embryoblast; CT = cytotrophoblast; ST = syncytiotrophoblast; EM = extraembryonic mesoderm; CP = primary chorionic plate; T = trabeculae and primary villi; L = maternal blood lacunae; TS = trophoblastic shell; EV = endometrial vessel; D = decidua; RF = Rohr's fibrinoid; NF = Nitabuch's or uteroplacental fibrinoid; G = trophoblastic giant cell; X = X cells or extravillous cytotrophoblast; BP = basal plate; PB = placental bed; J = junctional zone. (Modified from Kaufmann and Scheffen, 1992, with permission.)

ness of both epithelia (i.e., trophoblast and endometrium) is apparently achieved for only a short, specific phase, which has been called the implantation window (Psychoyos, 1988). This phase is used for attachment of the blastocyst. To find or to generate this window is the most important prerequisite for successful implantation after in vitro fertilization.

With the noninvasive types of implantation, that result in epitheliochorial placental placentation (e.g., pig, horse, some ruminants) is arrested at the stage of attachment. Invasion with destruction of either epithelial surface does not follow. In contrast, in most mammals more intimate types of maternofetal contacts are established by invasion. In the human, implantation is an invasive process as well. Knowledge of structural details, however, are largely lacking, as appropriate human material is rare; and when it is available it is usually poorly preserved. Numerous studies in animals have revealed the existence of three types of invasive implantation (Schlafke & Enders, 1975; Denker, 1990).

1. Displacement type. This type is observed in rodents. The blastocyst is attached to the apical plasma membrane of the uterine epithelium and degenerate thereafter, detaching from the basal lamina. The subsequent penetration of the basal lamina is initiated by the underlying decidual cells, rather than by penetrative activities of the trophoblast itself.
2. Fusion type. The apical plasma membrane of the attached trophoblast fuses with the apical membranes of the uterine epithelial cells and forms a mixed syncytium, derived from maternal and trophoblastic cells. This syncytium then actively penetrates the basal lamina and endometrial connective tissue, and it finally erodes the maternal blood vessels. This mode of invasion has been described for the rabbit. According to Larsen (1970), it may also be present in the human.
3. Intrusive type. This type is the usual one in carnivores. Small extensions of syncytiotrophoblast intrude into the intercellular clefts between the uterine epithelial cells, opening the intercellular junctions between the epithelial cells. At the same time, new junctions between trophoblast and uterine epithelium are formed. In some species, even local formation of mixed syncytia of maternal and trophoblastic origin has been observed. Based on the results of Larsen (1970), this mechanism of implantation may also pertain for the human.

Lacking respective human findings, further structural details and mechanisms of the implantation process are not discussed here. For this purpose, we refer to the comparative anatomy literature (for reviews see Finn, 1977; Denker, 1977, 1990; Pijnenborg et al., 1981; Denker & Aplin, 1990).

During attachment and after invasion of the endometrial epithelium, the trophoblastic cells of the implanting embryonic pole of the blastocyst display increased proliferation, resulting in a double-layered trophoblast (Heuser & Streeter, 1941). The outer of the two layers, directly facing the maternal tissue, is transformed to *syncytiotrophoblast* by fusion of neighboring trophoblast cells. The remaining cellular components of the blastocyst wall, which have not yet achieved contact to maternal tissues, remain temporally unfused and are

called *cytotrophoblast* (Figure 24a). Throughout the following days and with progressive invasion, additional parts of the blastocyst surface come into close contact with maternal tissues, followed by trophoblastic proliferation with subsequent fusion. The mass of syncytiotrophoblast increases and achieves considerable thickness at the implantation pole as the cytotrophoblast lying underneath continues to proliferate and to fuse syncytially. It increases further by expanding over the surface of the implanting blastocyst as implantation progresses. At the implantation pole, it is not a smooth-surfaced mass; rather, it is covered with branching, finger-like extensions that deeply invade the endometrium. This first stage, lasting from day 7 to day 8 p.c., during which time the syncytiotrophoblast (except for its basal extensions) is a rather solid mass, was defined as the prelacunar period by Wislocki and Streeter (1938).

The syncytiotrophoblast has lost its generative potency during fusion. The cytotrophoblast acts as a stem cell that guarantees growth of the trophoblast by continuous proliferation, with subsequent fusion (see Chapter 7). The syncytiotrophoblast is formed by cellular fusion (i.e., syncytium), rather than by nuclear division without subsequent cytoplasmic division (i.e., plasmodium). Bargmann and Knoop (1959) suggested that the term "plasmodiotrophoblast" (often used in the literature) be abandoned and be replaced by "syncytiotrophoblast."

The syncytiotrophoblast is a continuous system, not interrupted by intercellular spaces and composed of neither individual cells nor individual syncytial units. Terms such as syncytial cells or syncytiotrophoblasts, which are widely used in the literature, are inappropriate. The few available reports that point to the existence of vertical cell membranes, which subdivide the syncytium into syncytial units (e.g., Tedde et al., 1988a,b) have an accidental rather than a real basis (see Chapter 7).

Lacunar Stage

At day 8 p.c., small intrasyncytial vacuoles appear in the increasing syncytiotrophoblastic mass at the implantation pole. The vacuoles quickly grow and become confluent, forming a system of *lacunae* (Figures 24b,c). The separating lamellae and pillars of syncytiotrophoblast are called the *trabeculae*. Their appearance marks the beginning of the lacunar or trabecular stage of placentation, which lasts from day 8 to day 13 p.c. Lacuna formation starts at the implantation pole. With advancing implantation, the syncytiotrophoblastic mass expands over the entire blastocystic surface. In all those places where it exceeds a certain critical thickness, new lacunae become evident, so the lacunar system extends over the entire blastocyst within a few days.

This process lasts until day 12 p.c., when the blastocyst is so deeply implanted that the uterine epithelium closes over the implantation site (Boyd & Hamilton, 1970). At this time the outer surface of the blastocyst is completely transformed to syncytiotrophoblast. At its inner surface, it is covered by a locally incomplete layer of cytotrophoblast. Because trophoblastic proliferation and syncytial fusion have started at the implantation pole, the trophoblastic wall is considerably thicker at this point than at the antiimplantation pole. This difference in thickness is never made up by the thinner parts during the subsequent developmental steps. The thicker trophoblast of the implantation pole is later transformed to the placenta, whereas the opposing thinner trophoblastic circumference only initially attempts to establish the same structure; later it shows regressive transformation to the smooth chorion, the membranes. All data of placental development in this volume refer to the situation at the implantation pole.

Lacunar formation subdivides the trophoblastic covering of the blastocyst into three layers (Figures 24c,d): (1) primary chorionic plate, facing the blastocystic cavity; (2) lacunar system together with the trabeculae; and (3) trophoblastic shell, facing the endometrium.

The *primary chorionic plate* is composed of a more or less continuous stratum of cytotrophoblast, which in some places is double- or even triple-layered. Toward the lacunae, the cytotrophoblast is covered by syncytiotrophoblast (Figure 24d). At day 14 p.c. mesenchymal cells spread around the inner surface of the cytotrophoblast layer. There they transform into a loose network of branching cells, the *extraembryonic mesenchyme*. In the older literature, this mesenchyme has been thought to be of trophoblastic origin (Hertig, 1935; Wislocki & Streeter, 1938; Hertig & Rock, 1941, 1945, 1949). When reevaluating the Carnegie collection of early human ova, Luckett (1978) found proof that these primitive connective tissue cells were derived from the embryonic disk. Later, Luckett's findings were supported by Enders and King (1988), who studied mesenchyme development during early macaque development.

Below the primary chorionic plate is the *lacunar system*. The lacunae are separated from each other by septa or pillars of syncytiotrophoblast, the trabeculae (Figure 24c). Originally, these trabeculae were merely syncytiotrophoblastic in nature. At around day 12 p.c., however, they are invaded by cytotrophoblastic cells (Figure 24d), which are derived from the primary chorionic plate. Within a few days the cytotrophoblast spreads over the entire length of the trabeculae. Where the peripheral ends of the trabeculae join together, they

form the outermost layer of the trophoblast, the *trophoblastic shell* (Hertig & Rock, 1941; Boyd & Hamilton, 1970). At the beginning it is a merely syncytiotrophoblastic structure, but as soon as the cytotrophoblast reaches the shell via the trabeculae (about day 15 p.c.) the former achieves a more heterogeneous structure (Figure 24e). The syncytiotrophoblast establishes the bottom of the lacunae. It is followed by a more or less complete, sometimes multilayered zone of cytotrophoblast. Below the latter and facing the endometrial connective tissue, one again can find discontinuous syncytiotrophoblastic elements.

During the early stages of implantation, erosion of the maternal tissues occurred under the lytic influence of the syncytial trophoblast. Now the existence of cytotrophoblast at the bottom of the shell changes this situation. The proliferative activity of the cytotrophoblast and its rapid migration into the depth of the endometrium appear to be responsible for the further invasion and thus for the further expansion of the implantation area (Boyd & Hamilton, 1970; Pijnenborg et al., 1981). During the course of this process, numerous syncytial elements can be observed far removed from the trophoblastic shell, in the depth of the uterine wall. Boyd and Hamilton (1970) suggested that they were remnants of the originally merely syncytiotrophoblastic shell. More recent reports have provided evidence that these so-called syncytiotrophoblastic or multinuclear giant cells are derived from invading cytotrophoblast that later fused (Park, 1971; Robertson & Warner, 1974; Pijnenborg et al., 1981).

The endometrial stroma undergoes remarkable changes throughout this process. The presence of eroding trophoblast, by being a mechanical irritant and by hormonal activity, causes the endometrial stromal cells to proliferate and to enlarge, thus giving rise to the *decidual cells* (Kaiser, 1960; Dallenbach-Hellweg & Sievers, 1975; Welsh & Enders, 1985). Further structural and functional details are presented in Chapter 11.

The invasive activities of the basal syncytiotrophoblast from day 12 p.c. onward cause disintegration of the maternal endometrial vessel walls. Blood cells, leaving the leaky capillaries at that time, are found inside the lacunae (Boyd & Hamilton, 1970). The detailed mechanisms of this phenomenon are still a mystery of early implantation. Studies on rabbit implantation showed subepithelial capillary coiling and dilatation as the initial process, resulting in increased capillary permeability and stromal edema (Hafez & Tsutsumi, 1966; Finn, 1977; Hoos & Hoffman, 1980). This phase is followed by disintegration of the walls of capillary loops, a process that is likely to be induced by the trophoblast nearby (Larsen, 1961; Denker, 1980; Steven, 1983). At the same time, the disintegrating capillaries are surrounded by the basally expanding syncytiotrophoblast, which in stepwise fashion replaces the capillary walls (Leiser & Beier, 1988). It thus forms new lacunae.

At the next developmental step, the newly formed lacunae fuse with the preexisting lacunae and thus establish maternal perfusion of the entire lacunar system. Further invasion of the trophoblast, with progressive incorporation of the capillary limbs down to their arteriolar beginnings and their venular endings, provides the anatomical basis for the final formation of separate arterial inlets into the lacunar system as well as venous outlets.

Throughout the first steps of development, the maternal blood in the lacunae, which is propelled only by capillary pressure, moves sluggishly. With deeper invasion of the endometrium, the spiral arteries are also eroded, resulting in a higher intralacunar blood pressure and the first maternal circulation of the placenta.

Note that these views are largely based on studies performed in animals with labyrinthine placentas. Morphological (Hustin et al., 1988) and clinical (Doppler ultrasound, endoscopy) (Schaaps & Hustin, 1988) studies in the human suggest that true maternal blood flow in the normal human placenta is established only after the 12th week of pregnancy (see Chapter 11). This finding is surprising, in particular because the structural processes of lacuna formation look similar to those in labyrinthine placentas. Further studies are required to solve this problem.

Early Villous Stages

Shortly after the first appearance of maternal erythrocytes in the lacunae, at about day 13 p.c., increased cytotrophoblastic proliferation with subsequent syncytial fusion in the trabeculae takes place. As a result, not only can longitudinal trabecular growth be observed but blindly ending syncytial side branches form and protrude into the lacunae (Figures 24d,e). With increasing length and diameter, these *primary villi* are invaded by cytotrophoblast. Both processes mark the beginning of the villous stages of placentation. Further proliferative activities, with branching of the primary villi, initiate the development of primitive *villous trees*, the stems of which are derived from the former trabeculae (Figure 24e). When the latter keep their contact to the trophoblastic shell, they are called *anchoring villi*. At the same time, the lacunar system, by definition, is transformed into the *intervillous space*.

Only 2 days later mesenchymal cells derived from the extraembryonic mesenchyme layer of the primary chorionic plate begin to invade the villi, transforming them to *secondary villi* (Figure 24e). Within a few days the mesenchyme expands peripherally to the villous tips and near the base of the anchoring villi (Wislocki & Streeter, 1938; Hertig & Rock, 1945; Boyd & Hamilton, 1970).

The expanding villous mesenchyme does not reach the trophoblastic shell, which during these early stages of placentation remains free of fetal connective tissue. Rather, the basal segments of the trabeculae, until late stages of pregnancy, persist on the primary villous stage; they consist of clusters of cytotrophoblast surrounded by a thin, partly incomplete sheet of syncytiotrophoblast. These cytotrophoblastic "feet" of the trabeculae or anchoring villi (Figures 24e,f) are called *cell columns*. They are sites of longitudinal growth of anchoring villi as well as sources of extravillous trophoblast (see Chapter 11). A similar phenomenon is found in some free-floating villi. If the villous tips are not invaded by villous mesenchyme, they too persist on the primary villous stage as merely trophoblastic structures. The cytotrophoblast within short time shows nearly explosive proliferation, transforming the villous tips into *trophoblastic cell islands* (see Chapter 11). The function of these cell islands is still uncertain.

Early theories of an additional in situ delamination of mesenchyme from villous cytotrophoblast (Hertig, 1935; Wislocki & Streeter, 1938; Hertig & Rock, 1945) have been refuted by Dempsey (1972), King (1987), and Demir et al. (1989). Their electron microscopic studies, performed on human and rhesus monkey placentas, showed that cytotrophoblast and villous mesenchyme are always clearly separated from each other by a complete basal lamina, which is never transgressed by delaminating cytotrophoblast that might transform to mesenchyme.

With a few days delay and beginning between days 18 and 20 p.c., the first *fetal capillaries* can be observed in the mesenchyme. They are derived from hemangioblastic progenitor cells (Figure 61), which locally differentiate from the mesenchyme (King, 1987; Demir et al., 1989). The same progenitor cells give rise to groups of *hematopoietic stem cells*, which are always surrounded by the early endothelium and are thus positioned within the primitive capillaries (Figure 61e). The appearance of capillary cross sections in the villous stroma marks the development of the first *tertiary villi*. Until term, all fetally vascularized villi (comprising most of the villi) can be subsumed under this term. Henceforth, only cell columns, cell islands (see above), and transitory developmental stages of new villous formation (trophoblastic and villous sprouts) correspond to primary or secondary villi.

At about the same time the fetal vascularization of the villi starts, the fetally vascularized allantois (Figure 25) reaches the chorionic plate and fuses with the latter. Allantoic vessels develop into the chorionic plate and,

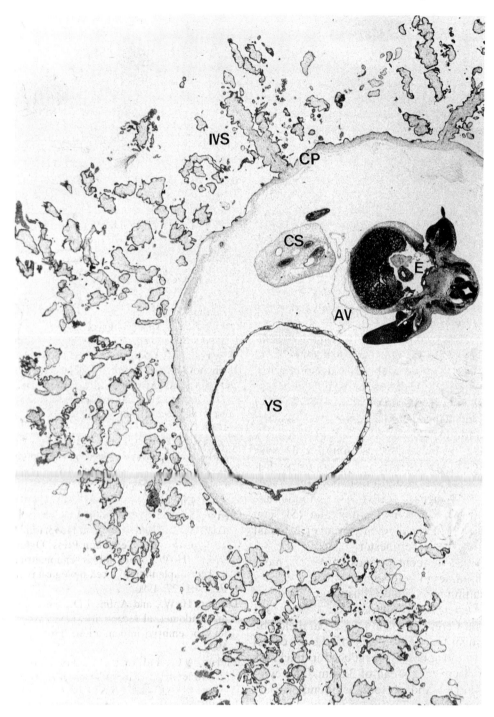

FIGURE 25. Semithin section across an embryo and placenta of the fourth week after conception. Underneath the embryo (E) one can identify the connective stalk (CS) as precursor of the cord, the yolk sac (YS), and a small amnionic vesicle (AV). The chorionic cavity is surrounded by the chorionic plate (CP); from the latter, numerous placental villi protrude into the surrounding intervillous space (IVS). The basal plate is missing in this specimen, as it remained in utero, attached to the endometrium. ×9.5 (From Kaufmann, 1990, with permission.)

according to Benirschke (1965), even into the larger villi. There they come into contact with the locally formed intravillous capillary segments. A complete fetoplacental circulation is established at around the beginning of the 5th week p.c., as soon as enough capillary segments fuse with each other to form a regular capillary bed. Intravascular hematopoiesis can be observed during the following weeks, restricted to newly sprouting villi with de novo produced capillaries in most cases.

The expansion of the early villous trees takes place in the following way (Castellucci et al., 1990): At the surfaces of the larger villi, local cytotrophoblast proliferation with subsequent syncytial fusion causes the production of syncytial (trophoblastic) sprouts (Figure 72). These sprouts are structurally comparable to the early primary villi and are composed of only trophoblast. Most of the syncytial sprouts degenerate, probably owing to inappropriate local conditions; but some are invaded by villous mesenchyme and are thus transformed into the so-called villous sprouts (Figure 72). They correspond structurally to the secondary villi of the first steps of placentation. Formation of fetal vessels within the stroma (Figures 61, 73), with subsequent growth in length and width, is characteristic for the transformation to new mesenchymal villi. Along their surfaces, new sprouts are again produced. (For further details, see Chapter 8.)

Assuming that there is already an intervillous circulation in the human placenta, fetal and maternal blood come into close contact with each other as soon as an intravillous (i.e., fetal) circulation is established. The two bloodstreams are always separated by the *placental barrier* (Figure 26d), which is composed of the following layers: (1) a continuous layer of syncytiotrophoblast covering the villous surface and thus lining the intervillous space; (2) an initially (first trimester) complete, but later (second and third trimesters) discontinuous, layer of cytotrophoblast (Langhans' cells); (3) a trophoblastic basal lamina; (4) connective tissue; and (5) fetal endothelium, which is surrounded only by an endothelial basal lamina during the last trimester.

Throughout the subsequent periods of development the tertiary villi undergo a complex process of differentiation, resulting in various villous types that differ from each other in terms of structure and function (see Chapter 8). This differentiation process is paralleled by qualitative and quantitative changes of the placental barrier: The syncytiotrophoblast is reduced in thickness from more than $20\,\mu m$ to a mean of $3.5\,\mu m$. The cytotrophoblast is rarefied and at term is found in only 20% of the villous surface. The mean villous diameter decreases, as the newly formed villous types are generally smaller than those preceding them. Because of the latter process, the intravillous position of the fetal capillaries comes closer to the villous surface with advanced maturation. In many places the capillary basal lamina may even fuse with that of the trophoblast (Figure 33), considerably reducing the barrier in terms of thickness and number of layers.

In summary, all these factors result in a reduction of the mean maternofetal diffusion distance from 50 to $100\,\mu m$ during the second month, to between 4 and $5\,\mu m$ at term. The evident functional and pathogenetic importance of these phenomena makes it advisable to deal with the villous differentiation in more detail (see Chapter 8).

References

Bargmann, W., and Knoop, A.: Elektronenmikroskopische Untersuchungen an Plazentazotten des Menschen: Bemerkungen zum Synzytiumproblem. Z. Zellforsch. 50:472–493, 1959.

Beck, L., and Heywinkel, E.: Berechtigte und unberechtigte Befürchtungen in der Reproduktionsmedizin. Gynakologe 23:249–251, 1990.

Benirschke, K.: In, Fetal Homeostasis. Vol. I . R.M. Wynn, ed., p. 328. New York Academy of Sciences, New York, 1965.

Boyd, J.D., and Hamilton, W.J.: The Human Placenta. Heffer & Sons, Cambridge, 1970.

Castellucci, M., Scheper, M., Scheffen, I., Celona, A., and Kaufmann, P.: The development of the human placental villous tree. Anat. Embryol. (Berl.) 181:117–128, 1990.

Dallenbach-Hellweg, G., and Sievers, S.: Die histologische Reaktion des Endometrium auf lokal applizierte Gestagene. Virchows Arch. Pathol. Anat. 368:289–298, 1975.

Demir, R., Kaufmann, P., Castellucci, M., Erbengi, T., and Kotowski, A.: Fetal vasculogenesis and angiogenesis in human placental villi. Acta Anat. (Basel) 136:190–203, 1989.

Dempsey, E.W.: The development of capillaries in the villi of early human placentas. Am. J. Anat. 134:221–238, 1972.

Denker, H.-W.: Implantation: the role of proteinases, and blockage of implantation by proteinase inhibitors. Adv. Anat. Embryol. Cell Biol. 53:3–123, 1977.

Denker, H.-W.: Embryo implantation and trophoblast invasion. In, Cell Movement and Neoplasia. M. de Brabander, ed., pp. 151–162. Pergamon Press, Oxford, 1980.

Denker, H.-W.: Trophoblast-endometrial interactions at embryo implantation: a cell biological paradox. Trophoblast Res. 4:1–27, 1990.

Denker, H.-W., and Aplin, J.D., eds.: Trophoblast invasion and endometrial receptivity: novel aspects of the cell biology of embryo implantation. Trophoblast Res. 4:1–462, 1990.

Enders, A.C., and King, B.F.: Formation and differentiation of extraembryonic mesoderm in the rhesus monkey. Am. J. Anat. 181:327–340, 1988.

Finn, C.A.: The implantation reaction. In, Biology of the Uterus. R.M. Wynn, ed., pp. 245–308. Plenum Press, New York, 1977.

Hafez, E.S.E., and Tsutsumi, Y.: Changes in endometrial vascularity during implantation and pregnancy in the rabbit. Am. J. Anat. 118:249–282, 1966.

Hertig, A.T.: Angiogenesis in the early human chorion and in the primary placenta of the macaque monkey. Contrib. Embryol. Carnegie Inst. 25:37–81, 1935.

Hertig, A.T.: La nidation des oeufs humains fecondes normaux et anormaux. In, Les Fonctions de Nidation Uterine et Leurs Troubles. J. Ferin and M. Gaudefroy, eds., pp. 169–213. Masson, Paris, 1960.

Hertig, A.T., and Rock, J.: Two human ova of the previllous stage having an ovulation age of about eleven and twelve days respectively. Contrib. Embryol. Carnegie Inst. 29: 127–156, 1941.

Hertig, A.T., and Rock, J.: Two human ova of the pre-villous stage, having a developmental age of about seven and nine days respectively. Contrib. Embryol. Carnegie Inst. 31: 65–84, 1945.

Hertig, A.T., and Rock, J.: Two human ova of the pre-villous stage, having a developmental age of about eight and nine days respectively. Contrib. Embryol. Carnegie Inst. 33: 169–186, 1949.

Heuser, C.H., and Streeter, G.L.: Development of the macaque embryo. Contrib. Embryol. Carnegie Inst. 29: 15–55, 1941.

Hoos, P.G., and Hoffman, L.H.: Temporal aspects of rabbit uterine vascular and decidual responses to blastocyst stimulation. Biol. Reprod. 23:453–459, 1980.

Hustin, J., Schaaps, J.P., and Lambotte, R.: Anatomical studies of the uteroplacental vascularization in the first trimester of pregnancy. Trophoblast Res. 3:49–60, 1988.

Kaiser, R.: Über die Rückbildungsvorgänge in der Decidua während der Schwangerschaft. Arch. Gynecol. 192:209–220, 1960.

Kaufmann, P.: Placentation und Placenta. In, Humanembryologie. K.V. Hinrichsen, ed., pp. 159–204. Springer-Verlag, Heidelberg, 1990.

Kaufmann, P., and Scheffen, I.: Placental development. In, Neonatal and Fetal Medicine—Physiology and Pathophysiology. R. Polin and W. Fox, eds., pp. 47–56. Saunders, Orlando, FL, 1992.

King, B.F.: Ultrastructural differentiation of stromal and vascular components in early macaque placental villi. Am. J. Anat. 178:30–44, 1987.

Larsen, J.F.: Electron microscopy of the implantation site in the rabbit. Am. J. Anat. 109:319–334, 1961.

Larsen, J.F.: Electron microscopy of nidation in the rabbit and observations on the human trophoblastic invasion. In, Ovo-Implantation, Human Gonadotrophins and Prolactin. P.O. Hubinont, F. Leroy, C. Robyn, and P. Leleux, eds., pp. 38–51. S. Karger, Basel, 1970.

Leiser, R., and Beier, H.M.: Morphological studies of lacunar formation in the early rabbit placenta. Trophoblast Res. 3:97–110, 1988.

Luckett, W.P.: Origin and differentiation of the yolk sac and extraembryonic mesoderm in presomite human and rhesus monkey embryos. Am. J. Anat. 152:59–97, 1978.

Mossman, H.W.: Comparative morphogenesis of the fetal membranes and accessory uterine structures. Carnegie Contrib. Embryol. 26:129–246, 1937.

Mossman, H.W.: Vertebrate Fetal Membranes: Comparative Ontogeny and Morphology; Evolution; Phylogenetic Significance; Basic Functions; Research Opportunities. Macmillan, London, 1987.

Park, W.W.: Choriocarcinoma: A Study of its Pathology, pp. 13–27. Heinemann, London, 1971.

Pijnenborg, R., Robertson, W.B., Brosens, I., and Dixon, G.: Trophoblast invasion and the establishment of haemochorial placentation in man and laboratory animals. Placenta 2: 71–92, 1981.

Psychoyos, A.: The "implantation window": can it be enlarged or displaced? Excerpta Med. Int. Congr. Ser. 768:231–232, 1988.

Robertson, W.B., and Warner, B.: The ultrastructure of the human placental bed. J. Pathol. 112:203–211, 1974.

Schaaps, J.P., and Hustin, J.: In vivo aspect of the maternal-trophoblastic border during the first trimester of gestation. Trophoblast Res. 3:3–48, 1988.

Schlafke, S., and Enders, A.C.: Cellular basis of interaction between trophoblast and uterus in implantation. Biol. Reprod. 12:41–65, 1975.

Steven, D.H.: Interspecies differences in the structure and function of trophoblast. In, Biology of Trophoblast. Y.W. Loke and A. Whyte, eds., pp. 111–136. Elsevier, Amsterdam, 1983.

Tedde, G., Tedde-Piras, A., and Berta, R.: A new structural pattern of the human trophoblast: the syncytial units. In, Abstracts of the 11th Rochester Trophoblast Conference, abstract 117, 1988a.

Tedde, G., Tedde-Piras, A., and Fenu, G.: Demonstration of an intercellular pathway of transport in the human trophoblast. In, Abstracts of the 11th Rochester Trophoblast Conference, abstract 77, 1988b.

Welsh, A.O., and Enders, A.E.: Light and electron microscopic examination of the mature decidual cells of the rat with emphasis on the antimesometrial decidua and its degeneration. Am. J. Anat. 172:1–29, 1985.

Wislocki, G.B., and Streeter, G.L.: On the placentation of the macaque (Macaca mulatta) from the time of implantation until the formation of the definitive placenta. Contrib. Embryol. Carnegie Inst. 27:1–66, 1938.

7
Basic Structure of the Villous Trees

M. Castellucci* and P. Kaufmann

Nearly all maternofetal and fetomaternal exchange takes place in the placental villi. There is only a limited contribution by the extraplacental membranes. In addition, most metabolic and endocrine activities of the placenta have been localized in the villi (for review see Gröschel-Stewart, 1981; Miller & Thiede, 1984; Knobil & Neill, 1993).

Throughout placental development, types of villi emerge that have differing functional specializations. Despite this diversification, all villi exhibit the same basic structure (Figure 26). They are covered by trophoblast, an epithelium-like surface layer that separates the maternal blood that flows around the villi from the villous interior. The trophoblast is composed of syncytiotrophoblast and cytotrophoblast. The former, unlike other epithelia, is not composed of individual cells but consists of a continuous, uninterrupted, multinucleated layer of syncytiotrophoblast without separating cell borders (Figures 26c and 71). Between syncytiotrophoblast and its basement membrane are single or aggregated cytotrophoblastic cells, the Langhans' cells, which are the stem cells of the syncytium; they support the growth and regeneration of the latter. The trophoblastic basement membrane separates the trophoblast from the stromal core of the villi. The stroma is composed of varying numbers and types of connective tissue cells, connective tissue fibers, ground substance, and fetal vessels of various kind and caliber. In the larger stem villi the vessels are mainly arteries and veins; in the peripheral branches most fetal vessels are capillaries, or sinusoids.

Syncytiotrophoblast

Syncytium or Multinucleated Giant Cells?

The syncytiotrophoblast is a continuous, normally uninterrupted layer that extends over the surfaces of all

*Istituto Morfologia Umana Normale, Facolta Medicina e Chirurgia, Via Ranieri, 60131 Ancona, Italy.

villous trees as well as over parts of the inner surfaces of chorionic and basal plates. It lines the intervillous space. Systematic electron microscopic studies of the syncytial layer (e.g., Bargmann & Knoop, 1959; Schiebler & Kaufmann, 1969; Boyd & Hamilton, 1970; Schweikhart & Kaufmann, 1977; Wang & Schneider, 1987) have revealed no evidence that the syncytiotrophoblast is composed of separate small or large units. Without a doubt, it is a single continuous structure for every placenta if we disregard some isolated syncytial elements at the surfaces of chorionic and basal plates that have lost contact with the syncytial continuum due to fibrinoid degeneration and some syncytial streamers that have invaded deeply into the junctional zone. Therefore terms such as syncytial cells and syncytiotrophoblasts, widely used in experimental disciplines, are inappropriate and must be avoided. Their use points to a basic misunderstanding of the real nature of the syncytiotrophoblast.

Where the syncytiotrophoblast is interrupted by degeneration, the gap is filled by fibrin-type fibrinoid (see Chapter 11). A few reports (Tedde et al., 1988a,b) pointed to the existence of vertical cell membranes that may subdivide the syncytium into syncytial units. These findings have an accidental rather than a real basis. They represent the likely results of a syncytiotrophoblastic repair mechanism (Figures 27b, 28). That is, after syncytial rupture apical and basal plasmalemmas fuse at either side of the wound, avoiding further loss of syncytioplasm. Afterward the wound is closed by a fibrinoid plug, or the disconnected parts of the syncytium again come into close contact to form a lateral intercellular cleft bridged by desmosomes. Later, fusion may occur by disintegration of the separating membranes (Figure 27). Transitory stages of this process may be misinterpreted as borders of syncytial units.

Many authors have described various types of intercellular junction within the syncytiotrophoblast (Carter,

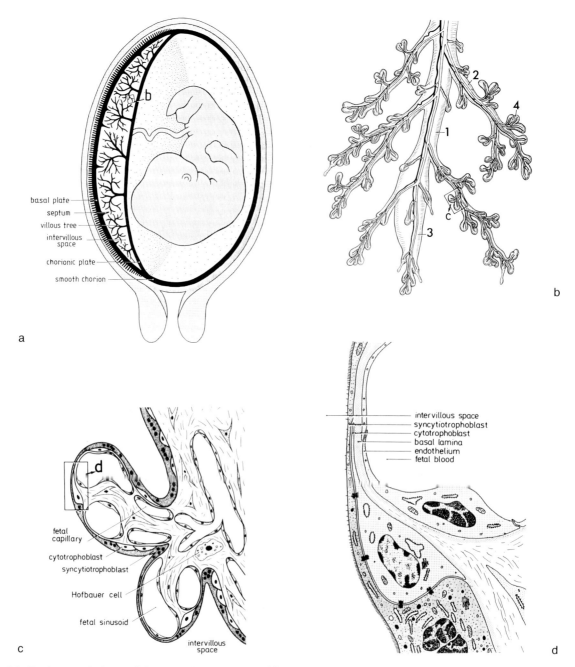

FIGURE 26. Basic morphology of human placental villi. (a) Simplified longitudinal section across the uterus, placenta, and membranes in the human. The chorionic sac, consisting of placenta (left half) and membranes (right half), is black. (b) Peripheral ramifications of the mature villous tree, consisting of a stem villus (1), which continues in a bulbous immature intermediate villus (3); the slender side branches (2) are the mature intermediate villi, the surface of which is densely covered with grape-like terminal villi (4). (c) Highly simplified light microscopic section of two terminal villi, branching off a mature intermediate villus (right). (d) Representation of an electron microscopic section of the placental barrier, demonstrating its typical layers. (Modified after Kaufmann, 1983, with permission.)

1963, 1964; Boyd & Hamilton, 1966; Burgos & Rodriguez, 1966; Metz et al., 1979; Reale et al., 1980; Wang & Schneider, 1987). Some have interpreted these junctions as vestiges of a former cellular state of the syncytium or as proof for recent cytotrophoblastic contribution to the syncytiotrophoblast (Carter, 1963, 1964; Boyd & Hamilton, 1966). In a systematic study of these junctions, Metz et al. (1979) described zonulae and maculae occludentes that were mostly located in apical membrane infoldings, as well as numerous isolated desmosomes, without contact to any surface membranes. These authors hypothesized that the various

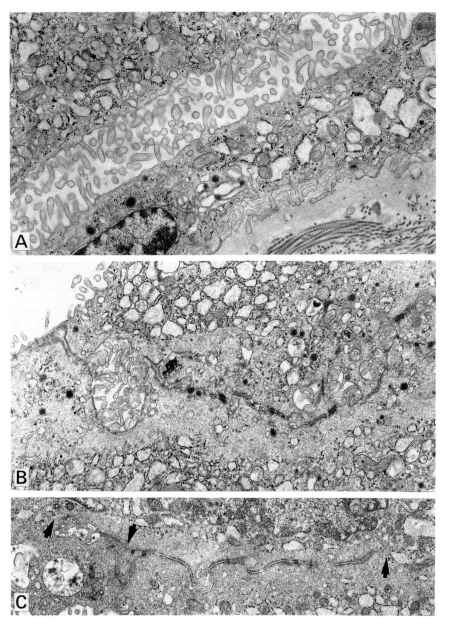

FIGURE 27. Remains of cell membranes in the syncytiotrophoblast result from two mechanisms: fusion of neighboring villous surfaces forming bridges and repair of disrupted syncytial surfaces. (A) As a first step of repair, the wound surfaces are covered by microvillous membranes. The latter interdigitate. The identical initial step occurs with surfaces of neighboring villi prior to fusion and the formation of bridges. ×14,500. (B) Follow-up stage of that depicted in (A). The interdigitating syncytial surfaces have largely lost their micro-villi and now establish a smooth intercellular cleft bridged by numerous desmosomes, which vertically traverse the syncytiotrophoblast (see Figure 28). ×11,000. (C) As the next step of repair the newly developed separating cell membranes show disintegration (arrows), so the newly formed intrasyncytial cleft becomes focally bridged by syncytioplasm. After complete disintegration of membranes and desmosomes, the syncytial villous cover is again continuous. ×13,800. (From Cantle et al., 1987, with permission.)

junctions represent stages of several dynamic processes (e.g., establishment of intervillous contacts by partial or complete syncytiotrophoblastic surface fusion, repair of syncytial disruption, or decomposition of temporary surface invagination of the syncytiotrophoblast). The syncytiotrophoblast must be seen as a highly dynamic layer that is qualified for ameboid movements. Moreover, traumatic disconnection and subsequent refusion and the formation of invaginations and bridges for stabilization of the villous tree seem to be regular phenomena. We do not observe such processes but find their ultrastructural remains.

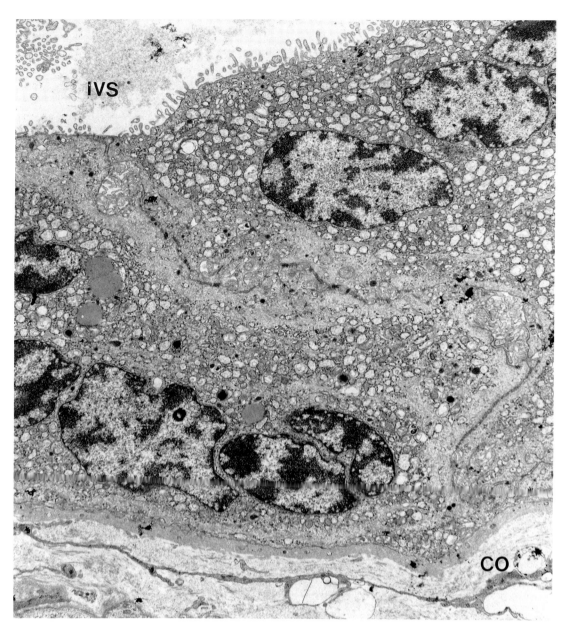

FIGURE 28. Survey electron micrograph of the section shown in Figure 27B. It demonstrates that during intermediate stages of syncytial repair the villous syncytial trophoblast can be traversed by vertical "intercellular" clefts connecting the inter- villous space (IVS) with the connective tissue core (CO) of the villi. Such intrasyncytial membranes must not be misinter- preted as stable intercellular clefts subdividing the syncytium in smaller syncytial units. ×7,000.

Syncytial Plasmalemmas and Microvilli

With deference to the intentions of this monograph, we deal only briefly with some aspects of the plasma membranes of the syncytiotrophoblast. Sideri et al. (1983) have pointed to differences between the apical plasmalemma (facing the maternal blood) and the basal plasmalemma (facing the basal lamina and the stromal core) of the syncytiotrophoblast. They exhibit different densities of intramembranous particles that are likely to represent mostly proteins. These differences have been studied in more detail by Vanderpuye and Smith (1987) who, in addition, presented a useful review of the relevant literature. These authors found that the fol- lowing proteins were common to preparations of both membranes: actin, alkaline phosphatase, albumin, human placental lactogen, transferrin, transferrin recep- tor, and immunoglobulin G. Particular attention was paid to the content of glycosaminoglycans and sialoglycoproteins by Kelley et al. (1979) and Wasserman et al. (1983a,b).

Independent of the type of syncytial specialization, the syncytiotrophoblastic surface is nearly completely covered by microvilli, which represent an enormous maternofetal contact zone (Figure 47); at term, the presence of microvilli multiplies the total villous surface area of about $12\,m^2$ (Table 6) by a factor of about 7.67 (Teasdale & Jean-Jacques, 1986; see also Mayhew, 1985). Because of their immunological importance and the basic cell biological implications, the microvilli have engendered much interest. Two summarizing articles provide detailed reviews of all biological aspects of syncytiotrophoblastic microvilli (Smith et al., 1977; Truman & Ford, 1984).

Morphological studies of microvillous structure and their functional significance have been reported by Boyd et al. (1968b), Herbst and Multier (1970), Wainwright and Wainwright (1974), Truman et al. (1981), King (1983), and Al-Zuhair et al. (1983, 1987). Most of the histochemical studies concerning the composition of the microvillous membrane have focused on the glycocalyx; they described its polysaccharide composition and discussed the immunological relevance of the polysaccharides (Bradbury et al., 1969, 1970; Rovasio & Monis, 1973; Liebhart, 1974; Martin et al., 1974; Okudaira & Hayakawa, 1975; Nelson et al., 1976; Wada et al., 1977, 1979; King, 1981; Wasserman et al., 1983a,b; Fisher et al., 1984; Parmley et al., 1984). Various lectin-binding sites have been described by Whyte (1980) and Gabius et al. (1987). Cytochemical demonstration of surface enzymes, mostly bound to the microvilli, have provided the morphological impression of transmembranous transfer processes. The enzymes studied by transmission electron microscopy (TEM) are alkaline phosphatase (Hempel & Geyer, 1969; Borst et al., 1973; Hulstaert et al., 1973; Kameya et al., 1973; Jemmerson et al., 1985; Matsubara et al., 1987d), galactosyltransferase (Nelson et al., 1977), α-amylase (Fisher & Laine, 1983), protein kinases (Albe et al., 1983), Ca-ATPase (Matsubara et al., 1987b), cyclic 3,5-nucleotide phosphodiesterase (Matsubara et al., 1987c), and 5-nucleotidase (Matsubara et al., 1987a).

The analysis of surface receptors involved in transplacental transfer (King, 1976; Ockleford & Menon, 1977; Wood et al., 1978a,b; Galbraith et al., 1980; Johnson & Brown, 1980; Brown & Johnson, 1981; Green & Ford, 1984; Malassine et al., 1984, 1987; Alsat et al., 1985; Parmley et al., 1985; Bierings, 1989; Yeh et al., 1989) has contributed importantly to our understanding of transplacental transport. Finally, the identification of receptors for hormones and growth factors is one of the most intriguing chapters of modern pla-

centology. The vast literature has been discussed elsewhere (Mitchell et al., 1993) and is not reviewed here. For further reading on particular subjects we refer to the following publications: insulin receptor (Nelson et al., 1978; Jones et al., 1993; Desoye et al., 1994); insulin-like growth factor II (Daughaday et al., 1981); interleukin-6 receptor (Nishino et al., 1990); parathyroid hormone receptor (Lafond et al., 1988); epidermal growth factor and its receptor (Rao et al., 1984, 1985; Chegini & Rao, 1985; Maruo & Mochizuki, 1987; Maruo et al., 1987; Morrish et al., 1987; Chen et al., 1988; Yeh et al., 1989; Mühlhauser et al., 1993); proto-oncogen protein products with the quality of growth factor receptors (Adamson, 1987; Mühlhauser et al., 1993).

Syncytiotrophoblastic Cytoskeleton

Ockleford et al. (1981a) have speculated that there must be other factors responsible for maintenance of the complex shape of the villus in addition to the skeletal structures of the villous stroma. They described a superficially arranged complex system of intrasyncytial filaments that largely occupies the superficial layer of the syncytiotrophoblast. Ockleford et al. (1981a) suggested the name syncytioskeletal layer for this zone. Numerous other authors have contributed to our knowledge of the syncytial cytoskeleton as well (Vacek, 1969; Scheuner et al., 1980; Ockleford et al., 1981a,b,c; King, 1983; Khong et al., 1986; Beham et al., 1988).

The syncytial cytoskeleton is composed of actin, tubulin, and intermediate filament proteins as cytokeratins and desmoplakin (Ockleford et al., 1981a; King, 1983; Beham et al., 1988). The microtubules are arranged in a coarse, open lattice-like network that is oriented parallel to the syncytial surface. They are intermingled with microfilaments that form an apparently disordered meshwork. Actin filaments of this meshwork pass into the microvilli, where they display a distinct polarity, with their S1 arrowheads pointing away from the microvillous tips. Different from intestinal microvilli, the rootlets of the microvillous filaments are short and interact with other filaments of the terminal web almost immediately after emergence from the microvilli. The overall impression of this system, reported by King (1983), is one of a poorly developed terminal web. Beham et al. (1988) found immunohistochemical evidence for the presence of cytokeratin and desmoplakin in the apical zone. The presence of the latter intermediate filament protein is in agreement with the occasional appearance of desmosomes in this zone. Both intermediate filaments were also found in the basal zone of the syncytioplasm

(Beham et al., 1988), where King (1983) also detected actin.

Specialized Regions of the Villous Surface

Dempsey and Zergollern (1969), and Dempsey and Luse (1971) have subdivided the syncytiotrophoblast into three zones: an outer absorptive zone in which organelles related to vesicular uptake and large parts of the cytoskeleton are accumulated (syncytioskeletal layer) (Ockleford et al., 1981a); a middle secretory zone containing most organelles; and a basal zone with few organelles. Structural changes and variations in thickness of the middle zone are responsible for regional specializations that become evident during the second half of pregnancy.

During earlier stages of pregnancy, the syncytiotrophoblast is a mostly homogeneous layer with evenly distributed nuclei (Figure 46) (Boyd & Hamilton, 1970; Kaufmann & Stegner, 1972). The distribution of cellular organelles is homogeneous, which indicates that there is no particular structural or functional differentiation inside this layer. Beginning at the 15th week this situation gradually changes (Kaufmann & Stegner, 1972), and at term there is a highly variable pattern of mosaic areas of different structure and histochemical attributes (Figures 29–32). The various types of syncytiotrophoblastic specialization have been described in numerous publications (Amstutz, 1960; Fox, 1965; Burgos & Rodriguez, 1966; Hamilton & Boyd, 1966; Schiebler & Kaufmann, 1969; Alvarez et al., 1970; Dempsey & Luse, 1971; Kaufmann & Stark, 1973; Martin & Spicer, 1973b; Kaufmann et al., 1974a; Jones & Fox, 1977). It must be pointed out, however, that these specialized areas lack sharp demarcations because they are part of a syncytium. The various types of syncytiotrophoblast described in the following sections can be differentiated by taking into account the thickness of the syncytiotrophoblast, the distribution of its nuclei, the kind and number of its organelles, and its enzymatic activities.

Epithelial Plates

Epithelial plates, or vasculosyncytial membranes (Figures 29, 32–34), were first identified by Bremer

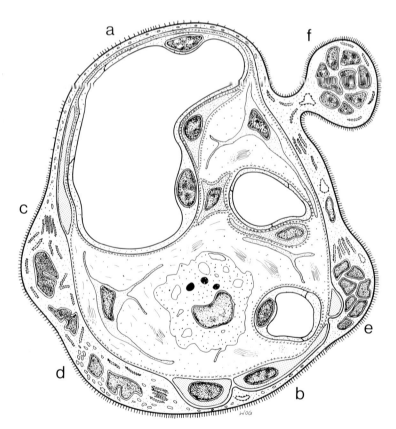

FIGURE 29. Cross section of a terminal villus demonstrating the structural variability of its syncytiotrophoblastic cover. a = Epithelial plate (vasculosyncytial membrane) (see Figures 32–34); b = thin syncytial lamella covering villous cytotrophoblast (see Figures 30, 37, 38); c = syncytiotrophoblast with well developed rough endoplasmic reticulum (see Figure 35); d = syncytiotrophoblast with well developed smooth endoplasmic reticulum (see Figure 36); e = syncytial knot (compare Figures 32, 39); f = syncytial sprout (see Figures 40–43).

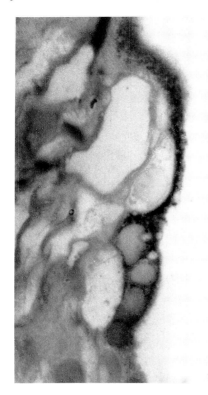

FIGURE 30. Semithin section demonstrating the histochemical activity of 17β-hydroxysteroid dehydrogenase. As an indicator of syncytiotrophoblastic specialization, this enzyme has maximum activity in and around a syncytial lamella covering villous cytotrophoblast. ×1,000. (From Kaufmann et al., 1974a, with permission.)

(1916) and later defined in more detail by Amstutz (1960). They are thin syncytiotrophoblastic lamellae measuring 0.5 to about 1.0 μm in thickness; they are free of nuclei and poor in organelles and are directly apposed to sinusoidally enlarged parts of the fetal capillaries (Schiebler & Kaufmann, 1969; Fox & Blanco, 1974). One can conclude from the structural features that the enlarging sinusoids bulge against the villous surface and completely displace the syncytial nuclei and most of the syncytial organelles. Capillary basement membrane and trophoblastic basement membrane may come into such close contact that they fuse (Figures 26, 33). In agreement with this view, accumulations of nuclei and most of the organelles may be observed directly lateral to the epithelial plates; they are called syncytial knots (Figures 29, 32, 39). The density of microvilli at the surface of the vasculosyncytial membranes sometimes is considerably reduced (Figures 33, 34) (Leibl et al., 1975; however, compare King & Menton, 1975). High activities of hexokinase and glucose-6-phosphatase are present histochemically, whereas enzymes involved in energy metabolism are largely inactive (Figure 31). Regarding structure and

endorsement with enzymes, we conclude that these areas are especially involved in diffusional transfer of gases and water, as well as in facilitated transfer of glucose.

Slightly thicker vasculosyncytial membranes are equipped with more organelles. In addition, they show hydrolytic enzymes such as alkaline phosphatase (Kameya et al., 1973), 5-nucleotidase, and ATPase (Schiebler & Kaufmann, 1981). These sites are presumably concerned with active transfer rather than merely passive transfer processes (e.g., amino acids, electrolytes).

When studying optimally fixed terminal villi of the term placenta, the epithelial plates (vasculosyncytial membranes) amount to 25% to 40% of the villous surface (Sen et al., 1979), depending on the maturational status of the villi. After delayed fixation this value may be considerably smaller owing to fetal vessel

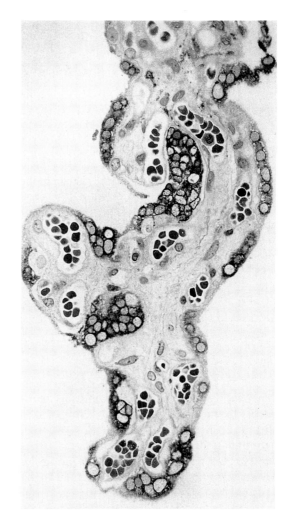

FIGURE 31. Semithin section with histochemical demonstration of lactate dehydrogenase. The enzyme activity is bound to the vicinity of syncytial nuclei, whereas syncytium devoid of nuclei does not exhibit enzyme activity. ×420. (From Schiebler & Kaufmann, 1981, with permission.)

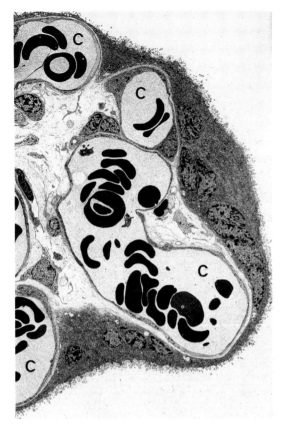

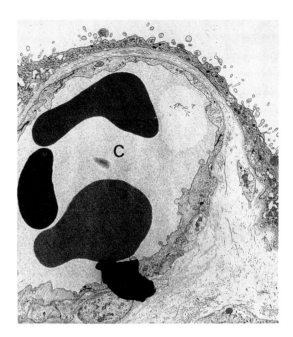

FIGURE 33. Transmission electron micrograph of an epithelial plate (vasculosyncytial membrane). Note the extremely thin syncytial lamella that extends over the fetal capillary (C), the former being characterized by only a few organelles and a reduced number of microvilli. ×4,800.

FIGURE 32. Transmission electron microscopic section of a terminal villus. Note that the structural specialization of the syncytiotrophoblast depends on its spatial relation to the fetal capillaries (C). In nearly all places where the capillaries bulge against the villous surface, the syncytiotrophoblast is attenuated to thin lamellae (epithelial plates, vasculosyncytial membranes) devoid of nuclei. The nuclei accumulate between the lamellae and form syncytial knots. ×1,350. (From Castellucci & Kaufmann, 1982a, with permission.)

collapse and trophoblastic shrinkage (Tables 7, 10) (Voigt et al., 1978).

Syncytial Lamellae Covering Langhans' Cells

The syncytial lamellae covering Langhans' cells are comparable to the epithelial plates in terms of structure and thickness. In many or even most cases, they are direct continuations of the epithelial plates, as the thin syncytial lamellae of the latter extend from the bulging capillaries to the neighboring bulging Langhans' cells (Figures 29, 30, 37, 38). The lamellae are normally characterized by increased numbers of dense bodies (lysosomes? secretory granules?) that are found in both, the syncytium and the Langhans' cell, underneath. Histochemically, they often show an intense reaction for 17β-hydroxysteroid dehydrogenase (Figure 30) (Kaufmann & Stark, 1973; Kaufmann et al., 1974a). It

has been speculated that the development of these specialized zones from the 15th week postmenstruation (p.m.) on is related to increased concentrations of that enzyme in the maternal serum and to increased maternal urinary estriol excretion (Kaufmann & Stark, 1973).

Syncytiotrophoblast with Prevailing Rough Endoplasmic Reticulum

Syncytiotrophoblast with prevailing rough endoplasmic reticulum is the most common type of syncytium represented at the term villous surface. The thickness varies between 2 and about 10 μm. It may contain nuclei or be devoid of them. The surface is covered by more or less densely packed microvilli. In addition to vesicles and all types of lysosomes, the cytoplasm is characterized by numerous mitochondria, Golgi fields, and ample rough endoplasmic reticulum. After conventional postpartum fixation, the latter is vesicular (Figures 27, 28) (Boyd et al., 1968a). With optimal fixation (e.g., aspiration biopsy during cesarean section from a placenta in situ that is still maternally perfused) (Schweikhart & Kaufmann, 1977), the rough endoplasmic reticulum is composed of slender cisternae oriented in parallel (Figure 35). The degree of dilatation depends on the delay of fixation (Kaufmann, 1985).

Several reports have dealt with structural aspects of this type of syncytiotrophoblast (Boyd et al., 1968a;

Dempsey & Zergollern, 1969; Schiebler & Kaufmann, 1969; Dempsey & Luse, 1971; Martin & Spicer, 1973a; Ockleford, 1976). Histochemically, numerous enzymes have been demonstrated, for example, enzymes related to energy metabolism (Figure 31), glutamate dehydrogenase, α-glycerophosphate dehydrogenase, nonspecific esterase, acid phosphatase, alkaline phosphatase, and proteases (Wielenga & Willighagen, 1962; Velardo & Rosa, 1963; Wachstein et al., 1963; Lister, 1967; Hoffman & Di Pietro, 1972; Hulstaert et al., 1973; Kaufmann et al., 1974a; Gossrau et al., 1987). These studies make it likely that this type of syncytium is involved in more complex, active maternofetal transfer mechanisms, including catabolism and resynthesis of proteins and lipids. Some immunocytochemical studies have provided evidence that synthesis of several proteo- and peptide hormones takes place here, including human chorionic gonadotropin (hCG) (Dreskin et al., 1970; Hamanaka et al., 1971; Genbacev et al., 1972; Kurman et al., 1984; Beck et al., 1986; Frauli & Ludwig, 1987b; Morrish et al., 1987; Sakakibara et al., 1987; Hay, 1988); human chorionic somatotropin or placental lactogen (hCS or hPL) (Kim et al., 1971; De Ikonicoff & Cedard, 1973; Dujardin et al., 1977; Kurman et al., 1984; Beck et al., 1986; Fujimoto et al., 1986; Morrish et al., 1988); other human growth hormones, such as hGH-V and HGH-N (Liebhaber et

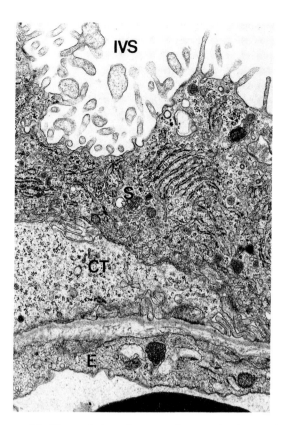

FIGURE 35. Transmission electron micrograph of syncytiotrophoblast with well developed rough endoplasmic reticulum, probably active in protein metabolism. IVS = intervillous space; S = syncytiotrophoblast; CT = cytotrophoblast; E = fetal endothelium. ×14,000. (From Schiebler & Kaufmann, 1981, with permission.)

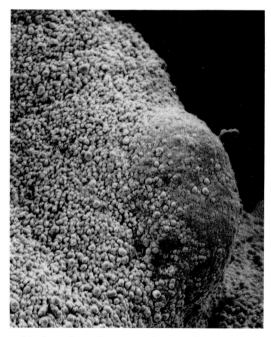

FIGURE 34. Scanning electron micrograph of an epithelial plate comparable to that depicted in Figure 33. It is viewed here from the intervillous space (black area) at the villous surface. The protrusion of the villous surface caused by the underlying capillary is clearly visible. It is largely devoid of microvilli. ×3,300. (From Schiebler & Kaufmann, 1981, with permission.)

al., 1989); prolactin (hPRL) (Bryant-Greenwood et al., 1987; Sakbun et al., 1987; Unnikumar et al., 1988); oxytocin (Unnikumar et al., 1988); β-endorphin and β-lipotropin (Laatikainen et al., 1987); and various placental proteins, such as SP1 (Gosseye & Fox, 1984; Beck et al., 1986).

Syncytiotrophoblast with Prevailing Smooth Endoplasmic Reticulum

Syncytiotrophoblast with prevailing smooth endoplasmic reticulum comprises small spot-like areas dispersed in the syncytium equipped with rough endoplasmic reticulum (Figures 29, 36–38). It is usually present near mitochondria of the tubular type. The structural similarity to endocrine cells active in steroid metabolism (Gillim et al., 1969; Crisp et al., 1970) allows speculation that it is specialized in the metabolism of steroid hormones. Focally increased activity of 3β-hydroxysteroid dehydrogenase and of 17β-hydroxysteroid dehydrogenase has been found by enzyme histochemistry

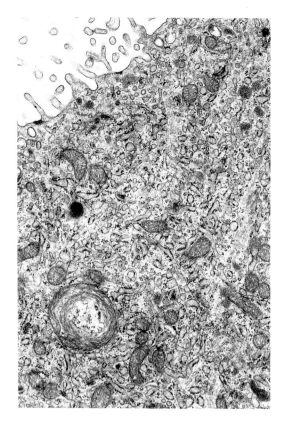

FIGURE 36. Electron micrograph of syncytiotrophoblast with well developed smooth endoplasmic reticulum. Such areas are probably involved in steroid metabolism. ×14,800.

(Figure 30) (Kaufmann & Stark, 1973; Kaufmann et al., 1974a).

Syncytial Knots, Sprouts, Bridges, and Stromal Trophoblastic Buds

Syncytial knots, sprouts, bridges, and stromal trophoblastic buds are the names for a group of syncytiotrophoblastic specializations characterized by accumulation of nuclei (Hamilton & Boyd, 1966; Boyd & Hamilton, 1970). Studies by Küstermann (1981), Burton (1986a,b), Cantle et al. (1987), and Kaufmann et al. (1987a) provided evidence that most of these structures in fact are results of tangential sectioning of the villous surfaces. There is, however, a limited amount of true syncytiotrophoblastic outgrowth, characterized by aggregated nuclei.

Syncytial knots are characterized by a multilayered group of aggregated nuclei that bulge only slightly on the trophoblastic surface. If they exhibit the same structural and histochemical features as the surrounding syncytiotrophoblast, they are likely to be only representations of tangential sections. A few are characterized by densely packed nuclei, separated from each other by slender strands of cytoplasm devoid of most

organelles. The small nuclei show a more or less condensed chromatin and sometimes severe pyknosis (Figure 39) (Martin & Spicer, 1973b; Jones & Fox, 1977; Schiebler & Kaufmann, 1981). The surrounding cytoplasm usually exhibits degenerative changes. In many cases the changes are found directly lateral to epithelial plates, suggesting that they are the site of accumulation of displaced nuclei from the thin trophoblastic lamellae.

Larger aggregates of syncytial nuclei, those protruding into the intervillous space in a mushroom-like fashion, are usually called syncytial sprouts (Figures 40–43) (Langhans, 1870; Boyd & Hamilton, 1970). It is a historical and in most cases inappropriate name, as it implies that these structures are structural correlates of villous sprouting. During early pregnancy (Figures 42, 43, 72) this interpretation is often correct (Cantle et al., 1987). In the term placenta, most of the "sprouts" are sectional artifacts that represent tangential sections of the villous surface (Küstermann, 1981; Burton, 1986a; Cantle et al., 1987). The few remaining true syncytiotrophoblastic protrusions are composed of two completely different groups. Most exhibit the same degenerative changes as described for the syncytial knots (Figure 40). The functional interpretations com-

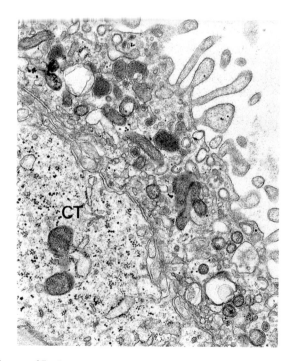

FIGURE 37. Transmission electron micrograph of a thin syncytiotrophoblastic lamella covering villous cytotrophoblast (CT). Syncytiotrophoblast of this type is well equipped with dense bodies and vesicles. As can be deduced from its enzymatic activity, such areas are probably involved in endocrine activity. ×22,000.

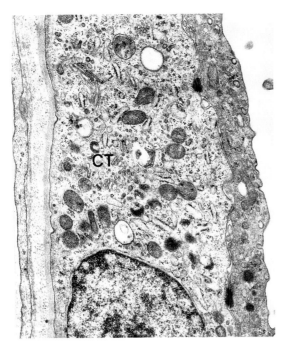

FIGURE 38. Transmission electron micrograph of a thin syncytiotrophoblastic lamella covering cytotrophoblast (CT). This lamella is devoid of microvilli and dense bodies. Its cytoplasm is characterized only by vesicles. After enzyme histochemical reactions (see Figure 30) it exhibits high activities of 17β-hydroxysteroid dehydrogenase and thus participates in steroid metabolism. ×14,500.

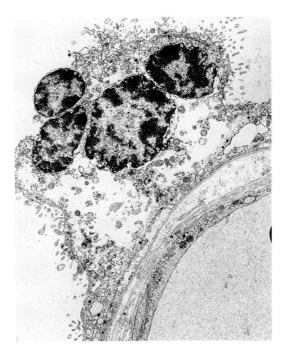

FIGURE 40. Electron micrograph of a syncytial sprout that shows obvious signs of degeneration and extrusion of its nuclei. It must be interpreted as a later stage of the process depicted in Figure 39. ×5,100.

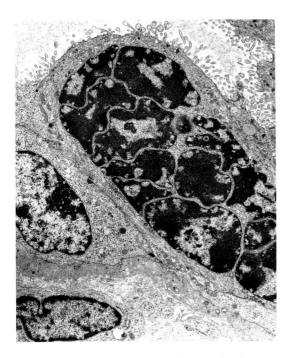

FIGURE 39. Transmission electron micrograph of a syncytial knot characterized by clustered nuclei that are rich in pyknotic heterochromatin, suggesting a degenerative character. In between, there are only narrow bands of syncytioplasm. ×5,000. (From Cantle et al., 1987, with permission.)

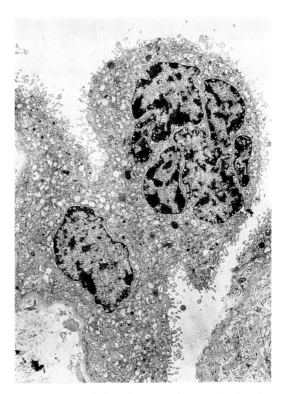

FIGURE 41. Transmission electron micrograph of a "syncytial sprout" from a mature placenta that, because of its appearance, is likely to represent a tangential section of the villous surface (see Figures 94–98). Most "knots" and "sprouts" observed in the mature placenta belong to this type of sectional artifact. ×4,600. (From Schiebler & Kaufmann, 1981, with permission.)

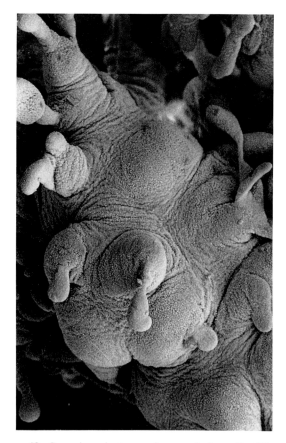

FIGURE 42. Scanning electron micrograph from the 8th week p.m. of gestation, showing local accumulations of mushroom-like true syncytial sprouts arising from broad villous protrusions. The latter probably represent the initial steps of the formation of new villi; they are common features in the early placenta but are rare at term. ×180. (From Cantle et al., 1987, with permission.)

prise local hyperplasia of the syncytium (Baker et al., 1944), results of trophoblastic degeneration (Tenney & Parker, 1940; Merrill, 1963), structural expression of placental insufficiency (Becker & Bleyl, 1961; Kubli & Budliger, 1963; Werner & Bender, 1977), structural expression of ischemia, hypoxia, or hypertension (Wilkin, 1965; Tominaga & Page, 1966; Alvarez, 1970; Alvarez et al., 1972; Gerl et al., 1973), and results of fetal malperfusion of placental villi (Fox, 1965; Myers & Fujikura, 1968).

Martin and Spicer (1973b) and Dorgan and Schultz (1971) demonstrated that the life-span of syncytiotro-phoblast is limited. Thus the presence of local degenera-tive changes due to normal aging must be expected. Based on such views, Martin and Spicer (1973b), Jones and Fox (1977), Schiebler and Kaufmann (1981), and Cantle et al. (1987) described the last group of "sprouts" as sites where aged syncytial nuclei are accumulated and are later pinched off, together with some surrounding cytoplasm (Figures 39–41, 52). Iklé

(1964) found such segregated parts of the syncytiotro-phoblast in the maternal circulation.

Occasional sprouts, however, can be found that are characterized by loosely distributed, large ovoid nuclei. They possess little heterochromatin and are surrounded by ample free ribosomes and well developed rough endoplasmic reticulum. They resemble the true sprouts of the early placenta. Normally, they are found only in small groups on the surfaces of immature intermediate and mesenchymal villi in the centers of the villous trees. From studies of villous development (Castellucci et al., 1990c) it has become evident that sprouts of this type are an expression of villous sprouting. Their concentra-tion in the centers of the villous trees is in agreement with Schuhmann's view (1981) that the centers are growth zones for the villous trees.

It is likely that the syncytial buds or stromal tropho-blastic buds (Boyd & Hamilton, 1970) are, without exception, tangential sections of indenting villous surfaces or places of villous branching (Küstermann,

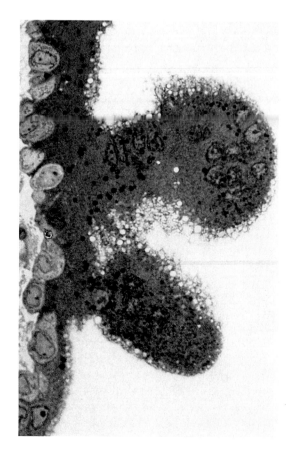

FIGURE 43. Semithin section from the 9th week of gestation, showing two real syncytial sprouts, comparable to those depicted in Figure 42. Note the unevenly dispersed nuclei and compare with the aggregated and pyknotic nuclei of the false sprouts depicted in Figures 39–41. ×870. (From Cantle et al., 1987, with permission.)

1981). Therefore the old question whether these trophoblastic elements may "invade" fetal vessels (Salvaggio et al., 1960; Boyd & Hamilton, 1970) is no longer relevant.

There has been intense discussion concerning syncytial bridges. It began with their first description by Langhans (1870) and continued with the reports of Stieve (1936, 1941), Ortmann (1941), Peter (1943, 1951), Hörmann (1953), Schiebler and Kaufmann (1969), Boyd and Hamilton (1970), Kaufmann and Stegner (1972), and Jones and Fox (1977). Most are sectional artifacts that must be interpreted as results of tangential sectioning of villous branchings (Figures 94– 99) (Küstermann, 1981; Burton, 1986a; Cantle et al., 1987). Placentas with tortuously malformed villi, as those seen with severe preeclampsia, may exhibit so many bridges in histological sections that a net-like appearance is achieved (Figure 105). In the light of these findings, one may argue that reports on villi, arranged as a three-dimensional network (Stieve, 1941; Schiebler & Kaufmann, 1981), have been three-dimensional misinterpretations of tangential sections of tortuous villi. The famous diagram by Stieve (1941) of the human placenta with villi in a net-like arrangement was refuted by Peter (1951) based on reconstructions of wax plates.

Only the studies of Burton (1986a,b, 1987) and Cantle et al. (1987) made clear that there are real bridges in addition to those of artifactual genesis (Figures 44, 45). Hörmann (1953), Kaufmann and Stegner (1972), Jones and Fox (1977), and Cantle et al. (1987) presented evidence that real bridges are the result of fusion of adjacent villous surfaces, which occurs as soon as those surfaces come into prolonged intimate contact. Intermediate stages can be found as soon as slender intercellular gaps are formed between neighboring villous surfaces and become bridged by desmosomes. Later, the separating membranes disintegrate, causing the formation of a real syncytial bridge. Using radioangiographic and morphological methods, vascularization of such bridges has been observed resulting in fetal intervillous vascular connections (Peter, 1951; Lemtis, 1955; Boyd & Hamilton, 1970). Unlike Stieve (1941), who postulated a net-like fetal vascular system that connects all villi, the authors cited above provided evidence that such connections are rare exceptions. Whether the syncytial bridges have any mechanically supporting effects on the villous tree or are accidental structures without significance is a matter of speculation.

Transtrophoblastic Channels

The syncytium has been thought to be an uninterrupted barrier composed of two plasmalemmas with an intermediate layer of syncytial cytoplasm. Therefore every

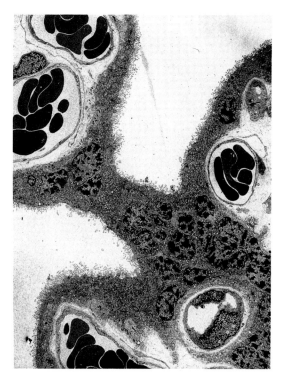

FIGURE 44. Transmission electron micrograph of a syncytial bridge connecting two neighboring villi. ×1,500. (From Cantle et al., 1987, with permission.)

substance passing the syncytiotrophoblast from the maternal to the fetal circulation was thought to do so under the control of this trophoblast layer. The existence of pericellular pathways was unacceptable to many placentologists. Discussions during a 1986 workshop on transtrophoblastic channels, held on the occasion of the 2nd Meeting of the European Placenta Group, caused considerable controversy.

Transport experiments by Stulc et al. (1969) provided the first evidence for the existence of water-filled routes, so-called pores or channels, across the rabbit placenta. Their radius was calculated to be approximately 10 nm. This finding has been confirmed for the guinea pig placenta by Thornburg and Faber (1977) and Hedley and Bradbury (1980). Morphological studies of various placental types, however, have long failed to demonstrate such structural correlates. There are now some results that make the existence of membrane-lined transtrophoblastic channels likely.

Application of lanthanum hydroxide as an extracellular tracer via the maternal or fetal circulation resulted in the demonstration of membrane-lined channels in the isolated guinea pig placenta (Kaufmann et al., 1987b, 1989) and the postpartally perfused human placenta (Kertschanska & Kaufmann, 1992; Kertschanska et al., 1994); these channels have a luminal diameter of 15 to 25 nm and extend as winding, branching structures from

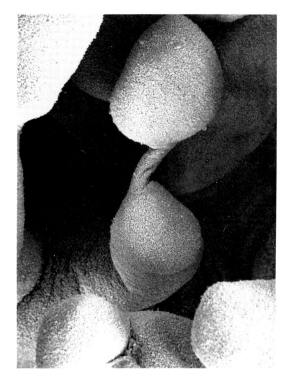

FIGURE 45. Scanning electron micrograph of a syncytial bridge similar to that depicted in Figure 44. It demonstrates that not all bridges seen in sections are artifacts and caused by tangential sectioning. Such real bridges are probably caused by local contacts of neighboring villous surfaces with subsequent syncytial fusion. ×890. (From Cantle et al., 1987, with permission.)

the apical or basal surface into the syncytiotrophoblast. Because of their winding structure, they could never be traced in full length across the trophoblast. The release of the tracer into the maternal circulation, when applied via the fetal circulation and vice versa, make it likely that at least some of these channels pass the syncytiotrophoblast in full length.

These results are in agreement with earlier findings obtained in the guinea pig placenta. In the fully isolated, artificially perfused organ, hydrostatic and colloid osmotic forces cause fetomaternal fluid shifts (Schröder et al., 1982). Fetal venous pressure elevation of 5 to 17 mm Hg were enough to shift 30% to 50% of the arterial perfusion volumes into the maternal circulation. We detected ultrastructurally initially slender and later bag-like dilated channels that passed the syncytiotrophoblast in full length, as routes for the fluid shift (Kaufmann et al., 1982). As soon as the fetal venous pressure was reduced to normal, the fluid shift ceased and the bag-like channels disappeared. These experiments have been successfully repeated in the isolated human placental lobule (Kertschanska & Kaufmann, 1992). The reversibility of the events refuted the possibility that they were of traumatic origin. The only

possible explanation is the existence of channels that can be dilated under conditions of pressure increase. It is likely that the channels traced with lanthanum hydroxide are identical to those dilated experimentally under the conditions of fluid shift and those postulated in transfer experiments by the physiologists mentioned above (for review see Stulc, 1989).

Similar basal invaginations or intrasyncytial vacuoles such as those found under the experimental conditions of fluid shift are sometimes observed in freshly delivered human placentas. It is still open to question if this phenomenon is an expression of active fetomaternal fluid shift during labor.

Functionally, the transtrophoblastic channels are possible sites of transfer for water-soluble, lipid-insoluble molecules with an effective molecular diameter of about 1.5 nm (Thornburg & Faber, 1977; Stulc, 1989). Under the conditions of fetomaternal fluid shift due to fetal venous pressure increase or fetal decrease of osmotic pressure, the channels may dilate to such an extent that all molecules, independent of size and solubility, may pass (Kaufmann et al., 1982; Schröder et al., 1982; Kertschanska & Kaufmann, 1992; Kertschanska et al., 1994).

Another functional aspect may be important. The embryo and fetus have problems of eliminating surplus water. Simple renal filtration with subsequent urination does not necessarily solve this problem, as the urine is delivered into the amnionic fluid and is still inside the fetoplacental unit. On the other hand, excessive fetal hydration causes an increase of fetal venous pressure and a decrease of fetal osmotic pressure. Both factors have been experimentally proved to open narrow channels so they are widely dilated, allowing fetomaternal fluid shift and equilibration of the surplus water. Because electrolytes, nutrients, proteins, and so on follow the water from the fetal circulation into the maternal circulation, the fluid shift itself does not correct the fetal osmotic pressure. As in renal tubules, these substances may become resorbed by the maternal surface of the trophoblast and transferred back into the fetal circulation. Thus pressure-dependent dilatation and closure of the channels may act as an important factor in fetal osmoregulation and water balance.

Plasma Protrusions or Blebs

After studying the syncytiotrophoblastic surface of human placental villi electron microscopically, many authors have reported the existence of fungiform, membrane-lined protrusions of the apical syncytioplasm. These structures are largely or completely devoid of organelles. Their diameter normally ranges from 2 to about 15 μm (Ikawa, 1959; Hashimoto et al., 1960a,b; Arnold et al., 1961; Geller, 1962; Rhodin & Terzakis, 1962; Lister, 1964; Nagy et al., 1965; Strauss et al., 1965; Herbst et al., 1968, 1969; Knoth, 1968; Kaufmann, 1969). Numerous studies have shown that these protrusions are not a specific feature of syncytiotrophoblast but, rather, common features of most epithelia and sometimes of other cellular types (for review see Kaufmann, 1975b). They are produced under degenerative conditions (Kaufmann, 1969; Stark & Kaufmann, 1971, 1972). Blockage of glycolysis by several enzyme inhibitors results in increased development of protrusions; experimental substitution of glycolysis below the point of blockage results in suppression of their formation (Kaufmann et al., 1974b; Thorn et al., 1974). Hypoxia or experimental blockage of oxidative phosphorylation does not induce their production (Thorn et al., 1976).

After the protrusions have reached a certain size, they are pinched off into the maternal circulation. The only pathological importance attributed to the plasma protrusions is related to placental infarction. Pronounced production of plasma protrusions in the guinea pig placenta was induced by experimental blockage of glycolysis, which led to obstruction of the maternal placental blood spaces by released masses of protrusions (Kaufmann, 1975a). Their disintegration induced blood clotting. The final result was experimental infarction. Similar events have been described for the human placenta (Stark & Kaufmann, 1974).

Villous Cytotrophoblast (Langhans' Cells)

Langhans' Cells as Precursors of the Syncytiotrophoblast

The Langhans' cells form a second trophoblastic layer underneath the syncytiotrophoblast. During early pregnancy, this layer is nearly complete (Figure 46) and later becomes discontinuous (Figures 57, 71; Table 4). In contrast to early reports that described the villous cytotrophoblast to be absent from the mature placenta (Hörmann, 1948; Clavero-Nunez & Botella-Llusia, 1961), it is now well established that the Langhans' cells persist until term. In the mature placenta they can be found underneath 20% of the villous syncytiotrophoblast (Figure 71); the exact figure depends on the villous type, the kind of tissue preservation, and the pathological state of the organ (Table 7).

One should not deduce from these figures that the number of Langhans' cells decreases toward term. When one multiplies the relative number of Langhans' cells per volume of villous tissue (Table 7) with the villous volume per placenta (Table 3) during the 12th week p.m. and compares the figure to that for the term placenta, one arrives at surprising results. The total Langhans' cell volume during the 12th week p.m. amounts to about 2 g, in contrast to 12 g at term. Stereological studies have shown that the total number of cells increases steadily until term (Simpson et al., 1992). The situation is that as the villous surface rapidly expands the cytotrophoblast cells become widely separated and so less numerous in sectioned material. This point has important consequences for maternofetal immunoglobulin transfer, because unlike the syncytiotrophoblast and endothelial cells cytotro-

phoblast cells do not express Fc-γ receptors (Bright & Ockleford, 1993). Transport of immunoglobulins may therefore be possible only during later pregnancy, when the cytotrophoblastic layer becomes incomplete.

Earlier authors (Spanner, 1941; Stieve, 1941) considered a syncytiotrophoblastic origin of the Langhans' cells. This idea was refuted by Ortmann as early as 1942, however, who pointed out that formation of a syncytium must be regarded as differentiation from cellular precursors, an irreversible process. First proof for this assumption was presented by Richart (1961) using ^{3}H-thymidine incorporation to demonstrate the absence of DNA synthesis from syncytiotrophoblastic nuclei but its existence in cytotrophoblastic nuclei. These data were supported by Galton (1962), who simultaneously carried out microspectrophotometric DNA measurements of trophoblastic nuclei. The cytotrophoblastic contribution to the formation of syncytiotrophoblast has been generally accepted since the detailed ultrastructural evaluation of human placental villi from early pregnancy until full term by Boyd and Hamilton (1966) also structurally demonstrated this process. The vast literature of the subsequent studies was reviewed in much detail by Hörmann et al. (1969); and the early autoradiographic findings were supported and extended by many authors (Pierce & Midgley, 1963; Fox, 1970; Weinberg et al., 1970; Kim & Benirschke, 1971; Geier et al., 1975; Kaufmann et al., 1983). The authors found that ^{3}H-thymidine is incorporated only into the cytotrophoblastic nuclei, never into those of syncytiotrophoblast (Figure 53). This fact excludes nuclear replication within the syncytiotrophoblast. The only conflicting results have been reported by Moe (1971), who described mitoses of syncytiotrophoblastic nuclei following in vitro application of colchicine. Because his results have never been reproduced they must be regarded as misinterpretation.

Langhans' Cell Types

During all stages of pregnancy, most of the Langhans' cells possess light-microscopic and ultrastructural features that clearly distinguish them from overlying syncytiotrophoblast, the characteristic features of undifferentiated, proliferating stem cells (Figure 47). The undifferentiated cytotrophoblast is characterized by a well developed Golgi field, few mitochondria, few dilated rough endoplasmic cisternae, and numerous polyribosomes (Figures 47, 48) (Schiebler & Kaufmann, 1969; Kaufmann, 1972; Martin & Spicer, 1973b). The large, ovoid nucleus has ample euchromatin, which light-microscopically results in faint staining of easily identifiable cells (Figure 46). Histochemically, enzymes of aerobic and anaerobic glycolysis stain largely negative (Figures 55, 56) (Kaufmann & Stark, 1972).

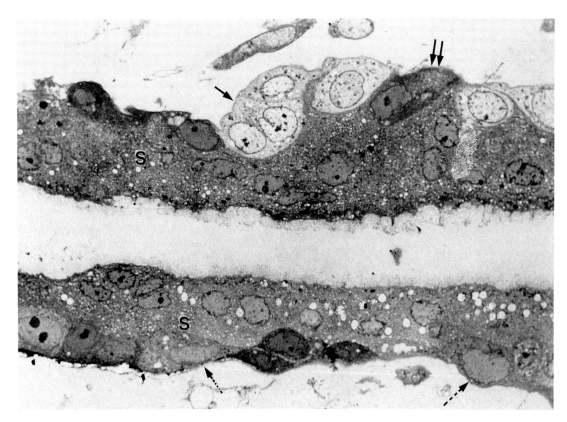

FIGURE 46. Semithin section showing two opposing villous surfaces, from the 9th gestational week p.m. Underneath the thick syncytiotrophoblast (S) are nearly complete layers of cytotrophoblast. Its varying staining intensities indicate different stages of differentiation from undifferentiated, proliferating cytotrophoblast (arrow) to highly differentiated cytotrophoblast with signs of syncytial fusion (interrupted arrows). Some of the cytotrophoblastic cells are obviously degenerating (double arrow). ×1,270. (From Kaufmann, 1972, with permission.)

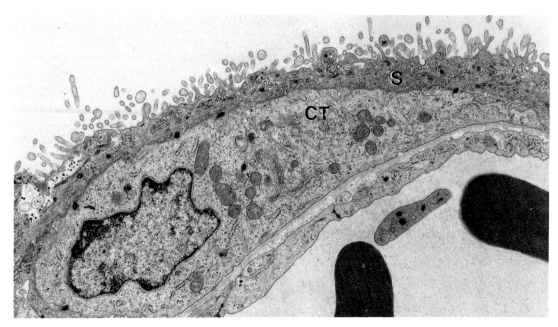

FIGURE 47. Transmission electron micrograph of mature placenta. Note the undifferentiated cytotrophoblastic cell (CT) lying underneath a thin syncytiotrophoblastic lamella (S). During all stages of pregnancy, most of the villous cytotrophoblast belongs to this type of proliferating or resting stem cell. ×9,800. (From Schiebler & Kaufmann, 1981, with permission.)

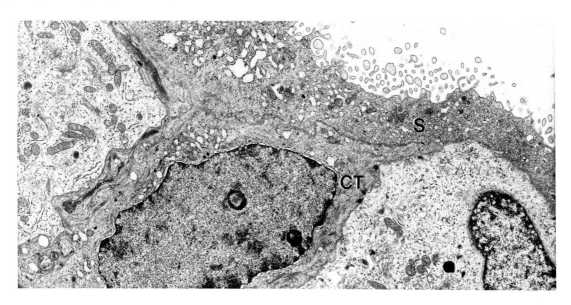

FIGURE 48. Transmission electron micrograph of mature placenta. Note the highly differentiated Langhans' cell (CT), shortly before its syncytial fusion with the neighboring syncytiotrophoblast (S), and the ultrastructural similarity of the two. ×7,400.

Occasional mitoses, ^{3}H-thymidine incorporation, and Ki-67/MIB-1 positivity demonstrate that the cell is the proliferating stem cell (Tedde & Tedde-Piras, 1978; Arnholdt et al., 1991; Kohnen et al., 1993b).

A few Langhans' cells show higher degrees of differentiation, expressed by large amounts of free ribosomes, rough endoplasmic reticulum, and mitochondria (Figure 48). This finding has usually been interpreted as a sign of differentiation toward a later syncytial state (Boyd & Hamilton, 1966; Hörmann et al., 1969; Schiebler & Kaufmann, 1969; Kaufmann, 1972). Light-microscopically, these cells may show staining patterns similar to those of syncytiotrophoblast (Figure 46). Increasing activities are expressed by the enzymes of aerobic and anaerobic glycolysis (Figure 55).

As soon as the cytotrophoblast reaches an electron density that is comparable to that of the neighboring syncytium, the first signs of syncytial fusion may be observed (Boyd & Hamilton, 1966; Hörmann et al., 1969; Kemnitz, 1970; Kaufmann, 1972; Kaufmann et al., 1977a). Only in severely damaged areas of the villous trees are Langhans' cells observed with an organellar density exceeding that of the overlying syncytiotrophoblast (Figures 50, 51) (Kaufmann et al., 1977a).

Syncytial fusion begins with the disintegration of separating cell membranes (Figure 52). This process has been studied in detail by Contractor et al. (1977) in humans and by Firth et al. (1980) in the guinea pig. The fusion seems to be initiated by establishment of gap junctions that bridge the intercellular space. Thus far, the respective gap junction molecules, connexins, have not been identified in humans. Their identification

should enable us to analyze this process in more detail. It is proposed that the major role of the gap junctions is to bring the adjacent plasma membranes into close contact so as to become starting points for cell fusion. Experimental studies in pseudopregnant rabbits have shown that the formation of a uterine epithelial syncytium, characteristic for implantation in this species, is also introduced by formation of gap junctions; they establish intercellular coupling and finally induce dissolution of the membranes (Winterhager, 1985). As a second step, plasma bridges between syncytium and cytotrophoblast are formed. From the gap junctions, this process spreads over the contact surface between Langhans' cell and syncytiotrophoblast. According to Contractor (1969) and Contractor et al. (1977), increased numbers of secondary lysosomes are actively involved in disintegration of the plasma membranes.

Former Langhans' cells, those that are freshly incorporated into the syncytium, can easily be identified by electron microscopy, enzyme histochemistry, and immunohistochemistry (Figures 49, 52, 56). They are characterized by a compact area of accumulated organelles, such as mitochondria, rough endoplasmic reticulum, and free ribosomes. These structures surround a large, ovoid nucleus rich in euchromatin. Such nuclei still may show immunoreactivity for PCNA, a protein related to DNA polymerase δ and usually expressed in proliferating cells (Kohnen et al., 1993b); the molecule has a half-life of about 24 hours and may thus persist from the last mitosis, through syncytial fusion, to the syncytial state. Its presence in syncytiotrophoblast must not be misinterpreted as a sign of proliferative activity of the latter.

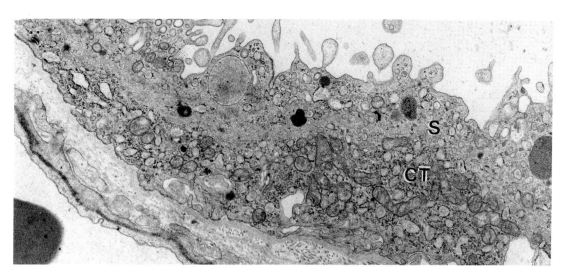

FIGURE 49. Transmission electron micrograph of mature placenta. Even after syncytial fusion with complete disappearance of the separating cell membranes, the area of the original cytotrophoblast (CT) can be clearly distinguished from the overlying syncytium (S) because of the marked difference in the density of the cell organelles. Note the accumulation of mitochondria and endoplasmic reticulum transferred into the syncytium by this kind of organellar transplantation into the syncytium. ×14,700.

In accordance with the ultrastructural appearance, maximal activities of all aerobic and anaerobic glycolytic enzymes have been shown (Kaufmann & Stark, 1972). The density of organelles and the activities of enzymes considerably exceeds that of the overlying syncytiotrophoblast. The density of organelles and enzyme activities decrease soon with spreading over the neighboring parts of the syncytium. Even then, the "new" syncytial area can easily be detected by the unusual size of its nucleus; and it indicates structural and functional regeneration of this segment of syncytiotrophoblast.

According to the results of Martin and Spicer (1973b), the nuclei are the most reliable indicators for the syncytial "age," which is the time elapsed since syncytial fusion. The prevalence of small, densely stained, obviously pyknotic syncytial nuclei together with reduced numbers of Langhans' cells indicate degenerative changes of the syncytiotrophoblast due to reduced syncytial fusion.

Nematosomes

Many authors have described nematosomes as regular features of undifferentiated Langhans' cells. They have also been found within other embryonic tissues and in neurons. The most detailed review of the relevant literature is that by Ockleford et al. (1987). Nematosomes are spherical to ovoid, non-membrane-bound organelles with a diameter of about 1 μm. They consist of helically arranged central strands of filaments to which small electron-dense conglomerates are attached. The latter are thought to consist of storage forms of RNA (Grillo, 1970; Ockleford et al., 1987). No evidence has thus far been found of any relation between nematosomes and overt gestational pathology and between nematosomes and virus infections in the placenta (Ockleford et al., 1987).

Endocrine Activity of the Langhans' Cells

There has been much speculation concerning the function of Langhans' cells because of their prominence. Among other functions, endocrine activity has been attributed to them, with several authors suggesting that Langhans' cells are the source of hCG. Two arguments have been stressed: (1) The number of Langhans' cells and their proliferative activity seem to parallel the urinary and serum levels of hCG (Gey et al., 1938; Wislocki & Bennett, 1943; Tedde & Tedde-Piras, 1978); and (2) trophoblast cultures continue to produce hCG when only cytotrophoblast survives (Stewart et al., 1948). The first deduction is inconclusive, as it is only the relative amount of villous cytotrophoblast that is so impressive during early pregnancy. As discussed above, the absolute number of Langhans' cells increases steadily until term. Also, it can no longer be argued that cytotrophoblast produces hCG because we know that these cells behave differently under culture conditions. Here they acquire stages of differentiation that are not reached during normal pregnancy, including hCG production (Nelson et al., 1986; Kao et al., 1988). Localization of hCG production has been obtained by many immunohistochemical studies. For example, Midgley and Pierce (1962), Dreskin et al. (1970), Hamanaka et al. (1971), and Kim et al. (1971) described the immunoreactivity to be concentrated within the villous syncytiotrophoblast. Outside the villi (i.e., in extravillous trophoblast, where syncytial fusion is absent) the cellular form of trophoblast may synthesize this hormone (see Chapter 11).

Gaspard et al. (1980) first pointed out that there may be some secretory activity for α-hCG and β-hCG in the villous cytotrophoblast. The latter hormonal subunit was detected in cytotrophoblast only underlying heavily damaged syncytium. More recent molecular biological studies by Hoshina et al. (1982, 1983, 1984) and Kliman et al. (1986, 1987) produced evidence that the ability to secrete hormones, such as hCG and hPL, is related to trophoblastic differentiation, including syncytial fusion. Boime et al. (1988) proposed a model for hCG and hPL expression that associates subsequent activation of α-hCG, β-hCG, and hPL genes at different stages of differentiation. These events were correlated with syncytial fusion in such a way that α-hCG is secreted directly before fusion, β-hCG directly afterward in transitory form, and hPL as early as in the syncytial state of the trophoblast. Having compared the results with our own experience and evaluated discussions with the authors during meetings, we believe that this hypothesis may be generally correct; we suppose, however, that this cascade of gene activation is not tied to the syncytial fusion itself, as proposed by Boime, but rather to the process of trophoblastic differentiation. Under normal in vivo conditions, syncytial fusion takes place at such an early stage of differentiation that all steps of hormonal synthesis are performed in the syncytial state (see the highly differentiated, freshly fused trophoblastic area depicted in Figure 49). In pathological conditions (β-hCG expression by cytotrophoblast, reported by Gaspard et al., 1980), in tissue culture, and under normal conditions in extravillous cytotrophoblast, syncytial fusion seems to be inhibited or delayed. Thus expression of one or several of the above genes may take place at the usual stage of differentiation but still in the cellular form.

Few reports deal with additional secretory activity of the villous cytotrophoblast. Nishihira and Yagihashi (1978, 1979) reported the production of somatostatin in Langhans' cells. Somatostatin is an intensive inhibitor of pituitary tropic hormones, such as growth hormone and thyroid-stimulating hormone (TSH). These authors discussed a suppressive role of somatostatin on hCG and hPL production by the syncytiotrophoblast.

Other peptides with alleged origin in the villous cytotrophoblast are corticotropin-releasing factor (CRF) (Petraglia et al., 1987; Saijonmaa et al., 1988), gonadotropin-releasing hormone (GnRH, placental LRF) (Khodr & Siler-Khodr, 1978), neuropeptide Y (NPY) (Petraglia et al., 1989), and inhibin (Petraglia et al., 1987). Not all of these reports are acceptable. Thus when one studies the papers on inhibin (Petraglia et al., 1987) and neuropeptide Y localization (Petraglia et al., 1989) carefully, one realizes that the immunoreactivity was not localized within the cytotrophoblast. Rather, it was in the villous capillary walls. In cooperation with the authors and using their antibodies, we have repeated the experiments on immune reactions and found inhibin immunoreactivity in villous endothelium and in the trophoblastic layer, the exact localization depending on the inhibin subunit. Korhonen and coworkers (1991) arrived at similar conclusions. In later reports Petraglia et al. (1991, 1992) specified their findings for the various inhibin subunits, and the regulatory effects of inhibin on hCG secretion were discussed by the same group (Petraglia et al., 1987, 1990; Petraglia, 1991).

Functional Aspects of Syncytial Fusion

It is evident that the syncytiotrophoblast differs appreciably from undifferentiated Langhans' cells. The latter are normally associated with syncytium that is equipped with rough endoplasmic reticulum and numerous mitochondria (Figures 35, 47). With the increasing degree of differentiation of the Langhans' cells, the number of ribosomes and mitochondria in the syncytiotrophoblast decreases, to the benefit of smooth endoplasmic reticulum or degenerative features (Figures 49, 52). Similar relations are seen in autoradiographic enzyme histochemical preparations (Figures 53–56). Decreasing activity of enzymes related to the energy metabolism of syncytium are associated with increasing activities in the cytotrophoblast (Figures 55, 56) (Kaufmann & Stark, 1972).

We have concluded that degenerative changes within the syncytiotrophoblast induce cytotrophoblastic differentiation and subsequent syncytial fusion (Kaufmann, 1972; Kaufmann & Stark, 1972). It can then be deduced that syncytial fusion is a prerequisite not only for syncytial growth but for regeneration of aging syncytiotrophoblast as well. Martin and Spicer (1973b) have described several stages of maturation and aging within the villous trophoblast, and Dorgan and Schultz (1971) described "programmed death" in multinucleated giant cells of the rat placenta. From experimental studies in the rhesus monkey placenta (Panigel & Myers, 1972), it has become evident that loss of villous cytotrophoblast and degenerative changes of the syncytiotrophoblast are usually associated. On the other hand, maximal villous cytotrophoblast proliferation without syncytial fusion, as observed with severe hypoxia, is accompanied by syncytial degeneration; this view is supported by tissue culture experience (Fox, 1970; Castellucci et al., 1990a). Syncytiotrophoblast, without cytotrophoblastic fusion, shows steeply decreasing hormonal production rates and finally dies within a few days. These results lead to the conclusion that survival of syncytiotrophoblast depends on cytotrophoblastic fusion.

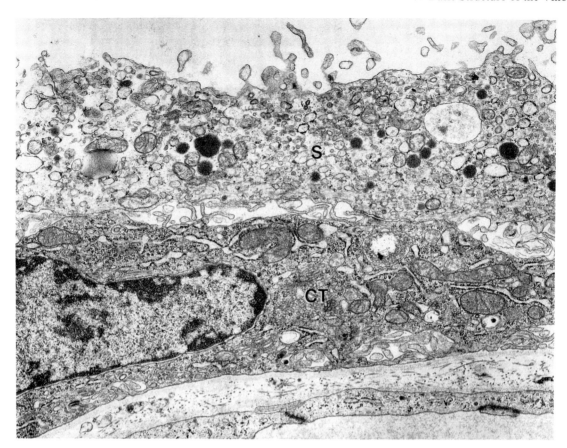

FIGURE 50. Transmission electron micrograph of mature placenta. Highly differentiated cytotrophoblast (CT) sometimes fails to fuse with the neighboring syncytiotrophoblast (S). Because it lacks regeneration, the latter shows obvious signs of degeneration, such as vesicular hydrops of most organelles, absence of ribosomes, and disintegration of the plasmalemma. There is continuous differentiation, so the nonfusing cytotrophoblast has an unusually large accumulation of organelles. Similar pictures can be seen in extravillous cytotrophoblast, which also lacks syncytial fusion. ×16,800.

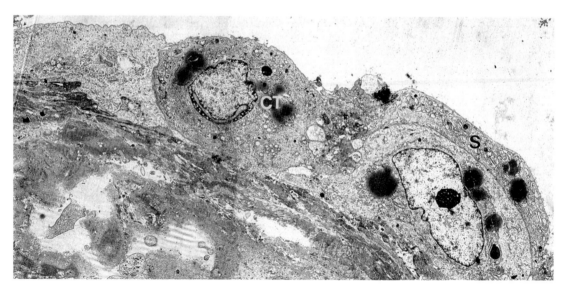

FIGURE 51. Survey transmission electron micrograph in the presence of preeclampsia. If the cytotrophoblast (CT) fails definitely to fuse syncytially, the syncytiotrophoblast (S) degenerates, as demonstrated in Figure 50. As a final stage, the syncytiotrophoblast may disappear locally, so hypertrophic cellular trophoblast makes up the villous surface and directly borders the intervillous space (above). In this case the villous stroma (below) also exhibits severe degenerative changes. ×2,800.

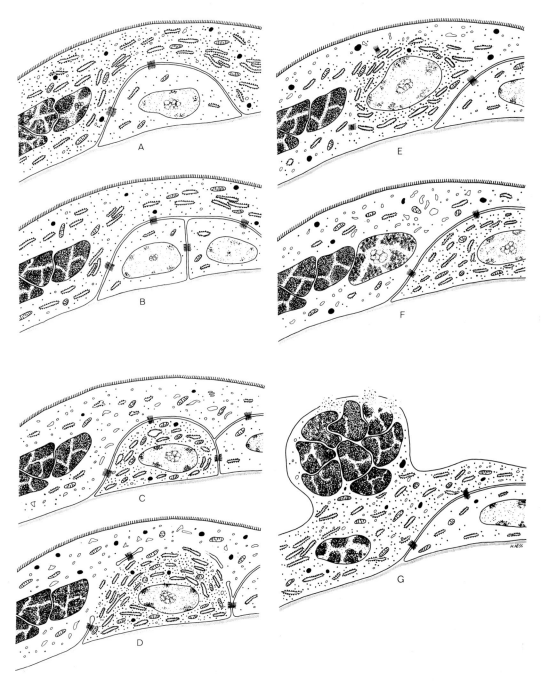

FIGURE 52. Cytotrophoblastic contribution to the regeneration of the villous syncytiotrophoblast. As soon as the syncytiotrophoblast shows its first signs of degeneration (loss of ribosomes, degranulation of rough endoplasmic reticulum), the cytotrophoblast begins to proliferate (A,B). Some of the daughter cells develop large numbers of organelles (C). After disintegration of the separating membranes, these organelles are transferred into the syncytium (D) and thus regenerate the latter. The freshly incorporated nucleus can easily be identified for a certain period because of its size and low quantity of heterochromatin (E,F). As soon as the syncytial organelles degenerate, this process starts anew (F). In this way, large numbers of trophoblastic nuclei accumulate in the syncytiotrophoblast. The oldest are clustered as syncytial knots, protrude as "syncytial sprouts," and extrude into the intervillous space (G) (see Figures 39 and 40). (From Kaufmann, 1983, with permission.)

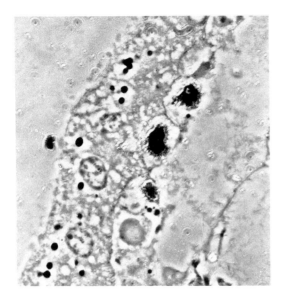

FIGURE 53. ³H-thymidine incorporation into the villous trophoblast. The black silver grains indicate active DNA synthesis. They have accumulated over the cytotrophoblastic nuclei only (large black spots in the center). Syncytiotrophoblast shows no signs of DNA synthesis. ×1,400. (Courtesy Dr. W. Nagl.)

To test this interpretation, ³H-uridine incorporation into villous trophoblast was studied, with results that largely resemble those of ³H-thymidine incorporation. This RNA precursor was incorporated only into

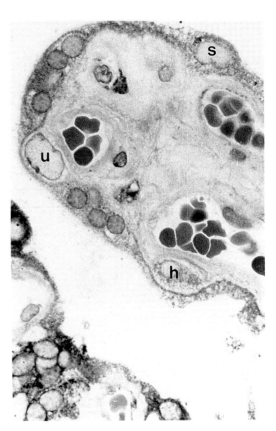

FIGURE 55. Semithin section with enzyme histochemical demonstration of lactate dehydrogenase. Cytotrophoblast shows increasing enzyme activities from the undifferentiated form (u), through the highly differentiated form (h), to the syncytial fusing form (s). ×840. (From Kaufmann & Stark, 1972, with permission.)

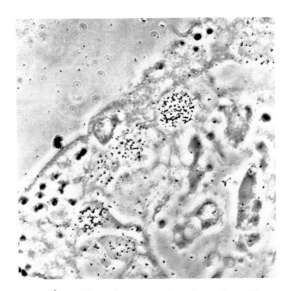

FIGURE 54. ³H-uridine incorporation into the villous trophoblast. Similar to the ³H-thymidine incorporation, ³H-uridine, as a precursor of RNA, is mostly incorporated into the cytotrophoblast (fine black grains), indicating that RNA metabolism is also concentrated in the cellular trophoblast. ×1,400. (Courtesy Dr. W. Nagl.)

Langhans' and stromal cells (Figure 54) (Kaufmann, 1983; Kaufmann et al., 1983). It appears that syncytiotrophoblast requires syncytial fusion of Langhans' cells for the maintenance of its functional and structural integrity. This mechanism at work may be a sort of transplantation of new organelles, fresh enzyme systems, and perhaps simply RNA (Figure 52).

As a consequence of syncytial fusion of Langhans' cells, which considerably exceeds the syncytial needs for growth, aged syncytioplasm and aged nuclei become accumulated within the syncytium. This material is extruded into the maternal circulation as "syncytial sprouts" (Figures 40, 52) (Martin & Spicer, 1973b; Jones & Fox, 1977; Schiebler & Kaufmann, 1981; Cantle et al., 1987).

Regulation of Cytotrophoblastic Proliferation and Fusion

Increased villous cytotrophoblast is a striking feature in several pathological conditions related to hypoxia. Among these conditions are maternal anemia

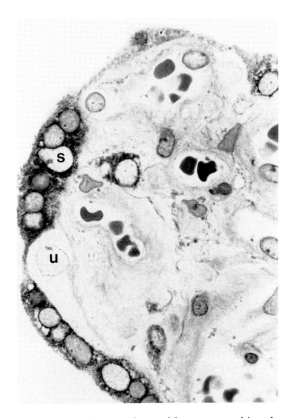

FIGURE 56. Semithin section with enzyme histochemical demonstration of lactate dehydrogenase. Note the complete absence of this enzyme in an undifferentiated cytotrophoblastic cell (u) compared to the high activity in a cell in syncytial fusion (s). The large, bright nucleus of the latter can be easily distinguished from the smaller nuclei of the surrounding older syncytiotrophoblast. ×840. (From Kaufmann & Stark, 1972, with permission.)

(Piotrowicz et al., 1969), maternal hypertensive disorders (Wigglesworth, 1962), preeclampsia (Jeffcoate & Scott, 1959; Wigglesworth, 1962; Fox, 1964, 1978), and pregnancies at high altitude (Jackson et al., 1985; Mayhew et al., 1990; Mayhew, 1991). This increase has been proved also in tissue culture (Fox, 1964; Amaladoss & Burton, 1985; Burton et al., 1989; Castellucci et al., 1990a; Ong & Burton, 1991).

We conclude from these findings that oxygen is an important regulator for cytotrophoblastic proliferation and syncytial fusion. A common finding from normal villous histology supports the regulatory influence of local oxygen partial pressure on the proliferative activity of Langhans' cells. With the reduction of Langhans' layer during the course of pregnancy, the remaining Langhans' cells accumulate in the neighborhood of fetal capillaries, situated near the trophoblastic surface (Figure 57) (Kaufmann, 1972). Finally, in the term placenta most Langhans' cells are located at the epithelial plates (Figures 26d, 29, 30, 35, 47, 71). This associa-

tion appears illogical, as this localization increases the maternofetal diffusion distances at the main sites of diffusional exchange. With the use of some simple physiological consideration, this structural situation may be related to the local behavior of the oxygen partial pressures (Kaufmann, 1972). As can be seen in Figure 58, the PO_2 gradient is much steeper in places where the fetal capillaries directly face the trophoblast. In this location, Langhans' cells are exposed to much lower PO_2 levels than those that are far from the capillaries, indicating that decreased PO_2 stimulates proliferation. Consequently, far from the capillaries in zones of higher PO_2, the poorly proliferating Langhans' cells fuse and finally disappear. In contrast, increased proliferation near the capillaries helps some of the Langhans' cells to persist, even if syncytial fusion is increased. This kind of regulation makes sense if we assume that hypoxic conditions damage the syncytiotrophoblast functionally and structurally. The need for regeneration by increased syncytial fusion can be fulfilled by the elevated number of Langhans' cells.

In most placentas one observes villi with obstructed fetal vessels. If the maternal circulation is not impaired in these areas, loss of villous cytotrophoblast is the normal finding, proved experimentally by Panigel and

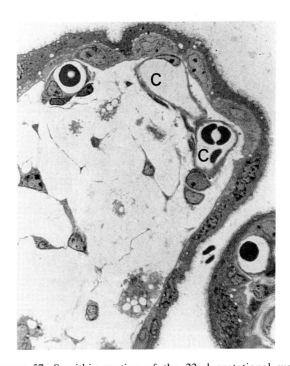

FIGURE 57. Semithin section of the 22nd gestational week p.m. In contrast to earlier stages of pregnancy, from this stage onward the fetal capillaries (C) come into a more peripheral position and establish close contact with the trophoblastic surface of the villus owing to the reduced villous diameter. Cytotrophoblast is concentrated in the neighborhood of the capillaries. ×820. (From Kaufmann, 1972, with permission.)

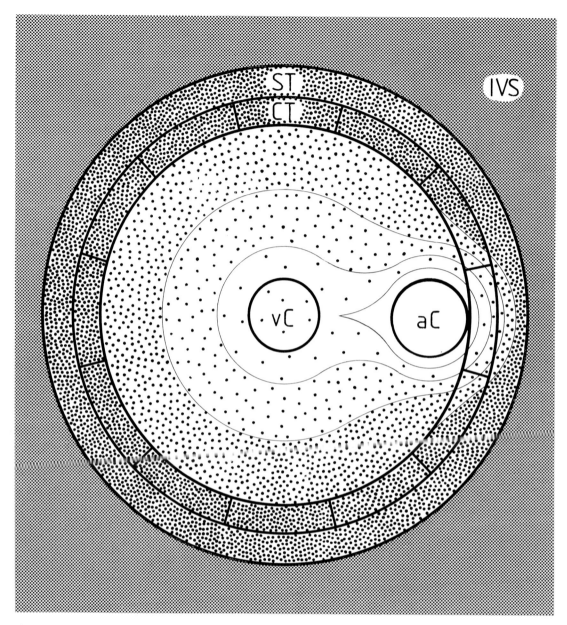

FIGURE 58. Why is cytotrophoblast concentrated near the fetal capillaries? This idealized cross section of a placental villus demonstrates the distribution of the villous cytotrophoblast related to the oxygen tension. The PO_2 is symbolized by the density of dots. The basic assumption is that the PO_2 of the intervillous space (IVS, densely dotted) is highest, and the PO_2 in the arterial capillary limb (aC, not dotted) is lowest; despite unlimited oxygen diffusion, this gradient is kept constant so long as the maternal and fetal circulations are intact. If this assumption is true, one expects a steeper PO_2 gradient near the arterial capillary limb (aC) than far from it, as symbolized by the dotting patterns. As becomes evident in this figure, the cytotrophoblast near a capillary is located in zones of lower PO_2, because of its steep gradient, compared to cytotrophoblast, which is far from fetal capillaries and lying in zones of a moderate PO_2 gradient. The stimulating influence of low oxygen tension on cytotrophoblastic mitoses explains the persistence of cytotrophoblast near the capillaries. On the other hand, in zones of elevated PO_2 far from capillaries, retarded mitotic activity and continuous loss of cytotrophoblast by syncytial fusion lead to the disappearance of cytotrophoblast, as depicted in Figure 57. ST = syncytiotrophoblast; CT = cytotrophoblast; vC = venous capillary limb. (Modified from Kaufmann, 1972, with permission.)

Myers (1972). These authors ligated the umbilical vessels of one placental disk of the bidiscoidal rhesus monkey placenta. The fetus survived. After disintegration of the fetal villous capillaries in the ligated disk, the authors observed an involution of the Langhans' cells and, finally, degenerative changes of the syncytiotrophoblast. Because the maternal circulation was intact, the changes could not be explained as being a consequence of deficient nutrition. Rather, it must be the result of deficient proliferation of cyto-trophoblast due to abnormally high intravillous PO_2 and subsequently deficient regeneration of the syncytiotrophoblast.

It is likely that the hypoxic regulation is more complex than discussed. The endocrinological findings discussed above may act as starting points for future research. It must be noted that the functional importance of hCG and hPL secretion during advanced stages of pregnancy is still a mystery (Chard, 1993). The secretion of both hormones into the maternal circulation has been interpreted as a kind of "placental radar" (Chard, 1993) regulating placental functions. If inhibin, as a potent regulator of hCG secretion, is produced by the fetal endothelium and if hCG and hPL secretion are related to syncytial fusion (Boime et al., 1988), all three hormones may well be involved in complex maternofetal endocrine interactions that regulate trophoblastic growth.

Trophoblastic Basement Membrane

The trophoblastic basement membrane separates the trophoblastic epithelium from the villous stroma. It forms a supportive matrix for the cytotrophoblast and, where the latter is lacking, for the syncytiotrophoblast (Figures 26, 29). Polarization optical methods and fluorescence microscopy, reported by Scheuner (1972, 1975), Scheuner and Hutschenreiter (1972, 1977), and Pfister et al. (1989), have provided information of the structural organization. Under normal conditions the average thickness of the trophoblast basement membrane ranges from 20 to 50 nm.

Collagen IV, laminin, and heparan sulfate are the main components in any basement membrane and so are expressed in the basement membrane of the trophoblast (Ohno et al., 1986; Autio-Harmainen et al., 1991; Castellucci et al., 1993a,b). Fibronectin was also detected but was considered not to be an integral part of the trophoblastic basement membrane; rather, it seems to be instrumental in the cell attachment to it (Virtanen et al., 1988). This molecule has binding sites for various collagens and proteoglycans (Bray, 1978; Duance & Bailey, 1983). On the other hand, fibronectin plays an important role in the adhesion of cells to the extracellular environment.

The basement membrane acts as a support for the trophoblastic epithelium and allows a certain amount of movement. The attachment of cytotrophoblast cells can possibly be unlocked by matrix proteins, such as tenascin, which counteracts the action of fibronectin (Aufderheide & Ekblom, 1988). This effect could enable postmitotic Langhans' cells to migrate along the basal lamina to those places where they are needed for syncytial fusion. Accordingly, tenascin is regularly expressed in places of Langhans' cell mitosis and degenerative syncytiotrophoblastic foci (Castellucci et al., 1991). Another important function of the basal lamina is to act as a filtration barrier between maternal and fetal circulations. Whether the trophoblastic basal lamina plays a role as a molecular sieve, as reported for the glomerular basal lamina, remains to be studied.

Connective Tissue

The basic architecture of the villous stroma is constructed of fixed connective tissue cells that form a network. They enmesh connective tissue fibers, free connective tissue cells (Hofbauer cells), and fetal vessels. Depending on the age of the placenta and on the type of villus, various types of fixed stromal cells have been described (Boyd & Hamilton, 1967; Kaufmann et al., 1977b; Castellucci et al., 1980; Castellucci & Kaufmann, 1982a; Martinoli et al., 1984; King, 1987).

Mesenchymal Cells

Mesenchymal cells, or undifferentiated stromal cells, are the prevailing cell type until the end of the second month (Kaufmann et al., 1977b; Martinoli et al., 1984). At all later stages of pregnancy they are found only in newly formed villi, the mesenchymal villi. They are usually small (10–20 μm long, 3–4 μm wide) spindle-shaped cells with little cytoplasm. They are connected to each other by a few thin, long processes. Polyribosomes are the prevailing organelles. Mitotic mesenchymal cells may have much more cytoplasm and form nearly epithelioid cells (Figure 73). These cells make up the mesenchymal stroma, which is the primitive forerunner of all other stromal types. As cytoskeletal filaments they express usually only vimentin (Kohnen, 1994). The cells are enmeshed in a loose, spongy meshwork of reticular and collagen fibrils. Because the processes of the mesenchymal cells are filiform rather than sail-like, they do not delimit stromal channels (Figures 72, 82, 83).

Reticulum Cells

At the end of the second month, dramatic changes in stromal architecture and cellular composition take place (Kaufmann et al., 1977b; Martinoli et al., 1984). King (1987) reported similar changes for the rhesus monkey placenta. Within a few days, numerous small reticulum cells form that represent the prevailing cell type in the immature intermediate villi until the end of pregnancy (Figure 59). The first of these villi are developed at the

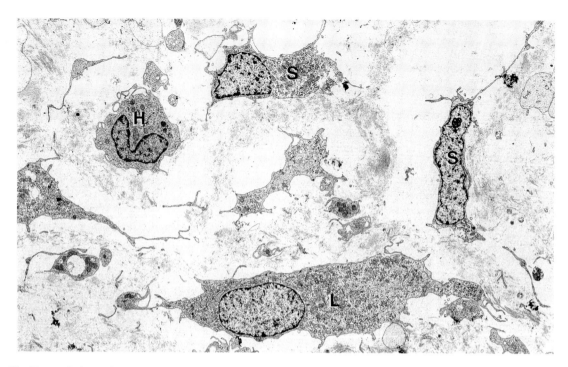

FIGURE 59. Transmission electron micrograph shows the typical variety of connective tissue cells in a mature intermediate villus at the 36nd week p.m. Small reticulum cells (S) with long, slender, richly branched cytoplasmic extensions, a large reticulum cell (L, below), and a macrophage, or Hofbauer cell (H), are seemingly scattered irregularly among loosely arranged connective tissue fibers. ×2,500. (From Kaufmann et al., 1977a, with permission.)

beginning of the 3rd month p.m. The small reticulum cells have large, elongated, bizarre-shaped cell bodies that measure about 20 to 30 µm in length. From the cell bodies, several long, thin branching cytoplasmic processes take off. Also, reticulum cells are different immunohistochemically from mesenchymal cells, as they express not only vimentin but desmin as cytoskeletal protein (Kohnen, 1994).

Transmission electron microscopically studied serial sections and scanning electron microscopy revealed that these processes are flat sails of cytoplasm (Kaufmann et al., 1977b; Castellucci & Kaufmann, 1982a; Martinoli et al., 1984). They branch in a cone-like pattern, the apex of the cone pointing to the cell body. In sections, these extensions are seen to form nets by establishing contacts to the extensions of neighboring cells (Figure 67c). In three-dimensional preparations, it can be demonstrated that these sail-like processes make up longitudinally-oriented stromal channels that, in cross sections, appear as rounded compartments or chambers of 20 to 50 µm diameter (Figures 65, 67).

Fetal vessels and the connective tissue fibers are fitted into the spaces between the channels, as well as between channels and trophoblastic basement membrane. This reticular structure has been described in detail by Castellucci and Kaufmann (1982a,b), Castellucci et al. (1984), and Martinoli et al. (1984).

In immature intermediate villi, the small reticulum cells form most of the fixed connective tissue cells. In mature intermediate villi, an additional group of large reticulum cells can be found (Figure 59) that are characterized by fewer processes but abundant perinuclear cytoplasm. Their voluminous bodies have a length of 20 to 40 µm and a width of 10 to 15 µm.

In the classical histological literature, the term reticulum cell was used for a stellate cell, which makes up a loose reticular stroma that is poor in collagen fibrils and contains abundant argyrophilic (reticular) fibers. This type of tissue was identified in lymphatic organs and in the lamina propria of the digestive tract. It is well equipped with free connective tissue cells. In later publications, the term reticulum cell was reserved for a stellate cell within the lymphatic organs. Despite this situation, we suggest that the term be used in its classical sense for this villous connective tissue, which shows much similarity with the classical "reticular connective tissue," considering the shape, number of reticular fibers, and number of free connective tissue cells.

Fibroblasts

Villi with fibrosed stroma are characterized by a third type of connective tissue cell that is structurally and immunohistochemically different from mesenchymal reticulum cells. We have therefore restricted use of the broadly applied term "fibroblast" to this peculiar cell type. They are found in stem villi and in smaller numbers in terminal villi and immature intermediate villi surrounding the larger vessels. The cells have much cytoplasm and are 30 to 50 μm long but only 5 to 8 μm wide. In contrast to the reticulum cells, they have only a few short, filiform or thick processes (Figure 60). The cytoplasm is rich in rough endoplasmic reticulum, which is usually concentrated on only one side of the nucleus; other parts of the cell body may be completely devoid of it.

Myofibroblasts

Spanner (1935) and Krantz and Parker (1963) have described extravascular contractile cells in large stem villi. Feller et al. (1985) provided histochemical evidence that myofibroblasts can be found among the stromal cells. The latter authors concluded that, except for the vessels and a negligible number of macrophages, myofibroblasts make up nearly all of the cellular constituents of human villous stroma. As arguments for their contention, they found a strong positivity for dipeptidylpeptidase IV, the isoenzyme pattern of which was identical with that of myofibroblasts of other origin.

Electron microscopically, cells having the structure typical of myofibroblasts (e.g., areae densae and incom-plete basal laminae) can be found only in stem villi (Demir et al., 1992). Immunohistochemical analysis of the cytoskeleton of the villous stromal cells (Kohnen et al., 1993a; Kohnen, 1994) revealed a heterogeneous population of cells that exhibit advancing differentiation to myofibroblasts (1) from early to later stages of pregnancy, (2) from mesenchymal to stem villi, and (3) from the subtrophoblastic stromal layer to the perivascular stroma. In immature intermediate and stem villi, all stages of differentiation arranged from the periphery to the center can be observed (Kohnen, 1994). The peripheral cells express vimentin and desmin as described for reticulum cells. Slightly more centrally they are followed by cells with the typical shape of fibroblasts and expressing vimentin, α-smooth muscle actin, and desmin. Near the larger vessels, typical myofibroblasts can be seen that, in addition to the aforementioned antigens, express GB 42 antigen, an actin isoform that is likely to represent γ-enteric actin (Kohnen et al., 1993a). Directly surrounding the stem vessels, the myofibroblasts reach the highest degree of differentiation; they express smooth muscle myosin in addition to the aforementioned cytoskeletal proteins; hence immunohistochemically they correspond largely to smooth muscle cells.

Different from the vascular smooth muscle cells, the myofibroblasts are arranged parallel to the longitudinal axis of the villi. It has been suggested that the contraction of extravascular contractile cells is important for

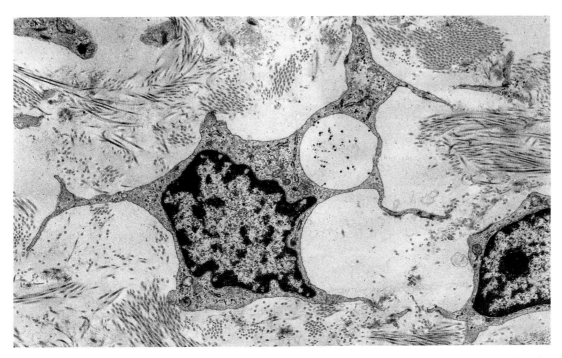

FIGURE 60. Electron micrograph of a fibroblast with sparse cytoplasm and short but richly branched cytoplasmic extensions, surrounded by bundles of collagen fibers. ×9,300.

the turgor of the villi (Krantz & Parker, 1963; Castellucci & Kaufmann, 1982a), and that it may influence the width of the intervillous space, thus regulating maternal intravillous blood pressure (Kohnen et al., 1992, 1993a). Some of the myofibroblasts are positive for nitric oxide (NO) synthase (Schönfelder et al., 1993), an enzyme involved in the production of nitric oxide, a potent vasodilator. NO synthase inhibition in guinea pigs and rats has been shown to result in preeclamptic symptoms, including intrauterine growth retardation (Yallampalli & Garfield, 1993; Chwalisz et al., 1994; Garfield et al., 1994).

Matrix Components of the Villous Stroma

Various types of collagen (e.g., collagens I, III, IV, and VI) have been identified in the core of the placental villi by immunohistochemistry (Autio-Harmainen et al., 1991; Nanaev et al., 1991a; Rukosuev, 1992; Castellucci et al., 1993a,b; Frank et al., 1994). In addition, laminin, some fibronectin isoforms, and tenascin have been detected in the villous stroma (Pfister et al., 1988; Autio-Harmainen et al., 1991; Rukosuev, 1992; Castellucci et al., 1991, 1993a,b; Frank et al., 1994). Collagen IV and laminin are considered to be molecules specific for basement membrane; however, their presence in the villous core suggests an important role for these molecules in morphogenetic processes and tissue remodeling that take place in the stroma of the villi.

Ultrastructural data concerning reticular (precollagen) and collagen fibers have been reported (Enders & King, 1970; Vacek, 1970; Kaufmann et al., 1977b). Precollagen or reticular fibers have a diameter of 5 nm or less. They form seemingly nonoriented meshworks without predominant fiber direction. In mesenchymal connective tissue, they are the prevailing fiber type.

The thicker collagen fibers have diameters of 20 to 60 nm. They show the typical 64.9 nm cross-striation. Usually grouped in twisted bundles of around 100 parallel fibers, they are arranged as a coarse meshwork, running in spiral courses around the fetal vessels (Kaufmann et al., 1977b). The amount of collagenous fibers increases from mesenchymal stroma, to reticular sinusoidal to fibrous stroma (Figures 66c, 67c). Histologically, collagen fibers can be stained with the usual connective tissue stains; reticular fibers cannot.

Hofbauer Cells

It is now generally agreed that Hofbauer cells are fetal tissue macrophages of the human placenta. Statements concerning their macrophage character are based on morphological, cytochemical, histochemical, immunological, and immunohistochemical studies (for reviews

see Bourne, 1962; Boyd & Hamilton, 1970; Castellucci & Zaccheo, 1989; Castellucci et al., 1990b). Here, we review the main aspects of these cells.

First Descriptions

From the middle of the nineteenth century, several authors have reported the presence of large cells in the stroma of chorionic villi of the human placenta (Müller, 1847; Schröder van der Kolk, 1851; Virchow, 1863, 1871; Langhans, 1877; Merttens, 1894; Ulesko-Stroganowa, 1896; Marchand, 1898). Their precise location in the villous stroma was first described by Kastschenko (1885). Virchow (1871) and later Chaletzky (1891) and Neumann (1897) first commented on the particular association of hydatidiform mole with large isolated cells having clear cytoplasm. This observation led to the term Chaletzky-Neumann cells, used in the past by several pathologists. Hofbauer, whose name has come to be associated with these cells, comprehensively described these cells in normal villi at the beginning of the twentieth century (1903, 1905). It is probably because of these detailed morphological studies that the name Hofbauer cell has been widely accepted in the literature and is currently used.

Morphology

In some of the first descriptions and in later studies, the Hofbauer cells were described as pleomorphic cells of the villous stroma with round, fusiform, or stellate appearance (Langhans, 1877; Hofbauer, 1903, 1905; Schmidt, 1956; for a review see Bourne, 1962). Their size depends on the length of their processes. The cells vary from 10 to 30 μm in diameter. Early investigations had pointed out that the most striking aspects of the Hofbauer cells are their highly vacuolated appearance and their granulated cytoplasm (Virchow, 1863, 1871; Langhans, 1877; Minot, 1889; Merttens, 1894; Hofbauer, 1903, 1905; Graf Spee, 1915; Meyer, 1919; Lewis, 1924). Indeed, more recent light-microscopic and transmission electron microscopic studies have pointed out that these cells are characterized by numerous membrane-bound, electron-lucent vacuoles of different size, possessing amorphous material of varying density, dense granules (presumably lysosomes), and short profiles of endoplasmic reticulum (Figures 63, 67a,c) (Hörmann, 1947; Boyd & Hughes, 1955; Rodway & Marsh, 1956; Geller, 1957; Bargmann & Knoop, 1959; Rhodin & Terzakis, 1962; Panigel & Anh, 1964; Boyd & Hamilton, 1967; Wynn, 1967a,b, 1973, 1975; Fox 1967b, 1978; Enders & King, 1970; Tedde, 1970; Vacek, 1970, 1978; Demir & Erbengi, 1984; King, 1987; Katabuchi et al., 1989; for reviews see Snoeck, 1958; Bourne, 1962; Boyd & Hamilton, 1970; Castellucci & Zaccheo, 1989). Enders and King (1970), in an elegant investigation, pointed out that the large intracytoplasmic vacuoles, containing varying amounts of flocculent precipitate, are numerous and large during the first half of pregnancy (Figures 63a,b, 67a). As pregnancy progresses, the vacuoles decrease in number and size, and the Hofbauer cells show an increase of intracytoplasmic granules (Figures 67c, 71) that are presumably lysosomes (Enders & King, 1970; Castellucci et al., 1980). This granulated type of Hofbauer cell can easily be differentiated from the rare mast cells (Figure 63C). Hofbauer cells with few or no vacuoles are, however, also present during early pregnancy and have been considered immature Hofbauer cells (Castellucci et al., 1987; Katabuchi et al., 1989). This finding is in agreement with immunological investigations that have considered the vacuolated Hofbauer cells to be the morphologically obvious and fully differentiated member of a much larger mononuclear phagocyte population (Wood, 1980; Frauli & Ludwig, 1987a).

The first three-dimensional visualization of Hofbauer cells, their intracytoplasmic vacuoles, surface aspects, and relations with other components of the villous core (Figure 67b) was possible by combining the cryofracture method with scanning electron microscopy (Castellucci et al., 1980; Martinoli et al., 1984). The surface morphology of Hofbauer cells was found to be characterized by spherical or elongated blebs, or microplicae (Figure 67b). These features were irregularly distributed. Other Hofbauer cells showed a ruffled surface, characterized by lamellipodia, which were large, smooth-surfaced, and well developed. They sometimes overlapped one another, creating cups or funnel-like structures. Sometimes Hofbauer cells bearing both lamellipodia and blebs were observed (Castellucci et al., 1980, 1984; Martinoli et al., 1984). In addition, scanning electron microscopy of chorionic villous stroma during the first half of pregnancy revealed that most of the Hofbauer cells were inside collagen-free intercommunicating stromal channels (Figure 67b) composed of large sail-like processes of fixed stromal cells (Castellucci et al., 1980, 1984; Castellucci & Kaufmann, 1982a). These channels were particularly well developed in the central region of the core of the chorionic villi and were oriented mostly parallel to the major axis of the villus. Some Hofbauer cells inside the channels had an elongated shape and extended their cellular bodies between intercommunicating channels or between channels and intercellular substance outside the channels (Castellucci et al., 1980, 1984). These morphological features strongly suggest motility of Hofbauer cells in the villous core.

The channels characterized most of the chorionic villi of the first half of pregnancy (Figures 63a,b, 67a,b). Their number was decreased toward term. In the mature placenta they were found only in villi at the center of the placentones (Figure 67c) (Schuhmann, 1981; Castellucci & Kaufmann, 1982a,b; Castellucci et al., 1990c). During the last trimester of gestation, Hofbauer cells present in villi outside the placentone centers (i.e.,

villi characterized by a core with large amounts of collagen fibers and narrow or absent channels) showed mostly blebs, or microplicae, at their surface but rarely lamellipodia (Figures 59, 71) (Castellucci & Kaufmann, 1982a; Martinoli et al., 1984).

The intracytoplasmic vacuoles and large lamellipodia of the Hofbauer cells have been considered to be structures involved in the reduction of fetal serum proteins contained in the villous stroma and in the water balance of the early placenta. This function was also likely because the placenta lacks a lymphatic system to return proteins from the interstitial space to the blood vascular system (Enders & King, 1970). Closely related to these concepts is the presence of stromal channels that could allow relatively easy movement of Hofbauer cells along the villous cores of chorionic villi and thus function as a substitute for the lymphatic system (Enders & King, 1970; Castellucci & Kaufmann, 1982a). Moreover, the motility of Hofbauer cells inside the stromal channels might allow these macrophages to: (1) exert their role in maintaining host defense (Castellucci et al., 1980; Wood, 1980); and (2) influence the remodeling of the villous core by stimulating or inhibiting the proliferation of other mesenchymal cells (Castellucci et al., 1980; Martinoli et al., 1984; King, 1987). It must be considered, however, that the motility of Hofbauer cells is hindered, at least in part, in the villi during the last trimester. Here the stromal channels are mostly narrow or absent (Figures 59, 71). It is therefore conceivable that the Hofbauer cells assume additional tasks in these villi (Martinoli et al., 1984).

Several authors have speculated on endocrine activities of Hofbauer cells (Acconci, 1925; Pescetto, 1952; Rodway & Marsh, 1956). Prosdocimi (1953) suggested hCG synthesis by these cells, and we detected hCG immunohistochemically within Hofbauer cells (Kaufmann & Stark, 1973). It was unlikely that this glycoprotein was synthesized in the cells; rather, it was probably phagocytosed from the surrounding environment. Still, the regular presence of hCG proves to be a useful marker for villous macrophages (Frauli & Ludwig, 1987c); on the other hand, phagocytic activity must be considered when interpreting immunohistochemical findings concerning the presence of proteins in these macrophages (e.g., hormones and placental proteins).

Occurrence and Distribution

Although some initial reports of Hofbauer cells described them to be present in villi that had undergone hydatid degeneration (Virchow, 1871; Chaletzky, 1891; Neumann, 1897), it was early established that these cells are present in both normal and pathological conditions (Hofbauer, 1903, 1905, 1925; Graf Spee, 1915; Lewis, 1924; for reviews see Bourne 1962; Boyd & Hamilton, 1970; Fox, 1978; Becker & Röckelein, 1989).

Hofbauer cells are first seen in placental villi on day 18 p.c. (Boyd & Hamilton, 1970). They are always present in the villi of immature placentas (Figures 67a,b). It has been claimed that in placentas from uncomplicated pregnancies, Hofbauer cells either disappear or become scanty after the 4th to 5th month of gestation (see Fox, 1967b, 1978). Geller (1957), Bleyl (1962), Fox (1967b), and several electron microscopic studies have demonstrated, however, that Hofbauer cells are present until term, and not only in immature villi of the center of the placentone (compare Figures 67c and 71). The apparent reduction in number as pregnancy progresses is due to their being compressed and masked by the condensation of the villous stroma (Figure 71) during placental maturation (Fox, 1967b). Strongly supporting this interpretation is the finding by Bleyl (1962) that many Hofbauer cells are found in villi in which edema is produced by postpartum saline perfusion through the umbilical artery.

Numerous Hofbauer cells can easily be recognized in term placentas only in pathological conditions in which most villi have a wide-meshed stroma (stromal channels, immature intermediate villi), that is, in placentas with failure or delay of villous maturation, which is the case in villi of prematurely delivered placentas and in cases of maternal diabetes (Horky, 1964; Fox, 1967b, 1978) and rhesus incompatibility (Hörmann, 1947; Thomsen & Berle, 1960; De Cecco et al., 1963; for review see Fox, 1978). Fox (1967b, 1978) emphasized that villous edema, occurring in the two latter pathological conditions, can also unmask the numerous Hofbauer cells by distension of the villous stroma. Hofbauer cells have also been described in human amnion and chorion laeve (Meyer, 1919; Bautzmann & Schröder, 1955; Schmidt, 1956; Bourne, 1962; for review see Boyd & Hamilton, 1970).

Origin

The origin of Hofbauer cells has received much attention, starting with the first descriptions (for historical details and reviews see Geller, 1957; Snoeck, 1958; Bourne, 1962; Wynn, 1967a; Boyd & Hamilton, 1970; Vacek, 1970; Schiebler & Kaufmann, 1981). Numerous theories have been abandoned, for example, those proposed by Chaletzky (1891), who derived them from cells of maternal decidua. Similarly, the suggestions by Neumann (1897), who considered them to be derivatives of the syncytium and an expression of malignancy, and by ten Berge (1922), who supposed them to be derivatives of endothelial cells, are not valid.

An important finding for establishing the origin of these cells was the observation by Wynn (1967b), based on sex chromatin staining, that Hofbauer cells are fetal cells. Most authors now consider Hofbauer cells to be of chorionic mesenchymal origin; that is, these cells gradually differentiate from the fixed stromal cells of the villous core (Fox, 1967b; Wynn, 1967a; Vacek, 1970; Kaufmann et al., 1977b). Morphological investigations have questioned this concept (Martinoli et al., 1984; King, 1987), as no transitional forms between the two cell types have been clearly recognized. Nevertheless, according to other observations on Hofbauer cells (Demir et al., 1989) and data obtained from macrophages and macrophage precursors of various organs (Sorokin & Hoyt 1987; Naito et al., 1989; Mebius et al., 1991; Sorokin & Hoyt, 1992; Sorokin et al., 1992a,b), this concept must be taken into consideration because Hofbauer cells possibly originate from mesenchymal cells during the early stages of pregnancy (i.e., before the fetal circulation is established) (Figure 61). Later, once the fetal circulation is established (Figure 62), Hofbauer cells may originate, as do other macrophages of various tissues, from fetal bone marrow-derived monocytes (van Furth, 1982; Castellucci et al., 1987). Indeed, Moskalewski et al. (1975) observed transitional forms between Hofbauer cells and monocytes. Concerning this hypothesis, it must be emphasized that human cord blood contains at the end of pregnancy almost three times as many monocytes as does adult blood (Khansari & Fudenberg, 1984; Santiago-Schwarz & Fleit, 1988). These monocytes show subpopulations with considerable functional heterogeneity (Khansari & Fudenberg, 1984).

It has been proposed that Hofbauer cells may have different origins throughout gestation, and that they may represent a heterogeneous group of cells (Castellucci et al., 1987). These data relate to in vivo (Figure 63b) and in vitro observations that Hofbauer cells can undergo mitotic division (Hofbauer, 1903; Hörmann, 1947; Geller, 1957; Boyd & Hamilton, 1970; Castellucci et al., 1985, 1987; Frauli & Ludwig, 1987c). Mitosis of Hofbauer cells (Figure 63b) may be important for the permanent presence of cell subpopulations with different origins and functions. In addition, the mitotic activity suggests that they may be, in part, an independent self-replicating population, allowing a rapid increase in number when required by the local microenvironment (Castellucci et al., 1987).

Immunological Aspects

Immunological data indicate that Hofbauer cells are numerous in the chorionic plate and the villous stroma throughout pregnancy (Wood, 1980; Goldstein et al., 1988). Studies on isolated Hofbauer cells, and immuno-

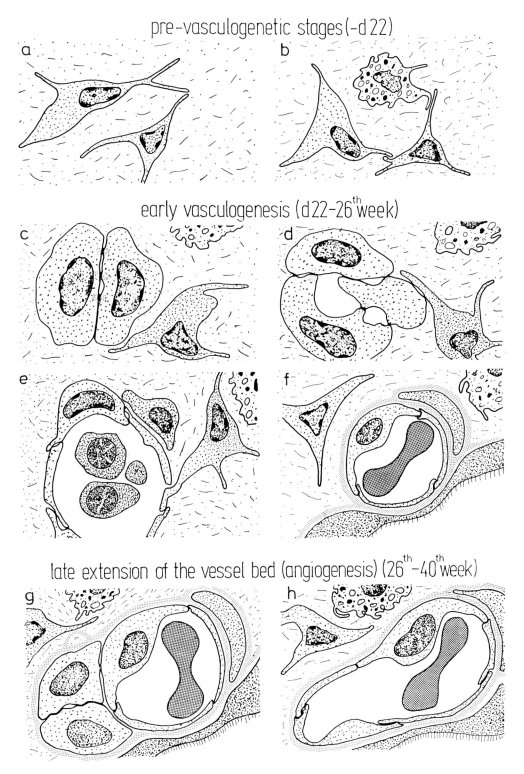

FIGURE 61. Vasculogenesis and angiogenesis in early and late placental villi. For further details see text. (From Demir et al., 1989, with permission.)

histochemical investigations have provided data that have furthered our knowledge concerning the immunological role of this cell population. Isolation of Hofbauer cells has usually employed proteolytic enzymes (Moskalewski et al., 1975; Wood et al., 1978a,b; Flynn et al., 1982; Loke et al., 1982; Frauli & Ludwig, 1987a) and a combination of enzymatic digestion and density gradient centrifugation (Wilson et al., 1983; Uren &

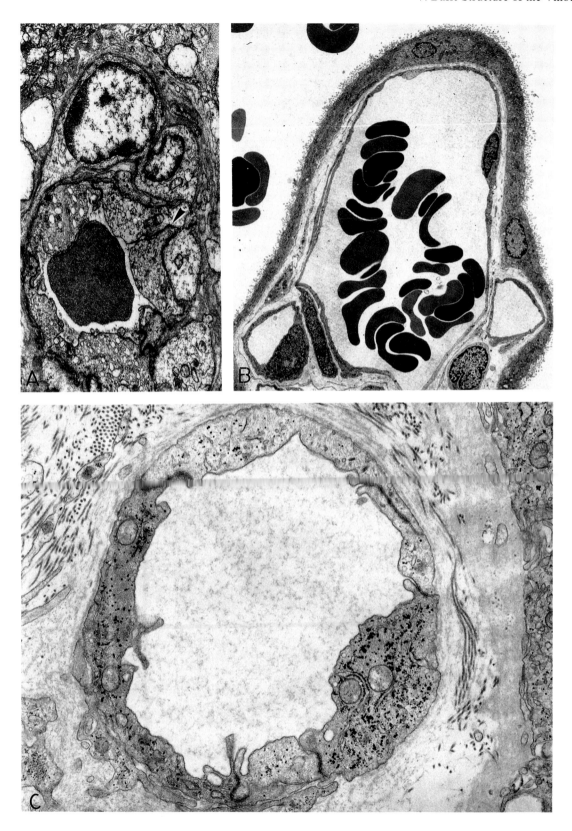

Boyle, 1985; Sutton et al., 1989). Additionally, cell separation methods, based on mechanical action with (Zaccheo et al., 1989) or without (Oliveira et al., 1986) density gradient centrifugation, have been used. It has been demonstrated that Hofbauer cells possess Fc receptors (FcR) for immunoglobulin G (Moskalewski et al., 1975; Wood et al., 1978a,b; Wood, 1980; Johnson & Brown, 1981; Loke et al., 1982; Zaccheo et al., 1982; Uren & Boyle, 1985; Oliveira et al., 1986; Goldstein et al., 1988).

Three subtypes of leukocyte FcR have been identified on the basis of molecular and chemical analysis and cloning of cDNA: FcRI (CD64), FcRII (CD32), and FcRIII(CD16) (Stengelin et al., 1988). The three subtypes are expressed on Hofbauer cells (Goldstein et al., 1988; Kristoffersen et al., 1990; Kameda et al., 1991; Sedmak et al., 1991). These receptors have been postulated to serve a protective function by binding maternal anti-fetal antigen-antibody complexes (Wood, 1980; Johnson & Brown, 1981; Goldstein et al., 1988).

C3b receptor activity has been demonstrated on isolated Hofbauer cells by some authors (Wood, 1980; Loke et al., 1982; Oliveira et al., 1986), whereas others have failed to detect C3b receptors in human placental sections using tissue hemadsorption techniques with C3b-coated erythrocytes (Faulk et al., 1980), or monoclonal antibodies against C3b receptor (CR1) (Bulmer & Johnson, 1984; Goldstein et al., 1988). By applying monoclonal antibodies to tissue sections, Goldstein et al. (1988) demonstrated that the receptor for the C3bi component of complement (CR3) is expressed by Hofbauer cells. Moreover, Hofbauer cells are capable of immune and nonimmune phagocytosis (Moskalewski et al., 1975; Wood, 1980; Loke et al., 1982; Wilson et al., 1983; Uren & Boyle, 1985; Oliveira et al., 1986; Zaccheo et al., 1989) and elimination of exogenous antigen-antibody complexes (Wood & King, 1982).

Braunhut et al. (1984) provided evidence for the presence of α_1-antichymotrypsin in Hofbauer cells but failed to demonstrate lysozyme in the cells derived from term placentas using immunohistochemical methods. Zaccheo et al. (1989) showed that Hofbauer cells from first trimester placentas are capable of secreting lysozyme in vitro. It is not clear whether these discrepant results are due to the different techniques used or they reflect a functional heterogeneity in lysozyme production between Hofbauer cells from the first trimester and those at term.

It has been established that Hofbauer cells can express class I and II major histocompatibility complex (MHC) determinants (Bulmer & Johnson, 1984; Uren & Boyle, 1985; Sutton et al., 1986; Bulmer et al., 1988). It is well known that class II MHC determinants include at least three well defined subregions: DR, DP, and DQ. First trimester Hofbauer cells are rarely DR- and DP-positive, and DQ antigens are not expressed (Bulmer & Johnson, 1984; Sutton et al., 1986; Bulmer et al., 1988; Goldstein et al., 1988; Lessin et al., 1988; Zaccheo et al., 1989). It may be important that DQ antigens, missing on first trimester cells, are restriction elements for T cell clones (Thorsby, 1984) and have been implicated in the generation of cytotoxic cells (Corte et al., 1982).

Class II MHC antigens are acquired by increasing numbers of placental macrophages beginning during the second trimester (Edwards et al., 1985; Sutton et al., 1986; Bulmer et al., 1988; Goldstein et al., 1988; Lessin et al., 1988). In term placental tissues, DR-positive villous stromal macrophages are often observed within groups of closely associated chorionic villi (Bulmer & Johnson, 1984; Bulmer et al., 1988). On the other hand, DP and DQ antigens are detected on a small number of Hofbauer cells, mostly located in villi immediately adjacent to the basal plate (Bulmer et al., 1988). In addition, such DP or DQ antigens are not detected in the absence of DR antigens on any placental macrophage (Bulmer et al., 1988). The patchy expression of class II MHC antigens in chorionic villi

---

FIGURE 62. Comparison of fetal capillaries in delayed versus immediately fixed terminal villi. (A) Fetal capillaries with endothelial cells protrude into the lumen and compress the erythrocytes. This phenomenon is best explained by postpartal capillary collapse due to delayed fixation. In such cases, the tight junctions (arrow) are restricted to the basal parts of the endothelial cell bodies. ×10,300. (From Demir et al., 1989, with permission.) (B) Distended terminal villi are characterized by a mixture of dilated fetal sinusoids with an extremely thin endothelium and neighboring smaller capillary cross sections with the same thin endothelial lining. Such pictures usually can be obtained only from immediately fixed specimens obtained at cesarean section. Even in this well preserved specimen, angular shapes of the smaller capillaries point to early capillary collapse. ×2,000. (From Demir et al., 1989, with permission.) (C) Transmission electron micrograph of fetal vessel cross section at high magnification to demonstrate that the endothelial lining may be composed of differently structured endothelial cells. The functional meaning of this finding is uncertain. The darker cells, containing numerous filaments, may be contractile and may be involved in peripheral blood flow regulation. It is uncertain whether this vessel is a capillary or a small collecting venule. ×18,000.

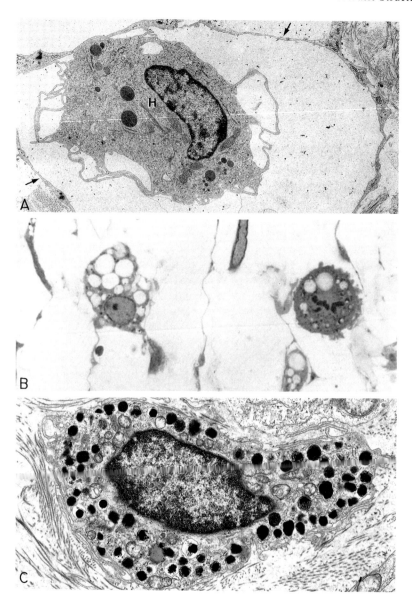

FIGURE 63. (A) Transmission electron micrograph of sail-like cytoplasmic processes (arrows) of the small reticulum cells line channel-like stromal cavities within immature intermediate villi. They are filled with some fluid but are devoid of connective tissue fibers. The latter can be found only in the vicinity of the channels. Suspended in the fluid of the channels one finds the macrophages, or Hofbauer cells (H). ×5,300. (B) Light microscopic, semithin section of reticular stroma of an immature intermediate villus from the 12th week p.m., showing two Hofbauer cells. Both are located in longitudinally sectioned stromal channels, delimited by long, thin cytoplasmic extensions of fixed stromal cells. The left Hofbauer cell is the highly vacuolated type that prevails during early pregnancy. The right cell shows fewer vacuoles and is characterized by its rounded appearance and numerous bleb-like protrusions on its surface. This cell is in mitosis. ×1,000. (C) Transmission electron micrograph. As a second type of free connective tissue cells, mast cells are observed in villous tissues. Their prevailing location is in the vicinity of larger fetal vessels of stem villi. This cell type is easily identified by its typical secretory granules. ×16,000.

and the accumulation of DR-, DP-, and DQ-positive cells at the villous—decidual tissue junction may indicate areas of enhanced immune stimulation. Although clear evidence is still lacking, these data (particularly the increasing expression of DR antigens as gestation proceeds) may represent acquisition of antigen-presenting capacity by the Hofbauer cells to

fetal lymphocytes. This point may be relevant for fetal responses to transplacental infection.

Goldstein et al. (1988) and Nakamura and Ohta (1990) have shown that Hofbauer cells react strongly with antibodies to the CD4 antigen throughout gestation. This antigen is a cell surface glycoprotein that is thought to interact with nonpolymorphic determinants of class II MHC molecules (Lamarre et al., 1989). The antigen is present on the T-helper subset of lymphocytes and has been shown to be expressed weakly by blood monocytes, some tissue macrophages, and dendritic cells (Wood et al., 1983, 1985; Buckley et al., 1987). It also functions as the membrane "receptor" for infection of cells by the human immunodeficiency virus (HIV). Lewis et al. (1990) have identified HIV-1 antigen and nucleic acid by immunohistochemical and in situ hybridization techniques in Hofbauer cells of placentas from seropositive patients. Thus the Hofbauer cells could serve as the portal of entry or reservoir for HIV in fetuses of HIV-positive women. The CD4 antigen is not being expressed on the surfaces of syncytiotrophoblast (Cuthbert et al., 1992).

One of the most consistent immunohistological markers of Hofbauer cells throughout gestation is the monoclonal antibody anti-leu-M3 (Bulmer & Johnson, 1984; Zaccheo et al., 1989). It has been pointed out that this antibody detects the CD14 monocyte differentiation antigen (Goyert et al., 1986), which is a 55 kilodalton (kDa) glycoprotein, expressed primarily by monocytes and macrophages (Goyert et al., 1988); it is anchored to the cell membrane by a phosphatidylinositol linkage (Haziot et al., 1988). Its restricted expression on mature cells suggests an important effector function (Goyert et al., 1988). In addition, it has been shown that the gene encoding CD14 is located in a region of chromosome 5 (Goyert et al., 1988) that is known to encode several growth factors or receptors, including interleukin-3 (IL-3), granulocyte-macrophage colony-stimulating factor (GM-CSF), CSF-1, CSF-1 receptor, and the platelet-derived growth factor receptor. It has been suggested that the CD14 antigen may also serve as some type of growth factor receptor (Goyert et al., 1988; Ziegler-Heitbrock, 1989) that could be involved in regulating the activity of the Hofbauer cells related to the process of villous morphogenesis (Castellucci et al., 1980; Martinoli et al., 1984; King, 1987). CD14 has been found to bind complexes of lipopolysaccharide and lipopolysaccharide-binding protein (Wright et al., 1990). These data suggest that CD14 could play an important role in infections.

Type I interferons (IFN-α, IFN-β) are molecules with multiple biological activities (reviewed by Russell and Pace, 1987). IFN-α has been found (by immunohistochemical methods) in Hofbauer cells of 50% of placentas tested (Howatson et al., 1988). However, these data do not demonstrate that Hofbauer cells really synthesize IFN-α. On the other hand, IFN-β has been demonstrated to be produced by isolated Hofbauer cells, particularly in large amounts after priming (Toth et al., 1991). Thus in vivo the interferon produced by the trophoblast (Toth et al., 1990) could prime placental macrophages and induce these cells to secrete large amounts of interferon.

Type I interferons may play important roles in protecting the fetus against intrauterine infection and in several differentiative processes; they can also interact with IFN-γ and other cytokines (Wang et al., 1981; Taylor-Papadimitriou & Rozengurt, 1985; Hunt, 1989; Toth et al., 1991).

Flynn et al. (1982, 1985) and Glover et al. (1987) showed that placental villous macrophages produce IL-1. Because the antigen presentation correlates with class II antigen expression and IL-1 secretion, the authors suggested that fetal placental macrophages function nearly as efficiently as adult cells for antigen presentation (Glover et al., 1987), which could present a hazard for maintenance of the fetal allograft. They hypothesized that competence for antigen presentation may be regulated by tissue-specific factors or other mediators (Glover et al., 1987). In support of this idea is the study by Yagel et al. (1987), which showed that physiological concentrations of progesterone induced a significant increase in fetal placental macrophage prostaglandin E_2, a potent immunosuppressant. This finding suggested a functional role for fetal placental macrophages in immunosuppression at the fetomaternal surface. Isolated Hofbauer cells consistently demonstrated inhibition or suppression of both mixed lymphocyte reaction and cell-mediated lympholysis (Uren & Boyle, 1990). Therefore Hofbauer cells may in fact exert a sentinel function that would prevent strong, destructive maternal T cell responses against the fetus. These data are also in agreement with the observation of Mues et al. (1989), who detected a large number of Hofbauer cells positive for the monoclonal antibody RM3/1. This antibody recognizes an antigen that is strongly induced by dexamethasone but down-regulated by IFN-γ, lipopolysaccharide, and triphorbolacetate on in vitro cultured monocytes. In vivo, RM3/1 macrophage populations are the predominant cells in liver and heart allografts from patients receiving high dose corticosteroid medication (Mues et al., 1989). The dominance of a corticosteroid-induced antiinflammatory macrophage phenotype within the placental villous core suggests localized immunosuppression, and it is probably related to the fact that cortisone is a prominent steroid in the human placenta (Murphy, 1979).

Interleukin-1 is a well known stimulus for T lymphocyte IL-2 production; therefore placental macrophage-derived IL-1 may stimulate the expression of IL-2 by placental components. Indeed, Boehm et al. (1989b) pointed out that the IL-2 gene is expressed in the syncytiotrophoblast of the human placenta. IL-2 is an important regulator of immune function. If it is produced by the syncytiotrophoblast, it would most certainly play a major role in any scheme of immune interaction(s) postulated to exist between the mother and the fetoplacental graft.

Other Free Connective Tissue Cells

Most free connective tissue cells of the human placental villi have been identified to be macrophages. There are a few cells, however, without macrophage character, among which are mast cells and plasma cells. Pescetto (1950), Latta and Beber (1953), Mahnke and Jacob (1972), and Durst-Zivkovic (1973) have dealt with the structural peculiarities of mast cells (Figure 63C). According to these reports, mast cells are found mainly in the walls of the large fetal blood vessels of stem villi. Structurally, they correspond to mast cells of other origins. The same is true for plasma cells, the occasional appearance of which in the stroma of stem villi of immature placentas has been reported by Benirschke and Bourne (1958); the plasma cell is often seen in a variety of chronic villitides.

Development and Structure of Fetal Villous Vessels

Origin of the Hemangioblastic Cells

There is only one systematic report that deals with early development of villous vessels, and it was based on exactly defined and exactly dated placental material (King, 1987). It describes the macaque placenta. In this primate, the first steps of vasculogenesis can be observed on day 19 p.c. or even earlier. The corresponding dates for the human placenta are probably similar. It became evident from the reports of Dempsey (1972) and Demir et al. (1989), however, that it is impossible to collect a similar series of exactly defined early human specimens under appropriate conditions for electron microscopy. Thus our information is based on a few specimens obtained by chance in good preservation. Knoth (1968) described primitive capillaries in a four-somite human embryo (approximately 21–22 days p.c.). Hertig (1935) stated that the fetal circulation is not established until the seven-somite stage (approximately 22nd day p.c.). According to our own material (Demir et al., 1989), the dates given by Hertig are too early. In the placental villi associated with a six-somite embryo (21–22 days p.c.), we identified hemangioblastic cell cords and primitive capillary sprouts without blood cells. On day 28 p.c., developing blood cells were present in the primitive capillary lumens. There were no convincing signs of a continuous vessel system that allows fetal villous circulation.

Hertig (1935) formulated the classical theory that villous mesenchymal cells and hemangioblastic cells are derived from villous cytotrophoblast by in situ delamination. This view has been refuted by all subsequent authors (Dempsey, 1972; Luckett, 1978; King, 1987; Demir et al., 1989), who found that the villous mesenchyme is directly derived from the fetus and invades the villi. The hemangioblastic cells differentiate locally from the mesenchymal cells. The two cell types are structurally similar. The results confirm a step-by-step differentiation of mesenchymal cells into endothelium (Demir et al., 1989). As a first step, the hemangioblastic cells form cell cords, the cells of which are connected to each other by primitive tight junctions (Figure 61). Dilatations of the intercellular clefts can be interpreted as forerunners of the capillary lumen. As soon as the latter has been formed, at around day 28 p.c., the first hematopoietic stem cells develop by delamination from the primitive vessel wall into the early lumen.

Capillary Formation During Early Pregnancy

Davidoff and Schiebler (1970) described the apposition of mesenchymal cells in the guinea pig placenta with the subsequent enlargement of scattered intercellular dilations forming a capillary lumen (Figure 61). This description differed from other observations, which suggested that lumen formation takes place by fusion of intraendothelial vacuoles (Folkman & Haudenschild, 1980). Davidoff and Schiebler's description was later confirmed by King (1987) for the rhesus monkey placenta and by Demir et al. (1989) for human villi. At the same time, some cells that are attached to the endothelial cells on the abluminal side acquire the characteristics of pericytes (Figure 61e). These cells were interpreted to be the "principal progenitors of fetal blood vessels" by Dempsey (1972). He assumed that only pericytes showed mitotic activity and were incorporated into the endothelial lining to support its growth. The findings by King (1987) and Demir et al. (1989) do not rule out this possibility, although we doubt that it is the only path of differentiation, as Castellucci et al. (1987) described endothelial mitoses in immature villi. In addition, an important role for platelet-derived growth factor B (PDGF-B) and PDGF-β-receptor in placental angiogenesis has been emphasized by Holmgren et al. (1991). The presence of PDGF-B and its receptor in most microvascular endothelial cells and the absence of the latter (PDGF-β-receptor mRNA) in macrovascular endothelial cells suggest the formation of an autostimulatory loop in capillary endothelium to promote cell proliferation and angiogenesis. Ogawa et al. (1991) and Shreeniwas et al. (1991) have reported experimental evidence that the endothelial proliferation under hypoxic conditions is controlled by basic fibroblast growth factor (bFGF); the expression of this cytokine in macrophages and the expression of its receptor on endothelial cells were considerably increased under hypoxic conditions. Even though the mode of deliberation of bFGF from macrophages is unknown, increased amounts of bFGF could be detected in the culture medium of hypoxic macrophages; and hypoxic endothelial cells reacted to incubation in this medium with stimulated proliferation. Also the presence of insulin receptor in second and third trimester endothelial cells of both capillaries and stem vessels has been interpreted as an expression of growth-promoting activities of insulin (Jones et al., 1993; Desoye et al., 1994); fetal insulin secretion must be discussed as a regulator of placental villous capillarization according to fetal demands during transplacental nutrient transfer.

The endothelial basement membrane, which in later stages separates endothelial cells and pericytes, cannot now clearly separate the two cell types because the former is absent during early stages of pregnancy. In the rhesus monkey the basement membrane is not established until day 57 of gestation (Luckett, 1970). In the human placenta, the complete basement membrane has not been observed until the beginning of the last trimester (Demir et al., 1989).

Basic Structure of the Vessel Walls

Generally speaking, the fetal placental vessels vary little from vessels of other organs. They show some peculiarities, however, that must be briefly noted (for details see Kaufmann & Miller, 1988). The composition of arterial and venous walls of stem villi largely corresponds to that of the vessels of the chorionic plate and the umbilical cord (Nanaev et al., 1991b) (see Chapter 13). In both vessel types, elastic membranes are largely absent. The muscular coats are thinner, and the muscle cells are more dispersed than in corresponding arteries and veins of other organs (Figure 66a). Nikolov and Schiebler (1973) reported more numerous and more stretched intercellular junctions. In addition, they described numerous myoendothelial contacts. Extensions of smooth muscle cells and of endothelial cells pass through gaps in the basal lamina into the neighboring layer, where they establish intense intercellular contacts. The attached parts of either cell type are characterized by increased amounts of plasmalemmal vesicles. Nikolov and Schiebler (1973) have interpreted it as a "musculoendothelial system" that may have importance for autonomous, local vasoregulation. Such local regulatory mechanisms of fetal intravillous blood flow must exist, as nerves are absent in the fetoplacental vessel system.

Fetal vasoactivity, however, has been described by several authors. Mayer et al. (1959), Sakata (1960), Freese (1966), and Panigel (1968) reported fetal vessel constriction, as seen by cinematographic methods. Lemtis (1970) found experimental proof for an uneven blood supply of the various villous trees and interpreted it to result from autonomous regulation and an attempt of adaptation to changing functional demands.

Several substances have been shown to participate in the vasomotor control of the fetoplacental vessels. The most potent vasodilator is endothelial-derived relaxing factor (EDRF) (Pinto et al., 1991) which is thought to be identical with nitric oxide (NO) (Myatt et al., 1991; for review see Macara et al., 1993). NO is formed from the conversion of L-arginine to citrulline by NO synthase. The activity of the latter enzyme has been found enzyme histochemically (NADPH diaphorase) and immunohistochemically in the fetal endothelium, the syncytiotrophoblast (Myatt et al., 1993), and villous myofibroblasts (Schönfelder et al., 1993). Another vasodilator is atrial natriuretic peptide, the receptors of which have been detected in smooth muscle cells of placental stem vessels (Salas et al., 1991).

Concerning vasoconstrictors, endothelin-1 has been demonstrated biochemically in the human placenta (Hemsen et al., 1991) and localized to the trophoblast (Malassine et al., 1993). Endothelin-1 receptor sites have been demonstrated on smooth muscle cells within stem villi (Wilkes et al., 1990).

The endothelium of arteries and arterioles in conventional histological sections appears often to be columnar. The hydropic endothelial cell bodies partly obstruct the lumens. Deep herniation of muscle cells through gaps in the basal lamina, between or into the endothelial cells, is a usual finding. Such features have been interpreted as results of pathological processes, for example, in placentas of HIV-infected mothers (Jimenez et al., 1988). Röckelein and Hey (1985) and Hey and Röckelein (1989) opposed this interpretation. They found endothelial hydrops and myoendothelial herniation to be the results of delayed immersion fixation. It could have been avoided by perfusion fixation of the fetal vascular system. We have shown wide vascular lumens surrounded by flat endothelium in large vessels after fetal or maternal perfusion fixation (Figure 66A,B). Compare them with the occluded arteriole in the lower right of Figure 67A, obtained from an immersion-fixed specimen.

These considerations, of course, do not rule out the possibility that in vivo constrictions or occlusions of the major fetal arteries and arterioles may occur and influence fetal hemodynamics of the placenta. Ample evidence exists that they do occur frequently. These findings have achieved major importance for the interpretation of Doppler measurements of umbilical artery flow velocity waveforms (Trudinger et al., 1985; Jimenez et al., 1988; Nessmann et al., 1988). The influence of fixation artifacts must be carefully considered when evaluating factors such as arterial lumen width, endothelial hydrops, and myoendothelial herniation.

Note that the distribution of major fetal vessels throughout the villous trees is not homogeneous. Its density (number of vessel cross sections per surface unit of histological section) is highest in the centers of the villous trees near the chorionic plate, where the large trunci chorii and rami chorii and their branches prevail; it is lowest in the periphery of the villous trees (placentones), where we find predominantly mature, intermediate, and terminal villi. Thus without a careful sampling regimen, meaningful results cannot be obtained (Mayhew & Burton, 1988). The principles of sampling, tissue preservation, and structural heterogeneity of the organ with artifacts that bias central findings are further explored in Tables 7, 9, 10, and 11.

The endothelial cells of capillaries and sinusoids are arranged as a monolayer (Figure 62B,C). During the last trimester they rest on a basal lamina. The cells are connected to each other by intercellular junctions. Whereas the rat and the mouse placenta display a fenestrated endothelium (Metz et al., 1976; Heinrich et al., 1977), a continuous endothelium is found in the human, guinea pig, and rabbit placenta (Becker & Seifert, 1965; Heinrich et al., 1976, 1977; Kaufmann et al., 1982, Orguero de Gaisan et al., 1985). Whether it is valid for all segments—from the arterial beginning to the venous end of the long capillary loops—of both the perivascular capillaries and the terminal capillary bed is unresolved. In humans, two types of endothelial cells have been described that differ ultrastructurally (Nikolov & Schiebler, 1973, 1981; Heinrich et al., 1976). Normally, these cell types can be found in the same capillary cross section (Figure 62C). Also the lectin-binding patterns point to considerable heterogeneity of the fetal villous endothelium (Lang et al., 1993b).

The lateral intercellular spaces that separate the single endothelial cells are bridged by intercellular junctions (Figure 62C), which serve as mechanical links between apposed cells and as gates that limit permeability for the paracellular transfer route. In human placental capillaries and sinusoids, most of these junctions are zonulae occludentes (Heinrich et al., 1988). They are known to limit paracellular transfer along the intercellular clefts to molecules with molecular weight about 40 kDa (molecular diameter about 6 nm) or less. Therefore, the transendothelial transport of immunoglobulin G takes place via plasmalemmal vesicles (Leach et al., 1989). As a second parameter, the molecular charge influences the permeability: The

above molecular size is valid for cationic probes, whereas anionic molecules of even smaller size may not pass (Firth et al., 1988).

There exist some hints that transplacental traffic of smaller molecules is influenced by the capillary endothelium. Mühlhauser et al. (1994) found immunoreactivity of carbonic anhydrase isoenzymes I and II in fetal villous endothelium, suggesting that the capillaries are actively involved in fetomaternal bicarbonate transfer and thus in carbon dioxide removal and fetal pH regulation. During the second and third trimesters, the human villous endothelium acquires insulin receptors that were present during the first trimester only at the intervillous surface of the syncytiotrophoblast (Jones et al., 1993; Desoye et al., 1994). It is still an open question whether the endothelial receptors bind fetal insulin in order to regulate maternofetal glucose transfer. Another explanation would be that fetal insulin acts as a growth factor regulating endothelial proliferation and villous angiogenesis according to the fetal demands.

Fibrinoid of the Villous Tree

Disseminated fibrinoid deposition in the intervillous space and the villous trees is a regular finding in every normal term placenta. Different from most other types of localization of fibrinoid, excess amounts are obviously pathological events. They are often incompatible with normal fetal outcome. It is not surprising, then, that pathologists have classified and made an attempt to define the fibrinoid deposits in this area (Wilkin, 1965; Benirschke & Driscoll, 1967; Fox, 1967a, 1968, 1975; Oswald & Gerl 1972; Becker, 1981). From an anatomical point of view, the nomenclature used by Fox (1967a, 1968, 1975) seems to be the most appropriate. He differentiated between perivillous fibrin(oid), which surrounds more or less altered but still identifiable villi, and intravillous or subsyncytial fibrinoid (villous fibrinoid necrosis), which primarily affects the villous interior. Although the two processes may later mix, they appear to have a different pathogenesis, at least at the beginning.

Perivillous Fibrinoid

The perivillous fibrinoid or perivillous fibrin defined by Fox (1967a, 1975) is probably identical with the microfibrinoid of Oswald and Gerl (1972) and with the *gitterinfarct* designated by Becker (1981). It probably partly overlaps with the fibrinoid found in the maternal floor infarction, discussed in Chapter 11.

Microscopically, perivillous fibrinoid can be found in every term placenta, but Fox (1967a) identified macroscopically such deposits in only 22.3% of normal placentas after 37 weeks of pregnancy. In our own experience, this figure is much too low. A mature placenta, free from macroscopically identifiable perivillous fibrinoid, is a rare exception. Problems may exist only insofar as it might be impossible to differentiate macroscopically between perivillous fibrinoid, intravillous fibrinoid, and old intervillous hematomas. The diameter of perivillous deposits in most cases is between a few hundred micrometers and some millimeters. Larger deposits that reach a few centimeters represent usually intervillous hematomas and displace villi rather than encasing them. The "placental floor infarction" is easily differentiated because of its large size and normally basal position, being directly connected to the basal plate.

Histologically, perivillous fibrinoid is lamellar in structure (Toth et al., 1973). Immunohistochemically, its superficial layer always represents fibrin-type fibrinoid (see Chapter 11). This layer may directly contact the trophoblastic lamina of the villi, or it may be followed by the more homogeneous matrix-type fibrinoid (see Chapter 11) that embeds a few large trophoblast cells.

Perivillous fibrinoid either fills gaps in the syncytiotrophoblastic cover of villi, or it encases entire villi or even groups of villi. The syncytiotrophoblast of these villi degenerates during the early stages of fibrinoid formation. In later stages it disappears completely. A thickened trophoblastic basal lamina surrounds the fibrotic villous stroma. Their fetal vessels sometimes remain intact, but in most cases they obliterate.

The villous cytotrophoblast perivillous fibrinoid may disappear, or it may show increased proliferation. Like the extravillous trophoblast cells of the basal plate, cell islands, and septa, these cells grow to considerable size. Immunohistochemically, they cannot be distinguished from extravillous trophoblast cells of other localizations. They partly lose their connection to the basal lamina and develop in strings or as single cells deep in the fibrinoid (Figure 148a) (Villee, 1960; Wilkin, 1965; Fox, 1967a), adding by secretion and degeneration additional matrix-type fibrinoid. This finding suggests that villous cytotrophoblast (Langhans' cells) and extravillous cytotrophoblast do not represent two completely different lines of trophoblast differentiation that separate during the early stages of placentation. Rather, it implies that villous trophoblast cells even during late pregnancy can be transformed into extravillous cells, losing their polarization and secreting matrix-type fibrinoid instead of a basal lamina, as soon as these cells are covered by fibrin-type fibrinoid rather than by villous syncytiotrophoblast.

Moe and Joergensen (1968) electron microscopically studied aggregates of platelets at the villous syncytial surfaces and described these aggregates as representing the initial stages of fibrinoid deposition. According to Fox (1967a), syncytiotrophoblastic degeneration is only a secondary phenomenon that is introduced by platelet aggregation on the intact syncytial surfaces. The latter process is thought to be caused by a disturbed intervillous circulation. On the other hand, it is known that collagens (Kunicki et al., 1988), fibronectins (Piotrowicz et al., 1988), and laminin (Sonnenberg et al., 1988) are able to initiate blood clotting. These molecules are constituents of the trophoblastic basal lamina. Thus it is reasonable to assume that focal degeneration of syncytiotrophoblast with free exposure of the basal lamina to the intervillous blood results in local blood clotting and closure of the trophoblastic defect by a fibrinoid plug. As has been demonstrated by Edwards et al. (1991), it must be discussed how far such fibrinoid plugs are sufficient barriers controlling maternofetal macromolecule transfer.

Statistical results published by Fox (1967a, 1975) suggested that perivillous fibrinoid is a more frequent phenomenon in placentas from normal pregnancies than in those involved in pathological processes. This finding may be an indicator that it is just the maximal maternal perfusion of the intervillous space that predisposes to perivillous fibrin deposition. In agreement with this conclusion, the same author failed to find any local or statistical correlation between perivillous fibrinoid and placental infarction. In general, there seemed to be no influence on fetal well-being.

Even though these findings and theories by Fox are supported by early publications (Siddall & Hartman, 1926; Huber et al., 1961), there are many reports that point in another direction. Eden (1897), who was probably the first author to state that infarcts are the result of maternal vascular occlusion, considered derivation from blood coagulation and degeneration; Sala et al. (1982) found, with stereological techniques, that significantly more fibrin was deposited in "venous" ("hypoxic") areas of the placenta, where there is stasis of blood. Huguenin (1909), Wilkin (1965), Boyd and Hamilton (1970), and Toth et al. (1973) considered perivillous fibrinoid to be the result of trophoblastic degeneration. Boyd and Hamilton (1970) and Wilkin (1965) described fibrinoid deposition below the syncytiotrophoblast, preceding intervillous clotting. Thomsen (1954) reported cases of villous rupture with fetal bleeding into the intervillous space as being responsible for this process.

Our experimental studies in the pregnant guinea pig (Kaufmann et al., 1974a; Kaufmann, 1975a) caused us to assume that, in addition to mere intervillous (i.e., circulatory) factors, there are intrasyncytial causes for perivillous fibrinoid deposition, including maternal acidosis induced by intravenous lactate infusion. This situation resulted within hours in intrasyncytial degenerative changes, including intrasyncytial deposition of fibrillar material. These changes were immediately followed by platelet aggregates wrapped in fine fibrillar fibrin at the syncytial surface. This finding is in agreement with older findings by Hörmann (1965), who considered that hypoxia and acidosis may induce "fibrinoid secretion" by the trophoblast. Zacks and Blazar (1963) have also described the deposition of intrasyncytial filamentous material that may lead to syncytial degeneration and eventually result in replacement of the syncytium by fibrinoid. Inhibition of intrasyncytial energy metabolism in the guinea pig, using monoiodine acetate or sodium fluoride (Kaufmann et al., 1974a; Kaufmann, 1975a), induced a similar process. Focal intrasyncytial degenerative changes were observed by electron microscopy within minutes after application of the drugs, followed by intrasyncytial accumulation of fibrillar products and later by fibrin/fibrinoid deposition in the neighboring maternal blood.

Fox (1978) objected, stating that it seems difficult to accept that a metabolic disturbance affects only a localized area of villous tissue. One must bear in mind, however, that it is accepted for other parts of our vascular system that metabolic disorders (e.g., diabetes mellitus), cooperating with other pathogenic factors, may result in localized tissue damage. Why cannot the same situation pertain to the placenta? Corresponding experimental results are not absolute proof for the intrasyncytial genesis of forerunners of fibrinoid. For instance, it has been demonstrated by B.L. Sheppard (personal communication, 1979) and Kaufmann (1981) that maternal fibrin may be internalized by the trophoblast. The above experimental findings, however, strongly suggest that syncytial degeneration may initiate perivillous fibrin deposition. In summary, this controversy indicates that multiple and only poorly understood interactions between syncytiotrophoblast and maternal blood are involved in the production of perivillous fibrinoid.

Intravillous Fibrinoid

Fox (1968) first described and defined a separate kind of fibrinoid that appears in the subtrophoblastic space and finally occupies the entire villous stroma. According to his views, up to 3% of the villous cross sections may be partially or completely replaced by intravillous fibrinoid after a normal pregnancy. The intravillous deposition is increased during pregnancies complicated by maternal diabetes, Rh incompatibility, and preeclampsia.

The process is thought to be initiated by small, subsyncytially positioned, electron microscopically heterogeneous (Figure 123), periodic acid-Schiff-positive nodules that later increase in size and finally replace the stroma. This view has been supported by Wilkin (1965) and Boyd and Hamilton (1970). As stated by these authors, the originally intact syncytium degenerates only secondarily if at all. Liebhart (1971) has described degeneration of the villous cytotrophoblast as the initial process. Some immunological studies have supported the idea of an extracellular fibrinoid deposition in the villous stroma, independent from cellular degeneration (Gille et al., 1974; Faulk et al., 1975). Although probably of secondary importance only, there has been ample discussion whether this process is completely independent from the genesis of perivillous fibrinoid (Fox, 1967a) or it may be complicated by it (Wilkin, 1965; Boyd & Hamilton, 1970; Burstein et al., 1973).

The derivation of the intravillous fibrinoid is not as clear as one may suppose. Based on Liebhart's description (1971) of a primarily intracytotrophoblastic deposition, Fox (1975) concluded that this material cannot be fibrin. In contradistinction to what he has defined to be perivillous "fibrin," he proposed the term intravillous "fibrinoid." It seems obvious that an intact syncytiotrophoblastic barrier and an intact fetal capillary wall prevent maternal or fetal fibrin imbibition of the villous interior. On the other hand, Moe (1969a,b,c) immunohistochemically demonstrated fibrinogen and fibrin in the cytotrophoblast. Moreover, several immunohistochemical studies found proof for an intravillous existence of fibrin, fibrinogen, or both: for example, in the trophoblastic basal lamina (McCormick et al., 1971) and the intravillous fibrinoid (Gille et al., 1974; Faulk et al., 1975). This possibility had already been suggested by early publications, such as those of Kline (1951), McKay et al. (1958), and Wigglesworth (1964). Finally, our studies concerning the immunohistochemistry of fibrinoids (Frank et al., 1994) provided clear evidence that intravillous fibrinoid may contain both fibrin (fibrin-type fibrinoid) and extracellular matrix molecules, such as oncofetal fibronectin, laminin, and collagen IV (matrix-type fibrinoid) (see Chapter 11). The question as to a maternal or fetal derivation of this fibrin is still open.

Concerning the etiology of the formation of the intravillous fibrinoid, Fox (1968) discussed an immunological attack against the villous cytotrophoblast as a possibility. Wislocki and Bennett (1943) proposed villous degeneration as a result of placental aging to be the primary agent. The histological and histochemical studies by Burstein and coworkers (1973) have provided some evidence that intravillous fibrinoid and amyloid might be identical, whereas perivillous fibrinoid showed staining patterns that were different from those of amyloid. In agreement with the extraplacental genesis of amyloid, these authors suggested that intravillous fibrinoid is a result of placental degeneration induced by aging and by immunological processes.

Intravillous fibrinoid, involved in immunological processes, has been discussed on many occasions. McCormick et al. (1971) described this type of fibrinoid as a result of antigen-antibody reactions in the villous stroma and as resulting in an immunological barrier between maternal and fetal circulations. Burstein et al. (1963) even named the villous stroma an immunological battlefield, as they found a specific stromal binding of insulin in cases of maternal diabetes mellitus and of anti-D antibodies in cases of Rh incompatibility. Slightly different from the foregoing and based on experimental studies in healthy pregnant women, Gille et al. (1974) came to the conclusion that immunological diseases may affect the syncytiotrophoblastic barrier. As a consequence, the latter was thought to become permeable for antigen-antibody complexes, which then may become enriched and are finally deposited as fibrinoid in the villous stroma.

CELL BIOLOGICAL TRENDS

Some of the cell biological trends in modern placental research may become important for understanding villous pathology in the near future. The aim of this section is to act as a guide to the recent literature of this area

Cell Isolation and Culture

An important step toward applying modern cell biology to any organ is the possibility of isolating its cells and performing in vitro studies. It is now possible to culture cells from most organs of the body under conditions in which they continue to express at least some of their differentiated traits. Fundamental for the human placenta was the development of a technique to isolate the cyto-trophoblast. Such a technique was established by Kliman et al. (1986). At present, most laboratories use this technique, in some cases with certain modifications (Douglas & King, 1989; Bischof et al., 1991). Several methods have been reported that isolate the Hofbauer cells using proteolytic enzymes (Flynn et al., 1982; Frauli & Ludwig, 1987a) by a combination of enzymatic digestion and density gradient centrifugation (Uren & Boyle, 1985) or by using mechanical action and density gradient centrifugation without the use of enzymes (Zaccheo et al., 1989). Lang et al. (1993a) and Leach et al. (1993) have established a technique to isolate and culture endothelial cells from fetal villous vessels. Placental fibroblasts have been separated by Fant (1991). The possibility of isolating and culturing the various placental cells and developing co-culture systems opens fascinating perspectives to obtain better insights in cellular interactions during morphogenesis of the organ.

Growth Factors, Growth Factor Receptors, Oncogenes

The human placenta undergoes dramatic structural reorganization and remodeling during villous development. Growth factor genes and proto-oncogenes are generally linked to such processes. It has been established that the placenta produces a large number of polypeptide growth factors, has a complex array for their receptors, and expresses several proto-oncogene protein products (for reviews see Adamson, 1987; Blay & Hollenberg, 1989;

Ohlsson, 1989). Here we provide a brief survey for some of them.

It has been demonstrated that epidermal growth factor receptor (EGF receptor), a product of the proto-oncogene c-erbB-1, is present in the syncytiotrophoblast as well as in the villous and extravillous cytotrophoblast (Bulmer et al., 1989; Ladines-Llave et al., 1991; Mühlhauser et al., 1993). EGF is detectable in amnionic fluid, umbilical vessels, and placental tissue (Scott et al., 1989). The question of placental production sites is still open. Morrish et al. (1987) pointed out that this growth factor induces morphological differentiation together with increased production of hCG and hPL in vitro.

Structurally related to the protein product of c-erbB-1 is that of the proto-oncogene c-erbB-2, which encodes a receptor protein for an as yet unknown ligand, although some candidate ligands have been identified (Lupu et al., 1992; Peles et al., 1992). The latter proto-oncogene seems to play a role in human cancer. In some malignant tumors, c-erbB-2 protein product and EGF-R are both overexpressed, which correlates with a reduction in patient relapse-free and overall survival (Slamon et al., 1987; Wright et al., 1989). These data suggest that the two receptors may contribute to the development and maintenance of the malignant phenotype. It is interesting that in the human placenta, which shares some aspects with invasive tumors, this co-expression is present in villous syncytiotrophoblast, which in contrast to invasive tumor cells is nonproliferative; on the other hand, in the proliferating cells of the extravillous trophoblast, only EGF-R is expressed, whereas c-erbB-2 characterizes the differentiating and no longer proliferating cells (Mühlhauser et al., 1993).

Insulin-like growth factors (IGF-1 and IGF-2) and their receptors are also expressed in the human placenta (Boehm et al., 1989a; Ohlsson, 1989; Ohlsson et al., 1989). In particular, IGF-2 is expressed primarily in highly proliferative cytotrophoblastic structures, as for example in cell islands and cell columns, whereas other cellular components (e.g., villous cytotrophoblast or mesenchymal stromal cells) harbor less active IGF-2 genes (Ohlsson et al., 1989). Because numerous IGF receptors are expressed in villous cytotrophoblast, it has been suggested that IGF mediates autocrine or short-range paracrine growth control of placental development (Ohlsson et al., 1989).

Platelet-derived growth factor (PDGF) and its receptors (PDGF-R) are expressed in the human placenta (Goustin et al., 1985; Marez et al., 1987; Taylor & Williams, 1988; Holmgren et al., 1991). PDGF is a potent mitogen for a variety of cells, particularly for mesenchymal cells, and there is evidence that it plays a role in angiogenetic processes (Holmgren et al., 1991; Risau et al., 1992) and in stimulating cell movement through chemotaxis (Westermark et al., 1990). PDGF consists of homodimers and heterodimers of two subunits, PDGF-A and PDGF-B, the latter encoded by the cellular equivalent of the v-sis oncogene (Doolittle et al., 1983). It has been shown that PDGF is coexpressed with the myc proto-oncogene in proliferative cytotrophoblast, and it has been suggested that PDGF influences the "pseudomalignant" phenotype of the early human placenta (Goustin et al., 1985). In addition, Holmgren et al. (1991) have proposed an important role for PDGF-B and its receptors in placental angiogenic processes.

Another growth factor detected in the human placenta and related to but different from PDGF is the platelet-derived endothelial cell growth factor (PD-ECGF). By immunohistochemistry, it is mainly detected in the stromal cells of the chorionic villi (Usuki et al., 1990). Ishikawa et al. (1989) have established that PD-ECGF stimulates growth and chemotaxis of endothelial cells in vitro and angiogenesis in vivo.

Transforming growth factor β (TGF-β) and TGF-β messenger RNA have been isolated from the human placenta (Frolik et al., 1983). This growth factor is a multifunctional peptide involved in immunosuppressive activities and, depending on the cell type, in stimulation or inhibition of cell growth (Miller et al., 1990; Sporn & Roberts, 1990). Concerning the human placenta, Morrish et al. (1991) have shown that it acts as a major inhibitor of trophoblast differentiation and concomitant peptide secretion.

Proteases

Remodeling of the villous stroma during placental development could also be related to the secretion of matrix-degrading proteolytic enzymes by the various stromal cells. It has been shown that trophoblast expresses interstitial and type IV collagenolytic activities (Emonard et al., 1990; Moll & Lane, 1990; Librach et al., 1991), and the former has also been detected in villous fibroblasts (Moll & Lane, 1990). Autio-Harmainen et al. (1992) detected 70 kDa type IV collagenase in endothelial cells and fibroblasts of the villi.

Plasminogen activators (uPA and tPA) and their inhibitors have been shown to be present in amnionic fluid (Kjaeldgaard et al., 1989) and to be produced by the trophoblast (Åstedt et al., 1986; Feinberg et al., 1989; Radtke et al., 1990; Librach et al., 1991; for reviews see Lala & Graham, 1990; Bischof & Martelli, 1992). It is interesting that plasminogen activator inhibitor type 1 (PAI-1) is mainly present in invading cytotrophoblast cells, whereas PAI-2 is prominent in the villous syncytiotrophoblast (Feinberg et al., 1989).

Extracellular Matrix

Research concerning the extracellular matrix in the human placenta has strongly emphasized the role of its molecular constituents in morphogenetic and invasive processes. Tenascin (Castellucci et al., 1991; Damsky et al., 1992) has been shown to be expressed in fetal stroma and is related to proliferative trophoblast and to trophoblastic defects covered by fibrinoid.

Fibronectins are well known to be expressed in the villous stroma (Yamada et al., 1987; Virtanen et al., 1988; Earl et al., 1990). They are also expressed in the cytotrophoblastic cell columns (Earl et al., 1990; Damsky et al., 1992; Castellucci et al., 1993a,b); in this area, the oncofetal isoform (absent in the villous stroma) is specifically expressed (i.e., at the fetomaternal border of the basal plate) (Feinberg et al., 1991). Fibronectins are involved in attaching cells to extracellular matrix through such integrins as α5/β1 (Damsky et al., 1992; for a review see Akiyama et al., 1990). In vitro studies have demonstrated that extracellular matrix-integrin interactions involve cytoskeletal structures transmitting extracellular signals that regulate various programs of gene expression; these findings imply that cell shape may be a primary regulator of phenotypic expression (Ben-Ze'ev, 1986; Werb et al., 1986).

In the human placenta, different from most other organs, molecules such as laminin, collagen IV, and heparan sulfate are detectable not only in the basement membrane but also weakly throughout the villous stroma (Yamada et al., 1987; Nanaev et al., 1991a; Rukosuev, 1992). The universal presence of these molecules in the extracellular matrix may facilitate remodeling of basement membranes and thus increase morphogenetic and functional flexibility of the various villous cell populations. Moreover, collagen types I, III, V, and VI have been found by immunohistochemistry in the stroma of the chorionic villi (Amenta et al., 1986; Nanaev et al., 1991a; Rukosuev, 1992). Decorin, a small leucine-rich proteoglycan that seems to have a primary function in the organization of the extracellular matrix (Hardingham & Fosang, 1992), has been also detected in the villous stroma (Bianco et al., 1990). It is interesting that the core protein of decorin (whose synthesis is induced by TGF-β) binds and neutralizes TGF-β (Yamaguchi et al., 1990).

There is an increasing use of extracellular matrix molecules in in vitro studies of the trophoblast. It has been demonstrated that such molecules influence trophoblast differentiation (Kao et al., 1988; Nelson et al., 1990); they can play a pivotal role in repair mechanisms (Nelson et al., 1990), may participate in modulating hormone and protein production (Castellucci et al., 1990a), and can influence the morphology and proteolytic activity of the trophoblast (Kliman & Feinberg, 1990; Bischof et al., 1991).

References

Acconci, G.: Mola vesicolare destruente e corioepitelioma. Folia Ginecol. (Genoa) 21:253–268, 1925.

Adamson, E.D.: Review article: expression of proto-oncogenes in the placenta. Placenta 8:449–466, 1987.

Akiyama, S.K., Nagata, K., and Yamada, K.M.: Cell surface receptors for extracellular matrix components. Biochim. Biophys. Acta 1031:91–110, 1990.

Albe, K.R., Witkin, H.J., Kelley, L.K., and Smith, C.H.: Protein kinases of the human placental microvillous membrane. Exp. Cell Res. 147:167–176, 1983.

Alsat, E., Mondon, F., Rebourcet, R., Berthelier, M., Ehrlich, D., Cedard, L., and Goldstein, S.: Identification of specific binding sites for acetylated low density lipoprotein in microvillous membranes from human placenta. Mol. Cell. Endocrinol. 41:229–235, 1985.

Alvarez, H.: Proliferation du trophoblaste et sa relation avec l'hypertension arterielle de la toxemie gravidique. Gynecol. Obstet. (Paris) 69:581–588, 1970.

Alvarez, H., Benedetti, W.L., Morel., R.L., and Scavarelli, M.: Trophoblast development gradient and its relationship to placental hemodynamics. Am. J. Obstet. Gynecol. 106:416–420, 1970.

Alvarez, H., Medrano, C.V., Sala, M.A., and Benedetti, W.L.: Trophoblast development gradient and its relationship to placental hemodynamics. II. Study of fetal cotyledons from the toxemic placenta. Am. J. Obstet. Gynecol. 114:873–878, 1972.

Al-Zuhair, A.G.H., Ibrahim, M.E.H., Mughal, S., and Mohammed, M.E.: Scanning electron microscopy of maternal blood cells and their surface relationship with the placenta. Acta Obstet. Gynecol. Scand. 62:493–498, 1983.

Al-Zuhair, A.G.H., Ibrahim, M.E.A., Mughal, S., and Abdulla, M.A.: Loss and regeneration of the microvilli of human placental syncytiotrophoblast. Arch. Gynecol. 240:147–151, 1987.

Amalados, A.S., and Burton, G.J.: Organ culture of human placental villi in hypoxic and hyperoxic conditions: a morphometric study. J. Dev. Physiol. 7:113–118, 1985.

Amenta, P.S., Gay, S., Vaheri, A., and Martinez-Hernandez, A.: The extracellular matrix is an integrated unit: ultrastructural localization of collagen types I, III, IV, V, VI, fibronectin, and laminin in human term placenta. Collagen Relat. Res. 6:125–152, 1986.

Amstutz, E.: Beobachtungen über die Reifung der Chorionzotten in der menschlichen Placenta mit besonderer Berücksichtigung der Epithelplatten. Acta Anat. (Basel) 42:122–130, 1960.

Arnholdt, H., Meisel, F., Fandrey, K., and Löhrs, U.: Proliferation of villous trophoblast of the human placenta in normal and abnormal pregnancies. Virchows Arch B Cell Pathol. 60:365–372, 1991.

Arnold, M., Geller, H., and Sasse, D.: Beitrag zur elektronenmikroskopischen Morphologie der menschlichen Plazenta. Arch. Gynecol. 196:238–253, 1961.

Åstedt, B., Hägerstrand, I., and Lecander, I.: Cellular localisation in placenta of placental type plasminogen activator inhibitor. Thromb. Haemost. 56:63–65, 1986.

Aufderheide, E., and Ekblom, P.: Tenascin during gut development: appearance in the mesenchyme, shift in molecular forms, and dependence on epithelial-mesenchymal interactions. J. Cell Biol. 107:2341–2349, 1988.

Autio-Harmainen, H., Sandberg, M., Pihlajaniemi, T., and Vuorio, E.: Synthesis of laminin and type IV collagen by trophoblastic cells and fibroblastic stromal cells in the early human placenta. Lab. Invest. 64:483–491, 1991.

Autio-Harmainen, H., Hurskainen, T., Niskasaari, K., Höyhtyä, M., and Tryggvason, K.: Simultaneous expression of 70 kilodalton type IV collagenase and type IV collagen α1(IV) chain genes by cells of early human placenta and gestational endometrium. Lab. Invest. 67:191–200, 1992.

Baker, B.L., Hook, S.J., and Severinghaus, A.E.: The cytological structure of the human chorionic villus and decidua parietalis. Am. J. Anat. 74:291–325, 1944.

Bargmann, W., and Knoop, A.: Elektronenmikroskopische Untersuchungen an Plazentarzotten des Menschen: Bemerkungen zum Synzytiumproblem. Z. Zellforsch. 50:472–493, 1959.

Bautzmann, H., and Schröder, R.: Über Vorkommen und Bedeutung von "Hofbauerzellen" ausserhalb der Placenta. Arch. Gynecol. 187:65–76, 1955.

Beck, T., Schweikhart, G., and Stolz, E.: Immunohistochemical location of hPL, SP1 and β-hCG in normal placentas of varying gestational age. Arch. Gynecol. 239:63–74, 1986.

Becker, V.: Gefäße der Chorionplatte und Stammzotten. In, Die Plazenta des Menschen. V. Becker, Th.H. Schiebler, and F. Kubli, eds., Thieme Verlag, Stuttgart, 1981.

Becker, V., and Bleyl, U.: Placentarzotte bei Schwangerschaftstoxicose und fetaler Erythroblastose im fluorescenzmikroskopischen Bilde. Virchows Arch. Pathol. Anat. 334:516–527, 1961.

Becker, V., and Röckelein, G., eds.: Pathologie der weiblichen Genitalorgane. Springer-Verlag, Heidelberg, 1989.

Becker, V., and Seifert, K.: Die Ultrastruktur der Kapillarwand in der menschlichen Placenta zur Zeit der Schwangerschaftsmitte. Z. Zellforsch. 65:380–396, 1965.

Beham, A., Denk, H., and Desoye, G.: The distribution of intermediate filament proteins, actin and desmoplakins in human placental tissue as revealed by polyclonal and monoclonal antibodies. Placenta 9:479–492, 1988.

Benirschke, K., and Bourne, G.L.: Plasma cells in immature human placenta. Obstet. Gynecol. 12:495–503, 1958.

Benirschke, K., and Driscoll, S.G.: The Pathology of the Human Placenta. Springer-Verlag, New York, 1967.

Ben-Ze'ev, A.: The relationship between cytoplasmic organization, gene expression and morphogenesis. Trends Biochem. Sci. 11:478–481, 1986.

Bianco, P., Fisher, L.W., Young, M.F., Termine, J.D., and Robey, P.G.: Expression and localization of the two small proteoglycans biglycan and decorin in developing human skeletal and non-skeletal tissues. J. Histochem. Cytochem. 38:1549–1563, 1990.

Bierings, M.B.: Placental iron uptake and its regulation. Medical thesis, University of Rotterdam, 1989.

Bischof, P., and Martelli, M.: Proteolysis in the penetration phase of the implantation process. Placenta 13:17–24, 1992.

Bischof, P. Friedli, E., Martelli, M., and Campana, A.: Expression of extracellular matrix degrading metalloproteinases by cultured human cytotrophoblast cells: effects of cell adhesion and immunopurification. Am. J. Obstet. Gynecol. 165:1791–1801, 1991.

Blay, J., and Hollenberg, M.D.: The nature and function of polypeptide growth factor receptors in the human placenta. J. Dev. Physiol. 12:237–248, 1989.

Bleyl, U.: Histologische, histochemische und fluoreszenzmikroskopische Untersuchungen an Hofbauer-Zellen. Arch. Gynecol. 197:364–386, 1962.

Boehm, K.D., Kelley, M.F., and Ilan, J.: Expression of insulin-like growth factors by the human placenta. In, Molecular and Cellular Biology of Insulin-Like Growth Factors and Their Receptors. D. Leroith and M.K. Raizada, eds., pp. 179–193. Plenum, New York, 1989a.

Boehm, K.D., Kelley, M.F., Ilan, J., and Ilan, J.: The interleukin 2 gene is expressed in the syncytiotrophoblast of the human placenta. Proc. Natl. Acad. Sci. U.S.A. 86:656–660, 1989b.

Boime, I., Otani, T., Otani, F., Daniels-McQueen, S., and Bo, M.: Factors regulating peptide hormone biosynthesis in human placenta. In, Abstracts of the 11th Rochester Trophoblast Conference, Rochester, N.Y., p. 1, 1988.

Borst, R., Kussäther, E., and Schuhmann, R.: Ultrastrukturelle Untersuchungen zur Verteilung der alkalischen Phosphatase im Placenton (maternofetale Strömungseinheit) der menschlichen Placenta. Arch. Gynecol. 215:409–415, 1973.

Bourne, G.: The Human Amnion and Chorion. Lloyd-Luke, London, 1962.

Boyd, J.D., and Hamilton, W.J.: Electron microscopic observations on the cytotrophoblast contribution to the syncytium in the human placenta. J. Anat. 100:535–548, 1966.

Boyd, J.D., and Hamilton, W.J.: Development and structure of the human placenta from the end of the 3rd month of gestation. J. Obstet. Gynaecol. Br. Commonw. 74:161–226, 1967.

Boyd, J.D., and Hughes, A.F.W.: Etude des villosites placentaires au moyen du microscope electronique. In, 6th Congress, International Federation of Anatomists. Abstract 32, Masson, Paris, 1955.

Boyd, J.D., and Hamilton, W.J.: The Human Placenta. Heffer & Sons, Cambridge, 1970.

Boyd, J.D., Boyd, C.A.R., and Hamilton, W.J.: Observations on the vacuolar structure of the human syncytiotrophoblast. Z. Zellforsch. 88:57–79, 1968a.

Boyd, J.D., Hamilton, W.J., and Boyd, C.A.R.: The surface of the syncytium of the human chorionic villus. J. Anat. 102:553–563, 1968b.

Bradbury, S., Billington, W.D., Kirby, D.R.S., and Williams, E.A.: Surface mucin of human trophoblast. Am. J. Obstet. Gynecol. 104:416–418, 1969.

Bradbury, S., Billington, W.D., Kirby, D.R.S., and Williams, E.A.: Histochemical characterization of the surface muco-protein of normal and abnormal human trophoblast. Histochem. J. 2:263–274, 1970.

Braunhut, S.J., Blanc, W.A., Ramanarayanan, M., Marboe, C., and Mesa-Tejada, R.: Immunocytochemical localization of lysozyme and alpha-1-antichymotrypsin in the term human placenta: an attempt to characterize the Hofbauer cell. J. Histochem. Cytochem. 32:1204–1210, 1984.

Bray, B.A.: Presence of fibronectin in basement membranes and acidic structural glycoproteins from human placenta and lung. Ann. N. Y. Acad. Sci. 312:142–150, 1978.

Bremer, J.L.: The interrelations of the mesonephros, kidney and placenta in different classes of mammals. Am. J. Anat. 19:179–209, 1916.

Bright, N.A., and Ockleford, C.D.: Fc-τ receptor bearing cells in human term amniochorion. J. Anat. 183:187–188, 1993.

Brown, P.J., and Johnson, P.M.: Isolation of a transferrin receptor structure from sodium deoxycholate-solubilized human placental syncytiotrophoblast plasma. Placenta 2:1–10, 1981.

Bryant-Greenwood, G.D., Rees, M.C.P., and Turnbull, A.C.: Immunohistochemical localization of relaxin, pro-lactin and prostaglandin synthetase in human amnion, chorion and decidua. J. Endocrinol. 114:491–496, 1987.

Buckley, P.J., Smith, M.R., Broverman, M.F., and Dickson, S.A.: Human spleen contains phenotypic subsets of macrophages and dendritic cells that occupy discrete microanatomic locations. Am. J. Pathol. 128:505–520, 1987.

Bulmer, J.N., and Johnson, P.M.: Macrophage populations in the human placenta and amniochorion. Clin. Exp. Immunol. 57:393–403, 1984.

Bulmer, J.N., Morrison, L., and Smith, J.C.: Expression of class II MHC gene products by macrophages in human uteroplacental tissue. Immunology 63:707–714, 1988.

Bulmer, J.N., Thrower, S., and Wells, M.: Expression of epidermal growth factor receptor and transferrin receptor by human trophoblast populations. Am. J. Reprod. Immunol. 21:87–93, 1989.

Burgos, M.H., and Rodriguez, E.M.: Specialized zones in the trophoblast of the human term placenta. Am. J. Obstet. Gynecol. 96:342–356, 1966.

Burstein, R., Berns, A.W., Hirata, Y., and Blumenthal, H.T.: A comparative histo- and immunopathological study of the placenta in diabetes mellitus and in erythroblastosis fetalis. Am. J. Obstet. Gynecol. 86:66–76, 1963.

Burstein, R., Frankel, S., Soule, S.D., and Blumenthal, H.T.: Ageing in the placenta: autoimmune theory of senescence. Am. J. Obstet. Gynecol. 116:271–274, 1973.

Burton, G.J.: Intervillous connections in the mature human placenta: instances of syncytial fusion or section artifacts? J. Anat. 145:13–23, 1986a.

Burton, G.J.: Scanning electron microscopy of intervillous connections in the mature human placenta. J. Anat. 147:245–254, 1986b.

Burton, G.J.: The fine structure of the human placental villus as revealed by scanning electron microscopy. Scanning Electron Microsc. 1:1811–1828, 1987.

Burton, G.J., Mayhew, T.M., and Robertson, L.A.: Stereo-logical re-examination of the effects of varying oxygen tensions on human placental villi maintained in organ culture for up to 12 h. Placenta 10:263–273, 1989.

Cantle, S.J., Kaufmann, P., Luckhardt, M., and Schweikhart, G.: Interpretation of syncytial sprouts and bridges in the human placenta. Placenta 8:221–234, 1987.

Carter, J.E.: The ultrastructure of the human trophoblast. Transcript 2nd Rochester Trophoblast Conference. C.J. Lund and H.A. Thiede, eds., 1963.

Carter, J.E.: Morphologic evidence of syncytial formation from the cytotrophoblastic cells. Obstet. Gynecol. 23:647–656, 1964.

Castellucci, M., and Kaufmann, P.: A three-dimensional study of the normal human placental villous core. II. Stromal architecture. Placenta 3:269–285, 1982a.

Castellucci, M., and Kaufmann, P.: Evolution of the stroma in human chorionic villi throughout pregnancy. Bibl. Anat. 22:40–45, 1982b.

Castellucci, M., Zaccheo, D., and Pescetto, G.: A three-dimensional study of the normal human placental villous core. I. The Hofbauer cells. Cell Tissue Res. 210:235–247, 1980.

Castellucci, M., Schweikhart, G., Kaufmann, P., and Zaccheo, D.: The stromal architecture of immature in-termediate villus of the human placenta: functional and clinical implications. Gynecol. Obstet. Invest. 10.55–99, 1984.

Castellucci, M., Richter, A., Steininger, B., Celona, A., and Schneider, J.: Light and electron microscopy identification of mitotic Hofbauer cells in the human placenta. Arch. Gynecol. 237(Suppl.):235, 1985.

Castellucci, M., Celona, A., Bartels, H., Steininger, B., Benedetto, V., and Kaufmann, P.: Mitosis of the Hofbauer cell: possible implications for a fetal macrophage. Placenta 8:65–76, 1987.

Castellucci, M., and Zaccheo, D.: The Hofbauer cells of the human placenta: morphological and immunological aspects. Prog. Clin. Biol. Res. 269:443–451, 1989.

Castellucci, M., Kaufmann, P., and Bischof, P.: Extracellular matrix influences hormone and protein production by human chorionic villi. Cell Tissue Res. 262:135–142, 1990a.

Castellucci, M., Mühlhauser, J., and Zaccheo, D.: The Hofbauer cell: the macrophage of the human placenta. In, Immunobiology of Normal and Diabetic Pregnancy. D. Andreani, G. Bompiani, U. Di Mario, W.P. Faulk, and A. Galluzzo, eds., pp. 135–144. Wiley & Sons, Chichester, 1990b.

Castellucci, M., Scheper, M., Scheffen, I., Celona, A., and Kaufmann, P.: The development of the human placental villous tree. Anat. Embryol. (Berl.) 181:117–128, 1990c.

Castellucci, M., Classen-Linke, I., Mühlhauser, J., Kaufmann, P., Zardi, L., and Chiquet-Ehrismann, R.: The human placenta: a model for tenascin expression. Histochemistry 95:449–458, 1991.

Castellucci, M., Crescimanno, C., Mühlhauser, J., Frank, H.G., Kaufmann, P., and Zardi, L.: Expression of extracellular matrix molecules related to placental development. Placenta 14:A9, 1993a.

Castellucci, M., Crescimanno, C., Schroeter, C.A., Kaufmann, P., and Mühlhauser, J.: Extravillous trophoblast: immunohistochemical localization of extracellular matrix molecules. In, Frontiers in Gynecologic and Obstetric Investigation. A.R. Genazzani, F. Petraglia, A.D. Genazzani, eds., pp. 19–25. Parthenon, New York, 1993b.

Chaletzky, E.: Hydatidenmole. Thesis, University of Bern, 1891.

Chard, T.: Placental radar. J. Endocrinol. 138:177–179, 1993.

Chegini, N., and Rao, CH.V.: Epidermal growth factor binding to human amnion, chorion, decidua, and placenta from mid- and term pregnancy: quantitative light microscopic autoradiographic studies. J. Clin. Endocrinol. Metab. 61:529–535, 1985.

Chen, C.-F., Kurachi, H., Fujita, Y., Terakawa, N., Miyake, A., and Tanizawa, O.: Changes in epidermal growth factor receptor and its messenger ribonucleic acid levels in human placenta and isolated trophoblast cells during pregnancy. J. Clin. Endocrinol. Metab. 67:1171–1177, 1988.

Chwalisz, K., Ciesla, I., and Garfield, R.E.: Inhibition of nitric oxide (NO) synthesis induces preterm parturition and preeclampsia-like conditions in guinea pigs. Society for Gynecologic Investigation Meeting, 1994.

Clavero-Nunez, J.A., and Botella-Llusia, J.: Measurement of the villus surface in normal and pathologic placentas. Am. J. Obstet. Gynecol. 86:234–240, 1961.

Contractor, S.F.: Lysosomes in human placenta. Nature 223:1274–1275, 1969.

Contractor, S.F., Banks, R.W., Jones, C.J.P., and Fox, H.: A possible role for placental lysosomes in the formation of villous syncytiotrophoblast. Cell Tissue Res. 178:411–419, 1977.

Corte, G., Moretta, A., Cosulich, M.E., Ramarli, D., and Bargellesi, A.: A monoclonal anti-DC1 antibody selectively inhibits the generation of effector T cells mediating specific cytolytic activity. J. Exp. Med. 156:1539–1544, 1982.

Crisp, T.M., Dessouky, D.A., and Denys, F.R.: The fine structure of the human corpus luteum of early pregnancy and during the progestational phase of the menstrual cycle. Am. J. Anat. 127:37–70, 1970.

Cuthbert, P., Sedmak, D., Morgan, C., Lairmore, M., and Anderson, C.: Placental syncytiotrophoblasts do not express CD4 antigen or MRNA [abstract]. Mod. Pathol. 5:91A, 1992.

Damsky, C.H., Fitzgerald, M.L., and Fisher, S.J.: Distribution patterns of extracellular matrix components and adhesion receptors are intricately modulated during first trimester cytotrophoblast differentiation along the invasive pathway, in vivo. J. Clin. Invest. 89:210–222, 1992.

Daughaday, W.H., Mariz, I.K., and Trivedi, B.: A preferential binding site for insulin-like growth factor II in human and rat placental membranes. J. Clin. Endocrinol. Metab. 53:282–288, 1981.

Davidoff, M., and Schiebler, T.H.: Über den Feinbau der Meerschweinchenplacenta während der Entwicklung. Z. Anat. Entwicklungsgesch. 130:234–254, 1970.

De Cecco, L., Pavone, G., and Rolfini, G.: La placenta umana nella isoimmunizzazione anti Rh. Quad. Clin. Ostet. Ginecol. 18:675–682, 1963.

De Ikonicoff, L.K., and Cedard, L.: Localization of human chorionic gonadotropic and somatomammotropic hormones by the peroxidase immunohisto-enzymologic method in villi and amniotic epithelium of human placenta (from six weeks to term). Am. J. Obstet. Gynecol. 116:1124–1132, 1973.

Demir, R., and Erbengi, T.: Some new findings about Hofbauer cells in the chorionic villi of the human placenta. Acta Anat. (Basel) 119:18–26, 1984.

Demir, R., Kaufmann, P., Castellucci, M., Erbengi, T., and Kotowski, A.: Fetal vasculogenesis and angiogenesis in human placental villi. Acta Anat. (Basel) 136:190–203, 1989.

Demir, R., Demir, N., Kohnen, G., Kosanke, G., Mironov, V., Üstünel, I., and Kocamaz, E.: Ultrastructure and distribution of myofibroblast-like cells in human placental stem villi. Electron Microsc. 3:509–510, 1992.

Dempsey, E.W.: The development of capillaries in the villi of early human placentas. Am. J. Anat. 134:221–238, 1972.

Dempsey, E.W., and Luse, S.A.: Regional specializations in the syncytial trophoblast of early human placentas. J. Anat. 108:545–561, 1971.

Dempsey, E.W., and Zergollern, L.: Zonal regions of the human placenta barrier. Anat. Rec. 163:177, 1969.

Desoye, G., Hartmann, M., Blaschitz, A., Dohr, G., Hahn, T., Kohnen, G., and Kaufmann, P.: Insulin receptors in syncytiotrophoblast and fetal endothelium of human placenta. Immunohistochemical evidence for developmental changes in distribution pattern. Histochemistry 101:277–285, 1994.

Doolittle, R.F., Hunkapiller, M.W., Hood, L.E., Devare, S.G., Robbins, K.C., Aaronson, S.A., and Antoniades, H.N.: Simian sarcoma virus oncogene, v-sis, is derived from the gene (or genes) encoding a platelet derived growth factor. Science 221:275–277, 1983.

Dorgan, W.J., and Schultz, R.L.: An in vitro study of programmed death in rat placental giant cells. J. Exp. Zool. 178:497–512, 1971.

Douglas, G.C., and King, B.F.: Isolation of pure villous cytotrophoblast from term human placenta using immunomagnetic microspheres. J. Immunol. Methods 119:259–268, 1989.

Dreskin, R.B., Spicer, S.S., and Greene, W.B.: Ultrastructural localization of chorionic gonadotropin in human term placenta. J. Histochem. Cytochem. 18:862–874, 1970.

Duance, V.C., and Bailey, A.J.: Structure of the trophoblast basement membrane. In, Biology of Trophoblast. Y.W. Loke and A. Whyte, eds. Elsevier, Amsterdam, 1983.

Dujardin, M., Robyn, C., and Wilkin, P.: Mise en evidence immuno-histoenzymologique de l'hormone chorionique somatomammotrope (HCS) au niveau des divers constituants cellulaires du placenta humain normal. Biol. Cell 30:151–154, 1977.

Durst-Zivkovic, B.: Das Vorkommen der Mastzellen in der Nachgeburt. Anat. Anz. 134:225–229, 1973.

Earl, U., Estlin, C., and Bulmer, J.N.: Fibronectin and laminin in the early human placenta. Placenta 11:223–231, 1990.

Eden, T.W.: A study of the human placenta, physiological and pathological. J. Pathol. Bacteriol. 4:265–283, 1897.

Edwards, D., Jones, C.J.P., Sibley, C.P., Farmer, D.R., and Nelson, D.M.: Areas of syncytial denudation may provide routes for paracellular diffusion across the human placenta. Placenta 12:383, 1991.

Edwards, J.A., Jones, D.B., Evans, P.R., and Smith, J.L.: Differential expression of HLA class II antigens on human fetal and adult lymphocytes and macrophages. Immunology 55:489–500, 1985.

Emonard, H., Christiane, Y., Smet, M., Grimaud, J.A., and Foidart, J.M.: Type IV and interstitial collagenolytic activities in normal and malignant trophoblast cells are specifically regulated by the extracellular matrix. Invasion Metastasis 10:170–177, 1990.

Enders, A.C., and King, B.F.: The cytology of Hofbauer cells. Anat. Rec. 167:231–252, 1970.

Fant, M.E.: In vitro growth rate of placental fibroblasts is developmentally regulated. J. Clin. Invest. 88:1697–1702, 1991.

Faulk, P., Trenchev, P., Dorling, J., and Holborow, J.: Antigens on post-implantation placentae. In, Immunobiology of Trophoblast. R.G. Edwards, C.W.S. Howe, and M.H. Johnson, eds. Cambridge University Press, Cambridge, 1975.

Faulk, W.P., Jarret, R., Keane, M., Johnson, P.M., and Boackle, R.J.: Immunological studies of human placentae: complement components in immature and mature chorionic villi. Clin. Exp. Immunol. 40:299–305, 1980.

Feinberg, R.F., Kao, L.-C., Haimowitz, J.E., Queenan, J.T., Jr., Wun, T.-C., Strauss, J.F., III and Kliman, H.J.: Plasminogen activator inhibitor types 1 and 2 in human trophoblasts. PAI-1 is an immunocytochemical marker of invading trophoblasts. Lab. Invest. 61:20–26, 1989.

Feinberg, R.F., Kliman, H.J., and Lockwood, C.J.: Is oncofetal fibronectin a trophoblast glue for human implantation? Am. J. Pathol. 138:537–543, 1991.

Feller, A.C., Schneider, H., Schmidt, D., and Parwaresch, M.R.: Myofibroblast as a major cellular constituent of villous stroma in human placenta. Placenta 6:405–415, 1985.

Firth, J.A., Farr, A., and Bauman, K.: The role of gap junctions in trophoblastic cell fusion in the guinea-pig placenta. Cell Tissue Res. 205:311–318, 1980.

Firth, J.A., Bauman, K., and Sibley, C.P.: Permeability pathways in fetal placental capillaries. Trophoblast Res. 3:163–177, 1988.

Fisher, S.J., and Laine, R.A.: High alpha-amylase activity in the syncytiotrophoblastic cells of first-trimester human placentas. J. Cell Biochem. 22:47–54, 1983.

Fisher, S.J., Leitch, M.S., and Laine, A.: External labelling of glycoproteins from first-trimester human placental microvilli. Biochem. J. 221:821–828, 1984.

Flynn, A., Finke, J.H., and Hilfiker, M.L.: Placental mononuclear phagocytes as a source of interleukin-1. Science 218:475–477, 1982.

Flynn, A., Finke, J.H., and Loftus, M.A.: Comparison of interleukin-1 production by adherent cells and tissue pieces from human placenta. Immunopharmacology 9:19–26, 1985.

Folkman, J., and Haudenschild, C.: Angiogenesis in vitro. Nature 288:551–556, 1980.

Fox, H.: The villous cytotrophoblast as an index of placental ischaemia. J. Obstet. Gynaecol. Br. Commonw. 71:885–893, 1964.

Fox, H.: The significance of villous syncytial knots in the human placenta. J. Obstet. Gynaecol. Br. Commonw. 72:347–355, 1965.

Fox, H.: Perivillous fibrin deposition in the human placenta. Am. J. Obstet. Gynecol. 98:245–251, 1967a.

Fox, H.: The incidence and significance of Hofbauer cells in the mature human placenta. J. Pathol. Bacteriol. 93:710–717, 1967b.

Fox, H.: Fibrinoid necrosis of placental villi. J. Obstet. Gynaecol. Br. Commonw. 75:448–452, 1968.

Fox, H.: Effect of hypoxia on trophoblast in organ culture. Am. J. Obstet. Gynecol. 107:1058–1064, 1970.

Fox, H.: Morphological pathology of the placenta. In, The Placenta and Its Maternal Supply Line: Effects of Insufficiency on the Fetus. P. Gruenwald, ed. Medical Technical Publications, Lancaster, 1975.

Fox, H.: Pathology of the Placenta. Saunders, Philadelphia, 1978.

Fox, H., and Blanco, A.A.: Scanning electron microscopy of the human placenta in normal and abnormal pregnancies. Eur. J. Obstet. Gynecol. 4:45–50, 1974.

Frank, H.G., Malekzadeh, F., Kertschanska, S., Crescimanno, C., Castellucci, M., Lang, I., Desoye, G., and Kaufmann, P.: Immunohistochemistry of two different types of placental fibrinoid. Acta Anat. (Basel) 150:55–68, 1994.

Frauli, M., and Ludwig, H.: Demonstration of the ability of Hofbauer cells to phagocytose exogenous antibodies. Eur. J. Obstet. Gynecol. Reprod. Biol. 26:135–144, 1987a.

Frauli, M., and Ludwig, H.: Identification of human chorionic gonadotropin (HCG) secreting cells and other cell types using antibody to HCG and a new monoclonal antibody (mABlu-5) in cultures of human placental villi. Arch. Gynecol. Obstet. 241:97–110, 1987b.

Frauli, M., and Ludwig, H.: Immunocytochemical identification of mitotic Hofbauer cells in cultures of first trimester human placental villi. Arch. Gynecol. Obstet. 241:47–51, 1987c.

Freese, U.E.: The fetal-maternal circulation of the placenta. I. Histomorphologic, plastoid injection, and x-ray cinematographic studies on human placentas. Am. J. Obstet. Gynecol. 94:354–360, 1966.

Frolik, C.A., Dart, L.L., Meyers, C.A., Smith, D.M., and Sporn, M.B.: Purification and initial characterization of a type β transforming growth factor from human placenta. Proc. Natl. Acad. Sci. U.S.A. 80:3676–3680, 1983.

Fujimoto, S., Hamasaki, K., Ueda, H., and Kagawa, H.: Immunoelectron microscope observations on secretion of human placental lactogen (hPL) in the human chorionic villi. Anat. Rec. 216:68–72, 1986.

Gabius, H.-J., Debbage, P.L., Engelhardt, R., Osmers, R., and Lange, W.: Identification of endogenous sugar-binding proteins (lectins) in human placenta by histochemical localization and biochemical characterization. Eur. J. Cell Biol. 44:265–272, 1987.

Galbraith, G.M.P., Galbraith, R.M., Temple, A., and Faulk, W.P.: Demonstration of transferrin receptors on human placental trophoblast. Blood 55:240–242, 1980.

Galton, M.: DNA content of placental nuclei. J. Cell Biol. 13:183–191, 1962.

Garfield, R.E., Yallampalli, C., Buhimschi, I. and Chwalisz, K.: Reversal of preeclampsia symptoms induced in rats by nitric oxide inhibition with L-arginine, steroid hormones and an endothelin antagonist. Presented at the Society for Gynecologic Investigation Meeting, 1994.

Gaspard, U.J., Hustin, J., Reuter, A.M., Lambotte, R., and Franchimont, P.: Immunofluorescent localization of placental lactogen, chorionic gonadotrophin and its alpha and beta subunits in organ cultures of human placenta. Placenta 1:135–144, 1980.

Geier, G., Schuhmann, R., and Kraus, H.: Regional unterschiedliche Zellproliferation innerhalb der Plazentone reifer menschlicher Plazenten: autoradiographische Untersuchungen. Arch. Gynecol. 218:31–37, 1975.

Geller, H.F.: Über die sogenannten Hofbauerzellen in der reifen menschlichen Placenta. Arch. Gynecol. 188:481–496, 1957.

Geller, H.F.: Elektronenmikroskopische Befunde am Synzytium der menschlichen Plazenta. Geburtshilfe Frauenheilkd. 22:1234–1237, 1962.

Genbacev, O., Robyn, C., and Pantic, V.: Localization of chorionic gonadotropin in human term placenta on ultrathin sections with peroxidase-labeled antibody. J. Microsc. 15:399–402, 1972.

Gerl, D., Eichhorn, H., Eichhorn, K.-H., and Franke, H.: Quantitative Messungen synzytialer Zellkernkonzentrationen der menschlichen Plazenta bei normalen und pathologischen Schwangerschaften. Zentralbl. Gynäkol. 95:263–266, 1973.

Gey, G.O., Seegar, G.E., and Hellman, L.M.: The production of a gonadotrophic substance (prolan) by placental cells in tissue culture. Science 88:306–307, 1938.

Gille, J., Börner, P., Reinecke, J., Krause, P.-H., and Deicher, H.: Über die Fibrinoidablagerungen in den Endzotten der menschlichen Placenta. Arch. Gynecol. 217:263–271, 1974.

Gillim, S.W., Christensen, A.K., and McLennan, Ch.E.: Fine structure of the human menstrual corpus luteum at its stage of maximum secretory activity. Am. J. Anat. 126:409–428, 1969.

Glover, D.M., Brownstein, D., Burchette, S., Larsen, A., and Wilson, C.B.: Expression of HLA class II antigens and secretion of interleukin-1 by monocytes and macrophages from adults and neonates. Immunology 61:195–201, 1987.

Goldstein, J., Braverman, M., Salafia, C., and Buckley, P.: The phenotype of human placental macrophages and its variation with gestational age. Am. J. Pathol. 133:648–659, 1988.

Gosseye, S., and Fox, H.: An immunohistological comparison of the secretory capacity of villous and extravillous trophoblast in the human placenta. Placenta 5:329–348, 1984.

Gossrau, R., Graf, R., Ruhnke, M., and Hanski, C.: Proteases in the human full-term placenta. Histochemistry 86:405–413, 1987.

Goustin, A.S., Betsholtz, C., Pfeifer-Ohlsson, S., Persson, H., Rydnert, J., Bywater, M., Holmgren, G., Heldin, C.-H., Westermark, B., and Ohlsson, R.: Coexpression of the sis and myc proto-oncogenes in developing human placenta suggests autocrine control of trophoblast growth. Cell 41:301–312, 1985.

Goyert, S.M., Ferrero, E.M., Seremetis, S.V., Winchester, R.J., Silver, J., and Mattison, A.C.: Biochemistry and expression of myelomonocytic antigens. J. Immunol. 137:3909–3914, 1986.

Goyert, S.M., Ferrero, E.M., Rettig, W.J., Yenamandra, A.K., Obata, F., and Le Beau, M.M.: The CD14 monocyte differentiation antigen maps to a region encoding growth factors and receptors. Science 239:497–500, 1988.

Graf Spee, F.: Anatomie und Physiologie der Schwangerschaft. In, Handbuch der Geburtshilfe. Vol. 1. A. Doederlein, ed., pp. 3–152. Bergmann, Wiesbaden, 1915.

Green, T., and Ford, H.C.: Human placental microvilli contain high-affinity binding sites for folate. Biochem. J. 218:75–80, 1984.

Grillo, M.A.: Cytoplasmic inclusions resembling nucleoli in sympathetic neurones of adult rats. J. Cell Biol. 45:100–117, 1970.

Gröschel-Stewart, U.: Plazenta als endokrines Organ. In, Die Plazenta des Menschen. V. Becker, Th.H. Schiebler, and F. Kubli, eds., pp. 217–233. Thieme Verlag, Stuttgart, 1981.

Hamanaka, N., Tanizawa, O., Hashimoto, T., Yoshinari, S., and Okudaira, Y.: Electron microscopic study on the localization of human chorionic gonadotropin (HCG) in the chorionic tissue by enzyme labeled antibody technique. J. Electron Microsc. 20:46–48, 1971.

Hamilton, W.J., and Boyd, J.D.: Specializations of the syncytium of the human chorion. B.M.J. 1:1501–1506, 1966.

Hardingham, T.E., and Fosang, A.J.: Proteoglycans: many forms and many functions. FASEB J. 6:861–870, 1992.

Hashimoto, M., Kosaka, M., Mori, Y., Komori, A., and Akashi, K.: Electron microscopic studies on the epithelium of the chorionic villi of the human placenta. I. J. Jpn. Obstet. Gynecol. Soc. 7:44, 1960a.

Hashimoto, M., Shimoyama, T., Hirasawa, T., Komori, A., Kawasaki, T., and Akashi, K.: Electron microscopic studies on the epithelium of the chorionic villi of the human placenta. II. J. Jpn. Obstet. Gynecol. Soc. 7:122, 1960b.

Hay, D.L.: Placental histology and the production of human choriogonadotrophin and its subunits in pregnancy. Br. J. Obstet. Gynaecol. 95:1268–1275, 1988.

Haziot, A., Chen, S., Ferrero, E., Low, M.G., Silber, R., and Goyert, S.M.: The monocyte differentiation antigen, CD14, is anchored to the cell membrane by a phosphatidylinositol linkage. J. Immunol. 141:547–552, 1988.

Hedley, R., and Bradbury, M.B.W.: Transport of polar nonelectrolytes across the intact and perfused guinea-pig placenta. Placenta 1:277–285, 1980.

Heinrich, D., Metz, J., Raviola, E., and Forssmann, W.G.: Ultrastructure of perfusion fixed fetal capillaries in the human placenta. Cell Tissue Res. 172:157–169, 1976.

Heinrich, D., Weihe, E., Gruner, C., and Metz, J.: Vergleichende Morphologie der Placentakapillaren. Anat. Anz. 71:489–491, 1977.

Heinrich, D., Aoki, A., and Metz, J.: Fetal capillary organization in different types of placenta. Trophoblast Res. 3:149–162, 1988.

Hempel, E., and Geyer, G.: Submikroskopische Verteilung der alkalischen Phosphatase in der menschlichen Placenta. Acta Histochem. 34:138–147, 1969.

Hemsen, A., Gillis, C., Larson, O., Haegerstrand, A., and Lundberg, J.M.: Characterization, localization and actions of endothelin in umbilical vessels and placenta of man. Acta Physiol. Scand. 43:395–404, 1991.

Herbst, R., and Multier, A.M.: Les microvillosites a la surface des villosites chorioniques du placenta humain. Gynecol. Obstet. 69:609–616, 1970.

Herbst, R., Multier, A.M., and Hörmann, G.: Die menschlichen Plazentazotten des 2. Schwangerschaftstrimenon im elektronenoptischen Bild. Z. Geburtshilfe Gynäkol. 169:1–16, 1968.

Herbst, R., Multier, A.M., and Hörmann, G.: Elektronenoptische Untersuchungen an menschlichen Placentazotten. Zentralbl. Gynäkol. 91:465–475, 1969.

Hertig, A.T.: Angiogenesis in the early human chorion and in the primary placenta of the macaque monkey. Contrib. Embryol. Carnegie Inst. 25:37–81, 1935.

Hey, A., and Röckelein, G.: Die sog. Endothelvakuolen der Plazentagefäße—Physiologie oder Krankheit? Pathologe 10:66–67, 1989.

Hofbauer, J.: Über das konstante Vorkommen bisher unbekannter zelliger Formelemente in der Chorionzotte der menschlichen Plazenta und über Embryotrophe. Wien. Klin. Wochenschr. 16:871–873, 1903.

Hofbauer, J.: Grundzüge einer Biologie der menschlichen Plazenta mit besonderer Berücksichtigung der Fragen der fötalen Ernährung. Braumüller, Vienna, 1905.

Hofbauer, J.: The function of the Hofbauer cells of the chorionic villus particularly in relation to acute infection and syphilis. Am. J. Obstet. Gynecol. 10:1–14, 1925.

Hoffman, L.H., and Di Pietro, D.L.: Subcellular localization of human placental acid phosphatases. Am. J. Obstet. Gynecol. 114:1087–1096, 1972.

Holmgren, L., Glaser, A., Pfeifer-Ohlsson, S., and Ohlsson, R.: Angiogenesis during human extraembryonic development involves the spatiotemporal control of PDGF ligand and receptor gene expression. Development 113:749–754, 1991.

Horky, Z.: Beitrag zur Funktionsbedeutung der Hofbauer-Zellen (Beobachtungen in der Placenta bei Diabetes mellitus). Zentralbl. Gynäkol. 86:1621–1626, 1964.

Hörmann, G.: Haben die sogenannten Hofbauerzellen der Chorionzotten funktionelle Bedeutung? Zentralbl. Gynäkol. 69:1199–1205, 1947.

Hörmann, G.: Die Reifung der menschlichen Chorionzotte im Lichte ökonomischer Zweckmäßigkeit. Zentralbl. Gynäkol. 70:625–631, 1948.

Hörmann, G.: Ein Beitrag zur funktionellen Morphologie der menschlichen Placenta. Arch. Gynecol. 184:109–123, 1953.

Hörmann, G.: Die Fibrinoidisierung des Chorionepithels als Konstruktionsprinzip der menschlichen Plazenta. Z. Geburtshilfe Gynäkol. 164:263–269, 1965.

Hörmann, G., Herbst, R., and Ullmann, G.: Die Transformation des Zytotrophoblasten in den Synzytiotrophoblasten. Z. Geburtshilfe. Gynäkol. 171:171–182, 1969.

Hoshina, M., Boothby, M., and Boime, I.: Cytological localization of chorionic gonadotropin and placental lactogen mRNAs during development of the human placenta. J. Cell Biol. 93:190–198, 1982.

Hoshina, M., Hussa, R., Patillo, R., and Boime, I.: Cytological distribution of chorionic gonadotropin subunit and placental lactogen messenger RNA in neoplasms derived from human placenta. J. Cell Biol. 97:1200–1206, 1983.

Hoshina, M., Boime, I., and Mochizuki, M.: Cytological localization of hPL and hCG mRNA in chorionic tissue using in situ hybridization. Acta Obstet. Gynecol. Jpn. 36:397–404, 1984.

Howatson, A.G., Farquharson, M., Meager, A., McNicol, A.M., and Foulis, A.K.: Localization of alpha-interferon in the human feto-placental unit. J. Endocrinol. 119:531–534, 1988.

Huber, C.P., Carter, J.E., and Vellios, F.: Lesions of the circulatory system of the placenta: a study of 243 placentas with special reference to the developments of infarcts. Am. J. Obstet. Gynecol. 81:560–572, 1961.

Huguenin, B.: Über die Genese der Fibringerinnungen und Infarktbildungen der menschlichen Placenta. Beitr. Geburtshilfe Gynäkol. 13:339–357, 1909.

Hulstaert, C.E., Torringa, J.L., Koudstaal, J., Hardonk, M.J., and Molenaar, I.: The characteristic distribution of alkaline phosphatase in the full-term human placenta. Gynecol. Invest. 4:24–30, 1973.

Hunt, J.S.: Cytokine networks in the uteroplacental unit: macrophages as pivotal regulatory cells. J. Reprod. Immunol. 16:1–17, 1989.

Ikawa, A.: Observations on the epithelium of human chorionic villi with the electron microscope. J. Jpn. Obstet. Gynecol. Soc. 6:219, 1959.

Iklé, F.A.: Trophoblastzellen im strömenden Blut. Schweiz. Med. Wochenschr. 91:934–945, 1964.

Ishikawa, F., Miyazono, K., Hellman, U., Drexler, H., Wernstedt, C., Hagiwara, K., Usuki, K., Takaku, F., Risau, W., and Heldin, C.-H.: Identification of angiogenic activity and the cloning and expression of platelet-derived endothelial cell growth factor. Nature 338:557–562, 1989.

Jackson, M.R., Joy, C.F., Mayhem, T.M., and Haas, J.D.: Stereological studies on the true thickness of the villous membrane in human term placentae: a study of placentae from high-altitude pregnancies. Placenta 6:249–258, 1985.

Jeffcoate, T.N.A., and Scott, J.S.: Some observations on the placental factor in pregnancy toxemia. Am. J. Obstet. Gynecol. 77:475–489, 1959.

Jemmerson, R., Klier, F.G., and Fishman, W.H.: Clustered distribution of human placental alkaline phosphatase on the surface of both placental and cancer cells. J. Histochem. Cytochem. 33:1227–1234, 1985.

Jimenez, E., Vogel, M., Arabin, B., Wagner, G., and Mirsalim, P.: Correlation of ultrasonographic measurement of the utero-placental and fetal blood flow with the morphological diagnosis of placental function. Trophoblast Res. 3:325–334, 1988.

Johnson, P.M., and Brown, P.J.: The IgG and transferrin receptors of the human syncytiotrophoblast microvillous plasma membrane. Am. J. Reprod. Immunol. 1:4–9, 1980.

Johnson, P.M., and Brown, P.J.: Fc gamma receptors in the human placenta. Placenta 2:355–369, 1981.

Jones, C.J.P., and Fox, H.: Syncytial knots and intervillous bridges in the human placenta: an ultrastructural study. J. Anat. 124:275–286, 1977.

Jones, C.J.P., Hartmann, M., Blaschitz, A., and Desoye, G.: Ultrastructural localization of insulin receptors in human placenta. Am. J. Reprod. Immunol. 30:136–145, 1993.

Kameda, T., Koyama, M., Matsuzaki, N., Taniguchi, T., Fumitaka, S., and Tanizawa, O.: Localization of three subtypes of Fc gamma receptors in human placenta by immunohistochemical analysis. Placenta 12:15–26, 1991.

Kameya, T., Watanabe, K., Kobayashi, T., and Mukojima, T.: Enzyme- and immuno-histochemical localization of human placental alkaline phosphatase. Acta Histochem. Cytochem. 6:124–136, 1973.

Kao, L.-C., Caltabiano, S., Wu, S., Strauss, J.F., III, and Kliman, H.J.: The human villous cytotrophoblast: interactions with extracellular matrix proteins, endocrine function, and cytoplasmic differentiation in the absence of syncytium formation. Dev. Biol. 130:693–702, 1988.

Kastschenko, N.: Das menschliche Chorionepithel und dessen Rolle bei der Histogenese der Placenta. Arch. Anat. Physiol. (Leipzig), 451–480, 1885.

Katabuchi, H., Naito, M., Miyamura, S., Takahashi, K., and Okamura, H.: Macrophages in human chorionic villi. Prog. Clin. Biol. Res. 296:453–458, 1989.

Kaufmann, P.: Über polypenartige Vorwölbungen an Zell- und Syncytiumoberflächen in reifen menschlichen Plazenten. Z. Zellforsch. 102:266–272, 1969.

Kaufmann, P.: Untersuchungen über die Langhanszellen in der menschlichen Placenta. Z. Zellforsch. 128:283–302, 1972.

Kaufmann, P.: Experiments on infarct genesis caused by blockage of carbohydrate metabolism in guinea pig placenta. Virchows Arch. Pathol. Anat. Histol. 368:11–21, 1975a.

Kaufmann, P.: Über die Bedeutung von Plasmaprotrusionen an reifenden und alternden Zellen. Anat. Anz. 69:307–312, 1975b.

Kaufmann, P.: Fibrinoid. In, Die Plazenta des Menschen. V. Becker, Th.H. Schiebler, and F. Kubli, eds. Thieme, Stuttgart, 1981.

Kaufmann, P.: Vergleichend-anatomische und funktionelle Aspekte des Placenta-Baues. Funkt. Biol. Med. 2:71–79, 1983.

Kaufmann, P.: Influence of ischemia and artificial perfusion on placental ultrastructure and morphometry. Contrib. Gynecol. Obstet. 13:18–26, 1985.

Kaufmann, P., and Miller, R.K., eds.: Placental vascularization and blood flow: basic research and clinical applications. Trophoblast Res. 3:1–370, 1988.

Kaufmann, P., and Stark, J.: Enzymhistochemische Untersuchungen an reifen menschlichen Placentazotten. I. Reifungs- und Alterungsvorgänge am Trophoblasten. Histochemistry 29:65–82, 1972.

Kaufmann, P., and Stark, J.: Semidünnschnitt-cytochemische und immunautoradiographische Befunde zum Hormonstoffwechsel der reifen menschlichen Placenta. Anat. Anz. 67: 245–249, 1973.

Kaufmann, P., and Stegner, H.E.: Über die funktionelle Differenzierung des Zottensyncytiums in der menschlichen Placenta. Z. Zellforsch. 135:361–382, 1972.

Kaufmann, P., Schiebler, Th.H., Ciobotaru, C., and Stark, J.: Enzymhistochemische Untersuchungen an reifen menschlichen Placentazotten. II. Zur Gliederung des Syncytiotrophoblasten. Histochemistry 40:191–207, 1974a.

Kaufmann, P., Thorn, W., and Jenke, B.: Die Morphologie der Meerschweinchenplacenta nach Monojodacetat- und Fluorid-Vergiftung. Arch. Gynecol. 216:185–203, 1974b.

Kaufmann, P., Gentzen, D.M., and Davidoff, M.: Die Ultrastruktur von Langhanszellen in pathologischen menschlichen Placenten. Arch. Gynecol. 22:319–332, 1977a.

Kaufmann, P., Stark, J., and Stegner, H.E.: The villous stroma of the human placenta. I. The ultrastructure of fixed connective tissue cells. Cell Tissue Res. 177:105–121, 1977b.

Kaufmann, P., Schröder, H., and Leichtweiss, H.-P.: Fluid shift across the placenta. II. Fetomaternal transfer of horseradish peroxidase in the guinea pig. Placenta 3:339–348, 1982.

Kaufmann, P., Nagl, W., and Fuhrmann, B.: Die funktionelle Bedeutung der Langhanszellen der menschlichen Placenta. Anat. Anz. 77:435–436, 1983.

Kaufmann, P., Luckhardt, M., Schweikhart, G., and Cantle, S.J.: Cross-sectional features and three-dimensional structure of human placental villi. Placenta 8:235–247, 1987a.

Kaufmann, P., Schröder, H., Leichtweiss, H.-P., and Winterhager, E.: Are there membrane-lined channels through the trophoblast? A study with lanthanum hydroxide. Trophoblast Res. 2:557–571, 1987b.

Kaufmann, P., Firth, J.A., Sibley, C.P., and Schröder, H.: Feto-maternal protein permeability of the placenta-tracer studies using various haeme proteins and lanthanum hydroxide. Gegenbaurs Morphol. Jahrb. 135:305, 1989.

Kelley, L.K., King, B.F., Johnson, L.W., and Smith, C.H.: Protein composition and structure of human placental microvillous membrane. Exp. Cell Res. 123:167–176, 1979.

Kemnitz, P.: Die Morphogenese des Zottentrophoblasten der menschlichen Plazenta—Ein Beitrag zum Synzytiumproblem. Zentralbl. Allg. Pathol. 113:71–76, 1970.

Kertschanska, S., and Kaufmann, P.: Morphological evidence for the existence of transtrophoblastic channels in human placental villi. Placenta 13:A33, 1992.

Kertschanska, S., Kosanke, G., and Kaufmann, P.: Is there morphological evidence for the existence of transtrophoblastic channels in human placental villi? Trophoblast Res. 8 (1994, in press).

Khansari, N., and Fudenberg, H.H.: Functional heterogeneity of human cord blood monocytes. Scand. J. Immunol. 19: 337–342, 1984.

Khodr, G.S., and Siler-Khodr, T.M.: Localization of luteinizing hormone releasing factor (LRF) in the human placenta. Fertil. Steril. 29:523–526, 1978.

Khong, T.Y., Lane, E.B., and Robertson, W.B.: An immunocytochemical study of fetal cells at the maternal-placental interface using monoclonal antibodies to keratins, vimentin and desmin. Cell Tissue Res. 246:189–195, 1986.

Kim, Ch.K., and Benirschke, K.: Autoradiographic study of the "X cells" in the human placenta. Am. J. Obstet. Gynecol. 109:96–102, 1971.

Kim, Ch.K., Naftolin, F., and Benirschke, K.: Immunohistochemical studies of the "X cell" in the human placenta with anti-human chorionic gonadotropin and anti-human placental lactogen. Am. J. Obstet. Gynecol. 111:672–676, 1971.

King, B.F.: Localization of transferrin on the surface of the human placenta by electron microscopic immunocyto-chemistry. Anat. Rec. 186:151–159, 1976.

King, B.F.: The distribution and mobility of anionic sites on the surface of human placental syncytial trophoblast. Anat. Rec. 199:15–22, 1981.

King, B.F.: The organization of actin filaments in human placental villi. J. Ultrastruct. Res. 85:320–328, 1983.

King, B.F.: Ultrastructural differentiation of stromal and vascular components in early macaque placental villi. Am. J. Anat. 178:30–44, 1987.

King, B.F., and Menton, D.N.: Scanning electron microscopy of human placental villi from early and late in gestation. Am. J. Obstet. Gynecol. 122:824–828, 1975.

Kjaeldgaard, A., Pschera, H., Larsson, B., Gaffney, P., and Åstedt, B.: Plasminogen activators and inhibitors in amniotic fluid. Fibrinolysis 3:203–206, 1989.

Kliman, H.J., and Feinberg, R.F.: Human trophoblast-extracellular matrix (ECM) interactions in vitro: ECM thickness modulates morphology and proteolytic activity. Proc. Natl. Acad. Sci. U.S.A. 87:3057–3061, 1990.

Kliman, H.J., Nestler, J.E., Sermasi, E., Sanger, J.M., and Strauss, J.F., III: Purification, characterization and in vitro differentiation of cytotrophoblasts from human term placenta. Endocrinology 118:1567–1582, 1986.

Kliman, H.J., Feinman, M.A., and Strauss, J.F., III: Differentiation of human cytotrophoblasts into syncytiotro-phoblasts in culture. Trophoblast Res. 2:407–421, 1987.

Kline, B.S.: Microscopic observations of development of human placenta. Am. J. Obstet. Gynecol. 61:1065–1074, 1951.

Knobil, E., and Neill, J.D., eds.: The Physiology of Reproduction. Vol. 2. Raven Press, New York, 1993.

Knoth, M.: Ultrastructure of chorionic villi from a four-somite human embryo. J. Ultrastruct. Res. 25:423–440, 1968.

Kohnen, G.: Immunhistochemische Charakterisierung extravaskulärer kontraktiler Zellen in menschlichen Placentazotten. Medical thesis, Technical University of Aachen, 1994.

Kohnen, G., Mironov, V., Demir, R., Castellucci, M., and Kaufmann, P.: Immunhistochemische Klassifizierung von Stammzotten in der menschlichen Plazenta. Anat. Anz. 174 (Suppl.):127, 1992.

Kohnen, G., Castellucci, M., Graf, R., and Kaufmann, P.: Contractile filaments of extravascular stromal cells in human placental villi. Placenta 14:A38, 1993a.

Kohnen, G., Kosanke, G., Korr, H., and Kaufmann, P.: Comparison of various proliferation markers applied to human placental tissue. Placenta 14:A38, 1993b.

Korhonen, M., Ylanne, J., Laitinen, L., Cooper, H.M., Quaranta, V., and Virtanen, I.: Distribution of the alpha 1–alpha 6 integrin subunits in human developing and term placenta. Lab. Invest. 65:347–356, 1991.

Krantz, K.E., and Parker, J.C.: Contractile properties of the smooth muscle in the human placenta. Clin. Obstet. Gynecol. 93:253–258, 1963.

Kristoffersen, E.K., Ulvestad, E., Vedeler, C.A., and Matre, R.: Fc-gamma receptor heterogeneity in the human placenta. Scand. J. Immunol. 31:561–564, 1990.

Kubli, F., and Budliger, H.: Beitrag zur Morphologie der insuffizienten Plazenta. Geburtshilfe Frauenheilkd. 23:37–43, 1963.

Kunicki, T.J., Nugent, D.J., Staats, S.J., Orchekowski, R.P., Wayner, E.A., and Carter, W.G.: The human fibroblast class II extracellular matrix receptor mediates platelet adhesion to collagen and is identical to the platelet Ia-IIa complex. J. Biol. Chem. 263:4516–4519, 1988.

Kurman, R.J., Young, R.H., Norris, H.J., Main, C.S., Lawrence, W.D., and Scully, R.E.: Immunocytochemical localization of placental lactogen and chorionic gonado-tropin in the normal placenta and trophoblastic tumors, with emphasis on intermediate trophoblast and the placental site trophoblastic tumor. Int. J. Gynecol. Pathol. 3:101–121, 1984.

Küstermann, W.: Über "Proliferationsknoten" und "Syn-cytialknoten" der menschlichen Placenta. Anat. Anz. 150:144–157, 1981.

Laatikainen, T., Saijonmaa, O., Salminen, K., and Wahlström, T.: Localization and concentrations of beta-endorphin and beta-lipotrophin in human placenta. Placenta 8:381–387, 1987.

Ladines-Llave, C.A., Maruo, T., Manalo, A.S., and Mochizuki, M.: Cytologic localization of epidermal growth factor and its receptor in developing human placenta varies over the course of pregnancy. Am. J. Obstet. Gynecol. 165:1377–1382, 1991.

Lafond, J., Auger, D., Fortier, J., and Brunette, M.G.: Parathyroid hormone receptor in human placental syn-cytiotrophoblast brush border and basal plasma membranes. Endocrinology 123:2834–2840, 1988.

Lala, P.K., and Graham, C.H.: Mechanisms of trophoblast invasiveness and their control: the role of proteases and protease inhibitors. Cancer Metastasis Rev. 9:369–379, 1990.

Lamarre, D., Ashkenazi, A., Fleury, S., Smith, D.H., Sekaly, R.-P., and Capon, D.J.: The MHC-binding and gp 120-binding functions of CD4 are separable. Science 245:743–746, 1989.

Lang, I., Dohr, G., and Desoye, G.: Isolation and culture of fetal vascular endothelial cells derived from human full term placenta. Placenta 14:A40, 1993a.

Lang, I., Hartmann, M., Blaschitz, A., Dohr, G., Skofitsch, G., and Desoye, G.: Immunohistochemical evidence for the heterogeneity of maternal and fetal vascular endothelial cells in human full-term placenta. Cell Tissue Res. 274:211–218, 1993b.

Langhans, T.: Zur Kenntnis der menschlichen Placenta. Arch. Gynäkol. 1:317–334, 1870.

Langhans, T.: Untersuchungen über die menschliche Placenta. Arch. Anat. Physiol. Anat. Abt. 188–267, 1877.

Latta, J.S., and Beber, C.R.: Cells with metachromatic granules in the stroma of human chorionic villi. Science 117:498–499, 1953.

Leach, L., Eaton, B.M., Firth, J.A., and Contractor, S.F.: Immunogold localisation of endogenous immunoglobulin-G in ultrathin frozen sections of the human placenta. Cell

Tissue Res. 257:603–607, 1989.

Leach, L., Bhasin, Y., Clark, P., and Firth, J.A.: Isolation and characterisation of human microsvascular endothelial cells from chorionic villi of term placenta. Placenta 14:A41, 1993.

Leibl, W., Kerjaschki, D., and Hörandner, H.: Mikrovillusfreie Areale an Chorionzotten menschlicher Placenten. Gegenbaurs Morphol. Jahrb. 121:26–28, 1975.

Lemtis, H.: Über die Architektonik des Zottengefäßapparates der menschlichen Plazenta. Anat. Anz. 102:106–133, 1955.

Lemtis, H.: Physiologie der Placenta. Bibl. Gynaecol. (Basel) 54:1–52, 1970.

Lessin, D.L., Hunt, J.S., King, C.R., and Wood, G.W.: Antigen expression by cells near the maternal-fetal interface. Am. J. Reprod. Immunol. Microbiol. 16:1–7, 1988.

Lewis, S.H., Reynolds-Kohler, C., Fox, H.E., and Nelson, J.A.: HIV-1 in trophoblastic and villous Hofbauer cells, and haematological precursors in eight-week fetuses. Lancet 335:565–568, 1990.

Lewis, W.H.: Hofbauer cells (clasmatocytes) of the human chorionic villus. Bull. Johns Hopkins Hosp. 35:183–185, 1924.

Librach, C.L., Werb, Z., Fitzgerald, M.L., Chiu, K., Corwin, N.M., Esteves, R.A., Grobelny, D., Galardy, R., Damsky, C.H., and Fisher, S.J.: 92-kD Type IV collagenase mediates invasion of human cytotrophoblasts. J. Cell Biol. 113:437–449, 1991.

Liebhaber, S.A., Urbanek, M., Ray, J., Ruan, R.S., and Cooke, N.E.: Characterization and histologic localization of human growth hormone-variant gene expression in the placenta. J. Clin. Invest. 83:1985–1991, 1989.

Liebhart, M.: Some observations on so-called fibrinoid necrosis of placental villi: an electron-microscopic study. Pathol. Eur. 6:217–220, 1971.

Liebhart, M.: Polysaccharide surface coat (glycocalix) of human placental villi. Pathol. Eur. 9:3–10, 1974.

Lister, U.M.: Ultrastructure of the early human placenta. J. Obstet. Gynaecol. Br. Commonw. 71:21–32, 1964.

Lister, U.M.: The localization of placental enzymes with the electron microscope. J. Obstet. Gynaecol. Br. Commonw. 74:34–49, 1967.

Loke, Y.W., Eremin, O., Ashby, J., and Day, S.: Characterization of the phagocytic cells isolated from the human placenta. J. Reticuloendothel. Soc. 31:317–324, 1982.

Luckett, W.P.: The fine structure of the placental villi of the rhesus monkey (Macaca mulatta). Anat. Rec. 167:141–164, 1970.

Luckett, W.P.: Origin and differentiation of the yolk sac and extraembryonic mesoderm in presomite human and rhesus monkey embryos. Am. J. Anat. 152:59–97, 1978.

Lupu, R., Colomer, R., Kannan, B., and Lippman, M.E.: Characterization of a growth factor that binds exclusively to the erbB-2 receptor and induces cellular responses. Proc. Natl. Acad. Sci. U.S.A. 89:2287–2291, 1992.

Macara, L.M., Kingdom, J.C.P., and Kaufmann, P.: Control of fetoplacental circulation. Fetal Maternal Med. Rev. 5:167–179, 1993.

Mahnke, P.F., and Jacob, C.: Histologische, histochemische und papierchromatographische Untersuchungen an Mastzellen (MZ) der menschlichen Plazenta. Z. Mikrosk. Anat.

Forsch. 85:105–122, 1972.

Malassine, A., Goldstein, S., Alsat, E., Merger, Ch., and Cedard, L.: Ultrastructural localization of low density lipoprotein bindings site on the surface of the syncytial microvillous membranes of the human placenta. IRCS Med. Sci. 12:166–167, 1984.

Malassine, A., Besse, C., Roche, A., Alsat, E., Rebourcet, R., Mondon, F., and Cedard, L.: Ultrastructural visualization of the internalization of low density lipoprotein by human placental cells. Histochemistry 87:457–464, 1987.

Malassine, A., Cronier, L., Mondon, F., Mignot, T.M., and Ferre, F.: Localization and production of immunoreactive endothelin-1 in the trophoblast of human placenta. Cell Tissue Res. 271:491–497, 1993.

Marchand, F.: Über das maligne Chorionepitheliom. Berl. Klin. Wochenschr. 35:249–250, 1898.

Marez, A., Nguyen, T., Chevallier, B., Clement, G., Dauchel, M.C., and Barritault, D.: Platelet derived growth factor is present in human placenta: purification from an industrially processed fraction. Biochimie 69:125–129, 1987.

Martin, B.J., and Spicer, S.S.: Multivesicular bodies and related structures of the syncytiotrophoblast of human term placenta. Anat. Rec. 175:15–36, 1973a.

Martin, B.J., and Spicer, S.S.: Ultrastructural features of cellular maturation and aging in human trophoblast. J. Ultrastruct. Res. 43:133–149, 1973b.

Martin, B.J., Spicer, S.S., and Smythe, N.M.: Cytochemical studies of the maternal surface of the syncytiotrophoblast of human early and term placenta. Anat. Rec. 178:769–786, 1974.

Martinoli, C., Castellucci, M., Zaccheo, D., and Kaufmann, P.: Scanning electron microscopy of stromal cells of human placental villi throughout pregnancy. Cell Tissue Res. 235:647–655, 1984.

Maruo, T., and Mochizuki, M.: Immunohistochemical localization of epidermal growth factor receptor and myc oncogene product in human placenta: implication for trophoblast proliferation and differentiation. Am. J. Obstet. Gynecol. 156:721–727, 1987.

Maruo, T., Matsuo, H., Oishi, T., Hayashi, M., Nishino, R., and Mochizuki, M.: Induction of differentiated trophoblast function by epidermal growth factor: relation of immunohistochemically detected cellular epidermal growth factor receptor levels. J. Clin. Endocrinol. Metab. 64:744–750, 1987.

Matsubara, S., Tamada, T., Kurahashi, K., and Saito, T.: Ultracytochemical localizations of adenosine nucleotidase activities in the human term placenta, with special reference to 5'-nucleotidase activity. Acta Histochem. Cytochem. 20:409–419, 1987a.

Matsubara, S., Tamada, T., and Saito, T.: Cytochemical study of the electron microscopical localization of Ca ATPase activity in the human trophoblast. Acta Obstet. Gynecol. Jpn. 39:1080–1086, 1987b.

Matsubara, S., Tamada, T., and Saito, T.: Ultracytochemical localizations of adenylate cyclase, guanylate cyclase and cyclic 3',5'-nucleotide phosphodiesterase activity on the trophoblast in the human placenta. Histochemistry 87:505–509, 1987c.

Matsubara, S., Tamada, T., and Saito, T.: Ultracytochemical

localizations of alkaline phosphatase and acid phosphatase activities in the human term placenta. Acta Histochem. Cytochem. 20:283–294, 1987d.

Mayer, M., Panigel, M., and Tozum, R.: Observations sur l'aspect radiologique de la vascularisation fetale du placenta humain isole mainten en survie par perfusion de liquides physiologiques. Gynecol. Obstet. (Paris) 58:391–397, 1959.

Mayhew, T.M.: The problem of ambiguous profiles of microvilli between apposed cell surfaces: a stereological solution. J. Microsc. 139:327–330, 1985.

Mayhew, T.M.: Scaling placental oxygen diffusion to birth-weight: studies on placentae from low- and high-altitude pregnancies. J. Anat. 175:187–194, 1991.

Mayhew, T.M., and Burton, G.J.: Methodological problems in placental morphometry: apologia for the use of stereology based on sound sampling practice. Placenta 9:565–581, 1988.

Mayhew, T.M., Jackson, M.R., and Haas, J.D.: Oxygen diffusive conductances of human placentae from term pregnancies at low and high altitudes. Placenta 11:493–503, 1990.

McCormick, J.N., Faulk, W.P., Fox, H., and Fudenberg, H.H.: Immunohistological and elution studies of the human placenta. J. Exp. Med. 91:1–13, 1971.

McKay, D.G., Hertig, A.T., Adams, E.C., and Richardson, M.V.: Histochemical observations on the human placenta. Obstet. Gynecol. 12:1–36, 1958.

Mebius, R.E., Martens, G., Breve', J., Delemarra, F.G.A., and Kraal, G.: Is early repopulation of macrophage-depleted lymph node independent of blood monocyte immigration? Eur. J. Immunol. 21:3041–3044, 1991.

Merrill, J.A.: Common pathological changes of the placenta. Clin. Obstet. Gynecol. 6:96–109, 1963.

Merttens, I.: Beiträge zur normalen und pathologischen Anatomic der menschlichen Placenta. Z. Geburtshilfe Gynakol. 30:1–22, 1894.

Metz, J., Heinrich, D., and Forssmann, W.G.: Ultrastructure of the labyrinth in the rat full term placenta. Anat. Embryol. 149:123–148, 1976.

Metz, J., Weihe, E., and Heinrich, D.: Intercellular junctions in the full term human placenta. I. Syncytiotrophoblastic layer. Anat. Embryol. 158:41–50, 1979.

Meyer, A.W.: On the nature, occurrence and identity of the plasma cells of Hofbauer. J. Morphol. 32:327–349, 1919.

Midgley, A.R., and Pierce, G.B.: Immunohistochemical localization of human chorionic gonadotropin. J. Exp. Med. 115:289–297, 1962.

Miller, R.K., and Thiede, H.A., eds.: Fetal nutrition, metabolism, and immunology: the role of the placenta. Trophoblast Res. 1:1–387, 1984.

Miller, D., Pelton, R., Deryick, R., and Moses, H.: Transforming growth factor-β: a family of growth regulatory peptides. Ann. N. Y. Acad. Sci. 593:208–217, 1990.

Minot, C.S.: Uterus and embryo. I. Rabbit. II. Man. J. Morphol. 2:341–460, 1889.

Mitchell, M.D., Trautman, M.S., and Dudley, D.J.: Cytokine networking in the placenta. Placenta 14:249–275, 1993.

Moe, N.: Deposits of fibrin and plasma proteins in the normal human placenta. Acta Pathol. Microbiol. Scand. 76:74–88, 1969a.

Moe, N.: Histological and histochemical study of the extracellular deposits in the normal human placenta. Acta Pathol. Microbiol. Scand. 76:419–431, 1969b.

Moe, N.: The deposits of fibrin and fibrin-like materials in the basal plate of the normal human placenta. Acta Pathol. Microbiol. Scand. 75:1–17, 1969c.

Moe, N.: Mitotic activity in the syncytiotrophoblast of the human chorionic villi. Am. J. Obstet. Gynecol. 110:431, 1971.

Moe, N., and Joergensen, L.: Fibrin deposits on the syncytium of the normal human placenta: evidence of their thrombogenic origin. Acta Pathol. Microbiol. Scand. 72:519–541, 1968.

Moll, U.M., and Lane, B.L.: Proteolytic activity of first trimester human placenta: localization of interstitial collagenase in villous and extravillous trophoblast. Histochemistry 94:555–560, 1990.

Morrish, D.W., Bhardwaj, D., Dabbagh, L.K., Marusyk, H., and Siy, O.: Epidermal growth factor induces differentiation and secretion of human chorionic gonadotropin and placental lactogen in normal human placenta. J. Clin. Endocrinol. Metab. 65:1282–1290, 1987.

Morrish, D.W., Marusyk, H., and Bhardwaj, D.: Ultrastructural localization of human placental lactogen in distinctive granules in human term placenta: comparison with granules containing human chorionic gonadotropin. J. Histochem. Cytochem. 36:193–197, 1988.

Morrish, D.W., Bhardwaj, D., and Paras, M.T.: Transforming growth factor β1 inhibits placental differentiation and human chorionic gonadotropin and placental lactogen secretion. Endocrinology 129:22–26, 1991.

Moskalewski, S., Ptak, W., and Czarnik, Z.: Demonstration of cells with IgG receptor in human placenta. Biol. Neonate 26:268–273, 1975.

Mues, B., Langer, D., Zwadlo, G., and Sorg, C.: Phenotypic characterization of macrophages in human term placenta. Immunology 67:303–307, 1989.

Mühlhauser, J., Crescimanno, C., Kaufmann, P., Höfler, H., Zaccheo, D., and Castellucci, M.: Differentiation and proliferation patterns in human trophoblast revealed by c-erbB-2 oncogene product and EGF-R. J. Histochem. Cytochem. 41:165–173, 1993.

Mühlhauser, J., Crescimanno, C., Rajaniemi, H., Parkkila, S., Milovanov, A.P., Castellucci, M., and Kaufmann, P.: Immunohistochemistry of carbonic anhydrase in human placenta and fetal membranes. Histochemistry 101:91–98, 1994.

Müller, H.: Abhandlung über den Bau der Molen. Bonitas-Bauer, Würzburg, 1847.

Murphy, B.E.P.: Cortisol and cortisone in human fetal development. J. Steroid Biochem. 11:509–513, 1979.

Myatt, L., Brewer, A., and Brockman, D.E.: The action of nitric oxide in the perfused human fetal-placental circulation. Am. J. Obstet. Gynecol. 164:687–692, 1991.

Myatt, L., Brockman, D.E., Eis, A.L.W., and Pollock, J.S.: Immunohistochemical localization of nitric oxide synthase in the human placenta. Placenta 14:487–495, 1993.

Myers, R.E., and Fujikura, T.: Placental changes after experimental abruptio placentae and fetal vessel ligation of rhesus monkey placenta. Am. J. Obstet. Gynecol. 100:846–851, 1968.

Nagy, T., Boros, B., and Benkoe, K.: Elektronenmikroskopische Untersuchungen junger und reifer menschlicher Plazenten. Arch. Gynecol. 200:428–440, 1965.

Naito, M., Yamamura, F., Nishikawa, S., and Takahashi, K.: Development, differentiation, and maturation of fetal mouse yolk sac macrophages in cultures. J. Leukocyte Biol. 46:1–10, 1989.

Nakamura, Y., and Ohta, Y.: Immunohistochemical study of human placental stromal cells. Hum. Pathol. 21:936–940, 1990.

Nanaev, A.K., Rukosuev, V.S., Shirinsky, V.P., Milovanov, A.P., Domogatsky, S.P., Duance, V.C., Bradbury, F.M., Yarrow, P., Gardiner, L., D'Lacey, C., and Ockleford, C.D.: Confocal and conventional immunofluorescent and immunogold electron microscopic localization of collagen types III and IV in human placenta. Placenta 12:573–595, 1991a.

Nanaev, A.K., Shirinsky, V.P., and Birukov, G.: Immunofluorescent study of heterogeneity in smooth muscle cells of human fetal vessels using antibodies to myosin, desmin, and vimentin. Cell Tissue Res. 266:535–540, 1991b.

Nelson, D.M., Smith, C.H., Enders, A.C., and Donohue, T.M.: The non-uniform distribution of acidic components on the human placental syncytial trophoblast surface membrane: a cytochemical and analytical study. Anat. Rec. 184:159–182, 1976.

Nelson, D.M., Enders, A.C., and King, B.F.: Galactosyltransferase activity of the microvillous surface of human placental syncytial trophoblast. Gynecol. Invest. 8:267–281, 1977.

Nelson, D.M., Smith, R.M., and Jarett, L.: Nonuniform distribution and grouping of insulin receptors on the surface of human placental syncytial trophoblast. Diabetes 27:530–538, 1978.

Nelson, D.M., Meister, R.K., Ortman-Nabi, J., Sparks, S., and Stevens, V.C.: Differentiation and secretory activities of cultured human placental cytotrophoblast. Placenta 7:1–16, 1986.

Nelson, D.M., Crouch, E.C., Curran, E.M., and Farmer, D.R.: Trophoblast interaction with fibrin matrix: epithelialization of perivillous fibrin deposits as a mechanism for villous repair in the human placenta. Am. J. Pathol. 136:855–865, 1990.

Nessmann, C., Huten, Y., and Uzan, M.: Placental correlates of abnormal umbilical Doppler index. Trophoblast Res. 3:309–323, 1988.

Neumann, J.: Beitrag zur Kenntnis der Blasenmolen und des malignen Deciduoms. Monatsschr. Geburtshilfe Gynakol. 6:17–36, 1897.

Nikolov, Sp.D., and Schiebler, T.H.: Über das fetale Gefäßsystem der reifen menschlichen Placenta. Z. Zellforsch. 139:333–350, 1973.

Nikolov, Sp.D., and Schiebler, T.H.: Über Endothelzellen in Zottengefäßen der reifen menschlichen Placenta. Acta Anat. (Basel) 110:338–344, 1981.

Nishihira, M., and Yagihashi, S.: Immunohistochemical demonstration of somatostatin-containing cells in the human placenta. Tohoku J. Exp. Med. 126:397, 1978.

Nishihira, M., and Yagihashi, S.: Simultaneous detection of immunoreactive hCG- and somatostatin-containing cells and their gestational changes in the human placental villi and decidua. Acta Histochem. Cytochem. 12:434–442, 1979.

Nishino, E., Matsuzaki, N., Masuhiro, K., Kameda, T., Taniguchi, T., Tagagi, T., Saji, F., and Tanizawa, O.: Trophoblast-derived interleukin-6 (IL-6) regulates human chorionic gonadotropin release through IL-6 receptor on human trophoblasts. J. Clin. Endocrinol. Metab. 71:436–441, 1990.

Ockleford, C.D.: A three dimensional reconstruction of the polygonal pattern on placental coated vesicle membranes. J. Cell Sci. 21:83–91, 1976.

Ockleford, C.D., and Menon, G.: Differentiated regions of human placental cell surface associated with exchange of materials between maternal and foetal blood: a new organelle and the binding of iron. J. Cell Sci. 25:279–291, 1977.

Ockleford, C.D., Wakely, J., and Badley, R.A.: Morphogenesis of human placental chorionic villi: cytoskeletal, syncytioskeletal and extracellular matrix proteins. Proc. R. Soc. Lond. [Biol.] 212:305–316, 1981a.

Ockleford, C.D., Wakely, J., and Badley, R.A.: The human placental chorionic villous tree. Presented at the International SEM Symposium, Nijmegen, The Netherlands, 1981b.

Ockleford, C.D., Wakely, J., Badley, R.A., and Virtanen, I.: Intermediate filament proteins in human placenta. Cell Biol. Int. Rep. 5:762, 1981c.

Ockleford, C.D., Nevard, C.H.F., Indans, I., and Jones, C.J.P.: Structure and function of the nematosome. J. Cell Sci. 87:27–44, 1987.

Ogawa, S., Leavy, J., Clauss, M., Koga, S., Shreeniwas, R., Joseph-Silverstein, J., Furie, M., and Stern, D.: Modulation of endothelial cell (EC) function in hypoxia: alterations in cell growth and the response to monocyte-derived mitogenic factors. J. Cell. Biochem. Suppl. 15F: 213, 1991.

Ohlsson, R.: Growth factors, protooncogenes and human placental development. Cell Diff. Dev. 28:1–16, 1989.

Ohlsson, R., Holmgren, L., Glaser, A., Szpecht, A., and Pfeifer-Ohlsson, S.: Insulin-like growth factor 2 and short-range stimulatory loops in control of human placental growth. EMBO J. 8:1993–1999, 1989.

Ohno, M., Martinez-Hernandez, A., Ohno, N., and Kefalides, N.A.: Laminin M is found in placental basement membranes, but not in basement membranes of neoplastic origin. Connect. Tissue Res. 15:199–207, 1986.

Okudaira, Y., and Hayakawa, K.: Electron microscopic study on the surface coat of the human placental trophoblast. J. Electron Microsc. 24:279–281, 1975.

Oliveira, L.H.S., Leandro, S.V., Fonseca, M.E.F., and Dias, L.M.S.: A new technique for the isolation of placental phagocyte cells and a description of their macrophage properties after in vitro culture. Braz. J. Med. Biol. Res. 19:249–255, 1986.

Ong, P.J., and Burton, G.J.: Thinning of the placental villous membrane during maintenance in hypoxic organ culture:

structural adaptation or syncytial degeneration? Eur. J. Obstet. Gynäkol. Reprod. Biol. 39:103–110, 1991.

Orgnero de Gaisan, E., Aoki, A., Heinrich, D., and Metz, J.: Permeability studies of the guinea pig placental labyrinth. II. Tracer permeation and freeze fracture of fetal endothelium. Anat. Embryol. 171:297–304, 1985.

Ortmann, R.: Zur Frage der Zottenanastomosen in der menschlichen Placenta. Z. Anat. Entwicklungsgesch. 111: 173–185, 1941.

Ortmann, R.: Untersuchungen an einer in situ fixierten menschlichen Placenta vom 4.—5. Schwangerschaftsmonat. Arch. Gynäkol. 172:161–172, 1942.

Oswald, B., and Gerl, D.: Die Mikrofibrinoidablagerungen in der menschlichen Placenta. Acta Histochem. 42:356–359, 1972.

Panigel, M.: Comparative physiological and pharmacological aspects of placental permeability and hemodynamics in the non-human primate placenta and in the isolated perfused human placenta. Excerpta Med. 170:13, 1968.

Panigel, M., and Anh, J.N.H.: Ultrastructure des villosites placentaires humains. Pathol. Biol. (Paris) 12:927–949, 1964.

Panigel, M., and Myers, R.E.: Histological and ultrastructural changes in rhesus monkey placenta following interruption of fetal placental circulation by fetectomy or interplacental umbilical vessels ligation. Acta Anat. (Basel) 81:481–506, 1972.

Parmley, R.T., Takagi, M., and Denys, F.R.: Ultrastructural localization of glycoaminoglycans in human term placenta. Anat. Rec. 210:477–484, 1984.

Parmley, R.T., Barton, J.C., and Conrad, M.C.: Ultrastructural localization of transferrin, transferrin receptor, and iron-binding sites on human placental and duodenal microvilli. Br. J. Haematol. 60:81–89, 1985.

Peles, E., Bacus, S.S., Koski, R.A., Lu, H.S., Wen, D., Ogden, S.G., Levy, R.B., and Yarden, Y.: Isolation of the neu/HER-2 stimulatory ligand: a 44 kd glycoprotein that induces differentiation of mammary tumor cells. Cell 69: 205–216, 1992.

Pescetto, G.: Sulla presenza di elementi granulosi basofili metacromatici nella placenta fetale umana. Biol. Lat. (Milan) 2:744–757, 1950.

Pescetto, G.: Osservazioni istologiche e istochimiche sulle cellule di Hofbauer del villo coriale umano. Riv. Biol. 44:231–241, 1952.

Peter, K.: Placenta-Studien. 1. Zotten und Zwischen-Zottenräume zweier Placenta aus den letzten Monaten der Schwangerschaft. Z. Mikrosk. Anat. Forsch. 53:142–174, 1943.

Peter, K.: Placenta-Studien. 2. Verlauf, Verzweigung und Verankerung der Chorionzottenstämme und ihrer Äste in geborenen Placenten. Z. Mikrosk. Anat. Forsch. 56:129–172, 1951.

Petraglia, F.: Placental neurohormones: secretion and physiological implications. Mol. Cell. Endocrinol. 78:C109–C112, 1991.

Petraglia, F., Sawchenko, P., Lim, A.T.W., Rivier, J., and Vale, W.: Localization, secretion, and action of inhibin in human placenta. Science 237:187–189, 1987.

Petraglia, F., Calza, L., Giardino, L., Sutton, S., Marrama, P., Rivier, J., Genazzani, A.R., and Vale, W.: Identification of immunoreactive neuropeptide-y in human placenta: localization, secretion, and binding sites. Endocrinology 124:2016–2022, 1989.

Petraglia, F., Volpe, A., Genazzani, A.R., Rivier, J., Sawchenko, P.E., and Vale, W.: Neuroendocrinology of the human placenta. Front. Neuroendocrinol. 11:6–37, 1990.

Petraglia, F., Garuti, G., Calza, L., Roberts, V., Giardino, L., Genazzani, A.R., and Vale, W.: Inhibin subunits in human placenta: localization and messenger ribonucleic acid levels during pregnancy. Am. J. Obstet. Gynecol. 165: 750–758, 1991.

Petraglia, F., Woodruff, T.K., Botticelli, G., Botticelli, A., Gernazzani, A.R., Mayo, K.E., and Vale, W.: Gonadotropin-releasing hormone, inhibin, and activin in human placenta: evidence for a common cellular localization. J. Clin. Endocrinol. Metab. 74:1184–1188, 1992.

Pfister, C., Scheuner, G., Bahn, H., and Stiller, D.: Immunhistochemischer Nachweis von Fibronectin in der menschlichen Placenta. Acta Histochem. 84:83–91, 1988.

Pfister, C., Scheuner, G., and Städtler, N.: Fluorescenz- und polarisationsoptische Untersuchungen zur qualitativen und quantitativen Erfassung neutraler Carbohydrate in Basalmembranen menschlicher Placenta Zotten. Acta Histochem. 85:29–37, 1989.

Pierce, G.B., and Midgley, A.R.: The origin and function of human syncytiotrophoblast giant cells. Am. J. Pathol. 43: 153–173, 1963.

Pinto, A., Sorrentino, R., Sorrentino, P., Guerritore, T., Miranda, L., Biondi, A., and Martinelli, P.: Endothelial-derived relaxing factor released by endothelial cells of human umbilical vessels and its impairment in pregnancy-induced hypertension. Am. J. Obstet. Gynecol. 164:507–513, 1991.

Piotrowicz, B., Niebroj, T.K., and Sieron, G.: The morphology and histochemistry of the full term placenta in anaemic patients. Folia Histochem. Cytochem. 7:435–444, 1969.

Piotrowicz, R.S., Orchekowski, D.J., Nugent, D.J., Yamada, K.Y., and Kunicki, T.J.: Glycoprotein Ic-IIa functions as an activation-independent fibronectin receptor on human platelets. J. Cell Biol. 106:1359–1364, 1988.

Prosdocimi, O.: Richerche istochimiche per la localizzazione delle sostanze gonadotrope nel tessuto coriale normale, nella mola vescicolare e corioepitelioma. Riv. Ostet. Ginecol. 35:133, 1953.

Radtke, K.-P., Wenz, K.-H., and Heimburger, N.: Isolation of plaminogen activator inhibitor-2 (PAI-2) from human placenta: evidence for vitronectin/PAI-2 complexes in human placenta extract. Biol. Chem. Hoppe Seyler 371: 1119–1127, 1990.

Rao, C.V., Carman, F.R., Chegini, N., and Schultz, G.S.: Binding sites for epidermal growth factor in human fetal membranes. J. Clin. Endocrinol. Metab. 58:1034–1042, 1984.

Rao, C.V., Ramani, N., Chegini, N., Stadig, B.K., Carman, F.R., Jr., Woost, P.G., Schultz, G.S., and Cook, C.L.:

Topography of human placental receptors for epidermal growth factor. J. Biol. Chem. 260:1705–1710, 1985.

Reale, E., Wang, T., Zaccheo, D., Maganza, C., and Pescetto, G.: Junctions on the maternal blood surface of the human placental syncytium. Placenta 1:245–258, 1980.

Rhodin, J., and Terzakis, J.: The ultrastructure of the human fullterm placenta. J. Ultrastruct. Res. 6:88–106, 1962.

Richart, R.: Studies of placental morphogenesis. I. Radio-autographic studies of human placenta utilizing tritiated thymidine. Proc. Soc. Exp. Biol. Med. 106:829–831, 1961.

Risau, W., Drexler, H., Mironov, V., Smits, A., Stegbahn, A., Funa, K., and Heldin, C.-H.: Platelet-derived growth factor is angiogenic in vivo. Growth Factors 7:261–266, 1992.

Röckelein, G., and Hey, A.: Ultrastrukturelle Untersuchungen der Vakuolenbildung in arteriellen Choriongefäßen der reifen menschlichen Plazenta. Z. Geburtshilfe Perinatol. 189:65–68, 1985.

Rodway, H.E., and Marsh, F.: A study of Hofbauer's cells in human placenta. J. Obstet. Gynaecol. Br. Emp. 63: 111–115, 1956.

Rovasio, R.A., and Monis, B.: Cytochemical changes of a glycocalix of human placenta with maturation. Experientia 29:1115–1118, 1973.

Rukosuev, V.S.: Immunofluorescent localization of collagen types I, III, IV, V, fibronectin, laminin, entactin, and heparan sulphate proteoglycan in human immature placenta. Experientia 48:285–287, 1992.

Russel, S.W., and Pace, J.L.: The effects of interferons on macrophages and their precursors. Vet. Immunol. Immunopathol. 15:129–165, 1987.

Saijonmaa, O., Laatikainen, T., and Wahlström, T.: Corticotrophin-releasing factor in human placenta: localization, concentration and release in vitro. Placenta 9:373–385, 1988.

Sakakibara, R., Yokoo, Y., Yoshikoshi, K., Tominaga, N., Eida, K., and Ishiguro, M.: Subcellular localization of intracellular form of human chorionic gonadotropin in first trimester placenta. J. Biochem. 102:993–1001, 1987.

Sakata, M.: The study on the fetal placental circulation. Shikoku Acta Med. 16:796–812, 1960.

Sakbun, V., Koay, E.S.C., and Bryant-Greenwood, G.D.: Immunocytochemical localization of prolactin and relaxin C-peptide in human decidua and placenta. J. Clin. Endocrinol. Metab. 65:339–343, 1987.

Sala, M.A., Matheus, M., and Valeri, V.: Regional variation in the frequency of fibrinoid degeneration in the human term placenta. Z. Geburtshilfe Perinatol. 186:80–81, 1982.

Salas, S.P., Power, R.F., Singleton, A., Wharton, J., Polak, J.M., and Brown, J.: Heterogeneous binding sites for α-atrial natriuretic peptide in human umbilical cord and placenta. Am. J. Physiol. 261:R633–R638, 1991.

Salvaggio, A.T., Nigogosyan, G., and Mack, H.C.: Detection of trophoblast in cord blood and fetal circulation. Am. J. Obstet. Gynecol. 80:1013–1021, 1960.

Santiago-Schwarz, F., and Fleit, H.B.: Identification of non-adherent mononuclear cells in human cord blood that differentiate into macrophages. J. Leukocyte Biol. 43:51–59, 1988.

Scheuner, G.: Über die Verankerung der Nabelschnur an der Plazenta. Morphol. Jahr. 106:73–89, 1972.

Scheuner, G.: Zur Morphologie der materno-fetalen Stoffwechselschranke in der menschlichen Plazenta. Zentralbl. Gynäkol. 97:288–300, 1975.

Scheuner, G., and Hutschenreiter, J.: Strukturanalysen an Basalmembranen. Gefäßwand Blutplasma 4:217–218, 1972.

Scheuner, G., and Hutschenreiter, J.: Ergebnisse histophysikalischer Untersuchungen zur submikroskopischen Struktur von Basalmembranen. Anat. Anz. 71:1213–1216, 1977.

Scheuner, G., Ruckhäberle, K.-E., Flemming, G., and Reissig, D.: Submikroskopischer Nachweis orientierter Proteinfilamente im Plasmoditrophoblasten der menschlichen Plazenta. Anat. Anz. 147:145–151, 1980.

Schiebler, T.H., and Kaufmann, P.: Über die Gliederung der menschlichen Plazenta. Z. Zellforsch. 102:242–265, 1969.

Schiebler, T.H., and Kaufmann, P.: Reife Plazenta. In, Die Plazenta des Menschen. V. Becker, T.H. Schiebler, and F. Kubli, eds., pp. 51–100. Georg Thieme, Stuttgart, 1981.

Schmidt, W.: Der Feinbau der reifen menschlichen Eihäute. Z. Anat. Entwicklungsgesch. 119:203–222, 1956.

Schönfelder, G., Graf, R., and Schmidt, H.H.H.W.: A possible regulation of the extravascular contractile system in human placenta by nitric oxide synthase immunoreactive cells. Placenta 14:A69, 1993.

Schröder, H., Nelson, P., and Power, B.: Fluid shift across the placenta. I. The effect of dextran T40 in the isolated guinea pig placenta. Placenta 3:327–338, 1982.

Schroeder van der Kolk, J.L.C.: Waarnemigen over het Maaksel van de Menschlijke Placenta. Sulpke, Amsterdam, 1851.

Schuhmann, R.: Plazenton: Begriff, Entstehung, funktionelle Anatomie. In, Die Plazenta des Menschen. V. Becker, Th.H. Schiebler, and F. Kubli, eds., pp. 199–207. Thieme Verlag, Stuttgart, 1981.

Schweikhart, G., and Kaufmann, P.: Zur Abgrenzung normaler, artefizieller und pathologischer Strukturen in reifen menschlichen Plazentazotten. I. Ultrastruktur des Syncytiotrophoblasten. Arch. Gynecol. 222:213–230, 1977.

Scott, S.M., Buenaflor, G.G., and Orth, D.N.: Immunoreactive human epidermal growth factor concentrations in amniotic fluid, umbilical artery and vein serum, and placenta in full-term and preterm infants. Biol. Neonate 56:246–251, 1989.

Sedmak, D.D., Davis, D.H., Singh, U., van de Winkel, J.G.J., and Anderson, C.L.: Expression of IgG Fc receptor antigens in placenta and on endothelial cells in humans: an immunohistochemical study. Am. J. Pathol. 138:175–181, 1991.

Sen, D.K., Kaufmann, P., and Schweikhart, G.: Classification of human placental villi. II. Morphometry. Cell Tissue Res. 200:425–434, 1979.

Shreeniwas, R., Ogawa, S., Cozzolino, F., Torcia, G., Braunstein, N., Butura, C., Brett, J., Lieberman, H.B., Furie, M.B., and Joseph-Silverstein, J.: Macrovascular and microvascular endothelium during long-term hypoxia: alterations in cell growth, monolayer permeability, and cell surface coagulant properties. J. Cell. Physiol. 146:8–17, 1991

Siddall, R.S., and Hartman, F.W.: Infarcts of the placenta; study of seven hundred consecutive placentas. Am. J. Obstet. Gynecol. 12:683–699, 1926.

Sideri, M., de Virgiliis, G., Rainoldi, R., and Remotti, G.: The ultrastructural basis of the nutritional transfer: evidence of different patterns in the plasma membranes of the multilayered placental barrier. Trophoblast Res. 1:15–26, 1983.

Simpson, R.A., Mayhew, T.M., and Barnes, P.R.: From 13 weeks to term, the trophoblast of human placenta grows by the continuous recruitment of new proliferative units: a study of nuclear number using the dissector. Placenta 13:501–512, 1992.

Slamon, D.J., Clark, G.M., Wong, S.G., Levin, W.J., Ullrich, A., and McGuire, R.L.: Human breast cancer: correlation of relapse and survival with amplification of the HER-2/neu oncogene. Science 235:177–182, 1987.

Smith, C.H., Nelson, D.M., King, B.F., Donohue, T.M., Ruzycki, St.M., and Kelley, L.K.: Characterization of a microvillous membrane preparation from human placental syncytiotrophoblast: a morphologic, biochemical and physiologic study. Am. J. Obstet. Gynecol. 128:190–196, 1977.

Snoeck, J.: Le Placenta Humain. Masson, Paris, 1958.

Sonnenberg, A., Modderman, P.W., and Hogervorst, F.: Laminin receptor on platelets is the integrin VLA-6. Nature 336:487–489, 1988.

Sorokin, S.P., and Hoyt, R.F., Jr.: Pure population of non-monocyte derived macrophages arising in organ cultures of embryonic rat lungs. Anat. Rec. 217:35–52, 1987.

Sorokin, S.P., and Hoyt, R.F., Jr.: Macrophage development. I. Rationale for using Griffonia simplicifolia isolectin B4 as a marker for the line. Anat. Rec. 232:520–526, 1992.

Sorokin, S.P., Hoyt, R.F., Jr., Blunt, D.G., and McNelly, N.A.: Macrophage development. II. Early ontogeny of macrophage populations in brain, liver, and lungs of rat embryos as revealed by a lectin marker. Anat. Rec. 232:527–550, 1992a.

Sorokin, S.P., McNelly, N.A., Blunt, D.G., and Hoyt, R.F., Jr.: Macrophage development. III. Transformation of pulmonary macrophages from precursors in fetal lungs and their later maturation in organ culture. Anat. Rec. 232:551–571, 1992b.

Spanner, R.: Mütterlicher und kindlicher Kreislauf der menschlichen Placenta und seine Strombahnen. Z. Anat. Entwicklungsgesch. 105:163–242, 1935.

Spanner, R.: Zellinseln und Zottenepithel in der zweiten Hälfte der Schwangerschaft. Morphol. Jahr. 86:407–461, 1941.

Sporn, M., and Roberts, A.: The transforming growth factor-betas: past, present and future. Ann. N. Y. Acad. Sci. 593:1–6, 1990.

Stark, J., and Kaufmann, P.: Protoplasmatische Trophoblastabschnürungen in den mütterlichen Kreislauf bei normaler und pathologischer Schwangerschaft. Arch. Gynecol. 210:375–385, 1971.

Stark, J., and Kaufmann, P.: Trophoblastische Plasmapolypen und regressive Veränderungen am Zottentrophoblasten der menschlichen Placenta. Arch. Gynecol. 212:51–67, 1972.

Stark, J., and Kaufmann, P.: Infarktgenese in der Placenta. Arch. Gynecol. 217:189–208, 1974.

Stengelin, S., Stamenkovic, I., and Seed, B.: Isolation of cDNAs for two distinct human Fc receptors by ligand affinity cloning. EMBO J. 7:1053–1059, 1988.

Stewart, J.L., Jr., Sano, M.E., and Montgomery, T.L.: Hormone secretion by human placenta grown in tissue culture. J. Clin. Endocrinol. 8:175–188, 1948.

Stieve, H.: Neue Untersuchungen über die Placenta, besonders über die Entstehung der Placentasepten. Arch. Gynecol. 161:160–167, 1936.

Stieve, H.: Das Zottenraumgitter der reifen menschlichen Plazenta. Z. Geburtshilfe Gynakol. 122:289–316, 1941.

Strauss, L., Goldenberg, N., Hiroto, K., and Okudaira, Y.: Structure of the human placenta; with observations on ultrastructure of the terminal chorionic villus. Birth Defects 1:13–26, 1965.

Stulc, J.: Extracellular transport pathways in the haemochorial placenta. Placenta 10:113–119, 1989.

Stulc, J., Friederich, R., and Jiricka, Z.: Estimation of the equivalent pore dimensions in the rabbit placenta. Life Sci. 8:167–180, 1969.

Sutton, L., Gadd, M., Mason, D.Y., and Redman, C.W.G.: Cells bearing class II MHC antigens in the human placenta and amniochorion. Immunology 58:23–29, 1986.

Sutton, L.N., Mason, D.Y., and Redman, C.W.G.: Isolation and characterization of human fetal macrophages from placenta. Clin. Exp. Immunol. 78:437–443, 1989.

Taylor, R.N., and Williams, L.T.: Developmental expression of platelet-derived growth factor and its receptor in the human placenta. Mol. Endocrinol. 2:627–632, 1988.

Taylor-Papadimitriou, J., and Rozengurt, E.A.: Interferons as regulators of cell growth and differentiation. In, Interferons. Their Impact in Biology and Medicine. J. Taylor-Papadimitriou, ed., pp. 81–98. Oxford University Press, Oxford, 1985.

Teasdale, F., and Jean-Jacques, G.: Morphometry of the microvillous membrane of the human placenta in maternal diabetes mellitus. Placenta 7:81–88, 1986.

Tedde, G.: Ultrastruttura del villo placentare umano nella seconda meta della gravidanza. Arch. Ital. Anat. Embriol. 75:101–131, 1970.

Tedde, G., and Tedde Piras, A.: Mitotic index of the Langhans' cells in the normal human placenta from the early stages of pregnancy to the term. Acta Anat. (Basel) 100:114–119, 1978.

Tedde, G., Tedde Piras, A., and Berta, R.: A new structural pattern of the human trophoblast: the syncytial units [abstract 117]. 11th Rochester Trophoblast Conference, Abstract Booklet, 1988a.

Tedde, G., Tedde Piras, A., and Fenu, G.: Demonstration of an intercellular pathway of transport in the human trophoblast [abstract 77]. 11th Rochester Trophoblast Conference, Abstract Booklet, 1988b.

Ten Berge, B.S.: Merkwaardige cellen in chorionvlokken. Medical thesis, University of Utrecht, 1922.

Tenney, B., and Parker, F.: The placenta in toxemia of pregnancy. Am. J. Obstet. Gynecol. 39:1000–1005, 1940.

Thomsen, K.: Zur Morphologie und Genese der sogenannten Plazentarinfarkte. Arch. Gynecol. 185:221–247, 1954.

Thomsen, K., and Berle, P.: Placentarbefunde bei Rh-Inkompatibilität. Arch. Gynecol. 192:628–643, 1960.

Thorn, W., Kaufmann, P., and Müldener, B.: Kohlenhydrat-umsatz, Energiedefizit und Plasmapolypenbildung in der Placenta nach Vergiftung mit Monojodacetat und NaF. Arch. Gynecol. 216:175–183, 1974.

Thorn, W., Kaufmann, P., Müldener, B., and Freese, U.: Einfluß von 2,4–Dinitrophenol, Monojodacetat, Natrium-fluorid und Hypoxie auf Plasmapolypenbildung in der Placenta von Meerschweinchen. Arch. Gynecol. 221:203–210, 1976.

Thornburg, K., and Faber, J.J.: Transfer of hydrophilic molecules by placenta and yolk sac of the guinea pig. Am. J. Physiol. 233:C111–C124, 1977.

Thorsby, E.: The role of HLA in T cell activation. Hum. Immunol. 9:1–7, 1984.

Tominaga, R., and Page, E.W.: Accommodation of the human placenta to hypoxia. Am. J. Obstet. Gynecol. 94:679–685, 1966.

Toth, F., Paal, M., Nemeth, J., and Doemoetoeri, J.: Histo chemical studies of fibrinoid, mucopolysaccharides and chorionic gonadotrophin in the normal and pathologic human placenta. Acta Morphol. Acad. Sci. Hung. 21:89–104, 1973.

Toth, F.D., Juhl, C., Norskov-Lauritsen, N., Mosborg-Petersen, P., and Ebbesen, P.: Interferon production by cultured human trophoblast induced with double stranded polyribonucleotide. J. Reprod. Immunol. 17:217–227, 1990.

Toth, F.D., Norskov-Lauritsen, N., Juhl, C., and Ebbesen, P.: Human trophoblast interferon: pattern of response to priming and superinduction of purified term trophoblast and choriocarcinoma cells. J. Reprod. Immunol. 19:55–67, 1991.

Trudinger, B.J., Giles, W.B., Cook, C.M., Bombardieri, J., and Collins, L.: Uteroplacental blood flow velocity-time waveforms in normal and complicated pregnancy. Br. J. Obstet. Gynaecol. 92:23–30, 1985.

Truman, P., Wakerfield, J.St.J., and Ford, H.C.: Microvilli of the human term placenta. Biochem. J. 196:121–132, 1981.

Truman, P., and Ford, H.C.: The brush border of the human term placenta. Biochim. Biophys. Acta 779:139–160, 1984.

Ulesko-Stroganova, K.: Beitraege zur Lehre vom mikrosko-pischen Bau der Placenta. Monatsschr. Geburtshilfe Gynäkol. 3:207, 1896.

Unnikumar, K.R., Wegmann, R., and Panigel, M.: Immu-nohistochemical profile of the human placenta: studies on localization of prolactin, human chorionic gonadotropin, human placental lactogen, renin and oxytocin. Cell. Mol. Biol. 34:697–710, 1988.

Uren, S., and Boyle, W.: Isolation of macrophages from human placenta. J. Immunol. Methods 78:25–34, 1985.

Uren, S.J., and Boyle, W.: Class II MCH antigen-positive macrophages from human placentae suppress strong MLR and CML reations. Cell. Immunol. 125:235–246, 1990.

Usuki, K., Norberg, L., Larsson, E., Miyazono, K., Hellman, U., Wernstedt, C., Rubin, K., and Heldin, C.-H.: Localiza-tion of platelet-derived endothelial cell growth factor in human placenta and purification of an alternatively proces-sed form. Cell Regul. 1:577–584, 1990.

Vacek, Z.: Electron microscopic observations on the filaments in the trophoblast of the human placenta. Folia Morphol. (Praha) 17:382–388, 1969.

Vacek, Z.: Derivation and ultrastructure of the stroma cells of the human chorionic villus. Folia Morphol. (Praha) 18:1–13, 1970.

Vanderpuye, O., and Smith, C.H.: Proteins of the apical and basal plasma membranes of the human placental syncytiotrophoblast: immunochemical and electrophoretic studies. Placenta 8:591–608, 1987.

Van Furth, R.: Current view on the mononuclear phagocyte system. Immunobiology 161:178–185, 1982.

Velardo, J.T., and Rosa, C.: Female genital system. In, Handbuch der Histochemie. Vol. 7. 3rd Ed. W. Graumann and K. Neumann, eds. Fischer, Stuttgart, 1963.

Villee, C.A., ed.: The Placenta and Fetal Membranes. Wil-liams & Wilkins, Baltimore, 1960.

Virchow, R.: Die krankhaften Geschwülste. Vol. I. Hirsch-wald, Berlin, 1863.

Virchow, R.: Cellularpathologie in ihrer Begründung auf physiologische und pathologische Gewebelehre. 4th Ed. Hirschwald, Berlin, 1871.

Virtanen, I., Laitinen, L., and Vartio, T.: Differential ex-pression of the extra domain-containing form of cellular fibronectin in human placentas at different stages of matura-tion. Histochemistry 90:25–30, 1988.

Voigt, S., Kaufmann, P., and Schweikhart, G.: Zur Abgren-zung normaler, artefizieller und pathologischer Strukturen in reifen menschlichen Plazentazotten. II. Morphometrische Untersuchungen zum Einfluß des Fixationsmodus. Arch. Gynecol. 226:347–362, 1978.

Wachstein, M., Meagher, J.G., and Ortiz, J.: Enzymatic histochemistry of the term human placenta. Am. J. Obstet. Gynecol. 87:13–26, 1963.

Wada, H.G., Gornicki, S.Z., and Sussman, H.H.: The sialoglycoprotein subunits of human placental brush border membranes characterized by two-dimensional electro-phoresis. J. Supramol. Struct. 6:473–484, 1977.

Wada, H.G., Hass, P.E., and Sussman, H.H.: Characteriza-tion of antigenic sialoglycoprotein subunits of the placental brush border membranes: comparison with liver and kidney membrane subunits by two-dimensional electrophoresis. J. Supramol. Struct. 10:287–305, 1979.

Wainwright, S.D., and Wainwright, L.K.: Preparation of human placental villous surface membrane. Nature 252:302–303, 1974.

Wang, E., Pfeffer, L.M., and Tamm, I.: Interferon increases the abundance of submembranous microfilaments in HeLa-S3 cells in suspension culture. Proc. Natl. Acad. Sci. U.S.A. 78:6281–8285, 1981.

Wang, T., and Schneider, J.: Cellular junctions on the free surface of human placental syncytium. Arch. Gynecol. 240:211–216, 1987.

Wasserman, L., Abramovici, A., Shlesinger, H., Goldman, J.A., and Allalouf, D.: Histochemical localization of acidic glycosaminoglycans in normal human placentae. Placenta 4:101–108, 1983a.

Wasserman, L., Shlesinger, H., Goldman, J.A., and Allalouf, D.: Pattern of glycosaminoglycan distribution in tissue and blood vessels of human placenta. Gynecol. Obstet. Invest. 15:242–250, 1983b.

Weinberg, P.C., Cameron, I.L., Parmley, T., Jeter, J.R., and Pauerstein, C.J.: Gestational age and placental cellular replication. Obstet. Gynecol. 36:692–696, 1970.

Werb, Z., Hembry, R.M., Murphy, G., and Aggeler, J.: Commitment to expression of the metalloendopeptidases, collagenase and stromelysin: relationship of inducing events to changes in cytoskeletal architecture. J. Cell Biol. 102:697–702, 1986.

Werner, C., and Bender, H.G.: Phasenkontrastmikroskopie der Plazenta. In, Neue Erkenntnisse über die Orthologie und Pathologie der Plazenta. H.J. Födisch, ed., pp. 63–71. Enke, Stuttgart, 1977.

Westermark, B., Siegbahn, A., Heldin, C.-H., and Claesson, W.L.: B-Type receptor for platelet-derived growth factor mediates a chemotactic response by means of ligand-induced activation of the receptor protein-tyrosine kinase. Proc. Natl. Acad. Sci. U.S.A. 87:128–132, 1990.

Whyte, A.: Lectin binding by microvillous membranes and coated-pit regions of human syncytial trophoblast. Histochem. J. 12:599–607, 1980.

Wielenga, G., and Willighagen, R.G.J.: The histochemistry of the syncytiotrophoblast and the stroma in the normal full-term placenta. Am. J. Obstet. Gynecol. 84:1059–1064, 1962.

Wigglesworth, J.S.: The gross and microscopic pathology of the prematurely delivered placenta. J. Obstet. Gynaecol. Br. Commonw. 69:934–943, 1962.

Wigglesworth, J.S.: Morphological variations in the insufficient placenta. J. Obstet. Gynaecol. Br. Commonw. 71:871–884, 1964.

Wilkes, B.M., Mento, P.F., Hollander, A.H., Maita, M.E., Sung, S.Y., and Girardi, E.P.: Endothelin receptors in human placenta: relationship to vascular resistance and thromboxane release. Am. J. Physiol. 258:E864–E870, 1990.

Wilkin, P.: Pathologie du Placenta. Masson, Paris, 1965.

Wilson, C.B., Haas, J.E., and Weaver, W.M.: Isolation, purification and characteristics of mononuclear phagocytes from human placentas. J. Immunol. Methods 56:305–317, 1983.

Winterhager, E.: Dynamik der Zellmembran: Modellstudien während der Implantationsreaktion beim Kaninchen. Medical thesis, Technologic University of Aachen, 1985.

Wislocki, G.B., and Bennett, H.S.: Histology and cytology of the human and monkey placenta, with special reference to the trophoblast. Am. J. Anat. 73:335–449, 1943.

Wood, G., and King, G.R., Jr.: Trapping antigen-antibody complexes within the human placenta. Cell Immunol. 69:347–362, 1982.

Wood, G., Reynard, J., Krishnan, E., and Racela, L.: Immunobiology of the human placenta. I. IgGFc receptors in trophoblastic villi. Cell. Immunol. 35:191–204, 1978a.

Wood, G., Reynard, J., Krishnan, E., and Racela, L.: Immunobiology of the human placenta. II. Localization of macrophages, in vivo bound IgG and C3. Cell Immunol. 35:205–216, 1978b.

Wood, G.S., Warner, N.L., and Warnke, R.A.: Anti-Leu-3/T4 antibodies react with cells of monocyte/macrophage and Langerhans lineage. J. Immunol. 131:212–216, 1983.

Wood, G.S., Turner, R.R., Shiurba, R.A., Eng, L., and Warnke, R.A.: Human dendritic cells and macrophages: In situ immunophenotypic definition of subsets that exhibit specific morphologic and microenvironmental characteristics. Am. J. Pathol. 119:73–82, 1985.

Wood, G.W.: Mononuclear phagocytes in the human placenta. Placenta 1:113–123, 1980.

Wright, C., Angus, B., Nicholson, S., Sainsbury, J.R., Cairns, J.C., Gullick, W.J., Kelley, P., Harris, A.L., and Horne, C.H.W.: Expression of c-erbB-2 oncoprotein: a prognostic indicator in human breast cancer. Cancer Res. 49:2087–2090, 1989.

Wright, S.D., Ramos, R.A., Tobias, P.S., and Ulevitch, R.J.: CD 14, a receptor for complexes of lipopolysaccaride (LPS) and LPS binding protein. Science 249:1431–1433, 1990.

Wynn, R.M.: Derivation and ultrastructure of the so-called Hofbauer cell. Am. J. Obstet. Gynecol. 97:235–248, 1967a.

Wynn, R.M.: Fetomaternal cellular relations in the human basal plate: an ultrastructural study of the placenta. Am. J. Obstet. Gynecol. 97:832–850, 1967b.

Wynn, R.M.: Fine structure of the placenta. In, Handbook of Physiology, Section 7, Endocrinology. R.O. Greep and E.B. Astwood, eds., pp. 261–276. American Physiological Society, Washington, DC, 1973.

Wynn, R.M.: Fine structure of the placenta. In, The Placenta and Its Maternal Supply Line. P. Gruenwald, ed., pp. 56–79. Medical and Technical Publishing, Lancaster, 1975.

Yagel, S., Hurwitz, A., Rosenn, B., and Keizer, N.: Progesterone enhancement of prostaglandin E_2 production by fetal placental macrophages. Am. J. Reprod. Immunol. 14:45–48, 1987.

Yallampalli, C., and Garfield, R.E.: Inhibition of nitric oxide synthesis in rats during pregnancy produces signs similar to those of preeclampsia. Am. J. Obstet. Gynecol. 169:1316–1320, 1993.

Yamada, T., Isemura, M., Yamaguchi, Y., Munakata, H., Hayashi, N., and Kyogoku, M.: Imunohistochemical localization of fibronectin in the human placentas at their different stages of maturation. Histochemistry 86:579–584, 1987.

Yamaguchi, Y., Mann, D.M., and Ruoslahti, E.: Negative regulation of transforming growth factor-β by the proteoglycan decorin. Nature 346:281–284, 1990.

Yeh, C.-J., Mühlhauser, J., Hsi, B.-I., Castellucci, M., and Kaufmann, P.: The expression of receptors for epidermal growth factor and transferrin on human trophoblast. Placenta 10:459, 1989.

Zaccheo, D., Zicca, A., Cadoni, A., Leprini, A., Castellucci, M., and Kaufmann, P.: Preliminary observations on Hofbauer cells in short-term culture and. Bibl. Anat. 22:63–68, 1982.

Zaccheo, D., Pistoia, V., Castellucci, M., and Martinoli, C.: Isolation and characterization of Hofbauer cells from human placental villi. Arch. Gynecol. 246:189–200, 1989.

Zacks, S., and Blazar, A.S.: Chorionic villi in normal pregnancy, pre-eclamptic toxemia, erythroblastosis, and diabetes mellitus: a light- and electron-microscope study. Obstet. Gynecol. 22:149–167, 1963.

Ziegler-Heitbrock, H.-W.L.: The biology of the monocyte system. Eur. J. Cell Biol. 49:1–12, 1989.

8
Architecture of Normal Villous Trees

Structure of Villous Types

The ramifications of the villous trees can be subdivided into segments that differ mainly as to caliber, stromal structure, vessel structure, and position within the villous tree (Figure 64). Five villous types have been described (Kaufmann et al., 1979; Sen et al., 1979; Castellucci & Kaufmann, 1982a,b; Kaufmann, 1982; Castellucci et al., 1984, 1990; Burton, 1987), some of which can be further subdivided. As is discussed, all villous types derive from single precursors, the mesenchymal villi, which correspond to the tertiary villi of the early stages of placentation.

The following villous types have been described (Figure 65).

1. *Stem villi* are characterized by a condensed fibrous stroma, arteries and veins, or arterioles and venules with a light-microscopically identifiable media or adventitia. They comprise (Figures 66, 76a) the following structures: (a) the main stems (truncus chorii) of a villous tree, which connect the latter with the chorionic plate; (b) up to four generations of branchings (rami chorii of the first to fourth orders), which are short, thick branches derived from the truncus already in the vicinity of the chorionic plate; (c) 2 to 30 (mean 10) more generations of unequal dichotomous branchings (ramuli chorii of the first to tenth orders), which are more slender branches that extend into the periphery of the villous trees; and (d) a special group of stem villi represented by the anchoring villi; these villi are ramuli chorii, which connect to the basal plate by a cell column. The latter acts as a growth zone for this ramulus as well as for the basal plate.
2. *Mature intermediate villi* (Figures 68, 69) are long, slender, peripheral ramifications characterized by the absence of vessels with a light-microscopically identifiable media or adventitia.

3. *Terminal villi* (Figures 70, 71) are the final, grape-like ramifications of the mature intermediate villi, characterized by their high degree of capillarization and the presence of highly dilated sinusoids. They represent the main sites of fetomaternal exchange.
4. *Immature intermediate villi* (Figures 67, 86) are peripheral, immature, bulbous continuations of stem villi. They are in a position comparable to that of the mature intermediate villi (i.e., interposed between stem villi and peripheral branches) and prevail in immature placentas. Normally, this type persists in small groups within the centers of the villous trees (placentones) and represents the immature forerunners of stem villi.
5. *Mesenchymal villi* (Figures 72, 73) are the most primitive. They prevail during the first stages of pregnancy, where they are the forerunners of immature intermediate villi. During later stages of pregnancy these villi are inconspicuous, mostly small, slender structures that can be found along the surfaces of immature intermediate villi or at the tips of mature intermediate villi. Also at this stage they act as zones of villous proliferation and further branching.

The principal morphometric data of the various villous types are shown in Table 8 and Figure 75.

Stem Villi

Trunci chorii, rami chorii, ramuli chorii, and the anchoring villi are grouped as stem villi because they exhibit similar histological features and differ from each other only in caliber and position within the hierarchy of villous branching. The calibers vary from about $80\,\mu$m (smallest ramuli chorii) to about $3,000\,\mu$m (some trunci, near the chorionic plate). In the normal mature placenta, they make up 20% to 25% of the total villous volume (Table 8). Because of the typical branching

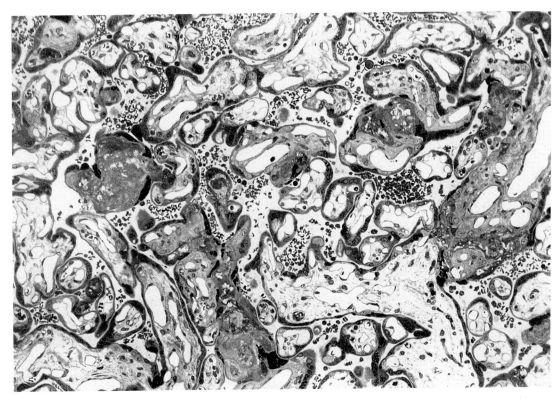

FIGURE 64. Semithin section from the 40th week p.m. demonstrating the structural and staining variability of villous cross sections. Such pictures suggest that the villous tree is composed of several villous types that differ from each other regarding size, stromal fibrosis, and density of fetal vascularization. ×165.

patterns of the villous trees, the volumetric share of the stem villi is the highest in the central subchorionic portion of the villous tree.

Histologically, stem villi have a uniformly thick trophoblastic cover and lack epithelial plates. Cytotrophoblastic cells, located below the superficial syncytiotrophoblast, can be found on about 20% of villous surfaces. In the mature placenta the trophoblast is often degenerated and largely replaced by perivillous fibrinoid (Figures 66A, 92, 93). Trophoblastic degeneration is more impressive in stem villi of large caliber than in the small peripheral villi. Moreover, there seems to be a certain positive correlation with intrauterine growth retardation (Ara et al., 1984; Macara et al., 1994).

The stroma is characterized by huge condensed bundles of collagen fibers that encase occasional fibroblasts and rare macrophages (Figure 66C). Within trunci, rami, and large ramuli, the fetal vessels are composed of arteries and veins that are accompanied by smaller arterioles and venules as well as superficially located paravascular capillaries (Figure 66A). The latter are comparable to the vasa vasorum of large-caliber vessels of other organs. In the smaller, more peripheral ramuli, arteries and veins are lacking; rather, the fetal vessels are represented by a few arterioles and venules

that typically have thin vessel walls and are accompanied by few paravascular capillaries (Figure 66B). The adventitia of arteries and veins continues without sharp demarcation into the surrounding fibrous stroma of the villous core (Figure 66A). The more centrally located connective tissue cells are myofibroblasts, whereas the more peripheral ones are fibroblasts (Demir et al., 1992; Kohnen et al., 1992). In stem villi that are not yet fully mature, a superficial rim of reticular stroma, deficient in fibers, may separate the fibrous stroma from the trophoblastic cover (Figures 86–89). Macrophages are evenly distributed throughout the stroma (Demir et al., 1992). Occasionally, mast cells are present in the vascular walls of the stem villi (Figure 63C).

Functionally speaking, stem villi serve to mechanically support the structures of the villous trees. Considering the low degree of fetal capillarization and degenerative changes of the trophoblast, their share in fetomaternal exchange and endocrine activity is presumably negligible. The presence of the large fetal vessels with thick muscular walls and the presence of extravascular myofibroblasts (Demir et al., 1992; Kohnen et al., 1992) makes their contribution to the autoregulation of the fetoplacental vascular system likely. Moreover, the myofibroblasts that are oriented

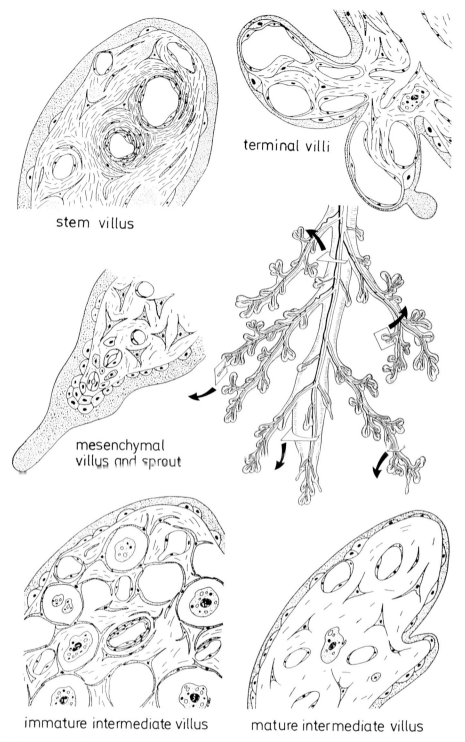

stem villus

terminal villi

mesenchymal
villus and sprout

immature intermediate villus   mature intermediate villus

FIGURE 65. Simplified representation of the peripheral part of a mature placental villous tree, and typical cross sections of the various villous types. For further details see text and Figures 66 to 71. (From Kaufmann & Scheffen, 1992, with permission.)

in parallel to the longitudinal axis of the villous stems may provide a regulating system for maternal circulation in the intervillous space. Because many of the larger villous stems are anchoring villi that connect the chorion and basal plate, their longitudinal contraction decreases intervillous volume (Krantz & Parker, 1963) and increases uteroplacental flow impedance. As has been demonstrated in vitro by Karimu and Burton

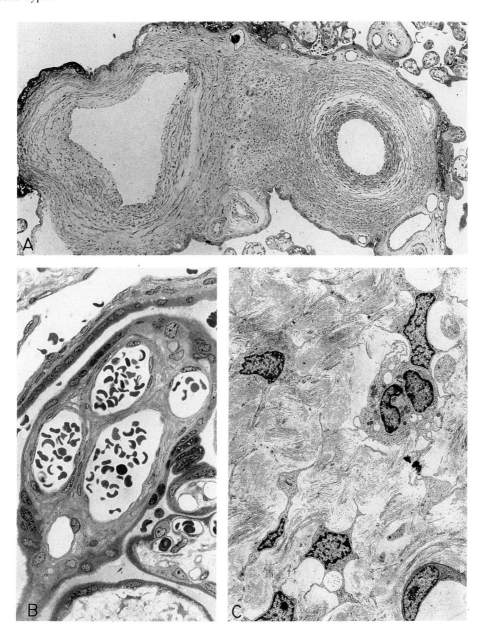

FIGURE 66. Structural features of stem villi. (A) Semithin cross section of a large stem villus. Note that the adventitias of the artery (right) and vein (left) continue directly into the surrounding dense fibrous stroma of the villus. Superficially, numerous smaller vessels of the paravascular capillary net are seen. As is typical for stem villi of the mature placenta, the trophoblastic covering of this villus has been replaced in many places by fibrinoid. ×115. (From Leiser et al., 1985, with permission.) (B) More peripherally positioned stem villi of small caliber can be identified by the condensed fibrous stroma located between the fetal arterioles and venules (large lumens). Fetal capillaries are rare. ×430. (C) Transmission electron micrograph of the fibrous stroma of a stem villus. The interstitial space between the various types of connective tissue cells is mostly occupied by dense bundles of collagen fibers. ×2,400.

(1994), pressure changes in the intervillous space affect the width of the fetoplacental capillaries and thus influence fetal perfusion of the placenta. In conclusion, myofibroblasts may act as an important link adapting maternal and fetal perfusion of the placenta to each other: An increase in fetoplacental blood flow impedance due to high pressure in the villous surround-

ing can be down-regulated by relaxation of the myofibroblasts (Kohnen et al., 1992; Kohnen, 1994).

Immature Intermediate Villi

The immature intermediate villi have been known as immature villi or immature terminal villi. We have

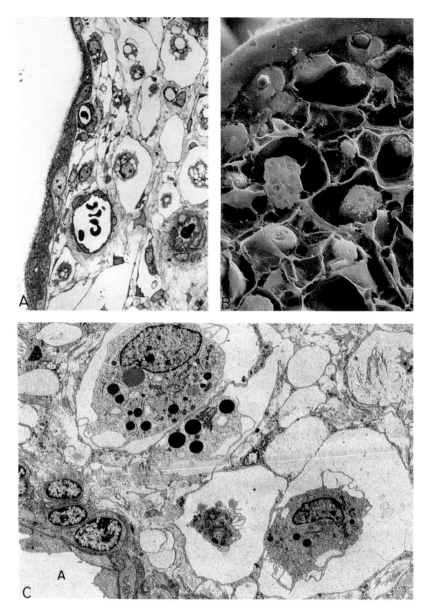

FIGURE 67. Typical structure of the immature intermediate villus. (A) Semithin section of an immature intermediate villus from the 22nd week p.m. with its typical reticular stroma. The rounded, vacuolated macrophages (Hofbauer cells) are located in stromal channels, which are devoid of connective tissue fibers and therefore appear as empty holes. In faintly stained histological sections, this feature can be misinterpreted as villous edema. ×520. (From Kaufmann, 1981, with permission.) (B) Scanning electron micrograph of a freeze-cracked immature intermediate villus shows the three- dimensional view of the reticular stroma with its characteristic stromal channels. ×1,050. (Courtesy M. Castellucci.) (C) Transmission electron micrograph of the reticular stroma of an immature intermediate villus at term. Several stromal channels, each containing a macrophage, can be identified. They are delimited from the surrounding connective tissue fibers by slender, sail-like extensions of fixed connective tissue cells (small reticulum cells, R). A small fetal arteriole (A) is seen in the lower left corner. ×2,700. (From Castellucci & Kaufmann, 1982a, with permission.)

suggested that the term immature intermediate is more appropriate because the villi are not the only immature villous type, nor are they immature forerunners of later terminal villi (Kaufmann et al., 1979; Kaufmann, 1982). Rather, both types of intermediate villi (immature and mature villi) are mature successors of mesenchymal villi.

1. The immature intermediate villi result from matura- tion of mesenchymal villi throughout the first two trimesters. Later they are transformed into stem villi.

2. The mature intermediate villi that derive from mesenchymal precursors during the last trimester produce the terminal villi.

Thus both "intermediate" villi are in an intermediate developmental position between mesenchymal and fully mature villi. Moreover, both are in an intermediate topographical position between stem villi and the most peripheral branches.

Histologically, immature intermediate villi have the same uniform, thick trophoblastic cover as stem villi (Figures 65, 67A). Epithelial plates are absent. During early pregnancy, Langhans' cells can be found below the syncytium on more than 50% of villous surfaces. During late pregnancy their prevalence is reduced to about 20%. The most characteristic feature of the immature intermediate villi is their reticular stroma. It is typified by numerous channels that are delimited by large, saillike processes of the fixed stromal cells (Kaufmann et al., 1977b) (Figure 67). Hofbauer cells are inside the channels (Enders & King, 1970; Castellucci & Kaufmann, 1982a) suspended in some fluid. Fetal vessels (e.g., capillaries, arterioles, and venules) together with scarce bundles of collagen fibers are positioned between the stromal channels. Collagen bundles and vessel walls are separated from the lumens of the channels by the sail-like extensions of the connective tissue cells (Figure 67C).

Transformation of immature intermediate villi into stem villi takes place during the first trimester. It is a gradual process that results in numerous intermediate steps. The starting point for the stromal fibrosis is the vascular wall. In the beginning, vessels acquire a distinct media and adventitia. The latter expands in later stages over the entire villous thickness. During this process the intercanalicular bundles of connective tissue fibers increase in diameter and thus compress the neighboring stromal channels. Finally, they disappear. Residues can be found in all stem villi when one studies the stroma carefully for Hofbauer cells (Figure 66C).

The first immature intermediate villi are formed around the 8th week post menstruation (p.m.). Between the 14th and 20th weeks (Figures 84–86) they comprise most of the villous cross sections. At term they may be completely absent; in most cases they can be found in small groups in the centers of the villous trees, the "placentones," where they still act as growth zones and produce new sprouts. At term a volumetric share of 0% to 5% is normal for immature intermediate villi. This figure is applicable only when all parts of a placentone are equally represented in the histological section. Sections restricted to the more central parts of a villous tree may show higher values and must thus be interpreted with care.

The immature intermediate villi can be regarded functionally as the growth centers of the villous trees. They produce the true sprouts (see Chapter 10) and, later, mesenchymal villi as forerunners of all other villous types. Because of the long maternofetal diffusion distances, these mesenchymal villi are the principal sites of exchange only during the first two trimesters, so long as other specialized villous types are not yet differentiated.

Immature intermediate villi may cause diagnostic problems, as their reticular stromal core has only a weak affinity for conventional stains owing to the lack of collagen. Typical features are depicted in Figures 67A and 84–86; the weak staining, however, often results in disappearance of the extensions of the sail-like connective tissue cells. The resulting histological picture is that of a seemingly edematous villus that had accumulated much interstitial fluid. Such true edematous villi indeed exist. They are particularly impressive in hydatidiform moles and may be found in association with maternal diabetes mellitus and some infections (e.g., syphilis, toxoplasmosis, cytomegalovirus infection). On the other hand, as experienced a pathologist as Fox expressed some doubt when he wrote: "This has long been recognized as one of the characteristic features of placentae from diabetic women and from cases of materno-fetal rhesus incompatibility, though in fact only a proportion of such placentae are edematous." For other cases, he simply stated that villous immaturity is the correct designation (Fox, 1978). We believe that many villi referred to as "edematous villi" in the literature are in fact normal, immature intermediate villi (e.g., in most cases of rhesus incompatibility) (Pilz et al., 1980; Kaufmann et al., 1987). Naeye et al. (1983) have dealt in much detail with the clinical significance of placental villous edema. We cannot exclude, based on their report, that these changes represent true edematous alterations, but at least one of the two examples they depicted (their Figure 2) is a normal, immature intermediate villus. They described it as follows: "Villous edema was recognized by the finding of open spaces in the interstitium of the villi," but they pointed to normal stromal channels.

This contradiction does not negate the existence of villous edema. It is probable that true generalized villous edema has functional significance, as it may compress the intervillous space and thus limit maternal blood flow (Alvarez et al., 1972; Fox, 1978); it also increases the maternofetal diffusion distances. Fox (1978) stated that "villous oedema is usually considered to be of no clinical significance," and that "there is, as yet, no clear evidence that villous oedema has, in itself, any effect on fetal growth or nutrition." Perhaps this negative conclusion is based on the interpretation that most cases of "villous edema" are misinterpretations of normal villous structures.

For further details regarding normal structure and function of immature intermediate villi, see the publications by Castellucci and Kaufmann (1982a,b), Castellucci et al. (1984), Highison and Tibbitts (1986), Kaufmann (1982), Kaufmann et al. (1977b, 1979), and Sen et al. (1979).

Mature Intermediate Villi

Mature intermediate villi are long slender villi with diameters of about 60 to 150 μm. As soon as their surfaces bear terminal villi, their shape is characterized by numerous slight bends at points where the terminal villi branch off, resulting in a typical zigzag course (Figure 70A,D). This course is absent when terminal side branches are not present (Figure 103a), features that may be of diagnostic importance. Mature intermediate villi have roughly the same diameters as terminal villi. Because of their zigzag courses, longitudinal histological sections are rare. When mature intermediate villi fail to produce terminal villi, they do not pursue the zigzag course but, rather, remain straight. In sections this appearance is one of groups of cross sections that alternate with bundles of slender longitudinal sections (Figure 103b). This pattern is often the only suggestion leading to the histological diagnosis of "terminal villi deficiency."

The stroma of mature intermediate villi is composed of seemingly unoriented, loose bundles of connective tissue fibers and fixed connective tissue cells. In some places it surrounds rudimentary narrow stromal channels that are usually devoid of macrophages (Figures 68, 69). The vessels comprise numerous capillaries, small terminal arterioles, and collecting venules. The media of the latter is usually too thin for light-microscopic identification. Because the terminal villi originate from the surface of the mature intermediate villi, there is a gradual transition. Cross sections are defined as mature intermediate villi, the stroma of which contains fewer than 50% vascular lumens (Table 7). Roughly one-fourth of the villous volume in the normal term placenta is comprised of this villous type (Table 8).

Functionally, the mature intermediate villi produce the terminal villi. The high degree of fetal vascularization and the large share in the exchange surface make them important for fetomaternal exchange. When studying the enzyme patterns and the localization of

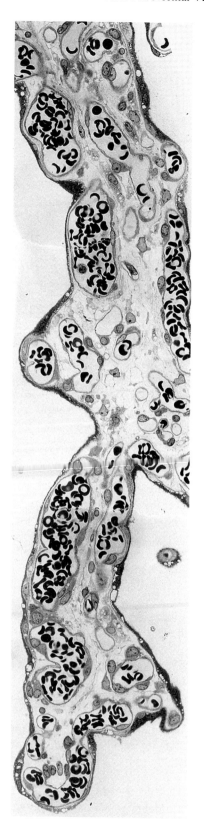

FIGURE 68. Semithin section of the richly vascularized peripheral end of a mature intermediate villus (upper half), with a terminal villus (lower half) arising at a narrow neck region (center). The fetal vessels show the typical composition of narrow capillaries and dilated sinusoids. The latter are closely related to the trophoblastic surface, forming thin epithelial plates. ×430. (From Kaufmann et al., 1979, with permission.)

FIGURE 69. Typical structure of mature intermediate villi. Semithin cross section of the poorly vascularized, more central portion of a mature intermediate villus. Note the peripheral position of the small fetal capillaries and the ample connective tissue, deficient in cells and fibers. The syncytiotrophoblastic covering of the villus is more uniform in structure than that of the terminal villi. ×730. (B) Transmission electron micrograph of the typical loose connective tissue of a mature intermediate villus. The seemingly unoriented mixture of small reticulum cells (R) with long processes, macrophages (M), and loosely arranged connective tissue fibers is highly characteristic for this villous type. ×2,150.

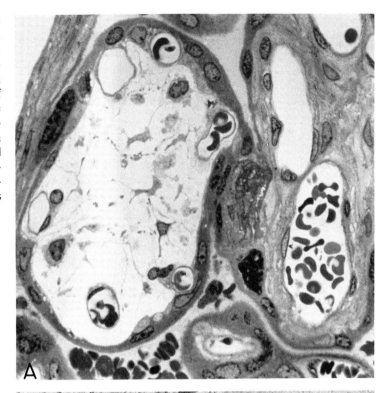

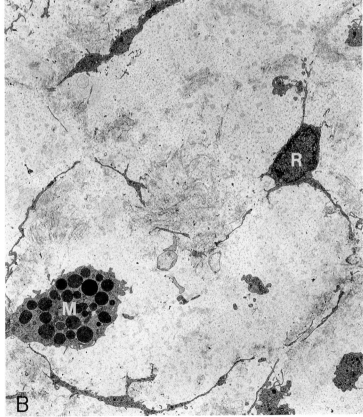

placental hormones, one gains the impression that they are prominent sites for hormone production. In analogy with the vascular bed of other organs, one may conclude that the presence of terminal arterioles allows participation in vasoregulation and thus intravillous blood distribution (Nikolov & Schiebler, 1973).

Terminal Villi

Terminal villi are the final ramifications of the villous tree during the last trimester. They are grape-like outgrowths of the mature intermediate villi, where they appear as single or poorly branched side branches (Figures 70A,D). The peripheral end of the mature intermediate villus normally branches into a larger aggregate of such terminal villi (Figure 70B). They usually connect to the mature intermediate villi by a narrow neck region (Figures 70C, 79A). Only a small proportion of the terminal villi are directly connected to stem villi or to immature intermediate villi.

Histologically, terminal villi are characterized by a thin trophoblastic cover and sinusoidally dilated capillaries. The latter occupy more than 50% of the stromal volume and more than 35% of the villous volume (Table 7; Figures 68, 71) (Kaufmann et al., 1979; Sen et al., 1979). The remaining connective tissue has scant fibers and cells. Macrophages are rare (Figure 71). The fetal sinusoids are in intimate contact with the trophoblastic surface and form the epithelial plates Depending on the quality of tissue preservation, they amount to 30% to 40% of the villous surface (Table 7; Figure 79).

The average diameter of terminal villi ranges from 30 to 80 µm. Their histological appearance differs, depending· on where they are sectioned. The slender neck region, containing mostly undilated capillaries, is easily differentiated from the bulbous tip and from flat sections across tips (Figure 79).

It must be pointed out that the light-microscopic appearance is heavily influenced by the mode of tissue preservation. Delayed fixation (Tables 7, 10), inappropriate osmolarity of the fixative (Table 11), and time and mode of cord clamping (Table 9) influence the villous structure. In particular, the highly dilated sinusoids respond to postpartal changes of fetal blood pressure. They tend to collapse within minutes, dramatically changing the villous proportions (Voigt et al., 1978; Burton & Palmer, 1988). An increase in pressure in the peripheral fetal vessels, such as during cord compression (knots, torsion, nuchal cord), leads to congestion in the terminal capillaries and results in seemingly "hypercapillarized" villi. We found this feature frequently with preterm rupture of membranes, and the correlation is highly significant. There was also an increase in villous blood volume, sometimes of more than 50%. It may be speculated that loss of amnionic fluid predisposes to compression of the umbilical veins and thus inhibits placental venous backflow (Paprocki, 1992).

The high degree of vascularization and minimal mean maternofetal diffusion distance of about 3.7 µm (Voigt et al., 1978; Sen et al., 1979; Feneley & Burton, 1991) (Table 7) make this villous type the most appropriate place for diffusional exchange (e.g., transfer of oxygen, carbon dioxide, and water). In the normal mature placenta, the terminal villi comprise nearly 40% of the villous volume. Because of their small diameters, the sum of their surfaces amounts to 50% of the total villous surface. They comprise about 60% of villous cross sections. These figures explain why a remarkable reduction of terminal villi (as with terminal villi deficiency) (Kaufmann et al., 1985) may lead to fetal hypoxia. Also, according to Fox (1978) there is a clear-cut inverse relation between the incidence of villous vasculosyncytial membranes and fetal hypoxia.

Mesenchymal Villi

The term mesenchymal villi has been proposed for the first generation of tertiary villi. They are characterized by a seemingly primitive stromal core (Castellucci & Kaufmann, 1982a). From the 5th to the 7th week p.m., these villi comprise the only vascularized villous type. At later stages, their number continuously decreases. Some of these villi are still found at term, indicating that expansion of the villous trees never comes to a standstill.

They comprise the first generation of newly formed villi, not only during the first trimester but also at later stages. They are derived from trophoblastic sprouts by mesenchymal invasion and vascularization and precede the formation of new intermediate villi (Figure 72). In accordance with their role as proliferating segments, the mesenchymal villi decrease in number as pregnancy advances. At term they are primarily found in small numbers on the surfaces of immature intermediate villi. They are located in the centers of the villous trees.

Histologically, mesenchymal villi have thick trophoblastic surfaces with large numbers of Langhans' cells, which are interposed between syncytium and the trophoblastic basal lamina on 50% to 100% of the villous surfaces (Castellucci et al., 1990). The stroma is characterized by loosely arranged collagen fibers that enmesh mesenchymal cells and some Hofbauer cells. Condensed collagen is sometimes observed. Fetal capillaries are poorly developed and never show sinusoidal dilatation. Near the villous tips capillary lumens may still be occluded and made up of a string of endothelium (Figure 73); several steps in the formation of lumens can be observed. We refer to this still

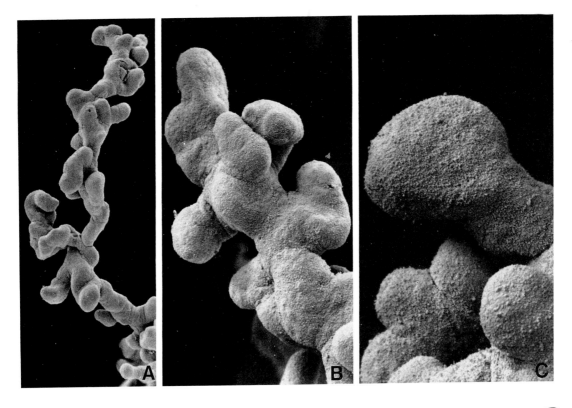

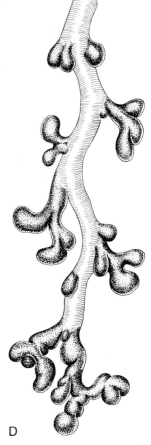

FIGURE 70. Scanning electron microscopic appearance of terminal villi. (A) Single, long, mature intermediate villus shows the characteristic bends of its longitudinal axis and multiple grape-like terminal villi. Note that the terminal villi largely have the same diameter as the mature intermediate villus from which they branch. ×180. (B) Tip of a mature intermediate villus with rich final branching into terminal villi. ×470. (C) Group of terminal villi, the central one showing a typical constricted neck region and a dilated final portion. ×500. (D) Mature intermediate villus (line shaded) and its branching terminal villi (point shaded). As is typical, most terminal villi arise from the convex sides of each bend, either directly or with a narrow neck region. They branch repeatedly, particularly at the end of the mature intermediate villus. (From Kaufmann et al., 1979, with permission.)

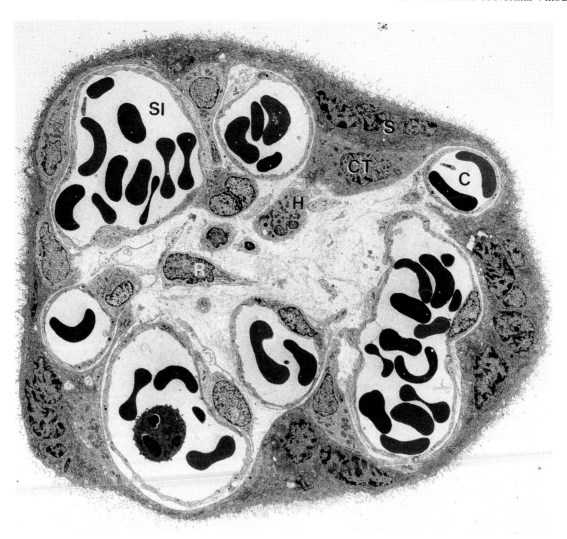

FIGURE 71. Survey electron micrograph of a typical, well fixed terminal villus. It illustrates the high degree of fetal capillarization, with some of the capillaries (C) narrow and others dilated, forming sinusoids (SI). The sparse connective tissue is composed of macrophages (H), fibroblasts or small reticulum cells (R), and a loose meshwork of connective tissue fibers. The stroma is surrounded by a structurally highly variable layer of syncytiotrophoblast (S) below which a few cytotrophoblastic cells (CT) can be seen. ×2,000. (From Schiebler & Kaufmann, 1981, with permission.)

unvascularized segment as a villous sprout. At the tip of the mesenchymal villus, the villous sprout continues into a trophoblastic sprout (Figures 65, 73). In summary the typical sequence of structures representing the process of villous sprouting is as follows: syncytial sprout, trophoblastic sprout with a central core of cytotrophoblast, villous sprout with some connective tissue, and mesenchymal villus with fetal capillaries (Figure 65).

During the first weeks of pregnancy mesenchymal villi are not only the places of villous proliferation (Figure 74), they are also sites of maternofetal exchange and nearly all endocrine activity. With advancing pregnancy and development of more advanced villous types, their functional importance is reduced to

villous growth. At term, their share in total villous volume is far below 1% (Figure 75) (Castellucci et al., 1990).

Immunohistochemical Characterization of Villous Types

The first parameters on which villous classification has been based were villous fibrosis and distribution of the various segments of the fetal vessel system (Kaufmann et al., 1979; see also above). The apparent differences in stromal structure (mesenchymal, reticular, fibrous) make it likely that the fixed connective tissue cells are different with respect to their patterns of expression of cytoskeletal proteins. Kohnen (1994) has described the cytoskeletal differentiation of villous connective tissue cells:

1. Undifferentiated mesenchymal cells express only vimentin.
2. Reticulum cells and fibroblasts express vimentin and desmin.

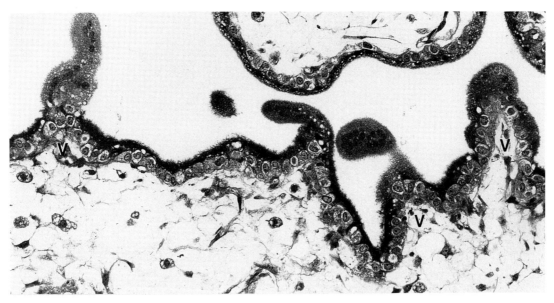

FIGURE 72. Structural features of villous sprouts and mesenchymal villi in a methacrylate section of placental villi from the 6th week p.m. From a larger mesenchymal villus (below), several sprouts protrude into the intervillous space. At their tips the latter consist merely of syncytiotrophoblast. Nearer the base they are invaded by cytotrophoblast and finally by loose connective tissue (villous sprout, V). The latter is the forerunner of new mesenchymal villi, which become established as soon as the sprouts are invaded by fetal vessels. ×390.

3. Myofibroblasts in addition to vimentin and desmin are characterized by the expression of α-smooth muscle.
4. At later stages of myofibroblast differentiation another actin isoform, γ-enteric actin, is added.
5. The highest stages of myofibroblast differentiation are characterized by the additional expression of smooth muscle myosin. The latter cells share most structural features with smooth muscle cells.

Because these fixed stromal cells are differentially distributed in the various villous types, immunohistochemistry of cytoskeletal proteins can help to identify the villous types (Table 12). It is hoped that further sophistication of such immunohistochemical staining patterns may be used in the not too distant future for an automatic and reproducible quantification of villous types as the basis for the diagnosis of villous maldevelopment (see Chapter 10).

Differentiation and Maturation of Villous Types

The mechanisms of villous maturation have attracted little attention, perhaps because they may seem to be unimportant to the understanding of placental pathology. This notion is supported by the experience that with conventional paraffin histology it is difficult to identify the various villous types and stages of villous differentiation. Direct structural evidence of villous differentiation and maturation are usually lacking. Only if one compares a mature placenta with early villous trees does there come some realization that important developmental steps must have occurred.

An improved histological and immunohistochemical methodology and easier availability of human material from most stages of pregnancy enabled us to deal with the mechanism of villous maturation and differentiation in some detail (Kaufmann, 1982; Castellucci et al., 1990; Kohnen et al., 1992; Kohnen, 1994). Further insights into the dynamics of the growth of the villous trees can be obtained from their topological analysis of the branching patterns and their later comparison with theoretical branching models (Kosanke et al., 1993). Our insight is still superficial, and conclusions are accordingly preliminary. We believe, however, that we must discuss this concern because clinical methods (e.g., chorion biopsy and Doppler studies) have caused renewed interest.

Development of Mesenchymal Villi

The first tertiary villi recognizable are the mesenchymal villi (Castellucci & Kaufmann, 1982a). They are derived from the following sources (Castellucci et al., 1990): Up to the 6th week p.m. the mesenchymal villi are formed from primary villi via secondary villi (Boyd & Hamilton, 1970). The numerous trophoblastic primary villi are transformed into secondary villi by invagination of extraembryonic mesenchyme. Immediately thereafter, the first capillaries form, giving rise to tertiary villi, the mesenchymal villi considered here. Beginning from the 6th week p.m., new mesenchymal villi are formed by vascularization of trophoblastic sprouts.

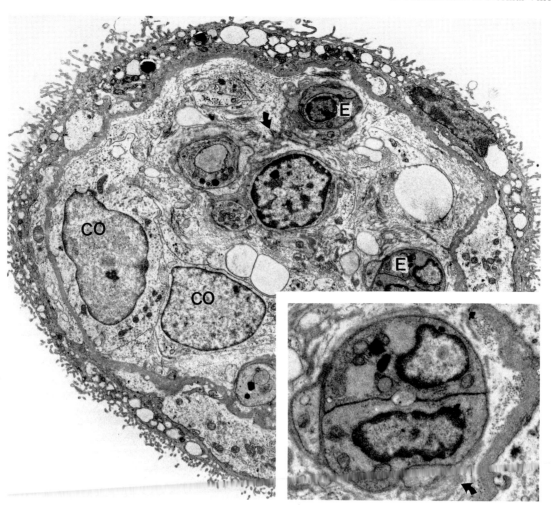

FIGURE 73. Transmission electron microscopic cross section of an intermediate stage between a villous sprout and a mesenchymal villus from a term placenta. This villus is characterized by large, epithelioid connective tissue cells (CO) and capillary sprouts. The latter consist of densely packed endothelial cells (E) connected to each other by tight junctions, showing no or only minimal lumens (inset) and surrounded by basal laminas. The latter form sometimes thick convolutions (arrow). It is interesting to note that many of the villous sprouts and mesenchymal villi observed exhibit degenerative signs (compare the highly vacuolated syncytiotrophoblast), which can be explained by the fact that not all sprouts survive, depending on the local circulatory conditions in the intervillous space. By this selection, the shape of the villous tree is adapted to the intervillous hemodynamics. ×5,200; inset ×13,000. (From Demir et al., 1989, with permission.)

These structures are trophoblastic outgrowths of the surfaces of mesenchymal and immature intermediate villi and result from trophoblastic proliferation (Figures 72, 74). Not all sprouts (i.e., fungiform outgrowths from the villous surface) are signs of trophoblastic sprouting. Some represent stages of expulsion of aged syncytial nuclei, and others are simply flat sections of villous surfaces (Cantle et al., 1987). The true trophoblastic sprouts correspond to the primary villi of the early stages of placentation. As the latter sprouts are invaded by mesenchyme and transformed into villous sprouts, the sprouts correspond to secondary villi of early development. The first signs of capillary formation mark the transformation to mesenchymal villi (Figure 73).

The concentration of Langhans' cells is greater in mesenchymal villi than in all other villi. In addition, the mitotic index of villous cytotrophoblast (counted from autoradioangiograms following ³H-thymidine incorporation and from immunohistochemical preparations using the antibodies KI 67, MIB 1, or PCNA) (Kohnen et al., 1993) considerably exceeds that of all other villi. This fact was not evident in previous publications (Moe, 1971; Tedde & Tedde-Piras, 1978; Kaufmann et al., 1983; Arnholdt et al., 1991) because the authors did not differentiate among the various villous types. The

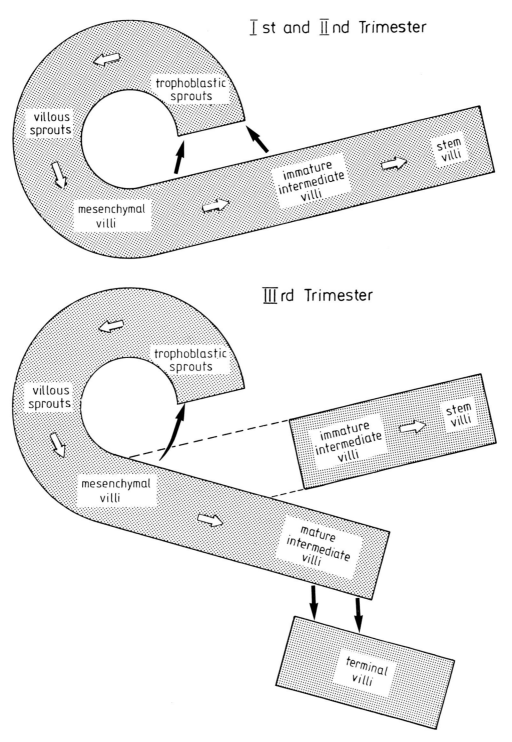

FIGURE 74. Routes of villous development during early and late pregnancy. White arrows = transformation of one villous type into another. Black arrows = new production of villi or sprouts along the surface of other villi. During the first and second trimesters trophoblastic sprouts are produced along the surfaces of mesenchymal and immature intermediate villi. Via villous sprouts, they are transformed into mesenchymal villi. The latter differentiate into immature intermediate villi, which produce new sprouts before they are transformed into stem villi. Throughout the third trimester, the mesenchymal villi are transformed into mature intermediate villi, which later produce terminal villi along their surfaces. There is no longer transformation of mesenchymal into immature intermediate villi. The remaining immature intermediate villi differentiate into stem villi, and so their number steeply decreases toward term. Hence the base for the formation of new sprouts is also reduced, and the growth capacity of the villous trees gradually slows.

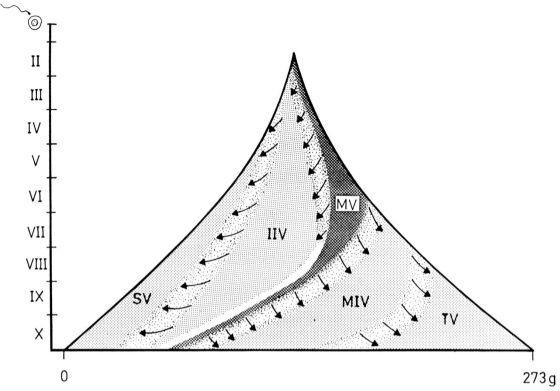

FIGURE 75. Development of the total villous weight and the weight of the various villous types (in grams), from the 2nd month p.m. until term. Abscissa: villous weight (in grams per placenta). Ordinate: gestational age p.m. (in months). The arrows demonstrate the routes of transformation, or the formation of villi. The lightly stippled areas around the arrows symbolize transitional stages between closely related villous types. At term the mean villous weight per placenta amounts to 273 g. After morphometric evaluation of representative histological sections, this weight can be assigned to the various villous types at term as follows: stem villi (SV), 31 g (11%); transitional stages to immature intermediate villi, 24 g (9%); immature intermediate villi (IIV), 9 g (3%); mesenchymal villi (MV), fewer than 1%; transitional stages to mature intermediate villi, 3 g (1%); mature intermediate villi (MIV), 77 g (28%); transitional stages to terminal villi, 31 g (11%); terminal villi (TV), 95 g (35%). Rough data for earlier stages of pregnancy can be deduced from the diagram. It must be pointed out that these data are preliminary, obtained from only a few placentas. There is a considerable local and inter-individual variation. It becomes evident that the sum of stem villi (SV) plus immature intermediate villi (IIV) decreases throughout the last 3 months of pregnancy; the decrease can be explained by a massive transformation of stem villi into fibrinoid. (Modified from Castellucci et al., 1990, with permission.)

postmitotic Langhans' cells migrate to the tips of trophoblastic sprouts. They are apparently responsible for longitudinal growth and branching of mesenchymal villi. Branching is introduced by the production of laterally positioned trophoblastic sprouts, which subsequently become vascularized.

Development and Fate of Immature Intermediate Villi

Beginning between the 7th and 8th weeks p.m., mesenchymal villi transform to immature intermediate villi. This process is characterized by: (1) a considerable increase in villous diameter; (2) the formation of the stromal channels (Figure 67) containing numerous macrophages (Enders & King, 1970; Kaufmann et al., 1979; Castellucci & Kaufmann, 1982a,b; Castellucci et al., 1984; King, 1987); (3) the transformation of mesenchymal cells in structurally and immunohisto-chemically different reticulum cells and fibroblasts (Kohnen, 1994); and (4) a decrease in thickness of syncytiotrophoblast and in the number of the Langhans' cells.

The reticular stroma is the most characteristic feature of immature intermediate villi. It seems to play an important role during transformation of these villi into fibrosed stem villi. According to G. Petry (personal communication, 1981), the accumulation of connective tissue fibers is preceded by a similar reticular architecture of connective tissue cells during the course of early

TABLE 12. Immunohistochemical classification of villous types using monoclonal antibodies directed against various cytoskeletal filaments.

Villous type and stroma	Immunohistochemical reactions[a]					Ultrastructure
	Vimentin	Desmin	α-sm-Actin	γ-Enteric-actin	sm-Myosin	
Mesenchymal villi						
Undifferentiated	+	0	0	0	0	Mesenchymal cells
Differentiated	+	+	0	0	0	Mesenchymal and reticulum cells
Immature intermediate villi						
Reticular stroma	+	+	0	0	0	Reticulum cells
Fibrosed stroma surrounding larger vessels	+	+	+	0	0	Fibroblasts or myofibroblasts
Inner adventitia of larger vessels	+	+	+	+	0	Myofibroblasts
Stem villi						
In general						
Superficial cellular rim	+	+	0	0	0	Reticulum cells or fibroblasts
Fibrous stroma	+	+	+	0	0	Fibroblasts or myofibroblasts
Adventitia of larger vessels	+	+	+	+	+[e]	Myofibroblasts
Type I (caliber >250 μm)						
Adventitia and media of arteries and veins	+	+	+	+[b]	+[f] +[g]	Myofibroblasts and smooth muscle cells
Type II (caliber 120–300 μm)						
Adventitia and media of arterioles and venules	+	+	+	+[c]	+[g]	Smooth muscle cells
Type III (caliber <150 μm)						
Adventitia and media of arterioles and venules	+	+	+	+[d]	+[g]	Smooth muscle cells
Mature intermediate villi	+	+	0	0	0	Fibroblasts or reticulum cells
Terminal villi	+	+	0	0	0	Fibroblasts or reticulum cells

For details see text. These results are based on the findings of Kohnen (1994).
[a] 0 = no immune reaction; + = positive immune reaction.
[b] In adventitia and media of arteries and veins.
[c] Only in media of arterioles and venules.
[d] Only in media of arterioles.
[e] Partly positive.
[f] Partly positive in adventitia.
[g] In media.

scar formation in the skin. The significance of this stromal type appears to be defined by the role of Hofbauer cells which, as macrophages, are probably involved in the remodeling of the connective tissue (Scott & Cohn, 1982; Werb, 1983; Castellucci et al., 1984; Takemura & Werb, 1984). There is presently no specific function for the immature intermediate villi, other than being a quickly growing developmental precursor for stem villi (Figure 74).

Development of additional immature intermediate villi from mesenchymal villi gradually ceases at the end of the second trimester. Their transformation into stem villi, however, continues to term. Therefore the number of immature intermediate villi decreases dramatically (Figure 75). Sometimes they completely disappear before term. It is common, however, that small numbers persist in the centers of the villous trees and serve as growth zones.

Development of Stem Villi

The development of stem villi is closely related to the formation of the immature intermediate villi. As early as the 8th week p.m., the central vessels of the proximal segments of immature intermediate villi, near the chorionic plate, commence constructing a compact adventitia. They thus slowly transform into arteries and veins. Centrifugal expansion of the adventitia, paralleled by transformation of reticulum cells and fibroblasts into myofibroblasts, leads to a reduction of the adjacent reticular connective tissue (Figures 85–89).

The transition of immature intermediate villi to stem villi is a gradual process. According to our definition, stem villi are established as soon as the superficial sheet of reticular connective tissue underneath the trophoblast is thinner than the fibrous center surrounding stem vessels (Figures 86, 87) (Castellucci et al., 1990). Stem vessels have then been transformed into arteries and veins or arterioles and venules. The persistence of a small rim of reticular connective tissue underneath the trophoblast in the term placenta can be regarded as a reliable sign of placental immaturity (Kaufmann, 1981).

The formation of additional stem villi depends on the availability of immature intermediate villi. Therefore the expansion of villous stems gradually ceases during the last trimester, as soon as most immature intermediate villi have been transformed and new ones are no longer produced.

Increased stromal fibrosis outside stem villi is considered to be a pathological phenomenon. Such villi are usually referred to as fibrotic. Fox (1978) reported several conditions that are commonly associated with fibrotic villi.

1. Stromal fibrosis is a regular finding of peripheral villi following fetal artery thrombosis.
2. It may also be found in inadequately vascularized villi adjacent to areas of infarction.
3. Increased numbers of fibrotic villi have been observed in placentas from macerated stillbirths. Fox (1978) concluded that it must be a postmortem change because this feature is absent from placentas in fresh stillbirths; however, this issue is still debatable and probably depends on the cause of the fetal demise.
4. A marked increase of fibrosed villi may be found in placentas of prolonged pregnancy.

Contrary to many other reports, Fox (1978) was unable to show an association between villous fibrosis and fetal complications, such as hypoxia or low birth weight. He thus refuted the theory that increased stromal fibrosis is a response to uteroplacental ischemia. In his opinion, it is more likely a result of reduced intravillous blood flow. This situation may result in intravillous hyperoxic conditions, as oxygen transfer from the villi to the fetus is impaired (Kaufmann et al., 1993; Macara et al., 1994; see below). We found a generally increased degree of stromal fibrosis within the mature intermediate villi associated with the condition known as terminal villi deficiency (Schweikhart & Kaufmann, 1983; Schweikhart, 1985; Kaufmann et al., 1987). This entity not only is often combined with prolonged pregnancy, but it appears to be the result of reduced fetal vascularization as well.

Development of Mature Intermediate Villi

One of the most important steps for an understanding of villous development occurs at the beginning of the last trimester. At this time, the transformation of newly formed mesenchymal villi into immature intermediate villi switches to a transformation into mature intermediate villi (Figures 74, 75, 88, 89) (Castellucci et al., 1990). Differing in this respect from immature intermediate villi, the mature villi do not transform into stem villi; only in pathological conditions do they acquire a larger amount of collagen fibers. They are responsible for the future development of terminal villi.

Development of Terminal Villi

The first terminal villi, as defined in the past (Kaufmann et al., 1979; Sen et al., 1979), are produced soon after the first mature intermediate villi are formed (Figure 75). The formation of terminal villi is closely related to the longitudinal growth of capillaries within the mature intermediate villi (Figure 80). As soon as longitudinal capillary growth exceeds longitudinal growth, the capillaries become coiled and form loops (Kaufmann et al., 1985, 1988). Because of the slender shape of these villi, the loops bulge on the trophoblastic surface and finally protrude as grape-like outgrowths into the intervillous space. This process is not accompanied by trophoblastic proliferation and therefore is accompanied by considerable stretching of the trophoblast. This process results in numerous epithelial plates of terminal villi. It follows that the terminal villi are not active outgrowths induced by proliferation; rather, they represent passive formations caused by capillary coiling. The slight bends of the mature intermediate villi, at points where terminal villi branch off (Figures 70A,D), illustrate the mechanical forces that have been active during capillary growth and coiling. Terminal villi, at the surfaces of stem villi and immature intermediate villi and derived from coiling of paravascular capillaries, are the exceptions. These particular capillaries show less impressive longitudinal growth (Leiser et al., 1985).

Angioarchitecture of Villi

Vascular Arrangement in Immature Villi

The first vascular nets formed in early placental villi show no differentiation into arteries, veins, or capillaries (Demir et al., 1989), a picture that changes around the 8th week p.m. As a consequence of fusion of locally developed intravillous vascular nets with the fetal vessels that invade the villous trees via the connective stalk (the forerunner of the umbilical cord), the fetoplacental circulation becomes established. Because of pressure gradients between arterial and venous limbs, differently structured vessel walls appear (Figure 84). Connective tissue cells that aggregate around the endothelial tubes in a circular fashion are the first steps in the formation of the walls of future arteries and veins. Normally, one artery and one vein are formed. The remaining capillary net that surrounds the larger vessels is referred to as paravascular net. An example of this phenomenon has been illustrated by Boe (1969) (Figure 78). When he traced single vessels, he found numerous capillaries that formed shortcuts between arteries and veins but also between neighboring arteries (arterioarterial anastomoses). Because of the low blood pressure in the vascular system, effective arteriovenous shunting is unlikely.

The villus depicted by Boe (Figure 78) is consistent with what we described as an immature intermediate villus. It is an undifferentiated, still growing villous type that can be found even in the mature placenta, although in only small restricted groups. The small branching-off villi described by Boe as terminal villi are likely newly formed mesenchymal villi (Figures 72, 78). As is typical for newly formed villi, their richly branched capillary nets are connected only with the paravascular net, rather than directly with arteries and veins. Only after further development, as soon as some of their capillaries have been transformed to arterioles and venules, are direct connections to the fetal stem vessel established.

Large Vessels of Stem Villi

Large stem villi normally contain one artery in a nearly central position. If not constricted or collapsed, the lumen accounts for about one-third of the villous caliber (Figure 66A). The endothelium is surrounded by a few layers of smooth muscle cells. The adventitia, which is two to three times as thick as the media, is continuous with the surrounding connective tissue, without a sharp line of demarcation. The artery is normally accompanied by a corresponding vein. Its luminal width does not much exceed that of the artery in most preparations owing to the collapse that occurs after delivery. In addition to the two main vessels, varying numbers of smaller arterioles and venules exist (Leiser et al., 1985; Kaufmann et al., 1988).

The most peripheral generations of stem villi branch or continue into mature intermediate villi and have diameters ranging from 80 to 150 µm (Figures 66B, 76). The stem vessels are arterioles and venules that are surrounded by one or two layers of smooth muscle cells. The inconspicuous venules have one, usually incomplete, layer of muscle cells. Some are surrounded only by pericytes and correspond to the collecting venules of Rhodin (1968), despite their different diameter. Frequently arterioles and venules of this segments are so similar they cannot be identified on cross-sectioning but only from reconstructions. For quantitative estimations of stem vessels we refer to a survey by Leiser et al. (1991).

Paravascular Capillary Net of Stem Villi

Underneath the trophoblast, numerous cross sections of capillaries with small calibers appear. They belong to the paravascular net (Boe, 1953) (Figure 76C). This system is derived from the paravascular net of the earlier immature villi. Because of vascular obstruction during transformation of the immature intermediate villi into stem villi, a rarefied and poorly branching system of slender capillary loops develops. It can be seen in most stem villi depicted in the literature (Arts, 1961; Thiriot and Panigel, 1978; Habashi et al., 1983; Leiser et al., 1985; Kaufmann et al., 1988). The paravascular capillaries follow a straight course, mostly parallel to the longitudinal axis of the villus. In our material of mature stem villi, net-like connections have been uncommon. We have seen such richly branched and dense paravascular capillary nets as depicted by Burton (1987) only in immature intermediate villi (Figure 78) and in not yet fully matured stem villi. We concede, however, that our impression may be incomplete. The paravascular capillaries are connected to the arteries and veins by short arteriolar and venular segments, measuring up to 100 µm in length. These capillaries often form hairpin-like loops, their connections to the larger vessels being close together.

Only in rare cases do the paravascular capillaries show focal sinusoidal dilatations. If it occurs, the dilated and coiling segments bulge on the surface of the stem villus and form a terminal villus that arises from the stem villus (Kaufmann et al., 1979; Burton, 1987) (Figure 76C, upper half). Such terminal villi are serially intercalated into the paravascular net. According to our experience, this occurrence is rare (less than 5% of all terminal villi), whereas Burton (1987) described it to be a regular finding.

When we traced individual paravascular capillaries from their arteriolar beginnings to their venular ends, we found an average length of 1,000 to 2,000 µm. Arteriovenous and arterioarterial shortcuts, as described by Boe (1953, 1969) for the earlier stages of development, could no longer be detected in mature stem villi. There is therefore no real basis for speculations that the paravascular net participates in the regulation of fetal blood flow impedance as an arteriovenous shunting system.

The functional relevance of the paravascular capillary net is still uncertain. Thiriot and Panigel (1978) suggested that it was the site for effective fetomaternal exchange. The long diffusion distances in these places, as well as the fact that the capillaries are often arranged in a hairpin-like manner, allowing reversed diffusion, make this interpretation implausible. Moreover, the assumption by Arts (1961) that the paravascular net may

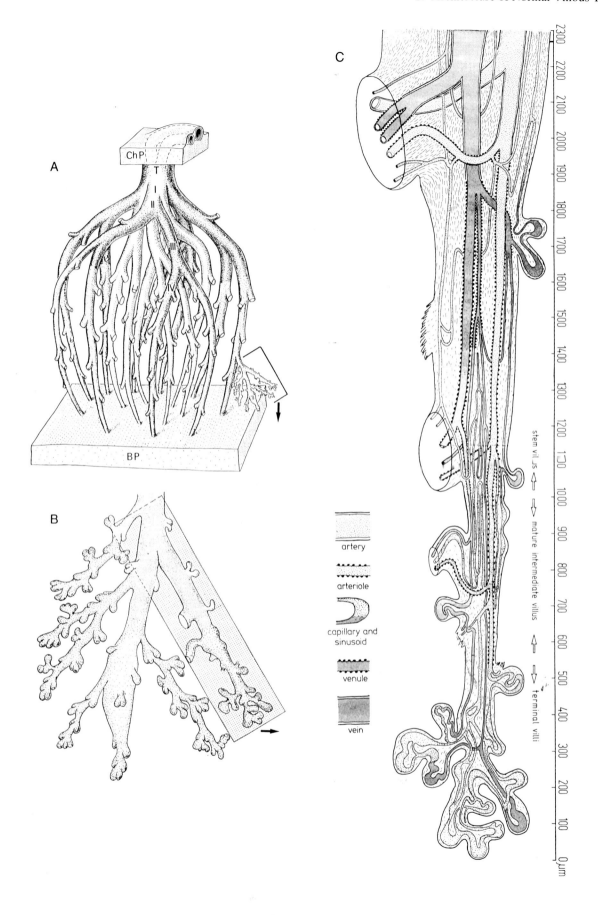

be of nutritional importance for the stem villi, acting as a kind of vasa vasorum, seems unlikely to us. The concentration of oxygen and most nutrients in the surrounding intervillous space considerably exceeds that in the fetal vessels. Thus the nutrition by direct diffusion from the maternal blood is probably more effective. This finding is in agreement with those of Zeek and Assali (1950) and of Fox (1978), who found not only survival of stroma but also increased fibroblast proliferation and collagen production within stem villi after fetal death.

Boyd and Hamilton (1970) described the paravascular net to be simply a residual indication of better vascularization during early stages of development. Keeping in mind that the developmental forerunners of the stem villi were immature intermediate villi with a well developed paravascular net (Kaufmann et al., 1988), the respective capillaries of the mature stem villi probably represent the remains of the immature state where terminal villi with their effective exchange system were absent and the paravascular net had to sustain maternofetal exchange. The development of better-vascularized terminal villi during the course of the last trimester renders the paravascular capillaries largely nonfunctional.

Arrangement of Vessels in Mature Intermediate and Terminal Villi

The mature intermediate villi serve as junctional segments between the most peripheral stem villi and most of the terminal villi. Their vessels are direct continuations of the smallest stem villous vessels (Figure 76C). One or two small arterioles, with luminal diameters ranging from 20 to 40 μm, appear histologically as bare endothelial tubes, accompanied by occasional muscle cells (Figures 66B, 69A). Precapillary sphincters, or narrow segments with complete muscular coats comparable to those described for other vascular beds (Rhodin, 1967), have not been identified. Rather,

the terminal ends of arterioles continue directly into one or two capillaries by a gradual reduction of their diameters and loss of smooth muscle (Kaufmann et al., 1985; Leiser et al., 1991).

Whereas the arterioles occupy a more central position in the villous stroma, one or two venules can be found more superficially. Surprisingly, their diameter usually appears to be considerably smaller than that of the arterioles, usually 15 to 20 μm. In agreement with the classification of Rhodin (1968), the term postcapillary venule seems to be most appropriate because of the absence of muscle cells and the existence of a nearly complete sheet of pericytes. The most peripheral loops of the paravascular capillaries of the stem villi surround the terminal arterioles and postcapillary venules. They extend to about the middle of the mature intermediate villi (Figure 76C).

In the distal one-half of the mature intermediate villi, the paravascular capillaries are absent. Histologically, the distal segment can easily be differentiated from the more proximal segments by the absence of large vessel cross sections and the absence of vessels in the center of the stromal core; most capillaries are located directly underneath the trophoblast (Figure 69A). In most cases, the abrupt end of the paravascular "net" causes a sharp line of demarcation between the more proximal segment, which is rich in capillaries, and the distal, less vascularized part (Figure 76C).

The terminal capillaries are different from the mostly straight paravascular capillaries and are characterized by the formation of loops and coilings. Focally dilated segments may bulge against the trophoblast and thus form epithelial plates, knob-like protrusions, or even terminal villi. As one approaches the peripheral end of the mature intermediate villus, the number and extent of capillary coilings increases and so does the number of terminal outgrowths that cover the surface of the mature intermediate villus (Figures 70A,B,D, 76, 79). At its end, the mature intermediate villus regularly branches into a cluster of terminal villi (Figure 70D).

FIGURE 76. Fetal vascularization of term placental villi based on the spatial reconstruction of serial sections. (A) Large stem villi of the villous tree. ChP = chorionic plate; BP = basal plate; T = truncus; I, II, III, IV = rami chorii of the first to the fourth order. The more peripheral branches depicted in this drawing are ramuli chorii of the first to the tenth order. The marked peripheral ramulus with its terminal branches refers to (B). (B) Higher magnification of peripheral branches of the villous tree. A peripheral stem branches into several mature intermediated villi (slender) and one immature intermediate villus (thick). The shaded rectangular area corresponds to the reconstructed branches depicted in (C). (C) Fetal vascular branching patterns of a peripheral stem villus

(above), continuing into a mature intermediate villus, extending into several terminal villi, reconstructed from a series of 2,300 semithin sections. Length and caliber of the villi are drawn on the same scale, whereas the diameter of the vessels is reduced to two-thirds (necessary because of two-dimensional representation of a three-dimensional system). Occasional spots of fibrinoid necrosis on the villous surface are marked by hatching. Note that the capillary loops of neighboring terminal villi are serially connected. They are normally not continuous with the straight paravascular capillaries of the stem and mature intermediate villi but form a second independent capillary bed. (Modified from Kaufmann et al., 1988, with permission.)

There is no sharp demarcation between mature intermediate and terminal villi. Increased capillary coiling, accompanied by increased sinusoidal dilatation and reduced stromal connective tissue is responsible for the structural differences. The descriptive name "terminal villus" is used for those villi (1) that contain no vessels other than capillaries and sinusoids; and (2) in which the vascular lumens comprise at least one-half of the stromal volume (Kaufmann et al., 1979, 1985).

Depending on the level at which such terminal villi are sectioned, their histological appearance is highly variable. An example is depicted in Figure 79. The capillary loops of the peripheral terminal villi are direct continuations of terminal arterioles. According to our experience, they only occasionally show cross-connections to peripheral loops of the paravascular capillaries, described as a regular feature by Arts (1961). It is of particular importance to note that the capillary loops of neighboring terminal villi are serially connected to each other (Figures 76C, 77, 79A). Fetal blood leaving a terminal arteriole and entering the terminal capillaries normally passes through the capillary loops of three to five terminal villi in series before entering a postcapillary venule. This passage is responsible for the length of terminal capillaries, which we measured as ranging from 3,000 to 5,000 μm (Kaufmann et al., 1985). Shortcuts at the base of terminal capillary loops are the exception, so that each erythrocyte has to pass the full length of the capillaries. As reported above, the paravascular capillary loops measure only 1,000 to 2,000 μm in length.

When one looks at casts of vessels such as those depicted in Figure 79, it seems that the terminal capillary bed is made up of a highly branching network, and it has usually been described as such (Boe, 1953,

1968; Arts, 1961; Boyd & Hamilton, 1970; Thiriot & Panigel, 1978; Habashi et al., 1983; Burton, 1987). In contrast, our reconstructions of terminal vessel beds revealed only a low degree of branching. When discussing this discrepancy, Burton (1987) stated that "the superimposition of SEM [scanning electron microscopy] images can lead to mistaken estimates of the incidence of vessels joining, but it cannot be denied that branching and union between capillaries does occur within terminal villi. The problem may be only one of degree...." We admit that our results were obtained from the reconstruction of only a few cases (Kaufmann et al., 1985); it is our opinion, however, that the more likely explanation for the discrepancy is one of definition. Branching, with directly subsequent union, is indeed a frequent feature (Figure 77). It must not be confused with the establishment of true, complex intravillous capillary nets, which offer the possibility of basal shortcuts. The latter possibility might considerably shorten the individual capillary length. On the other hand, a high degree of coiling with serially intercalated branching and direct fusion has no influence on the mean capillary length. This difference may have physiological importance for fetal blood flow impedance.

Boe (1968) described and illustrated "terminal villi" with impressive capillary nets that were directly connected to the paravascular net of their parent villus (Figure 78). We are convinced that the villi described by him were newly formed mesenchymal villi, derived from an immature intermediate villus. We interpret the figures of Burton (1987)—and described as terminal villi that originate from the paravascular net—in the same way. Such controversies indicate that much systematic research is needed in this area.

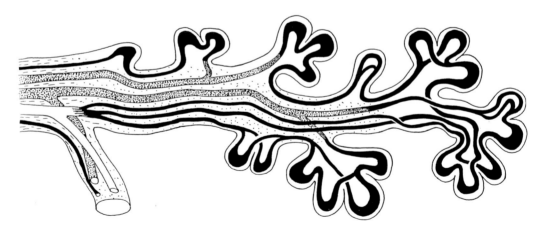

FIGURE 77. Arrangement of the fetal vessels in a group of terminal villi derived from one mature intermediate villus. Note the highly complex loop formation of the terminal fetal capillaries. Branching is usually followed shortly by refusion of the two capillary branches. Such a branching pattern avoids basal shortcuts. Each erythrocyte must pass the terminal capillaries of several terminal villi in their full length. Local dilatations, or sinusoids, reduce blood flow impedance.

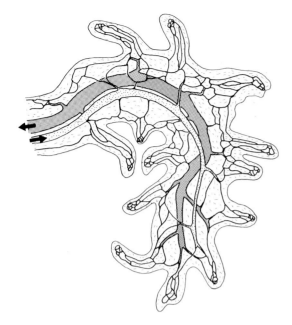

FIGURE 78. Classical representation of the villous vascularization by Boe (1969). It represents an immature intermediate villus with numerous mesenchymal side branches. The web-like arrangement of the fetal capillaries protruding from the paravascular net of the immature intermediate villus into its sprouting side branches is highly characteristic not only for early placentas but also for villous sprouting patterns in the term placenta. As depicted in the foregoing pictures, it is normally absent in the mature villous types. (Based on findings of Boe, 1969.)

Sinusoids of Terminal Villi

Sinusoids are focal capillary enlargements that attain diameters up to about 50 μm (Figures 62B, 71, 79). They are thought to be typical features of the mature placenta and are not comparable to the sinusoids of liver, spleen, and bone marrow, as the former possess a continuous endothelium and complete basal lamina. They thus differ from conventional capillaries only by their increased diameters. In semithin sections, the sinusoids are normally positioned near the villous tips. Vascular casts, however, reveal that they are randomly scattered over the full length of the terminal capillaries, rather than being dilatations of defined segments (Kaufmann et al., 1985). They may narrow and dilate serially several times (Figure 77). Statistically, they are found more frequently near the villous tips, along the venous limbs, and at points of branching and fusion. The grade of dilatation and the degree of tortuosity of the capillary loops seem to depend on each other.

We have measured the diameters of capillaries and sinusoids in semithin sections and compared them to casts of vessels (Kaufmann et al., 1985). The results, obtained with both methods, were largely consistent. The mean diameters of capillaries and sinusoids of the

mature placenta varied from 12.2 ± 0.58 μm in vessel casts to 14.4 ± 1.94 μm in semithin sections. The difference can be explained by different degrees of shrinkage of the resins used for preparation. In our experience, the higher values seem to be more appropriate. The maximum values were 39 μm in casts of vessels and 45 μm in semithin sections. Depending on the method applied, 60% to 80% of the vessel lumens had diameters larger than 10 μm. Our data are largely consistent with those reported by Becker (1962), Becker and Seifert (1965), and Boyd and Hamilton (1970).

The smaller diameters reported by Habashi et al. (1983) and O'Neill (1983), the latter author giving a range of only 4 to 7 μm, are probably due to incomplete filling of vessels of their casts and resin shrinkage. Even more contradictory are the physiological results published by Penfold et al. (1981). These authors perfused capillaries with microspheres of varying diameter. They concluded that as many as 25% of capillaries measure less than 4 μm in diameter, and virtually no capillary exceeds 11 μm in diameter. Their results were based on the erroneous assumption that narrow and dilated capillary loops are arranged in parallel; their results must be refuted (Habashi et al., 1983). In fact, the capillaries become narrow and dilate serially. Thus when using microsphere perfusion, the diameter for the narrowest segment of each capillary loop can only be estimated. Even so, the value of 4 μm for 25% of the capillary loops cannot be accepted.

The functional relevance of the sinusoids has caused ample speculation. It is evident from the above description that the sinusoidal dilatation cannot be regarded as dilated venous limbs of the capillary loops that allow retarded venous backflow, as was discussed by Nikolov and Schiebler (1973). The localization of most sinusoids near the villous tips supports the conclusion of Arts (1961) that the sinusoids locally decelerate blood flow, providing ample opportunity for fetomaternal exchange. This assumption is in agreement with the finding that the sinusoids are regularly situated in contiguity with the epithelial plates (Boyd & Hamilton, 1970; Nikolov & Schiebler, 1973, 1981; Schiebler & Kaufmann, 1981). These plates are thought to represent areas of maximal diffusional exchange (Amstutz, 1960; Kaufmann et al., 1974).

It is still a matter of dispute if the reduced blood flow velocity facilitates maternofetal exchange or if the increased diffusion distance from the center of the sinusoids to the villous surface negatively influences the diffusion capacity. Another explanation for the existence of sinusoids has been that they serve as functionally specialized segments devoted to specific transport processes. Nikolov and Schiebler (1981) described two types of endothelial cell. These findings,

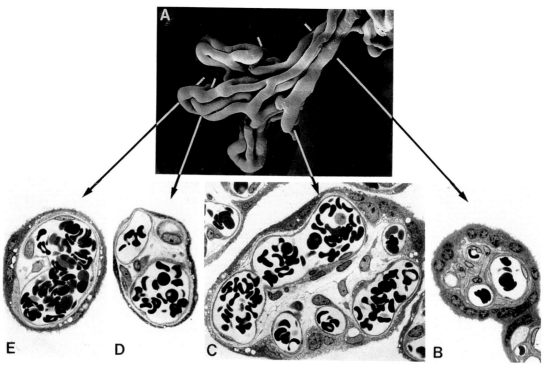

FIGURE 79. Fetal vascularization of terminal villi. (A) Cast of vessels from a neck region (right) branching into three terminal villi. Comparable to mature intermediate villi, the capillaries of the neck region are strikingly straight and arranged in parallel; however, the diameter of the villus is much smaller. ×520. Corresponding semithin sections of the neck region (B), the basis of the branching terminal villi (C), a single terminal villus near its tip (D), and a flat section of the terminal villous tip (E). The fetal capillaries and the highly dilated sinusoids amount to more than 50% of the stromal volume as long as postpartal collapse can be avoided by early fixation. Compare Figure 62a,b ×630. (From Kaufmann et al., 1988, with permission.)

however, cannot serve as arguments for a functional specialization of sinusoids compared to narrow capillaries, as they seem to be evenly distributed in both vessel segments (Figures 62B,C).

We discussed another explanation for the function of the sinusoids elsewhere (Kaufmann et al., 1985, 1987, 1988). It is remarkable that the sinusoids are produced at the end of pregnancy (Becker, 1981), as soon as the terminal villi achieve the highest degree of branching and twisting and as the terminal capillary loops reach their maximal length of 3,000 to 5,000 µm. On the other hand, sinusoids are largely absent in the short terminal capillary loops of immature placentas and in the short paravascular capillaries. Moreover, they are not found in labyrinthine placentas, such as those of the guinea pig (Kaufmann & Davidoff, 1977) and chinchilla (Dantzer et al., 1988), both of which are characterized by short (500–1,000 µm) fetal capillaries. We have studied some capybara placentas. This species is of the same suborder of caviomorph rodents as the guinea pig and chinchilla but has a much larger placenta, with fetal capillaries of about twice their lengths. Its placenta shows fetal sinusoids. The same is true for the goat placenta, which has long capillary loops comparable to those of the human placenta (Leiser, 1987; Dantzer et al., 1988).

According to the law of Hagen-Poiseuille, blood flow resistance is reduced by the fourth power of the vascular radius. It can be concluded that even limited and focal sinusoidal dilatation of the long terminal capillary loops may considerably decrease blood flow impedance to such a degree that it no longer exceeds that in the shorter paravascular capillaries. In this way, an even blood flow distribution is guaranteed for all capillaries, independent of their length and diameter. In addition, for this low-pressure fetal circulatory system, the perfusion of the huge extracorporeal organ becomes much easier.

Capillary Growth as Related to the Development of Terminal Villi

Thorough comparison of the capillary arrangement in normally and in abnormally matured terminal ramifications demonstrates that the development of terminal villi depends on capillary growth (Kaufmann et al., 1985). More than 95% of terminal villi arise from the surfaces of mature intermediate villi by bulging of coiled capillaries. "Hypermature villi" (Salvatore, 1968; Kaufmann, 1982; Kaufmann et al., 1987) show an increased number of terminal villi, together with longer, wider, more coiled capillaries (Figures 80, 104). In contrast, cases of terminal villi deficiency (Schweikhart & Kaufmann, 1983, 1987; Kaufmann et al., 1987) exhibit nearly naked mature intermediate villi that are almost devoid of terminal villi. The terminal capillaries are much shorter, usually uncoiled, with only a few sinusoidal dilatations (Figures 80, 103). We concluded from the observations shown in Figure 80 that the development of terminal villi is influenced by the balance of longitudinal growth of mature intermediate villi and that of their capillary loops. The more capillary growth exceeds the longitudinal villous growth, the more do the capillaries become coiled. The single coils bulge against the surfaces of the mature intermediate villi and thus produce the terminal villi. We interpret the terminal villi to be passive outpocketings, rather than the result of trophoblastic proliferation.

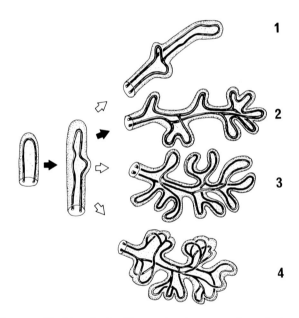

FIGURE 80. Terminal villous development in relation to capillary growth. So long as longitudinal capillary growth corresponds to the longitudinal growth of the mature intermediate villus (two left figures), the latter remains straight and does not form side branches. When longitudinal capillary growth exceeds the longitudinal villous growth, however, capillary loops are formed and bulge against the surface, thereby causing the development of terminal villi. Varying degrees of imbalance between villous and capillary growth result in different types of terminal villous development: 1 = Terminal villi deficiency (see Figure 103A); 2 = normal mature placenta (see Figures 70A,D and 100A); 3 = hypermaturity (see Figure 104A); 4 = hypoxic hypervascularization (see Figures 105A and 106A). (From Kaufmann et al., 1988, with permission.)

Because of the correlations discussed above, over- or understimulated capillary growth results in various types of villous maldevelopment. It is still uncertain whether such cases of maldevelopment result from abnormal conditions long before term or they can be induced during the last few weeks of pregnancy. Many authors have stated that villous growth comes to a standstill during the last weeks of pregnancy. Some morphological results provide evidence, however, that villous development is still in progress even at term. Vascular casts of term placentas show blindly ending outgrowths of capillaries (Thiriot & Panigel, 1978; Kaufmann et al., 1985). Such outgrowths may be interpreted as the result of incomplete filling of the casts. Reconstruction of serial sections revealed similar features (Figure 76C). Some continue into massive endothelial cords, indicating that the processes of capillary sprouting and terminal villous growth at term are still active.

Intervillous Space as Related to the Villous Trees

The human placenta is a hemochorial, villous placental type. After leaving the spiral arteries, the maternal blood circulates through the diffuse intervillous space and flows directly around the villi. The maternal blood is outside the confines of the endothelium of the maternal vascular system.

The anatomic investigations of the intervillous space suffer the disadvantage of having been made on delivered placentas, which have lost considerable amounts of maternal blood during delivery. They are also usually fixed without the in vivo maternal blood pressure distending the intervillous space. Therefore the usual appearance of the intervillous space of the delivered placenta is that of a system of narrow clefts. Hörmann (1951, 1953, 1958a,b) and Lemtis (1955) called it the intervillous cleft system. This view was supported by Becker (1963), who attempted to restablish in vivo pressure conditions prior to fixation and found the same narrow clefts. Becker described neighboring villi as clinging closely to one another, the tips of some fitting into notches of others, as in a jigsaw puzzle. Becker interpreted the occasional appearance of a wide intervillous space (in conventional histological material) as the result of shrinkage. Freese (1966) also failed to demonstrate an intervillous space of larger than capillary dimensions, except for the subchorial lake. Boyd and Hamilton (1970) contradicted these interpretations. According to their experience from in vivo radioangiograms, the rapid filling of the intervillous space is not compatible with a cleft system of capillary dimensions.

Using the data for postpartal intervillous blood volume (23.3–37.9% of the placental volume) and the villous surface (11.0–13.3 m²) (Tables 6, 9), we calculate the mean width of the intervillous space (blood volume ÷ villous surface/2) as ranging from 16.4 to 32.0 μm. The villous surface must be divided by 2 because it covers the clefts on both sides. Bouw et al. (1976) demonstrated that late cord clamping is responsible for a loss of intervillous volume, probably owing to the decreasing turgor of the villi that border the intervillous space (Table 9). If we calculate the mean width of the intervillous space with his data from term placentas obtained after early cord clamping, the width is 31.6 μm. One must bear in mind that there is a considerable subchorial lake, and wide spaces exist in the arterial inflow area as well. Thus the real "intervillous" volume is likely to be lower and the intervillous clefts narrower. On the other hand, when one adds the considerable loss of maternal blood during labor, we consider that these calculations may be near the truth.

Wigglesworth (1967) studied corrosion casts of fetal vessels and suggested that most villous trees are arranged as hollow-centered bud-like structures. When he injected the spiral arteries, Wigglesworth found the injection mass to collect in the loose centers of the villous trees. This finding is in agreement with most descriptions of the maternal arterial inlets as being located near the centers of the villous trees (Schuhmann & Wehler, 1971; Schuhmann, 1981) and directing the bloodstream into these centers (Panigel & Pascaud, 1968). The 50 to 200 maternal venous outlets of each placenta are thought to be arranged around the periphery of the villous trees. Thus each fetomaternal circulatory unit is composed of one villous tree with a corresponding, centrifugally perfused portion of the intervillous space (Figures 7, 81). This unit was called a placentone by Schuhmann and Wehler (1971).

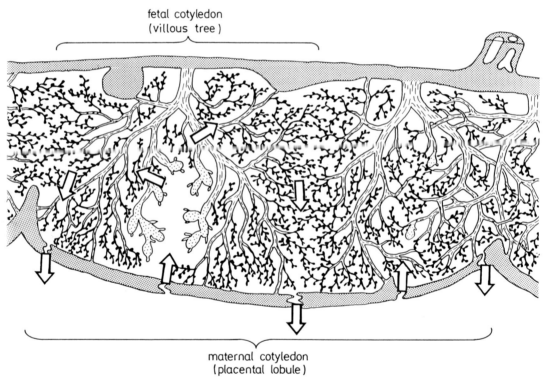

FIGURE 81. Typical spatial relations between villous trees, single villous types, and the maternal bloodstream. According to the placentone theory of Schuhmann (1981), a placentone is one villous tree plus the related part of the intervillous space. In the case of typical placentones (left half of figure), which prevail in the periphery of the placenta, the maternal blood (arrows) enters the intervillous space near the center of the villous tree and leaves the intervillous space near the clefts between neighboring villous trees. In the term placenta the larger stem villi (line-shaded), immature intermediate villi (point-shaded), and their tiny mesenchymal branches are concentrated in the centers of the villous trees, surrounding a central cavity as maternal inflow area. The mature intermediate villi (black) together with their terminal branches (black, grape-like) make up the periphery of the villous trees, near the venous outflow area. One or a few villous trees occupy one placental lobule (see Figure 17), which is delimited by grooves in the basal surface of the placenta (see Figure 16b). In the central parts of the placenta the villous trees, because of size and nearby location, may partly overlap (right half of figure) so the zonal arrangement of the placentone disappears. (Modified from Kaufmann, 1985, with permission.)

Most placentologists agree that under in vivo conditions most of the 40 to 60 placentones are in contact with each other and that they overlap more or less broadly. This supposition is highly probable, as structural borderlines, such as placental septa, are absent (Becker & Jipp, 1963). It is our experience that the peripheral placentones are more clearly separated from each other and thus exhibit typical structural differences between their central and peripheral zones. In the thicker, more central regions of the placenta, most villous trees overlap (Figure 81), causing less distinct differences between maternal inflow and outflow areas of the placentone.

According to studies of Schuhmann and Wehler (1971), the centers of typical placentones exhibit loosely arranged villi, mostly of the immature intermediate type, and provide a large intervillous space for the maternal arterial inflow. It is still uncertain if these large, loosely arranged villi regularly delineate a central cavity as described by Wilkin (1965). Schuhmann (1981) suggested that these cavities are pressure-dependent in vivo structures that rapidly collapse after delivery, and his suggestion is borne out by sonographic findings. If one accepts the considerations of Moll (1981), the existence of such a central cavity makes sense because it guarantees the rapid and homogeneous distribution of blood into the surrounding mantle of small, densely packed villi with little loss of pressure.

The surrounding mantle is composed mostly of small villi of the mature intermediate and terminal types. They are densely packed. Schmid-Schönbein (1988) described the intervillous space in this zone as a system of randomly shaped and oriented, interconnected clefts, or "connected voids." With respect to their topology, these clefts lack the regular connectivity seen in dichotomously branching vascular beds. The fixed relations of the latter vessels, which orient pressure gradients, are not found in randomly connected voids as in the intervillous space. This feature may be advantageous under normal conditions, but it may also cause hazards to the intervillous circulation.

The most peripheral zone of a placentone is the loosely arranged area that separates neighboring villous trees and that, subchorially, is connected to the subchorial lake. It is the venous outflow area that collects the maternal venous blood that has left the high impedance area of the fetomaternal exchange zone of the densely packed terminal villi. Moll (1981) called it the perilobular zone, which is functionally comparable to wide venules of other vascular beds. It allows venous backflow under conditions of low blood flow resistance.

The radioangiographic studies of Ramsey et al. (1963) in rhesus monkey placentas, and those of Borell et al. (1958) in human placentas are consistent with the placentone concept. They demonstrated rapid filling of the centers of the villous trees and called

them jets or spurts. More recent physiological concepts of intervillous circulation (Moll, 1981; Schmid-Schönbein, 1988) do not agree with these terms, as the actual filling velocities amount to only a few centimeters per second, which might not be enough to describe the driving forces of a fountain as implied by the terms jet or spurt. After passage of the central cavity, a subsequent, rather slow centrifugal spreading of the blood toward the subchorial and peripheral zone was observed. Wallenburg et al. (1973) ligated single spiral arteries in rhesus monkeys, which resulted in obliteration of the intervillous space and degeneration of the corresponding villous tree. This experiment demonstrated that each villous tree depends on its own spiral artery. Even though the intervillous space is a widely open, freely communicating system, villous arrangement and pressure gradients are coordinated in such a way that blood perfusion depends strictly on the original flow arrangement. Reversal of the direction is impossible.

If one accepts these considerations, the immature intermediate villi, together with their sprouting mesenchymal side branches (Figures 72, 81), are concentrated in the placentones' centers and are thus in the zones of highest PO_2 in the intervillous space. Schuhmann's group found that ^{3}H-thymidine incorporation, as an index for the mitotic rate, is twice as high in the center of the placentone as at the periphery (Geier et al., 1975). This finding is in seeming contrast to several experimental and histological findings. The latter authors also suggested that low oxygen concentration serves as a stimulus for trophoblastic proliferation and villous sprouting (Alvarez, 1967; Alvarez et al., 1970; Fox, 1970). The most likely explanation for this discrepancy is that oxygen delivery to the centrally located large villi—those in the central cavity and its close vicinity—is reduced owing to high blood flow velocity and long diffusion distances. The adjacent densely packed zones, though already located nearer the venous pole, probably have a much higher oxygen delivery, as blood flow velocity is reduced in the slender intervillous clefts and diffusion distances are short. This situation results in high mean PO_2 values at the villous surfaces, which is a prerequisite for effective maternofetal oxygen transfer. At the same time it inhibits villous proliferation and stimulates villous differentiation in the placentones' periphery.

These relations may be the basis for regulatory mechanisms. Wide intervillous clefts in the periphery of the villous trees of immature placentas, which lack fine and richly branched terminal villi, result in long diffusion distances and high blood flow velocities—and thus in reduced oxygen delivery. The resulting intravillous PO_2 in this area is low, which stimulates villous sprouting and especially capillary sprouting (Bacon et al., 1984; Scheffen et al., 1990). Increased capillary sprouting is followed by the production of new terminal villi. The latter narrow the intervillous space, reduce blood flow velocity and diffusion distances, and thus increase oxygen delivery. Finally, the elevated PO_2 inhibits further villous branching.

According to this hypothesis, the maternal bloodstream, oxygenation, and villous branching act as limbs of a simple feedback mechanism that regulates growth of the villous trees. As a further consequence, a functional diversity of the placentone is obtained. Whereas the centers act as proliferative zones that guarantee placental growth until term, the periphery is the functionally fully active exchange and secretory area. This situation has also been highlighted by the histochemically and biochemically higher activity of enzymes such as alkaline phosphatase (Schuhmann et al., 1976) and by the higher conversion rate of steroid hormones (Lehmann et al., 1973) in the placentones' periphery.

The zonal differences become evident only after the development of mature intermediate villi, at the end of the second trimester. Up to that time, the villous trees are largely homogeneous. In most placentas the immature placentone centers are present until term, at least in the more peripheral areas of the placenta. Only in cases of preterm maturation of the placenta (hypermaturity, maturitas praecox) do we regularly find mature placentone centers, resulting in a virtually homogeneous structure of the placentones. Such a placenta has lost its capacity to grow, as only the immature intermediate villi and their immediate mesenchymal branches are able to sprout and act as growth zones.

For the histopathologist, the inhomogeneity of the villous trees causes considerable problems of interpretation. Because the average diameter of a placentone is 1 to 4 cm, histological sections often do not cover a representative part of the placentone, which would comprise immature growth zones as well as highly differentiated, mature tissue. The prevalence of one or the other tissue may influence the diagnosis. This danger is even greater when one considers that placentones from various locations may show varying degrees of maturation. Even the careful study of several sections from a given placenta may lead to incorrect interpretations. This point is of particular importance when performing morphometric evaluations of the placenta. Burton (1987) remarked that "strict attention must be paid to the sampling regimen if meaningful results are to be obtained. Sadly this has not always been taken into consideration in the past, and so many of the published claims must be qualified accordingly."

This problem is greater still when one uses small tissue samples, such as semithin sections for light microscopy or ultrafine sections for electron microscopy. Neither section type allows a diagnosis concerning the degree of maturation on which one can rely. The same holds true for samples obtained by aspiration from the intact uterus (Alvarez et al., 1964; Aladjem, 1968), the placenta at cesarean section (Schweikhart & Kaufmann, 1977), and chorionic villus sampling. Although the latter samples are of greatest value for genetic purposes (Hugentobler et al., 1987), one must be careful with a histological evaluation of such material (Gerl et al., 1973; Ehrhardt et al., 1974), even during early stages of pregnancy. In these situations one does not have the problem of heterogeneity of the placentones but the problem of general heterogeneity.

CONTROL OF VILLOUS DEVELOPMENT

Little is known concerning the control of villous development. Not only genetic abnormalities but also numerous other pathological conditions, such as diabetes mellitus, maternal hypertension, maternal anemia or pregnancy in high altitude, rhesus incompatibility, and smoking while pregnant, severely affect villous

development. These facts suggest that the villous maturational processes are influenced not only by genes but also by metabolic and endocrine parameters. From the latter, only the role of oxygen has been studied in detail. Few data are available concerning the influences of hormones.

Oxygen as Regulator of Villous Development

Transplacental oxygen transfer is only one of many villous functions, but its particular importance becomes evident from the fact that it is nearly the only villous function that, upon disturbance, may cause fetal death. Therefore, it is not surprising that the maternal oxygen supply to the placenta affects villous growth and differentiation to a greater degree than any other known parameter.

Histopathological reports unanimously note that the amount of villous cytotrophoblast is increased in all those pathological conditions, that are thought to be related to intrauterine hypoxia (Fox, 1964, 1970; Piotrowicz et al., 1969; Beischer et al., 1970; Kaufmann et al., 1977a). Arnholdt and coworkers (1991) found evidence that it is due not only to an increased mitotic index but also to a reduction in the length of the cell cycle. In contrast, unusually good oxygenation of villi reduces the rate of proliferation and the quantity of villous cytotrophoblast (Panigel & Myers, 1971, 1972; Myers & Panigel, 1973; Kaufmann et al., 1977a).

In addition, the villous syncytiotrophoblast is affected by hypoxia, as was shown experimentally by Tominaga and Page (1966) and Ong and Burton (1991) as well as in pathological specimens (Alvarez et al., 1969, 1970). It is reduced in thickness, and increased numbers of syncytial knots are produced simultaneously, the nuclei of which show signs of chromatin clumping. Tominaga and Page (1966) interpreted it as a sign of adaptation by reducing diffusion distances. More stringent stereological studies have suggested, however, that the changes are more likely due to degenerative processes (Ong & Burton, 1991).

All in vitro studies on the effects of hypoxia have been performed on villous explants rather than on villous cytotrophoblast cultures. For that reason it is still an open question whether cytotrophoblast responds directly to variations of the oxygen partial pressure, or the response is mediated by factors released by other hypoxic tissue components such as syncytiotrophoblast or villous macrophages.

There are several factors that might mediate hypoxic signals: Epidermal growth factor (EGF) may be derived from maternal sources and is additionally produced by syncytiotrophoblast (for review see Prager et al., 1992); its mitogenic action on trophoblast has been shown by Lysiak and coworkers (1992), and its receptors have been detected on syncytiotrophoblastic surfaces (Rao et al., 1985) as well as on cytotrophoblastic membranes (Mühlhauser et al., 1993). Transforming growth factor α (TGF-α) (Lysiak et al., 1992), tumor necrosis factor α (TNF-α), the latter produced by macrophages (for review see Hunt, 1989), and colony–stimulating factor 1 (CSF-1) produced by mesenchymal cells (Jokhi et al., 1992; Shorter et al., 1992) are other candidates. Finally, TGF-β1 and TGF-β2, both produced by macrophages (for review see Hunt, 1989), and trophoblast (Graham & Lala, 1991) seem to be involved in the regulation of syncytial fusion of the postproliferative cytotrophoblast in order to regenerate the hypoxically damaged syncytiotrophoblast.

It is a common experience in pathological studies of the placenta that the villous connective tissue also responds to variations in the intrauterine oxygen supply. Chronic hypoxia results in minimal fibrosis of the villi (Fox, 1978); in contrast, higher levels of intravillous PO_2 increase villous fibrosis (Panigel & Myers, 1971, 1972; Fox, 1978). Related in vitro experiments with placental tissues are still to be done. Possible mediators are macrophage products, such as TGF-β, which stimulates collagen I transcription (Rossi et al., 1988), or interleukin-1, which among other functions regulates fibroblast proliferation (Schmidt et al., 1982).

Several histopathological studies have dealt with the reaction of fetal villous endothelium to hypoxia. Complicated pregnancies suffering from intrauterine hypoxia show villous hypercapillarization (Hölzl et al., 1974); the same is true for placentas obtained from pregnancies at high altitude (Jackson et al., 1987; Reshetnikova et al., 1993). It is difficult to find clear experimental evidence for this correlation using in vitro culture of villous explants (Tominaga & Page, 1966; Fox, 1970; Amaladoss & Burton, 1985; Ong & Burton, 1991), as the isolated fragments of fetal endothelial tubes tend to disintegrate in culture.

Experimental chronic hypoxia in pregnant guinea pigs resulted in increased fetal capillarization and CO diffusion capacity (Bacon et al., 1984). More detailed studies revealed that these increases were due to stimulated sprouting and branching of capillaries: The mean capillary length and diameter were reduced, and the number of parallel capillary loops was considerably increased (Scheffen et al., 1990). Because the trophoblastic thickness also decreased, the mean maternofetal diffusion distance was much shorter compared to that in normoxic placentas (Bacon et al., 1984).

The first evidence for cell biological regulations was obtained from experiments with endothelial cultures (Werb, 1983; Ogawa et al., 1991; Shreeniwas et al., 1991). Surprisingly, endothelial cells showed reduced mitotic rates and reduced motility when cultured under hypoxic conditions (Ogawa et al., 1991; Shreeniwas et al., 1991). The addition of conditioned medium obtained from hypoxic macrophages, however, stimulated endothelial proliferation (Ogawa et al., 1991). In the same report the authors showed that increased production of basic fibroblast growth factor (bFGF) by the hypoxic macrophages and enhanced expression of bFGF receptor by the hypoxic endothelium were responsible for the enhanced endothelial proliferation. The signal sequence for exocytosis of bFGF is missing, although several mechanisms of bFGF liberation from the cells producing the protein have been proposed (for review see Rifkin & Moscatelli, 1989). It is likely that bFGF is involved in the control of endothelial growth.

Other angiogenetic factors have been discussed to mediate hypoxic signals.

1. Platelet-derived endothelial cell growth factor (PDECGF), which is thought to be of trophoblastic origin (Jackson et al., 1992)
2. Platelet-derived growth factor B (PDGF-B) produced by villous cytotrophoblast, by endothelium, or both (Holmgren et al., 1991)
3. Amitogenic angiogenesis factor secreted by hypoxic macrophages (Werb, 1983)

There are few data concerning hypoxic influences on the maternal vascularization of the placenta. In the guinea pig, the volume and surface of maternal blood lacunae are reduced under hypoxic conditions (Bacon et al., 1984). In contrast, in human placentas from patients at high altitude the intervillous space was reported to be increased (Jackson et al., 1987). For the cow placenta, Reynolds and coworkers (1992) have demonstrated maternal endothelial mitogens of endometrial origin. Up to the present, however, these data have not provided a clear concept as to how uteroplacental oxygenation modulates maternal vascularization of the placenta. All of these regulatory mechanisms are paracrine or even autocrine in nature. To our knowledge, there is no convincing evidence thus far that the placenta can respond also to endocrine signals derived from a hypoxic mother or fetus. In particular, the latter type of signals (i.e., fetal cytokines or hormones that control fetoplacental capillarization) are likely to exist.

Summarizing the above data, we arrive at the following conclusions regarding villous reactions to hypoxia: Hypoxia damages villous syncytiotrophoblast, which in turn stimulates cytotrophoblastic proliferation and subsequent syncytial fusion. Despite these attempts to regenerate the damaged syncytiotrophoblast, the volume and thickness of the latter are reduced, facilitating maternofetal oxygen diffusion. Villous connective tissue, which is also reduced under these conditions, may add to the same effects. Fetal oxygen uptake is further facilitated by expansion of the villous capillary bed via sprouting and nonsprouting angiogenesis, both processes probably being stimulated by growth factors derived from hypoxic macrophages and hypoxic trophoblast. A widening of the capillary bed with reduction of the length of the individual capillaries causes the reduction of fetoplacental blood flow impedance and may thus be advantageous for the fetal cardiovascular system being exposed to hypoxic conditions.

Considering the results of hypoxic conditions in the fetoplacental unit often causes confusion, in particular if the hypoxic department is not exactly defined. Maternal hypoxemia (high altitude: Jackson et al., 1987; Reshetnikova et al., 1993; maternal anemia: Piotrowicz et al., 1969; Beischer et al., 1970) and maternal heart disease, which must also be considered, cause intraplacental and intrafetal hypoxic conditions. The same is true in normoxemic, hypertensive mothers if the placenta is maternally malperfused (Alvarez et al., 1970). In all of these cases, typical features of intraplacental hypoxia as described above are to be expected.

The situation becomes more confusing if the oxygen transfer from the placenta to the fetus is hampered, for instance by insufficient placental capillarization (terminal villous deficiency; see Chapter 10), fetal vessel obstruction (Panigel & Myers, 1971, 1972; Fox, 1978), or intraplacental stasis (Macara et al., 1994). Provided the mother is normoxemic, the fetus in such cases becomes hypoxic, and the maternally well perfused placental tissue even becomes relatively hyperoxic because it liberates less oxygen to the fetus. As a consequence, the placenta shows typical structural features of a normoxic or hyperoxic placenta (Panigel & Myers, 1971, 1972; Macara et al., 1994) even though the fetus may be severely hypoxic. We have found this condition in all cases of severe intrauterine growth retardation combined with absent enddiastolic blood flow within the umbilical arteries (Macara et al., 1994).

Hormones as Regulators of Villous Development

Even though it should be expected that villous development is controlled by maternal and fetal hormones, there are few clinical hints in this direction. Experimental proof is completely missing. We deal briefly here with the suggestions that look promising for future research.

Ovarian steroids are the most likely group of hormones to be involved in placental development and probably represent the only group of hormones that, in a few cases, have been used for the treatment of villous maldevelopment. Placentas from pregnancies complicated by intrauterine growth retardation and combined with decreased or absent end-diastolic blood flow are characterized by homogeneous features of villous maldevelopment (Macara et al., 1994): reduced trophoblastic proliferation rate, reduced number of terminal villi, reduced total villous volume, poor branching of terminal villous capillaries, increased terminal villous fibrosis, and increased differentiation of villous myofibroblasts. The functional consequences of these alterations are likely to be responsible for the impaired fetal nutrition and the increased fetoplacental blood flow impedance. Several groups of investigators have found evidence that third trimester treatment with gestagens (allylestrenol) decreased blood flow impedance and increased fetal birth weight and placental weight (Kaneoka et al., 1983; Kurjak & Pal, 1986; Marzolf et al., 1986). The only histological study of these placentas that we were able to find is that by Papierowski (1981), who described a stimulated development of villi. As far as we were able to see from Papierowski's data, an increase in immature, proliferating villous tissue was responsible for the overall increased villous growth rate. In contrast, P. Prahalada (personal communication, 1982) found that treatment of rhesus monkeys with high doses of estrogens during midpregnancy caused reduced placental and fetal growth rates. To our knowledge, these placentas have not been studied histologically. These findings were supported by the experimental data of Yallampalli and Garfield (1993), Chwalisz et al. (1994), and Garfield et al. (1994). These authors induced symptoms of preeclampsia in rats and guinea pigs, including intrauterine growth retardation (IUGR) by blockage of nitric oxide synthase, and reversed these effects by treatment with gestagens.

All the data suggest that gestagens and estrogens have antagonistic effects on villous development, including proliferation and differentiation. Because of the lack of convincing data it is tempting to speculate that both hormones control the switch of mesenchymal villous transformation into either continuously growing immature intermediate villi or differentiating mature intermediate villi. This switch usually takes place at the transition of the second to the third trimesters (Figure 74) (Castellucci et al., 1990). An earlier initiation of this switch results in small premature placentas (e.g., those in IUGR combined with absent end-diastolic umbilical blood flow); postponement of the switch results in persisting villous immaturity with abnormally large placentas (Kaufmann, 1982).

In addition to the above hormones, *insulin* is under discussion regarding its influence on villous development. The prevailing finding is an overall increased proliferation rate of villous trophoblast, villous stromal cells, and villous capillaries. This increase results in large placentas characterized by voluminous, seemingly immature villi with high cellular density (Widmaier, 1970; Werner & Schneiderhan, 1972; Fox, 1978).

So far all attempts have failed to demonstrate classical insulin effects on the maternal side of the placenta, such as stimulation of glucose (Challier et al., 1986) and amino acid transport (Montgomery & Young, 1982) and an increase in glycogen levels in trophoblast cells (Schmon et al., 1991). The results can be explained by the low levels of insulin receptors on the syncytiotrophoblastic surface during the second half of pregnancy (Jones et al., 1993; Desoye et al., 1994).

Because of this situation, direct growth-promoting effects of insulin (for review see Strauss, 1984) on the various placental tissues must be discussed. During the first trimester, insulin receptors are expressed mainly along the trophoblastic surfaces of sprouting segments of the villous trees (sprouts, mesenchymal villi) (Desoye et al., 1994), indicating that maternal insulin might be involved in first trimester villous growth, which is mainly a result of trophoblastic proliferation (Castellucci et al., 1990). During the last trimester, the highest immunoreactivities for insulin receptors are found in fetal villous endothelium (Jones et al., 1993), in particular in segments with capillary sprouting, such as mature intermediate villi and terminal villous necks (Desoye et al., 1994). During this period, expansion and differentiation of the villous trees are mainly a result of capillary sprouting (Kaufmann et al., 1988; Castellucci et al., 1990). A switch in villous growth control from maternal insulin (with trophoblastic insulin receptors) during early pregnancy to fetal insulin (with endothelial insulin receptors) during late pregnancy would make sense, as it would enable the fetus to control villous differentiation in accordance with his own nutritional needs.

Another group of hormones likely to be involved in villous development are the *thyroid hormones*. It is now recognized that during pregnancy maternal thyroid function is mediated by the placenta (Fisher, 1983). The placenta plays a major role in the synthesis and metabolism of the thyroid hormones; the putative trophoblastic thyrotropin (Hershman, 1972), as well as human chorionic gonadotropin (hCG) (Kennedy & Darne, 1991), stimulate maternal thyroid hormone production. Thyroid stimulating hormone (TSH), triiodothyronine (T_3), thyroxine (T_4), and thyroglobulin cannot pass the placental barrier, whereas thyroid hormone-releasing hormone (TRH), iodine, and thyroid-stimulating immunoglobulins can (Cappoen, 1989). Because placental tissue and decidua have a high nuclear-binding capacity for T_3, Banovac et al. (1986) suggested the placenta to be a thyroid hormone-dependent tissue. Maruo et al. (1991) have described stimulatory effects of maternal T_3 and T_4 on trophoblastic endocrine functions; moreover, they found that T_3 enhances trophoblastic production of epidermal growth factor, a potent trophoblastic mitogen; they concluded that thyroid hormone, in synergy with EGF, regulates villous growth (Matsuo et al., 1993).

There are fewer data concerning the correlation of thyroid malfunction with placental function or development. According to experiments in rats (Kumar & Chaudhuri, 1989) the levels of maternal thyroid hormone secretion are positively correlated with fetal growth. Thorpe Beeston et al. (1991) found significantly reduced maternal T_4 levels in small-for-gestational-age fetuses combined with fetal hypoxemia and acidemia.

All these data suggest that maternal thyroid hormones are involved in villous development and thus influence placental transfer functions for nutrients and gases. Unfortunately, no relevant histological data of the placentas are available. We have seen some placentas of hypothyroid mothers, all of which were characterized by decreased capillarization and reduced formation of terminal villi [the terminal villi deficiency of Schweikhart and Kaufmann (1987)]. These data, however, were difficult to interpret, as all mothers were medicated with thyroid hormones.

Fetomaternal Flow Interrelations

The efficiency of diffusional exchange (e.g., oxygen, carbon dioxide, water), among other factors, depends on the arrangement of fetal and maternal blood flows to each other. As early as in 1926 Mossman described countercurrent flow conditions in the rabbit placenta; that is, neighboring maternal and fetal bloodstreams were thought to be arranged in parallel but with opposite flow directions. Later, this author found the same condition to be valid for the human placenta (Mossman, 1965). This finding, however, is not supported by anatomical or physiological results. Rather, it has been recognized for many years that the anatomic arrangement of placental vascular pathways differ from one species to another. For humans we have described three major morphological objections to the existence of countercurrent flow conditions (Kaufmann, 1985).

1. All villi would have to be oriented in the same direction, parallel to the maternal bloodstream. They are, in fact, arranged at varying angles to each other because of the structure of the villous tree.

2. Only one limb of the hairpin-like fetal capillary loops is allowed to have interchange contact with the maternal blood; in fact, both limbs normally exhibit the same structure and the same diffusion distance to the maternal blood.

3. According to the results of Lemtis (1969), one must consider the possibility that considerable amounts of venous maternal blood are recirculated by the arterial "jet" before leaving the intervillous space. Thus intraplacental circulatory "orbits" are formed.

The anatomical situation and the physiological effectiveness of the human placenta is much more in agreement with the concept of a multivillous flow arrangement (Bartels & Moll, 1964; Moll, 1981). In this condition, the maternal bloodstream crosses subsequent villi with hairpin-like arranged fetal capillaries. It seems to be of minor importance with which angle the maternal bloodstream crosses the individual villi or whether the vessels of the villi are serially connected to each other or arranged in parallel. The multivillous blood flow is less effective for diffusional transfer than the countercurrent flow (Moll, 1981).

This explanation may be the reason 1 g of human placenta supplies only 6 g of fetus at term, compared to a ratio of 1:20 in the guinea pig with a countercurrent flow placenta (Table 1) (Dantzer et al., 1988). On the other hand, the multivillous arrangement is structurally more flexible. It allows rearrangement and adaptation to changing developmental conditions and the continuous growth to a much greater extent. In this respect, it is worthy of note that the highly effective guinea pig placenta is small (about 5 g) and functions for only 68 days. The capybara, which belongs to the same suborder of rodents, has a structurally closely related placenta but a much longer pregnancy (150 days) and a much higher placental weight (150 g), but the capybara placenta is less effective than the guinea pig placenta (1 g of placenta at term supplies 10 g of fetus).

References

Aladjem, S.: Morphopathology of the human placental villi and the fetal outcome. J. Obstet. Gynaecol. Br. Commonw. 75:1237–1244, 1968.

Alvarez, H.: Syncytial proliferation in normal and toxemic pregnancies. Obstet. Gynecol. 29:637–643, 1967.

Alvarez, H., De Bejar, R., and Aladjem, S.: La placenta human: aspectos morfologicos y fisio-patologicos. In, 4th Uruguayan Congress for Obstetrics and Gynecology. Vol. 1, pp. 190–261, 1964.

Alvarez, H., Morel, R.L., Benedetti, W.L., and Scavarelli, M.: Trophoblast hyperplasia and maternal arterial pressure at term. Am. J. Obstet. Gynecol. 105:1015–1021, 1969.

Alvarez, H., Benedetti, W.L., Morel, R.L., and Scavarelli, M.: Trophoblast development gradient and its relationship to placental hemodynamics. Am. J. Obstet. Gynecol. 106: 416–420, 1970.

Alvarez, H., Medrano, C.V., Sala, M.A., and Benedetti, W.L.: Trophoblast development gradient and its relationship to placental hemodynamics. II. Study of fetal cotyledons from the toxemic placenta. Am. J. Obstet. Gynecol. 114:873–878, 1972.

Amaladoss, A.S.P., and Burton, G.J.: Organ culture of human placental villi in hypoxic and hyperoxic conditions: a morphometric study. J. Dev. Physiol. 7:13–118, 1985.

Amstutz, E.: Beobachtungen über die Reifung der Chorionzotten in der menschlichen Placenta mit besonderer Berücksichtigung der Epithelplatten. Acta Anat. (Basel) 42:122–30, 1960.

Ara, G., Bari, M.A., and Siddiquey, A.K.: Effects of age, parity and length of pregnancy on the morphology and histology of human placenta. Bangladesh Med. Res. Counc. Bull. 10:53–58, 1984.

Arnholdt, H., Meisel, F., Fandrey, K., and Löhrs, U.: Proliferation of villous trophoblast of the human placenta in normal and abnormal pregnancies. Virchows Arch. B Cell Pathol. 60:365–372, 1991.

Arts, N.F.T.: Investigation on the vascular system of the placenta. Am. J. Obstet. Gynecol. 82:147–166, 1961.

Bacon, B.J., Gilbert, R.D., Kaufmann, P., Smith, A.D., Trevino, F.T., and Longo, L.D.: Placental anatomy and diffusing capacity in guinea pigs following long-term maternal hypoxia. Placenta 5:475–488, 1984.

Banovac, K., Ryan, E.A., and O'Sullivan, M.J.: Triiodothyronine (T3) nuclear binding sites in human placenta and decidua. Placenta 7:543–549, 1986.

Bartels, H., and Moll, W.: Passage of inert substances and oxygen in the human placenta. Pflugers Arch. Ges. Physiol. 280:165, 1964.

Becker, V.: Mechanismus der Reifung fetaler Organe. Verh. Dtsch. Pathol. Ges. 46:309–314, 1962.

Becker, V.: Funktionelle Morphologie der Plazenta. Arch. Gynecol. 198:3–28, 1963.

Becker, V.: Pathologie der Ausreifung der Plazenta. In, Die Plazenta des Menschen. V. Becker, T.H. Schiebler, and F. Kubli, eds., pp. 266–281. Thieme, Stuttgart, 1981.

Becker, V., and Jipp, P.: Über die Trophoblastschale der menschlichen Plazenta. Geburtshilfe Frauenheilkd. 23:466–474, 1963.

Becker, V., and Seifert, K.: Die Ultrastruktur der Kapillarwand in der menschlichen Placenta zur Zeit der Schwangerschaftsmitte. Z. Zellforsch. 65:380–396, 1965.

Beischer, N.A., Sivasamboo, R., Vohra, S., Silpisornkosal, S., and Reid, S.: Placental hypertrophy in severe pregnancy anaemia. J. Obstet. Gynaecol. Brit. Commonw. 77:398–409, 1970.

Boe, F.: Studies on the vascularization of the human placenta. Acta Obstet. Gynecol. Scand. Suppl. 5 32:1–92, 1953.

Boe, F.: Studies on the human placenta. II. Gross morphology of the fetal structures in the young placenta. Acta Obstet. Gynecol. Scand. 47:420–435, 1968.

Boe, F.: Studies on the human placenta. III. Vascularization of the young fetal placenta. A. Vascularization of the chorionic villus. Acta Obstet. Gynecol. Scand. 48:159–166, 1969.

Borell, U., Fernstroem, I., and Westman, A.: Eine arteriographische Studie des Plazentarkreislaufs. Geburtshilfe Frauenheilkd. 18:1–9, 1958.

Bouw, G.M., Stolte, L.A.M., Baak, J.P.A., and Oort, J.: Quantitative morphology of the placenta. 1. Standardization of sampling. Eur. J. Obstet. Gynecol. Reprod. Biol. 6:325–331, 1976.

Boyd, J.D., and Hamilton, W.J.: The Human Placenta. Heffer & Sons, Cambridge, 1970.

Burton, G.J: The fine structure of the human placental villus as revealed by scanning electron microscopy. Scanning Electron Microsc. 1:1811–1828, 1987.

Burton, G.J., and Palmer, M.E.: Eradicating fetomaternal fluid shift during perfusion fixation of the human placenta. Placenta 9:327–332, 1988.

Cantle, S.J., Kaufmann, P., Luckhardt, M., and Schweikhart, G.: Interpretation of syncytial sprouts and bridges in the human placenta. Placenta 8:221–234, 1987.

Cappoen, J.P.: Physiology of the thyroid during pregnancy: various exploratory tests. Rev. Fr. Gynecol. Obstet. 84: 893–897, 1989.

Castellucci, M., and Kaufmann, P.: A three-dimensional study of the normal human placental villous core. II. Stromal architecture. Placenta 3:269–286, 1982a.

Castellucci, M., and Kaufmann, P.: Evolution of the stroma in human chorionic villi throughout pregnancy. Bibl. Anat. 22:40–45, 1982b.

Castellucci, M., Schweikhart, G., Kaufmann, P., and Zaccheo, D.: The stromal architecture of the immature intermediate villus of the human placenta. Gynecol. Obstet. Invest. 18:95–99, 1984.

Castellucci, M., Scheper, M., Scheffen, I., Celona, A., and Kaufmann, P.: The development of the human placental villous tree. Anat. Embryol. (Berl.) 181:117–128, 1990.

Challier, J.C., Hauguel, S., and Desmaizieres, V.: Effect of insulin on glucose uptake and metabolism in the human placenta. J. Clin. Endocrinol. Metab. 62:803–807, 1986.

Chwalisz, K., Ciesla, I., and Garfield, R.E.: Inhibition of nitric oxide (NO) synthesis induces preterm parturition and preeclampsia-like conditions in guinea pigs. Presented at the Society for Gynecologic Investigation Meeting, 1994.

Dantzer, V., Leiser, R., Kaufmann, P., and Luckhardt, M.: Comparative morphological aspects of placental vascularization. Trophoblast Res. 3:221–244, 1988.

Demir, R., Kaufmann, P., Castellucci, M., Erbengi, T., and Kotowski, A.: Fetal vasculogenesis and angiogenesis in human placental villi. Acta Anat. (Basel) 136:190–203, 1989.

Demir, R., Demir, N., Kohnen, G., Kosanke, G., Mironov, V., Üstünel, I., and Kocamaz, E.: Ultrastructure and distribution of myofibroblast-like cells in human placental stem villi. Electron Microsc. 3:509–510, 1992.

Desoye, G., Hartmann, M., Blaschitz, A., Dohr, G., Hahn, T., Kohnen, G., and Kaufmann, P.: Insulin receptors in syncytiotrophoblast and fetal endothelium of human placenta: immunohistochemical evidence for developmental changes in distribution pattern. Histochemistry 101:277–285, 1994.

Ehrhardt, G., Gerl, D., Estel, C., Kadner, J., and Günther, M.: Morphologische Auswertbarkeit von in vitro gewonnenen Punktionszylindern der Plazenta. Zentralbl. Gynakol. 96:705–711, 1974.

Enders, A.C., and King, B.F.: The cytology of Hofbauer cells. Anat. Rec. 167:231–252, 1970.

Feneley, M.R., and Burton, G.J.: Villous composition and membrane thickness in the human placenta at term: a stereological study using unbiased estimators and optimal fixation techniques. Placenta 12:131–142, 1991.

Fisher, D.A.: Maternal-fetal thyroid function in pregnancy. Clin. Perinatol. 10:615–626, 1983.

Fox, H.: The villous cytotrophoblast as an index of placental ischaemia. J. Obstet. Gynaecol. Br. Commonw. 71:885–893, 1964.

Fox, H.: Effect of hypoxia on trophoblast in organ culture: a morphologic and autoradiographic study. Am. J. Obstet. Gynecol. 107:1058–1064, 1970.

Fox, H.: Pathology of the Placenta. Saunders, London, 1978.

Freese, U.E.: The fetal-maternal circulation of the placenta. I. Histomorphologic, plastoid injection, and x-ray cinematographic studies on human placentas. Am. J. Obstet. Gynecol. 94:354–360, 1966.

Garfield, R.E., Yallampalli, C., Buhimschi, I., and Chwalisz, K.: Reversal of preeclampsia symptoms induced in rats by nitric oxide inhibition with L-arginine, steroid hormones and an endothelin antagonist. Presented at the Society for Gynecologic Investigation Meeting, 1994.

Geier, G., Schuhmann, R., and Kraus, H.: Regional unterschiedliche Zellproliferation innerhalb der Plazentone reifer menschlicher Plazenten; autoradiographische Untersuchungen. Arch. Gynecol. 218:31–37, 1975.

Gerl, D., Eichhorn, H., Eichhorn, K.-H., and Franke, H.: Quantitative Messungen synzytialer Zellkernkonzentrationen der menschlichen Plazenta bei normalen und pathologischen Schwangerschaften. Zentralbl. Gynakol. 95:263–266, 1973.

Graham, C.H., and Lala, P.K.: Mechanism of control of trophoblast invasion in situ. J. Cell Physiol. 148:228–234, 1991.

Habashi, S., Burton, G.J., and Steven, D.H.: Morphological study of the fetal vasculature of the human placenta: scanning electron microscopy of corrosion casts. Placenta 4: 41–56, 1983.

Hershman, J.M.: Hyperthyroidism induced by trophoblastic thyrotropin. Mayo Clin. Proc. 47:913–918, 1972.

Highison, G.J., and Tibbitts, F.D.: Ultrasonic microdissection of immature intermediate human placental villi as studied by scanning electron microscopy. Scanning Electron Microsc. 2:679–685, 1986.

Holmgren, L., Glaser, A., Pfeifer-Ohlsson, N.S., and Ohlsson, R.: Angiogenesis during human extraembryonic development involves the spatiotemporal control of PDGF ligand and receptor gene expression. Development 113:749–754, 1991.

Hölzl, M., Lüthje, D., and Seck-Ebersbach, K.: Placentaveränderungen bei EPH-Gestose. Arch. Gynecol. 217:315–334, 1974.

Hörmann, G.: Lebenskurven normaler und entwicklungsfähiger Chorionzotten; Ergebnisse systematischer Zottenmessungen. Arch. Gynecol. 181:29–43, 1951.

Hörmann, G.: Ein Beitrag zur funktionellen Morphologie der menschlichen Placenta. Arch. Gynecol. 184:109–123, 1953.

Hörmann, G.: Versuch einer Systematik plazentarer Entwicklungsstörungen. Geburtshilfe Frauenheilkd. 18:345– 349, 1958a.

Hörmann, G.: Zur Systematik einer Pathologie der menschlichen Placenta. Arch. Gynecol. 191:297–344, 1958b.

Hugentobler, W., Binkert, F., Haenel, A.F., and Schaetti, D.: Die Chorionzotten-(Plazenta-)Biopsie im II. und III. Trimenon: Neue Perspektiven der Pränataldiagnostik. Geburtshilfe Frauenheilkd. 47:729–732, 1987.

Hunt, J.S.: Macrophages in human uteroplacental tissues: a Review. Am. J. Reprod. Immunol. 21:119–122, 1989.

Jackson, M.R., Mayhew, T.M., and Haas, J.D.: Morphometric studies on villi in human term placentae and the effects of altitude, ethnic grouping and sex of newborn. Placenta 8:487–495, 1987.

Jackson, M.R., Carney, E.W., Lye, S.J., and Ritchie, J.W.K.: Immunolocalisation of two angiogenic factors (PDECGF and VEGF) in human placental villi throughout gestation. Placenta 13:A27, 1992.

Jokhi, P., Chumbley, G., King, A., Gardner, L., and Loke, W.: Expression of the colony stimulating factor-1 receptor by cells at the uteroplacental interface. Placenta 13:A29, 1992.

Jones, C.J.P., Hartmann, M., Blaschitz, A., and Desoye, G.: Ultrastructural localization of insulin receptors in human placenta. Am. J. Reprod. Immunol. 30:136–145, 1993.

Kaneoka, T., Taguchi, S., Shimizu, H., and Shirakawa, K.: Prenatal diagnosis and treatment of intrauterine growth retardation. J. Perinat. Med. 11:204–212, 1983.

Karimu, A.L., and Burton, G.J.: The effects of maternal vascular pressure on the dimensions of the placental capillaries. Br. J. Obstet. Gynaecol. 101:57–63, 1994.

Kaufmann, P.: Entwicklung der Plazenta. In, Die Plazenta des Menschen. V. Becker, T.H. Schiebler, and F. Kubli, eds., pp. 13–50. Thieme Verlag, Stuttgart, 1981.

Kaufmann, P.: Development and differentiation of the human placental villous tree. Bibl. Anat. 22:29–39, 1982.

Kaufmann, P.: Basic morphology of the fetal and maternal circuits in the human placenta. Contrib. Gynecol. Obstet. 13:5–17, 1985.

Kaufmann, P., and Davidoff, M.: The guinea pig placenta. Adv. Anat. Embryol. Cell Biol. 53:1–90, 1977.

Kaufmann, P., and Scheffen, I.: Placental development. In, Neonatal and Fetal Medicine—Physiology and Pathophysiology. Vol. I. R.A. Polin and W.W. Fox, eds., pp. 47–55. Saunders, Orlando, FL, 1992.

Kaufmann, P., Schiebler, T.H., Ciobotaru, C., and Stark, J.: Enzymhistochemische Untersuchungen an reifen menschlichen Placentazotten. II. Zur Gliederung des Syncytiotrophoblasten. Histochemistry 40:191–207, 1974.

Kaufmann, P., Gentzen, D.M., and Davidoff, M.: Die Ultrastruktur von Langhanszellen in pathologischen menschlichen Placenten. Arch. Gynecol. 222:319–332, 1977a.

Kaufmann, P., Stark, J., and Stegner, H.-E.: The villous stroma of the human placenta. I. The ultrastructure of fixed connective tissue cells. Cell Tissue Res. 177:105–121, 1977b.

Kaufmann, P., Sen, D.K., and Schweikhart, G.: Classification of human placental villi. I. Histology and scanning electron microscopy. Cell Tissue Res. 200:409–423, 1979.

Kaufmann, P., Nagl, W., and Fuhrmann, B.: Die funktionelle Bedeutung der Langhanszellen der menschlichen Plazenta. Verh. Anat. Ges. 77:435–436, 1983.

Kaufmann, P., Bruns, U., Leiser, R., Luckhardt, M., and Winterhager, E.: The fetal vascularization of term human placental villi. II. Intermediate and terminal villi. Anat. Embryol. (Berl.) 173:203–214, 1985.

Kaufmann, P., Luckhardt, M., Schweikhart, G., and Cantle, S.J.: Cross-sectional features and three-dimensional structure of human placental villi. Placenta 8:235–247, 1987.

Kaufmann, P., Luckhardt, M., and Leiser, R.: Threedimensional representation of the fetal vessel system in the human placenta. Trophoblast Res. 3:113–137, 1988.

Kaufmann, P., Kohnen, G., and Kosanke, G.: Wechselwirkungen zwischen Plazentamorphologie und fetaler Sauerstoffversorgung. Versuch einer zellbiologischen Interpretation pathohistologischer und experimenteller Befunde. Gynakologe 26:16–23, 1993.

Kennedy, R.L., and Darne, J.: The role of hCG in regulation of the thyroid gland in normal and abnormal pregnancy. Obstet. Gynecol. 78:298–307, 1991.

King, B.F.: Ultrastructural differentiation of stromal and vascular components in early macaque placental villi. Am. J. Anat. 178:30–44, 1987.

Kohnen, G.: Immunhistochemische Charakterisierung extravaskulärer kontraktiler Zellen in menschlichen Placentazotten. Medical thesis, Technical University of Aachen, 1994.

Kohnen, G., Mironov, V., Demir, R., Castellucci, M., and Kaufmann, P.: Immunhistochemische Klassifizierung von Stammzotten in der menschlichen Plazenta. Anat. Anz. 174(Suppl.):127, 1992.

Kohnen, G., Kosanke, G., Korr, H., and Kaufmann, P.: Comparison of various proliferation markers applied to human placental tissue. Placenta 14:A38, 1993.

Kosanke, G., Castellucci, M., Kaufmann, P., and Mironov, V.A.: Branching patterns of human placental villous trees: perspectives of topological analysis. Placenta 14:591–604, 1993.

Krantz, K.E., and Parker, J.C.: Contractile properties of the smooth muscle in the human placenta. Clin. Obstet. Gynecol. 93:253–258, 1963.

Kumar, R., and Chaudhuri, B.N.: Altered maternal thyroid function: fetal and neonatal development of rat. Indian J. Physiol. Pharmacol. 33:233–238, 1989.

Kurjak, A., and Pal, A.: The effect of gestanon on the fetal and uteroplacental blood flow. Acta Med. Jugosl. 40:121–131, 1986.

Lehmann, W.D., Schuhmann, R., and Kraus, H.: Regionally different steroid biosynthesis within materno-fetal circulation units (placentones) of mature human placentas. J. Perinat. Med. 1:198–204, 1973.

Leiser, R.: Microvascularisation der Ziegenplazenta dargestellt mit rasterelektronisch untersuchten Gefäßausgüssen. Schweiz. Arch. Tierheilkd. 129:59–74, 1987.

Leiser, R., Luckhardt, M., Kaufmann, P., Winterhager, E., and Bruns, U.: The fetal vascularisation of term human placental villi. I. Peripheral stem villi. Anat. Embryol. (Berl.) 173:71–80, 1985.

Leiser, R., Kosanke, G., and Kaufmann, P.: Human placental vascularization. In, Placenta: Basic Research for Clinical

Application. H. Soma, ed., pp. 32–45. Karger, Basel, 1991.

Lemtis, H.: Über die Architektonik des Zottengefäß apparates der menschlichen Plazenta. Anat. Anz. 102:106–133, 1955.

Lemtis, H.: New insights into the maternal circulatory system of the human placenta. In, The Foetoplacental Unit. A. Pecile and D. Finzi, eds. Excerpta Medica, Amsterdam, 1969.

Lysiak, J., Khoo, N., Conelly, I., Stettler-Stevenson, W., and Peeyush, L.: Role of transforming growth factor (TGF) and epidermal growth factor (EGF) on proliferation, invasion, and hCG production by normal and malignant trophoblast. Placenta 13:A41, 1992.

Macara, L., Kingdom, J.C.P., Hair, J., More, I.A.R., Lyall, F., Kohnen, G., Greer, I.A., and Kaufmann, P.: Placental terminal villi from pregnancies complicated by intrauterine growth retardation: immunohistochemical and ultrastructural aspects. (1994, submitted).

Maruo, T., Matsuo, H., and Mochizuki, M.: Thyroid hormone as a biological amplifier of differentiated trophoblast function in early pregnancy. Acta Endocrinol. (Copenh.) 125: 58–66, 1991.

Marzolf, G., Lobstein, J.F., Dillmann, J.C., Spizzo, M., Eberst, B., and Gandar, R.: Double blind comparison of the effects of Gestanon versus placebo in intra-uterine growth retardation. Presented at the 4th Asia Oceanic Congress on Perinatology, Tokyo, 1986.

Matsuo, H., Maruo, T., Murata, K., and Mochizuki, M.: Human early placental trophoblasts produce an epidermal growth factor-like substance in synergy with thyroid hormone. Acta Endocrinol. (Copenh.) 128:225 229, 1993.

Moe, N.: Mitotic activity in the syncytiotrophoblast of the human chorionic villi. Am. J. Obstet. Gynecol. 110:431, 1971.

Moll, W.: Physiologie der maternen plazentaren Durchblutung. In, Die Plazenta des Menschen. V. Becker, T.H. Schiebler, and F. Kubli, eds., pp. 172–194. Thieme, Stuttgart, 1981.

Montgomery, D., and Young, M.: The uptake of naturally occurring amino acids by the plasma membrane of the human placenta. Placenta 3:13–20, 1982.

Mossman, H.W.: The rabbit placenta and the problem of placental transmission. Am. J. Anat. 37:433–497, 1926.

Mossman, H.W.: The principal interchange vessels of the chorioallantoic placenta of mammals. In, Organogenesis. R.L. DeHann and H. Ursprung, eds., pp. 771–786. Holt, Rinehart & Winston, New York, 1965.

Mühlhauser, J., Crescimanno, C., Kaufmann, P., Höfler, H., Zaccheo, D., and Castellucci, M.: Differentiation and proliferation patterns in human trophoblast revealed by c-erbB-2 oncogene product and EGF-R. J. Histochem. Cytochem. 41:165–173, 1993.

Myers, R.E., and Panigel, M.: Experimental placental detachment in the rhesus monkey: changes in villous ultrastructure. J. Med. Primatol. 2:170–189, 1973.

Naeye, R.L., Maisels, J., Lorenz, R.P., and Botti, J.J.: The clinical significance of placental villous edema. Pediatrics 71:588–594, 1983.

Nikolov, S.D., and Schiebler, T.H.: Über das fetale Gefäßsystem der reifen menschlichen Plazenta. Z. Zellforsch. 139:333–350, 1973.

Nikolov, S.D., and Schiebler, T.H.: Über Endothelzellen in Zottengefäßen der reifen menschlichen Plazenta. Acta Anat. (Basel) 110:338–344, 1981.

Ogawa, S., Leavy, J., Clauss, M., Koga, S., Shreeniwas, R., Joseph-Silverstein, J., Furie, M., and Stern, D.: Modulation of endothelial cell (EC) function in hypoxia: alterations in cell growth and the response to monocyte-derived mitogenic factors. J. Cell. Biochem. Suppl. 15F:213, 1991.

O'Neill, J.E.G.: Vascularizacao da placenta humana. Thesis, Universidade Nova de Lisboa, Portugal, 1983.

Ong, P.J., and Burton, G.J.: Thinning of the placental villous membrane during maintenance in hypoxic organ culture: structural adaptation or syncytial degeneration? Eur. J. Obstet. Gynecol. Reprod. Biol. 39:103–110, 1991.

Panigel, M., and Myers, R.E.: The effect of fetectomy and ligature of the interplacental fetal vessels on the ultrastructure of placental villosities in Macaca mulatta. C. R. Acad. Sci. Hebd. Seances. Acad. Sci. D 272:315–318, 1971.

Panigel, M., and Myers, R.E.: Histological and ultrastructural changes in rhesus monkey placenta following interruption of fetal placental circulation by fetectomy or interplacental umbilical vessel ligation. Acta Anat. (Basel) 81:481–506, 1972.

Panigel, M., and Pascaud, M.: Les orifices artériels d'entrée du sang maternel dans la chambre intervilleuse du placenta humain. Bull. Assoc. Anat. 142:1287 1298, 1968.

Papierowski Z.: Effects of selected progestagens used for the protection of high-risk pregnancy on the clinical course, morphological changes and proliferative activity of the trophoblast. Ginekol. Pol. 52:298–303, 1981.

Paprocki, M.: Morphologie und Morphometrie der Zottengefäße der reifen menschlichen Plazenta nach vorzeitigem Blasensprung. Medical thesis, Technical University of Aachen, 1992.

Penfold, P., Wootton, R., and Hytten, P.E.: Studies of a single placental cotyledon in vitro. III. The dimensions of the villous capillaries. Placenta 2:161–168, 1981.

Pilz I., Schweikhart, G., and Kaufmann, P.: Zur Abgrenzung normaler, artefizieller und pathologischer Strukturen in reifen menschlichen Plazentazotten. III. Morphometrische Untersuchungen bei Rh-Inkompatibilität. Arch. Gynecol. Obstet. 229:137–154, 1980.

Piotrowicz, B., Niebroj, T.K., and Sieron, G.: The morphology and histochemistry of the full term placenta in anaemic patients. Folia Histochem. Cytochem. 7:436–444, 1969.

Prager, D., Weber, M.M., and Herman-Bonert, V.: Placental growth factors and releasing/inhibiting peptides. Semin. Reprod. Endocrinol. 10(2):83–94, 1992.

Ramsey, E.M., Corner, G.W., and Donner, M.W.: Serial and cineradioangiographic visualization of maternal circulation in the primate (hemochorial) placenta. Am. J. Obstet. Gynecol. 86:213, 1963.

Rao, C.V., Ramani, N., Chegini, N., Stadig, B.K., Carman, F.R., Jr., Woost, P.G., Schultz, G.S., and Cook, C.L.: Topography of human placental receptors for epidermal growth factor. J. Biol. Chem. 260:1705–1710, 1985.

Reshetnikova, O.S., Burton, G.J., and Milovanov, A.P.: The effects of hypobaric hypoxia on the terminal villi of the human placenta. J. Physiol. (Lond.) 459:308P, 1993.

Reynolds, L.P., Killilea, S.D., and Redmer, D.A.: Angiogenesis in the female reproductive system. FASEB J. 6: 886–892, 1992.

Rhodin, J.A.G.: The ultrastructure of mammalian arterioles and precapillary sphincters. J. Ultrastruct. Res. 18:181–223, 1967.

Rhodin, J.A.G.: Ultrastructure of mammalian venous capillaries, venules and small collecting veins. J. Ultrastruct. Res. 25:452–500, 1968.

Rifkin, D.B., and Moscatelli, D.: Recent developments in the cell biology of basic fibroblast growth factor. J. Cell Biol. 109:1–6, 1989.

Rossi, P., Karsenty, G., Roberts, A.B., Roche, N.S., Sporn, M.B., and De Crombrugghe, B.: A nuclear factor 1 binding site mediates the transscriptional activation of a type I collagen promoter by transforming growth factor-β. Cell 52:405–414, 1988.

Salvatore, C.A.: The placenta in acute toxemia. Am. J. Obstet. Gynecol. 102:347–352, 1968.

Scheffen, I., Kaufmann, P., Philippens, L., Leiser, R., Geisen, C., and Mottaghy, K.: Alterations of the fetal capillary bed in the guinea pig placenta following long-term hypoxia. In, Oxygen Transfer to Tissue, XII. J. Piiper, T.K. Goldstick, and D. Meyer, eds., pp. 779–790. Plenum Press, New York, 1990.

Schiebler, T.H., and Kaufmann, P.: Reife Plazenta. In, Die Plazenta des Menschen. V. Becker, T.H. Schiebler, and F. Kubli, eds., pp. 51–111, Thieme, Stuttgart, 1981.

Schmid-Schönbein, H.: Conceptional proposition for a specific microcirculatory problem: maternal blood flow in hemochorial multivillous placentae as percolation of a "porous medium." Trophoblast Res. 3:17–38, 1988.

Schmidt, J.A., Mizel, S.B., Cohen, D., and Green, I.: Interleukin 1: a potential regulator of fibroblast proliferation. J. Immunol. 128:2177–2182, 1982.

Schmon, B., Hartmann, M., Jones, C.J., and Desoye, G.: Insulin and glucose do not affect the glycogen content in isolated and cultured trophoblast cells of human term placenta. J. Clin. Endocrinol. Metab. 73:888–893, 1991.

Schuhmann, R.: Plazenton: Begriff, Entstehung, funktionelle Anatomie. In, Die Plazenta des Menschen. V. Becker, T.H. Schiebler, and F. Kubli, eds., pp. 199–207. Thieme Verlag, Stuttgart, 1981.

Schuhmann, R., and Wehler, V.: Histologische Unterschiede an Plazentazotten innerhalb der materno-fetalen Strömungseinheit: ein Beitrag zur funktionellen Morphologie der Plazenta. Arch. Gynecol. 210:425–439, 1971.

Schuhmann, R., Kraus, H., Borst, R., and Geier, G.: Regional unterschiedliche Enzymaktivität innerhalb der Placentone reifer menschlicher Placenten: histochemische und biochemische Untersuchungen. Arch. Gynecol. 220: 209–226, 1976.

Schweikhart, G.: Morphologie des Zottenbaumes der menschlichen Plazenta—orthologische und pathologische Entwicklung und ihre klinische Relevanz. Thesis, Medical Faculty, University of Mainz, 1985.

Schweikhart, G., and Kaufmann, P.: Zur Abgrenzung normaler, artefizieller und pathologischer Strukturen in reifen menschlichen Plazentazotten. I. Ultrastruktur des Syncytiotrophoblasten. Arch. Gynecol. 222:213–230, 1977.

Schweikhart, G., and Kaufmann, P.: Histologie und Morphometrie der Plazenta bei intrauteriner Mangelentwicklung des Feten. Arch. Gynecol. 235:566–567, 1983.

Schweikhart, G., and Kaufmann, P.: Endzottenmangel und klinische Relevanz. Gynäkol. Rundsch. 27(Suppl. 2):147–148, 1987.

Scott, W.A., and Cohn, Z.A.: Secretory products of mononuclear phagocytes. In, Pathobiology of the Endothelial Cell. H.L. Nossel and H.J. Vogel, eds. Raven Press, New York, 1982.

Sen, D.K., Kaufmann, P., and Schweikhart, G.: Classification of human placental villi. II. Morphometry. Cell Tissue Res. 200:425–434, 1979.

Shorter, S., Clover, L., and Starkey, P.: Evidence for both an autocrine and paracrine role for the colony-stimulating factors in regulating placental growth and development. Placenta 13:A58, 1992.

Shreeniwas, R., Ogawa, S., Cozzolino, F., Torcia, G., Braunstein, N., Butura, C., Brett, J., Lieberman, H.B., Furie, M.B., and Joseph-Silverstein, J.: Macrovascular and microvascular endothelium during long-term hypoxia: alterations in cell growth, monolayer permeability, and cell surface coagulant properties. J. Cell. Physiol. 146:8–17, 1991.

Strauss, D.S.: Growth-stimulatory actions of insulin in vitro and in vivo. Endocr. Rev. 5:356–369, 1984.

Takemura, R., and Werb, Z.: Secretory products of macrophages and their physiological functions. Am. J. Physiol. 246:C1–C9, 1984.

Tedde, G., and Tedde-Piras, A.: Mitotic index of the Langhans' cells in the normal human placenta from the early stages of pregnancy to the term. Acta Anat. (Basel) 100:114–119, 1978.

Thiriot, M., and Panigel, M.: Microcirculation: la microvascularisation des villosites placentaires humaines. C. R. Acad. Sci. [D] 287:709–712, 1978.

Thorpe Beeston, J.G., Nicolaides, K.H., Snijders, R.J., Felton, C.V., and McGregor, A.M.: Thyroid function in small for gestational age fetuses. Obstet. Gynecol. 77: 701–706, 1991.

Tominaga, T., and Page, E.W.: Accommodation of the human placenta to hypoxia. Am. J. Obstet. Gynecol. 94: 679–691, 1966.

Voigt, S., Kaufmann, P., and Schweikhart, G.: Zur Abgrenzung normaler, artefizieller und pathologischer Strukturen in reifen menschlichen Plazentazotten. II. Morphometrische Untersuchungen zum Einfluss des Fixationsmodus. Arch. Gynecol. 226:347–362, 1978.

Wallenburg, H.C.S., Hutchinson, D.L., Schuler, H.M., Stolte, L.A.M., and Janssens, J.: The pathogenesis of placental infarction. II. An experimental study in the rhesus monkey. Am. J. Obstet. Gynecol. 116:841–846, 1973.

Werb, Z.: How the macrophage regulates its extracellular environment. Am. J. Anat. 166:237–256, 1983.

Werner, C., and Schneiderhan, W.: Plazentamorphologie und Plazentafunktion in Abhängigkeit von der diabetischen Stoffwechselführung. Geburtshilfe Frauenheilkd. 32:959–966, 1972.

Widmaier, G.: Zur Ultrastruktur menschlicher Placentazotten beim Diabetes mellitus. Arch. Gynecol. 208:396–409, 1970.

Wigglesworth, J.S.: Vascular organization of the human placenta. Nature 216:1120–1121, 1967.

Wilkin, P.: Pathologie du Placenta. Masson, Paris, 1965.

Yallampalli, C., and Garfield, R.E.: Inhibition of nitric oxide synthesis in rats during pregnancy produces signs similar to those of preeclampsia. Am. J. Obstet. Gynecol. 169:1316–1320, 1993.

Zeek, P.M., and Assali, N.S.: Vascular changes in the decidua associated with eclamptogenic toxemia of pregnancy. Am. J. Clin. Pathol. 20:1099–1109, 1950.

9
Characterization of Developmental Stages

This chapter is a synopsis and presents brief descriptions of the average data of placenta and membranes throughout the single stages of placental development. Embryological data concerning the embryo and fetus are given only insofar as they are of importance for the definition of the stage. The data concerning villous development are summarized in Table 13.

It is not the intention of this chapter to compare data of various sources on a scientific level but, rather, to present data that are directly applicable to the pathological and histological examination of human material. For this purpose, all data have been extrapolated and were standardized where necessary.

The data are based on the following publications: embryonic staging according to O'Rahilly (1973) and Boyd and Hamilton (1970); crown-rump length (CRL), embryonic and fetal weight, mean diameter of the chorionic sac, placental diameter and thickness, placental weight: Boyd and Hamilton (1970), O'Rahilly (1973), and Kaufmann (1981); placental and uterine thickness in vivo: Johannigmann et al. (1972); length of umbilical cord: Winckel (1893); villous surfaces, villous volumes, villous diameters: Hörmann (1951), Knopp (1960), Clavero-Nunez and Botella-Llusia (1961, 1963), Aherne and Dunnill (1966), Kaufmann (1981), Schiemer (1981), and Gloede (1984); mean trophoblastic thickness, distribution of villous cytotrophoblast, mean maternofetal diffusion distance: Kaufmann (1972), Kaufmann and Stegner (1972), Gloede (1984), and Kaufmann (1981). For further details see the summarizing tables in Chapter 5.

Stages of Development

Day 1 p.c. (p.c. = post coitum) Carnegie stage 1: one fertilized cell; diameter 0.1 mm.

Day 2 p.c. Carnegie stage 2a: from 2 to 4 cells; diameter 0.1 to 0.2 mm.

Day 3 p.c. Carnegie stage 2b: from 4 to ±16 cells; diameter 0.1 to 0.2 mm.

Day 4 p.c. Carnegie stage 3: free blastocyst, from 16 to ±64 cells; diameter about 0.2 mm.

Day 5 to early day 6 p.c. Carnegie stage 4: blastocyst attached to the endometrium, from about 128 to ±256 cells; diameter 0.2 to 0.3 mm.

Late day 6 to early day 8 p.c. Carnegie stage 5a: implantation, prelacunar stage of the trophoblast; the flattened blastocyst measures about $0.3 \times 0.3 \times 0.15$ mm. The blastocyst is partially implanted. The implanted part of the blastocyst wall is considerably thickened, largely consisting of solid syncytiotrophoblast. The still not implanted, thin part of the blastocyst wall consists of a single layer of cytotrophoblast. The embryonic disk measures about 0.1 mm in diameter.

Late day 8 to day 12 p.c. Lacunar or trabecular stage.

Late day 8 to day 9 p.c. Carnegie stage 5b: diameter of chorionic sac $0.5 \times 0.5 \times 0.3$ mm; embryonic disk about 0.1 mm. The syncytiotrophoblast at the implantation pole exhibits vacuoles as forerunners of the lacunar system.

Day 10 to day 12 p.c. Carnegie stage 5c: diameter of chorionic sac $0.9 \times 0.9 \times 0.6$ mm. The vacuoles in the syncytiotrophoblast fuse to form the lacunar system; first lacunae at the antiimplantation pole. First contact of the lacunar system with eroded endometrial capillaries. Some maternal erythrocytes may be observed in the lacunae. Around day 11, implantation is complete; the defect in the endometrial epithelium is closed by a blood coagulum and is covered by epithelium on day 12. At the implantation site the endometrium measures 5 mm in thickness; first signs of decidualization.

Day 13 to day 14 p.c. Carnegie stage 6, villous stage (first free primary villi).

Day 13 p.c. The nearly round chorionic sac has a diameter of 1.2 to 1.5 mm; length of embryonic disk is 0.2 mm.

Day 14 p.c. Diameter of chorionic sac 1.6 to 2.1 mm; length of embryonic disk 0.2 to 0.4 mm. First appearance of primitive streak and of yolk sac.

With the expansion of the lacunar system, the syncytiotrophoblast becomes reduced to radially oriented trophoblastic trabeculae, the forerunners of the stem villi. After invasion of cytotrophoblast into the trabeculae, free trophoblastic outgrowths into the lacunae, the "free primary villi," are formed. The trabeculae are now called villous stems. By definition, from this date onward the lacunae are transformed into the intervillous space. Cytotrophoblast from the former trabeculae penetrates the trophoblastic shell and invades the endometrium.

Days 15 to 18 p.c. Villous stage (secondary villi).

Days 15 to 16 p.c. Carnegie stage 7: diameter of chorionic sac about 5 mm; length of embryonic disk less than 0.9 mm; appearance of notochordal process and primitive node (Hensen).

Days 17 to 18 p.c. Carnegie stage 8: diameter of embryonic sac less than 8 mm; length of chorionic disc less than 1.3 mm. On the germinal disk, the notochordal and neurenteric canals and the primitive pit can be discerned.

Starting at the implantation pole and continuing all around the circumference to the antiimplantation pole, mesenchyme (derived from the extraembryonic mesoderm in the chorionic cavity) invades the villi, transforming them into secondary villi. The basal feet of the villous stems, connecting the latter with the trophoblastic shell, and some villous tips remain free of mesenchyme and thus persist in the primary villous stage (forerunners of the cell columns and cell islands).

Days 19 to 23 p.c. This is the beginning of the 2nd month post menstruation (p.m.), villous stage (early tertiary villi).

Days 19 to 21 p.c. Carnegie stage 9: diameter of chorionic sac less than 12 mm; length of embryonic disk equals the crown-rump length of the embryo, 1.5 to 2.5 mm; 1 to 3 somites. Neural folds appear; first cardiac contractions.

Days 22 to 23 p.c. Carnegie stage 10: diameter of chorionic sac less than 15 mm; crown-rump length 2.0 to 3.5 mm; 4 to 12 somites. Neural folds start to fuse; two visceral arches.

The villous mesenchyme is characterized by the appearance of the first fetal capillaries (formation of first tertiary villi). The villous diameters are largely homogeneous, presenting two different-sized groups of villi. The larger villous stems and their branches exhibit diameters of 120 to 250 μm. Histologically, the stroma of both is mesenchymal in nature. Along their surfaces, one finds numerous small (diameters 30–60 μm) trophoblastic and villous sprouts.

Days 23 to 29 p.c. Early tertiary villus stage.

Days 23 to 26 p.c. Carnegie stage 11: diameter of the chorionic sac less than 18 mm; crown-rump length 2.5 to 4.5 mm; 13 to 20 somites; closure of the rostral neuropore; optic vesicles identifiable.

Days 26 to 29 p.c. Carnegie stage 12: diameter of chorionic sac less than 21 mm; crown-rump length 3 to 5 mm; 21 to 29 somites; closure of the caudal neuropore; three visceral arches; upper limb buds appear.

The length of villous stems between the chorionic plate and trophoblastic shell varies from 1 mm (antiimplantation pole) to 2 mm (implantation pole). The central two-thirds is supplied with mesenchyme and capillaries (Figure 82); the peripheral one-third remains in the primary villous stage (cell columns). The villous calibers are similar to those described for the previous stage. The amount of trophoblastic and villous sprouts is reduced. Most villi contain loose mesenchyme together with centrally positioned fetal capillaries (mesenchymal villi). Peripherally, they continue via villous sprouts (with unvascularized mesenchymal core) into massive trophoblastic sprouts. In the villous stems, vessels of larger caliber acquire the first signs of a surrounding adventitia (start of formation of typical stem villi characterized by fibrous stroma). The villous trophoblastic surface is composed of an outer syncytiotrophoblast and complete inner layer of cytotrophoblast. Together they measure 20 to 30 μm in thickness.

The chorionic plate, consisting of fetal mesenchyme, cytotrophoblast, and syncytiotrophoblast still lacks fibrinoid. The trophoblastic shell is transformed into the basal plate by intense mixing of decidual and trophoblastic cells. Secretory activities or tissue necrosis of both cell types causes the appearance of the first foci of Nitabuch fibrinoid. The superficial syncytiotrophoblastic layer of the basal plate, bordering the intervillous space, becomes locally replaced by Rohr fibrinoid.

Days 29 to 42 p.c. Late 2nd month p.m.

Days 29 to 32 p.c. Carnegie stage 13: diameter of chorionic sac less than 25 mm; crown-rump length 4 to 6 mm; 30+ somites; four limb buds and otic vesicle.

Days 32 to 35 p.c. Carnegie stage 14: diameter of chorionic sac less than 28 mm; crown-rump length 5 to 8 mm; first appearance of lens pit and optic cup.

Days 35 to 37 p.c. Carnegie stage 15: diameter of chorionic sac less than 31 mm; crown-rump length 7 to

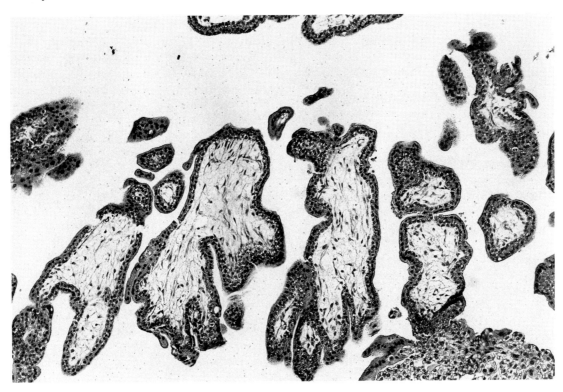

FIGURE 82. Placental villi of the 6th week p.m. Note the thick trophoblastic covering consisting of complete layers of cytotrophoblast and syncytiotrophoblast. Fetal capillaries are poorly developed or, in some places, still lacking. In the lower right corner, an early step of the formation of a cell island can be seen attached to the villous surface. Paraffin section. ×125.

10 mm; closure of lens vesicle; clear evidence of cerebral vesicles; hand plates.

Days 37 to 42 p.c. Carnegie stage 16: diameter of chorionic sac less than 34 mm; crown-rump length 8 to 12 mm; embryonic weight about 1.1 g; retinal pigment visible; foot plates.

The net weight of the chorionic sac in stage 16 is about 6 to 10 g; the thickness of the chorion at the implantation pole is about 6 mm and at the antiimplantation pole about 3 mm. The uterine lumen is still open, and parietal and capsular decidua are not yet in contact.

The range of villous calibers changes slightly from the previous stage (Figure 83). The largest stems reach diameters of less than 400 μm. A variety of medium-sized mesenchymal villi are found between the stem villi that measure about 200 μm in diameter and the small sprouts. The mean villous caliber is about 200 μm. The total placental villous surface is about 0.08 m². The connective tissue layer of the chorionic plate is completely fibrosed, the fibrous tissue partly extending in the initial parts of the villous stems. The overwhelming share of the villous stroma is still mesenchymal in nature. The villous cytotrophoblastic layer is incomplete; 85% of the villous surface is double-layered (cytotrophoblast plus syncytium). The thickness of the villous trophoblast varies between 10 and 30 μm (mean 15.4 μm). Near the end of this period most of the mesenchymal villi show increased numbers of macrophages, as well as the first signs of reticular transformation of their stroma toward immature intermediate villi. Only 2.7% of the villous volume is occupied by fetal vascular lumens. The mean maternofetal diffusion distance is more than 50 μm.

The villous stems are almost completely occupied by connective tissue; basal segments, persisting in the primary villous stage, are the exception. Those segments now show the typical appearance of cell columns. Short portions of villous side branches, persisting in the primary villous stage and that are positioned somewhere between chorionic and basal plate, may increase in size by continuous cell proliferation with subsequent fibrinoid degeneration; they thus establish the first cell islands.

Third month p.m. 9th to 12th weeks p.m.; days 43 to 70 p.c.

Days 43 to 44 p.c. Carnegie stage 17: maximum diameter of chorionic sac 38 mm; crown-rump length 10 to 14 mm; finger rays.

Days 44 to 48 p.c. Carnegie stage 18: maximum diameter of chorionic sac 42 mm; crown-rump length 12 to 16 mm. Elbow region, toe rays, nipples, and eyelids appear.

Days 48 to 51 p.c. Carnegie stage 19: maximum

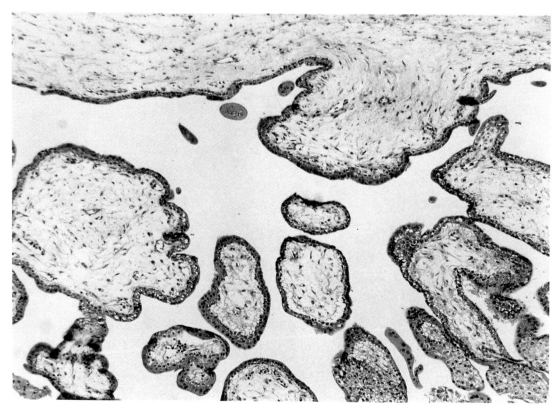

FIGURE 83. Placental villi of the 8th week p.m. All villi are vascularized. As can be seen from the diffuse stromal structure, the villi still belong to the mesenchymal type. Paraffin section. ×125. (From Kaufmann, 1981, with permission.)

diameter of chorionic sac 44 mm; crown-rump length 14 to 18 mm.

Days 51 to 53 p.c. Carnegie stage 20: maximum diameter of chorionic sac 47 mm; crown-rump length 17 to 22 mm. Upper limbs bent at the elbow region; first signs of finger separation.

Days 53 to 54 p.c. Carnegie stage 21: maximum diameter of the oval chorionic sac 51 mm; crown-rump length 20 to 24 mm.

Days 54 to 56 p.c. Carnegie stage 22: maximum diameter of the oval chorionic sac 58 mm; crown-rump length 23 to 28 mm.

Days 56 to 60 p.c. Carnegie stage 23: maximum diameter of the oval chorionic sac 63 mm; crown-rump length 26 to 31 mm.

Days 61 to 70 p.c. Maximum diameter of the oval to irregular chorionic sac 68 mm; crown-rump length 30 to 40 mm.

The embryonic weight increases throughout the 3rd month from 2 g to 17 g and the net weight of the chorionic sac from 10 g to 30 g. The chorionic sac is covered by villi over its surface; it is not yet subdivided into smooth chorion and placenta.

All villi are vascularized. Around the antiimplantation pole, the increased degenerative changes of villi and fibrinoid deposition in the intervillous space indicate that the formation of the smooth chorion will commence soon. Parietal and capsular decidua may come into contact locally, but they remain unfused.

The heterogeneity of villous diameters and villous structure increases. Fibrosis of the villous stems slowly extends into the more peripheral parts of the largest villi (diameters <500 μm). During the course of the 3rd month, most of the villi measuring between 100 and 400 μm establish the typical reticular appearance of immature intermediate villi (Figure 84), characterized by numerous macrophages (Hofbauer cells). Small villi with diameters less than 100 μm show mesenchymal stroma. Trophoblastic and villous sprouts are numerous. Total villous surface is about 0.3 m². The trophoblastic thickness varies from 10 to 20 μm. Eighty percent of the villous surfaces are covered by cytotrophoblast. Fetal vessel lumens occupy about 4% of the villous volume. Some of the larger fetal vessels achieve a thick adventitia, consisting of fibrous stroma, which occupies larger parts of the villous stroma. The reticular stroma, as a sign of immaturity of the stem villi, is restricted to the superficial parts of the stroma positioned under the trophoblast.

Whereas in the previous stages fibrinoid was restricted to the cell islands and the basal plate, spot-like fibrinoid deposition at some of the villous surfaces can now be

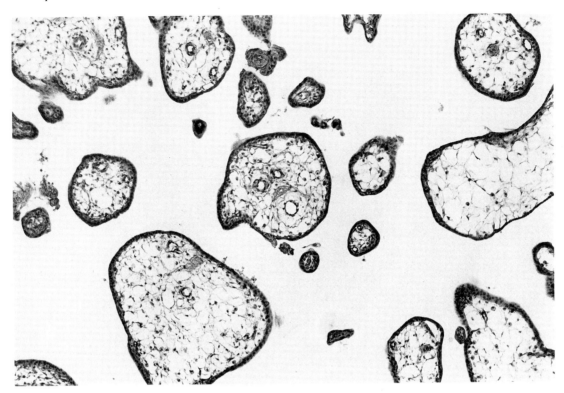

FIGURE 84. Placental villi of the 12th week p.m. The larger villi have achieved the reticular stroma of typical immature, intermediate villi. The smaller villi are mesenchymal in structure. The first small fetal arteries and veins can be seen. Paraffin section. ×125.

observed. Fibrinoid deposition at the intervillous surface of the chorionic plate is still an exception. The amnionic cavity has extended to such a degree that the amnionic mesoderm comes into contact with the connective tissue layer of the chorionic plate in many places.

Fourth month p.m.   13th to 16th week p.m.; 11th to 14th weeks p.c. The shape of the chorionic sac becomes more and more irregular because of compression between uterine wall and fetus. Its maximum diameter increases throughout this period from 68 mm to 80 to 90 mm. The crown-rump length grows from 45 mm to 80 mm and the fetal weight from 20 g to 70 g. The length of the umbilical cord is between 160 and 200 mm.

The continuous degeneration of placental villi at the antiimplantation pole, which is free of villi from the middle of the 4th month onward, as well as the villous proliferation at the implantation pole, initiate the differentiation of the chorionic sac into smooth chorion and placenta. The placental diameter increases from 50 mm to 75 mm at the end of this month and the placental weight from 30 g to 70 g. The maximal placental thickness in the delivered specimens is 10 to 12 mm. Numerous placental septa become visible. The cell columns become more deeply incorporated into the basal plate by fibrinoid deposition in their surrounding. The chorionic plate is in close contact with the amnion over its entire surface, giving it definite shape and layering. It consists of amnionic epithelium, amnionic mesoderm, chorionic mesoderm, a cytotrophoblast layer, and superficial syncytiotrophoblast.

The distribution of the villous calibers (Figure 85) is similar to that described for the preceding month. The inhomogeneous mixture of villi is composed of stem villi with diameters of 300 to 500 μm (the vascular adventitia of which occupies at least 75% of the villous stroma) and immature intermediate villi with diameters of 100 to about 300 μm. Mesenchymal villi and sprouts, 40 to 80 μm in diameter, are numerous; but because of their size they occupy only a small proportion of the total villous volume. Because the immature intermediate villi have the most characteristic reticular stroma in this stage and comprise the highest proportion of villi, one observes more villous macrophages (Hofbauer cells) than at all other stages of placental development. The total villous surface was measured to be 0.5 to 0.6 m². The share of fetal vessel lumens is increased to about 6%. Some of the capillaries establish contact with the villous trophoblast. In such places the syncytial nuclei are moved aside, resulting in the first epithelial plates. Therefore the trophoblastic thickness varies between 2 and 12 μm (mean 9.6 μm). As during the previous month, one observes cytotrophoblast on about 80% of the villous surface. Fibrinoid deposition becomes a usual finding on the villous surfaces.

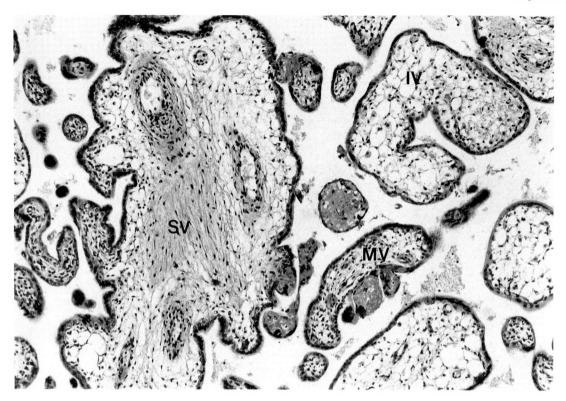

FIGURE 85. Placental villi of the 15th week p.m. The larger immature intermediate villi exhibit the first signs of central stromal fibrosis, originating from the larger fetal vessels, thus establishing the first stem villi (SV). Several typical immature intermediate villi (IV) and mesenchymal villi (MV) can be seen. As is typical for mesenchymal villi of the second and third trimester, they are associated with degenerating villi being more or less transformed into intravillous fibrinoid. Paraffin section. ×125.

Fifth month p.m. 17th to 20th week p.m.; 15th to 18th week p.c. Because of the geometrically irregular outer shape of the fetus, the diameter of the chorionic sac cannot be estimated from this period onward. Over the course of the 5th month the crown-rump length increases from 80 mm to 130 mm and the fetal weight from 70 g to 290 g. The placenta is clearly separated from the smooth chorion. The placental diameter is between 75 mm and 100 mm, and the placental weight increases from 70 g to 120 g. The maximum placental thickness after delivery is about 12 to 15 mm; measured by ultrasonography and in situ, including the uterine wall, it is approximately 28 mm. The length of the umbilical cord varies between 200 and 315 mm.

The structure of the stem villi is nearly the same as during the previous month; however, their number is considerably increased throughout this month (Figure 86). During the 20th week p.m., most of the large-caliber villi (those exceeding 300 μm) have achieved the fibrous stroma of stem villi. The number of slender, long mesenchymal villi with diameters around 80 to 100 μm increases. The mean diameter of the remaining immature intermediate villi is slightly reduced to around 150 μm. The mean villous diameter is 108 μm.

The total villous surface is about 1.5 m². Because the amount of villous cytotrophoblast is reduced to about 60% of the villous surface, the extent of thin trophoblastic areas from 1 to 2 μm thickness increases. Continuous development of fetal capillaries causes the reduction of mean maternofetal diffusion distance to about 22 μm.

Septa and cell islands, which originally consisted mainly of accumulations of cells, now grow considerably by apposition of fibrinoid. Cysts are often found in their centers.

Sixth month p.m. 21st to 24th week p.m.; 19th to 22nd week p.c. The fetus grows from 130 mm to 180 mm crown-rump length. Its weight increases from 290 g to 600 g. The placental diameter is between 100 and 125 mm, and the placental weight increases from 120 g to 190 g. Placental thickness after delivery is 15 to 18 mm, and ultrasonographic measurements in situ, including the uterine wall, indicate a thickness of about 34 mm. The mean length of the cord is between 315 and 360 mm.

The histological features change considerably. Most of the immature intermediate villi become transformed into stem villi of large caliber. Most of the stem villi

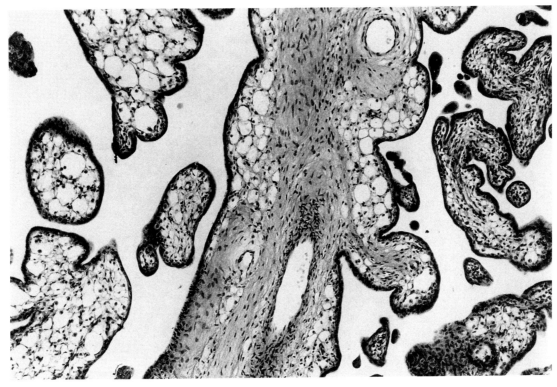

FIGURE 86. Placental villi of the 18th week p.m. The picture is comparable to that of the preceding stage. Formation of stem villi with stromal fibrosis is somewhat more expressed. Paraffin section. ×125.

measure around 200 μm in thickness, some achieving diameters of more than 1,000 μm. Their fibrous stroma still exhibits a small superficial rim of reticular connective tissue, indicating their immaturity (Figure 87). Different from all earlier stages, increasing numbers of newly formed intermediate villi exhibit small calibers (only 100–150 μm). Some of these villi are reticular in stromal structure, as their parent villi, whereas others are slender, mature intermediate villi with poorly vascularized and poorly fibrosed, nonreticular stroma (80–120 μm) (Figure 88). At their surfaces, the first richly capillarized terminal villi are formed. They are difficult to identify in the large group of smallest villi, measuring 50 to 80 μm, as the other members of this group, the small mesenchymal villi and villous sprouts, exhibit structural features similar to those of the terminal villi in paraffin sections. The total villous surface amounts to 2.8 m². The mean trophoblastic thickness is reduced to 7.4 μm, and the mean maternofetal diffusion distance is about 22 μm.

Seventh month p.m. 25th to 28th week p.m.; 23rd to 26th week p.c. Compared to the 6th month, there are only quantitative changes. The crown-rump length increases from 180 mm to 230 mm and the fetal weight from 600 g to 1,050 g. The placental diameter is 125 to 150 mm, and the placental weight is increased to 190 to 260 g. The thickness of the delivered placenta is 18 to 20 mm; by ultrasonography, including the uterine wall, it is 38 mm. The mean length of the umbilical cord increases from 360 mm to 410 mm.

The total villous surface of the placenta exceeds 4 m². The structure and the caliber of the villi are similar to what was seen during the 6th month. Only 45% of the villous surface is covered by cytotrophoblast. The trophoblastic thickness varies between 0.5 and 8 μm (mean 6.9 μm). The number of immature intermediate villi decreases in favor of stem villi and mature intermediate and terminal villi. The lumens of fetal vessel amount to 9.1% of the villous volume.

Cell columns are surrounded by increasing amounts of fibrinoid and become deeply invaginated in the basal plate. The syncytiotrophoblastic covering of the chorionic plate begins to degenerate. It becomes replaced by an initially thin layer of fibrinoid that grows in thickness throughout the following weeks and forms the Langhans' stria.

Eighth month p.m. 29th to 32nd week p.m.; 27th to 30th week p.c. Crown-rump length is 230 to 280 mm, and fetal weight is 1,050 to 1,600 g. The placental diameter normally varies between 150 and 170 mm; the placental weight increases from 260 g to 320 g. The placental thickness after delivery is about 20 to 22 mm;

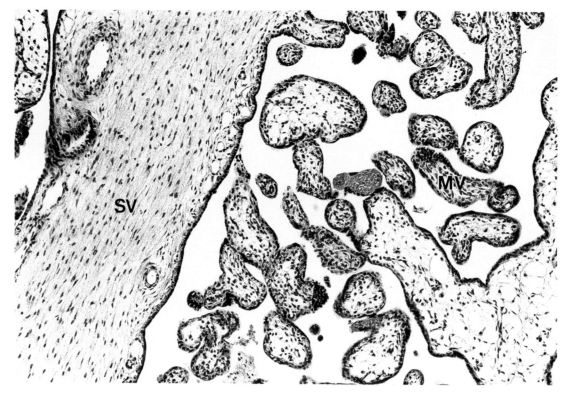

FIGURE 87. Placental villi of the 21st week p.m. The stroma of the stem villi (SV) is largely fibrous. Only a discontinuous thin superficial rim of reticular connective tissue is reminiscent of their derivation from immature intermediate villi. Paraffin section. ×125.

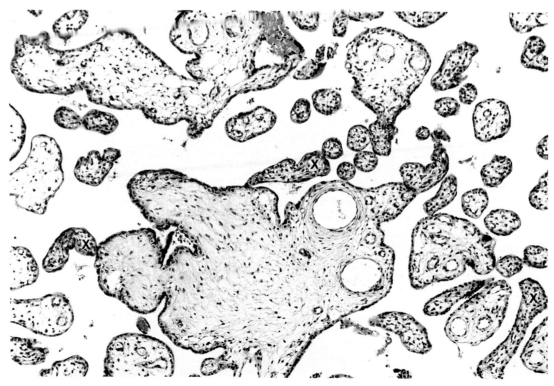

FIGURE 88. Placental villi of the 24th week p.m. Compared to the preceding stages, the variability in villous shapes and diameters is sharply increasing. The population of small slender villi (X), originally referred to as mesenchymal villi, has achieved structural characteristics of mature intermediate villi. Paraffin section. ×125.

measured by ultrasonography in situ and including the uterine wall it is 43 mm. The umbilical cord has a mean length of between 410 and 455 mm.

Steeply increasing numbers of mature intermediate villi and terminal villi, both of which exhibit calibers of 40 to 100 μm, are the reason for considerably increased numbers of villous cross sections per square millimeter of histological sections (Figure 89). The total villous surface is increased to a mean of about 7 m². In addition to the villi of small caliber, which comprise most of the villi, there are mainly stem villi of large caliber. Intermediate calibers of 100 to 200 μm are rare, causing a typical gap in the range of calibers. At times this gap is evident as early as the second half of the 7th month. The few existing villi of this particular caliber, mostly immature intermediate villi, are grouped together in the centers of the villous trees. Villous cytotrophoblast is reduced to about 35% of the villous surface. As a result of the beginning sinusoidal dilatation of the fetal capillaries in the newly formed terminal villi, the amount of vasculosyncytial membranes (epithelial plates) is increased, and the mean trophoblastic thickness reduced to about 6 μm.

Ninth month p.m. 33rd to 36th week p.m.; 31st to 34th week p.c. The crown-rump length is 280 to 330 mm, fetal weight is 1,600 to 2,400 g, placental diameter is 170 to 200 mm, and placental weight is 320 to 400 g. The placental thickness postpartum is 22 to 24 mm; by ultrasonography in situ, including the uterine wall, it is 45 mm. The mean cord length increases from 455 mm to 495 mm.

Histologically, the developmental processes described for the preceding month become even more prominent: The total villous surface of the placenta is increased to about 10 m². Capillary growth and continuous sinusoidal dilatation cause the mean maternofetal diffusion distance to decrease to less than 12 μm, and the mean trophoblastic thickness to about 5 μm. Cytotrophoblast is found on only 25% of the villous surfaces. The largest stem villi reach 500 to 1,500 μm in diameter. The small stromal rim, consisting of reticular connective tissue and indicating their immaturity, has normally disappeared to the credit of fibrous stroma, which completely occupies the villous core (Figure 90). The originally reticular superficial zone of the stroma shows an increased number of connective tissue cells for a few weeks, compared to the more central parts of the stem villi. This difference usually is no longer observed at term. Larger parts of the syncytiotrophoblast of the stem villi are replaced by fibrinoid. Most villi are mature intermediate and terminal villi (Figure 91). Small groups

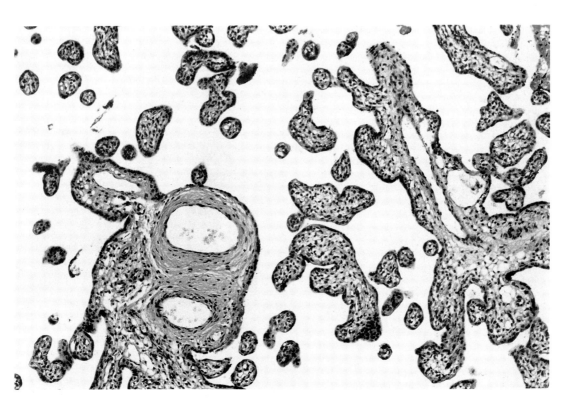

FIGURE 89. Placental villi of the 29th week p.m. During this period the mature intermediate villi and the stem villi (lower left) are the prevailing villous types. Immature intermediate villi with typical reticular stroma (lower right) are less common. Paraffin section. ×125.

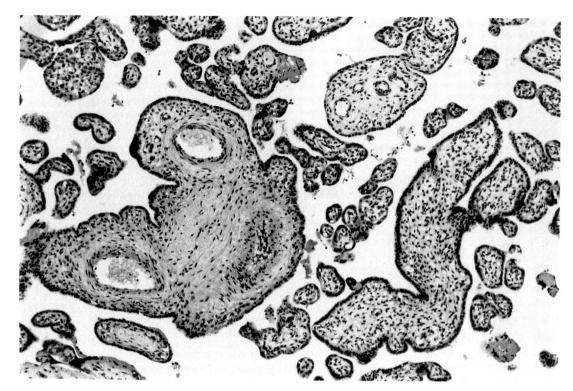

FIGURE 90. Placental villi of the 33rd week p.m. The number of immature intermediate villi is further decreasing. Most villi are stem villi and mature intermediate villi; the latter are intermingled with the first few terminal villi, which in paraffin sections (because of their similar diameters) are difficult to differentiate from mature intermediate villi. The stem villi are still not fully fibrosed; rather, they show a thin superficial stromal layer that has few fibers and is rich in connective tissue cells. Paraffin section. ×125.

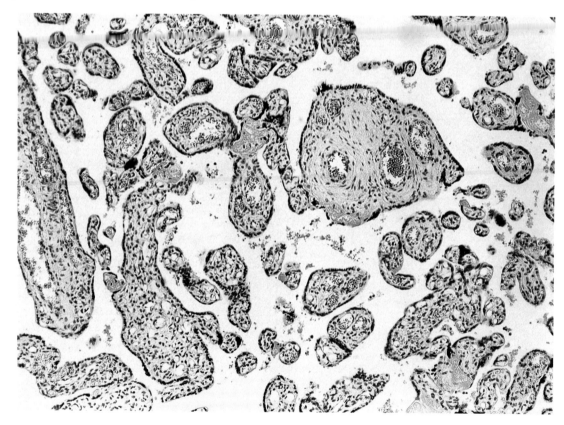

FIGURE 91. Placental villi of the 35th week p.m. The distribution of villous types is largely comparable to that demonstrated for the preceding stage. Paraffin section. ×125.

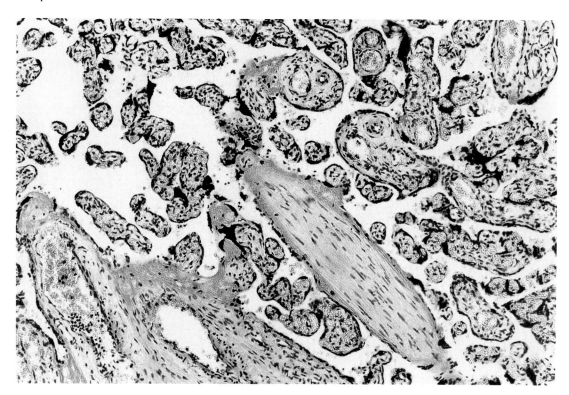

FIGURE 92. Placental villi of the 38th week p.m. Dominating villous types are mature intermediate villi and terminal villi, both of small caliber. Several stem villi of varying caliber can be seen in between. As is typical for near-term placentas, the trophoblastic cover of the stem villi is partly replaced by fibrinoid. The stromal core is completely fibrosed. Reticular stroma or cellular connective tissue (which, as a typical sign of immaturity, was visible below the trophoblast in earlier stages) is absent throughout the last few weeks. Paraffin section. ×125.

of immature intermediate villi, with calibers of 100 to 200 µm, can regularly be found in the centers of the villous trees, indicating still active placental growth.

Tenth month p.m. 37th to 40th week p.m.; 35th to 38th week p.c. The mean crown-rump length is increased from 330 mm to its final value of 380 mm and the mean fetal weight from 2,400 g to 3,400 g. The placental diameter during the last month of pregnancy varies between 200 and 220 mm, and the mean placental weight increases from 400 g to 470 g. There are considerable individual variations. Early clamping of the cord after delivery of the baby may even increase placental weight by as much as 100 g. The final maximal placental thickness postpartum is about 25 mm; measured by ultrasonography in situ, the uterine wall and placenta amount to 45 mm. The mean cord length at term is 495 to 520 mm.

The kind and amount of villous types differ from the foregoing stage in several aspects. There are considerably increased numbers of terminal villi (about 40% of the total villous volume of the placenta) (Figure 92) and a higher degree of capillarization of the latter, mainly due to the fact that many of the capillary cross sections are dilated sinusoidally to maximally 40 µm. In well preserved, early fixed placentas that are not suffering from fetal vessel collapse, the terminal fetal villous capillary lumens amount to 40% or more of the villous volume. About 20% of the villi are stem villi. In the fully matured placenta, the fibrous stroma reaches the trophoblastic or fibrinoid surface of the stem villi everywhere; a superficial reticular rim, or a superficial accumulation of fibroblasts, as during the 9th month, is usually absent at term. If not, it has to be interpreted as a sign of persisting immaturity. The syncytiotrophoblastic cover of the stem villi is degenerated in most places and often it is replaced by fibrinoid (Figure 93). About 30% to 40% of the villous volume is made up of mature intermediate villi, which can be differentiated histologically from the terminal villi by their reduced degree of fetal capillarization and from the stem villi by the absence of large fetal vessels with light microscopically identifiable media and adventitia. Maximally, only 10% of the total villous volume is of the immature, intermediate variety; they normally appear as small, loosely arranged groups in the centers of the villous trees, sometimes surrounding a central cavity.

The total villous volume of the placenta is about

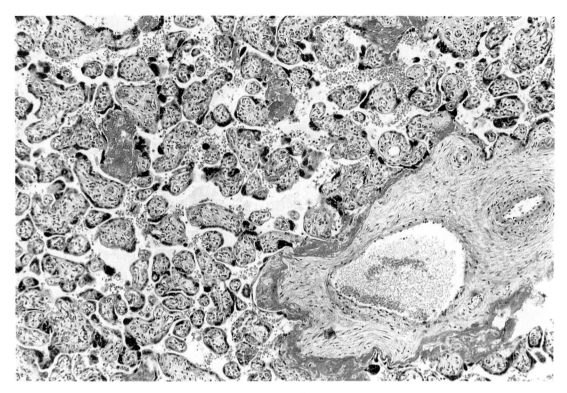

FIGURE 93. Placental villi of the 40th week p.m. The caliber distribution is little different from that of the 38th week. Despite this fact, some remarkable changes do exist: The fibrinoid deposits (homogeneously gray) around the larger stem villi and the number of terminal villi are considerably increased; also, because of the irregular shapes of terminal villi at term, numerous flat sections of villous surfaces can be seen. Here these structures appear as dark spots of seemingly accumulated nuclei (trophoblastic knotting). Paraffin section. ×125.

$12.5 \, \mathrm{m}^2$. The mean trophoblastic thickness is reduced to about $4 \, \mu\mathrm{m}$ and the mean maternofetal diffusion distance to less than $5 \, \mu\mathrm{m}$. Around 20% of the villous surfaces are double-layered, consisting of cytotrophoblast and syncytiotrophoblast. The remaining 80% are covered by only syncytium of highly varying thickness (0.5–10.0 $\mu\mathrm{m}$). The cell bodies of the existing villous cytotrophoblast, however, are so thin at times that they may be difficult to identify; thus many investigators tend to underestimate their quantity and sometimes even deny their existence. The amount of fibrinoid in and around the villi is variable. We have never observed a complete absence of fibrinoid. Amounts exceeding 10% of the total placental villous volume are an exception and are likely to be a sign of pathological processes. The amount of fibrinoid, inside and at the surfaces of the chorionic and the basal plate, is even more variable.

NUCLEATED RED BLOOD CELLS

There is considerable confusion about the normal numbers of nucleated red blood cells (NRBCs) in neonatal blood, and it is for this reason that this information is here included. In the truly normal term pregnancy, few if any RBCs with nuclei are visible in the fetal blood during the microscopic placental examination. When NRBCs are seen in the fetal blood at term (and it is important that they be correctly diagnosed as such), it is a distinctly abnormal finding. The pathologist should endeavor to ascertain the reason for the presence of the NRBCs when they are seen in placental sections, which is most conveniently done by making a blood smear of neonatal blood.

An extensive literature exists on this topic, and the findings in these contributions are not always in agreement. They have indeed led to considerable controversy as to how many NRBCs may be found in truly normal neonates. Most studies are based on neonatal blood smears, rather than placental sections. It is difficult to estimate the number accurately by studying placental slides. One reason for the results to be discrepant is, especially in the early references, that the authors have not always stated the exact age of the neonates they studied. They have also not excluded infants who suffered from any of the many causes of hypoxia. Most papers made no reference to the possible existence of growth retardation and many other factors that are only now becoming known as causing fetal erythropoietin release, the main reason for secretion of NRBCs.

One of the earliest contributions to this topic is that by Geissler and Japha (1901), who stated emphatically that, "contrary to the dogma," NRBCs are not found in young children; it is possible, however, that they occur rarely in premature infants. These authors were adamant in their opinion that the presence of NRBCs is to be viewed as "showing disease." Similar to many others, they did not specify the children's ages or the clinical conditions of their births. Lippman (1924) enumerated the NRBCs of neonatal blood, followed the children up to 5 days of life, and reviewed all prior literature. Lippman concluded that term neonates have an average of 3.2 NRBCs/100 white blood cells (WBCs). (To express the number of NRBCs per total WBCs is a convenient and widely practiced way of enumerating these cells, but an alternate method is referred to below.) The number of NRBCs was found to fall rapidly after birth, and at the age of 5 days there were none left. The condition of the newborns is again not clearly stated in this paper, except that children with congenital syphilis were excluded; but mothers with preeclampsia were not.

Ryerson and Sanes (1934) undertook one of the more incisive studies of placentally contained NRBCs. They were anxious to ascertain parameters that allowed specifying the age of a gestation by histological examination of the placenta. They concluded that virtually all NRBCs had disappeared at the end of the third month of pregnancy. They suggested also that if more than 1% NRBCs are found it indicates prematurity. Anderson (1941) made the next significant contribution and more or less confirmed the previous findings. He indicated that in approximately 16.5% of term placentas one or two NRBCs could be found among 1,000 RBCs; in the remaining 83.5% there were none at term. Stillborns were observed to have greater numbers, and he stated that a "decided increase... points to pathologic states." Fox (1967) next published on this phenomenon and related it to hypoxia or asphyxia. We concur with this interpretation of a relation to fetal tissue hypoxia, and it is our practice to always take special note of the presence of NRBCs when examining placentas microscopically.

Most recently, Green and Mimouni (1990) have addressed the question of NRBCs in newborns of diabetic mothers; their observation was that normative data are lacking in the literature. These authors stated the desirability to express NRBCs in absolute numbers, rather than as NRBCs/WBCs, as has been the common practice. One reason for so doing is that elevated WBC counts would lead to artificially low numbers of NRBCs when the usual method of enumeration (NRBC/100 WBCs) is employed. Green and Mimouni also provided rigid criteria for the selection and suggested that "a value greater than 1×10^9/L should be considered as a potential index of intrauterine hypoxia." Normally, there were no NRBCs in term neonates, and the 95th percentile had 1.7 in absolute counts. Diabetic mothers' babies had increased numbers, as did infants with hypoxia and growth-retarded neonates. Shurin (1987) concluded that there are about 200 to 600 NRBCs/mm^3 and 10,000 to 30,000 WBCs; she also stated that the normal infant has 4 or 5 NRBCs/100 WBCs in cord blood samples, which is higher than is our experience. Shurin reflected that this number indicates the erythroid hyperplasia due to high levels of erythropoietin (EPO) production.

Erythropoietin, initially made in liver and later in kidneys (Eckardt et al., 1992), is the principal agent in the secretion of NRBCs from the sites of hematopoiesis. It is now being measured with greater frequency in cord blood, and correlations are beginning to be made to perinatal circumstances. Maier et al. (1993) found that elevated levels of EPO in cord blood indicates prolonged fetal hypoxia and advocated that the determination of EPO levels might indicate the exact time course of events. The EPO levels did not correlate with gestational age, meconium staining, or Apgar scores, but they related to umbilical arterial pH level and were elevated in the presence of intrauterine growth retardation (IUGR); Maier et al. also quoted authors who found a relation

to fetal death and cerebral palsy. These findings are of great significance to the perinatologist and pathologist with an interest in ascertaining more precisely than is now possible the time of possible fetal hypoxia, especially its relation to possible labor problems. It is hoped that the rapidity (or sluggishness) of the EPO response and the appearance of NRBCs will be further defined in the future so as to allow a better analysis of perinatal hypoxia. Because these phenomena require some significant metabolic steps in fetal performance one would expect that many hours must pass from a hypoxic event to significantly elevate the levels of EPO and NRBCs of the fetus; but we do not presently know the exact number of hours. We also do not know whether the fetal response with EPO and numbers of NRBCs secreted in response to different amounts of acute blood loss is the same or if it is a graded response. There are, however, occasionally specific cases that allow some insight into these questions. They need to be recorded for a better understanding of the response. It is then essential that the precise status of the gestation and the well-being of the fetus be known for accurate assessment. Thus it would be impossible to compare accurately the levels of NRBCs found after a hemorrhage in a neonate with IUGR and those of a normal neonate; the former may have started at a higher baseline. Experimental observations (presently known only from sheep) are insufficient for the clinical setting. Quantitative and temporal sequences by Shields et al. (1993) have reviewed what is known of this aspect of RBC restoration after experimental hemorrhage in sheep. Despite an initial rise in the EPO level, a significant hemorrhage (40%) is not followed by a significant increase in reticulocyte count, nor are the former blood volume and hematocrit restored before birth. Thus the ovine model may not be adequate to settle these important questions.

Phelan et al. (1993) studied NRBCs in asphyxiated and normal neonates. They found that normal infants do not have NRBCs, but that in asphyxiated newborns the NRBC count is elevated. The most elevated NRBC counts were explicable only by assuming hypoxia to have occurred long before birth. Nicolini et al. (1990) observed that IUGR fetuses have elevated NRBC counts in cordocentesis samples.

The following observation may have relevance in this context. A patient at term whom we have known had a major "gush of bright red blood" (later identified as fetal blood from disrupted velamentous vessels) upon insertion of an intrauterine pressure catheter. She was delivered by cesarean section 48 minutes later; the infant was pale but the placenta otherwise entirely normal. The cord arterial pH was 7.05, the fetal hemoglobin 14.6 g, hematocrit 44.8%, WBC 28,000, platelets 120,000/mm^3 falling to 71,000/mm^3. Three transfusions of packed RBCs were given to the newborn, and the hemoglobin level was then only 10.3 g, hematocrit 29.9%. The NRBCs were first enumerated at 1.5 hours: 19 NRBCs/100 WBCs; 6 hours later the count was 32 NRBCs/100 WBCs. Thus there was a continued hematologic response after delivery of the anemic child, and the initial NRBC response was detectable within an hour. This finding is contrary to the rapid decline of NRBCs postnatally when the hypoxic event has been more remote; under those circumstances most NRBCs are gone on the second day.

Another relevant case concerns a woman who had a car accident while wearing a lap belt and was at 28 weeks' gestation. Approximately 12 ± 1 hours later the fetus was born with a hematocrit of 25% and an estimated 40 to 50 ml fetal blood in the maternal circulation. A count of 45 NRBCs/100 WBCs were then found. Moreover, villous edema indicated some degree of early fetal heart failure. This finding is surprising with a hematocrit of 25% and suggests that final adjustment of the blood volume had not yet been made.

TABLE 13. Structural characteristics of the five villous types from the 4th to the 40th week p.m.

	Stem villi	Immature intermediate villi	Mesenchymal villi	Mature intermediate villi	Terminal villi
4			Only mesenchymal villi (120–250 µm) and trophoblastic sprouts (30–60 µm) are present.		
5		%	Large mesenchymal villi (>200 µm) may show diffuse, moderate stromal fibrosis.		%
6					
7					
8		The first stromal channels appear within the mesenchymal villi.			
9		Numerous immature intermediate villi (100–200 µm) with reticular stroma; caliber of the largest vessels is 20–30 µm.	Numerous short mesenchymal villi (60–100 µm) partly continuous with slim trophoblastic sprouts, branch from the surfaces of immature intermediate villi.	%	
10	%				
11					
12		Increasing amount and size of immature intermediate villi (100–400 µm); caliber of stem vessels increased up to 100 µm; vessel walls with two to three concentric layers of cells.			
13					
14					
15		Light microscopically apparant bundles of collagen fibers arranged around vessel walls.			
16					
17	About 50% of all villi with calibers >150 µm show fusion of the fibrosed adventitial sheaths around the primitive arteries with those of the veins. This is the first step toward formation of the fibrosed stromal core of stem villi.		The numbers of mesenchymal villi and trophoblastic sprouts are slowly decreasing.		
18					
19					

No.	Stem villi	Immature intermediate villi	Mesenchymal / Mature intermediate villi	Terminal villi
20 21 22 23	First true stem villi appear. Smaller ones (150–300 μm) show centrally fibrosed core with arterial and venous adventitia being fused. Those >300 μm show a largely fibrosed core.	Immature intermediate villi are still the dominating villous type. Those with calibers of 100–150 μm show no stromal fibrosis. The larger ones fibrosis of the walls of larger vessels.	The number of mesenchymal villi with poorly fibrosed and poorly vascularized stroma, rich in cells, increases considerably. They grow in length and in width (calibers 80–150 μm) and show a continuous transition into mature intermediate villi.	Local spot-like groups of first typical terminal villi appear; they show calibers of about 60 μm, about half of their stromal volume being occupied by capillary lumens.
24 25 26 27 28 29	Caliber >300 μm: completely fibrosed stroma; caliber <300 μm: superficial layer of reticular stroma below the trophoblast.	Number and size of immature intermediate villi is decreasing.	Typical mesenchymal villi are rare and mostly located in the surrounding of immature intermediate villi. Mature intermediate villi with dense stroma, rich in stromal cells and poor in fibers, with calibers of 100–150 μm, comprise the dominating villous type.	Increasing amount of evenly distributed terminal villi with sinusoidally dilated capillaries and few epithelial plates.
30 31 32 33 34	Caliber >200 μm: completely fibrosed stroma; caliber <200 μm: incomplete superficial rim of reticular stroma.	Only a few evenly distributed immature intermediate villi can be found; the stroma is only partly reticular in nature.	Mesenchymal villi are histologically inconspicuous; the few identifiable ones are usually located around the central cavities.	Terminal villi are the dominating villous type; they amount to about 40% of the total villous volume.
35 36 37 38 39 40	Usually, all stem villi are void of reticular stroma; however, below the trophoblast still is a less densely fibrosed rim, rich in fibroblasts. All stem villi (except a few around the central cavity) are completely fibrosed. The trophoblast of the larger ones is often replaced by fibrinoid.	The few remaining immature intermediate villi are no longer evenly dispersed but, rather, concentrated as small groups in the centers of the villous trees lining the central cavities. The extremely loose reticular stroma shows only a few typical stromal channels.	The relative number of mature intermediate villi is decreasing to about 25% of total villous volume. The caliber is reduced to 80–120 μm.	

Reproduced with permission of Kaufmann and Castellucci. Development and anatomy of the placenta. In: Haines's and Taylor's Textbook of Obstetrical and Gynaecological Pathology, 4th ed. H. Fox and M. Wells (eds.). Churchill Livingstone, Edinburgh, 1994.

References

Aherne, W., and Dunnill, M.S.: Morphometry of the human placenta. Br. Med. Bull. 22:5–8, 1966.

Anderson, G.W.: Studies on the nucleated red cell count in the chorionic capillaries and the cord blood of various ages of pregnancy. Am. J. Obstet. Gynecol. 42:1–14, 1941.

Boyd, J.D., and Hamilton, W.J.: The Human Placenta. Heffer & Sons, Cambridge, 1970.

Clavero-Nunez, J.A., and Botella-Llusia, J.: Measurement of the villus surface in normal and pathologic placentas. Am. J. Obstet. Gynecol. 86:234–240, 1961.

Clavero-Nunez, J.A., and Botella-Llusia, J.: Ergebnisse von Messungen der Gesamtoberfläche normaler und krankhafter Placenten. Arch. Gynecol. 198:56–60, 1963.

Eckardt, K.-U., Ratcliffe, P.J., Tan, C.C., Bauer, C., and Kurtz, A.: Age-dependent expression of the erythropoietin gene in rat liver and kidneys. J. Clin. Invest. 89:753–760, 1992.

Fox, H.: The incidence and significance of nucleated erythrocytes in the foetal vessels of the mature human placenta. J. Obstet. Gynaecol. Br. Commonw. 74:40–43, 1967.

Geissler, D., and Japha, A.: Beitrag zu den Anämien junger Kinder. Jahrb. Kinderheilkd. 56:627–647, 1901.

Gloede, B.: Morphometrische Untersuchungen zur Reifung menschlicher Placentazotten. Medical thesis, University of Hamburg, 1984.

Green, D.W., and Mimouni, F.: Nucleated erythrocytes in healthy infants and in infants of diabetic mothers. J. Pediatr. 116:129–131, 1990.

Hörmann, G.: Lebenskurven normaler und entwicklungsfähiger Chorionzotten, Ergebnisse systematischer Zottenmessungen. Arch. Gynecol. 181:29–43, 1951.

Johannigmann, J., Zahn, V., and Thieme, V.: Einführung in die Ultraschalluntersuchung mit dem Vidoson. Elektromedica 2:1–11, 1972.

Kaufmann, P.: Untersuchungen über die Langhanszellen in der menschlichen Placenta. Z. Zellforsch. 128:283–302, 1972.

Kaufmann, P.: Entwicklung der Plazenta. In, Die Plazenta des Menschen. V. Becker, T.H. Schiebler, and F. Kubli, eds., pp. 13–50. Thieme Verlag, Stuttgart, 1981.

Kaufmann, P., and Castellucci, M.: Development and anatomy of the placenta. In, Haines' and Taylor's Textbook of Obstetrical and Gynaecological Pathology, 4th ed. H. Fox and M. Wells, eds. Churchill Livingstone, Edinburgh, 1994 (in press).

Kaufmann, P., and Stegner, H.E.: Über die funktionelle Differenzierung des Zottensyncytiums in der menschlichen Placenta. Z. Zellforsch. 135:361–382, 1972.

Knopp, J.: Das Wachstum der Chorionzotten. Monatsschr. Z. Anat. Entwicklungsgesch. 122:42–59, 1960.

Lippman, H.S.: A morphologic and quantitative study of the blood corpuscles in the new-born period. Am. J. Dis. Child. 27:473–536, 1924.

Maier, R.F., Böhme, K., Dudenhausen, J.W., and Obladen, M.: Cord blood erythopoietin in relation to different markers of fetal hypoxia. Obstet. Gynecol. 81:575–580, 1993.

Nicolini, U., Nicolaidis, P., Fisk, N.M., Vaughn, J.I., Fusi, L., Gleeson, R., and Rodeck, C.H.: Limited role of fetal blood sampling in prediction of outcome in intrauterine growth retardation. Lancet 336:768–772, 1990.

O'Rahilly, R.: Developmental stages in human embryos. Part A. Publication 631. Carnegie Institute, Washington, D.C., 1973.

Phelan, J.P., Ahn, N.O., Korst, L., and Martin, G.I.: Nucleated red blood cells: a marker for fetal asphyxia [abstracts 49]. Am. J. Obstet. Gynecol. 170:286, 1993.

Ryerson, C.S., and Sanes, S.: The age of pregnancy. histologic diagnosis from percentage of erythroblasts in chorionic capillaries. Arch. Pathol. 17:548–651, 1934.

Schiemer, H.G.: Mass und Zahl der Plazenta. In, Die Plazenta des Menschen. V. Becker, T.H. Schiebler, and F. Kubli, eds., pp. 112–122. Thieme Verlag, Stuttgart, 1981.

Shields, L.E., Widness, J.A., and Brace, R.A.: Restoration of fetal red blood cells and plasma proteins after a moderately severe hemorrhage in the ovine fetus. Am. J. Obstet. Gynecol. 169:1472–1478, 1993.

Shurin, S.B.: The blood and the hematopoietic system. In, A.A. Fanaroff and R.J. Martin, eds. Neonatal-Perinatal Medicine. Mosby, St. Louis, 1987, pp. 826–827.

Winckel, F.K.L.W.: Lehrbuch der Geburtshilfe, 2nd ed. Veit, Leipzig, 1893.

10
Three-Dimensional Aspects of Villous Maldevelopment

Villous Cross-Sectional Features

Placental histopathology is based on the light microscopy of paraffin sections. Thus the normal and pathological features of the placenta are usually described in terms of the two dimensions apparent by light microscopy.

The studies by Küstermann (1981) using reconstructions of serial paraffin sections, by Burton (1986a,b, 1987) who worked with plastic serial sections, and by Cantle et al. (1987) and Kaufmann et al. (1987) who compared light microscopic findings of villous sections with scanning electron microscopic results of comparable and identical material (Figure 94) revealed that the two-dimensional impression does not always reflect the three-dimensional structure. This point is particularly true for histopathologically meaningful findings such as syncytial knots, syncytial sprouts, and syncytial bridges (for definitions see Chapter 7), most of which prove to be only tangential sections of the villous surface. The true interpretation is of considerable importance for aspects of placental pathology, as the histological appearance of syncytial sprouts, for example, is widely accepted as a diagnostic indicator of placental ischemia (e.g., in preeclampsia) (Tenney & Parker, 1940; Alvarez et al., 1964, 1969, 1970; Schuhmann & Geier, 1972).

Küstermann's (1981) statement that all sprouts, knots, and bridges of the mature placenta must be interpreted as sectional artifacts brought about the question whether the histopathological experience should be abandoned. Küstermann's results were largely corroborated by the studies of Burton (1986a) and Cantle et al. (1987). At the same time, it became apparent (Kaufmann et al., 1987) that despite this new interpretation the diagnostic value of the sprouts, even though in most cases representing artifacts, was still useful. As is described below, they are significant artifacts that point to a characteristic deformation of the terminal villi. This deformation is usually caused by ischemia (Figures 98, 99). Therefore

the final conclusions drawn by Alvarez et al. (1969, 1970) are generally correct: The diagnostic value of the two-dimensional findings of syncytial sprouts remains.

Küstermann (1981) and Burton (1986a) used three-dimensional reconstructions of serial sections to verify that most knots, sprouts, and bridges are only flat sections (Figure 97), a point that can be demonstrated even more impressively in two other ways. Cantle et al. (1987) prepared 10 μm epoxy resin sections stained with toluidine blue. This dye does not infiltrate the resin and stains it only superficially. The light microscopic picture corresponds to that of a semithin section of 0.5 to 1.0 μm (Figure 95A). When studying the same section with phase contrast microscopy, one gets the picture of the complete 10 μm section of the identical material (Figure 95B). When comparing the two pictures of the same section, one easily realizes that the "thin section" does not show any sprouts, whereas the "thick section" reveals three apparent sprouts that were obviously tangential sections of the trophoblastic surface.

This finding is in agreement with the experience of all electron microscopists who have studied the placenta: that knots, sprouts, and bridges are common in paraffin sections (5–10 μm), rare in semithin sections (0.5–1.0 μm), and mostly absent in the ultrathin sections (0.05–0.1 μm) prepared for electron microscopy. The situation is depicted in Figure 96.

Similar conclusions were deduced when we prepared semithin sections for light microscopy and subsequently removed the epoxy resin from the rest of the tissue block. The remaining villi were studied with the scanning electron microscope and compared to the semithin section (Figure 94) (Cantle et al., 1987). Using this method, real sprouts and bridges as well as flat-sectioned villous surfaces can be easily identified and compared to the sectional picture of this tissue. It became evident from such material that branching, twisting, and coiling of villi (e.g., as a result of hypoxia) enhances the chance of tangential sectioning of trophoblastic surfaces and

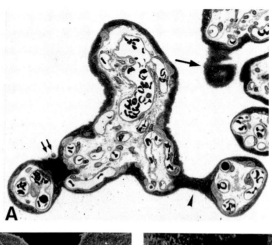

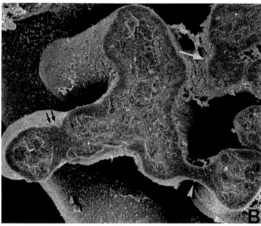
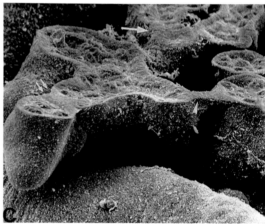

FIGURE 94. Term placenta. After preparing a semithin section (A), the epoxy resin was removed from the remaining tissue block. The latter was prepared for scanning electron microscopy. Identical villi are shown in a semithin section (A) and scanning electron micrographs in vertical (B) and nearly horizontal orientations (C). The arrowhead points to a true syncytial bridge, histologically characterized by its smooth surface, whereas the other "bridge" (double arrow), characterized by its irregular histological appearance, proves to be a tangential section of a curved villous portion. The large arrow marks an artifactual "sprout" that can easily be identified as a tangential section. ×265. (From Cantle et al., 1987, with permission.)

thus increases the number of artificial "knots," "sprouts," and "bridges" (Figures 98, 99).

On the other hand, scanning electron microscopic proof was presented by Schiebler and Kaufmann (1981), Burton (1986b, 1987), and Cantle et al. (1987) for the existence of real sprouts, knots, and bridges. These trophoblastic specializations may serve (1) as first steps of villous sprouting, that is, formation of new villi (trophoblastic or syncytial sprouts) (Boyd & Hamilton, 1970; Cantle et al., 1987; Castellucci et al., 1989); (2) as mechanism of extrusion of old syncytial nuclei (syncytial knots) (Martin & Spicer, 1973; Jones & Fox, 1977); or (3) as simple mechanical aids to establish junctions between neighboring villi (syncytial bridges) (Cantle et al., 1987).

Cantle et al. (1987) suggested criteria for discriminating between true trophoblastic specializations and tangential sections: True sprouts and bridges usually show smooth surfaces (Figure 94A), whereas tangentially sectioned surfaces tend to be irregularly shaped and notched. True sprouts show loosely scattered, ovoid nuclei. Degenerative syncytial knots have pyknotic nuclei forming condensed clusters. Flat sections of every shape are characterized by the usual heterogeneity of nuclear shapes; the apparent numerical density of nuclei depends on the sections' thickness.

Generally, in the young placenta most sprouts are true trophoblastic outgrowths. In paraffin sections of the mature placenta, almost all of these structures are artifacts caused by thick sectioning.

The question how to interpret knots, sprouts, and bridges relates to the more relevant question of how to interpret villous shapes and branching patterns three-dimensionally. Figure 97, based on a drawing by Burton

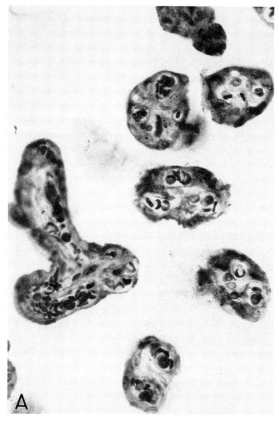
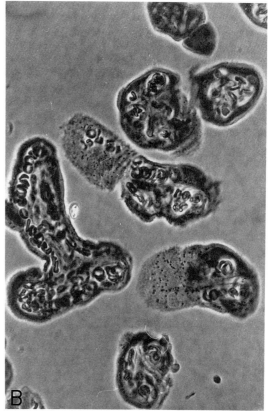

FIGURE 95. Term placenta from a patient with preeclampsia. (A) A 10 μm epoxy resin section is stained only superficially with toluidine blue, comparable to a semithin section of about 1 μm thickness. (B) Same section as in (A) is observed with phase contrast microscopy and now represents the full-section thickness of 10 μm. It shows three "syncytial sprouts," obvi- ously tangential sections of the trophoblastic surface and not visible in the "thinner" section. It demonstrates the influence of the thickness of the section on the appearance of so-called sprouts, caused by trophoblastic tangentional sectioning. ×380. (From Cantle et al., 1987, with permission.)

(1986a), shows that three factors increase the chance of tangential sectioning of villi: branching, curving, and superficial notching.

1. Long, slender, stretched villi [e.g., derived from a slightly immature placenta of about 32–36 weeks' menstrual age (Figures 90, 91) or from the condition of terminal villi deficiency (Figure 103)] have a low incidence of tangential sectioning.

2. Thicker, bulbous villi, as during the early stages of pregnancy (Figure 101), gestational diabetes mellitus, persisting immaturity at term, and rhesus incompatibility (Figure 102), show a few more tangential sections.

3. The normal mature placenta, which has numerous short terminal villi branching from the surfaces of the mature intermediate villi (Figure 100), has a higher incidence of tangential sectioning.

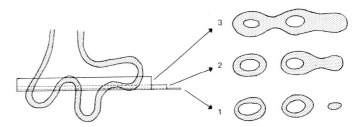

FIGURE 96. Influence of section thickness on the structural appearance of villi in the microscope. 1 = electron micro- scopic, ultrafine section that normally shows only few sprouts; 2 = light-microscopie semithin section; 3 = light microscopic paraffin section in which, because of its thickness, sprouts are frequent features.

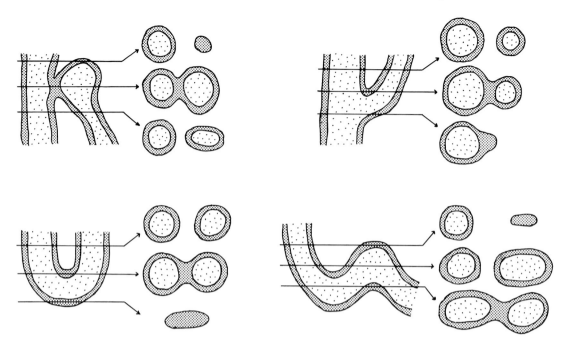

FIGURE 97. Ways by which the appearance of apparent syncytial fusion between villi may arise. Only in the first case (top left) is there true syncytial fusion, whereas in the other three cases the histological appearance of sprouting and bridging is of artifactual nature. (Adapted from Burton, 1986a, with permission.)

4. The number of trophoblastic flat sections as sectional artifacts in the hypermature placenta or in cases of preterm maturity [intrauterine growth retardation (IUGR) with absent end-diastolic umbilical blood flow] with large numbers of long, poorly branched terminal villi (Figures 99, 104) is low.

5. The hypoxic, hypercapillarized placenta, which is characterized by multiply branched, short, fist-like terminal villi (Figures 98, 105), shows such a degree of flat sectioning that the two-dimensional picture may achieve a net-like appearance in which most terminal villi are seemingly connected to each other by syncytial "bridges."

Villous Maldevelopment

Based on these considerations, the following sections deal briefly with typical cases of villous maldevelopment and their three-dimensional branching patterns and with the diagnostic problems they cause in histological sections. The findings reported here are largely based on those from another report (Kaufmann et al., 1987).

Normal Mature Placenta

In the normal, term placenta, the dominant structures are long, slender, mature intermediate villi from which short, grape-like terminal villi branch (Figures 70, 100A). So long as the terminal villi are short and only poorly branched, as in the cases depicted, the incidence of tangentional sectioning is low. Most of the peripheral villous cross sections are uniform in caliber (Figure 100B), except for some occasional immature intermediate and stem villi. Usually, the latter villi accumulate in the centers of the villous trees and nearer the chorionic plate. Trophoblastic tangentional sectioning resulting in the incorrect impression of sprouting is a rare event in thin plastic sections (Figure 100B); this picture is seen somewhat more frequently in the thicker paraffin sections (Figures 92, 93) (Fox, 1978; Becker, 1981). Only some of these "typical signs of villous maturation" (*Reifezeichen* of Becker, 1981) have a real structural basis. We estimate that about 5% of sprouts seen in paraffin sections are true trophoblastic outgrowths (i.e., signs of trophoblastic sprouting or extrusion of pyknotic nuclei); the remaining 95% are artifacts due to sectioning. Despite this fact, they can be regarded as reliable signs of full maturation in paraffin sections (Figure 93). Their artifactual genesis points to the existence of mature villous shapes. When studying the thinner semithin sections (1 μm) (Figure 100B), one must exercise care because to the unexperienced observer the reduced incidence of artificial sprouting may wrongly suggest an organ that is not yet fully mature.

FIGURE 98. Comparison of capillary branching patterns and their appearance in histological cross sections. Hypercapillarization is present due to hypoxia. Note the highly branching capillary nets in short, knob-like, multiply indented villi. Histologically, they appear as web-like connected small villous cross sections, having numerous "sprouts" and "bridges" as the result of tangentional sectioning.

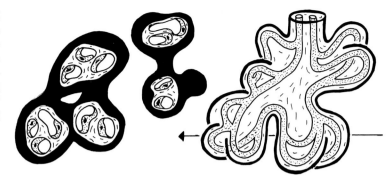

Synchronous Villous Immaturity

The term "synchronous" is used for histological features of the immature villous trees that correspond to what we expect to be normal for the pregnancy stage (Schweikhart et al., 1986). For a normal baseline, we refer to the pictures and data provided by Boyd and Hamilton (1970), Kaufmann (1981), Vogel (1986), Stoz et al. (1988), Vogel (1992), and to the data presented in Chapter 9.

From the 8th to 20th week post menstruation (p.m.), the immature villous trees are composed of uniformly thick, bulbous, immature intermediate villi. Their trophoblastic surface is unevenly curved and distended (Figure 101A). Terminal villi are virtually absent. The numerous side branches of small caliber are composed of sprouts and newly produced mesenchymal villi. For geometrical reasons, the chance of obtaining flat sections depends on the villous diameter and decreases with

increasing villous caliber. Therefore the rare event of tangential sectioning of such immature cases with prevailing large villi does not give an incorrect impression of sprouting.

Persisting Villous Immaturity and Rhesus Incompatibility

It is generally considered that villous maturation is retarded in the presence of rhesus incompatibility (Wentworth, 1967; Werner et al., 1973; Fox, 1978; Pilz et al., 1980), but it is still disputed whether the villous features are further complicated by edema. In our experience, the villous features are influenced by a delay in villous maturation at an unduly early stage of development. Thus immature intermediate villi of large caliber persist (Figure 102A). As is characteristic for this villous type, terminal branches are uncommon and

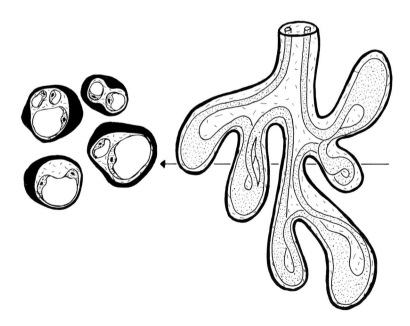

FIGURE 99. Preterm maturation or hypermaturity. Note the long, poorly branched capillaries in correspondingly long terminal villi with prominent sinusoidal dilatation. Histologically, the result is mostly separate villous cross sections. Compare with Figure 98.

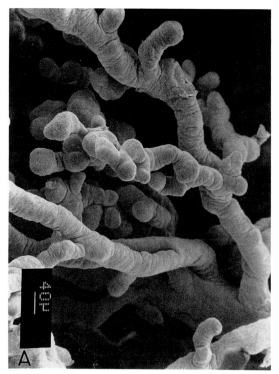

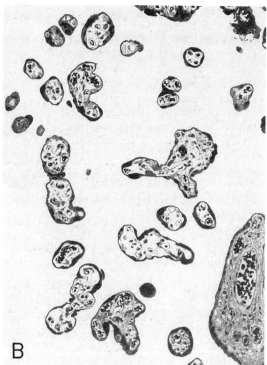

FIGURE 100. Normal mature placenta, 40th week of gestation. (A) In this scanning electron micrograph, long, slender, slightly curved mature intermediate villi with a moderate number of grape-like terminal villi are the dominating features. (B) In the corresponding semithin section, the incidence of trophoblastic tangential sectioning, causing artificial sprouts and bridges, is low. In contrast to the early placenta (Figure 101A), true sprouting is a rare event during this stage of pregnancy. ×120. (From Kaufmann et al., 1987, with permission.)

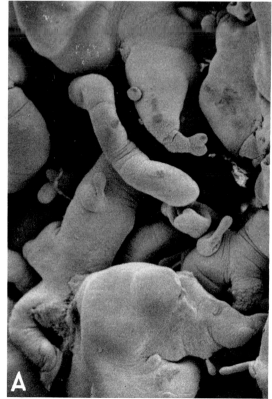

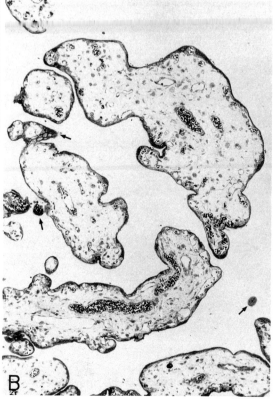

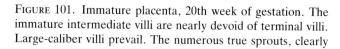

FIGURE 101. Immature placenta, 20th week of gestation. The immature intermediate villi are nearly devoid of terminal villi. Large-caliber villi prevail. The numerous true sprouts, clearly visible in the scanning electron micrograph (A), are rarely seen (arrows) in the corresponding cross-sectional picture (B). ×66. (A: from Kaufmann et al., 1987, with permission.)

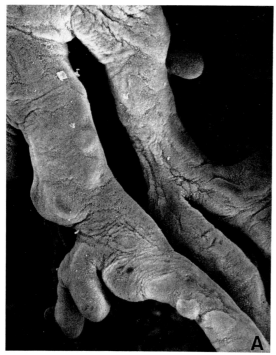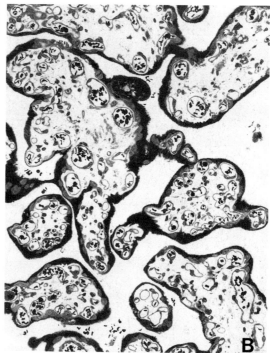

FIGURE 102. Placenta from a case of severe rhesus incompatibility, near term. Immature intermediate villi with a large caliber prevail. Only a few smaller side branches (terminal or mesenchymal villi) arise from the surfaces (A). True syncytial sprouting comparable to that seen in normal immature intermediate villi (Figure 101) is rare. The occasional "sprouts" and "bridges" visible in semithin sections (B) are artifacts caused by tangential sectioning of the irregular, notched outer surface of the immature intermediate villi. These villi are much better vascularized in the presence of rhesus incompatibility than are those of normal early pregnancy. In well stained, thin histological sections, one can easily identify that the large caliber of the villi is the result of villous immaturity rather than of villous edema. ×195. (From Kaufmann et al., 1987, with permission.)

depend on the degree of isoimmunization. There are, however, some differences when compared to cases of synchronous villous immaturity. True syncytial sprouts are largely absent. This finding is in agreement with the pathogenetic concept that villous maturation, and thus the formation of new villi, is decelerated in this condition. Moreover, cases of persisting immaturity at term or of severe maturational arrest in patients with erythroblastosis exhibit better fetal vascularization (Figure 102B) than cases of synchronous immaturity. In accordance with the straight course of the large villi and their intensively notched surfaces seen on scanning electron micrographs (Figure 102A), the histological sections (Figure 102B) usually reveal large-caliber villi of varying size, with only occasional sprouting and bridging. Most of them are caused by tangential sectioning.

Terminal Villi Deficiency

We have previously reported that in many cases of imminent fetal asphyxia the placenta exhibits typical scanning electron microscopic patterns (Schweikhart & Kaufmann, 1983, 1987; Schweikhart et al., 1986; Kaufmann et al., 1987) (Figure 103A). The peripheral parts of the villous trees are composed mainly of naked mature intermediate villi, the terminal side branches of which are lacking. We therefore refer to this abnormality as terminal villi deficiency.

The villous trees are composed of long, poorly branched mature intermediate villi arranged in loose bundles of usually striking parallel arrangement. Because mature intermediate villi and terminal villi are of nearly the same diameters, this condition is easy to identify on scanning electron micrographs but difficult to diagnose on histological sections. The lack of terminal villi becomes evident only on sections of sufficient quality to allow assessment of the finer structural characteristics of both villous types (e.g., sinusoidal dilatation in terminal villi and poor capillarization in mature intermediate villi) (Figure 103B).

As these structures cannot always be judged in paraffin sections with the postpartal vessel collapse having occurred, the straight course of the mature intermediate villi—the arrangement as either cross, oblique, or longitudinally sectioned bundles—often remains the only characteristic feature of this abnormality. Large

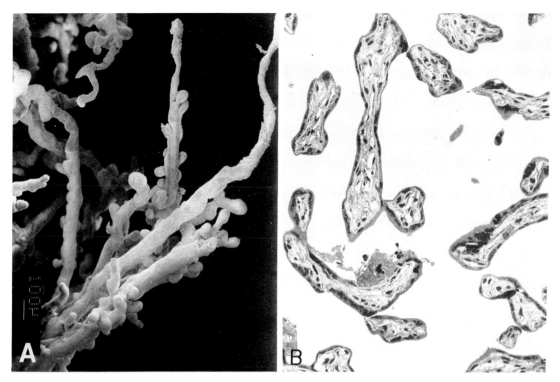

FIGURE 103. Terminal villi deficiency, 40th week of gestation. (A) Scanning electron micrograph (A) shows long, straight, poorly branched bundles of mature intermediate villi but only a few terminal villi. (B) Histological section resembles that of a normal term placenta (Figure 100), but the homogeneity of villous caliber, the dominance of mature intermediate villi, and the small number of terminal villi may lead to the correct diagnosis. ×55. (From Kaufmann et al., 1987, with permission.)

groups of small-caliber villi that do not show the normal mixture of villous sections of different shape but are composed of homogeneous groups of villous sections of similar shape and orientation always arouse suspicion regarding this condition. Artificial trophoblastic sprouting and bridging are virtually absent because of the remarkably straight course of the prevailing villous type, the mature intermediate villi. Other characteristic features are the paucity of villous cytotrophoblast, an unusual homogeneity of trophoblastic thickness with evenly distributed nuclei of similar shape, size, and orientation, and the scarcity of vasculosyncytial membranes and syncytial knots.

If one bears these features in mind, it is not difficult to identify the typical histological picture of a placenta with terminal villi deficiency as being different from that of a normal placenta. For the experienced placentologist, the lack of trophoblastic flat sectioning in this abnormality can provide hints that lead to the correct diagnosis. We are not certain if this condition has been previously described. It may correspond to the street-like villous arrangement described by Emmrich and Mälzer (1968).

Clinically, terminal villi deficiency is often combined with prolonged pregnancy (Mikolajczak et al., 1987; Schweikhart & Kaufmann, 1987); sometimes we found it combined with cases of abnormal thyroid function (hormone-treated hypothyroidism) (see p. 144). It is the prevailing structural feature in cases of acute peripartal hypoxia. It is also often combined with IUGR. Both clinical findings can be explained by the reduced exchange surface and increased maternofetal diffusion distance due to the lack of terminal villi.

Terminal villi deficiency has been interpreted as a result of reduced fetal capillary growth in the villous periphery (Figure 80) (Kaufmann et al., 1988); hypercapillarization is induced by chronic hypoxia (Bacon et al., 1984; Scheffen et al., 1990). Accordingly, one might propose that hyperoxic conditions initiate the terminal villi deficiency, but we are uncertain that such a condition exists. It is interesting to note, however, that the severest cases of terminal villi deficiency we have observed so far, most of which resulted in peripartal fetal death, were combined with maternal hyperthyroidism or were seen in patients treated with thyroid hormones without evidence of hypothyroidism (Kaufmann et al., 1988).

Maternal Diabetes Mellitus

The villi associated with maternal diabetes mellitus have usually been described as immature (Fox, 1978; Greco et al., 1989; Vogel, 1992). A more detailed evaluation reveals several differences when compared to synchronous immature villi or to those of persisting immaturity and rhesus incompatibility. Werner and Schneiderhan (1972), Emmrich et al. (1975), Gödel and Emmrich (1976), and Fox (1978) have all described characteristic features in diabetes, including stromal fibroblastic proliferation, an excess of Langhans' cells, and decreased fetal vascularization. We agree with Vogel (1992), who pointed to the local and interindividual variability of the villous patterns, which can be only partly explained by various degrees of illness or success of treatment.

The scanning electron microscopic appearance is similar to that of cases of synchronous immaturity but different from that of persisting immaturity and rhesus incompatibility. The number of drumstick-shaped trophoblastic sprouts increases with increasing diameter of the immature villi, suggesting considerable proliferative activity. Because of their small size, the incidence of true sprouts is low in histological sections, but the diagnosis can be based on the large caliber of the villi in combination with unusual amounts of villous cytotrophoblast and voluminous stromal cells.

Villous Hypermaturity and Preterm Villous Maturation

In 50% of placentas from babies of the 29th to 32nd week of pregnancy and in 32% of the placentas from the 33th to the 37th week, Schweikhart et al. (1986) found a villous maturational state corresponding to that of the normal mature placenta. It may even display hypermature villous patterns (Salvatore, 1968). Becker (1981) used the term maturitas precox placentae when the villous maturation was accelerated and reached normal term features considerably before the 40th week. He concluded that the prematurely matured placenta may induce labor. According to the results of Schweikhart et al. (1986), hypermaturity is an even more common finding in cases of preterm delivery than is maturitas precox. Sometimes structurally similar cases of hypermaturity were observed after prolonged pregnancy; however, the more common finding after the 42nd week is a persisting immature villous pattern (Mikolajczak et al., 1987).

Hypermaturity is structurally characterized by numerous, long, branched and twisted terminal villi that largely hide the central mature intermediate villus from which they branch (Figure 104A). The relative or absolute scarcity of mature intermediate villi has led Vogel (1992) to call this entity deficiency of intermediate villi; in fact, histologically well fibrosed stem villi and perfectly capillarized terminal villi are the prevailing structures.

In an earlier publication we correlated this scanning electron microscopic feature with the histological appearance of increased trophoblastic flat sectioning (Kaufmann et al., 1987). This correlation, however was a misinterpretation, probably caused by an admixture of cases with IUGR combined with absent end-diastolic umbilical blood flow (see below). After a comparative evaluation of several new cases, we arrived at the conclusion that the histological picture of hypermaturity without IUGR is different. It is characterized by numerous cross sections of large, highly vascularized terminal villi (Figure 104B). Because of the immature state of pregnancy, the villous stroma sometimes shows a loose, sometimes mesenchymal or reticular appearance and is deficient in fibers. This picture is in striking contrast to the sinusoidal dilatation of the fetal capillaries.

IUGR Combined with Absent End-Diastolic Umbilical Blood Flow

A great variety of pathological correlates has been found in cases of IUGR, such as small placenta, persisting placental immaturity, high degree of placental infarction, fetoplacental vasculopathy, villous hypermaturity, and terminal villus deficiency (for reviews see Chapter 19; also Fox, 1978; Vogel, 1992).

When we selected cases, however, in which IUGR was combined with absent end-diastolic umbilical blood flow as judged by Doppler examination, the histopathological findings were surprisingly homogeneous (Macara et al., 1994). In general, they resembled those (described above) for villous hypermaturity. However, there were some additional findings that are uncommon in cases of hypermaturity without severe reduction of umbilical blood flow.

As is the case in preterm maturity and hypermaturity, most of the villi are stem villi with signs of immaturity (superficial rim of reticular stroma) and abnormally slender terminal villi. Scanning electron microscopy and occasional longitudinal paraffin sections revealed that the terminal villi are long, largely unbranched, filiform structures. The capillaries are sometimes slender, sometimes highly dilated.

Further findings, according to Macara et al. (1994), comprised the following features: (1) paucity of villous trophoblast; (2) reduction of cytotrophoblastic proliferation; (3) increased incidence of pyknotic nuclei and syncytial knotting with extrusion of nuclei due to reduced cytotrophoblastic regeneration of the syncytiotrophoblast; and (4) increased amounts of stromal collagen I, collagen IV, and laminin. In agreement with the experimental findings by Panigel and Myers (1972), all these features were interpreted as signs of intraplacental hyperoxia, possibly due to decreased oxygen

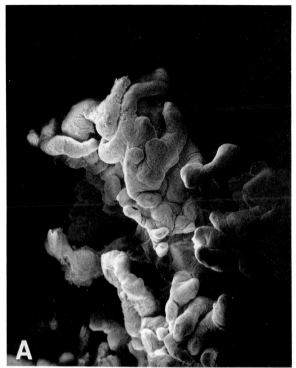
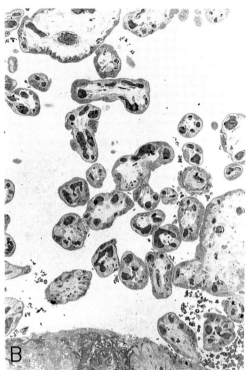

FIGURE 104. Placentas from patients with severe preeclampsia from the 37th (A) and 31st (B) weeks of pregnancy combined with IUGR. (A) Scanning electron micrograph shows the typical feature of preterm maturation (or hypermaturity) with long, twisted, partly branched terminal villi that are aggregated around the mature intermediate villus. (B) Histologically, it results in the appearance of numerous small cross sections of highly capillarized terminal villi with sinusoidal dilatation. Sometimes increased flat sectioning across the twisted villous surfaces can also be seen. Doppler high resistance results in similar features. ×125. (A: from Kaufmann et al. 1987, with permission.)

liberation from the villi into the reduced fetoplacental circulation (see Chapter 8).

Although one would expect histological features similar to those in hypermaturity (numerous small villous cross section, scarcity of trophoblastic flat sections), reality is more confusing, as the increase in syncytial knotting (described above) is difficult to discriminate from trophoblastic flat sectioning. All cases with minimum calibers of numerous and well vascularized terminal villi, combined with knotting and a paucity of mature intermediate villi, are likely to belong to this group of IUGR combined with reduced umbilical blood flow.

Casts of the fetoplacental villous vessels, prepared from such specimens and studied in the scanning electron microscope, revealed long, poorly branched, highly coiled capillaries (Leiser, personal communication, 1994) (compare item 3 in Figure 80 and Figure 109). The sinusoidal dilatation can be interpreted as an attempt at compensation for the increase in blood flow resistance in these long capillary loops. The Doppler measurement cited above provided evidence that the resulting blood flow resistance was considerably increased despite sinusoidal dilatation. In some parts of the fetoplacental vascular bed the flow of blood obviously came to a standstill; histologically, we found aggregation of fetal erythrocytes due to stasis (Figure 104B). Ultrastructurally, the erythrocytes had damaged membranes and were partially lysed, which can be interpreted as signs of fetal circulatory decompensation. Clinically, the Doppler findings were considered in all these cases as evidence of fetal compromise with a need for immediate termination of pregnancy (Fendel, personal communication, 1989; Macara et al., 1994).

Preeclampsia, Hypertensive Disorders, and Placentas at High Altitude

There is general agreement that hypoxia is responsible for the placental changes in women with anemia, preeclampsia, or hypertension and for those who live at a high altitude (Mohr, 1950; Alvarez et al., 1964, 1970; Piotrowicz et al., 1969; Beischer et al., 1970; Kemnitz & Theuring, 1974; Fox, 1978; Jackson et al., 1987, 1988a,b; Reshetnikova et al., 1993). This view has been corroborated by tissue culture studies of the influence of hypoxia on villous explants (Tominaga & Page, 1966; Fox, 1970; Amaladoss & Burton, 1985; Burton et al.,

1989; Ong & Burton, 1991) and experimental studies on long-term effects of hypoxia on pregnant guinea pigs (Bacon et al., 1984; Geisen et al., 1990; Scheffen et al., 1990).

All these studies indicate that increased trophoblastic proliferation and increased villous capillary growth and branching are the typical placental responses to long-term hypoxia (Figure 80). The capillary response to hypoxia is characterized by capillary branching (Scheffen et al., 1990) and is thus different from the fetal capillaries of hypermature villi. Hypoxia results in richly branched, net-like capillary beds that are easy to perfuse, as their structure provides less flow resistance than comparably large capillary beds composed of longer, less branched capillaries. This situation is compatible with the decrease in capillary diameter that was found in related animal experiments (Bacon et al., 1984; Scheffen et al., 1990) and that seemed to be highly characteristic for hypoxic villi in the studies on human placentas from high altitude performed by Jackson et al. (1987, 1988a,b). It must be pointed out, however, that Reshetnikova et al. (1993) arrived at opposite conclusions; among their group of placentas from women who lived and delivered at high altitude, they observed a general increase in capillary diameters compared to lowland pregnancies.

The richly branched capillaries from hypoxic placentas (Figures 80, 98) are responsible for a characteristic deformation of the outer shape of the terminal villi (Figures 98, 105A). The trophoblast directly covers the capillary surface, as the connective tissue is usually reduced. It results in short, knob-like, multiply indented villi that resemble fists. Preparation of histological sections of such villi unavoidably results in increased flat sectioning. Groups of villi are connected to each other by syncytial bridges (Figure 105B). Often a net-like appearance is achieved, the extent of which depends on the thickness of the section. The section depicted in Figure 105B is at 1 μm. One can easily imagine the amount of bridging in the thicker paraffin section.

Prolonged Pregnancy

For decades most "prolonged pregnancies" have actually been miscalculated term pregnancies (Fox, 1978); however, careful ultrasound examination throughout preg-

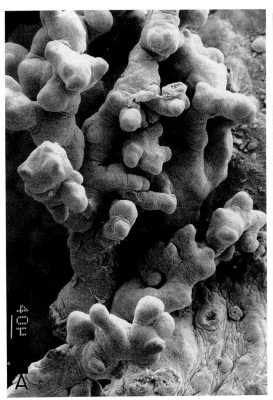
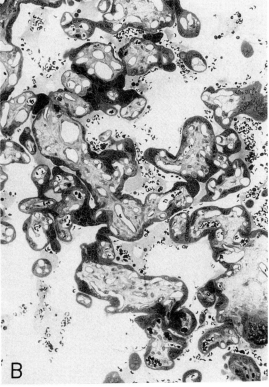

Figure 105. Placenta from a patient with severe preeclampsia, near term. Because of long-lasting hypoxia, the branching pattern of the villi in this case is different from that depicted in Figure 104. (A) The multiply branched, highly coiled, short capillary loops (Figure 80) cause short knob-like, indented villous surfaces. (B) Corresponding semithin section shows a conglomeration of terminal villi with apparent syncytial "bridging" and "sprouting" artifactually caused by tangential sectioning. Sometimes it results in a net-like appearance. ×125. (B: from Kaufmann et al., 1987, with permission.)

nancy now has allowed more precise dating. Placentas from true 42 and 43 weeks' gestations show many abnormal maturational features, among which are terminal villi deficiency (Kaufmann et al., 1987) and persisting immaturity (Mikolajczak et al., 1987). Many pathologists had pointed to these correlation even before ultrasound confirmation of pregnancy length was available (Beckcr, 1963; Emmrich & Mälzer, 1968; Kemnitz & Theuring, 1974; Kloos & Vogel, 1974; Fox, 1978) These changes seem to be the usual finding in prolonged pregnancy.

Only a few cases, 12% according to Schweikhart (1985), show signs of hypermaturity, as reported earlier by Essbach and Röse (1966) and Emmrich and Mälzer (1968). In our material, these placentas were different from the typical villous hypermaturity observed in cases of premature delivery (Figure 104). They showed increased capillarization but exhibited features of both hypoxia and hypermaturity. Complicated networks of narrow capillaries were paralleled by long, winding, dilated capillaries. The corresponding branching patterns of the terminal villi, as seen by scanning electron microscopy (Figure 106A), showed some long winding and some short multiply indented villi. In histological

sections this situation results in complex pictures, with partly isolated villous sections having dilated capillaries and some net-like villous conglomerates (Figure 106B).

CLASSIFICATION OF VILLOUS MALDEVELOPMENT

The primary finding in placentas from most of these conditions is an abnormal numerical composition of otherwise largely normal villous types (Kaufmann et al., 1987), which is valid for synchronous immaturity, persisting immaturity, rhesus incompatibility, hypoxic hypercapillarization, hypermaturity, and terminal villi deficiency. The villous trees of these conditions differ from the mature villous trees at term by predominance of only one villous type at the expense of others. The structure and number of stem villi are usually not altered in these conditions. We observe mainly numerical shifts among terminal villi, mature intermediate villi, and immature intermediate villi.

Figure 107 is an attempt to simplify these relations. Each corner represents the predominance of one villous type. The upper part of the triangle comprises all cases with marked immaturity, expressed by the predominance of immature intermediate villi and the simultaneous lack of mature intermediate and terminal villi. The base of the triangle represents villous ramification patterns characterized by largely absent immature intermediate villi, to the advantage of mature intermediate and terminal villi. These cases comprise terminal villi deficiency (lower left corner), normal

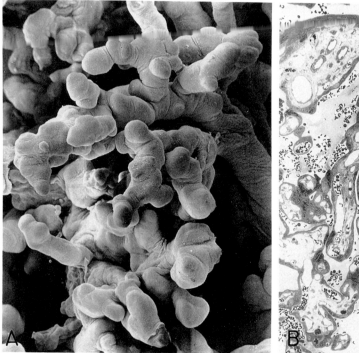 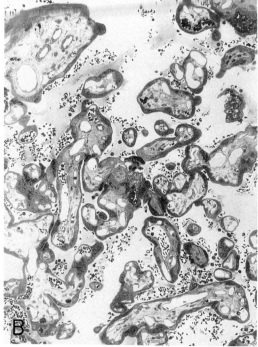

FIGURE 106. Placenta in prolonged pregnancy, 43rd week of gestation. This case shows a mixture of hypermature and hypoxic changes of the terminal villi, both resulting in hypercapillarization and overproduction of terminal branches. (A) Scanning electron micrograph shows complicated convolutions of long, branched, multiply notched and indented terminal

villi, completely hiding the central mature intermediate axis. (B) Semithin section is a mixture of small terminal villus cross sections (as in the case of hypoxia; see Figure 105) with a tangentially sectioned, web-like arrangement of villi (as in hypermaturity; see Figure 104). ×115. (From Kaufmann et al., 1987, with permission.)

basal trophoblast, trophoblastic giant cells, trophocytes, and spongiotrophoblast-like cells). Among these names, the term intermediate trophoblast has caused particular confusion. This term was introduced by Tighe et al. (1967) for a group of cells that appear to be intermediate between cytotrophoblast and syncytium. A few years later, within the cell columns, Okudaira et al. in 1971 reported various cell types, such as proliferating and differentiating cytotrophoblast and intermediate trophoblast. He also considered the latter to be an intermediary step of transformation into syncytiotrophoblast. Later, this term was used as a general heading for all extravillous trophoblast cells by Kurman et al. (1984a,b). These authors did not even mention the different use of the same name in the previous papers.

Meanwhile, this name (intermediate trophoblast) is widely employed in histopathological and clinical articles, although often it is not evident to which of the above three definitions the authors refer. Descriptions such as "intermediate trophoblasts of the villous sprouts" (Pampfer et al., 1992) or "intermediate trophoblast cells at both villous and extravillous sites" (Riley et al., 1992) illustrate this confusion.

We believe that the term *extravillous* describes the situation of trophoblast cells residing outside the villi much better than the term intermediate. Also, among cell biologists the term extravillous trophoblast is in use as the most general heading for all types of trophoblast occurring outside of villi. When syncytial elements can be excluded, the name extravillous cytotrophoblast may be more appropriate. The extravillous cytotrophoblast may be further subdivided into (1) intraarterial (or intravascular) trophoblast (Beck & Beck, 1967), infiltrating the uteroplacental vessels; and (2) interstitial trophoblast (Pijnenborg et al., 1980) comprising all extravillous trophoblast outside the uteroplacental vessel walls.

Historical Aspects

Placentologists have known for a long time that different cell types exist in the nonvillous parts of the placenta and that they differ markedly in shape and staining patterns (Figures 108, 109, 118). The derivation of the so-called X cells (i.e., the large, intensely staining extravillous cells) was uncertain until 1973. For this reason the cells of placental septa and cell islands, those in the basal plate and the cellular layer underneath the chorionic plate, and those in the membranes came under intense investigation. Their name, X cell, first employed by Scipiades and Burg (1930), implied that their origin was in dispute. Depending on the location at which the cells were prevalent, investigators alternately considered the origin to be maternal or fetal.

In efforts to differentiate between these cells, several authors (Klinger & Ludwig, 1957; Serr et al., 1958; Sohval et al., 1959) studied the prevalence of Barr bodies (sex chromatin, the heterochromatic second X chromosome of females) in cells of placental septa from male conceptuses. Klinger (1957) had earlier shown that this characteristic accurately reflects the genotype of placental cells when he applied this methodology to amnion and chorion. All the studies suggested that the large, darkly staining cells of septa were derived from maternal tissues. Only Zhemkova (1960), using the same methodology, had declared the X cells to be of fetal origin.

Electron microscopic findings of glycogen and other decidua-like features also initially indicated a maternal origin (Ruffolo et al., 1967) and thus differed from the results of Zhemkova (1960) and Wynn (1967a). Radioautographic investigation with ^{3}H-thymidine as precursor showed that X cells incorporate thymidine, indicating replicative activity. Only cytotrophoblast had a similar, albeit more pronounced, capacity (Kim & Benirschke, 1971). This finding led to a chromosome study, which again suggested a maternal origin of carefully collected cells (Kim et al., 1971a). Moreover, first immunohistochemical attempts with fluorescent antibodies to human chorionic gonadotropin (hCG) and placental lactogen (hPL) resulted in a hormone localization in syncytium but not in the X cells (Kim et al., 1971b).

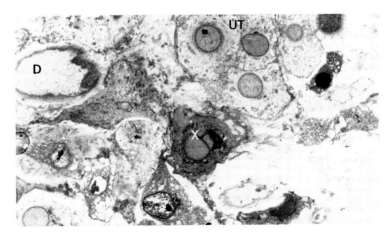

FIGURE 108. Basal plate at term. Enzyme histochemical proof of β-glucuronidase to demonstrate the typical mixture of cell types in the basal plate. D = decidua cell with its clearly visible surrounding basal lamina; X = highly differentiated extravillous cytotrophoblast, so-called X cells; UT = undifferentiated extravillous cytotrophoblast. Semithin section. ×810. (From Stark & Kaufmann, 1973, with permission.)

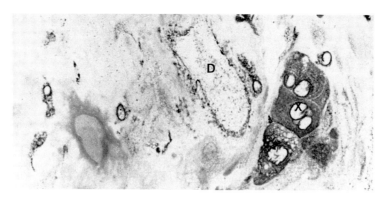

FIGURE 109. Mature basal plate. Enzyme histochemical proof of glucose-6-phosphate dehydrogenase. As is typical for this enzyme, extravillous trophoblast cells (X) exhibit intense reaction patterns, whereas decidua cells (D) stain largely negative, except slight granular staining along their surfaces. Semithin section. ×360. (See Figure 135.)

Detailed structural analysis undertaken at that time (Kaufmann & Stark, 1971) (Figure 108) and enzyme histochemical studies (Stark & Kaufmann, 1971) (Figure 109) gave evidence that the X cells are trophoblastic in nature. Their intense reaction for glucose-6-phosphate dehydrogenase made them clearly different from decidual cells (Figures 109, 135). Decidual cells largely lack the expression of this enzyme. Moreover, it was structurally and histochemically easy to trace these cells throughout several developmental stages from their main proliferating source, the cytotrophoblast of the cell columns.

The trophoblastic, fetal origin of the X cells was finally proved by Y-specific fluorescence in X cells of placentas from male infants (Faller & Ferenci, 1973; Khudr et al., 1973; Maidman et al., 1973; Steininger, 1978). Decidual cells lack this marker. By application of these methods it was easy to demonstrate that the septa and basal plate are composed of an admixture of maternal and trophoblastic cells. Wislocki (1951), Boyd and Hamilton (1966), and Hörmann (1966) had expressed this opinion many years earlier. As though additional proof for a fetal origin of these cells were needed, Powell et al. (1976) showed that, in a case of fetal I-cell disease, the X cells had the same cytoplasmic vacuolation that was exhibited by the syncytium. The decidual cells lacked this feature.

Today it is generally acknowledged that antibodies against cytokeratin, an epithelial intermediate filament, can be used as an easily applicable immunohistochemical marker for trophoblast (Khong et al., 1986b; Yeh et al., 1988, 1990; Daya & Sabet, 1991). This antigen seems to be the most sensitive marker for the distinction of extravillous trophoblast cells from decidual cells. Another immunohistochemical marker that is said to react specifically with extravillous trophoblast is an antibody against placental protein 19 (PP19) (Takayama et al., 1989). The antibody BC-1 (Loke et al., 1992a) can differentiate between villous and extravillous trophoblast, binding specifically to the latter.

Composition of the Extravillous Trophoblast Population

Depending on the localization and the structure, many types of extravillous cytotrophoblast have been described (Figure 110); and among these descriptions were several findings that suggest the existence of various independent lines of differentiation. On the other hand, it is tempting to speculate that there is only one pathway of extravillous trophoblast differentiation (King & Loke, 1988; Fisher et al., 1989; Loke, 1990; Damsky et al., 1992; Genbacev et al., 1993c) producing a broad variety of structurally and functionally different stages. And also this view is supported by several findings.

Most studies concerning the extravillous trophoblast have been performed on trophoblastic cell columns, and these studies present convincing evidence that the cell columns represent the growth zones for the interstitial and intravascular trophoblast of basal plate and septa (Wakuda & Yoshida, 1990, 1992; Damsky et al., 1992; Genbacev et al., 1992, 1993a; Loke et al., 1992a,b; Castellucci et al., 1993; Fisher & Damsky, 1993; Mühlhauser et al., 1993).

Regarding the *proliferation patterns*, as early as 1971 autoradiographic studies had shown that the extravillous trophoblast cells take up thymidine and that they can be cultured in vitro (Kim & Benirschke, 1971), but the cells apparently do not fuse syncytially. It has also become clear that not all cells behave the same. Many authors (Wakuda & Yoshida, 1990, 1992; Castellucci et al., 1991; King & Blankenship, 1993; Mühlhauser et al., 1993) have noted that only the proximal cells of the cell columns neighboring the basal lamina of the anchoring villus represent the proliferating entity (Figures 111B, 112). Moreover, they are immunoreactive for epidermal growth factor receptor (Wang et al., 1992; Mühlhauser et al., 1993). These two reports disprove older findings that described extremely low epidermal growth factor receptor (EGF-R) expression for the proliferating cells (Tavare & Holmes, 1989) or a diffuse presence of this receptor throughout the entire population of extravillous trophoblast cells (Bulmer et al., 1989).

The presence of EGF-R in this area is usually taken as an indicator of proliferative activity, as EGF is a well known epithelial mitogen. Its mitogenic activity has also been proved for the trophoblast (Lysiak et al., 1992). Other stimulators of extravillous trophoblastic prolifer-

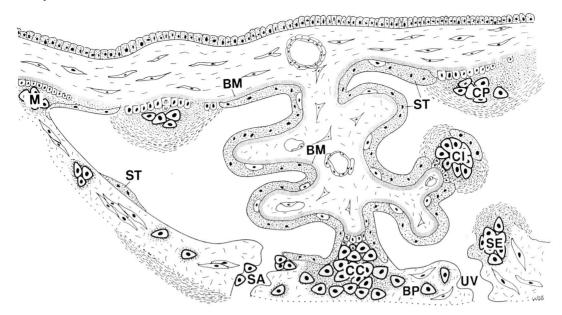

FIGURE 110. Distribution of three trophoblast populations of the human placenta (see Figure 112). All those trophoblast cells that rest on the trophoblastic basal lamina (BM) of membranes, chorionic plate, villi, cell columns, and cell islands represent the proliferating trophoblastic stem cells (Langhans' cells). Where these cells are close to the intervillous space they differentiate and fuse to form the syncytiotrophoblast (ST). Usually this event takes place in the placental villi. Without contact to the intervillous space, the daughter cells of the proliferating stem cells do not fuse syncytially but, rather, differentiate and become invasive, forming the extravillous trophoblast cells. The latter can be found in cell columns (CC), cell islands (CI), chorionic plate (CP), membranes (M), septa (SE), basal plate (BP), and spiral arteries (SA). The respective cells are derived from the next proliferating source. Uteroplacental veins (UV) are usually not invaded by extravillous trophoblast. Matrix-type fibrinoid is point-shaded; fibrin-type fibrinoid is line-shaded.

ation are the members of the colony-stimulating factor (CSF) family, potent mitogens of hematopoietic cells. The receptor of this cytokine, the protein product of the c-*fms* proto-oncogene, has been found in extravillous trophoblast (Pampfer et al., 1992); and Loke and coworkers (1992b) have shown an increased proliferation rate of this population in vitro after treatment with granulocyte-macrophage CSF.

The more distal cells that invade the basal plate no longer proliferate (Figures 111, 112); rather, they begin to differentiate. In the course of this process they lose the EGF-R and express c-*erb*B-2 protein product (Wang et al., 1992; Mühlhauser et al., 1993), which is thought to represent the receptor for an unknown growth factor. It is interesting that mRNA transcripts of c-*erb*B-2 could also be detected in the proliferating extravillous trophoblast cells; however, expression of the respective protein seemed to be blocked until the cells leave the mitotic cycle (Mühlhauser et al., 1993). This point represents an interesting difference between the extravillous trophoblast with its controlled invasiveness and many invasive tumors that continuously express c-*erb*B-2 protein product (for review see Mühlhauser et al., 1993).

There are no convincing indications that trophoblast cells that have left the cell columns can still proliferate. Conflicting results obtained in the rhesus monkey with antibodies directed against polymerase-δ-associated antigen (PCNA) (Blankenship et al., 1993; King & Blankenship, 1993) are not convincing because, owing to its long biological half-life, PCNA is also immunoreactive in trophoblast that has already left the mitotic cycle (Kohnen et al., 1993). When applying this "proliferation marker" one should always bear in mind that even nuclei of the clearly nonproliferative syncytiotrophoblast may stain (Wolf & Michalopoulos, 1992).

It is not only proliferation markers and growth factor receptors that suggest extravillous trophoblast cells emanate from the cell columns and deeply invade the junctional zone and even the uteroplacental vessels. The distribution of adhesion molecules, their extracellular matrix ligands, matrix degrading metalloproteinases, and class I major histocompatibility complex (MHC) molecules also support this view (Damsky et al., 1992; for review see Fisher & Damsky, 1993).

The process of extravillous trophoblast differentiation starting at the cell columns has also been studied in vitro using explants of anchoring villi (Genbacev et al.,

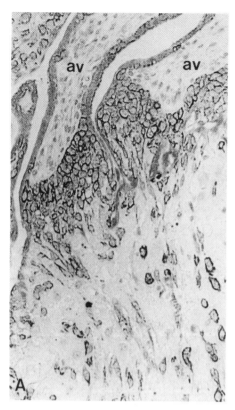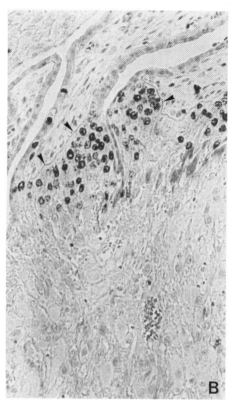

FIGURE 111. Two anchoring villi (av) are attached to the basal plate (below) by cell columns at the 16th week p.m. (A) Stained with anti-cytokeratin, which binds to all villous and extravillous trophoblast cells. (B) Stained with the monoclonal antibody MIB-1, which stains only proliferating cells. Note that the invasive trophoblast cells (lower half) are non-proliferative, whereas those cells facing the basal lamina of the anchoring villus (arrowheads) and villus cytotrophoblast are MIB-1-positive. These cells make up the proliferating stem cells (Langhans' cells). Serial paraffin sections. ×100. (Courtesy Dr. Gaby Kohnen, Aachen.)

1991, 1992, 1993a; Vicovac et al., 1993). Application of proliferation markers and antibodies directed against class I MHC, hPL, integrins, and extracellular matrix molecules has beautifully illustrated the differentiation process that takes place after the cells have left the proliferation zone near the basal lamina and begin to invade the surrounding matrix.

Questions concerning the *homogeneity of the extravillous trophoblast* population are difficult to resolve. We have compared the cell columns with other sites of extravillous trophoblast (septa, cell islands, chorionic plate, membranes) in terms of proliferation patterns and the expression of EGF-R and c-*erb*B-2 protein product (Castellucci et al., 1991; Mühlhauser et al., 1993; Nanaev et al., 1993a,b). The not unexpected result was that in all cases the proliferating cells that express EGF-R were either resting on the basal lamina, which delimits trophoblast from villous or chorionic stroma, or they were separated from the basal lamina only by other proliferating trophoblast cells. On the other hand, those extravillous trophoblast cells located far from the basal lamina no longer proliferated. They also no longer expressed EGF-R but, rather, c-*erb*B-2. Regarding the expression of extracellular matrix molecules (collagen IV, collagen VI, laminin, heparan sulfate, oncofetal fibronectin), the various stages of differentiation of extravillous trophoblast of all these sites behaved the same (Hearn et al., 1992; Nanaev et al., 1993a,b; Frank et al., 1994) (see below, under Fibrinoid). This report agrees with the findings of Aplin and Campbell (1985) and those of Malak et al. (1993), who described the distribution patterns of various extracellular matrix molecules around the extravillous trophoblast cells of the chorion laeve. Finally, Genbacev et al. (1993b) cultured explants of cell islands and found no differences when comparing them to cell columns. They concluded that cell islands represent free-floating cell columns. All these findings make it likely that extravillous trophoblast of all intraplacental sites represent one homogeneous population of cells that differ only in terms of their stage of differentiation.

This concept suggests the presence of two trophoblast populations: a villous and an extravillous one. This

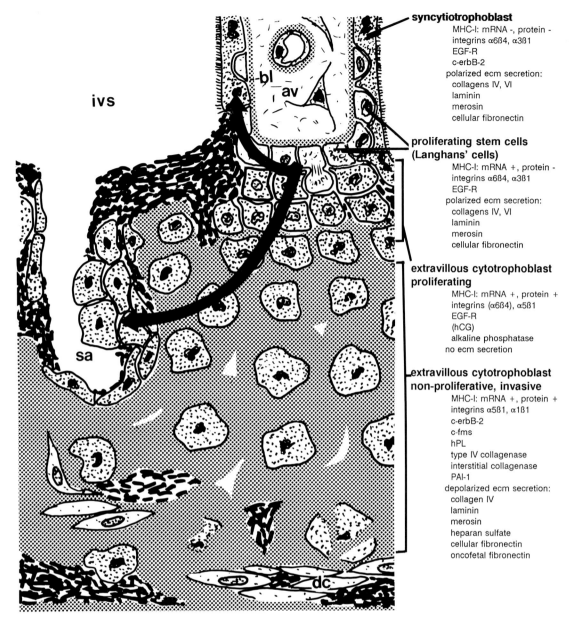

ivs

syncytiotrophoblast
MHC-I: mRNA -, protein -
integrins α6β4, α3β1
EGF-R
c-erbB-2
polarized ecm secretion:
collagens IV, VI
laminin
merosin
cellular fibronectin

**proliferating stem cells
(Langhans' cells)**
MHC-I: mRNA +, protein -
integrins α6β4, α3β1
EGF-R
polarized ecm secretion:
collagens IV, VI
laminin
merosin
cellular fibronectin

**extravillous cytotrophoblast
proliferating**
MHC-I: mRNA +, protein +
integrins (α6β4), α5β1
EGF-R
(hCG)
alkaline phosphatase
no ecm secretion

**extravillous cytotrophoblast
non-proliferative, invasive**
MHC-I: mRNA +, protein +
integrins α5β1, α1β1
c-erbB-2
c-fms
hPL
type IV collagenase
interstitial collagenase
PAI-1
depolarized ecm secretion:
collagen IV
laminin
merosin
heparan sulfate
cellular fibronectin
oncofetal fibronectin

FIGURE 112. Anchoring villus (av) attached to the basal plate (below) by a cell column (center). Proliferation of the trophoblastic stem cells (light) takes place near the basal lamina (bl). It follows either differentiation and fusion to syncytiotrophoblast (above) or differentiation and invasion into the maternofetal junctional zone. The arrows indicate these two routes of differentiation and invasion. The expression patterns of several matrix molecules, integrins, and surface antigens are summarized. ivs = intervillous space; sa = spiral artery; dc = decidual cells; dark point shading = basal laminas and matrix-type fibrinoid; black patches = fibrin-type fibrinoid. For further details see text. Based on findings by Feinberg et al. (1989), Moll and Lane (1990), Castellucci et al. (1991, 1993a), Korhonen et al. (1991), Damsky et al. (1992), Aplin (1993), Mühlhauser et al. (1993), and Frank et al. (1994).

view is supported by the immunohistochemical findings presented by Hsi and coworkers. These authors have raised two monoclonal antibodies, the first directed against villous trophoblast (GB 25) and the other against extravillous trophoblast (GB 36) (Hsi & Yeh, 1986; Hsi et al., 1987).

One Stem Cell Origin for Villous Syncytiotrophoblast and the Extravillous Trophoblast?

The immunohistochemical results obtained by Hsi and coworkers (Hsi & Yeh, 1986; Hsi et al., 1987) with the antibodies GB 25 and GB 36 allow an even more precise definition of the differences between the two populations of cells: GB 25 not only recognizes villous trophoblast in the narrow sense but also those trophoblast cells of the membranes that rest on the basal lamina (i.e., the proliferating subpopulation). GB 36 binds only to those extravillous trophoblast cells that are not polarized (i.e., that have lost contact with the basal lamina of their proliferation zone, e.g., anchoring villi). These findings are supported by another antibody (BC-1), produced by the same investigators, that identifies extravillous trophoblast including the intravascular cells rather than villous trophoblast (Loke et al., 1992a). As can be seen from Figure 1 of their publication, the most proximal layer of polarized, columnar cytotrophoblast that rests on the basal lamina of the anchoring villus remains unstained and behaves like villous cytotrophoblast.

In agreement with views presented by Wakuda and Yoshida (1990), we then come to the following conclusion: The trophoblast cells (Langhans' cells) that rest on the basal lamina of villi, including the columnar part of the anchoring villi, cell island, chorionic plate, and chorion laeve, represent a proliferating population of stem cells (Figure 110). Where they contact villous syncytiotrophoblast, the daughter cells fuse with the syncytium. In all those places where these proliferating stem cells (Langhans' cells) do not join syncytiotrophoblast but, rather, villous or extravillous fibrinoid or extravillous trophoblast, the cells lose polarity as soon as they have lost contact with the basal lamina; they now represent the point of origin of the extravillous pathway of differentiation.

These findings are supported by in situ hybridization studies on class I MHC antigen (Hunt et al., 1990, 1991). These studies also point to the existence of a separate Langhans' cell population and two differentiated trophoblast populations: the villous syncytiotrophoblast and the extravillous trophoblast (see below, Extravillous Trophoblast and Maternofetal Immune Interactions, p. 190).

The concept of Langhans' cells as precursors of both villous syncytiotrophoblast and extravillous trophoblast, requires two special pathways of trophoblast differentiation.

1. Langhans' cells in a villous position, but underlying perivillous fibrinoid should behave like extravillous trophoblast. This hypothesis is obviously true, as may be seen when one observes the large, basophilic trophoblast cells that spread from these fibrinoid deposits. Immunohistochemically, it has been demonstrated that they express the same pattern of extracellular matrix molecules (matrix type fibrinoid) as the extravillous trophoblast cells in other locations

(Frank et al., 1994). Also, in vitro experiments with villous explants show that villous Langhans' cells can achieve an extravillous phenotype, expressing no further syncytial fusion (Castellucci et al., 1990) but, rather, an invasive behavior that includes degradation of the surrounding matrix (Fisher et al., 1985).

2. The proliferating, polarized cells of the cell columns that rest on the basal lamina of the anchoring villi should have two options for differentiation (Figure 112): As soon as they leave the basal lamina without contacting the syncytiotrophoblast they differentiate into extravillous trophoblast. On the other hand, they become incorporated into syncytiotrophoblast when they come into contact with the latter (see Genbacev et al., 1993c). In fact, there are convincing arguments that growth of the stem villi cannot be explained by the low proliferation rate of the dispersed Langhans' cells along their surfaces (Kosanke, 1994). Rather, many or even most of the stem villi extend peripherally into cell columns or cell islands with their highly active trophoblastic growth zones. Stromal tenascin expression in these transitional areas only (Castellucci et al., 1991) suggests migration of some of the postmitotic trophoblast cells into the lateral villous walls. According to this concept, cell columns and cell islands serve as trophoblastic growth zones for the adjacent stem villi.

This explanation leaves open still the question whether the intravascular trophoblast cells represent the final stage of differentiation of this homogeneous population of extravillous trophoblast, as was suggested by Damsky et al. (1992), Fisher and Damsky (1993), and Genbacev et al. (1993c). Another possibility is that they constitute an independent route of extravillous differentiation. Blankenship and colleagues (1993a) have demonstrated proliferating intraarterial trophoblast cells in rhesus monkey placentas that were thought to be a self-replicating population. According to the authors' meticulous studies, these cells seem to enter the arteries via the lumens rather than being derived from columnar trophoblast invading the junctional zone and finally penetrating the arterial walls. The latter route, though, has been confirmed for the minimal trophoblastic invasion of uteroplacental veins (Blankenship et al., 1993b). Lectin-binding studies (Thrower et al., 1991) resulted in different lectin-binding patterns of intravascular and interstitial extravillous trophoblast and is thus supportive of the concept of two separate routes of development.

These findings are in partial contrast to our results in the human placenta (Figure 137). They did not reveal any proliferation of intravascular trophoblast cells; rather, our studies suggested that the intraarterial cells were final stages of invasion of columnar extravillous trophoblast, in agreement with the views presented by Fisher and Damsky (1993) and Genbacev et al. (1993c). One thus must question whether the PCNA antibodies used by Blankenship et al. (1993a,b) are reliable proliferation markers in the placenta (Kohnen et al., 1993).

Invasive Properties of the Extravillous Trophoblast

Implantation, placental development, and adhesion of the placenta to the uterine wall are mediated by invasion of extravillous trophoblast into the endometrium. This process has been studied during implantation (review see Denker, 1990) and in later stages of placentation in vitro (Kliman et al., 1990). The extravillous trophoblast simulates a malignant neoplasm by virtue of penetrating maternal tissues, invading uterine vessels, and embolizing into the maternal circulation. This process shares many aspects with tumor invasion. The principal difference is that, at any stage, this invasion is controlled and time-limited (Kliman & Feinberg, 1990).

According to Liotta and coworkers (1991) invasion of tumor cells involves three main steps: (1) binding of cell surface receptors to matrix molecules such as laminin and fibronectin; (2) activation of proteases and pericellular degradation of extracellular matrix; and (3) migration of the cells into this matrix. Similar events appear to take place during the invasion of extravillous cytotrophoblast (Bischof & Martelli, 1992).

The distribution of *adhesion molecules and their extracellular ligands* in the junctional zone has been studied in detail. Villous cytotrophoblast, as well as villous syncytiotrophoblast, is characterized by the presence of integrins $\alpha6\beta4$ and $\alpha3\beta1$ (Aplin, 1993; Korhonen et al., 1991) (Figure 112). These membranous adhesion molecules play a role in anchoring trophoblast to its basal lamina, integrin $\alpha6\beta4$ probably representing a laminin receptor and $\alpha3\beta1$ being a collagen IV receptor (Damsky et al., 1992). In agreement with our earlier statement that the basal cellular layer of the columnar trophoblast is comparable to villous cytotrophoblast (Langhans' cells), this layer also expresses the identical integrins (Damsky et al., 1992; Aplin, 1993).

As soon as the cells have lost contact with the basal lamina, the expression of these integrins becomes weaker and finally switches to the expression of $\alpha5\beta1$ (Figure 112), a fibronectin receptor, and finally to $\alpha1\beta1$, which binds to fibronectins and collagens (Korhonen et al., 1991; Damsky et al., 1992; Aplin, 1993). This switch in extracellular matrix binding properties has also been supported experimentally (Loke et al., 1989b).

Burrows et al., 1993) and is thought to enable the cells to invade the maternal tissue compartment.

This process is controlled by EGF of probably maternal origin, as local sources for EGF in the junctional zone have not been described so far according to Fisher et al. (1992). This point sheds new light on the already mentioned presence of EGF receptor in the proliferative but still noninvasive subpopulation of extravillous trophoblast cells in the proximal part of the columns.

The extravillous trophoblast cells change their expression patterns of extracellular matrix molecules in parallel with the modification of their adhesion molecules. This change makes sense, as the integrins represent the receptors to which the matrix molecules are bound in order to anchor the cell in its surrounding (Burrows et al., 1993).

Villous cytotrophoblast and the basal layer of the columnar trophoblast secrete laminin, collagen IV (Castellucci et al., 1993; Frank et al., 1994), and possibly merosin (Damsky et al., 1992), a laminin-related protein (Ehrig et al., 1990). The secretion occurs in a polarized manner toward the villous stroma, thus assembling the basement membrane. In addition, immunoreactivity for collagen VI and cellular fibronectin is found along the base of these cells (Frank et al., 1994) (Figure 112).

As soon as the cells lose contact with the basal lamina, but while still proliferating, they stop expressing these molecules for two or three cell cycles. Thereafter a nonpolarized secretion commences that embeds the cells in increasing amounts of extracellular matrix (matrix-type fibrinoid) (Frank et al., 1994) (Figure 112). This new secretory pattern comprises merosin (Leivo et al., 1989), collagen IV, laminin, and cellular fibronectin; and it no longer contains collagen VI. As new trophoblastic secretory products, heparan sulfate, oncofetal fibronectin (Borsi et al., 1987), and a special oncofetal fibronectin subtype, the trophouteronectin, may be detected in this matrix as a specific marker (Feinberg et al., 1991b; Castellucci et al., 1993; Feinberg & Kliman, 1993; Frank et al., 1994). Sunderland and coworkers (1985) found evidence that hyaluronic acid is also among the matrix molecules of this region. There are immunohistochemical suggestions that the facts cited above are also valid for the intravascular trophoblast (Earl et al., 1990). The possible importance of oncofetal fibronectins for trophoblastic invasion as well as the regulation of their expression have been discussed by Feinberg and Kliman (1993).

As previously stated, invasive processes are dependent on the production of *proteolytic enzymes and their activators and inhibitors* to degrade the surrounding extracellular matrix during the course of invasion (Bischof & Martelli, 1992). The balance in secretion of these substances is modified as soon as cells become invasive. As soon as the trophoblast cells leave the proliferation zone and achieve an invasive phenotype, they begin to secrete matrix metalloproteinases, which are involved in degrading the extracellular matrix. Subclasses of these metalloproteinases described in invasive extravillous trophoblast comprise interstitial collagenase (Moll & Lane, 1990) and type IV collagenase (gelatinase) (Fisher et al., 1989, 1992; Bischof et al., 1991; Librach et al., 1991). Autio-Harmainen et al. (1992) have pointed out that the invasive extravillous cytotrophoblast expresses the 72-kilodalton (kDa) gelatinase A, whereas neither enzyme nor mRNA could be detected in villous cytotrophoblast. Moreover, urokinase-type plasminogen activator has been found in much higher concentration in the invasive extravillous trophoblast cells than in all other types of trophoblast (Hofmann et al., 1994).

These enzymes are inhibited by specific tissue inhibitors (TIMPs) that have been shown to block invasion of extravillous trophoblast in vitro (Librach et al., 1991). In addition, the presence of other proteases, such as dipeptidyl peptidase IV (Gossrau et al., 1987), and of other protease inhibitors, such as plasminogen activator inhibitors 1 (PAI-1) and 2 (PAI-2), have been shown in invasive extravillous trophoblast (Feinberg et al., 1989; Hofmann et al., 1994) and in the surrounding fibrinoid (Kyodo et al., 1986). It is only matrix molecules such as collagen IV and laminin that modulate the expression and activity of metalloproteinases (Emonard et al., 1990); cytokines such as interleukin-1β (Fisher et al., 1992) have shown a stimulating effect.

Extravillous Trophoblast and Maternofetal Immune Interactions

It is generally accepted that trophoblast interposed between maternal blood and villous stroma (villous cyto- and syncytiotrophoblast) does not express class I and class II antigens of the MHC (for review see Loke, 1989). The same is true for at least most of the trophoblast that is deported into the maternal circulation (Iklé, 1964). Only for the intravascular trophoblast, those cells that line the maternal arterial blood vessels, are the expression patterns still uncertain. It has been deduced that the lack of allogeneic recognition molecules in this exposed site (fetal tissues opposed to maternal blood) must play an important role in placental survival (Loke, 1989).

The proliferating extravillous trophoblast cells of the cell columns behave like villous cytotrophoblast and are class I MHC-negative; in contrast, invasive extravillous trophoblast cells express class I MHC but not class II MHC antigens (Butterworth et al., 1985; Shorter et al., 1993).

From the morphological point of view, the situation becomes even more interesting when one compares the class I MHC expression with the distribution of the class I MHC mRNA (Hunt et al., 1990, 1991). Hunt and coworkers were able to divide placental trophoblast into three populations:

1. Villous cytotrophoblast (Langhans' cells) that contain class I mRNA but do not express the class I MHC antigen
2. Villous syncytiotrophoblast that neither contains class I mRNA nor expresses class I MHC antigen
3. Invasive extravillous cytotrophoblast that contains the mRNA message and expresses the class I MHC antigen.

These findings support the view that Langhans' cells (all trophoblast cells resting on villous and extravillous basal laminas) are the proliferating stem cells for both villous syncytiotrophoblast and extravillous cytotrophoblast.

The question of how extravillous trophoblast cells that bear fetal class I MHC antigens can survive in a maternal environment (uterus or extrauterine implantation sites) has caused much speculation (for review see Loke, 1989; Loke & King, 1991). One possible explanation is that the trophoblast expresses an unusual form of class I MHC molecule (Earl et al., 1985; Ellis et al., 1986, 1990; Shorter et al., 1993)—one that is considered to be unlikely to provoke immune responses even at the maternofetal interface. Moreover, it has been shown that the extravillous trophoblast cells do not express surface structures that can be recognized by natural killer cells from the endometrial population of large granular lymphocytes (King et al., 1989, 1990) (see below, Endometrial Large Granular Lymphocytes).

Secretory Activities of Extravillous Cytotrophoblast

Extravillous trophoblast is a rich source of *proteohormones and placental proteins*. Speculations along these lines have a long history. In 1957 Latta and Beber described a special form of extravillous trophoblast, the "transitional stages." They noted that originally chromophobic cells of the cell columns differentiate into chromophilic cells, and they assumed them to have a secretory function and conjectured that the cells may produce hCG, ACTH, or both. As early as 1963 Thiede and Choate studied the extravillous trophoblast immunohistochemically. They found some evidence for hCG synthesis in these cells. Kaufmann and Stark (1973), however, who used immunoautoradiography, could not verify this finding. Some reactivity detected in basal plate macrophages was interpreted as representing phagocytosed hCG, rather than as a sign of synthesis in these cells. Beck (1970) found hPL in the syncytiotrophoblast of an 18-day ovum, whereas it had not made its appearance in a 12-day specimen. Cytotrophoblast did not stain, and the intensity of the staining in the syncytium increased with advancing gestational age.

Beck et al. (1986) studied the localization of the several proteohormones in 64 placentas of varying gestational age. They confirmed the same results concerning hPL as noted above and pointed out that larger amounts of hCG occurred only in the extravillous trophoblast cells of cell islands.

Kurman et al. (1984a,b) provided much new information on the localization of hCG, hPL, and SP1 (pregnancy-specific β_1-glycoprotein) to the various forms of trophoblast. Not only were details provided for term placentas, but the report embraced all stages of placentation. The findings are abbreviated in Table 14. Also, Gosseye and Fox (1984) found that the villous syncytiotrophoblast was the principal source of hCG, hPL, PAPP-A, PP5, and SP1; in the infiltrating extravillous trophoblast, only hPL was present. The intensity of cellular hPL staining increased progressively with deeper penetration of the extravillous trophoblast. According to the findings by Hoshina et al. (1983, 1985) in villous cytotrophoblast this reaction pattern may be an expression of higher cytotrophoblastic differentiation. SP1 and hPL were also detected in some cell populations of trophoblastic tumors (Kurman et al., 1984b; Manivel et al., 1987).

The results concerning hPL and hCG distribution were largely corroborated by other investigators (Sasagawa et al., 1987; Zeng & Fu, 1991), however, Sakbun and coworkers (1990b), who measured mRNA concentrations of hPL, pointed out that villous trophoblast is the major source and that the extravillous

trophoblast adds only minor amounts to total placental hPL production.

Klopper (1980) reviewed the nature and origin of all newly described placental proteins and was skeptical that the precise origin had been proved. Despite the histochemical localization of many proteins to trophoblast, Klopper weighed alternatives that have not always been rigorously excluded.

Studies have now shown that extravillous trophoblast cells also produce substantial quantities of *major basic protein* (MBP), a protein similar to that contained in the granules of eosinophilic granulocytes (Wasmoen et al., 1989, 1991). Eosinophil MBP is highly toxic to parasites as well as to cells (Maddox et al., 1984; Kephart et al., 1988). It was found to circulate in the blood of pregnant women at levels 10 to 20 times higher than in nonpregnant women in the absence of eosinophilia (Maddox et al., 1983), and maternal MBP levels decreased rapidly after delivery. The concentration of this nonglycosylated protein, however, increases significantly before the onset of labor (Wasmoen et al., 1987b).

Immunofluorescence studies and extraction of placentas, particularly of cyst fluid, showed MBP to be derived from the extravillous trophoblast cells in the placenta (Maddox et al., 1984). The protein was found as early as the 6th week of pregnancy and was confined to trophoblast cells in anchoring villi, septa, basal plate, and "placental site giant cells" (Figure 113). No staining was observed in villous Langhans' cells, syncytium, or the "fibrinoid" of the placenta; decidual cells did not stain with these specific antibodies. The trophoblast of ectopic pregnancies and hydatidiform moles stained positively, whereas only one of two choriocarcinomas stained weakly. Immunohistochemistry showed the protein to be present in small granules (Figure 114) and to be packaged in membranes. These granules may be

TABLE 14. Approximate localization of placental proteins in various trophoblastic cells as identified by immunocytochemistry.

Trophoblast type	First trimester			Second trimester			Third trimester		
	hCG	hPL	SP1	hCG	hPL	SP1	hCG	hPL	SP1
Cytotrophoblast	−	−	−	−	−	−	−	−	−
X cells (intermediate)	+	+	±	±	+	+	−	+	±
Syncytiotrophoblast	+	+	+	+	+	+	+	+	+
Syncytial giant cells	+	+	±	−	+	±	−	+	±
Syncytial knots	+	+	+	+	+	+	+	+	+
Placental site trophoblast	±	+	±	−	+	±	−	+	±
Membranous trophoblast		+	+	−	+	+	−	+	±
Intravascular trophoblast	−	+	±	−	+	±	−	+	±

Modified from Kurman et al. (1984a).
hCG = human chorionic gonadotropin; hPL = human placental lactogen; SP1 = pregnancy-specific β_1-glycoprotein.

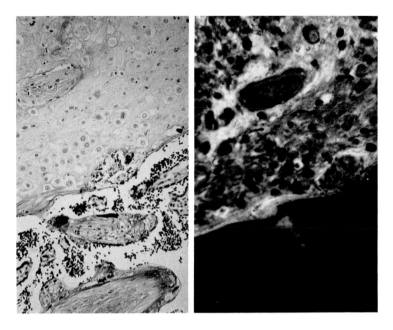

FIGURE 113. Intercotyledonary septum with extravillous trophoblast cells above. There is immunofluorescent localization of MBP between septal extravillous trophoblast cells but not in chorionic villi (below). Left: H&E. ×100. Right: Antieosinophil granule MBP stain. ×100. (Courtesy Dr. G. J. Gleich, Mayo Clinic, Rochester, Minnesota.)

the same ones that were detected by Dallenbach-Hellweg and Nette (1964) in placental site cells by cytochemistry and that were also observed by Steininger (1978). These investigators had already suggested a secretory activity of X cells.

Physicochemical comparison between the MBP from placentas and eosinophils showed only minor differences; the placental MBP was found to be more polymerized or bound to a carrier protein than was the MBP from eosinophils (Wasmoen et al., 1985). Indeed, the MBP derived from the placenta is indistinguishable from that contained in eosinophilic granulocytes (Wasmoen et al., 1988). MBP was also found in a wide variety of nonhuman primate placentas, but it was

absent from those of tamarins and lemurs (Wasmoen et al., 1987a).

The initial results of these studies suggested that the presence of an abundant amount of MBP in the invasive trophoblast may relate to the infiltrative function of trophoblast. This idea was thought plausible because MBP had previously been found to be toxic to cells. Such a role is made less likely, however, by the finding that the levels of this protein increase until the end of pregnancy, long beyond an invasive quality of trophoblast is exhibited. Also, when reviewing all of the functions of eosinophils and their proteins, Weller and Götzl (1980) concluded that "a causal relationship of the infiltrating eosinophils to the tissue damage has not

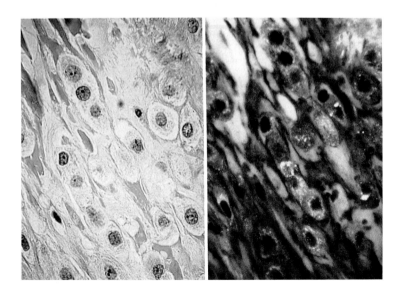

FIGURE 114. Placental septum composed of extravillous trophoblast cells. Note the intense immunofluorescence among and between cells. Left: H&E. ×400. Right: Antieosinophil granule MBP stain. ×400. (Courtesy Dr. G. J. Gleich, Mayo Clinic, Rochester, Minnesota.)

been established." Moreover, no placental MBP was found in Callithrichidae (tamarins) with a hemochorial placenta; the great phylogenetic distance of tamarins from other simians may be reflected by the absence of MBP from their eosinophils. It may thus be premature to engage in speculations until more is known about the physiology of this protein. Lemurs, having an epithelio-chorial placenta, as expected, had no MBP in their placentas. For a complete consideration of all functions of eosinophils, their granules, and related phenomena, the reader is referred to the review by Gleich and Adolphson (1986).

As early as 1973 Ermocilla and Altshuler speculated that extravillous trophoblast cells may suppress labor. Products of the cells that have been discussed more recently to be involved in *control of labor*, comprise 15-hydroxyprostaglandin dehydrogenase (type I-PGDH), pregnancy-associated prostaglandin synthetase inhibitor (PAPSI), and corticotropin-releasing hormone. Type I-PGDH was found not only in villous syncytiotropho-blast but also in invasive extravillous trophoblast (Cheung et al., 1990, 1992), where it is ideally localized to metabolize and maintain low concentrations of prostaglandins, in particular in close vicinity of the myometrium.

The PAPSI was detected in amnionic epithelium, villous macrophages, and extravillous trophoblast throughout pregnancy (Mortimer et al., 1989). Its importance for the maintenance of pregnancy and for the control of the onset of parturition is discussed by the authors.

Corticotropin-releasing hormone has been described to be present not only in villous cytotrophoblast (Petraglia et al., 1987; Saijonmaa et al., 1988) but in extravillous trophoblast as well (Riley et al., 1991). The authors suggested that this releasing hormone locally affects paracrine–autocrine interactions, and that it may be involved in the maturation of the fetal hypothalamic-pituitary-adrenal axis. Finally, its stimula-tory effects on labor are under discussion.

Placental Site Giant Cells

Another cell that plays an important role in the litera-ture on placental pathology is the placental site giant cell (Figures 115, 116). These cells are of great diag-nostic value for the histopathologist studying curettings. Their fetal/trophoblastic origin was proved by Khudr et al. (1973), but it remains an open question whether these cells are mononuclear (as extravillous cytotro-phoblast) or, in part at least, multinucleated cells (Pijnenborg et al., 1980). They thus overlap with the large group of multinucleated masses present in the junctional zone, primarily during the early stages of pregnancy. They are then often called the

chorionic giant cells, wandering cells, migratory cells, or megalokaryocytes (for review see Boyd & Hamilton, 1970).

Sauramo (1961) had characterized these cells, from histological and histochemical studies, as cell popu-lations that undergo frequent degeneration and that form, within the extraplacental membranes and placental floor, a separate compartment of cytotropho-blast. Bühler (1964) reviewed them extensively in a study of the margin of the placenta. He concluded that they represent decidua, despite the fact that the cells have a morphology different from that of typical decidual elements.

Typical placental site giant cells are often vacuolated (Figure 117), and they sometimes appear degenerative. These cells may be construed as being intermediate to cyst formation, which so often takes place in large accumulations of extravillous trophoblast cells (Figure 145). They may also be identical with what Yeh et al. (1989) described as a separate trophoblastic entity, the vacuolated cytotrophoblast. Thliveris and Speroff (1977) found an increased amount of fibrinoid deposition around these cells in membranes from preeclamptic women. Wynn (1967a) also noted their frequent, or regular, association with eosinophilic fibrin-like deposits.

Aside from presenting excellent illustrative material, Robertson and Warner (1974) reviewed the opinions concerning the ultimate origin of the placental site giant cells, cells that had long been known as being charac-teristic for the implantation site. Despite this know-ledge, pathologists are generally reluctant to make the diagnosis of intrauterine pregnancy merely from the presence of extravillous trophoblast cells (X cells) and in the absence of villi. To satisfy this demand for characterization of the placental site, O'Connor and Kurman (1988a,b) used the presence of hPL contained within placental site cells and thus demonstrated in relevant cases that an intrauterine gestation existed in curettings when an ectopic gestation needed to be ruled out.

In our opinion, placental site giant cells are highly differentiated, possibly already degenerative extra-villous trophoblast cells. This view is further supported by several publications dealing with the placental site trophoblastic tumor (PSTT) (Berger et al., 1984; Young et al., 1988; Duncan & Mazur, 1989; Larsen et al., 1991). This rare variant of trophoblastic disease derives from placental site giant cells and was univocally described to be composed of so-called intermediate tro-phoblast, equivalent to extravillous cytotrophoblast.

Multinucleated Trophoblastic Giant Cells

It is interesting to note that most villous trophoblast is syncytial in nature, whereas the extravillous trophoblast

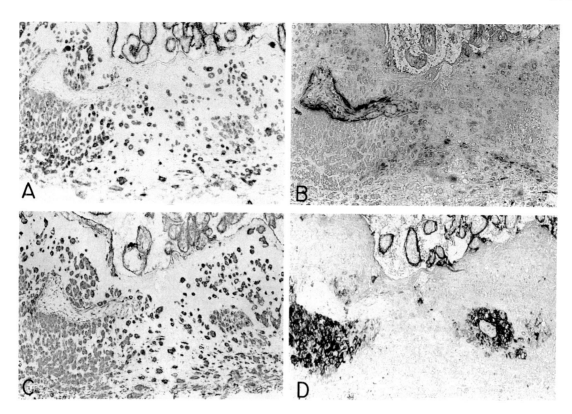

FIGURE 115. Basal plate containing the remains of cell columns deeply buried in the fibrinoid. (A) Isocitrate dehydrogenase. (B) Aminopeptidase. (C) Malate dehydrogenase. (D) Alkaline phosphatase. It becomes evident from this series of pictures that the aminopeptidase (B) stains mostly fetal connective tissue cells, whereas the alkaline phosphatase (D) stains only trophoblast cells derived from the cell columns (proliferating and early invasive stages). The numerous more highly differentiated, invasive (darker) extravillous trophoblast cells visible in the two left pictures no longer express alkaline phosphatase. Serial cryostat sections. ×45. (From Stark & Kaufmann, 1971, with permission.)

is composed mainly of cytotrophoblast. The relative amount of extravillous syncytiotrophoblast decreases toward term. Extravillous syncytiotrophoblast is found in few locations only as largely degenerative syncytial plaques covering the chorionic plate, the basal plate, and sometimes even parts of cell columns, cell islands, and septa. In addition, some syncytial elements can be found in the depth of the basal plate. These elements are usually referred to as multinucleated trophoblastic giant cells.

Attention was first directed to these elements by Kölliker (1861), who called them *Riesenzellen* and *vielkernige Riesenzellen*. Similar multinucleated trophoblastic masses have been described in the junctional zone of several mammals. Terms such as multinuclear giant cells, wandering cells, migratory cells, megalokaryocytes, and diplokaryocytes were employed (for reviews see Mossman, 1937, 1987; Boyd & Hamilton, 1970). Despite the fact that some authors have questioned the fetal origin of these structures (Keiffer, 1928; Park, 1959), there is agreement concerning their trophoblastic nature based on their immunoreactivity for cytokeratin.

Several investigators have described their derivation as arising by outward migration of the early syncytiotrophoblast ("syncytial streamers") (Boyd & Hamilton, 1960). In the guinea pig placenta, Uhlendorf and Kaufmann (1979), who used serial sections, were able to trace such "giant cells" from the placental syncytiotrophoblast peripherally via the junctional zone to the myometrium. Although most of these syncytial streamers had lost their connection to the placenta, some were still in continuity with it and formed rootlike extensions. For further details we refer to the beautifully illustrated reports and reviews by Boyd and Hamilton (1970) and Pijnenborg and coworkers (1980, 1981).

The relative reduction of multinucleated trophoblastic giant cells in the basal plate throughout gestation makes it unlikely that syncytial fusion of extravillous trophoblast to form these syncytial elements plays a major role during the later stages of pregnancy. Rather,

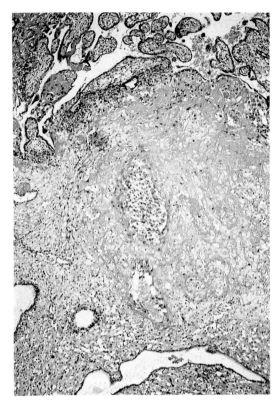

FIGURE 116. Basal plate of mature placenta. Above is the intervillous space: The decidua is covered with Rohr's fibrin stria and placental site giant cells; basophilic extravillous trophoblast cells are diffusely scattered throughout the paler decidual cells. Atrophied glandular spaces and small maternal vessels are also present. H&E. ×100.

it can be speculated that most are nonfunctional remains of the implantation period that no longer grow but gradually degenerate.

Syncytiogenesis

It is presently impossible to decide clearly whether all of the extravillous multinucleated trophoblastic masses are residues of the invading blastocyst syncytium that persist to term or there is some syncytiogenesis still active outside villi even during later pregnancy. Pijnenborg et al. (1981) favored the latter idea, but convincing proof is difficult to obtain.

This question is of interest as it is evident that, at least in most places, extravillous trophoblast cells do not fuse despite their high degree of differentiation and the presence of immediate intercellular contacts. The same is valid for villous cytotrophoblast. Except during the early stages of implantation, it has never been observed that neighboring villous trophoblast cells fuse syncytially in vivo. Rather, they fuse only with the covering syncytiotrophoblast. Therefore one may question whether cytotrophoblast cells in vivo are able to fuse at all syncytially with each other; rather, they may be able to fuse only with syncytiotrophoblast to increase the mass of the latter.

On the other hand, several investigators who have cultured trophoblast, have described in vitro fusion of the cells (Kliman et al., 1985, 1987; Bierings et al., 1988; Bullen & Bloxam, 1988;

Logothetou Rella et al., 1989; Douglas & King, 1990a; Farmer & Nelson, 1992). Sophisticated techniques have been developed to exclude cells of nontrophoblastic origin (Loke & Day, 1984; Kliman et al., 1985; Loke et al., 1986; Douglas & King, 1989, 1990b, 1993; Shorter et al., 1990) and even to enrich extravillous trophoblast cells (Loke & Burland, 1988; Loke et al., 1989a).

The methods applied during trophoblast isolation, however, did not exclude an admixture of syncytial fragments to the cultures that were retained as impurities during separation of the cytotrophoblast. According to our experience, such fragments are produced during the course of every cytotrophoblast isolation procedure and may be presumed to be the origin of syncytial fusion. In villous explant culture (i.e., composed of villous syncytiotrophoblast with underlying Langhans' cells), syncytial fusion of Langhans' cells with the neighboring syncytiotrophoblast is a common phenomenon (Castellucci et al., 1988, 1990).

In conclusion, one must consider that syncytial fusion of cytotrophoblast with cytotrophoblast may occur only during the first stages of placentation, during implantation. During all later stages of pregnancy, cytotrophoblast fusion with the basal surface of syncytiotrophoblast is a common phenomenon but obviously not with neighboring cytotrophoblast. Sophisticated co-culture systems of cytotrophoblast, with and without syncytiotrophoblast, are necessary to elucidate this problem. It may be one of the key phenomena for our understanding of syncytial fusion.

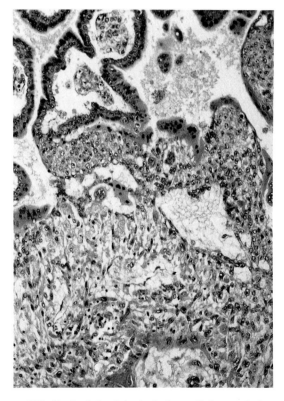

FIGURE 117. Early "physiological change" in a spiral artery (bottom) in the placental floor of a normal 33-day twin pregnancy. Few Nitabuch's and Rohr's fibrin striae are present as yet. Anchoring villi attach with columns, and the intervillous space is lined mostly with syncytium. The basal plate decidua (pale cells) is densely infiltrated with extravillous trophoblast cells, and the arterial wall (bottom) has undergone fibrinoid necrosis. H&E. ×100.

Decidua

The changes that occur in the human endometrium and that of many animals in response to either blastocyst implantation or to an artificial, (i.e. hormonal or mechanical) stimulation are collectively called decidualization. The modified endometrium after implantation is the decidua; that occurring after an artificial stimulus is called a deciduoma.

Vesalius is credited with having first used the term "decidua." John Hunter labeled the structure membrana decidua (Damjanov, 1985), and anyone who has seen a "decidual cast" shed after progesterone withdrawal knows the reason for its being called a membrane.

There is a long history of confusion between decidual cells (i.e., transformed endometrial stromal cells) and X cells. In a doctoral dissertation, Kühler (1890) decided that the placental septa and subchorial cells were decidua. The fact that the "decidua" of the membranes and of the placental floor is composed of an admixture of fetal and maternal cells has often led to erroneous interpretations of research findings. As recently as 1986 Angel and colleagues challenged these findings (inappropriately it might be added), noting that the deductions of Wewer et al. (1985) were perhaps erroneous because of the mixed cell population they studied. This point cannot be made too strongly because over and over again investigators have taken material from the placental floor and the outside the membranes for biochemical study and declared their results to reflect "decidual" activity.

Even more confusion regarding the nomenclature is caused by the fact that only one of the cell types involved in decidualization should properly be called a decidual cell (i.e., the transformed endometrial stromal cell). The endometrial reaction, however, includes not only decidualization of the endometrial stroma but also an accumulation of considerable numbers of bone marrow-derived cells. They comprise macrophages, B and T lymphocytes, eosinophilic granulocytes and considerable numbers of large granular lymphocytes (the former endometrial granular cells, or K cells) (Enders 1991; Khan et al., 1991; Dietl et al., 1992; Haller et al., 1993). Padykula and Driscoll (1978) described the mononuclear infiltration to occur specifically from the, 6th to the 11th week of pregnancy. In addition to lymphocytes and monocytes, they found plasma cells (not necessarily a regular finding, as these elements are generally held to be indicative of chronic infection).

Although decidualization is characteristic of the endometrium, similar changes occur focally over the ovarian surface in the stromal cells and occasionally in peritoneal foci and pelvic lymph nodes. This development of "pseudodecidua" merely betrays the similarity of the tissues, as the müllerian duct is derived from infolding of primitive pelvic peritoneum. Other endometrial responses, such as epithelial plaque reaction and hypertrophy of vascular endothelial cells (Enders, 1991), are not known in humans.

Endometrial Stromal Cells and Decidual Cells

Under the influence of progesterone, the endometrium is changed into decidua, a structurally different tissue. Faint signs of decidualization first become visible on day 23 of the endometrial cycle. They commence around the spiral arteries, from where they spread throughout the tissue. The youngest human implantation stage (Carnegie stage 5a, late day 6 to early day 8 p.c.) (see Chapter 9) does not show decidualization (Enders, 1991), and within the following 2 to 3 days it is barely beginning (Carnegie stage 5b). Electron microscopic studies have not been performed on these early human cases from the first 2 weeks of pregnancy, so the exact commencement of decidualization is difficult to describe.

Decidualization is characterized by the enlargement of endometrial stromal cells, which eventually assume an epithelioid appearance. This process has been described in detail by Kaiser (1960), Schmidt-Matthiesen (1963), Stegner et al. (1971), Dallenbach-Hellweg and Sievers (1975), Iwanaga (1983), and Welsh and Enders (1985). The final result includes cellular hypertrophy and an increase in number and complexity of cytoplasmic organelles, including the rough endoplasmic reticulum and Golgi complexes; it indicates an increase in synthetic and secretory activities. The cells accumulate glycogen and sometimes lipids and large areas with perinuclear bundles of intermediate filaments that are immunohistochemically positive for vimentin. This intermediate filament can be used as an immunohistochemical marker for decidual cells (Figures 20B, 21B, 138C). One to three nuclei per cell become fully euchromatic with prominent nucleoli. The localization of a variety of enzymes in the decidua was summarized by Kearns and Lala (1983) and Lapan and Friedman (1965). Their considerations are beyond the scope of the present discussion.

One of the most characteristic features of the mature decidual cells is the presence of club-shaped processes that extend into the surrounding external fibrillar lamina. The tips of these processes contain dense granular bodies about 0.5 μm diameter (Wynn, 1965; Lawn et al., 1971; Kisalus & Herr, 1988). The base of these processes is histochemically positive for glucose-6-phosphate dehydrogenase (Figure 109) and isocitrate dehydrogenase, the only part of the cell body where these enzymes can be detected in greater activities (Stark & Kaufmann, 1973). The apical granule was identified to contain heparan sulfate proteoglycan, which was also released into the surrounding fibrinoid (Kisalus & Herr, 1988). There it contributes to the acquisition of a pericellular lamina composed of argyrophilic, fibrillar material (Lawn et al., 1971; Wewer et al., 1985, 1988) that also stains with cresyl echt, aldehyde fuchsin, and other dyes (Waidl, 1963) and that resembles the basal lamina of epithelia. According to Kisalus et al. (1987) collagens are also secreted by decidual cells.

Although there have been many ultrastructural studies of rodent decidua, it was not until Wynn (1967b, 1974), Enders (1968), Lawn et al. (1971), and Spornitz & Ludwig (1984) studied this tissue in human uteri that further insight was gained of its structure. Gap junctions were found by several groups (Lawn et al., 1971; Wadsworth et al., 1980; Ono et al., 1989), and it was then discussed whether these structures synchronize decidual development or decidual function.

The epithelial appearance of decidual cells is evident from histological sections (Figures 18K, 19L). The cells have often been described as rounded to polygonal (Kisalus & Herr, 1988; Enders, 1991), but according to our experience this impression is incorrect. When we studied decidual cells in thick plastic sections (20–50 μm) after enzyme-histochemical reactions, we found large, branched cells (Figure 118) that resembled hypertrophied connective tissue cells. The length was 100 to 200 μm. At times they were arranged in elongated nets, the tips of their processes establishing intercellular contacts. Thus the typical epithelioid appearance is the result of cross-sectioning. When studying their structure more carefully, one can identify numerous cross sections that lack nuclei (Figures 18K, 108, 109). These sections are then taken across the slender processes of decidual cells. Also, the typical arrangement of the oval bodies of a group of obliquely sectioned decidual cells shown in Figures 131B and 19L is highly characteristic; it resembles a school of fish. The consequently low number of nuclear profiles, compared to the number of cellular cross sections, is one of the easiest available parameters for distinguishing decidual from trophoblastic cells (Figures 18K, 131B,C).

The structural variability of decidual cells may simply be a question of the sectional plane or of the stage of differentiation. For humans there are no suggestions that different localizations (basal, capsular, parietal decidua) show systematic differences in decidual structure and function in reference to rodents and lagomorphs. There is also no evidence that different types of decidual cells exist in one location (Enders, 1991).

The development of decidual cells was studied by Stark and Kaufmann (1973) with a variety of enzyme reactions. They were careful to differentiate the various cell types and observed numerous changes with advancing differentiation of the cells. Immature decidual cells were characterized by a high content of 17β-hydroxysteroid dehydrogenase, pointing to a particular importance of steroid hormones during this step of differentiation. The elaboration of estrone from precursors by the decidua, as shown in postpartum tissues from placentas by Romano et al. (1986), points into the same direction, even though it suffers from the investigators' inability to distinguish true decidual cells from trophoblastic invaders.

Few factors have been described that regulate decidualization. Progesterone is the most potent stimulator of this differentiation process (see above). Insulin-like growth factor (IGF) is also under discussion in the promotion of decidualization; its binding protein (IGF-BP) is expressed by decidual cells (Bell, 1989; Fazleabas et al., 1989; Rutanen et al., 1991) and appears to be involved in mitosis of endometrial stromal cells and their later differentiation into decidual cells.

It is not only maternal connective tissue cells and their decidualized analogues that are found in the maternofetal junctional zone; fetal connective tissue cells are also present. The latter enter the junctional zone via anchoring villi. Usually they are clearly separated from the other maternal tissues by columnar trophoblast or, if the latter have disappeared, at least by the remainders of its basal lamina (Figure 19I). Sometimes they are difficult to distinguish from

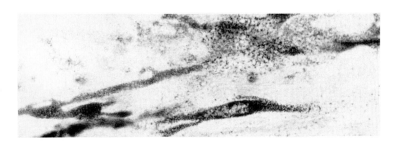

FIGURE 118. A 40-μm plastic section of the basal plate with enzyme histochemical proof of isocitrate dehydrogenase. The positively stained cells are decidua cells. The real structure of the elongated cells with long cytoplasmic extensions is revealed in such thick sections. ×450. (From Stark & Kaufmann, 1973, with permission.)

maternal stromal cells, despite the fact that they never undergo decidualization. Fetal stromal cells show a positive leucine aminopeptidase reaction enzyme-histochemically (Figure 115B), an enzyme that is largely absent from maternal connective tissue cells and its decidual derivatives (Stark & Kaufmann, 1971). High activities of aminopeptidases and various acid hydrolases have also been demonstrated, particularly in term rat decidual cells (Straatsburg & Gossrau, 1993). The authors suggested functions in connection with regression and degradation processes finally contributing to placental separation.

Kearns and Lala (1983) and Lala et al. (1984) deduced from experimenting with chimeric mice that the bone marrow was the "ultimate origin" of the "decidua," a position that is difficult to accept. Most probably only the decidual macrophage and lymphocyte populations stem from the migration of bone marrow elements (see Bulmer et al., 1988a,b,c).

Functional Relevance of Decidual Cells

Numerous studies have been performed concerning the functional importance of the decidua, and many speculations have been entertained. Even the more commonly suggested functions, such as limiting trophoblastic invasion and providing nourishment for the conceptus, still lack adequate supportive evidence (Enders, 1991). Despite this disillusioning statement, we will try to summarize some interesting findings that may stimulate further discussion.

Several publications ascribe *relaxin* secretion to decidual tissue (Bigazzi et al., 1982; Bryant-Greenwood et al., 1987; Hansell et al., 1991). Based on early immunohistochemical findings of Dallenbach and Dallenbach-Hellweg (1964), the endometrial granular cells had originally been favored. However, as their identity as large granular lymphocytes has now been established (see below), relaxin secretory activities are less likely and the probability that decidual cells themselves represent the source is given. The pictures shown by Sakbun et al. (1990a) support this view.

Early publications favored a decidual production of *human placental lactogen* (hPL); however, the decidua was taken from the membranes and placental floor for most of these studies. It was thus likely to be contaminated by extravillous trophoblast. Kurman et al. (1984a) immunostained specifically for hPL and other hormones in the basal plate, villous tissue, and membranes. They found that hPL was the principal product of what they chose to call the "intermediate trophoblast," the extravillous trophoblast cells. Wewer et al. (1986) also stated emphatically that decidua vera and the decidua found in the uterus of patients with ectopic pregnancy is unable to produce hPL.

Another possible explanation for the immunoreactivity of decidual cells for hPL is the fact that hPL and prolactin show considerable homology in their amino acid sequence. Correspondingly, during the early period of immunohistochemistry many antibodies were unsuitable for distinguishing between the two hormones and, as is discussed next, there is now convincing evidence that prolactin is a decidual product.

This proof was obtained not only by *prolactin* immunoreactivity in decidual cells (Golander et al., 1979; Rosenberg et al., 1980; Riddick & Daly, 1982; Andersen et al., 1987; Bryant-Greenwood et al., 1987). In vitro studies with isolated cells or tissues gave the same results (Daly et al., 1983; Fukamatsu et al., 1984; Hamaguchi et al., 1990). On the other hand, there are several reports that prolactin immunoreactivity was found in villous and extravillous trophoblast of the human placenta (Frame et al., 1979; Al Timimi & Fox, 1986). Prolactin immunofluorescence of the amnion (Healy et al., 1977) does not necessarily signify that it is being produced therein, as was inferred. In situ hybridization studies (Wu et al., 1991) indicated with high probability that only decidual cells are involved in the biosynthesis of prolactin; prolactin immunoreactivity found in amnion and trophoblast, as also described above, was likely to be due to receptor-mediated prolactin binding to the latter cells.

It was noted that prolactin production at various stages of pregnancy was closely related to prolactin concentrations in the amnionic fluid and concluded that prolactin is elaborated by decidual cells contained within the membranes and transported internally, a suggestion made by many investigators. Peak prolactin release into the amnionic fluid occurs during the 24th week of pregnancy (Neuberg, 1992).

The most important functions of decidual prolactin comprised regulatory effects on water and electrolyte transfer across the membranes, thereby controlling the fetal water balance: This effect has been observed in vitro when using amnionic fluid prolactin, although it was absent with human pituitary prolactin (de Bakker-Theunissen et al., 1988). Moreover, it was said to affect the synthesis of fetal surfactant and to influence calcium absorption in the fetal gut (for references see Neuberg, 1992).

Many factors have been described as regulators of decidual prolactin production: Intradecidual ion concentrations (potassium or chloride) are likely to control prolactin release (Andersen et al., 1984, 1986), a finding that is a reminder of the prolactin effects on fetoplacentomaternal water and electrolyte balance mentioned above. Not only have receptors for insulin-like growth factor I and for insulin been found on decidual cells, but the respective growth factors/hormones obviously have stimulatory effects on prolactin synthesis (Thrailkill et al., 1989).

Of even greater interest for the functional relations of decidua and trophoblast are the mutual effects of *chorionic gonadotropin* (hCG) and *epidermal growth factor* (EGF) on decidual and trophoblastic cells. The hCG is a secretory product not only of villous but also of extravillous trophoblast (Kurman et al., 1984a). EGF is secreted by villous trophoblast (Hofmann et al., 1992; Ladines Llave et al., 1993; Matsuo et al., 1993), and it may be of maternal origin as well (Fisher et al., 1992). EGF stimulates decidual cell proliferation but inhibits prolactin secretion of decidual cells in culture (Saji et al., 1990). Decidua produces a protein that inhibits hCG release from human trophoblast (Ren & Braunstein, 1991); according to other studies it is likely that prolactin inhibits hCG production (Yuen et al., 1986). On the other hand, not only do the decidual cells express hCG receptors (Reshef et al., 1990), but hCG (Rosenberg & Bhatnagar, 1984) and in particular αhCG (Blithe et al., 1991) stimulate decidual prolactin production in vitro. Moreover, tumor necrosis factor (TNF), a secretory product of decidual cells, inhibits trophoblast cell growth (for review see Briese & Müller, 1992). Finally, according to McWey et al. (1982), decidual cells express hPL receptors and may thus be a target for trophoblastic hPL. These complicated mutual relations illustrate only a small sector of the intimate endocrine and paracrine interactions between decidual cells and the invading extravillous trophoblast.

All these studies provide little evidence concerning the functional activity of the decidua. One must bear in mind that decidualization is not a general phenomenon related to placentation. Rather, it is found only in hemochorial placentation, which unavoidably is related to invasive processes. Consequently, most theories regarding decidual functions see the decidua in the light of trophoblastic invasion; classical descriptions see the decidual cells as being stuffed with glycogen and lipids, which serve as nutrients for the invading trophoblast.

A series of studies focused on the interactions between *decidualization and trophoblastic invasion* (for review see Bell, 1989). During the menstrual cycle, insulin-like growth factor binding protein (IGF-BP) appears to be associated with the stromal fibroblasts (Bell, 1989; Fazleabas et al., 1989; Rutanen et al., 1991). It was proposed that IGF-BP is involved in proliferation and decidualization of these cells. Possibly trophoblast cells stimulate the decidual stroma to produce IGF-BP. Moreover, the RGD tripeptide (Arg-Gly-Asp), which is known to be the recognition site in several adhesive matrix proteins for a range of cell receptors and which is part of the sequence of IGF-BP, has been shown to inhibit tumor cell invasion (Ruoslahti & Pierschbacher, 1987). IGF-BP can therefore be interpreted to be part of a paracrine loop by which the decidual cell and decidualization may

regulate local proliferation and invasion of trophoblast cells (Bell et al., 1988).

An interesting publication deals with the secretion of α_2-macroglobulin by the rat decidua (Gu et al., 1992). This potent protease inhibitor is specifically expressed by the mesometrial decidua, the site of trophoblastic invasion in the rat. Its expression is regulated in an autocrine loop by prolactin (Gu et al., 1992). On the other hand, the α_2-macroglobulin receptor is expressed by extravillous trophoblast cells (Coukos et al., 1994). Both groups of investigators have speculated that this protease inhibitor may limit tissue damage to decidual cells during extratrophoblastic protease secretion and invasion.

In accordance with all these findings, decidualization may be the answer of the endometrium to trophoblastic invasion, regulating the latter and solving problems posed by hemochorial placentation (Bell, 1989).

The increasing interest in the *immunological aspects* of pregnancy has led to numerous theories concerning the decidua. Lala et al. (1985) described an inhibitory effect of decidual cells on lymphocyte proliferation and T cell production. This effect, it is postulated, results in prevention of the production of anti-fetal antibodies (Globerson et al., 1976; Bell, 1983) and in modulation of immune reactions during pregnancy (Bell, 1983). The decidual prostaglandin E_2 (PGE_2) production has also been discussed in context with the immunology of gestation: PGE_2 secretion is said to block activation of maternal leukocytes in the decidua with potential anti-trophoblastic killer function by inhibiting interleukin-2 receptor generation and interleukin-2 production (Parhar et al., 1989).

Prostaglandins E_2 and $F_{2\alpha}$ have also been discussed in another context: During labor the production and release of these cytokines seems to be considerably increased in decidual cells (Khan et al., 1992); the authors discussed the functional relations to labor. The role of PGE_2 is still open, but it may play a role in prepartal ripening of the cervix, whereas $PGF_{2\alpha}$ is essential for the stimulation of uterine muscle during labor (Fuchs & Fuchs, 1984). Casey et al. (1989) proposed that prostaglandin dehydrogenase, resident in the decidua capsularis, regulates levels of prostaglandin therein as well as in amnionic fluid, uterus, and blood. Finally, endothelin-1, a potent vasoconstrictor, and its receptors are expressed in human decidual cells (Kubota et al., 1992). Their function during pregnancy and labor is still open.

Endometrial Large Granular Lymphocytes

The large granular lymphocytes of the endometrium have been described under various names, causing considerable confusion. The classical name is granular cell (*Körnchenzelle*, K cell) (Hamperl, 1954; Hellweg, 1957;

Dallenbach & Dallenbach-Hellweg, 1964; Dallenbach-Hellweg, 1971). Pijnenborg et al. (1980) used the term endometrial granulocyte for this cell type, which appeared to be confined to the endometrium. These cells are equivalent to the metrial gland cells of rodents for which an abundant literature exists (Bulmer & Peel, 1977; Peel & Bulmer, 1977; Bulmer, 1983; Bulmer et al., 1983; Tarachand, 1985, 1986).

Endometrial large granular lymphocytes are regular constituents of all implantation sites (Durst-Zivkovic, 1978). According to Kottsova et al. (1989) their number in the basal plate of normal pregnancies is rather low (0.5–1.0% of all cells of the decidual tissue); however, with severe forms of preeclampsia it increases to 12% (Kottsova et al., 1989). Histologically, they are rounded mononuclear cells of approximately 10 μm diameter with an eccentric, kidney-shaped nucleus. Their typical granular inclusions stain characteristically with phloxine tartrazine (Pijnenborg et al., 1980). During early pregnancy they form small, diffuse or focal infiltrates in the deep decidual layers and neighboring myometrium. They may be particularly impressively localized around the degenerating endometrial glands (Pijnenborg et al., 1980).

There is now general agreement that these cells are derived from the bone marrow (Pijnenborg et al., 1980; Bulmer & Sunderland, 1983; for reviews see Enders, 1991; Spornitz, 1992), rather than from stromal stem cells, as had been assumed by Dallenbach-Hellweg (1971). The cells have been well characterized immunohistochemically (Bulmer & Sunderland, 1984; Ritson & Bulmer, 1989). There has been some discussion whether they represent natural killer cells (Watanabe, 1987; Manaseki & Searle, 1989; King & Loke, 1991; Dietl et al., 1992; Saito et al., 1993; Welsh & Enders, 1993). It now seems to be clear that they belong to a special subgroup of T lymphocytes that can be found among the large granular lymphocytes of the peripheral blood (King & Loke, 1990). Among others, they express the T cell markers CD2 and CD7, but not natural killer cell markers such as CD16 and Leu7. The numbers of cells expressing the various lymphocyte markers change throughout pregnancy (Haller et al., 1993). It remains still to be established, however, whether these changes are of any importance for the mechanisms involved in fetal allograft protection.

Kawagoe (1985) analyzed 85 cases of tubal pregnancies and found that the nidatory site is often, but not always, surrounded by a band of lymphocytes. He discussed their immunological importance at this unusual implantation site (Kawagoe, 1985). As was demonstrated by Sengupta et al. (1990), the granular infiltration of the decidua is not restricted to pregnancy; rather, it was part of the hormone-induced decidual response in ovariectomized rhesus monkeys. Moreover,

Bulmer et al. (1988a) concluded from their studies on decidua in molar pregnancy and on choriocarcinomas that these cells are associated with the hormonal conditions of decidualization rather than with trophoblastic invasion. Correspondingly, they are also present in late proliferative and secretory endometrium (Bogaert, 1975) where they also may undergo mitosis (Pace et al., 1989).

Sengel and Stöbner (1972) gave a detailed ultrastructural account of these cells. They suggested that the K cells are involutive relaxin-secreting cells and that the actively relaxin-producing cells may have some different morphological features. In 1964 Dallenbach and Dallenbach-Hellweg showed that basal trophoblast and the granules of *Körnchenzellen* stained positively for relaxin immunoreactivity. They therefore inferred that granular cells produce relaxin. Trophoblast and decidual tissue are still considered the major sources for relaxin secretion during pregnancy (Bryant-Greenwood et al., 1987; Sakbun et al., 1990a). There are, however, no clear indications that the endometrial large granular lymphocytes contribute to this secretion. Rather, placental relaxin is likely to be synthesized by decidual and trophoblastic cells (Hansell et al., 1991). The same is true for the secretion of GM-CSF, a potent stimulator of myelopoiesis and trophoblastic growth; some findings point to secretion by the granular cells (Kanzaki et al., 1991), but most authors favor a decidual and trophoblastic origin (Duan, 1990; Shorter et al., 1992). Other definitive suggestions for a functional importance of these cells are still lacking (King & Loke, 1990).

Macrophages

Macrophages are regular constituents of each implantation site and later of the maternofetal junctional zone. They can be specifically stained by the monoclonal antibody anti-leu-M-3 (Bulmer & Johnson, 1984), which detects the CD14 monocyte differentiation antigen (see Chapter 7). They seem to represent a largely homogeneous population throughout all stages of pregnancy even though they are structurally heterogeneous (Bulmer et al., 1988b). Their role in maternofetal interactions has been discussed by Hunt (1990).

G Cells

Another cell found in the junctional zone, the G cell, has been described by Gladwell et al. (1974) as originating from the decidua. It is found when the portion of membrane that overlies the internal cervical os is sampled by amnioscopy. The cell has a huge polyploid, hyperchromatic nucleus. Its precise origin and nature are as yet undefined, although the relation to prostaglandin secretion and similarity to cells described by Gustavii (1975) have been considered. Sachs (1968) studied the ploidy of decidua cytophotometrically. He found that its cells were largely diploid in villus-free areas, and that octoploidy and polyploidy were common in the basal plate and in Arias-Stella cells. The G cells probably come from these areas. We were unable to find additional information regarding identity, derivation, or function of this cell in the recent literature. It cannot be excluded that the G cell represents a subpopulation of some other cell population described above.

Glandular Residues

During decidualization, the endometrial glands initially also enlarge, and they are often observed deep in the decidua of first trimester specimens (Figure 18M). Their epithelium actively secretes material that is discharged into the lumen ("uterine milk"). When pregnancy ensues, the epithelial cell nuclei undergo endomitosis, become polyploid, and acquire the feature known as the Arias-Stella (1973) change. Ultimately the glands atrophy, although remains can still be found in the basal plate and the placental bed. Due to the atypical structures of these residues they can usually be identified only by staining with immunohistochemical epithelial markers, such as cytokeratin (Bulmer et al., 1986) (see Chapter 4). Their regressive nature during these stages of pregnancy is also underlined by the absence of immunoreactivity of EGF (Hofmann et al., 1991).

Extracellular Matrix

Extracellular fibrillar material is characteristic of the decidual reaction. It is rich in laminin, type IV collagen, heparan sulfate proteoglycan, and fibronectin (Wewer et al., 1985). Decidual cells are embedded in a network of types I and III collagen, which is produced by the stromal cells. Type IV collagen and laminin surround the differentiated cells. Type V collagen and fibronectin are present throughout the extracellular matrix. Antibodies directed against osteonectin have shown that the surface of mature decidual cells stain heavily with this antibody and that young cells have this protein in their cytoplasm (Wewer et al., 1986). Based on their study of the invasion of the basal plate by trophoblast, Badarau et al. (1971) decided that the process of "fibrinoid necrosis" erects a barrier to further invasion.

Wewer et al. (1985) provided specific evidence that the extracellular matrix of the decidua is secreted by the decidual stromal cells and not by extravillous trophoblast cells. This concept, however, has been challenged by Angel et al. (1986). Study of their photographs suggests that the quality of cellular secretion of these proteins changes with advancing gestation but also that the

localization of basement membrane components is specific. In an even more detailed study of this secretory activity, Kisalus et al. (1987) showed club-shaped processes and secretory bodies on the cellular surfaces containing heparan sulfate that were exocytosed in a merocrine secretory fashion. From our own data we conclude that the extracellular matrix surrounding decidual cells in many places is similar in ultrastructure and in immunohistochemical composition to the extracellular matrix between extravillous trophoblast cells, the matrix-type fibrinoid (see Fibrinoid). Both seem to represent accumulated, modified basal lamina material that is secreted in an unpolarized fashion (Frank et al., 1994).

Decidual Degeneration

Degenerative changes and hemorrhages are frequent features of the decidua in the basal plate and the membranes. The "slowly progressive necrosis" of the decidua capsularis was believed to be the result of progressively decreasing vascularization (Grosser, 1927). The more likely explanation is endocrinological. One may presume that reduced concentrations of those steroid hormones that induced decidualization occur locally. It may be so because with increasing distance from the placenta decidual degeneration increases (Dallenbach-Hellweg & Sievers, 1975). This view has been supported by the findings of Welsh and Enders (1985), who found decidual involution at the mesometrial side of rodent uteri, opposite the placental site.

Hematomas of the basal plate were often considered to involve "histiotrophic substances." Grosser even suggested that such hemorrhages may be dangerous to the developing ovum, an aspect that has become important in medicolegal considerations. Decidual hemorrhages and necrosis have been linked to potential adverse effects on embryonic development. Ornoy et al. (1976) found an increase in severe congenital anomalies when prenatal bleeding had occurred, whereas Mau and Netter (1974), in their paired prospective analysis of 5,257 pregnancies, found no statistical difference of anomalies occurring in infants of mothers who bled and those who did not. Rutherford (1942) had suggested that prenatal bleeding was an ominous feature, an opinion that paved the way for future experimental decidual support with hormone "replacement." Javert (1955), who observed that expansion of the placenta lends itself to decidual bleeding, found administration of vitamin C to be helpful. It is perhaps of parenthetical interest to some readers that this author depicted a term placental basal plate in which the insertion of toothpicks delineates the orifices of maternal vessels.

Different conclusions were reached with respect to the occurrence of decidual necrosis by McCombs and Craig (1964). They reviewed the basal plates of 34 uteri from therapeutic hysterectomies and found decidual necrosis in 81%; in 52% the necrosis was present at some distance from the implantation site. They regarded it to be a normal phenomenon, which is also our opinion. At early implantation sites hemorrhages of the decidua are normal, although it may be a different matter when they become clinically evident by vaginal bleeding. The latter may be a sign of "decidual angiomatosis," according to Bittencourt and Sadigursky (1977). Their finding, however, may merely represent exaggerated dilatation of basal plate vessels with thrombosis. The regular finding of "fibrinoid necrosis" in the basal plate and its relation to the invading trophoblastic columns suggested to Badarau et al. (1971) that it becomes a barrier to further invasion, and that it is a normal phenomenon.

In the delivered placenta, one often finds small retromembranous hematomas. They appear as patches of adherent brown-yellow clot, which when they are old look as though they are comprised of fibrous tissue (Figure 119). Occasionally, this situation ensues after amniocentesis (Figure 120). Moreover, when an intrauterine device (IUD) remains in place during pregnancy, it is frequently locally associated with old hemorrhages (Figures 11, 12). These IUDs also lead to frequent placental "wandering" (trophotropism) with marginal or velamentous insertions of the umbilical cord.

Massive hemorrhage during early pregnancy was once reported to break into the amnionic sac, producing a sonographically apparent umbilical cord mass (Witter & Sanders, 1986). Retromembranous bleeding from "venous lakes" has also been described to occur,

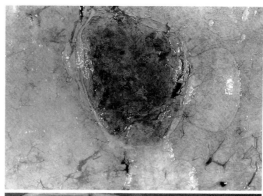

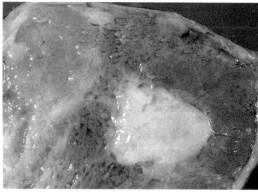

FIGURE 119. Localized retromembranous hematomas in an uncomplicated pregnancy. (Top) Note the brown patch of old blood in the decidua capsularis. (Bottom) There is an old, white retromembranous hematoma in an otherwise uncomplicated pregnancy at term. ×3.

according to Pozniak et al. (1988), following chorionic villous sampling. They found venous lakes to be uncommon in first trimester uteri and cautioned that they must be avoided in chorionic villous sampling (CVS).

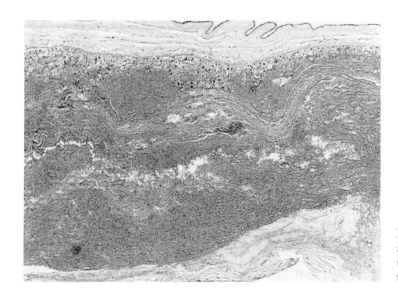

FIGURE 120. Retromembranous hematoma 4 weeks after amniocentesis. Note the vacuolated trophoblast underneath the chorion and the degenerating clot in the dead decidua capsularis (arrows). H&E. ×64.

Fibrinoid

Fibrinoid has always played a remarkable role in the literature of placental pathology. It is one of the most prominent substances when studying the placenta microscopically or even in its macroscopic parameters. Fibrin is prominently involved in pathological processes, such as intervillous thrombosis and placental infarction, its quantity steadily increasing throughout pregnancy. Although the pathogenetic mechanism and diagnostic value of fibrinoid are still under discussion, it is one of the most frequently mentioned "histopathological" findings and is therefore worthy of discussion in a special section.

Hörmann (1965) and Kretschmann (1967a,b) described fibrinoid as a "constructive principle" of the placenta, thus pointing to the view that it is not only a result of pathological events but a regular constituent of normal placentas as well. Many authors have discussed fibrinoid in the context of placental pathology and suggested its presence to be an indicator for pathological events. For example, it has been proposed that the intraplacental amount of fibrinoid correlates positively with the degree of atmospheric pollution (Bonashevskaia et al., 1985). Fox (1967a) made a thoughtful study of 715 placentas to determine if perivillous fibrin differed in quantity in placentas from preeclamptic gestations. He concluded that they contained less of the substance than did normal mature placentas. He thought that fibrin deposits are the result of eddies in turbulent flow. The more flow there is, he concluded, the more fibrin is deposited. Later he inferred that fibrin deposition results from previous immune interactions between mother and fetus (Fox, 1968). Fibrinoid may serve as a mechanically stabilizing factor in the placenta (Kaufmann, 1981b), as well as an immunological barrier, preventing fetus and placenta from maternal immunological attack (Kirby et al., 1964).

Definition of Fibrinoid

In paraffin sections of normal and pathological placentas of all stages of development, one finds a homogeneous material that preferably binds acid stains such as eosin (Figures 19C,F,H,I). This material was first described by Langhans (1877) at the intervillous surface of the chorionic plate, as a layer of "canalized fibrin." Soon thereafter Neumann (1880) introduced the term fibrinoid for a similar substance that was found in the blood vessel wall of atherosclerosis and had a certain resemblance to fibrin. In the placenta the term fibrinoid was not used until Hitschmann and Lindenthal (1903) proposed it when describing the "white infarcts." Fox

(1963) rejected the term white infarct, which had been in use since Rohr (1889) first described it.

The first attempt to clearly differentiate between "fibrin" and "fibrinoid" and to define the latter was made by Grosser (1925). He proposed that the name fibrin be used only for the precipitates of fibrinogen in blood and tissue fluids. The products of nonfibrous, noncellular, more or less homogeneous products in the placenta, possibly derived from heterogeneous sources such as cellular secretion, cellular degeneration, and blood clotting, were to be described as being fibrin-like (i.e., fibrinoid).

Local variations in the light microscopic structural appearance and staining behavior caused considerable discussion as to the homogeneity of fibrinoid. It also led to speculations whether fibrinoid is related to, or even identical with, fibrin (Kirby et al., 1964; Wynn, 1967a; Moe, 1969a,b,c,d; Robertson & Warner, 1974; Tekelioglu-Uysal et al., 1975). Because of conflicting results derived from different regions of the placenta and depending on the author, the material is sometimes called fibrin and sometimes fibrinoid. As a compromise, Wynn (1975) proposed that the term fibrinoid be used in all cases in which the exclusive derivation as a blood clotting product cannot be ascertained. Meanwhile, biochemical studies (Sutcliffe et al., 1982) and immunohistochemical studies (Frank et al., 1994; Lang et al., 1994) have contributed considerably to our knowledge of fibrinoid. The latter studies ascertained that there are two types of fibrinoid: a fibrin-type fibrinoid that is regarded to be a blood clot product, and a matrix-type fibrinoid that is a secretory product of extravillous trophoblast cells (Figures 121A,B). Because both substances are usually deposited close together and cannot easily be discriminated with every histological stain, we propose the more general term fibrinoid as appropriate for placental histology. The general use of the term fibrin is no longer justified.

There are no problems with the identification of fibrinoid. Intraplacental material of solid consistency and not composed of cells, syncytium, or connective tissue that shows special affinity to acid stains represents fibrinoid. Its light microscopic appearance changes from glossy and homogeneous to lamellar, fibrous, or reticular. In paraffin sections stained with hematoxylin and eosin, and depending on localization and staining conditions, the color of fibrinoid varies from slightly pink to intense red. When Mallory's connective tissue technique is used, the color is (ideally) a light blue but may vary from dark blue to lilac or even red. Using the PAF-Halmi stain, the orange staining fibrin-type fibrinoid can easily be differentiated from the blue-green staining matrix-type fibrinoid (Lang et al., 1994).

The following typical localizations of fibrinoid have been described:

1. Fibrinoid at the intervillous surface of the chorionic plate (subchorial fibrinoid, Langhans' stria) (Figures 127A,B)
2. Perivillous fibrinoid (Figure 19H)
3. Intravillous fibrinoid (Figure 19F)
4. Fibrinoid deposits in placental septa and cell islands (Figures 18G, 19J,K, 148A,B)
5. Superficial fibrinoid of the basal plate, facing the intervillous space (Rohr's stria) (Figures 19I, 131B)
6. Uteroplacental fibrinoid in the depth of the basal plate, where maternal and fetal cells come in close contact with each other (Nitabuch's stria) (Figures 19L, 131B)
7. Intramural fibrinoid of uteroplacental arteries and veins (Figure 18L)
8. Fibrinoid in the smooth chorion related to the obstructed intervillous space (Figure 169)

Unfortunately, most detailed histochemical, biochemical, immunohistochemical, and experimental studies have been performed at only one of these sites of fibrinoid localization. This selection may explain the considerable discrepancies concerning composition, proposed derivation, and functional interpretation. However, when comparing fibrinoid deposits from the various sites by means of immunohistochemistry (Frank et al., 1994) and lectin histochemistry (Lang et al., 1994) it is evident that fibrinoid from all these sites is directly comparable, the only differences being based on varying mixing rates of both components, the fibrin- and matrix-type fibrinoid.

Types of Fibrinoid

Throughout all stages of placental development and in all placental sites studied, two types of fibrinoid are apparent. Depending on their composition they are designated here as fibrin-type fibrinoid and matrix-type fibrinoid (Frank et al., 1994).

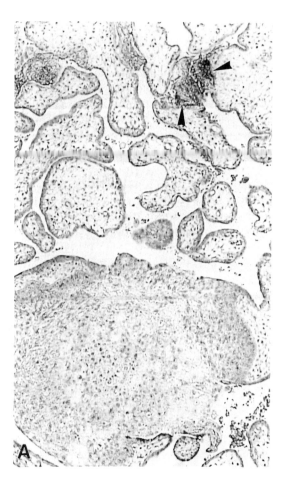
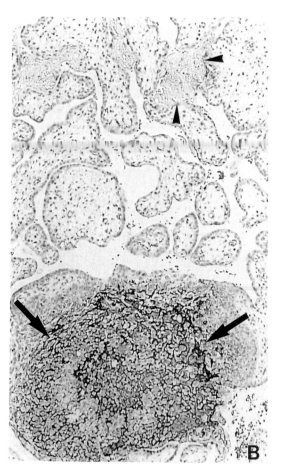

FIGURE 121. Placental villi and a cell island (below), 16th week p.m. (A) Stained with an antibody that detects fibrin but not fibrinogen; fibrin-type fibrinoid in a perivillous position is specifically stained (arrowheads) but not the matrix-type fibrinoid of the cell island. (B) Stained with an antibody directed against oncofetal fibronectin; this matrix molecule can be found specifically in matrix-type fibrinoid that encases the extravillous trophoblast cells of the cell island (arrows) but not in fibrin-type fibrinoid (arrowheads). Serial cryostat sections. ×50. (Courtesy Dr. Hans-Georg Frank, Aachen.)

Fibrin-type fibrinoid was characterized ultrastructurally by the presence of a dense meshwork of fibers measuring less than 10 nm in thickness, with the characteristic cross striation of fibrin filaments with an approximately 20 nm periodicity (Figures 122A,B). It never contains extravillous trophoblast cells. Immunohistochemically, it shows intense reactivity with fibrin antibodies (Figures 21C, 121A) that do not cross-react with fibrinogen (e.g., Immunotech fibrin antibody clone E8, directed against the β-peptide) (Hui et al., 1983). Moreover, the complete absence of matrix molecules, such as oncofetal fibronectin (antibody BC-1), collagen IV, collagen VI, laminin, and tenascin, is typical. For further details see Frank et al. (1994). Furthermore, fibrin-type fibrinoid can be characterized by binding *Ulex europaeus* lectin (UEA-I), indicating a reaction with encased and disintegrated remnants of endothelial and blood cells that usually bind this lectin (Lang et al., 1994); *Bandeiraea simplicifolia* lectin (BS-I) and *Lycopersicon esculentum* lectin (LEA) do not stain this type of fibrinoid.

Numerous other substances have been described to be present in fibrinoid. As far as we were able to interpret the findings that were not specified by parallel application of a fibrin-specific antibody, the following notes that likely to be valid for fibrin-type fibrinoid: Depending on the site of its deposition, various amounts of hyaluronic acid and sialic acid were found (Bradbury et al., 1965; Bagshawe & Lawler, 1975). Other authors have described the presence of immunoglobulins (IgG, IgA, IgM), complement C3 (Gille et al., 1974; Faulk et al., 1975), and albumins (Brzosko et al., 1965a,b; Moe, 1969a,b,d).

Matrix-type fibrinoid was regularly characterized by the presence of single or clustered trophoblast cells (Figures 148A,B), surrounded by a matrix that differs from the fibrin-type fibrinoid. It never stains with fibrin antibodies that do not cross-react with fibrinogen (Figure 121A; see above). Immunohistochemically, it contains only traces of fibrinogen. The most characteristic finding for matrix-type fibrinoid is its immunoreactivity for oncofetal fibronectin (antibody BC-1) (Figures 21D, 121B), which does not react with any other normal structure in the placenta (Frank et al., 1994). The presence of oncofetal fibronectin in the surroundings of extravillous trophoblast cells has been reported before (Feinberg et al., 1991b; Feinberg & Kliman, 1993); additionally, the basal lamina molecules collagen IV and laminin can be found only in this type of fibrinoid, usually showing a patchy pattern. When studying trophoblastic cell columns, Castellucci et al. (1993a) described the secretion of heparan sulfate proteoglycan by the distally located, more invasive cells into the surrounding extracellular matrix that, according to our findings, represents matrix-type fibrinoid.

Also, matrix-type fibrinoid is electron microscopically more or less devoid of fibrin fibers but contains a large variety of granular, fibrous, homogeneous materials (Figure 123). In preliminary communications Nanaev et al. (1993a,b) have also described the presence of matrix molecules in perivillous fibrin(oid) in addition to fibrin. These authors did not differentiate two types of fibrinoid, nor were they able to detect laminin. The immunohistochemical findings of Aplin and Campbell (1985) and those of Malak et al. (1993) show an accumulation of basal lamina molecules around extravillous trophoblast cells that represent what we call matrix-type fibrinoid, even though it is not explicitly attributed to (matrix-type) fibrinoid. According to the lectin-binding studies of Lang et al. (1994), matrix-type fibrinoid is further characterized by the presence of binding with LEA and BS-I, whereas UEA-I does not bind.

The quantitative proportion of matrix- and fibrin-type fibrinoids varies typically between the different locations. Chorionic plate (Langhans' stria) together with initial segments of large stem villi and deep parts of the basal plate (Nitabuch's fibrinoid) and cell islands are typical examples of a mixed composition. The thin perivillous fibrin sheets directly resting on the stromal core of most stem villi at term represent largely only fibrin-type fibrinoid. Almost pure deposits of matrix-type fibrinoid can be found in the centers of cell islands (Krönicher, 1975; Castellucci et al., 1993a,b) and in the depth of cell columns (Castellucci et al., 1993a,b; Mühlhauser et al., 1993). They are separated from the intervillous space by varying amounts of fibrin-type fibrinoid, especially where the syncytial layer is absent. Intravillous fibrinoid ("fibrinoid necrosis") (Fox, 1968) reveals highly variable mixtures of both fibrinoid types.

In conclusion, the subdivision into matrix-type and fibrin-type fibrinoid is independent of the well known topological nomenclatures (e.g., perivillous, villous, Langhans', Rohr's, and Nitabuch's fibrinoid). The matrix-type fibrinoid from different topological origins has always been homogeneous in its immunoreactivities; the same is true for the fibrin-type of fibrinoid.

Origin of Fibrinoid

The sources of the different types of fibrinoid are next to be considered. How are they derived, and why is their production in most placental sites linked so closely? It is only on first glance that the question of the origin of fibrin-type fibrinoid seems simple.

Fibrinoid has been shown to react with anti-fibrinogen antibodies in a variety of placental sites (Moe, 1969a, b,d; Gille et al., 1974; Faulk et al., 1975; Johnson & Faulk, 1978), a finding supported by the biochemical

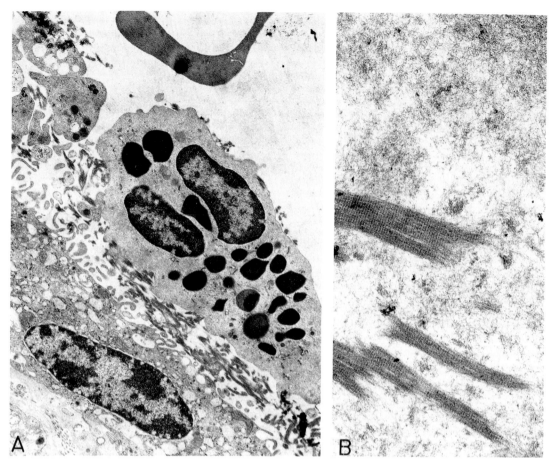

FIGURE 122. (A) Perivillous fibrin deposition on the tropho blastic surface of an obviously damaged villus (below). A maternal granulocyte (center) and several platelets (upper left corner) are attached to the bundles of fibrin. ×9,200.

(D) Higher magnification of fibrin-type fibrinoid from Nitabuch stria from the basal plate. The mixture of granular to fine filamentous material with larger bundles showing typical cross-striation is highly characteristic. ×35,000.

findings of Sutcliffe et al. (1982). According to our own experience with anti-fibrinogen binding it is likely that most of the fibrinogen-positive deposits represent fibrin-type fibrinoid, even though some immunoreaction for fibrinogen can be found also in matrix-type fibrinoid.

There is no doubt as to the importance of fibrinogen for the formation of fibrin-type fibrinoid. The local deposition of fibrin implies either local synthesis of fibrinogen or the deposition of blood fibrinogen. Although clear evidence for an extrahepatic fibrinogen synthesis has not yet been reported, it is still under discussion (Doolittle, 1975; Sutcliffe et al., 1982; for review see Faulk, 1989). Sutcliffe et al. (1982) failed to observe intracellular fibrinogen determinants in the vicinity of Nitabuch's fibrinoid. The local accumulation of hepatic or extrahepatic fibrinogen would imply local activation of blood clotting factors. Indeed, some authors have found enzymes in human trophoblast and uterine cells that were antigenically similar to the blood clotting factor XIII and that were able to polymerize fibrinogen (Chung, 1972; Bohn, 1978).

The typical distribution of most deposits of fibrin-type fibrinoid facing the intervillous space suggests their origin from maternal blood; however, one cannot exclude that fibrinogen derived from fetal plasma contributes to fibrinoid formation. In particular, in the villous tree matrix-type fibrinoid is often encapsulated with fibrin from both the intervillous and stromal sides, suggesting a derivation from both maternal and fetal fibrinogen.

The extracellular matrix molecules found in matrix-type fibrinoid are known to be secretory products of epithelial cells (Carnemolla et al., 1987; Castellucci et al., 1993a,b; Feinberg & Kliman, 1993; Hohn et al., 1993). The ED-B domain of fibronectin, which is detected by the antibody BC-1, is not present in plasma fibronectins (Carnemolla et al., 1989). Rather, it is expressed only in oncofetal fibronectin, which is secreted by some fetal and malignant cells but usually not by normal adult epithelial cells (Carnemolla et al., 1989). The secretory nature of matrix-type fibrinoid is further supported by the presence of substances such as collagen

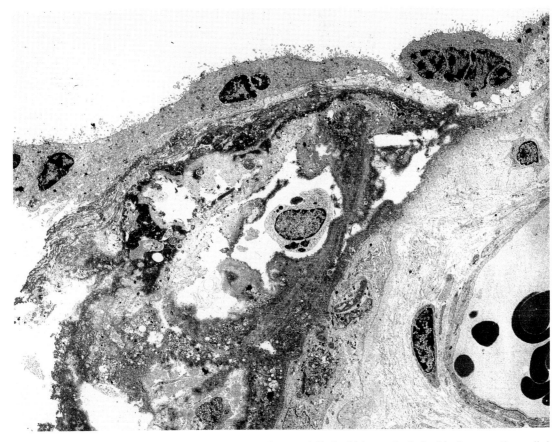

FIGURE 123. Intravillous fibrinoid. A large, heterogeneous plaque of fibrinoid intermingled with degenerative cellular remains and white blood cells is deposited between the syncytial covering of the villus and its stromal core. ×2,400.

IV, laminin, and heparan sulfate, which are well known secretory products of trophoblast cells (Castellucci et al., 1993a,b; Nanaev et al., 1993a,b).

Collagen IV, laminin, and cellular fibronectin are secreted also by villous cytotrophoblast together with collagen VI in a polarized manner at their basal surface, constituting the basement membrane (Rukosuev et al., 1990; Castellucci et al., 1993a,b; Nanaev et al., 1993a,b). As a consequence of highly active trophoblastic proliferation in cell columns and cell islands, some of the daughter cells of the proliferating stem cells (Langhans' cells) lose contact with the trophoblastic basal lamina (Figure 112). By definition, the latter are called extravillous trophoblast cells. At the same time, they stop secretion of the various matrix molecules (Castellucci et al., 1993a). As soon as the cells are located three or more layers distal to the basal lamina they start secreting extracellular matrix molecules anew, but in a non-polarized manner. At the same time, they change their secretory pattern by no longer secreting collagen VI but by adding oncofetal fibronectin (Frank et al., 1994) and, in deeper layers, heparan sulfate proteoglycan as well. These matrix molecules accumulate extracellularly as matrix-type fibrinoid, thereby increasingly separating

the extravillous trophoblast cells (Figures 21A,D, 111A). Electron microscopically, this material still has some structural similarity to basement membrane material, although disintegrated remains of degenerating trophoblast cells can also be found among the various secreted matrix components (Frank et al., 1994).

Secretion of heparan sulfate proteoglycan by decidual cells into the surrounding fibrinoid has also been described by Kisalus and Herr (1988). This finding raises the question whether extravillous trophoblast is the only source of matrix-type fibrinoid or if decidual cells also contribute to it by secretion and possibly by degeneration in the fetomaternal junctional zone.

Interactions Between Matrix-Type and Fibrin-Type Fibrinoid

Matrix-type fibrinoid deposits virtually never directly face the intervillous space; rather, the space is covered by thin layers of fibrin-type fibrinoid (Figure 123). On the other hand, fibrin-type fibrinoid usually does not directly cover cytotrophoblast but is separated from the latter by matrix-type fibrinoid. This typical co-localization suggests that the processes leading to formation of the two types are somehow linked.

The presence of collagens, laminin, and fibronectins in matrix-type fibrinoid may represent a possible link between the formation of the two types of fibrinoid. In general, collagens (Kunicki et al., 1988), fibronectins (Piotrowicz et al., 1988), and laminin (Sonnenberg et al., 1988) are able to initiate clotting by interaction with platelets (Coleman et al., 1987). Platelet antigens have been described in fibrinoid (for review see Coleman et al., 1987; Faulk, 1989). Thus it is likely that matrix-type fibrinoid initiates blood clotting and the formation of fibrin-type fibrinoid in all those positions where it is in contact with maternal or fetal blood.

In addition, it cannot be excluded that secreted proteases directly initiate fibrinogen cleavage with subsequent fibrin deposition. Such atypical pathways of fibrin formation do not involve the blood clotting cascade (Frank et al., 1994). The structural and immunohistochemical result is the same.

There are obvious relations between fibrin deposition and proliferation of extravillous trophoblast in perivillous fibrinoid. It is a common histopathological finding that villous cytotrophoblastic cells lose their contact with the trophoblastic basement membrane (Stark & Kaufmann, 1974). They are then transformed into extravillous trophoblast cells as soon as the covering syncytiotrophoblast is replaced by fibrin-type fibrinoid. Detailed investigation of such areas has revealed that these trophoblast cells are usually not in direct contact with the superficial fibrin-type fibrinoid but, rather, are embedded in their own matrix-type fibrinoid. The increasing diffusion distance for maternal oxygen due to fibrin deposition may stimulate trophoblastic proliferation (Fox, 1970) and the transformation into extravillous trophoblast followed by secretion of matrix-type fibrinoid.

Functional Conclusions

It is no longer justified to classify fibrinoid merely the result of degenerative processes, caused by placental aging or altered blood flow and nutrition (i.e., simply as an indicator for placental "degeneration"). Rather, most authors consider normal functional aspects and conclude that fibrinoid is an unavoidable constituent of the normal placenta. In this respect there are several aspects currently under active discussion.

1. Hörmann (1965) and Kretschmann (1967a,b) pointed to the mechanical importance as the *constructive principle*. Even though we believe that this aspect has never been studied in detail, it appears reasonable that perivillous fibrin, deposited on the stem villi, may increase their mechanical stability. In the same way,

mechanically supportive effects can be attributed to fibrinoid deposits lining the chorionic and basal plates (in most cases fibrin-type fibrinoid).

2. It is suggested that matrix-type fibrinoid represents, among other functions, the "glue" that guarantees *adhesiveness* of the placenta to the uterine wall. This type of fibrinoid fills most of the interstitium between extravillous trophoblast and decidual cells; it contains large amounts of basal lamina molecules (e.g., fibronectins, collagens) (Frank et al., 1994) for which receptors (integrins) have been found in the maternal and fetal cells of that region (Korhonen et al., 1991; Damsky et al., 1992; Aplin, 1993). Feinberg and coworkers (1991b) have suggested that oncofetal fibronectin, a regular constituent of the matrix-type fibrinoid of this area, acts as a "trophoblast glue" for human implantation and placental-uterine attachment throughout gestation. Matrix-type fibrinoid may constitute a three-dimensional net of a giant basal lamina to which all extravillous trophoblast cells and decidual cells of the maternofetal junctional zone are bound.

Jackson and coworkers (1993) have added another view. They found that the production of oncofetal fibronectins by trophoblast cells in vitro was stimulated by inflammatory products (endotoxin, lipopolysaccharide) and inflammatory mediators (interleukin-1β). These substances are known to mediate labor by stimulating prostaglandin secretion. The authors discussed secretion and metabolism of oncofetal fibronectin in relation to the initiation of preterm labor.

3. Additional importance may be attributed to fibrin-type fibrinoid as the *regulator of the intervillous circulation*. The intervillous space is an open, cleft-like communicating and continuously growing system. Problems in perfusion are to be expected during the establishment of its maternal circulation. One possibility to adapt the shape of the intervillous space to the maternal blood flow is to obstruct all poorly perfused areas by clotting of blood and fibrinoid deposits. If one were to accept this mechanism, it is then only of secondary importance whether it is achieved by hemostasis with subsequent coagulation or by trophoblastic malnutrition with subsequent degeneration and induction of fibrinoid deposition. In agreement with the findings and views of Stark and Kaufmann (1974), Becker (1981), and Kaufmann (1981b), the above mechanisms may be active in adapting the intervillous space to maternal hemodynamics during the formation of all fibrin-type fibrinoid lining the intervillous space.

4. The occurrence of fibrinoid at the maternofetal junction correlates with invasive placentation (Pijnenborg et al., 1981). This consideration has prompted several authors to discuss a functional role of fibrinoid as a *barrier to trophoblastic invasion*. The

nature of this influence remains an open question. Badarau and Gavrilita (1967), Wynn (1967a), and Moe (1969a,b,d) have suggested that fibrinoid plays a role as a barrier that limits the invasiveness of the trophoblast. This suggestion was supported by findings from tubal pregnancies (Kawagoe et al., 1981). For a long time, one had to counter by suggesting that this conclusion is not in agreement with histological findings: Considerable numbers of trophoblast cells can be found inside fibrinoid or even below Nitabuch's stria, sometimes even in the myometrium.

Our findings substantiate that the presence of trophoblast cells is related to only one type of fibrinoid, the matrix type. In contrast, the fibrin type is never invaded by extravillous cytotrophoblast (Frank et al., 1994) and may thus have the same barrier function against trophoblastic invasion that Dvorak et al. (1983) suggested existed for fibrin against tumor invasion.

5. Aplin and Foden (1982) described a placental extract, called the cell spreading factor, that contains fibronectin and fibrinogen. They speculated about its presence in the uteroplacental fibrinoid to restrict or perhaps even promote trophoblast migration and invasion. Their idea is one of the first to suggest the presence of *invasiveness-promoting activities*.

The presence of oncofetal fibronectin (BC-1), which is known to be present in the extracellular matrix of malignant tumors (Carnemolla et al., 1989), suggests interrelations of extravillous trophoblastic invasiveness with matrix-type fibrinoid. The invasive properties of these cells have been described and discussed for trophoblastic cell columns (Sutherland et al., 1988; Feinberg et al., 1989; Damsky et al., 1992; Mühlhauser et al., 1993). In cell columns the invasive phenotype of extravillous trophoblast correlates well with increasing amounts of matrix-type fibrinoid. Whereas fibrin-containing matrices have been discussed to act as a barrier against cellular invasion (Dvorak et al., 1983), the self-secreted matrix-type fibrinoid may provide the appropriate microenvironment for extravillous trophoblastic invasion. Numerous experimental and immunohistochemical results concerning extravillous trophoblast cells describe the expression of laminin receptors and integrins (Sutherland et al., 1988; Loke et al., 1989b; Damsky et al., 1992), tenascin (Castellucci et al., 1991; Damsky et al., 1992), and trophouteronectin (Feinberg & Kliman, 1993) and the secretion of proteases (Feinberg et al., 1989), in particular type IV collagenase (Librach et al., 1991). These substances are relevant when considering this topic.

The functions of matrix-type and fibrin-type fibrinoid described above may overlap. One example is the morphogenesis of the basal plate, where a barrier of fibrin-type fibrinoid is deposited continuously at the fetal surface. It possibly controls the invasion of trophoblast cells, which themselves secrete matrix-type fibrinoid as a supporting matrix along their invasive pathway.

6. Perivillous fibrinoid may be involved in *maternofetal transport processes*. The integrity and completeness of the syncytiotrophoblastic surface of the villi is not perfect. Where the syncytiotrophoblast is interrupted by degeneration or by mechanical forces, the gap is immediately filled by perivillous fibrin (fibrin-type fibrinoid) as a result of blood clotting. Corresponding fibrinoid spots locally replace the syncytiotrophoblast, a regular finding in every placenta. Such areas may serve as paratrophoblastic routes for maternofetal macromolecule transfer, bypassing the syncytiotrophoblast. Horseradish peroxidase (48,000 daltons; 3.0 nm molecular radius) was shown to pass through the fibrinoid foci from the maternal circulation into the fetal stroma (Edwards et al., 1991). According to Nelson et al. (1990), these foci of perivillous fibrinoid account for about 7% of the villous surface of the normal human term placenta.

7. Matrix-type fibrinoid and connective tissue related to both types of fibrinoid shows varying degrees of immunoreactivity for tenascin (Castellucci et al., 1991; Frank et al., 1994). Tenascin is a mesenchymal glycoprotein that facilitates epithelial cell migration during development and is thus involved in many embryonic formative processes (Chiquet-Ehrismann et al., 1986; Aufderheide & Ekblom, 1988). If the presence of tenascin is validated, one must consider if matrix-type fibrinoid also has a *formative character* during placental development. This action may be in cooperation with its incorporated extravillous trophoblast cells. Perhaps the spreading of these cells is linked to it.

Moreover, the presence of tenascin or other related molecules may be involved in reepithelialization of damaged villous surfaces. Nelson et al. (1990) found evidence that trophoblast fibrinoid interactions (fibrin-type or matrix-type?) modulate trophoblastic differentiation and proliferation.

8. Most of the discussion regarding the functional importance of fibrinoid is related to its possible *immunological significance*, with many authors discussing an immunologically protective function (Bardawil & Toy, 1959; Kirby et al., 1964; Currie & Bagshawe, 1967; McCormick et al., 1971; Azab et al., 1972; Faulk et al., 1975; Wynn, 1975). A particular immunoprotective role of sialic acid as normal constituent of fibrinoid has been stressed by Currie and Bagshawe (1967). This molecule may mask fetal antigens and thus prevent their recognition by maternal cells; moreover, it is thought to protect fetal cells from already sensitized maternal lymphocytes. It is known from several publications that experimental desialation of tumors by in vitro treatment with neuraminidase significantly increases their immunogenicity (for review see Bagshawe & Lawler, 1975).

Also, heparan sulfate proteoglycan, secreted by decidual cells into the surrounding uteroplacental fibrinoid (Kisalus & Herr, 1988), has been suggested as a molecule that provides immunoprotection. Immunoprotective functions must be considered for both fibrinoid types: heparan sulfate has been found in matrix-type fibrinoid (Castellucci et al., 1993a); sialic acid, the other immunoprotective molecule under discussion, is probably present in fibrin-type fibrinoid (see Bagshawe & Lawler, 1975).

A few publications have defined another immunoprotective function of fibrinoid, that is, its action as an immunoabsorptive sponge. This idea was first forward by Swinburne (1970). He proposed that the fibrinoid expresses target antigens that bind circulating maternal antibodies, and the resulting immune complexes are then thought to contribute to the deposition of fibrinoid. The same concept was later favored by Chaouat et al. (1983) and Hunziker and Wegmann (1987). Raghupathy et al. (1981, 1984) added two other findings that may be of interest in this context. They found that bound antibodies are internalized and degraded within 4 to 6 hours, and that the capacity of the antigen sponge is regenerated within 48 hours. Also, Montemagno (1967) opined that the fibrinoid derives from anti-fetal antibodies.

Only few findings negate the immunoprotective role of fibrinoid. Billington (1975) pointed to the immunological importance of sulfate groups. Because they are said to be present in the trophoblastic glycocalyx in high concentration, the immunoprotective function of the trophoblast was believed to be superior to that of the fibrinoid. According to the results of Kirby et al. (1964), some forms of fibrinoid in the rodent placenta contain locally produced, highly negatively charged mucoproteins that exhibit a protective effect against the maternal immune system. Sutcliffe et al. (1982) did not favor this idea for humans because of the relatively low carbohydrate levels in human uteroplacental fibrinoid. Ikonicoff (1971) also considered that the fibrin/fibrinoid/glycocalyx and other "noncellular components" of the placenta serve as a barrier against immunological recognition and rejection of the transplanted fetal organ. Important insight in this regard has been gained through the studies of Redline and Lu (1988). These authors showed that some of the molecules contained within the basal fibrinoid prevent macrophage movement, a subject that is fully discussed in the context of listeriosis (see Chapter 20).

Finally, a different view was presented by Bray (1978). He postulated an immunoprotective role of fibronectin, which is a regular constituent of basal laminas, such as that of the trophoblast; however, fibronectin isoforms are present also in both types of fibrinoid. In the noninvasive epitheliochorial placentas of Artiodactyla and Perissodactyla which largely lack fibrinoid, this basal lamina is uninterrupted and serves with the trophoblastic glycocalyx as a perfect double-layered immunobarrier. In contrast, the trophoblastic glycocalyx and basal lamina in hemochorial placentation are multiply interrupted and may thus raise the demand for an additional focal immunobarrier. Because fibrinoid is deposited in all sites where the trophoblast is discontinuous, the fibronectin-containing fibrinoids may serve as a substitute.

Calcification

The basal plate of the mature placenta often has finely divided deposits of calcium salts. They appear yellow and stippled and occur in irregular quantities. They may be detected by ultrasonography, and "placental grading" has been popular in prenatal sonographic studies. In rhesus monkeys the degree of calcification seems to be generally related to the stage of pregnancy (Bunton, 1986). In humans immature placentas rarely have any significant amount of grossly visible calcification, whereas postmature placentas often have a gritty sensation when the knife passes through the floor of the placenta. It is not a reliable sign of postmaturity, however, and sonographers have largely abandoned its grading. These calcium deposits occur not only in the placental floor but also within the internal structure of the placenta, generally accompanying the septa. Calcium deposits are blue in H&E preparations and, as seen in Figures 124, 125, and 126, the calcium deposits occur principally within accumulations of fibrin and fibrinoid. Occasionally, one finds calcifications in degenerated villi (see Chapter 15).

The quantity of placental calcium has been studied chemically by Jeacock et al. (1963), who also reviewed the older literature. These authors found the following calcium concentration in placentas.

Weeks of pregnancy	Mean conc. (mg/g dry tissue)
6–17	4.00
28–36	3.65
37–42	10.26
43–44	10.58

The increment found with postmaturity was small. Binovular twins did not always have the same concentrations. Patients with severe toxemia had higher values when they delivered prematurely but not at term. Stillbirth had no effect, and infarcts did not have a high calcium content. Rather than reflecting placental "aging," Jeacock et al. considered that the calcium deposits in the placenta serve fetal needs.

Fujikura (1963a,b) found that some 15% of placentas had moderate to marked calcification and that it tended to decrease with maternal age; it was most common

FIGURE 124. Focal fibrin deposit on the villous surface (with central calcification: dark) covers trophoblast defect on the villous surface. Note that such lesions in the placenta never have any fibrous ingrowth; they do not "organize" in the sense used by pathologists. H&E. ×200.

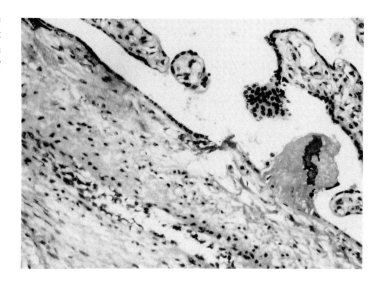

(in the United States) in placentas delivered between November and February. Fox (1964), who found a significant relation to primigravidity, classified 25% of the placentas as calcified and saw no relation to post-maturity. He emphatically stated that calcification is in no way related to degenerative changes, but that fetal distress and neonatal asphyxia were more common with calcified placentas.

Brown et al. (1988) found by ultrasonographic studies that increased calcification of the placenta occurred in smoking mothers irrespective of possible fetal weight reduction. When the placenta was studied by radiographic photography, 44% had slight, 30% moderate, and 2% severe calcification (Tindall & Scott, 1965). The manner of deposition varies (see also Hassler, 1969). The findings of Tindall and Scott indicate that calcium

deposits increase steadily from 29 to 43 weeks, and that the amounts are related to placental and fetal weights. Placentas of stillbirths had generally less calcification. In contrast to the observations of Fujikura (United States), the placentas of Tindall and Scott (England) had more calcification when delivered from June to October. These authors made reference to possible physiological mechanisms that regulate calcium deposition and did not consider the process to be a pathological event. Russell (1969) found calcium deposits most commonly in the spring and fall and in younger mothers; interestingly, prosperous women also had more calcium deposits in their placentas. The overall incidence, based on radiographic findings, was 18% of placentas after 38 weeks. Al-Zuhair et al. (1984) produced excellent scanning electron micrographs of irregular electron-dense

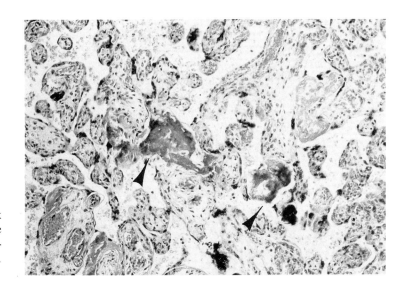

FIGURE 125. Irregular calcium salt deposits (dark black) in mature placenta. The dark areas are syncytial buds (knots); the light gray areas (arrowheads) represent fibrin in the intervillous space. H&E. ×160.

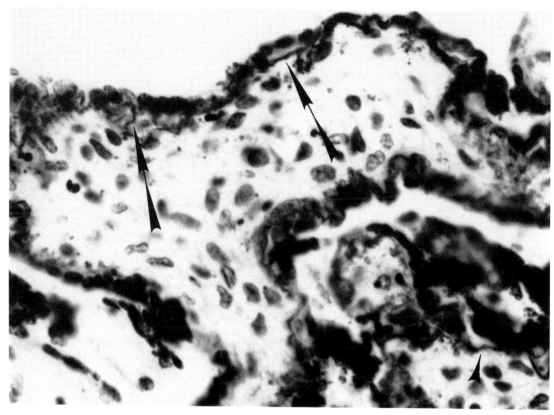

FIGURE 126. Mineral salt deposits (arrows) in basement membrane of immature placenta from a stillborn fetus. H&E. ×640.

attachments to the villous microvillous projections, but the inference that they are calcium deposits needs further proof.

In addition to the typical calcification that is grossly perceptible, the histopathologist often finds granular, purple deposits on the basement membrane of villous surfaces (Figure 126). They have been described by Avery and Aterman (1971) and are most common in abortions. We are uncertain that the purple granules they found also in fibrotic villi truly represent calcium. Pathologists have a tendency to assume something to be calcium when it is amorphous, purple, and stains with the von Kossa reaction. The fact is, however, that there is no specific stain for calcium; phosphorus and carbonate salts of all sorts stain with the von Kossa reaction. The murexide stain may be an exception; it may stain calcium more specifically (Kaufman & Adams, 1957).

That such "calcified" basement membranes may represent largely iron deposits has been shown by Birkenfeld et al. (1989) in a patient with β-thalassemia major whose pregnancy came to term. Krohn et al. (1967) addressed the relevance of these deposits when they showed that pregnancies complicated by hydramnios had an unusually high (67%) deposition rate

of "calcium" at the trophoblastic border. Iron and phosphates are intermixed and not readily separated by the usual methods. McKay et al. (1958) found it to be a feature of second trimester placentas.

From chemical analysis, Einbrodt et al. (1973) ascertained that, in a large city, the *lead* contamination of calcium in the placentas had increased from 45% to 65% between 1956 and 1961. In addition to these deposits of minerals, *melanin* has been demonstrated in the basement membranes of villi and in Hofbauer cells (Ishizaki & Belter, 1960). With special stains, these authors identified melanin in 85% of the placentas they examined. It was present as often in Caucasians as in Blacks. They suggested that these deposits occur more frequently in association with chronic skin lesions and called the condition dermatopathic melanosis of placenta. Melanin-containing macrophages in amnion have also been found in cases of prolonged amnion rupture (Bendon & Ray, 1986). Parmley et al. (1981) demonstrated the "aging pigment" *lipofuscin* in placentas beyond 32 weeks. They used fluorescence microscopy for its demonstration and saw it routinely in the trophoblast. In a discussion of that paper, Wynn remarked that one should not necessarily construe this finding as "aging." We agree with him and the many authors who believe that only maturation, not aging, occurs during normal gestation in placental tissue.

We have earlier stated that sonographers have used the presence of calcium and other structural features to "grade" the placenta before birth (Hobbins & Winsberg, 1977). Their grades I to III have been correlated with fetal maturity, as judged by the sphingomyelin/lecithin (L/S) ratio (Grannum et al., 1979). These studies have often shown that placental grading is not accurate enough to diagnose pulmonary maturity without determination of the L/S ratio (Harman et al., 1982; Petrucha & Platt, 1982). They are also not useful for delineating and monitoring postmature pregnancies (Hill et al., 1983; Monaghan et al., 1987). There has been a suggestion, however, that they may be useful for predicting IUGR (Kazzi et al., 1983).

This chapter is not the place for a detailed review of maternofetal calcium relations. Thoughtful reviews have been provided by Pitkin (1975) and Tsang et al. (1976). It has been said that pregnancy induces a maternal "physiological hyperparathyroidism" (Pitkin et al., 1979). High maternal calcitonin levels of pregnancy protect the mother against bone loss (Garel & Barlet, 1978). During the third trimester the fetus requires 100 to 150 mg calcium/kg fetal weight per day for bone apposition (Tsang et al., 1976), and there is evidence of placental production of vitamin D (Reddy et al., 1983). The paradox of higher serum levels of ionized calcium in the fetus than in the mother may relate to this finding. Despite many safeguards, abnormalities occur. Neonatal tetanus is not rare, particularly in premature infants, and may reflect secondary vitamin D deficiency (Rosen et al., 1974).

Although numerous investigations have been undertaken to clarify transplacental calcium/phosphorus transfer, none can be found that takes into consideration the simultaneous degree of placental calcium deposits. Are they related to homeostasis, or are they merely a reflection of dystrophic mineral deposits in extracellular matrix? Einbrodt and Schmid (1965) did not think that the excessive calcium deposits they found were the cause of an infant's death. They described two successive pregnancies with massive calcification of the placenta (20–30% in excess of normal) in a woman with latent pregnancy tetany. The first pregnancy had been medicated to alleviate these symptoms; the second pregnancy was not treated, yet excessive amounts of placental calcium accumulated. It is not clear that it was the result of the disturbance in maternal calcium homeostasis. The authors cited another case from the literature with similar pathology but without tetany. They identified the placental mineral deposits as hydroxyapatite, not carbonate. The authors made the point that the excessive calcification was not due to mere fibrin absorption of calcium. At present, then, we do not understand the normal mechanisms that lead to calcification of the placenta, let alone when it attains a seemingly pathological concentration.

CHORIONIC PLATE

Development

The development of the chorionic plate begins with formation of the primary chorionic plate. This process starts as soon as the first lacunae appear in the syncytiotrophoblast of the implanting blastocyst on day 8 p.c (see Chapter 6). Initially, this layer is composed only of syncytiotrophoblast and cytotrophoblast. It separates the early lacunar system from the blastocyst cavity (Figures 24c,d). As soon as the extraembryonic mesenchyme develops and spreads around the cytotrophoblastic surface of the blastocyst cavity (Figure 24d), the primary chorionic plate becomes triple-layered, consisting of mesenchyme, cytotrophoblast, and syncytiotrophoblast. At the same time, the trophoblastic trabeculae that separate the lacunae start proliferating and form the first villous outgrowths into the continuously expanding lacunar system (Figures 24d,e). The trabeculae are henceforth called villous stems; the lacunar system is transformed into the intervillous space. From this stage onward, the chorionic plate represents the "lid" of the intervillous space and at the same time serves as the base from which the villous trees are suspended into the intervillous space.

The layering of the primary chorionic plate described above is maintained until term (Kaufmann, 1981a). Multifocal tissue degeneration with subsequent fibrinoid deposition, however, may considerably disturb its architecture. Fibrinoid deposits within and along the surface of the chorionic plate are called Langhans' fibrinoid (Langhans, 1877; Bourne, 1962). Those parts of the fibrinoid that replace tissues of the chorionic plate are usually compact and largely homogeneous in appearance. Toward the intervillous space, it becomes mostly covered by an inhomogeneous material, fibrin-type fibrinoid, which is arranged in more or less net-like fashion. It is thought to be derived from blood clotting in the intervillous space (Bourne, 1962). The syncytiotrophoblastic cover of the chorionic plate is usually replaced by Langhans' fibrinoid, which occurs during early pregnancy.

In some places the cytotrophoblastic layer also degenerates, whereas in other places it proliferates, resulting in multilayered plaques. These plaques consist of either compact cytotrophoblast or scattered trophoblastic cells surrounded by fibrinoid. As was shown by enzyme histochemical studies (Weser & Kaufmann, 1978), the basal layer of cytotrophoblast, which rests on the chorionic mesenchyme, retains the characteristics of a proliferating layer of stem cells. Their highly differentiated, nonproliferative daughter cells (extravillous trophoblast cells) lose contact with the mesenchymal layer and migrate into the neighboring matrix-type fibrinoid. Here they grow in size and achieve the histochemical steroid dehydrogenases (Weser & Kaufmann, 1978) and ultrastructural (Wiese, 1975) characteristics of specialized, metabolically highly active cells. Continuous degeneration of these cells may serve as an important source for the accumulation of fibrinoid.

With advancing gestation, numerous small and large villi become attached to the fibrinoid. Through coagulation of blood in their surrounding, and with subsequent transformation into fibrinoid, they may become deeply incorporated into the Langhans' fibrinoid layer. The original Langhans' cells of the incorporated villi commence proliferation following degeneration of their syncytial layer. They then transform into extravillous trophoblast cells and migrate into the fibrinoid. In places that are devoid of such incorporated villi, the thickness of the chorionic plate rarely exceeds 200 μm, whereas conglomerates of encased villi, together with their derivatives, may measure up to more than 1 mm in thickness.

The extraembryonic mesenchyme that has formed after day 9 p.c. initially completely occupies the blastocyst cavity (Figure 208, day 13). During the course of the 3rd week p.c., the exocoelomic cavity is formed, reducing the extraembryonic mesenchyme to thin layers that cover the early embryo as well as the chorionic plate (Figure 208, day 18). In the latter position it establishes the chorionic mesoderm. Toward the exocoelomic cavity, the mesoderm is lined by a single layer of flat mesothelium.

During the course of the 2nd month p.m., fetal blood vessels derive from the allantois via the connecting stalk and establish contact with the chorionic plate (Figure 208; days 28 and 40). There they spread across the chorionic mesoderm and soon enter the early stem villi (Figures 24f, 25, 208). The vessels here come into contact with locally formed fetal villous capillaries, resulting in the completed fetoplacental circulatory system. The chorionic fetal vessels soon enlarge to form arteries and veins. It must be pointed out that all these vessels pass the chorionic plate and thus connect the villous trees with the umbilical cord. Capillaries for the nutrition of the various tissues of the chorionic plate are a rare, locally restricted exception.

At 17 weeks p.m. the amnionic vesicle has become so large that it comes into close contact with the chorionic plate (Grosser, 1927). At this time, the amnion is composed of an inner epithelial layer (amnionic epithelium) and an intermediate layer of amnionic mesoderm that, on its outer surface, is lined by amnionic mesothelium (see Chapter 12). Where amnion and chorion closely appose each other, their mesothelial layers slowly regress, resulting in mesodermal fusion. As in the membranes, this fusion is never perfect. Rather, it is a focal attachment, with the formation of net-like bridges between the layers (spongy layer). This structure establishes contact that allows easy gliding of the layers against each other. Attachment of the amnion to the primary chorionic plate transforms the latter into the definitive chorionic plate. Ample folding of the amnionic cover on the chorionic plate is a usual histological finding (Figure 127A). It is difficult to decide from histological preparations how extensively they reflect the in vivo situation and how much is a consequence of the collapse of the amnionic vesicle after delivery because of the easy gliding of the amnion.

Structure at Term

The structure of the chorionic plate at term has been poorly studied. Few publications deal only with aspects of this part of the placenta (Langhans, 1877; Grosser, 1927; Singer & Wislocki, 1948; Bourne, 1962; Boyd & Hamilton, 1970; Wiese, 1975; Weser & Kaufmann, 1978; Schiebler & Kaufmann, 1981). Studies especially devoted to the chorionic plate concern cord insertion (Scheuner, 1964), the subchorial Langhans' fibrinoid layer (Geller, 1959), and chorionic vessels (Nikolov & Schiebler, 1973). Aspects of its cellular composition have been studied twice: on the electron microscopic level by Wiese (1975) and histologically, including enzyme histochemistry, by Weser and Kaufmann (1978).

The layering of the term chorionic plate is consistent with that described during development. The following layers must be distinguished (Figure 128):

amnionic epithelium
compact layer
amnionic mesoderm
spongy layer, separating amnion and chorion
chorionic mesoderm
proliferating cytotrophoblast
langhans' fibrinoid layer encasing the extravillous cytotrophoblast

These are described in greater detail in the following sections.

Amnion

The three layers of the amnion (i.e., amnionic epithelium, compact layer, and amnionic mesoderm) are structurally largely identical with the respective layers described in Chapter 12. Bourne (1962) has given the most detailed review of these layers. Plaques of "squamous metaplasia" are common findings, especially surrounding the cord insertion. The usually columnar epithelium is here replaced by a squamous, keratinizing type. Sinha (1971) has dealt with this subject in more detail.

Wiese (1975) studied fiber arrangement in both connective tissue layers of the amnion by electron microscopy. The compact layer, devoid of cells, is composed of a condensed three-dimensional lattice of collagen fibers. The neighboring amnionic mesoderm differs in two aspects: Vertical collagen fibers are lacking; and the remaining two-dimensional loose network is composed only of fibers that are arranged parallel to the amnionic epithelium. Three or four thin layers of filaments alternate with layers of loosely arranged fibroblasts, forming an incomplete irregular network. Kratzsch and Grygiel (1972) have histochemically demonstrated the existence of diphosphoglucose dehydrogenase in these cells, an enzyme that is involved in the production of matrix proteoglycans. For further details see Chapter 12.

Spongy Layer

The spongy layer (Bourne, 1962) has also been called the intermediate layer (Petry, 1954a,b), jelly layer (Dohrn, 1865), or stratum intermedium (Bautzmann & Schröder, 1955). The layer is structurally similar to the corresponding layer of the free membranes (see Chapter 12). It is easier to study at the chorionic plate, however, because here it is less often dislocated by the forces of labor. The spongy clefts that separate amnion and chorion are normally less impressive. The clefts are partially lined by small, rounded cells. Because of their ultrastructural features, Wiese (1975) interpreted them to be macrophages. Histochemically, we were unable

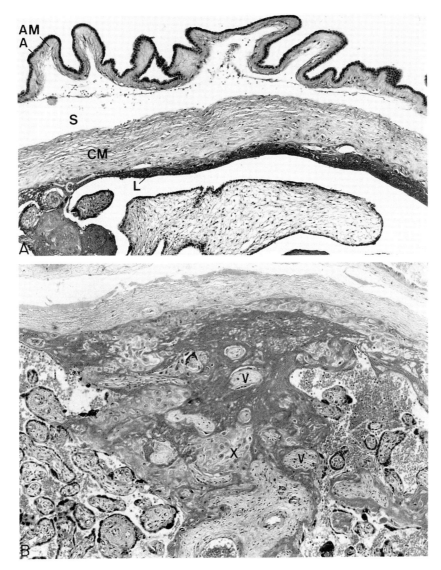

FIGURE 127. Comparison of the chorionic plate in the early and late stages of pregnancy. (A) At the 21st week p.m. (B) At the 40th week p.m. The typical layering of the chorionic plate with amnionic epithelium (A), amnionic mesenchyme (AM), spongy layer (S), chorionic mesenchyme (CM), chorionic (extravillous) cytotrophoblast (C), and Langhans' fibrinoid (L) is evident at both time points. The main difference between the two developmental stages is the increased deposition of Langhans' fibrinoid below the chorionic plate near term. Clusters of extravillous trophoblast cells (X) and residues of buried villi (V) are typically incorporated in the mature Langhans' fibrinoid. Paraffin sections. ×85.

to detect acid phosphatase in these cells (Weser & Kaufmann, 1978). On the other hand, immunohistochemical study makes it likely that they secret basal lamina molecules as is typical for epithelial, endothelial, mesothelial, and contractile cells (Malak et al., 1993; Ockleford et al., 1993, 1994). Because there are no immunohistochemical indications for the presence of contractile cells in this particular layer, it is likely that the cells are residues of the former amnionic and chorionic mesothelium, which once lined the exocoelomic cavity as "Heuser's membrane," prior to fusion of amnionic and chorionic mesoderms.

Chorionic Mesoderm

The chorionic mesoderm of the chorionic plate presents some peculiarities that have not been described in detail for the chorionic mesoderm of the membranes. Several authors (Scheuner, 1964; Wiese, 1975; Weser & Kaufmann, 1978) have described distinct layers, ranging from "oriented" connective tissue facing the spongy layer to "unoriented" connective tissue near the fibrinoid. In the unoriented layers, the collagen fibers seem to be irregularly arranged, with large polymorphic fibroblasts in between and nuclei rich in euchromatin.

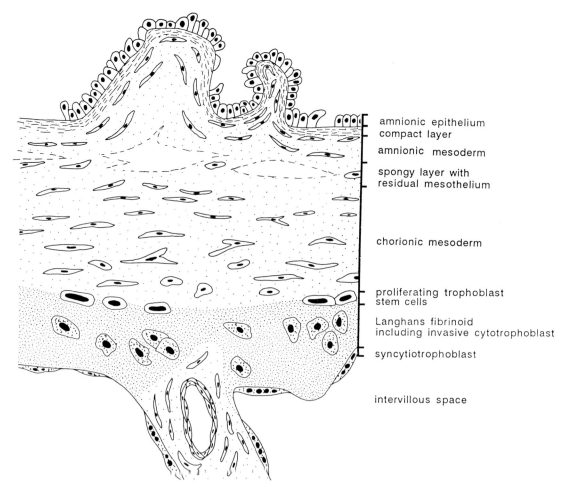

amnionic epithelium
compact layer
amnionic mesoderm

spongy layer with
residual mesothelium

chorionic mesoderm

proliferating trophoblast
stem cells

Langhans fibrinoid
including invasive cytotrophoblast

syncytiotrophoblast

intervillous space

FIGURE 128. Layering and cellular composition of mature chorionic plate.

The oriented layers, on the other hand, consist of thin strata with collagen fibers that are oriented in parallel. The layers are separated by small fibroblasts with long extensions and condensed nuclei. These authors suggested that the unoriented layers are the primitive precursors of the oriented layers, a suggestion supported by the fact that during early pregnancy the unoriented layers are prominent (Figure 127A) with a deficiency of oriented fibers. At term, only a thin unoriented layer remains as a kind of germinative zone.

Bertolini et al. (1969) reported the existence of smooth muscle cells within these layers, in agreement with the results of Spanner (1935). Later studies, in particular the detailed electron microscopic investigation by Wiese (1975), did not support this finding. Many of the cells, however, display typical immunohistochemical features of myofibroblasts.

The oriented layers of the mesoderm comprise the site of the chorionic vessels, which originate by branching from the umbilical vessels. These vessels have been described in greater detail in Chapter 13.

Extravillous Cytotrophoblast

The chorionic mesoderm is followed by an incomplete basal lamina. A layer of extravillous cytotrophoblast is found on its other side. In the central parts of the placenta it is a discontinuous layer of small groups of cells (Figures 128, 129). Near the placental margin, it becomes continuous and is finally multilayered. The location at the exact mesodermal–fibrinoid interface is characteristic for these cells. Where several cells lie close together, their cell membranes show intense interdigitations. They are fixed to each other by desmosomes. Foot-like extensions, equipped with hemidesmosomes, connect the cells to the basal lamina. The latter is absent where the chorionic mesoderm directly faces the Langhans' fibrinoid without interposed primary cytotrophoblast. Ultrastructurally, these cells are undifferentiated and resemble proliferating cells (Wiese, 1975). This view is supported by the demonstration of considerable glucose-6-phosphate dehydrogenase activity (Weser & Kaufmann, 1978), a key enzyme for the

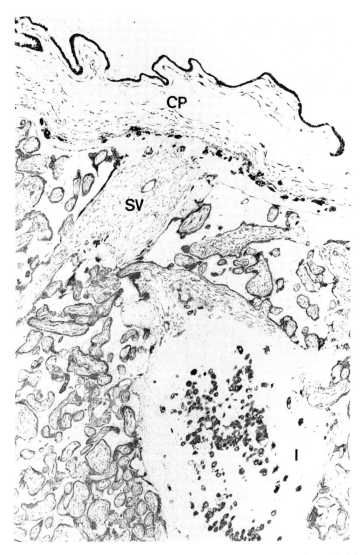

FIGURE 129. Cryostat survey picture at the 40th week p.m. showing the chorionic plate (CP) with a branching-off stem villus (SV), numerous small villous branches, and a cell island (I). Because of the histochemical reaction for malate dehydrogenase applied to this section, amnionic epithelium, cytotrophoblast, and syncytiotrophoblast show intense staining, whereas connective tissue cells are only weakly stained. Note the immediate relation of the cell island to a large stem villus. ×115. (From Schiebler & Kaufmann, 1981, with permission.)

pentose phosphate cycle that is particularly prominent in proliferating cells. Moreover, the proliferative activity of these cells can be demonstrated by application of immunohistochemical proliferation markers (MIB-1, PCNA).

Embryologically, these cells are thought to be residues of the layer of blastocyst cytotrophoblast that covers the primary chorionic plate from days 8 to 15 p.c. (Figure 24c). During early pregnancy all cytotrophoblast of the placenta is derived by proliferation and migration from this layer. In later stages, the residual cells serve as stem cells for the extravillous trophoblast cells, which are encased by Langhans' fibrinoid. Accumulations of this proliferating layer of extravillous cytotrophoblast, up to multilayered groups in the marginal zone of the placenta (Arnold, 1975a,b), account for particular growth activities at the placental margin.

The proliferative layer of cytotrophoblast expresses not only cytokeratins, as is typical for extravillous trophoblast, but sometimes also vimentin as revealed by immunohistochemistry (Lieder-Ochs, personal communication, 1991). The latter is an intermediate filament characteristic for mesenchymal cell lines. From this finding it may be possible to deduce the trophoblastic origin of the chorionic mesoderm as was postulated by Hertig (1935) and Wislocki and Streeter (1938). The studies by Luckett (1978), however, have clearly ruled out the possibility that chorionic cytotrophoblast contributes to the formation of the chorionic mesoderm; other experimental findings in chimeric mice support it as well (Rossant & Croy, 1985).

Langhans' Fibrinoid Layer

Langhans' fibrinoid layer is a rather constant feature, with a thickness and structure that increase continuously throughout pregnancy. In its early stages, the intervillous surface of Langhans' layer is still mostly covered by syncytiotrophoblast, which is completely replaced by additional fibrinoid during later pregnancy.

Abundant scattered or aggregated extravillous trophoblast cells can be seen in the fibrinoid. Ultrastructurally (Wiese, 1975), enzyme-histochemically (Weser & Kaufmann, 1978), and immunohistochemically the cells are comparable to the more highly differentiated invasive stages of extravillous trophoblast cells of other origin. The few undifferentiated, proliferating stem cells are located on the basal lamina separating chorionic mesenchyme from extravillous trophoblast or fibrinoid.

The assumption of Bertolini and Klinger (1966) that these cells are decidual cells is no longer tenable, but it must be pointed out that sometimes decidual cells are present in the chorionic plate, in particular near the placental margin (see below). They are the result of folding of basal plate tissue into chorionic plate tissue and can be interpreted as mild transitional stages toward placental circumvallation (see Chapter 14).

Nearly all of the early authors noted that the fibrinoid of the chorionic plate is normally composed of two distinct layers that differ in structure. The first is deep, compact layer that in the mature placenta that is nearly continuous and follows the chorionic connective tissue and, where present, the chorionic cytotrophoblastic layer (Figure 127). This compact fibrinoid represents matrix-type fibrinoid (Frank et al., 1994; Lang et al., 1994). It encases the extravillous trophoblast cells of the chorionic plate, which contribute to its growth by secretion and degeneration. This layer is covered either by syncytiotrophoblast bordering the intervillous space or, in those areas where the syncytium has degenerated, by a second fibrinoid layer of more reticulated fibrinoid that corresponds immunohistochemically to fibrin-type fibrinoid (Figure 127B) (Frank et al., 1994; Lang et al., 1994). The latter had been described as canalized fibrin by Langhans (1877).

Grosser (1927) interpreted the deep, compact layer as being the product of tissue degeneration of the chorionic plate, infiltrated by fibrin that is derived from interstitial fluids; the more superficial reticular layer was considered to be maternal fibrin, a mere blood clotting product from the intervillous space. This view has been corroborated by most later authors

(Geller, 1959; Arnold, 1975a,b; Wiese, 1975; Weser & Kaufmann, 1978; Frank et al., 1994; Lang et al., 1994).

The amount of subchorial fibrinoid at term varies considerably. According to our anatomical experience, it is impossible to define the amount that is compatible with normal pregnancy. Note, however, that the most impressive cases of subchorial fibrinoid deposition we have observed occurred in cases of Rh incompatibility. Here the Langhans' stria extended without identifiable demarcation into ample perivillous fibrinoid and numerous subchorial cell islands, occupying as much as one-half of the placental volume.

The subchorial fibrinoid is the basis for the "bosselations" and the laminated subchorial plaques that vary so much from one placenta to another. The latter are deposits resulting from eddying in the places where the intervillous blood is turned back towards the basal plate.

At times, large laminated hematomas are found underneath the chorionic surface. Such cases have been reported by Torpin (1960), Shanklin and Scott (1975), and Oláh et al. (1987), with the latter authors diagnosing it even during ultrasonographic examination. The 25 weeks' pregnant patient they described suffered a falling hemoglobin level and a rapidly enlarging abdomen. A fatally ill premature infant was delivered by cesarean section. The circumvallate placenta weighed 700 g (28 weeks) and had a 15 × 5 cm laminated thrombus under the chorionic plate. This case is not unlike the classical Breus' mole (tuberous subchorionic hematoma) of earlier abortions, except for the sacculations that Breus delineated (1892). Although Breus thought that these sacculations developed after fetal death, Oláh et al. (1987) cited evidence that the hematoma may be primary, albeit rare. A somewhat similar condition was reported by Howorka and Kapczynski (1971). In their patient, the hematoma was circumferential. It had disrupted the chorion laeve, much as in acute circumvallation. The authors included an interesting diagram that depicts their operative observations. It suggested to them that separate contractions, within sacculations of the uterine fundus, were the basis for the detachment. More extensive consideration is given these "thrombohematomas" in Chapter 12.

Marginal Zone

Subchorial Closing Ring

The marginal zone is not precisely defined. It consists of the transitional zone of the chorionic plate, the basal plate, and the membranes; and it has characteristics of all three regions. The internal margin, separating it by definition from the chorionic plate (Bühler, 1964), is the line connecting those points where the most peripheral branches of the chorionic plate vessels make their vertical bend to enter the most peripheral villous trees. The outer margin that separates it from the membranes represents the macroscopically visible transition from placenta to membranes (Bühler, 1964). It is largely identical with that line where the intervillous space is occluded by fusion of the chorionic plate with the basal plate. Macroscopically, the marginal zone is often represented by a slightly prominent opaque ring. It is about 1 cm in width and corresponds to the *schlussring* of the early German authors, the subchorial closing ring (Boyd & Hamilton, 1970). An increase in thickness of the marginal zone is represented by the designation placenta marginata (Kölliker, 1879). The transposition of the subchorial closing ring nearer to the cord, with origination of the membranes from the chorionic surface of the placenta rather than from the margin, is referred to as placenta circumvallata (see Chapter 14). In circumvallate placentas the intervillous space, together with smaller villous trees peripherally, exceeds the marginal zone. A complete, macroscopically identifiable subchorial closing ring was described by Bühler (1964) in 71% of placentas studied; in 21% it was incomplete, in 8% it was absent.

The structures of the marginal amnion and the marginal chorionic mesoderm are comparable to those of the neighboring zones: the chorionic plate and membranes (Arnold, 1975a,b). The structural basis for the prominence and the opaque appearance of the subchorial closing ring is the presence of an increased number of cells in the Langhans' fibrinoid, which normally forms a multilayered stratum. The origin of these cells, as those of all extravillous trophoblast cells, has led to some dispute. Winkler (1872) described them to be decidual cells, and Bühler (1964) supported this view when studying the distribution of the Barr bodies. Boyd and Hamilton (1970), however, came to the conclusion that Spanner (1935) and Ortmann (1960) were correct when they attributed a trophoblastic origin to these cells.

The ultrastructural results of Arnold (1975a,b) gave clear evidence that both cell types are present. A thick layer of extravillous cytotrophoblast accompanied by Langhans' fibrinoid crosses this region and then passes over to the trophoblast layer of the membranes (Arnold, 1975a,b; Wiese, 1975). In most cases, a hook-like extension of the basal decidua laterally surrounds the placental margin and protrudes into the Langhans' layer. The latter may be split in a Y-like fashion.

Trabeculae

In histological preparations of the marginal zone, rounded or elongated plaques of connective tissue or trabeculae become apparent. They are nearly uniformly scattered over the Langhans' fibrinoid and X cell layer. They must not be confused with the trabeculae of the early stages of previllous development. Histologically, the trabeculae are similar to villi that are encased in fibrinoid and that have lost their trophoblastic cover. Krafft (1973) studied these structures in serial sections and was able to demonstrate convincingly that they are continuous on the one side with encased branches of the most peripheral villous trees. Their peripheral ends extend far into the membranes, where they end blindly at the decidual layer. According to Krafft (1973), they are residues of villous branches that have been incorporated into the marginal zone during regression of the chorion frondosum to become the chorion laeve. They are thought to be important for the mechanical stability of the marginal zone and for anchoring the membranes to the placenta.

Marginal Sinus

Large maternal veins exist near the placental margin that open into the intervillous space. This coincidence has caused intense speculation regarding the intervillous circulation of blood. Spanner (1935, 1941) described it as the marginal sinus and concluded that this sinus drains more or less all of the maternal intervillous blood into the uterine veins. Ramsey (1956) and Arts (1961) called it the marginal lake. The beautiful studies of Ramsey (1956), Ramsey and Harris (1966), Ramsey et al. (1966), and Ramsey and Donner (1980) showed that it is indeed a prominent area of venous outflow, but also that it does not have the exclusive characteristics attributed to it by Spanner (1935, 1941). Numerous venous openings, scattered over the entire surface of the basal plate, offer sufficient venous drainage at the base of the placenta.

The wall of the initial part of the marginal uteroplacental veins is largely replaced by fibrinoid; in addition, numerous signs of cellular degeneration can be observed in the surrounding tissues (Arnold, 1975a,b). It has been speculated that it is the structural basis for the so-called marginal sinus hemorrhage (Schultze, 1953, 1968), as the peripheral decidual cover is thin.

BASAL PLATE

Trophoblastic Shell and Development of the Basal Plate

The basal plate is defined as the maternal aspect of the intervillous space. It is the most intimate and most important contact zone of maternal and fetal tissues (Figures 7, 24f). The definitive basal plate is a highly complex structure. It is composed of various tissues (e.g., extravillous trophoblast, endometrial stroma with its pregnancy-specific specialization, fibrinoid, residues of degenerating villi, and maternal vessels). General information concerning all of these tissues is provided separately at the beginning of this chapter.

The early precursor of the basal plate is the trophoblastic shell (Figure 130), a particular syncytiotrophoblastic layer that, in the implanting blastocyst, separates the lacunar system from the endometrial tissues (Figures 24c,d). Because of the intimate relation between the trophoblastic shell and the surrounding endometrium, the first steps in the formation of the basal plate are coupled with the mechanisms of implantation (see Chapter 6).

The trophoblastic shell of the blastocyst certainly actively invades the decidua at implantation. Many current animal studies have disclosed the existence of specific uterine secretions, with variable expression, during early development. For instance, Simmen et al. (1988) identified in the uterine luminal fluid of early pregnancy in pigs a heat-stable mitogen. It is distinct from that in mice and from EGF. It is probable that an active cross-talk exists between these proteins and the blastocyst, securing proliferation and nidation (for review see Denker & Aplin, 1990).

The morphological aspects of early human ovum invasion into the endometrium have been described in the numerous contributions of Hertig and his colleagues (for review see Hertig, 1960). These studies have shown that decidual cells are dissociated by these trophoblastic elements, and that trophoblastic cells actively incorporate glycoproteins and probably other substances from the decidual bed. Enders and Schlafke (1969) found junctional complexes between trophoblast and decidua in a variety of less invasive animal placentas. Although they discovered signs of phagocytic activity by the trophoblast, no cytolytic effect was identified.

Boeving was the most ardent student of the biochemical aspects that regulate implantation. In a large review of 1964, he lamented

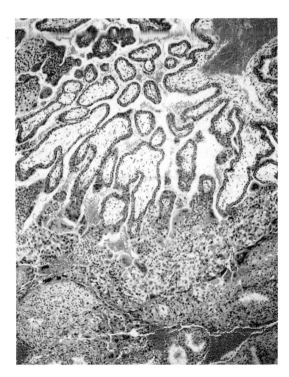

FIGURE 130. Trophoblastic shell of 13-day pregnancy. The cytotrophoblastic columns are covered with syncytium. Placental site giant cells are intermingled with decidua (right). H&E. ×300.

that the fixation of tissues for histology might produce some understanding of phylogeny and some helpful pictures, but he contended that it has been of little help in understanding the trophoblastic invasion. He favored the view (derived from his observations of high bicarbonate concentrations of the developing blastocyst) that this high pH was instrumental in dissociating the superficial decidual cells and thus securing access to the endometrial stroma.

Another view was expressed by Denker (1978), who based his ideas on the results of many other investigators. He proposed that implantation is secured by a variety of enzymes from the trophoblastic shell. Because it is difficult to work with human material, Denker used rabbit blastocysts. He showed that many enzymes become enriched on the trophoblastic surface and then wrote that "trypsin-like proteinase activity... plays a key role in initiation of implantation."

It is likely, however, that implantation is a complex process, and that analogies from animal observations have only limited value for understanding the human condition. Nevertheless, at a time when interspecific embryo transfer is often attempted, resolution of these considerations may be sought more actively.

As the invasive front of the blastocyst, the trophoblastic shell is not a flat, evenly curved plate as the name suggests. Rather, it has an irregular surface that interdigitates intensively with the endometrial connective tissue. During implantation the trophoblastic shell consists merely of syncytiotrophoblast. On day 13 p.c., cytotrophoblast reaches the shell via the trabeculae and splits the syncytiotrophoblast into an apical layer that faces the intervillous space and a basal layer that contacts the maternal tissues (Figures 24d,e). Within a few days the latter becomes incomplete. The surviving parts may invade deeply into the endometrium and finally reach the myometrium as "syncytial streamers." With human implantation, they appear as multinucleated trophoblastic giant cells (Figure 131A), first described by Kölliker (1861). We were able to demonstrate in the guinea pig that these "giant cells" are long, partially branched, root-like extensions of the placental base (Uhlendorf & Kaufmann, 1979) rather than isolated elements. It is uncertain whether this finding is valid also for the human placenta. According to the thorough evaluation of 48 pregnant human uteri by Pijnenborg et al. (1980), only a small amount of the invasive trophoblast is multinucleated (syncytial) in nature. The prevailing number of invasive cells are mononuclear. It is only in the vicinity of the myometrium that large numbers of multinucleated giant cells can be seen.

Because of the increasing incompleteness of the basal syncytial layer, increasing amounts of cytotrophoblast come into contact with the endometrium. As a typical sign of their invasive activity, these cells relinquish their closed epithelial formation and commence to invade the stroma as single cells or in small groups (Figures 24e,f, 131,133,134). It is the first time at which an exact border—one separating the trophoblastic shell and endometrium—can no longer be defined. An exactly dated, 22-day-old human specimen, described in detail by Larsen and Knoth (1971), illustrated this situation. From this date onward, the term trophoblastic shell has usually been replaced by the term basal plate, which includes the base of the intervillous space together with all placental and maternal tissues that adhere to it after parturition.

The deeper tissue layers of the placental site, which remain in utero and are later discharged as lochia, show a similar admixture of maternal and placental tissues, the placental bed. In situ the placental bed and basal plate cannot be delimited from each other because the demarcation zone becomes visible only shortly before delivery. Therefore they together comprise the "junctional zone" for in situ specimens. They encompass all regions of

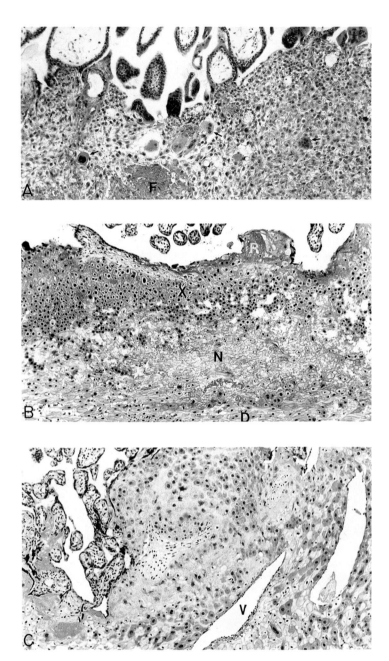

FIGURE 131. Developmental stages of the basal plate, paraffin sections. (A) At the 8th week p.m. The basal plate is composed of a dense mixture of extravillous trophoblastic and decidual cells intermingled with a few trophoblastic giant cells (arrows). There is little fibrinoid (F). ×75. (B) At the 23rd week of gestation. The typical layering of the basal plate is evident. Facing the intervillous space, it is covered by an interrupted layer of Rohr's fibrinoid (R), followed by a nearly complete layer of extravillous cytotrophoblast (X). The latter is largely separated from the decidua cells (D) by a loose layer of Nitabuch's fibrinoid (N). ×85. (C) At the 37th week p.m. During the last trimester of pregnancy the typical layering of the basal plate is again abolished by trophoblastic cells, and decidual cells penetrate the originally separating Nitabuch's layer in both directions. The result is a colorful mixture of fibrinoid and cells of maternal and fetal origin. A few cross sections of a fetal vein (V), lined by innocuous endothelium, can be seen. ×85.

admixed maternal and fetal composition that lie basal to the intervillous space (Figure 24f). Note that the term basal plate is applicable only to the delivered placenta.

During the first stages of pregnancy endometrial glands are still visible in the deep parts of the decidua of the implantation site (Figure 18M). So long as these remnants exist, trophoblastic invasion is largely limited to those parts of the compact and spongy layers of the decidua that overlie the glands (Pijnenborg et al., 1980). Only scattered trophoblast cells are found amid the glands, and they are only occasionally closely related to them. During the 15th to 18th weeks p.m. only occasional, isolated fragments of the glands are seen. Most are located in the lateral parts of the placental site, whereas in the central areas the glandular tissue is completely lost. The trophoblast invades the entire thickness of the decidua, down to the myometrium where glands are absent. One may speculate whether the existence of glands prevents trophoblastic invasion, or the invasive activities of the trophoblast contribute to the destruction of the glands. We believe the latter to be more likely.

Much tissue necrosis occurs where maternal and fetal cells come close together. This degeneration has been interpreted as the consequence of proteolytic activity of the invading trophoblast. Large necrotic foci of the decidua in this region may also be a consequence of obstruction of spiral arteries. The necrotic residues of decidua and trophoblast are transformed into fibrinoid, with a considerable admixture of fibrin being probable.

Two layers of fibrinoid exist. Rohr's fibrinoid is a superficial, multiply interrupted, more or less focal layer. It faces the intervillous space (Figures 24f, 131B), where it replaces the superficial layer of basal plate syncytiotrophoblast. Nitabuch's fibrinoid is a layer of uteroplacental fibrinoid. As is expressed by its name, this layer is believed to mark the border of the placental and maternal tissues (Figure 24f) and thus represents the immediate "battlefield" of the tissues (Kaufmann & Stark, 1971). Nitabuch's fibrinoid separates a superficial trophoblastic layer from a deeper decidual layer exactly in only a few areas (Figures 19L, 131B, 135). In other places the cell types may be intensely intermixed on one or both sides of the Nitabuch layer. Finally, the order of layers can be inverted in exceptional cases, with the decidua nearer the intervillous space and the X cells making up the base of the basal plate. A histologically identifiable uteroplacental fibrinoid layer is completely absent in many locations. Even then, immunohistochemically (Kisalus & Herr, 1988; Frank et al., 1994) or electron microscopically (Wiese, 1975), minor amounts of fibrinoid can be detected as surrounding the various cell types.

Growth of the basal plate laterally as well as in thickness is largely a consequence of extravillous cytotrophoblast proliferation of cell columns. The migration of their daughter cells into tissues of the basal plate can readily be demonstrated (for review see Extravillous Trophoblast).

The lateral growth of the basal plate probably is not always accompanied by a corresponding degree of local distension of the uterine wall. This lack may cause a lateral movement and enhance the folding of the basal plate and the uterine wall over each other. Such folding processes results in dislocation of basal plate tissues into the intervillous space, including all of its normal constituents. The placental septa are thus formed. Detached parts of the septa, which are connected to the villous trees only by some interposed fibrinoid, make up a subpopulation of the cell islands.

Layers of the Basal Plate at Term

The mature basal plate is of variable thickness, ranging from 100 μm to 1.5 mm. In most places it has lost its typical earlier layering (Figures 131C, 135). Only rarely can all of the following layers be identified in an undisturbed order (Hein, 1971; Kaufmann & Stark, 1971; Schiebler & Kaufmann, 1981).

1. The inner surface of the basal plate that faces the intervillous space shows residues of the former *syncytiotrophoblastic lining* in only a few places. These areas are small patches of largely degenerative syncytium, and an underlying cytotrophoblast is normally absent.

Wanner (1966) reported the existence of *endothelial cells* in the same location that were thought to be derived from the ostia of the uteroplacental vessels. According to recent immunohistochemical studies, maternal endothelium lines not only large parts of the intervillous surface of the basal plate (Figures 132, 138C,D) but also parts of the septa and of the marginal zone (Lang et al., 1993). Where syncytiotrophoblast and maternal endothelium are absent, the basal plate is superficially covered by Rohr's fibrinoid.

2. The syncytiotrophoblastic patches rest on a rudimentary, frequently interrupted basal lamina that separates the trophoblast from an inconsistent *connective tissue layer*. This layer, composed mostly of collagen fibers and intermingled with a few fibroblasts, measures 10 to 30 μm in thickness. It is usually present where syncytiotrophoblast covers the basal plate. It may be absent in other places. In most cases this superficial connective tissue stria can be traced to the stroma of anchoring villi that are deeply buried into basal plate fibrinoid. The enzyme-histochemically highly active leucine aminopeptidase in these cells is considered to be an indicator of fetal origin (Stark & Kaufmann, 1971).

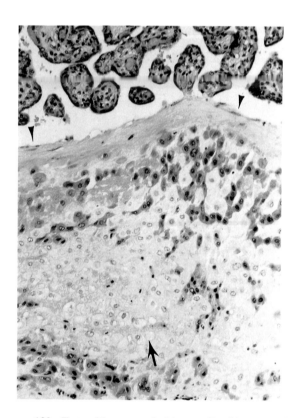

FIGURE 132. Extravillous trophoblast cells (dark cells) in decidua basalis of a near-term placenta. The arrow indicates a decidual stromal cell. The endothelial cells that are believed to line the basal portion of the intervillous space, above Rohr's fibrin layer, are indicated by arrowheads. H&E. ×240.

3. The superficial fibrinoid layer of the basal plate, *Rohr's stria*, was first described in 1888 by Wolska as superficially located, homogeneous or lamellar material in the basal plate (Figure 131B) that shows similarities to a deeper layer in the junctional zone (Figure 24); it was characterized by Nitabuch (1887) only 1 year earlier. A year later Rohr (1889) dealt with this superficial fibrinoid in some greater detail, pointing particularly to the fact that the superficial fibrinoid layer is less complete and more irregularly structured. His name was later connected with this layer. To our knowledge, no further studies deal with it.

Rohr's stria is basically similar to Langhans' stria of the chorionic plate. Like the latter, it is a highly inconsistent structure, appearing only in places where the covering syncytiotrophoblast has degenerated. Its thickness is highly variable, in some places enclosing numerous ghost villi, cell columns, and single cells and in other places being completely devoid of all cellular structures. Where villi are attached to Rohr's stria, it is continuous with perivillous fibrin, engulfing villi. Sometimes it is also continuous with the more deeply positioned Nitabuch's stria, so the striae cannot be separated from each other (Figure 131C).

Concerning the composition and derivation of Rohr' stria we refer to what has been said about fibrinoid in general (see Fibrinoid, above). All those deposits that directly face the intervillous space show immunohistochemical characteristics of fibrin-type fibrinoid (Frank et al., 1994). Only where Rohr's fibrinoid encases extravillous trophoblast cells, usually in the neighborhood of cell columns, can patches of matrix-type fibrinoid be found that are free of fibrin and rich in other extracellular matrix molecules.

4. A highly variable layer then follows that measures 50 μm to 1mm in thickness. It is composed of *extravillous cytotrophoblast*, patches of Rohr's fibrinoid, loosely arranged connective tissue, admixed *decidual cells*, remnants of encased anchoring villi, and "buried" cell columns (Figure 115). Most of the connective tissue of this region is of maternal origin. It is composed of endometrial stromal cells, small, highly branched fibroblast-like cells, and some macrophages. Because of the presence of maternal connective tissue in this layer, decidualization may also be present. Locally, there may be an admixture of fetal connective tissue cells that are derived from the stroma of encased and degenerating anchoring villi. Both lines of connective tissue cells can easily be distinguished by the application of the enzymatic histochemical reaction for leucine aminopeptidase. It results in positive staining of only the fetally derived connective tissue (Figure 115B) (Stark & Kaufmann, 1971).

A vast traditional descriptive literature deals in much detail with the structural, ultrastructural, histochemical,

and functional aspects of the extravillous trophoblast cells of the basal plate (Wislocki, 1951; Ortmann, 1955; McKay et al., 1958; Thomsen & Willemsen, 1959; Weber, 1961; Dallenbach-Hellweg & Nette, 1963a,b, 1964; Wachstein et al., 1963; Hein, 1971; Kaufmann & Stark, 1971; Stark & Kaufmann, 1971). It has now become clear that these cells represent the largely nonproliferative, invasive portion of the extravillous trophoblast cells emanating from the cell columns (Schindler et al., 1984; Eidelman et al., 1989; Feinberg et al., 1989, 1991a; Loke et al., 1989b, 1992a; Wakuda and Yoshida, 1990, 1992; Castellucci et al., 1991; Librach et al., 1991; Damsky et al., 1992; Burrows et al., 1993; Fisher and Damsky, 1993; Mühlhauser et al., 1993). We refer to the earlier section on Extravillous Trophoblast.

The number of decidual cells present in this layer varies greatly. These cells may be absent, or they may comprise most of the cells. For structural features of the decidual cells, see the section on Decidua. Cytotrophoblast and decidual cells may be intensively admixed (Figures 108, 133, 134, 135). According to Wynn (1967a), these cell types never establish direct intercellular contacts; rather, they are separated by fibrillar networks (external lamina of the decidual cells) (Kisalus & Herr, 1988), fibrinoid, or both. This finding is in partial disagreement with the results published by Hein (1971), who found the two types to be in intimate contact. The possibility of such contacts, even though established only occasionally in humans, is supported by findings in rats and mice (Martinek, 1970, 1971). In both rodents, cells of maternal and fetal origin establish intense interdigitations of their cell surfaces.

5. This heterogeneous but principal layer of the basal plate is followed by *Nitabuch's fibrinoid layer, the uteroplacental fibrinoid*, which is a net-like to lamellar structure that is variably interrupted (Figures 24, 131B). It is located in the immediate maternofetal "battlefield" of the junctional zone, the deeper part of the basal plate (Figure 24). Because of this location, it has commonly been regarded as the result of immunological processes.

This fibrinoid stria, first described by Nitabuch in 1887, is a rather consistent, more or less uninterrupted layer that is 20 μm to more than 100 μm thick. In many places the layer may split and rejoin, with trophoblastic and decidual cells or endometrial connective tissue interposed. In its most ideal, but rarely executed, situation Nitabuch's fibrinoid separates superficially positioned trophoblastic cells from more basally located decidual cells (Figures 24, 131B). In these cases it marks the exact maternofetal border (Wynn, 1967a). Usually, however, the arrangement of maternal and fetal cells is more irregular. Mixed populations of the two cell types on one or both sides of the stria are the commonest finding (Figure 135).

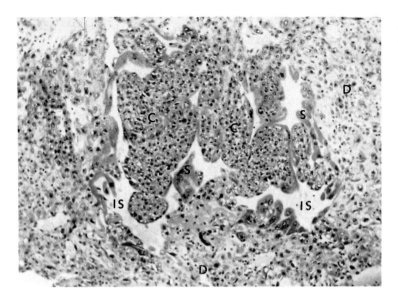

FIGURE 133. Implantation site of a 13-day human ovum showing the cytotrophoblastic cell columns (C), syncytium (S), intervillous space (IS) without maternal blood as yet, and the decidua (D) with infiltrating trophoblastic elements. H&E. ×260.

The thickness of this stria is usually related to the thickness of the basal plate: Thick parts of the basal plate, measuring up to 2,000 μm in thickness, exhibit the most prominent fibrinoid accumulations, whereas it may be completely absent in the thinnest part, measuring only 300 μm (Kaufmann & Stark, 1971; Stark & Kaufmann, 1971).

Electron microscopically, Nitabuch's fibrinoid is similar to that found in other places in the placenta; it is composed of an electron-dense meshwork of fibrin filaments with basal lamina material (see above) commonly ensheathing the trophoblast cells and plaques of amorphous electron-dense material with cellular debris (Wynn, 1967a; Hein, 1971). In many places, decidual and trophoblastic cells lie directly underneath each other

without interposed fibrinoid but also without establishing intercellular contacts (Hein, 1971). This description is in agreement with numerous reports demonstrating direct contacts between maternal and fetal tissue in epitheliochorial and endotheliochorial placental types characterized by the absence of separating fibrinoid layers (Dempsey et al., 1955; Björkman & Bloom, 1957; Ludwig, 1962; Björkman, 1965a,b, 1970; Kaufmann et al., 1985). Based on his own electron microscopic studies of these placental types, Wynn (1967a) postulated the existence of a thin separating layer of mucopolysaccharides. The junctional zone of hemochorial rodent placentas is characterized by the regular appearance of fibrinoid (Schiebler & Knoop, 1959; Bulmer & Dickson, 1961; Kirby et al., 1964; Bradbury et al., 1965;

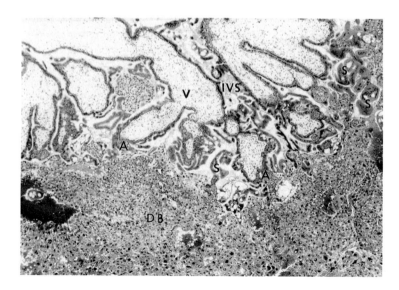

FIGURE 134. Very young placental floor with villi (V) containing connective tissue but no fetal vessels as yet, syncytium (S), intervillous space (IVS) with maternal blood, and the confusing intermixed population of cells in the decidua basalis (DB). The extravillous trophoblast cells and placental site giant cells are largely mononuclear but dark, in contrast to the lighter decidual cells. H&E. ×40.

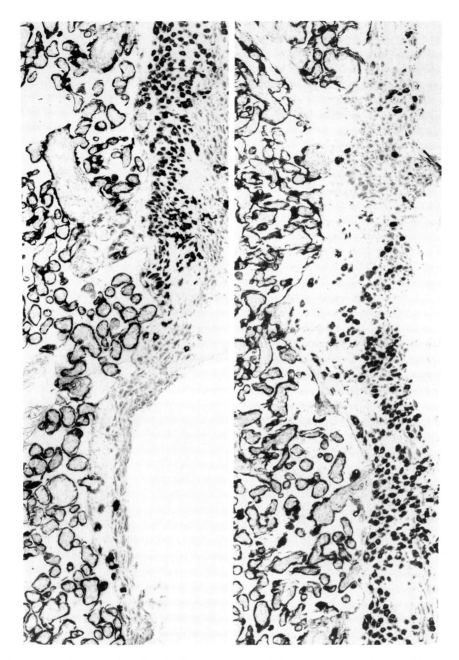

FIGURE 135. Cryostat survey section of the basal plate. Enzyme histochemical proof of glucose-6-phosphate dehydrogenase. The right half of the picture is the continuation of the upper end of the left half. At the left in each picture one can see the intervillous space with numerous villi. The ability of the glucose-6-phosphate dehydrogenase reaction to discriminate between extravillous trophoblast and decidua is used to illustrate the distribution of the two cell types in the basal plate. The extravillous cytotrophoblast cells can be identified as darkly stained polygonal cells, whereas the decidua is composed of slender, faintly stained cell bodies. Note that there are segments of the basal plate with perfect layering (upper left) but also segments consisting merely of decidua (left middle) or extravillous trophoblast cells (lower right). A colorful mixture of the two cell types is the most usual feature. ×65. (From Stark & Kaufmann, 1971, with permission.)

Martinek, 1970). This material largely (Martinek, 1970, 1971), or even completely (Kirby et al., 1964; Currie & Bagshawe, 1967), encloses the trophoblast cells.

The discussion regarding the derivation of Nitabuch's fibrinoid is as controversial as it is of fibrinoid deposits in other localizations. Kirby et al. (1964) described it as a result of trophoblastic secretion in the mouse placenta. Azab et al. (1972) found evidence for a decidual secretory origin, and Wigger (1977) suggested a trophoblastic origin. The fibrinoid has even been suggested to contain structures identical to Michaelis-Gutmann bodies of malakoplakia (Sala et al., 1982a,b). Dempsey et al. (1970) concluded that it was derived from maternal blood fibrinogen; fibrinogen derived from the interstitial fluid of the basal plate was thought to be the source according to Ludwig (1959). A more complex composition of fibrinogen and cellular secretory and degenerative products was favored by most authors (e.g., Grosser, 1927; Wynn, 1967a; Boyd & Hamilton, 1970; Burstein et al., 1973; Robertson & Warner, 1974).

The biochemical analysis of human Nitabuch's fibrinoid by Sutcliffe et al. (1982) showed a prevailing composition of proteins of 48,000 and 105,000 daltons, thus corresponding with components of blood fibrin. Whether other minor protein bands were of serum or local tissue origin remained open. The authors concluded that there is little support for the view that Nitabuch's fibrinoid is primarily a product of lysed trophoblast and uterine cells.

On the other hand, Kisalus and Herr (1988) found immunocytochemical proof for decidual secretion of heparan sulfate proteoglycan into the surrounding fibrinoid. This proteoglycan can also be detected in the uteroplacental fibrinoid for that reason. Immunohistochemical studies concerning the composition of Nitabuch' fibrinoid have confirmed its heterogeneity (Frank et al., 1994; Lang et al., 1994). Those parts that encase extravillous trophoblast or decidual cells represent largely pure matrix-type fibrinoid and thus support early theories of the secretory nature. Cell-free areas and in particular those layers that cover the basal surface of the delivered placenta are usually composed of fibrin-type fibrinoid. This point explains why Sutcliffe et al. (1982) biochemically detected mostly blood clot products because their material was derived from the basal surface.

Of the factors that are thought to initiate fibrinoid deposition at the maternofetal interface, primary importance has been attributed to immunological, enzymatic, and even mechanical aspects during trophoblast invasion into the genetically different decidua (Wynn, 1967a; Azab et al., 1972). Kirby et al. (1964) pointed to the interesting finding that large genetic differences between mother and fetus result in increasing amounts of uteroplacental fibrinoid. Consequently, a functionally protective immunological mechanism has been proposed. Bardawil and Toy (1959), Kirby et al. (1964), Currie and Bagshawe (1967), Azab et al. (1972), Wynn (1975), and Sutcliffe et al. (1982) suggested a barrier function that protects fetal antigens against identification by maternal cells so as to avoid direct contact of fetal tissues with sensitized maternal lymphocytes. The high concentration of sialic acid was believed to be important. Martinek (1970) and Robertson and Warner (1974) opposed this view. According to their

findings, the maternofetal intercellular contacts make a perfect immunological barrier an illusion.

Sutcliffe et al. (1982) have added another interesting view concerning the immunological importance. They pointed to the ample uteroplacental fibrinoid present in human and rodent placentas with invasive implantation, in contrast to the relative lack in artiodactyls and perissodactyls that are characterized by noninvasive implantation. This discrepancy does not imply the lack of a functional role of fibrinoid in the human. Rather, Sutcliffe and coworkers (1982) pointed to the finding that women homozygous for factor XIII deficiency have recurrent abortions if not treated by plasma transfusions (Ikkala et al., 1964; Fisher et al., 1966). If Nitabuch's fibrinoid is primarily a blood clotting product (Sutcliffe et al., 1982), it should be absent in the case of factor XIII deficiency. Regrettably, this point has not yet been studied.

6. The *separation zone* of the placenta from the placental bed is usually not identical with Nitabuch's stria, rather, separation occurs in most cases somewhat deeper. Therefore some additional tissues may be attached to the placental floor and form the deepest layer of the basal plate. Most cells in this layer are decidual cells and other components of the endometrial stroma, and a certain admixture of trophoblastic elements is a regular finding.

With increasing distance from the intervillous space, the number of multinucleated giant cells (Kölliker, 1861; Boyd & Hamilton, 1960; Hein, 1971) increases. These cells are large, highly differentiated, multinucleated elements with diameters up to 100 μm. With the use of serial sections, they appear as slender, branching streamers with syncytial character (Boyd & Hamilton, 1960; Uhlendorf & Kaufmann, 1979). As discussed earlier and considered to differ from the earlier views of Park (1959), these are not decidual elements but rather represent residues of invading syncytiotrophoblast.

This layer is the site of placental separation, a mechanism that is not fully understood. Even when separation is a rapid process, taking place within a few minutes, it must be assumed that tissue changes precede its occurrence. From clinical findings it seems likely that placental separation depends on the existence of decidua at the placental site. Where a decidual layer is lacking, as with an extrauterine pregnancy or placenta accreta, the placenta cannot separate spontaneously. We believe that placental separation occurs primarily on a mechanical basis, the contracting uterus shearing off the turgid placenta at the site of degeneration just discussed.

In human specimens of delivered placentas as well as of remaining placental beds, decidual changes can be observed morphologically in the future zone of separation. This phenomenon is also true of rodent placentas in situ. These changes comprise a reduction of collagen fibers, an accumulation of interstitial fluid, and many degenerative changes. Kaiser (1960) reported the preterm reduction in the thickness of the decidual spongy zone from an original 4.0 mm to 0.2 mm. In the guinea pig the prospective separation zone is completely devoid of intact cells 1 to 2 days before parturition. The latter has been replaced by a loosely arranged, net-like deposition of fibrin. It can be interpreted as an attempt to minimize the size of the postpartum wound of the placental bed. After placental separation, both surfaces—those of the placental bed and the basal plate—are covered by a thin layer of fibrin (Ludwig & Metzger, 1971). This covering was interpreted by these authors to be a peripartal or perhaps even postpartal phenomenon.

Development of Uteroplacental Vessels

The basal plate is traversed by maternal uteroplacental vessels, and numerous studies have been undertaken to delineate the maternal vascular supply of the placenta. The early literature, particularly the reports that describe the early connections of the intervillous space with the maternal vessels, are summarized in the large study of Harris and Ramsey (1966).

The first contacts between maternal endometrial vessels and the intraplacental lacunar system become established at around days 11 to 12 p.c. (Boyd & Hamilton, 1970). At this time the first maternal erythrocytes leave the eroded capillaries and enter the trophoblastic lacunae. For humans there is some doubt whether it results in an effective uteroplacental circulation. Boyd and Hamilton (1970) failed to find openings of spiral arteries into the intervillous space, even in the case of an embryo with 28 somites, which corresponds to the 28th to 29th day p.c. Their earliest specimen with such openings was around 40 days old (10 mm crown-rump length), whereas Harris and Ramsey (1966) reported this situation to exist as early as day 30 p.c. (5 mm crown-rump length).

The uteroplacental arteries are branches or direct continuations of myometrial arteries. As soon as they enter the decidua and the basal plate, they are called spiral arteries because of their spiral course. Some authors restrict the name spiral artery to the nonpregnant endometrium and rename the vessel after a placenta is established as the uteroplacental artery. In most publications the terms are used synonymously.

These arteries cross the uterine wall almost perpendicularly up to the 8th week p.m. (Pijnenborg et al., 1980). With advancing gestation, as the placental area enlarges the course of the peripheral arteries becomes more oblique, so that by 10 weeks distal segments are almost parallel to the basal plate. Invading trophoblast breaches these horizonal segments to form new openings into the intervillous space (Harris & Ramsey, 1966). Alteration of the blood flow, which is caused by these new openings, was thought to be the consequence in the most distal segments. Degeneration of the latter can be followed by necrosis of the surrounding decidua. This finding is common in the periphery of the placental site between 8 and 14 weeks of pregnancy. In most instances, obliterated arterial segments can be found within the areas of necrosis. Trophoblastic invasion of the necrotic areas is reduced (Pijnenborg et al., 1980).

The number of spiral arterial turns appears to decrease throughout pregnancy. Intense spiraling, with formation of large loops directly underneath the basal plate, may result in as many as seven openings, one after the other, in consecutive loops of one and the same spiral artery. On the other hand, multiple openings of one artery can also be produced by branching in the superficial layers of the basal plate. Both are common findings in early placentas. Near term, most of these additional openings and branches are apparently obstructed by blood clots, resulting in the final finding of one opening per artery. Some smaller branches (arterioles and venules) may branch off in the deeper layers of the junctional zone and in the superficial myometrial layers. They are nutritional vessels that result in only poorly developed capillary nets.

Number and Position of Uteroplacental Vessels

Comparative studies of the maternal circulations of rhesus monkey and human placentas have shown that they are similar. Thus appropriate deductions can be made from observations in monkeys (Freese, 1968). It is remarkable that, after all these studies, we still do not know the number of spiral arteries that perfuse the placenta. Panigel and Pascaud (1968) reviewed the topic; they wrote that in 1890 Klein found 53 arteries and 31 veins, whereas Spanner in 1934 and 1935 counted 80 to 90 arteries with 488 openings! Franken (1954) described 263 arterial and 79 venous openings. Marais (1962) counted 105 arterial ostia, Reynolds (1966) 40 to 50, and Boyd (1956) 102 to 156 at the end of the first trimester, and about 180 to 320 at term. Brosens (1988) reported 120 spiral arteries for the term placenta, each with a single opening. In contrast to Boyd's observations, Harris and Ramsey (1966) found decreasing numbers of arterial inlets during the course of pregnancy. The final density of arterial openings at term was reported to be one per square centimeter of basal plate surface (Harris & Ramsey, 1966) or 0.5 per square centimeter (Brosens, 1964). Haller (1968) found some 200 to 300 vascular openings in the floor of the delivered placenta; he described their morphology and stated that it was difficult to differentiate between arteries and veins.

Fewer figures have been given for the number of venous openings. Most authors agree that their number is considerably lower than that of the arterial ostia (Franken, 1954; Grünwald, 1966; Boyd & Hamilton, 1970). All these numbers are in disagreement with those of Borell et al. (1965), who, in cineradiographic studies of pregnant women, observed 25 arteries at term. These authors cautioned that erroneous enumeration of placental lobules causes false numbers of arteries.

Many authors now agree that a single decidual spiral artery delivers its blood into the center of a cotyledon, and on occasion lateral vessels add to the supply. This fact has been amply demonstrated by the injection studies of Freese (1968), Freese and Maciolek (1969), Wigglesworth (1969), Panigel and Pascaud (1968), Schuhmann and Wehler (1971), and Schuhmann (1981). Only Grünwald (1966), Nikolov and Schiebler (1973), and Brosens (1988) came to different conclusions. The latter authors found the arteries to open in the periphery of the cotyledons, at the base, or in the lower one-third of the septa. Even more controversial is the finding reported by Bumm in 1890, who believed that the arteries open at the tips of the placental septa. These opinions are not considered further because most authors believe them to be erroneous or functionally irrelevant. For example, Panigel and Pascaud (1968) stated that when an artery is found near the location of the septum the direction of flow from its mouth is toward the center of the cotyledon. The venous openings are thought to be in a more peripheral position of the cotyledons, which is in contrast to the views presented by Spanner (1934, 1935), who concluded that the intervillous venous blood is mainly drained via the marginal venous sinus. This opinion, in turn, has been contradicted by Arts (1961), who found the venous openings more evenly distributed over the basal plate.

It must be pointed out that the idealized arrangement, with one artery opening near the center of a villous tree (see Chapter 8), is rare. It is seen only at the placental periphery, where the average diameter of the cotyledons or lobules is small. Here the numerical relation of villous trees to basally visible lobes is 1:1 (Figure 17). Larger lobules, in particular those of the more central parts of the organ, normally contain two to four villous trees, which usually overlap partially at the margin (Figures 17, 81). Here the position of vascular openings, as they relate to the villous trees, is more confusing and this fact may have contributed to the above controversy.

The villous tissue within the central cotyledonary region, where the maternal "jet" enters, is forcefully separated. This mechanism is supported by the fact that the centers of the villous trees are composed of larger, more immature-appearing villous types. Here they are separated by wider intervillous clefts (Schuhmann & Wehler, 1971; Schuhmann, 1981; Kaufmann, 1985) (Figure 81). This result of pressure gradients is readily seen when a fresh placenta is sectioned. The area shows apparently empty spaces—the central cavities (Ramsey, 1962; Ramsey et al., 1963, 1966; Grünwald, 1966, 1971, 1973; Freese, 1968). Wigglesworth (1969) considered this area to be the site where intervillous thrombi most commonly occur, and we agree. Most intervillous thrombi are fresh and apparently result from local stasis of blood flow during labor. At times one can see that their triangular shape originates from vessels in the placental floor. The villous architecture is draped around these central cavities. Serial roentgenographic studies, with injection of radiopaque dyes, demonstrate them adequately. After these spaces are filled, the radiopaque material is dissipated peripherally, producing the familiar and oft-mentioned "smoke rings" (Freese, 1968).

Structure of Uteroplacental Arteries

The wall of the spiral arteries is characterized by considerable regressive changes that occur over the course of pregnancy. Most impressive is the reduction, or even loss, of elastic fibers (Ramsey & Harris, 1966; Boyd & Hamilton, 1970; Nikolov & Schiebler, 1973). Robertson (1976) and Robertson and Manning (1974) suggested that more elastic fibers develop in these vessels throughout gestation, but because of degenerative processes that are perhaps a consequence of the cytotrophoblast invasion most of these fibers seem to be lost again later.

The reduction of the media, another controversial aspect of placentation, has frequently been discussed. In the older literature the vessels were described as being devoid of smooth muscle cells (Wilkin, 1958; Brettner, 1964; Panigel & Pascaud, 1968). Nikolov and Schiebler (1973) described, via their electron microscopic studies, the existence of up to six layers of smooth muscle cells. A sphincter-like concentration around the arterial ostia, as reported by Spanner (1935), was absent. All subsequent authors reported the partial replacement of smooth musculature by trophoblastic cells (deWolf et al., 1973; Sheppard & Bonnar, 1974b; Brosens, 1988), which was more impressive in the decidual portion of the basal plate than at the more superficial levels (Nikolov & Schiebler, 1973).

According to Brosens et al. (1967), the loss of elastic tissue and muscle cells and the increase in intramural fibrinoid cause transformation of the originally flexible vessels into rigid channels. These channels then lack vasoregulation. The arterial wall becomes significantly altered by infiltrating extravillous trophoblast cells, which invade deeply. Ultrastructural studies have shown that the decidual portions of arteries, and less so the myometrial segments, undergo fibrinoid degeneration (Figure 136). The arteries are essentially destroyed by this infiltration of giant cells; and this tissue destruction contributes to the deposits of the fibrillar material (deWolf et al., 1973).

The accumulation of fibrinoid in the arterial walls has been discussed by Sheppard and Bonnar (1974a) in terms of being related to the presence of cytotrophoblast in this location. An antifibrinolytic activity of trophoblast (Kawano et al., 1968) is said to prevent the enzymatic digestion of fibrin. Wells et al. (1984) have examined the fibrinoid in basal plate vessels with antibodies directed against amnionic basement antigens. They found it to be present in the vascular bed at the site of invasion. Because the antigen was absent from normal trophoblastic cells, they believed it to have been produced by these specialized trophoblastic elements.

The loss of elasticity of the vessel walls, caused by a reduction of elastic fibers and musculature and by an increase in cytotrophoblast and fibrinoid, is paralleled by a considerable increase in their luminal width. The increase is particularly impressive near the intervillous space, where the spiral arteries may finally reach as much as five times their original luminal diameter. Panigel and Pascaud (1968), Boyd and Hamilton (1970), and Sheppard and Bonnar (1974a,b) reported arterial luminal diameters of about 200 μm in the myometrial segments, compared to 500 to 1,000 μm near their opening into intervillous space. The diameter of the arterial ostia may be as much as 2,000 μm. A terminal constriction of the lumens, and in particular a flow-regulating sphincter as described by Spanner (1935) and Debiasi et al. (1963), have been refuted by all subsequent authors.

When the placental bed was examined with antibodies directed against hCG and factor VIII-related antigens, interesting observations were made (Tuttle et al., 1985). Maternal vascular endothelium reacted for factor VIII, as expected, but not for hCG. Surprisingly, many large intravascular cells had factor VIII activity, which suggested that they are endothelium, rather than trophoblast.

The luminal lining of the arteries described by Nikolov and Schiebler (1973) based on electron microscopical observations, is a more or less continuous layer of endothelium. Sheppard and Bonnar (1974a,b, 1988) concluded that a considerable number of the "endothelium-like cells" lining the arterial lumens are in fact cytotrophoblastic in nature. Some of these cells may have reached the vessel surface by invasion across the vessel wall, and others may have entered the lumens from the intervillous space, actively migrating against the blood flow. This view has been supported by the studies of Blankenship et al. (1993a) in rhesus monkeys. The authors did not find any evidence for transmural infiltration of the vessel lumens. Rather, they described intraluminal cytotrophoblastic proliferation. This finding is in contrast to our findings in humans. We must admit, however, that the human material is never so perfectly preserved as macaque material can be. Moreover, as complete a series of stages in regular intervals as was available to Blankenship et al. (1993a) is impossible to obtain from humans. Our findings may therefore not be representative, and we may have missed decisive stages. Applying reliable proliferation markers such as Ki67 or MIB-1, however, we have never found any indication of intravascular trophoblastic proliferation (Figure 137). The only immunostained nuclei were those of endothelial cells. Our findings suggest that trophoblastic invasion of the uteroplacental arteries in humans takes place as the

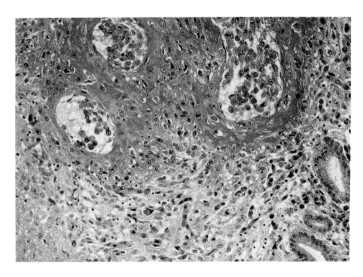

FIGURE 136. Arteries in the basal plate in the same placenta as shown in Figure 117. Note the fibrin in the wall, whose muscular coat is destroyed; the vessels are surrounded and thoroughly infiltrated by extravillous trophoblast cells. The paler cells at the bottom are decidual stromal cells; endometrial glands are at bottom right. H&E. ×160.

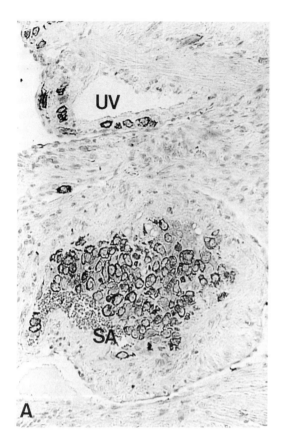

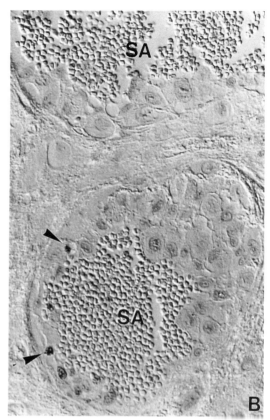

FIGURE 137. Uteroplacental vessels, paraffin sections, 16th week p.m. (A) Stained with an anti-cytokeratin antibody that detects extravillous trophoblast cells (black). The spiral artery (SA) is largely occluded by a plug of intraarterial trophoblast cells. The uteroplacental vein (UV) underneath shows only a few intramural trophoblast cells. ×100. (B) Stained with MIB-1, which binds to the nuclei of proliferating cells. The tropho-blastic plug protruding into the lumens is obviously nonpro-liferative, as are the trophoblast cells lining the upper vessel. The trophoblastic nature of these cells has been proved by anti-cytokeratin staining of a parallel section. The only positive (proliferating) nuclei (arrowheads) belong to cytokeratin-negative (endothelial) cells. ×250. (Courtesy Dr. Gaby Kohnen, Aachen.)

final step of trophoblastic invasion of the basal plate, emanating from the cell columns, as has also been suggested by Kurman et al. (1984a), Damsky et al. (1992), Loke et al. (1992a), and Fisher and Damsky (1993). It is interesting that this mode of transmural invasion was postulated by Blankenship et al. (1993b) for the utero-placental veins of the macaque.

The trophoblastic invasion of the vessels and the subsequent alterations have been designated "physio-logical change" to distinguish them from the changes seen in the placental bed vessels of patients with pre-eclampsia (Brosens et al., 1967). The process has been succinctly reviewed by Ramsey (1981), Brosens (1988), and Sheppard and Bonnar (1988). These significant changes are considered to have important ramifications for ensuring placental perfusion, and they are also seen in many other species with invasive placentation. The trophoblast remodels the spiral arteries into low-resistance vessels that are unable to constrict. Because

of the absence of local regulatory mechanisms in utero-placental vessels, the mother cannot reduce the nutrient supply to the placenta without reducing the nutrient supply to her own tissues (Haig, 1993). The absence of physiological changes of the spiral arteries has been demonstrated to be abnormal (Feinberg et al., 1991a). Often they represent a significant characteristic of hypertension during pregnancy. They are also typically associated with IUGR (Brosens et al., 1972, 1977; Sheppard & Bonnar, 1976; deWolf et al., 1980). Khong et al. (1986a) and Sheppard and Bonnar (1988) have even reported complete absence of such physiological change throughout the length of some of the spiral arteries in cases of preeclampsia and IUGR. Because the average number of spiral arteries entering the intervillous space is also reduced in such cases, Brosens (1988) concluded that it is caused by a general defect in the mechanism of placentation during the first half of pregnancy. It is interesting to note that such cases are characterized additionally by abnormal expression patterns of adhesion molecules by the interstitial extravillous trophoblast (Zhou et al., 1993). This finding also suggests intimate relations between the interstitial and intravascular extravillous trophoblast cells and does not favor the concept of an independent intravascular population.

The trophoblastic invasion of the uteroplacental arteries replacing the maternal endothelium was suggested to be responsible for a minimum nitric oxide synthase (NOS) activity found in these arteries (Morris et al., 1993). According to the authors, the significantly higher NOS activities found in placental villi and in the basal plate suggest that the regulation of uteroplacental blood flow is not dependent on NO production by uterine vessels but is controlled by either exogenous NO or NO produced by placental trophoblast.

In conclusion, even though severely pathological in appearance, these findings demonstrate that the pregnancy-induced vascular changes represent, in fact, the physiological state that is an unavoidable prerequisite for fetoplacental well-being. These vessel changes are typical enough to decide for an intrauterine pregnancy from curettings when villi cannot be found (O'Connor & Kurman, 1988a).

Structure of Uteroplacental Veins

The structure of the uteroplacental veins differs in some minor aspects from that of the spiral arteries. The muscular coat is even more reduced than that of the arteries; and smooth muscle cells are usually absent near the venous openings (Nikolov & Schiebler, 1973). The discontinuous endothelium is surrounded by some connective tissue. Trophoblast cells may be locally absent from the vessel walls (Figure 137A) or may show a low degree of infiltration. In the rhesus monkey, trophoblast cells sometimes have been observed even intraluminally replacing the endothelium in venous segments near the intervillous space (Blankenship et al., 1993b). We have not seen this infiltration in humans by means of immunohistochemistry. Electron microscopically, however, complete penetration of the wall by cytotrophoblast that reaches the venous lumen has been observed (Nikolov & Schiebler, 1973).

Different from the findings of Marais (1962) and Brettner (1964), and in contrast to the usual light microscopic impression (Figure 131C), Nikolov and Schiebler (1973) were unable to find signs of decidualization in the immediate vicinity of the endothelium by means of transmission electron microscopy. They denied direct deciduoendothelial contacts.

Wanner (1966) described that maternal endothelium may even leave the venous lumens and cover the surrounding parts of the basal plate. This finding has been supported immunohistochemically by applying a panel of endothelium-specific antibodies (Lang et al., 1993). Using an antibody directed against the factor VIII-related antigen we found maternal endothelium not only in the vicinity of the venous openings (Figure 138) but also covering other parts of the basal plate (Figure 20C), parts of septa, cell islands, and sometimes even perivillous fibrinoid deposits.

Intraarterial Trophoblast

The remarkable invasion of maternal blood vessels by intraluminal trophoblast has been studied by many investigators. The subject was particularly challenging because for many years the origin of this cellular component was in dispute (Figures 117, 136). Ortmann (1955) was probably the first author to affirm the fetal origin of the cells. He clearly stated that these cells are never found in the decidua vera of pregnant uteri. Proof for this assumption was obtained by Beck and Beck (1967), who, based on sex chromatin counts in rhesus monkey placentas, concluded that the cells are of fetal origin. Hamilton and Boyd (1966), based on their extensive and beautifully illustrated study of 1960, stated emphatically that only the arteries are invaded by trophoblast, whereas the veins are the site of deportation of syncytial buds and occasional villi. The latter, in fact, sometimes can be found histologically in uterine segments of the uteroplacental veins (Figure 139).

It is now no longer in doubt that the arteries of the maternal decidual bed are invaded by trophoblast (Blankenship et al., 1993a). Groups of the intraluminal cells are loosely attached to the vessel walls; most are found near the arterial ostia, and some may even reach the myometrial segments. They seem to be present in all spiral arteries of the basal plate until the end of the second trimester. Their number decreases steeply throughout the last trimester. According to Boyd and Hamilton (1970), these cells are largely absent at term. Although this picture is the histological impression, immunohistochemically we could identify nearly every cell that lines the arterial lumens as being a trophoblast cell, using cytokeratin antibodies (Figure 138B).

There are few immunohistochemical studies concerning functional aspects of the intravascular trophoblast. Most deal with the invasive properties of these cells. In this context it may be of interest that the two proteinase inhibitors, α_1-antitrypsin and α_1-antichymotrypsin, were found to be expressed only in the intraarterial trophoblast cells, whereas the interstitial subpopulation of invasive extravillous trophoblast cells was negative for both inhibitors (Earl et al., 1989). In contrast, however, the latter cells are characterized by considerable protease activity. On the other hand,

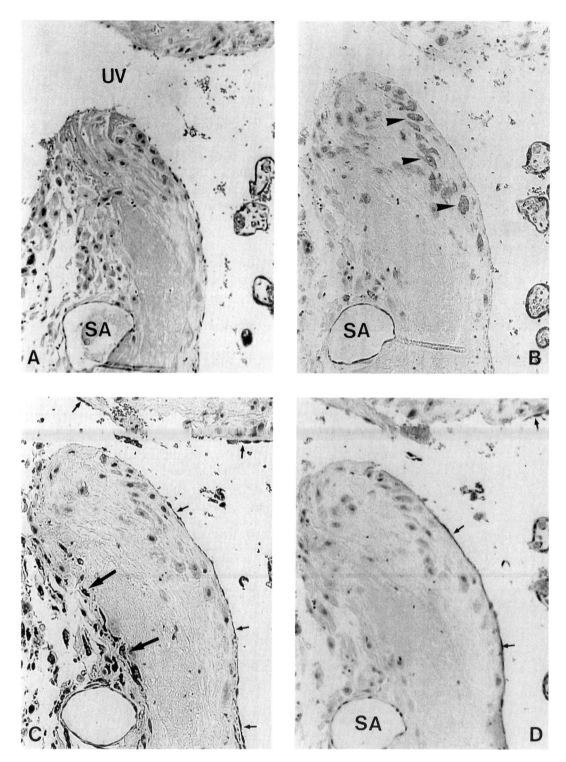

FIGURE 138. Cryostat serial sections of the basal plate of the mature placenta with a cross section of a spiral artery (SA); moreover, the basal plate is passed in full thickness by a uteroplacental vein (UV). (A) Stained with H&E, which does not allow specific identification of the various cellular components. (B) Stained with anti-cytokeratin, which binds to villous syncytiotrophoblast (right), extravillous trophoblast (arrowheads), and the trophoblastic lining of the spiral artery. (C) Stained with anti-vimentin, a marker for mesenchymal derivatives. It stains decidual cells (large arrows) and maternal endothelium lining the venous opening and spreading over the surface of the basal plate (small arrows). (D) Stained with anti-factor VIII-related antigen, a specific endothelial marker. Note the absence of staining from the wall of the spiral artery (SA) but the presence of maternal endothelium at the basal plate surface (small arrows). ×80. All sections are counterstained with hematoxylin so all nuclei appear dark. (Courtesy Dr. Sonya Kertschanska, Aachen.)

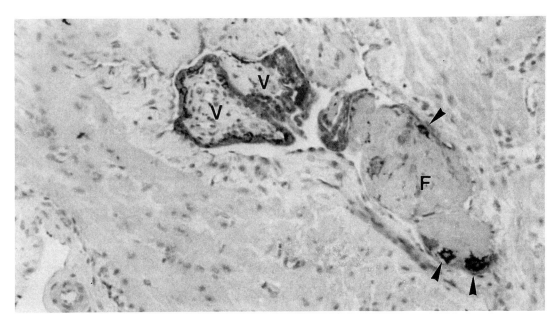

FIGURE 139. Myometrial vein from a 16th week pregnant uterus. The vein is blocked by two placental villi (V), which are lined by trophoblast (dark anti-cytokeratin staining), and by a large fibrinoid conglomerate (F) that contains three cytokeratin-positive extravillous trophoblast cells (arrowheads). Paraffin section. ×80. (Courtesy Dr. Gaby Kohnen, Aachen.)

interstitial collagenase was also present in the intra-arterial trophoblast (Moll & Lane, 1990).

Other immunohistochemical studies comprised the endocrine characterization of these cells. Gosseye and Fox (1984) found hPL expression but neither hCG nor secretory proteins such as PAPP-A, SP-1, or PP5.

In attempts to characterize the intraarterial cells by means of lectin histochemistry, Thrower et al. (1991) tested a large panel of such lectins. Among them, *Lens culinaris* A (LCH-A) reacted with columnar cytotrophoblast but not with the more highly differentiated extravillous trophoblast cells in the basal plate and in the arteries. On the other hand, *Griffonia simplicifolia* (GSI and GSII) bound preferentially to all types of extravillous trophoblast and only rarely to the villous trophoblast.

A provocative and challenging study with ultrasonography, histology, and barium injection of the maternal plate has come from Hustin and Schaaps (1987, 1988) and Schaaps and Hustin (1988). They had earlier observed that chorionic villous biopsies are always bloodless. They also found no echogenic evidence of intervillous blood flow before 13 weeks' gestation. Moreover, when they were able to observe the placenta in vivo during the first trimester it was pale, and barium could not be forced into the intervillous space. Furthermore, few maternal blood cells were ever observed histologically in this area. Hustin and Schaaps suggested that the intraarterial trophoblast so much obstructs the arterial lumen (Figure 136) that only filtered plasma reaches the intervillous space before 12 weeks' gestation. Careful inspection of sections from such immature placentas (Figures 113, 116, 117, 136) indeed showed a lack of red blood cells in our cases as well, at least those derived from normal pregnancies. Only in some pathological cases have we found erythrocytes in the intervillous space.

This novel hypothesis of uteroplacental circulation is one of the most interesting aspects of current histopathological investigations in the placenta. It necessitates reevaluation of the physiological implications that such plasma perfusion of the intervillous space might have for embryonic development. For instance, does plasma carry sufficient oxygen, or is relative hypoxia an important modulator of trophoblast behavior? Furthermore, because it is during these stages of embryonic development that most congenital anomalies are determined, how are teratogens transported to the embryo? Many more challenging avenues for investigations have been opened by this study.

Intramural Fibrinoid of Uteroplacental Arteries and Veins

Sheppard and Bonnar (1974a,b, 1988) and Bonnar and Sheppard (1977) described typical fibrin with a 200 Å cross-striation in all layers of these vessel walls. They observed intraluminal fibrin thrombi attached to the intimal lining and noted that muscular and elastic components of the vessel walls may be replaced by fibrin.

Whether the deposition is caused by increased fibrin polymerization or by decreased fibrinolytic activity is a matter of dispute. Endothelium is well known to have fibrinolytic activity. The endothelium of the utero-placental arteries, however, becomes largely replaced by trophoblast during pregnancy. According to Sheppard and Bonnar (1974a,b), trophoblast is suggested to be a potent source of antifibrinolytic activity.

Functional Aspects of Uteroplacental Vessels

It is difficult to assign a specific function to intraarterial cytotrophoblast. Boyd and Hamilton (1970) speculated that the arteries have lost their contractility owing to the physiological changes of their walls. The persistence of such cytotrophoblastic aggregates within the lumens suggests that the blood pressure cannot be high, otherwise the cytotrophoblast would be dislodged; and the authors speculated that the intravascular cell masses could conceivably dampen the arterial pressure.

This view is in partial agreement with the results of physiological experiments (Moll et al., 1988). During the course of pregnancy, the flow resistance is decreased by structural widening of the lumens of the uterine and terminal spiral arteries, so the maternal blood supply to the placenta is adjusted to fetal growth. When comparing parameters such as blood flow velocity, arterial widening, and timing of trophoblast invasion in rats and guinea pigs, it was found that the vascular changes proceed normally, even under conditions of reduced blood flow. They appeared earlier than the trophoblastic invasion, and they could be induced by long-term estradiol treatment. Moll et al. (1988) concluded that the changes in luminal width are not induced by the intraluminal trophoblast invasion but, rather, by hormonal factors.

The increased arterial diameters, together with trophoblastic aggregates, may guarantee sufficient uteroplacental blood flow volumes, thus preventing excessively high blood pressures in the intervillous space. Only a balance between the intervillous maternal blood pressure and the intravillous fetal blood pressure keeps the fetal vessels open and allows intravillous fetal circulation.

As is known from experimental studies in the guinea pig (Kaufmann et al., 1982) and in the isolated, dually perfused human cotyledon (Kaufmann, 1985), elevation of fetal blood pressure results in filtration through fetal vessels and finally in villous edema. A maternal intervillous blood pressure that considerably exceeds the fetal blood pressure leads to compression of villi. Thus the only realistic consequence is a reduction of the

intervillous blood pressure to that of the fetus. All pregnancy-induced physiological changes of the spiral arteries must be seen in the light of such considerations.

Septa

Placental septa are irregular structures composed of fibrinoid and various cell types (Figures 113, 114, 140) that arise from the basal plate and protrude into the intervillous space during the expansive growth of the placenta. Boyd and Hamilton (1966) provided a detailed historical and analytical description of these unusual structures. They found that the earliest formation of septa occurred late during the third month of development. In our opinion, this process may start even earlier. The septum depicted in Figure 141 was found in a placenta at the 8th week p.m. In specimens that were 2 weeks younger, we had already observed short basal plate protrusions into the intervillous space that were

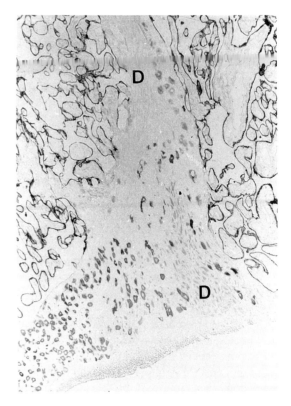

FIGURE 140. Placental septum (center and above) resting on the basal plate (below) at the 40th week p.m. From this glucose-6-phosphate dehydrogenase reaction it is evident that the faintly stained decidual cells (D) extend from the basal plate into the septum. Ample numbers of anchoring villi are attched to the septum. These similarities of basal plate and septum support the theory that the septa result from folding of the basal plate. Cryostat section. ×65.

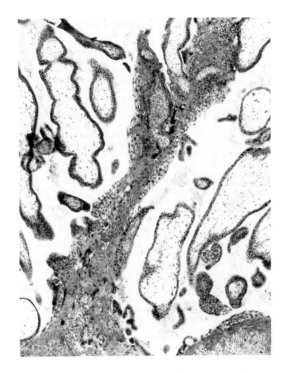

FIGURE 141. Early placental septum (middle) during the 8th week p.m. In this stage the septa have a cellular composition similar to that of the early basal plate (see Figure 131.) As in the latter, they are largely devoid of fibrinoid and can be interpreted as being extensions and folds of the early basal plate. Paraffin section. ×90.

composed of cytotrophoblastic cells, likely precursors of future septa.

Septa can be found in nearly every mature placenta. Absence of septa is a rare event that usually is linked to pathological conditions (Figure 142). The fetus of the placenta shown in Figure 142 had hygroma and X monosomy. True septa are also absent from abdominal pregnancies.

Structurally speaking, septa are irregular plates, or pillars, that partially subdivide the intervillous space. Their position normally corresponds to that of the grooves visible at the basal surface of the delivered placenta (Wilkin, 1958) (Figures 16, 143)—hence their designation "intercotyledonary septa." Many observers, such as Spanner (1935), Stieve (1940), Stieve and von der Heide (1941), have suggested that septa partly serve as subdivisions of intervillous blood flow, and these authors' famous drawings depicted chamber-like compartments of the intervillous space.

Based on dissection studies, Becker (1962) and Becker and Jipp (1963) rejected this concept. They found that septa never subdivide truly functional units of placental tissue. Moreover, most often they were found to be rather shallow "vela," measuring 12 to 18 mm in height, originating from the floor of the

placenta, and rarely reaching the fetal surface. They represent furrows or folds in the maternal surface or basal decidua, rather than complete septations of the villous tissue.

Inasmuch as there is only limited growth of decidual cells during placental development, Boyd and Hamilton (1966) suggested that septa probably result from buckling of the basal decidua. They envisaged this buckling to be induced by the pressures of expanding villous lobules and found further support for this idea from the relative paucity of villous attachments on only one side of the septa. When the septa are dissected, this side is found to be much smoother than the other.

When we studied early specimens from the 6th to 8th weeks p.m., which showed the first signs of septal formation (Figure 141), we found them to be composed of cytotrophoblast. Occasional multinucleated giant cells may be interspersed, and anchoring villi can often be observed near their tips (Figure 141). We concluded therefore that one of the initial causes of septum formation is traction of these anchoring villi combined with excessive proliferation of their cytotrophoblastic feet. Later, a considerable admixture of decidua can be found (Figures 140, 143). The latter cells prevail at the base of the septa. As was already discussed, it is likely that the combination of septa with groves in the basal plate (Figure 143) is a consequence of secondary folding of the basal plate along those points where the cytotrophoblastic septal precursors originate. This process can be induced by lateral movements between uterine wall and basal plate and is due to placental growth.

According to this concept of their genesis, it is understandable that septa in every respect resemble the basal

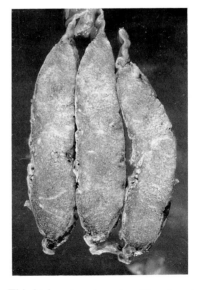

FIGURE 142. Third trimester placenta without septa or folds of the maternal floor. This placenta comes from a 45,X fetus with a hygroma.

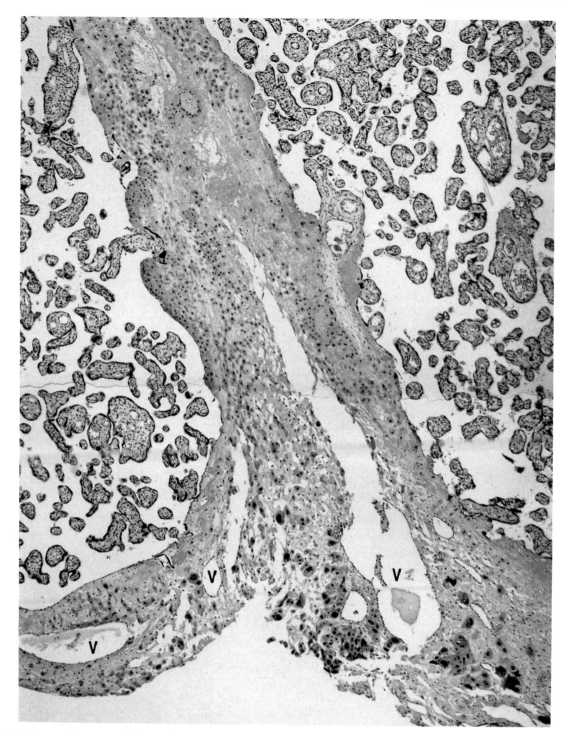

FIGURE 143. Placental septum, 37th week p.m. Note the numerous anchoring villi inserting at the septum. In its base several vessel cross sections (V) represent uteroplacental veins. Paraffin section. ×65.

plate. They are composed of both decidual cells and extravillous trophoblast cells embedded in matrix-type fibrinoid and are partly surrounded by fibrin-type fibrinoid. Anchoring villi are attached to the septa by means of cell columns, the latter representing the foci of extravillous trophoblastic proliferation. In addition,

the septa may contain all other basal plate constituents, such as glands (Figure 143) and vessels. Brosens (1988) interpreted the latter to be predominantly spiral arteries, which is in disagreement with current views. The vessels depicted in the septal base of Figure 143 are more likely veins.

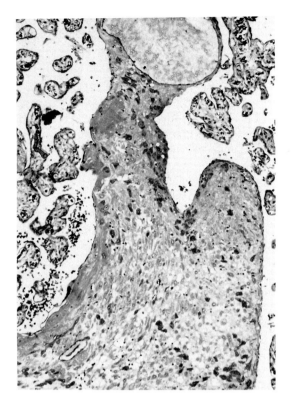

FIGURE 144. Intercotyledonary septum with a cyst at its tip (top center). The darker cells are extravillous trophoblast cells, which are intermingled with a larger number of decidua cells. Note that Rohr's fibrin stria (at left) follows the outline of the septum. H&E. ×80.

The ultrastructure of septa has been described in much detail by Glienke (1974). Another ultrastructural study of septa by Demir and Erbengi (1984) distinguished five cell types but did not draw conclusions as to their origin.

Whereas in the early stages of pregnancy (Figure 141) the septa are composed only of cells, with advancing gestation cellular degeneration occurs, resulting in the accumulation of much cellular debris, which is incorporated into fibrinoid. At term, the latter is normally the predominant element of septa.

Septa are a frequent site of placental cysts (Figures 144, 145). Macroscopically identifiable cysts are less common, but microscopically one finds septal cysts in nearly every placenta. Wieloch (1923) described such cysts as artifacts. Stieve and von der Heide (1941) identified trophoblastic necrosis in the walls of septa and concluded that it is the causal mechanism of cysts. Hörmann (1966) came to similar conclusions. In his studies of what he called "pseudocysts," however, the degenerating cell population is decidua. Schwartz et al. (1973) described the cysts to be the result of cellular necrosis and liquefaction. Additional transudation, as a result of hyperosmolar conditions inside these foci, may be responsible for further growth. In our material, large cysts are the exception. In many cases, particularly near the base, we found irregular clefts (Figure 143), which can be interpreted to have resulted from laceration of intercellular debris and fibrinoid during labor. On the other hand, cysts with well developed cellular walls and similar to the cysts of the cell islands (Figure 148B) are not mechanically induced artifacts.

Cell Islands

Cell islands are macroscopically round or irregularly shaped white structures connected to either the villous tree or the chorionic plate. Their diameter varies between several hundred micrometers and 3 mm. As the name implies, they are composed primarily of

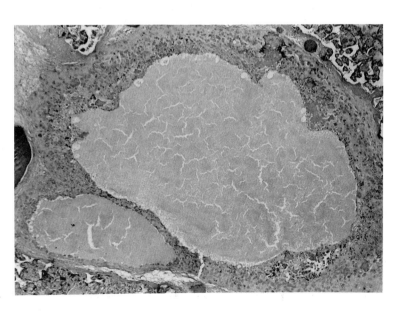

FIGURE 145. Septum with cystic centers. H&E. ×40.

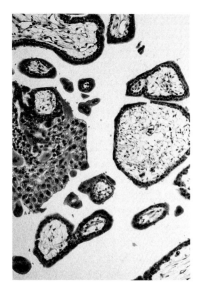

FIGURE 146. Placenta from a tubal ectopic pregnancy at 5 weeks' gestation. A cluster of extravillous trophoblast cells forming an early cell island is shown above, attached to villi and interspersed with syncytiotrophoblast. No interstitial "fibrinoid" is present as yet. H&E. ×240.

extravillous trophoblast cells (Figure 146) that with advancing gestation are encased in increasing amounts of fibrinoid (Figure 147). Fetal or maternal vessels are absent. They resemble septa in structure and composition. When one uses histological sections, it cannot be excluded that apparent cell islands are in fact tangential or cross sections of septa.

Most authors agree that cell islands are derived from trophoblast, without an admixture of decidual cells (Spanner, 1935, 1941; Stieve, 1936; Ortmann, 1955, 1960). A decidual origin had been considered only for a short time (Hörmann, 1966). This assumption was based mainly on the sex chromatin studies of Klinger and Ludwig (1957) and on the finding of reticular fibers that surround the cells (Waidl, 1963). As is discussed in much detail in this chapter, these results were revised when Steininger (1978) provided proof for their trophoblastic genesis using quinacrine fluorescence of the Y chromosome.

Steininger also described a small number of cell islands in which both decidual and trophoblast cells were present. It is likely that these islands represent either cross sectioned tips of septa or former portions of septa that during placental development by traction of anchoring villi have been be detached from the septum. Numerous intraseptal clefts indicate that such forces can be active.

The basophilia of the extravillous trophoblast cells, an expression of a richly developed rough endoplasmic reticulum, led investigators to believe that these cells are a potent source of protein hormones, such as hCG

(Ortmann, 1955, 1960; Bargmann, 1957). Boyd and Hamilton (1970) favored an endocrine function of the X cells as well. In this respect they are fully comparable to extravillous trophoblast cells of other origin.

Krönicher (1975) presented a detailed ultrastructural description of the cell islands from early to late pregnancy. He reported different stages of cytotrophoblastic differentiation in the trophoblastic islands. In particular, when studying cell islands from the second and third months, one does not get the impression that they are degenerative or useless groups of cells. Arnholdt and Löhrs (1989) demonstrated a high mitotic rate in the cells, and Boe (1967) had earlier pointed to their proliferative character. Boe studied the cell islands in placentas from therapeutic abortions. He believed that the extravillous trophoblast cells derive from the fusion of "erupted" proliferative masses of cytotrophoblast originating in anchoring villi. The process was well illustrated in his paper. The process of "eruption" removes the syncytial surface cells. Thereafter the X cells proliferate and aggregate to become islands. Only subsequently do they become progressively surrounded by "fibrinoid."

When we studied early placentas, we found such eruptive cytotrophoblast masses not only in and near the anchoring villi but also nearer the chorionic plate connected to villous tips (Figures 82, 83). They correspond to persistent primary villi that have not been occupied by villous stroma. They are comparable to the basal ends of the anchoring villi, the "cell columns."

This view has been supported by several cell biological and in vitro studies (e.g., Castellucci et al., 1991;

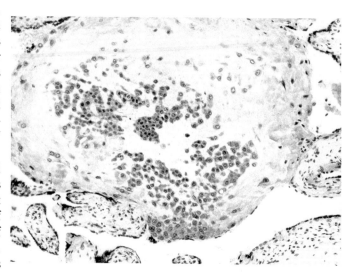

FIGURE 147. Cell island at 20 weeks' gestation. The mononuclear cells with dark cytoplasm in the center are the extravillous trophoblast cells. They are surrounded by "fibrinoid." Note that there is no differentiation to syncytium among the extravillous trophoblast cells. H&E. ×160.

Genbacev et al., 1993b; Mühlhauser et al., 1993). All these studies concluded that the major difference between a cell island and a cell column is the topographical relation: Cell islands are freely floating cell columns; cell columns in the narrow sense of the name are anchored to the basal plate or to septa. A further immunological difference may be derived from the fact that the proliferating extravillous trophoblast of cell columns invades decidual tissues, whereas that of the cell islands accumulates and finally degenerates under formation of cysts (Figure 148) without contact to maternal tissues. Otherwise both structures are comparable.

Cell Columns

The infiltration of primary villi by extraembryonic mesenchyme begins at around day 15 p.c. and originates from the chorionic plate (Figures 24e,f). It is followed by capillarization of the connective tissue, which then results in formation of the tertiary villi. Both processes spread from the chorionic plate peripherally but do not reach the basal plate via the anchoring villi. Rather, the basal feet of the villous stems, the anchoring villi, which connect the latter to the basal plate, persist in the primary villous stage. These segments of the anchoring villi are called cell columns. These developmental events are identical to those at some free-floating villous tips, leading to the formation of cell islands. The cell columns have been the topic of electron microscopic (Enders, 1968; Larsen & Knoth, 1971; Okudaira et al., 1971, 1991), enzyme-histochemical (Stark & Kaufmann, 1971), immuno-histochemical (Okudaira et al., 1971; Feinberg et al., 1989, 1991b; Castellucci et al., 1991, 1993a; Librach et al., 1991; Damsky et al., 1992; Fisher & Damsky, 1993; Mühlhauser et al., 1993; Zhou et al., 1993), and numerous in vitro studies (e.g., Genbacev et al., 1992, 1993a,c). This particular interest is due to the fact that they represent the most impressive proliferation zones of extravillous trophoblast, and that the various steps from trophoblastic proliferation via differentiation to invasion cannot be so easily studied anywhere else.

In this chapter we only briefly deal with their histological appearance. All cell biological and functional aspects have been dealt with earlier in the chapter.

Cell columns are composed of a multilayered core of cytotrophoblast surrounded by an incomplete sleeve of syncytiotrophoblast (Figures 18I, 206) (Enders, 1968; Boyd & Hamilton, 1970; Larsen & Knoth, 1971; Okudaira et al., 1971). As soon as cell columns are surrounded by fibrinoid and thus buried in the basal plate, their syncytiotrophoblastic cover becomes replaced by fibrinoid (Figure 150B) (Stark & Kaufmann,

1971). The cytotrophoblastic core continues without sharp demarcation into the Langhans' layer of the anchoring villus at one side (Figure 149); on the opposite side, it is connected to loose streamers of extravillous trophoblast.

There is a sharp demarcation against the stroma of the anchoring villus (Figure 149). Electron microscopically, it is represented by a basal lamina (Enders, 1968; Okudaira et al., 1971) that represents the indispensable pad for trophoblastic proliferation of this zone (Arnholdt et al., 1991; Castellucci et al., 1993a,b; Mühlhauser et al., 1993). Okudaira et al. (1971, 1991) pointed to the varying degrees of cytotrophoblastic differentiation. These authors used the term "intermediate trophoblast" for more highly differentiated cytotrophoblast that had not syncytially fused.

As has already been discussed, the cell columns function primarily as growth zones, the cytotrophoblast of which proliferates and subsequently migrates in either a chorionic direction (into the anchoring villi), or in a basal direction (into the basal plate). Thus it contributes to the growth of both adjacent tissues. With advancing gestation, the cellular layer of the cell columns is reduced by decreasing proliferative activity but continuous migration of the trophoblast (Figures 150A,B). Sometimes there are almost no trophoblast cells left, so anchoring villous stroma directly faces basal plate fibrinoid (Figure 19I). Because of this situation, Baker et al. (1944) and Ortmann (1960) reported that the cell columns disappear at the end of the third month of pregnancy, but this proposal is certainly incorrect.

Cysts and Breus' Mole

Placental cysts occur in many normal placentas. They may be found in the placental septa, in cell islands, and under the fetal surface. In addition, there are cystic structures in placental villi. The latter have a completely different pathogenesis and are largely ignored in this context; they are further considered in Chapters 21 and 22.

Also present and having a somewhat overlapping quality are liquefying hematomas (Breus' mole), which may occur in the subchorionic space of the placenta. They are included for discussion here merely for convenience, as they are not related to the common cysts of the mature placenta. Shipley and Nelson (1993) undertook a detailed chemical analysis of cyst fluid from a large (4 cm) prenatally diagnosed subchorionic cyst. They compared the content of many components with those of amnionic fluid, cord, and maternal serum. Unusually high concentrations of iron, aspartate and alanine aminotransferases, and lactic dehydrogenase were found in the fluid.

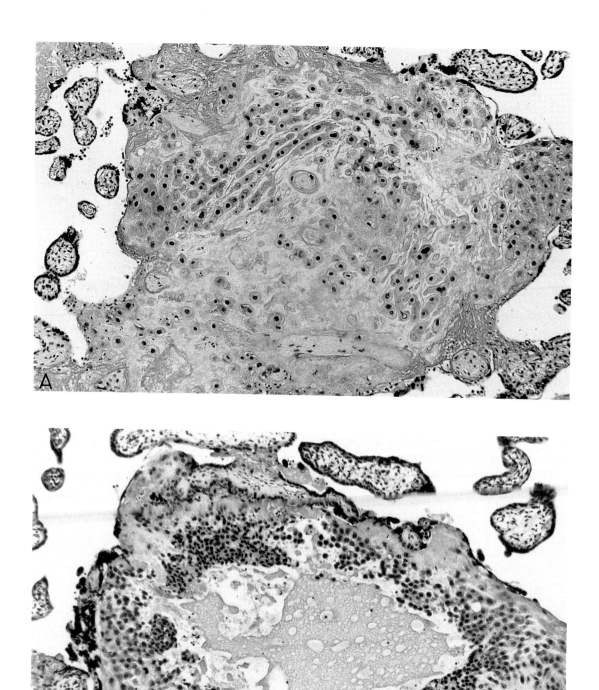

FIGURE 148. Cell islands. (A) At the 37th week p.m. the cell island is largely composed of a fibrinoid matrix in which strings of proliferating cytotrophoblastic cells are embedded. Incorporated decidual cells are rare findings. The surrounding placental villi may be attached to the surface; sometimes they are incorporated into the fibrinoid. Note the heterogeneous structure of the darker superficial patches of fibrin-type fibrinoid compared to the glossy, lighter matrix-type fibrinoid that makes up the center of the cell island. Paraffin section. ×110. (B) At the 19th week p.m. In the centers of large cell islands are central cavities, or "cysts." They must be considered to be the result of degeneration with subsequent liquefaction. Note two "anchoring villi" attached to this island (above and bottom right). The trophoblast cells lining the border from cell island to anchoring villus represent the proliferating subpopulation, comparable to cell columns. Paraffin section. ×120. (From Kaufmann, 1981, with permission.)

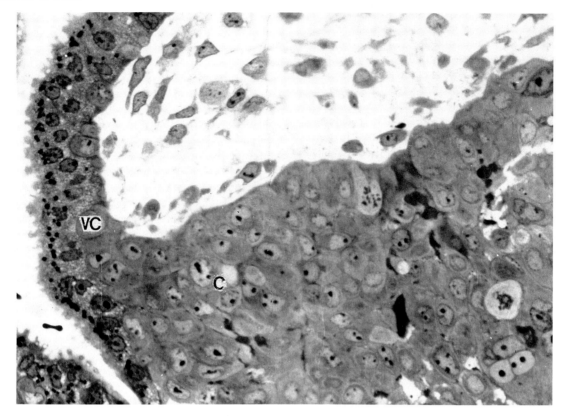

FIGURE 149. At the 22nd week p.m. Note the transition between the anchoring villus (above) and the cell column (below). The continuity of villous cytotrophoblast (VC) with the proliferating cluster of cytotrophoblast in the cell column (C) is clearly visible. Semithin section. ×800.

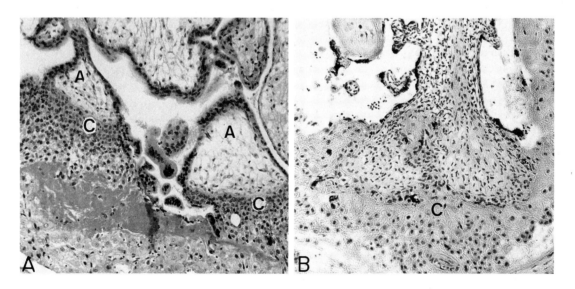

FIGURE 150. Histology of cell columns. (A) At the 15th week p.m. During the early stages of pregnancy the anchoring villi (A) are connected to the basal plate (below) by broad or slender feet consisting of cytotrophoblast, the so-called cell columns (C). They are proliferative zones for the villous trophoblast as well as for the trophoblast of the basal plate. Paraffin section. ×95. (B) At the 28th week p.m. During later stages of pregnancy the cell columns are deeply incorporated into the basal plate by surrounding fibrinoid deposition. Also, its cytotrophoblast is progressively replaced by fibrinoid, indicating reduced proliferative activity of these growth zones. A final stage of this process is depicted in Figure 19I. Paraffin section. ×95. (From Kaufmann, 1981, with permission.)

Placental cysts may be numerous and large (Figure 151). Although the cysts probably have no clinical significance—at least none is recognized as yet—their origin is interesting and has been a matter of controversy. The cells that produce the cysts have also had a varied nomenclature, as they were often mistaken for decidual cells. The cells that produce the cysts and the biochemical features of their viscid, mucin-like product have now been examined more closely. Grosser (1927) considered placental cysts to represent a special form of trophoblastic degeneration. He equated cyst formation with a process of fibrinoid degeneration. Bret et al. (1960) beautifully illustrated these structures in a study of 589 placental cysts and provided an extensive literature review. Cysts have been as large as a fetal head on rare occasion. Sanguineous material is often included, mixed with the normally "serous" content of cysts.

There are thus three principal types of cysts in the placenta. One is a *cystic "degeneration" of villi.* In this form (Figure 152) some villi distend remarkably with fluid. More commonly, however, the villous edema involves scattered areas of the placenta, and the process is related to a hydatidiform mole. It is also commonly found in triploid conceptuses and is then referred to as a "partial" mole. Partial moles are considered in Chapter 22.

Next, *cystic "degeneration" of subchorionic intervillous thrombi* occurs. Laminated thrombi form almost regularly and in small quantities in the subchorionic

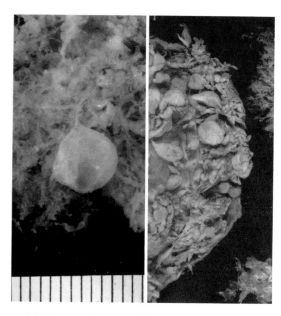

FIGURE 152. Two variants of villous "cysts," actually hydropic changes of villi. All are triploid conceptuses at different stages of gestation. The cysts are actually within villous tissue.

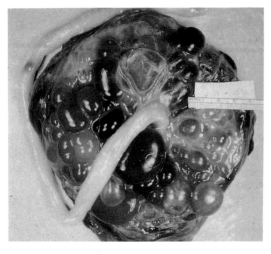

FIGURE 151. Multiple subchorionic cysts in a near-term placenta. Many cysts were discolored (red, brown, green) due to prior hemorrhage. The placenta had typical "maternal floor infarction." This was the fifth pregnancy in this patient that was so affected.

space. It is at this site that the intervillous (maternal) blood is deflected backward. Most likely, eddying of intervillous blood accounts for the deposition of the small amounts of fibrin that accumulate here. This process leads to the formation of some white patches of subchorionic fibrin and to the bosselation (tessellation) of the fetal surface of the placenta. The fibrin accumulations increase with maturation, and much more thrombotic material accumulates underneath the chorion in some abnormal placentas.

It is more often found when maternal circulatory disorders exist; we have seen it repeatedly, for instance, in mothers with complex heart disease. These large patches of subchorionic coagulation may protrude on the fetal surface; and when they contract, fluid may be extruded from the clot. In this way, cysts can develop that contain old clot (Figure 153). Some of these subchorionic cystic hematomas have been so large they were diagnosed antenatally by sonography (Kirkinen & Jouppila, 1986). In one of the cases reported by Kirkinen and Jouppila, Doppler velocimetry of blood flow in the umbilical cord identified that the hematoma, having dissected into the base of the cord, caused venous obstruction to blood flow. It was also the cause of furcate cord insertion.

On rare occasions, cysts with this macroscopic appearance contain a fetus papyraceus. This type of cyst is akin to the Breus mole (Figure 154). Breus (1892) had described these lesions in five cases of missed abortions. He interpreted them to be sacculations ("diverticula")

FIGURE 153. Term placenta with a large sub-chorionic intervillous thrombus that had liquefied and produced a protruding cyst. When the cyst was opened, it contained clot, contiguous with the intervillous space.

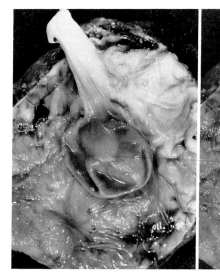

produced by the continued intervillous blood pressure against a decreased amniotic sac pressure. He believed that the membranous cover continues to grow after fetal death, and he called the lesion a subchorionic tuberous hematoma, wanting to differentiate it from hydatidiform moles.

The term Breus "mole," however, is confusing. It has to do with mass, rather than the process of molar degeneration as seen in hydatidiform moles. Torpin (1960, 1966) referred to these coagula as hematoma moles and related them to circumvallate placentas. He suggested that abnormally deep implantation is their cause. Linthwaite (1963) conjectured that this placental abnormality precedes fetal demise. This view and "excessive implantation" were upheld by Thomas (1964). He cited authors who disagreed with Breus' opinion, an aspect that was comprehensively discussed in the report by Shanklin and Scott (1975), who studied 10 cases past 25 weeks' gestation. Seven infants were liveborn, but only three survived the neonatal period. These findings argue strongly against the view that fetal death is primary in the development of the tuberous subchorionic hematoma. The authors also reviewed case reports that supported their opinion. Their incidence was 1:1,200 placentas. Many of their patients had various diseases, including diabetes and hypertension. Despite these observations and their meticulous illustrations, no unified etiology for subchorionic tuberous hematomas emerged from this study.

Breus mole apparently is more commonly associated with monosomy X (45,X, or Turner syndrome) (Figure 154) (see also Perrin, 1984). It is always a benign condition; and although it correlates with missed abortion, it is not limited to it, as Breus had suggested.

Finally, there are *true cysts* (Figures 155, 156) which are the principal focus of this discussion. These cysts

are often blood-tinged, frequently multiple, and most often found in mature placentas. Their frequency is more difficult to ascertain. In our experience, about 5% of mature placentas have surface cysts of varying size. We find a much higher percentage of septal and cell island cysts, provided the placentas are sliced at thin intervals. Paddock and Greer (1927) found 14% in a macroscopic study of 1,965 placentas; Carter et al. (1963) found 7% subchorial and 17% septal cysts in 400 mature placentas they examined for vascular lesions. Cysts may originate below chorial vessels and elevate them much above the rest of the fetal surface. There is no evidence, however, that it compromises the fetal circulation (Bret et al., 1960).

Subchorial cysts are rarely encountered at the margin of the placenta (Figure 157), and they have not been

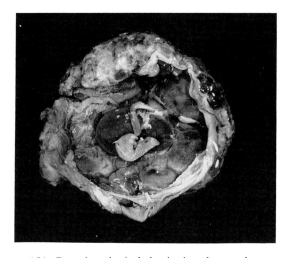

FIGURE 154. Breus' mole (subchorionic tuberous hematoma) in an immature placenta from a "missed abortion." Note the numerous blood-filled protrusions on the surface.

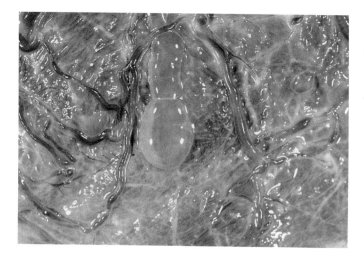

FIGURE 155. Multicameral subchorionic cysts issuing from subchorionic deposits of extravillous trophoblast cells in a mature placenta.

noted to occur on the extraplacental membranes. These cysts arise from the same extravillous trophoblast cells at the margin of the placenta that surrounds the entire membranous sac.

Cysts are most commonly found in placental septa (Figures 144, 145, 158–160) and in the cell islands (Figure 148B) of mature placentas. They contain a colorless, thin fluid that is frequently slightly mucinous in character. Real mucin, however, is not found. The fluid is a rich source of MBP. The rich protein content of these cysts is evident by the precipitate found in histological sections (Figure 161). Paddock and Greer (1927) likened the content of cysts to colloid, and Grosser (1927) wrote of "colliquation necrosis" as the origin of the cystic fluid. It has been the experience of many writers that X cell cysts are particularly often found in placentas that have "fibrinoid degeneration."

Thus in maternal floor infarction, an unusual condition to be discussed later in this chapter, an excessive number of cysts surrounded by extravillous trophoblast is typical (Figures 151, 161). Their lining is irregular and ragged. Spaces develop between the extravillous trophoblast cells during their expansion, and they ultimately coalesce to make cysts.

According to Soma et al. (1991) increased numbers of X cell cysts can be found in placentas from high altitude (Tibet and Nepal). This finding supports the view that cyst formation is a result of degenerative processes due to malnutrition and hypoxia in the centers of large accumulations of extravillous trophoblast. Further support is derived from the fact that cysts are formed within the extravillous trophoblast of the chorionic plate, septa, and cell islands, rather than in that of the basal plate, the difference being that in the basal plate the extravillous trophoblast cells are intermingled with macrophages. These macrophages might easily remove degenerative products by phagocytosis and thus avoid liquefaction of degenerative masses.

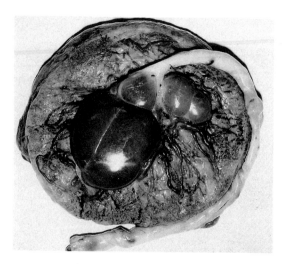

FIGURE 156. Large subchorial cysts, some discolored by blood, in a mature placenta. Note that one of the cysts dissects into the base of the umbilical cord. They may cause compression of vessels.

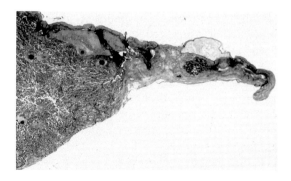

FIGURE 157. Subchorial cyst on membranes near the edge of the placental disk. It overlies an area of placental atrophy. H&E. ×2.

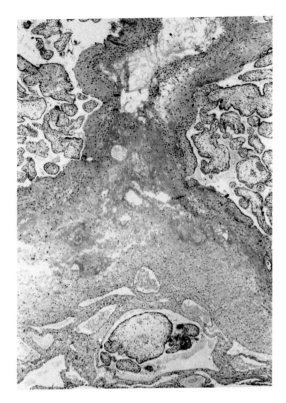

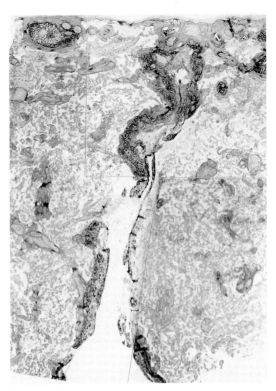

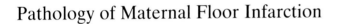

FIGURE 158. Placental floor with the origin of a septum of a near-term placenta. The septum shows cystic cavitation in extravillous trophoblast cell deposits. H&E. ×60.

Pathology of Maternal Floor Infarction

In maternal floor infarction (MFI), the floor of the placenta is thick, stiffened, and often yellow. The maternal surface has a corrugated appearance, and the placental septa are prominent (Figure 162). Often the lesion is associated with excessive proliferation of

FIGURE 159. Placental septum that reaches the chorionic surface (top). The intercellular substance has been stained dark (purple) with aldehyde fuchsin (Waidl, 1963). At top left and in the top portion of the septum are small cysts developing in subchorial deposits of extravillous trophoblast cells. Aldehydefuchsin. ×8. Montage.

extravillous trophoblast cells and cyst formation (Figure 163). Frequently, but not always, there is a massive net-like fibrin deposition throughout the placental tissue as well, occasionally referred to as *Gitterinfarkt* or *Netzinfarkt* in the German literature (Figures 164, 165)

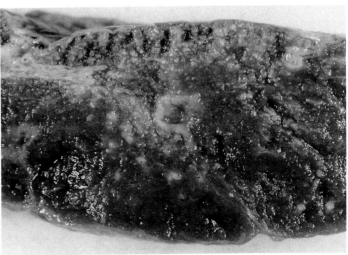

FIGURE 160. Typical septal cyst. Note that it is in the center of the placenta, at the tip of the partial septum.

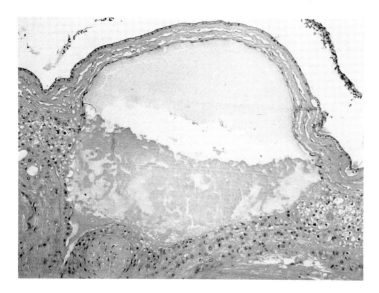

FIGURE 161. Subchorionic X cell cyst of the placenta. Note that the cyst contains precipitated protein. H&E. ×40.

(Becker, 1981). The same features occur also in association with villitis of unknown etiology (see Chapter 20). The placenta in MFI is often small and firm, and no other major pathological lesions are evident when it is sectioned. MFI is not associated with abruption, but IUGR is often a sequela. Most importantly, the condition may lead to fetal death, and it recurs frequently during subsequent pregnancies.

One patient seen by us had nine consecutive losses due to MFI. With other patients in whom the lesion had previously occurred, the anticipation of its recurrence has led to intense fetal monitoring, including an evaluation of estriol excretion. Twice, when fetal activity declined, Clewell and Manchester (1983) were able to obtain a living fetus by cesarean section. The placenta

had the same changes as those of the original descriptions of MFI (Benirschke, 1961; Benirschke & Driscoll, 1967), which strongly argues against the notion, expressed by Fox (1978), that MFI is a postmortem change of the placenta of stillborns. Likewise, Katz and colleagues (1987) found typical MFI in a patient whose baby survived and did well. That patient had previously had three abortions and one abruptio placentae with stillbirth. All of her placentas had excessive fibrin deposits. The patient had chronic hypertension; during the last pregnancy there was IUGR, and a 7.2-fold elevation of α-fetoprotein (AFP) was detected beginning at 17 weeks. She delivered at 34 weeks, and the growth-retarded infant eventually did well. The elevated AFP levels were interpreted to result from a disruption

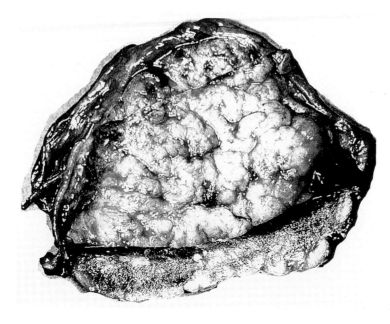

FIGURE 162. Maternal floor with maternal floor infarction. The entire decidual floor is thickened, yellowish, and infiltrated with fibrin. The cut section (below) shows the relatively shallow depth of fibrin infiltration.

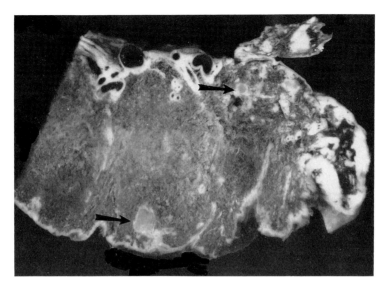

FIGURE 163. Typical maternal floor infarction (MFI) in the placenta of a premature infant who died with hyaline membrane disease. The infant had been reported to "never be active" in utero. The floor and septa have increased fibrin infiltrates, and there are two septal cysts (arrows) in this section. The entire placenta had a firm appearance.

at the maternofetal interface and at least once a fetal hemorrhage of 4 ml was detected by Kleihauer test. The MBP levels in maternal serum were significantly elevated in one of our patients with MFI, which had been established by elevated maternal serum AFP levels; the patient had had two previous stillbirths (Gleich, personal communication, 1989).

Subsequent evaluation of the possible utility of MBP levels in maternal serum for the anticipation of MFI were not productive (Vernof et al., 1992). Robinson et al. (1989) found a strong correlation between elevated AFP levels and poor pregnancy outcome, even when congenital anomalies and twins were excluded. Thus MFI and its variants must be entertained in the differential diagnosis of an unexplained elevation of AFP during pregnancy. Mandsager et al. (1993) established ultrasonographic criteria for the diagnosis of MFI and found it useful for anticipating the disease.

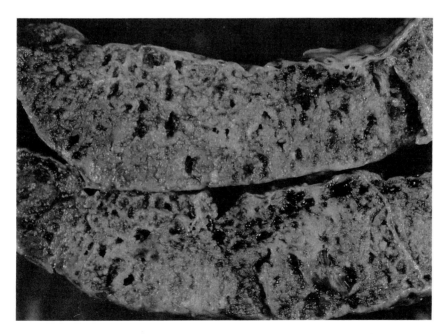

FIGURE 164. Massive intervillous fibrin deposition: *Gitterinfarct*. It was a 34 weeks' gestation placenta of a growth-retarded infant who did well. The previous pregnancy had also resulted in an infant with growth retardation.

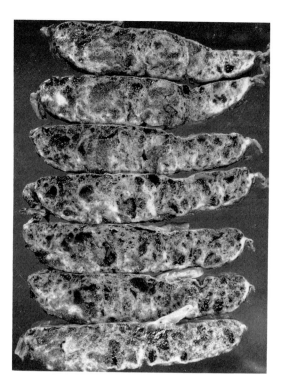

FIGURE 165. Case similar to that in Figure 164: massive diffuse fibrin encasement of villous tissue in MFI with *Gitterinfarct*. It was the third stillborn of a healthy mother; the maternal serum MBP levels were markedly elevated.

It is true that when a placenta has been retained for a long time after fetal death the organ accumulates fibrin and becomes firm. It is not the case, however, with most stillborns. Their placentas usually show no increased fibrin imbibition. Nor have the fetuses of some of the placentas with MFI been dead for especially long periods. As indicated earlier, this condition occurs with liveborn infants as well, especially with growth-retarded infants. MFI is a specific entity, but it is not always completely expressed; that is, in some placentas the characteristic fibrin deposition does not involve the entire floor. This variability occasionally makes the diagnosis difficult. One atypical case has been described in which the fetus ultimately developed microcephaly (Pfeiffer, 1974).

The histological findings of MFI include a marked increase in fibrin deposits of the decidual floor with encasement of many villous tips. Those villi then are sclerotic and avascular. The fibrin stains faintly with congo red, but electron microscopically it proves not to be amyloid. There is an increase of extravillous trophoblast (X cells) and septal cyst formation. Occasionally, many subchorionic cysts are found. Inflammation is usually not present, and the trophoblast in uninvolved areas is normal. The *Gitterinfarct* features are shown in Figures 164 and 165. Villi are encased in masses of

fibrin and appear to have been strangled, whereas adjacent villi are normal (Figures 166, 167). There is usually no inflammation. In some specimens of MFI, however, there is a moderate degree of lymphoid cell infiltration around the necrotic villi (Figure 168). Plasma cells are absent, and there is usually no villitis. These placentas are also not associated with the decidual vasculopathy (atherosis) of preeclampsia.

It must be emphasized that MFI is macroscopically and microscopically different from common infarcts. No large areas of villous infarction are present; the lesion is usually confined to the floor of the placenta, and the deposition of fibrinoid is an outstanding feature of this entity. Therefore when the nature and frequency of infarcts were studied (e.g., Fox, 1967b), this lesion was seen not to be encompassed. In considerations of the placenta in placental insufficiency, however, there is more often mention of fibrin encasement, lesions that apparently represent similar pathological features. Thus Wigglesworth (1964) found among the normotensive cases in his study that "the most extensive placental infarction was seen in cases of unexplained stillbirth. The lesions in those placentas were not always pure

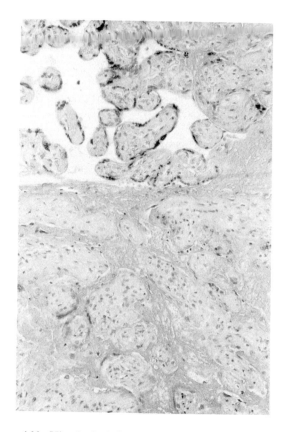

FIGURE 166. Histological features of *Gitterinfarct*. Villi are encased in masses of pale eosinophilic fibrin-like material. Adjacent villi are normal. The encasement usually begins, and is most severe, at the anchoring tips of the villi. H&E. ×160.

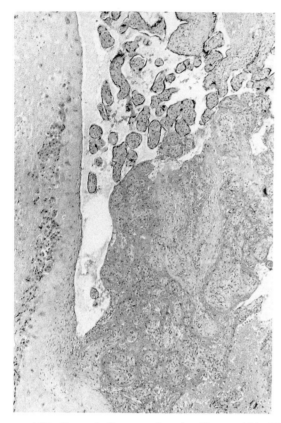

FIGURE 167. Case similar to that in Figure 166. Fibrin-engulfed clusters of mature villi exist adjacent to normally preserved villi. H&E. ×60.

infarcts but consisted of true infarction and massive arborescent fibrin deposits."

Kubli (1968), in a consideration of chronic placental insufficiency, mentioned that the lesions are variable and comprise cases with "disseminated ischemic necroses with fibrinoid degeneration ('essential' placental insufficiency, prolonged pregnancy)." Ermocilla and Altshuler (1973) found similar lesions, particularly a prominent proliferation of extravillous trophoblast cells (X cells) in three growth-retarded infants. They suggested that it would be better if we devoted our efforts to determining the function of X cells than be concerned with their origin. Davies et al. (1984), although not referring directly to MFI, also found an increased amount of fibrin in the placentas of growth-retarded infants.

The only author who has paid more attention to this lesion is Naeye (1985). He attempted to ascertain the incidence of MFI and its significance from the 39,215 placentas examined in the Collaborative Perinatal Study. He found that MFI was reported in 1 of 200 placentas. That figure is much higher than is our experience and may be related to the variability of observers. The fetuses were stillborn in 17%, and 50% of the patients (27% of controls) had had previous stillbirths or abortions. He also found chorioamnionitis and twice the expected frequency of IUGR. His experience of an increased incidence of preeclamptic decidual lesions is not supported by our cases. Smoking had no influence, but women with MFI had higher hemoglobin values. Nickel (1988) also described a case and discussed the recurrence and related diseases.

The etiology of MFI is unknown. We are convinced, partly because of its frequently recurrent nature, that MFI is a specific entity. Naeye (1985), on the other hand, believed that it represents the "final common pathway for a number of disorders, some of which are the result of damage to the decidua." He favored a relation to infection, with which we disagree. It is true that MFI and especially *Gitterinfarct* are seen in some cases of chronic villitis, but not all MFI placentas have villitis. We have suggested that MFI relates to an abnormal host–placenta interaction but not necessarily an immunological one. Because the lesion has generally been poorly recognized, no further support has been forthcoming for this notion. Be that as it may, it is important for the obstetrician to know of its existence

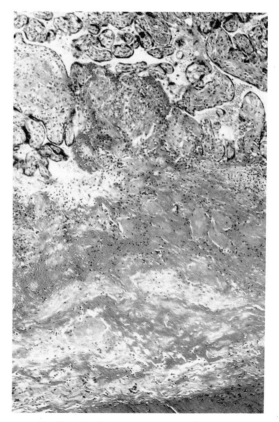

FIGURE 168. Histological appearance of a maternal floor infarction. There is an excessive amount of fibrin in the decidua. Many basal villi are dead and are surrounded by chronic inflammatory cells. H&E. ×100.

because, as the case reported by Clewell and Manchester (1983) clearly showed, subsequent pregnancies may be salvaged when the disease is recognized to have caused stillbirth or abortion.

We know nothing of the pathogenesis of MFI. The excessive fibrin (and perhaps other extracellular substances, such as fibronectin) deposits may reduce the flow into the intervillous space and thus be responsible for fetal malnutrition. We have not observed any specific maternal vascular disease in these patients, and lupus anticoagulants have not been present in the mothers. The few clinical correlations and histological observations have suggested that the fibrin deposition occurs relatively quickly. Usually this situation is the case during the second and third trimesters. With the exception of occasional diabetic patients, the mothers have been clinically normal.

One promising avenue for future study is based on the findings of Robb et al. (1986a,b). Using an immunohistochemical technique, these investigators located what was interpreted as herpes virus antigen in the floor of most specimens diagnosed as having MFI. They suggested that this deposition of antigen may represent a manifestation of latent herpes simplex virus infection.

References

Al Timimi, A., and Fox, H.: Immunohistochemical localization of follicle-stimulating hormone, luteinizing hormone, growth hormone, adrenocorticotrophic hormone and prolactin in the human placenta. Placenta 7:163–172, 1986.

Al-Zuhair, A.G.H., Ibrahim, M.E.A., and Mughal, S.: Calcium deposition on the maternal surface of the human placenta: a scanning electron microscopic study. Arch. Gynecol. 234:167–172, 1984.

Andersen, J.R., Borggaard, B., Schroeder, E., Olsen, E.B., Stimpel, H., and Nyholm, H.C.: The dependence of human decidual prolactin production and secretion on the osmotic environment in vitro. Acta Endocrinol. (Copenh.) 106:405–410, 1984.

Andersen, J.R., Borggaard, B., Olsen, E.B., Stimpel, H., Nyholm, H.C., and Schroeder, E.: Effect of ouabain and bumetanide on the basal and the osmolality-affected prolactin secretion from human decidual cells in vitro. Eur. J. Obstet. Gynecol. Reprod. Biol. 23:159–166, 1986.

Andersen, J.R., Borggaard, B., Olsen, E.B, Stimpel, H., Nyholm, H.C., and Schroeder, E.: Decidual prolactin content and secretion at term: correlations with the clinical data. Acta Obstet. Gynecol. Scand. 66:591–596, 1987.

Angel, E., Davis, J.R., and Nagle, R.B.: Correspondence: decidual cells. Lab. Invest. 55:120, 1986.

Aplin, J.D.: Expression of integrin alpha 6 beta 4 in human trophoblast and its loss from extravillous cells. Placenta 14:203–215, 1993.

Aplin, J.D., and Campbell, S.: An immunofluorescence study of extracellular matrix associated with cytotrophoblast of the chorion laeve. Placenta 6:469–479, 1985.

Aplin, J.D., and Foden, L.J.: A cell spreading factor, abundant in human placenta, contains fibronectin and fibrinogen. J. Cell Sci. 58:287–302, 1982.

Arias-Stella, J.: Gestational endometrium. In, The Uterus. H.J. Norris, A.T. Hertig, and M.R. Abel, eds., pp. 183–212. Williams & Wilkins, Baltimore, 1973.

Arnholdt, H., and Löhrs, U.: Proliferation and differentiation of Langhans' cells. Placenta 10:458, 1989.

Arnholdt, H., Meisel, F., Fandrey, K., and Löhrs, U.: Proliferation of villous trophoblast of the human placenta in normal and abnormal pregnancies. Virchows Arch. B Cell Pathol. 60:365–372, 1991.

Arnold, J.: Über den Schlussring reifer menschlicher Plazenten. Verh. Anat. Ges. 69:303–306, 1975a.

Arnold, J.: Über die Randzone der reifen menschlichen Plazenta. Inaugural Dissertation, Würzburg, 1975b.

Arts, N.F.T.: Investigations on the vascular system of the placenta. Am. J. Obstet. Gynecol. 82:147–166, 1961.

Aufderheide E., and Ekblom, P.: Tenascin during gut development: appearance in the mesenchyme, shift in molecular forms, and dependence on epithelial-mesenchymal interactions. J. Cell Biol. 107:2341–2349, 1988.

Autio Harmainen, H., Hurskainen, T., Niskasaari, K., Hoyhtya, M., and Tryggvason, K.: Simultaneous expression of 70 kilodalton type IV collagenase and type IV collagen alpha 1 (IV) chain genes by cells of early human placenta and gestational endometrium. Lab. Invest. 67:191–200, 1992.

Avery, C.R., and Aterman, K.: Calcification of the basement membrane of placental villi. J. Pathol. 103:199–200, 1971.

Azab, I., Okamura, H., and Beer, A.: Decidual cell production of human placental fibrinoid. Obstet. Gynecol. 40:186–193, 1972.

Badarau, L., and Gavrilita, L.: Intervillous fibrin deposition, the Rohr, Nitabuch and Langhans striae. Am. J. Obstet. Gynecol. 98:252–260, 1967.

Badarau, L., Gavrilita, L., Stratan, E., and Calinca, N.: Étude histologique de la caduque au cours de la grossesse normale: le mode de pénétration du trophoblaste dans la plaque basale; le processus de placentation. Gynecol. Obstet. (Paris) 70:273–290, 1971.

Bagshawe, K., and Lawler, S.: The immunogenicity of the placenta and trophoblast. In, Immunobiology of Trophoblast. R.G. Edwards, C.W.S. Howe, and M.H. Johnson, eds., pp. 171–182. Cambridge University Press, London, 1975.

Baker, B.L., Hook, J., and Severinghaus, A.E.: The cytological structure of the human chorionic villus and decidua parietalis. Am. J. Anat. 74:291–325, 1944.

Bardawil, W.A., and Toy, B.L.: The natural history of choriocarcinoma: problems of immunity and spontaneous regression. Ann. N.Y. Acad. Sci. 80:197–261, 1959.

Bargmann, W.: Über den Bildungsort der Choriongonadotropine und Plazentarsteroide. Geburtshilfe Frauenheilkd. 17:865–875, 1957.

Bautzmann, H., and Schröder, R.: Vergleichende Studien über Bau und Funktion des Amnions: Neue Befunde am menschlichen Amnion mit Einschluss seiner freien Bindegewebs- oder sog. Hofbauerzellen. Z. Anat. 119:7–22, 1955.

Beck, A.J., and Beck, F.: The origin of intra-arterial cells in the pregnant uterus of the macaque (Macaca mulatta). Anat. Rec. 158:111–113, 1967.

Beck, J.S.: Time of appearance of human placental lactogen in the embryo. N. Engl. J. Med. 283:189–190, 1970.

Beck, T., Schweikhart, G., and Stolz, E.: Immunohistochemical location of HPL, SP1 and β-HCG in normal placentas of varying gestational age. Arch. Gynecol. 239:63–74, 1986.

Becker, V.: Funktionelle Morphologie der Placenta. Arch. Gynecol. 198:3–28, 1962.

Becker, V.: Gefäße der Chorionplatte und Stammzotten. In, Die Plazenta des Menschen. V. Becker, T.H. Schiebler, and F. Kubli, eds., pp. 311–313. Thieme Verlag, Stuttgart, 1981.

Becker, V., and Jipp, P.: Über die Trophoblastschale der menschlichen Plazenta. Geburtshilfe Frauenheilkd. 23:466–474, 1963.

Bell, S.C.: Decidualization: regional differentiation and associated function. Oxford Rev. Reprod. Biol. 5:220–271, 1983.

Bell, S.C.: Decidualization and insulin-like growth factor (IGF) binding protein: implications for its role in stromal cell differentiation and the decidual cell in haemochorial placentation. Hum. Reprod. 4:125–130, 1989.

Bell, S.C., Patel, S.R., Jackson, J.A., and Waites, G.T.: Major secretory protein of human decidualized endometrium in pregnancy is an insulin-like growth factor binding protein. J. Endocrinol. 118:317–328, 1988.

Bendon, R.W., and Ray, M.B.: The pathologic findings of the fetal membranes in very prolonged amniotic fluid leakage. Arch. Pathol. Lab. Med. 110:47–50, 1986.

Benirschke, K.: Examination of the placenta. Obstet. Gynecol. 18:309–333, 1961.

Benirschke, K., and Driscoll, S.G.: The Pathology of the Human Placenta. Springer-Verlag, New York, 1967.

Berger, G., Verbaere, J., and Feroldi, J.: Placental site trophoblastic tumor of the uterus: an ultrastructural and immunohistochemical study. Ultrastruct. Pathol. 6:319–329, 1984.

Bertolini, R., and Klinger, M.: Über deziduaähnliche Zellnester in der Chorionplatte von geburtsreifen menschlichen Plazenten. Zentralbl. Gynäkol. 17:521–524, 1966.

Bertolini, R., Reissig, D., and Schippel, K.: Elektronenmikrokopische Befunde an den Zellen in der Chorionplatte der reifen menschlichen Plazenta. Z. Mikrosk. Anat. Forsch. 80:358–368, 1969.

Bierings, M.B., Adriaansen, H.J., and Van Dijk, J.P.: The appearance of transferrin receptors on cultured human cytotrophoblast and in vitro-formed syncytiotrophoblast. Placenta 9:387–396, 1988.

Bigazzi, M., Bruni, P., Nardi, E., Petrucci, F., Pollicino, G., Franchini, M., Scarselli, G., and Farnararo, M.: Human decidual relaxin. Ann. N. Y. Acad. Sci. 380:87–99, 1982.

Billington, D.: Organization, ultrastructure and histochemistry of the placenta: immunological considerations. In, Immunobiology of Trophoblast. R.G. Edwards, C.W.S. Howe, and M.H. Johnson, eds. Cambridge University Press, Cambridge, 1975.

Birkenfeld, A., Mordel, N., and Okon, E.: Direct demonstration of iron in a term placenta in a case of β-thalassemia major. Am. J. Obstet. Gynecol. 160:562–563, 1989.

Bischof, P., and Martelli, M.: Current topic: proteolysis in the penetration phase of the implantation process. Placenta 13:17–24, 1992.

Bischof, P., Friedli, E., Martelli, M., and Campana, A.: Expression of extracellular matrix-degrading metalloproteinases by cultured human cytotrophoblast cells: effects of cell adhesion and immunopurification. Am. J. Obstet. Gynecol. 165:1791–1801, 1991.

Bittencourt, A.L., and Sadigursky, M.: Decidual angiomatosis with abortion. Patologia (Mexico) 15:45–47, 1977.

Björkman, N.: On the fine structure of the porcine placental barrier. Acta Anat. (Basel) 62:334–342, 1965a.

Björkman, N.: The fine morphology of the area of foetal-maternal apposition in the equine placenta. Z. Zellforsch. 65:285–289, 1965b.

Björkman, N.: An Atlas of Placental Fine Structure. Baillière, London; Williams & Wilkins, Baltimore, 1970.

Björkman, N., and Bloom, G.: On the fine structure of the foetal-maternal junction on the bovine placentome. Z. Zellforsch. 45:649–659, 1957.

Blankenship, T.N., Enders, A.C., and King, B.F.: Trophoblastic invasion and the development of uteroplacental arteries in the macaque: immunohistochemical localization of cytokeratins, desmin, type IV collagen, laminin, and fibronectin. Cell Tissue Res. 272:227–236, 1993a.

Blankenship, T.N., Enders, A.C., and King, B.F.: Trophoblastic invasion and modification of uterine veins during placental development in macaques. Cell Tiss. Res. 274:135–144, 1993b.

Blithe, D.L., Richards, R.G., and Skarulis, M.C.: Free alpha molecules from pregnancy stimulate secretion of prolactin from human decidual cells: a novel function for free alpha in pregnancy. Endocrinology 129:2257–2259, 1991.

Boe, F.: Studies on the human placenta. I. The cell islands in the young placenta. Acta Obstet. Gynecol. Scand. 46:591–603, 1967.

Boeving, B.G.: Das Eindringen des Trophoblasten in das Uterusepithel. Klin. Wochenschr. 42:467–475, 1964.

Bogaert, L.J.: Endometrial granulocytes in proliferative endometrium. Br. J. Obstet. Gynaecol. 82:995–998, 1975.

Bohn, H.: The human fibrin-stabilizing factors. Mol. Cell. Biochem. 20:67–75, 1978.

Bonashevskaia, T.I., Lamentova, T.G., Shmakov, G.S., Nikolaeva, E.G., and Suslova, V.M.: Structuro-functional changes in the placenta as a result of exposure to atmospheric pollutants. Arkh. Anat. Gistol. Embriol. 88:72–76, 1985.

Bonnar, J., and Sheppard, B.L.: Treatment of poor intra-uterine fetal growth with heparin and dipyridamole. Minerva Med. 465–468, 1977.

Borell, U., Fernstroem, I., Ohlson, L., and Wiqvist, N.: Effect of uterine contractions on the uteroplacental blood flow at term. Am. J. Obstet. Gynecol. 93:44–57, 1965.

Borsi, L., Carnemolla, B., Castellani, P., Rossellini, C., Vecchio, D., Allemanni, G., Change, S.E., Taylor-Papadimitriou, J., Pande H., and Zardi, L.: Monoclonal antibodies in the analysis of fibronectin isoforms generated by alternative splicing of mRNA precursors in normal and transformed human cells. J. Cell Biol. 104:595–600, 1987.

Bourne, G.L.: The Human Amnion and Chorion. Lloyd-Luke, London, 1962.

Boyd, J.D.: Morphology and physiology of the utero-placental circulation. In, Gestation. C.A. Villee, ed., pp. 132–194, Macy. New York, 1956.

Boyd, J.D., and Hamilton, W.J.: The giant cells of the pregnant human uterus. J. Obstet. Gynaecol. Br. Emp. 67:208–218, 1960.

Boyd, J.D., and Hamilton, W.J.: Placental septa. Z. Zellforsch. 69:613–634, 1966.

Boyd, J.D., and Hamilton, W.J.: The Human Placenta. Heffer & Sons, Cambridge, 1970.

Bradbury, S., Billington, W.D., and Kirby, D.R.S.: A histochemical and electron microscopical study of the mouse placenta. J.R. Microsc. Soc. 84:199–211, 1965.

Bray, B.A.: Presence of fibronectin in basement membranes and acidic structural glycoproteins from human placenta and lung. Ann. N.Y. Acad. Sci. 312:142–150, 1978.

Bret, A.-J., Legros, R., and Toyoda, S.: Les kystes placentaires. Press Md. 68:1552–1555, 1960.

Brettner, A.: Zum Verhalten der sekundären Wand der Utero-Plazentargefässe bei der decidualen Reaktion. Acta Anat. (Basel) 57:367–376, 1964.

Breus, C.: Das Tuberöse Subchoriale Hämatom der Decidua. Eine typische Form der Molenschwangerschaft. F. Deuticke, Leipzig, 1892.

Briese, V., and Müller, H.: Fetomaternal signal transduction by growth factors. Zentralbl. Gynakol. 114:219–223, 1992.

Brosens, I.: A study of the spiral arteries of the decidua basalis in normotensive and hypertensive pregnancies. J. Obstet. Gynaecol. Br. Commonw. 71:222–230, 1964.

Brosens, I.: The utero-placental vessels at term—the distribution and extent of physiological changes. Trophoblast Res. 3:61–68, 1988.

Brosens, I., Robertson, W.B., and Dixon, H.G.: The physiological response of the vessels of the placental bed to normal pregnancy. J. Pathol. Bacteriol. 93:569–579, 1967.

Brosens, I., Robertson, W.B., and Dixon, H.G.: The role of the spiral arteries in the pathogenesis of preeclampsia. Obstet. Gynecol. Ann. 1:177–191, 1972.

Brosens, I., Dixon, H.G., and Robertson, W.B.: Fetal growth retardation and the arteries of the placental bed. Br. J. Obstet. Gynaecol. 84:656–663, 1977.

Brown, H.L., Miller, J.M., Khawli, O., and Gabert, H.A.: Premature placental calcification in maternal cigarette smokers. Obstet. Gynecol. 71:914–917, 1988.

Bryant-Greenwood, G.D., Rees, M.C.P., and Turnbull, A.C.: Immunohistochemical localization of relaxin, prolactin and prostaglandin synthase in human amnion, chorion and decidua. J. Endocrinol. 114:491–496, 1987.

Brzosko, W., Nowoslawski, A., and Pisarki, T.: Analiza immunohistochemiczna mas wloknikowatych w lozysku ludzkim. Ginekol. Polska 36:121–130, 1965a.

Brzosko, W., Nowoslawski, A., and Pisarski, I.: Immunohistochemical analysis of the fibrinoid masses in human placenta. Pol. Med. 5:114–123, 1965b.

Bühler, F.R.: Randbildungen der menschlichen Placenta. Acta Anat. (Basel) 59:47–76, 1964.

Bullen, B., and Bloxam, D.: Human placental trophoblast cultured on amnion basement membrane: a model for transport studies. In, Abstracts of the 11th Rochester Trophoblast Conference, p. 131, 1988.

Bulmer, D.: The metrial gland and endometrial granulocytes. J. Anat. 137:787–826, 1983.

Bulmer, D., and Dickson, A.D.: The fibrinoid capsule of the rat placenta and the disappearance of the decidua. J. Anat. 95:300–310, 1961.

Bulmer, D., and Peel, S.: The demonstration of immunoglobulin in the metrial gland cells of the rat placenta. J. Reprod. Fertil. 49:143–145, 1977.

Bulmer, D., Stewart, I., and Peel, S.: Endometrial granulocytes of the pregnant hamster. J. Anat. 136:329–337, 1983.

Bulmer, J.N., and Johnson, P.M.: Macrophage populations in the human placenta and amniochorion. Clin. Exp. Immunol. 57:393–403, 1984.

Bulmer, J.N., and Sunderland, C.A.: Bone-marrow origin of endometrial granulocytes in the early human placental bed. J. Reprod. Immunol. 5:383–387, 1983.

Bulmer, J.N., and Sunderland, C.A.: Immunohistological characterization of lymphoid cell populations in the early human placental bed. Immunology 52:349–357, 1984.

Bulmer, J.N., Wells, M., Bhabra, K., and Johnson, P.M.: Immunohistological characterization of endometrial gland epithelium and extravillous fetal trophoblast in third trimester human placental bed tissues. Br. J. Obstet. Gynaecol. 93:823–832, 1986.

Bulmer, J.N., Johnson, P.M., Sasagawa, M., and Takeuchi, S.: Immunohistochemical studies of fetal trophoblast and maternal decidua in hydatidiform mole and choriocarcinoma. Placenta 9:183–200, 1988a.

Bulmer, J.N., Morrison, L., and Smith, J.C.: Expression of class II MHC gene products by macrophages in human uteroplacental tissue. Immunology 63:707–714, 1988b.

Bulmer, J.N., Smith, J., Morrison, L., and Wells, M.: Maternal and fetal cellular relationships in the human placental basal plate. Placenta 9:237–246, 1988c.

Bulmer, J.N., Thrower, S., and Wells, M.: Expression of epidermal growth factor receptor and transferrin receptor by human trophoblast populations. Am. J. Reprod. Immunol. 21:87–93, 1989.

Bumm, E.: Zur Kenntnis der Uteroplacentargefässe. Arch. Gynäkol. 37:1–15, 1890.

Bunton, T.E.: Incidental lesions in nonhuman primate placentae. Vet. Pathol. 23:431–438, 1986.

Burrows, T.D., King, A., and Loke, Y.W.: Expression of integrins by human trophoblast and differential adhesion to laminin or fibronectin. Hum. Reprod. 8:475–484, 1993.

Burstein, R., Frankel, S., Soule, S.D., and Blumenthal, H.T.: Ageing in the placenta: autoimmune theory of senescence. Am. J. Obstet. Gynecol. 116:271–274, 1973.

Busanny-Caspari, W.: Zur Morphogenese des Fibrinoids in Placenta und Decidua. Virchows Arch. 322:452–460, 1952.

Busanny-Caspari, E.: Zur Morphologie des Fibrinoids in Placenta und Dezidua. Virchows Arch. [Pathol. Anat.] 322:452–460, 1956.

Busanny-Caspari, W.: Fibrin und Fibrinoid. Acta Histochem. 4:304–313, 1957.

Butterworth, B.H., Khong, T.Y., Loke, Y.W., and Robertson, W.B.: Human cytotrophoblast populations studied by monoclonal antibodies using single and double biotin-avidin-peroxidase immunocytochemistry. J. Histochem. Cytochem. 33:977–983, 1985.

Carnemolla, B., Borsi, L., Zardi, L., Owens, R.J., and Baralle, F.E.: Localization of the cellular-fibronectin-specific epitope recognized by the monoclonal antibody IST-9 using fusion proteins expressed in E. coli. FEBS Lett. 215:269–273, 1987.

Carnemolla, B., Balza, E., Siri, A., Zardi, L., Nicotra, M.R., Bigotti, A., and Natali, P.G.: A tumor associated fibronectin isoform generated by alternative splicing of messenger RNA precursors. J. Cell Biol. 108:1139–1148, 1989.

Carter, J.E., Vellios, F., and Huber, C.P.: Histologic classification and incidence of circulatory lesions of the human placenta, with a review of the literature. Am. J. Clin. Pathol. 40:374–378, 1963.

Casey, M.L., Delgadillo, M., Cox, K.A., Nisert, S., and MacDonald, P.C.: Inactivation of prostaglandins in human decidua vera (parietalis) tissue: substrate specificity of prostaglandin dehydrogenase. Am. J. Obstet. Gynecol. 160:3–7, 1989.

Castellucci, M., Kaufmann, P., and Bischof, P.: Extracellular matrix influences hormone and placental protein production by human chorionic villi. In, Abstracts of the 11th Rochester Trophoblast Conference, p. 49, 1988.

Castellucci, M., Kaufmann, P., and Bischof, P.: Extracellular matrix influences hormone and protein production by human chorionic villi. Cell Tissue Res. 262:135–142, 1990.

Castellucci, M., Classen Linke, I., Mühlhauser, J., Kaufmann, P., and Zardi, L.: The human placenta: a model for tenascin expression. Histochemistry 95:449–458, 1991.

Castellucci, M., Crescimanno, C., Schröter, C.A., Kaufmann, P., and Mühlhauser, J.: Extravillous trophoblast: immunohistochemical localization of extracellular matrix molecules. In, Frontiers in Gynecologic and Obstetric Investigation. A.R. Genazzani, F. Petraglia, and A.D. Genazzani, eds., pp. 19–25. Parthenon, New York, 1993a. (p. 297).

Castellucci, M., Crescimano, C., Mühlhauser, J., Frank, H.G., Kaufmann, P., and Zardi, L.: Expression of extracellular matrix molecules related to placental development. Placenta 14:A9, 1993b.

Chaouat, G., Kolb, J.P., and Wegmann, T.G.: The murine placenta as an immunological barrier between the mother and the fetus. Immunol. Rev. 75:31–60, 1983.

Cheung, P.Y., Walton, J.C., Tai, H.H., Riley, S.C., and Challis, J.R.: Immunocytochemical distribution and localization of 15-hydroxyprostaglandin dehydrogenase in human fetal membranes, decidua, and placenta. Am. J. Obstet. Gynecol. 163:1445–1449, 1990.

Cheung, P.Y., Walton, J.C., Tai, H.H., Riley, S.C., and Challis, J.R.: Localization of 15-hydroxy prostaglandin dehydrogenase in human fetal membranes, decidua, and placenta during pregnancy. Gynecol. Obstet. Invest. 33:142–146, 1992.

Chiquet-Ehrismann, R., Mackie, E.J., Pearson, C.A., and Sakakura, T.: Tenascin: an extracellular matrix protein involved in tissue interactions during fetal development and oncogenesis. Cell 47:131–139, 1986.

Chung, S.I.: Comparative studies on tissue transglutaminase and factor XIII. Ann. N.Y. Acad. Sci. 202:240–255, 1972.

Clewell, W.H., and Manchester, D.K.: Recurrent maternal floor infarction: a preventable cause of fetal death. Am. J. Obstet. Gynecol. 147:346–347, 1983.

Coleman, R.W., Marder, V.J., Salzman, E.W., and Hirsh, J.: Overview of hemostasis. In, Hemostasis and Thrombosis, 2nd ed. R.W. Coleman, J. Hirsh, V.J. Marder, and E.W. Salzman, eds., pp. 3–17. Lipincott, Philadelphia 1987.

Coukos, G., Gafvels, M.E., Wisel, S., Ruelaz, E.A., Strickland, D.K., Strauss, J.F., and Coutifaris, C.: Expression of alpha 2-macroglobulin receptor/low density lipoprotein receptor-related protein and the 39-kd receptor-associated protein in human trophoblasts. Am. J. Pathol.144:383–392, 1994.

Currie, C.A., and Bagshawe, K.D.: The masking of antigens on trophoblast and cancer cells. Lancet 1:708–710, 1967.

Dallenbach, F.D., and Dallenbach-Hellweg, G.: Immunohistologische Untersuchungen zur Lokalisation des Relaxins in menschlicher Placenta und Decidua. Virchows Arch. [Pathol. Anat.] 337:301–316, 1964.

Dallenbach-Hellweg, G.: Histopathology of the Endometrium. pp. 24–27. Springer-Verlag, Berlin, 1971.

Dallenbach-Hellweg, G., and Nette, G.: Über Glykoproteideinschlüsse in den Trophoblastzellen der menschlichen Plazenta und die Frage ihres Zusammenhangs mit der Bildung von Gonadotropin. Z. Zellforsch. 61:145–158, 1963a.

Dallenbach-Hellweg, G., and Nette, G.: Über Proteineinschlüsse in basalen Trophoblastzellen der reifen menschlichen Plazenta. Virchows Arch. [Pathol. Anat.] 336:528–543, 1963b.

Dallenbach-Hellweg, G., and Nette, G.: Morphological and histochemical observations on trophoblast and decidua of the basal plate of the human placenta at term. Am. J. Anat. 115:309–326, 1964.

Dallenbach-Hellweg, G., and Sievers, S.: Die histologische Reaktion des Endometrium auf lokal applizierte Gestagene. Virchows Arch. [Pathol. Anat.] 368:289–298, 1975.

Daly, D.C., Maslar, I.A., and Riddick, D.H.: Prolactin production during in vitro decidualization of proliferative endometrium. Am. J. Obstet. Gynecol. 145:672–678, 1983.

Damjanov, I.: Editorial: Vesalius and Hunter were right: decidua is a membrane. Lab. Invest. 53:597–598, 1985.

Damsky, C.H., Fitzgerald, M.L., and Fisher, S.J.: Distribution patterns of extracellular matrix components and adhesion receptors are intricately modulated during first trimester cytotrophoblast differentiation along the invasive pathway, in vivo. J. Clin. Invest. 89:210–222, 1992.

Davies, B.R., Casanueva, E., and Arroyo, P.: Placentas of small-for-dates infants: a small controlled series from Mexico City, Mexico. Am. J. Obstet. Gynecol. 149:731–736, 1984.

Daya, D., and Sabet, L.: The use of cytokeratin as a sensitive and reliable marker for trophoblastic tissue. Am. J. Clin. Pathol. 95:137–141, 1991.

De Bakker-Theunissen, O.J.G.B., Arts, N.F.T., and Mulder, G.H.: Fluid transport across human fetal membranes affected by human amniotic fluid prolactin: an in vitro study. Placenta 9:533–545, 1988.

Debiasi, E., Damiani, N., and Capodacqua, R.: Contributo allo studio della circolazione utero-placentare nelle donna. Minerva Ginecol. 15:539–545, 1963.

Demir, R., and Erbengi, T.: The cells of the intercotyledonary septae in full-term placenta. In, Proceedings of the 8th European Congress of Electron Microscopy. Vol. 3. pp. 2017–2018, 1984.

Dempsey, E.W., Wislocki, G.B., and Amoroso, E.C.: Electron microscopy of the pig's placenta, with especial reference to the cell membranes of the endometrium and chorion. Am. J. Anat. 96:65–102, 1955.

Dempsey, E.W., Lessey, R.A., and Luse, S.A.: Electron microscopic observations on fibrinoid and histiotroph in the junctional zone and villi of the human placenta. Am. J. Anat. 108:463–484, 1970.

Denker, H.W.: The role of trophoblastic factors in implantation. In, Novel Aspects of Reproductive Physiology. C.H. Spilman and J.W. Wilks, eds., pp. 181–212. Spectrum, New York, 1978.

Denker, H.-W.: Trophoblast-endometrial interactions at embryo implantation: a cell biological paradox. Trophoblast Res. 4:1–27, 1990.

Denker, H.-W., and Aplin, J.D. eds.: Trophoblast invasion and endometrial receptivity: novel aspects of the cell biology of embryo implantation. Trophoblast Res. 4:1–462, 1990.

DeWolf, F., DeWolf-Peeters, C., and Brosens, I.: Ultrastructure of the spiral arteries in the human placental bed at the end of normal pregnancy. Am. J. Obstet. Gynecol. 117. 833–848, 1973.

DeWolf, F., Brosens, I., and Renaer, M.: Fetal growth retardation and the maternal arterial supply of the human placenta in the absence of sustained hypertension. Br. J. Obstet. Gynaecol. 87:678–685, 1980.

Dietl, J., Ruck, P., Horny, H.P., Handgretinger, R., Marzusch, K., Ruck, M., Kaiserling, E., Griesser, H., and Kabelitz, D.: The decidua of early human pregnancy— immunohistochemistry and function of immunocompetent cells. Gynecol. Obstet. Invest. 33:197–204, 1992.

Dohrn, M.: Ein Beitrag zur mikroskopischen Anatomie der reifen menschlichen Eihüllen. Monatsschr. Geburtshilfe Frauenkr. 26:114–127, 1865.

Doolittle, R.F.: Fibrinogen and fibrin. In, The Plasma Proteins. 2nd Ed., Vol. 2. F.W. Putnam, ed., pp. 109–161. Academic Press, Orlando, FL, 1975.

Douglas, G.C., and King, B.F.: Isolation of pure villous cytotrophoblast from term human placenta using immuno-magnetic microspheres. J. Immunol. Methods 119:259–268, 1989.

Douglas, G.C., and King, B.F.: Differentiation of human trophoblast cells in vitro as revealed by immunocytochemical staining of desmoplakin and nuclei. J. Cell Sci. 96:131–141, 1990a.

Douglas, G.C., and King, B.F.: Isolation and morphologic differentiation in vitro of villous cytotrophoblast cells from rhesus monkey placenta. In Vitro Cell Dev. Biol. 26:754–758, 1990b.

Douglas, G.C., and King, B.F.: Colchicine inhibits human trophoblast differentiation in vitro. Placenta 14:187–201, 1993.

Duan, J.S.: Production of granulocyte colony stimulating factor in decidual tissue and its significance in pregnancy. Osaka City Med. J. 36:81–97, 1990.

Duncan, D.A., and Mazur, M.T.: Trophoblastic tumors: ultrastructural comparison of choriocarcinoma and placental-site trophoblastic tumor. Hum. Pathol. 20:370–381, 1989.

Durst-Zivkovic, B.: Endometrial granular cells in fetal membranes. Anat. Anz. 143:258–261, 1978.

Dvorak, H.F., Senger, D.R., and Dvorak, A.M.: Fibrin as a component of the tumor stroma: origins and biological significance. Cancer Metastasis Rev. 2:41–73, 1983.

Earl, U., Wells, M., and Bulmer, J.N.: The expression of major histocompatibility complex antigens by trophoblast in ectopic tubal pregnancy. J. Reprod. Immunol. 8:13–24, 1985.

Earl, U., Morrison, L., Gray, C., and Bulmer, J.N.: Proteinase and proteinase inhibitor localization in the human placenta. Int. J. Gynecol. Pathol. 8:114–124, 1989.

Earl, U., Estlin, C., and Bulmer, J.N.: Fibronectin and laminin in the early human placenta. Placenta 11:223–231, 1990.

Edwards, D., Jones, C.J.P., Sibley, C.P., Farmer, D.R., and Nelson, D.M.: Areas of syncytial denudation may provide routes for paracellular diffusion across the human placenta [abstract]. Placenta 12:383, 1991.

Ehrig, K., Leivo, I., Argraves, W.S., Ruoslahti, E., and Engvall, E.: Merosin, a tissue-specific basement membrane protein, is a laminin-like protein. Proc. Natl. Acad. Sci. U.S.A. 87:3264–3268, 1990.

Eidelman, S., Damsky, C.H., Wheelock, M.J., and Damjanov, I.: Expression of the cell-cell adhesion glyco-protein cell-CAM 120/80 in normal human tissues and tumors. Am. J. Pathol. 135:101–110, 1989.

Einbrodt, H.J., and Schmid, K.O.: Über abnorme Verkalkungen der menschlichen Placenta bei Maternitäts-tetanie. Arch. Gynecol. 200:327–339, 1965.

Einbrodt, H.J., Schiereck, F.W., and Kinny, H.: Über die Ablagerung von Blei in den Verkalkungen der menschlichen Placenta. Arch. Gynecol. 213:303–306, 1973.

Ellis, S.A., Sargent, I.L., Redman, C.W., and McMichael, A.J.: Evidence for a novel HLA antigen found on human extravillous trophoblast and a choriocarcinoma cell line. Immunology 59:595–601, 1986.

Ellis, S.A., Palmer, M.S., and McMichael, A.J.: Human trophoblast and the choriocarcinoma cell line BeWo express a truncated HLA Class I molecule. J. Immunol. 144:731–735, 1990.

Emonard, H., Christiane, Y., Smet, M., Grimaud, J.A., and Foidart, J.M.: Type IV and interstitial collagenolytic activities in normal and malignant trophoblast cells are specifically regulated by the extracellular matrix. Invasion Metastasis 10:170–177, 1990.

Enders, A.C.: Fine structure of anchoring villi of the human placenta. Am. J. Anat. 122:419–452, 1968.

Enders, A.C.: Current topic: structural responses of the primate endometrium to implantation. Placenta 12:309–325, 1991.

Enders, A.C., and Schlafke, S.: Cytological aspects of tropho-blast-uterine interaction in early implantation. Am. J. Anat. 125:1–30, 1969.

Ermocilla, R., and Altshuler, G.: The origin of "X cells" of the human placenta and their possible relationship to intrauterine growth retardation: an enigma. Am. J. Obstet. Gynecol. 117:1137–1140, 1973.

Faller, T., and Ferenci, P.: Der Aubau der Placenta-Septen: Untersuchungen mit Hilfe der Quinacrinfluorescenzfärbung des Y-Chromatins. Z. Anat. Entwicklungsgesch. 142:207–217, 1973.

Farmer, D.R., and Nelson, D.M.: A fibrin matrix modulates the proliferation, hormone secretion and morphologic differentiation of cultured human placental trophoblast. Placenta 13:163–177, 1992.

Faulk, W.P.: Placental fibrin. Am. J. Reprod. Immunol. 19:132–135, 1989.

Faulk, P., Trenchev, P., Dorling, J., and Holborow, J.: Antigens on post-implantation placentae. In, Immunobiology of Trophoblast. R.G. Edwards, C.W.S. Howe, and M.H. Johnson, eds., pp. 113–130. Cambridge University Press, Cambridge, 1975.

Fazleabas, A.T., Verhage, H.G., Waites, G., and Bell, S.C.: Characterization of an insulin-like growth factor binding protein, analogous to human pregnancy-associated secreted endometrial alpha 1-globulin, in decidua of the baboon (Papio anubis) placenta. Biol. Reprod. 40:873–885, 1989.

Feinberg, R.F., and Kliman, H.J.: Tropho-uteronectin (TUN): a unique oncofetal fibronectin deposited in the extracellular matrix of the tropho-uterine junction and regulated in vitro by cultured human trophoblast cells. Trophoblast Res. 7:167–181, 1993.

Feinberg, R.F., Kao, L.C., Haimowitz, J.E., Queenan, J.T., Jr., Wun, T.C., Strauss, J.F., and Kliman, H.J.: Plasminogen activator inhibitor types 1 and 2 in human trophoblasts: PAI-1 is an immunocytochemical marker of invading trophoblasts. Lab. Invest. 61:20–26, 1989.

Feinberg, R.F., Kliman, H.J., and Cohen, A.W.: Preeclampsia, trisomy 13, and the placental bed. Obstet. Gynecol. 78:505–508, 1991a.

Feinberg, R.F., Kliman, H.J., and Lockwood, C.J.: Is oncofetal fibronectin a trophoblast glue for human implantation? Am. J. Pathol. 138:537–543, 1991b.

Fisher, S., Rikover, M., and Naor, S.: Factor XIII deficiency with severe haemorrhagic diathesis. Blood 28:34–39, 1966.

Fisher, S.J., and Damsky, C.H.: Human cytotrophoblast invasion. Semin. Cell Biol. 4:183–188, 1993.

Fisher, S.J., Leitch, M.S., Kantor, M.S., Basbaum, C.B., and Kramer, R.H.: Degradation of extracellular matrix by the trophoblastic cells of first-trimester human placentas. J. Cell Biochem. 27:31–41, 1985.

Fisher, S.J., Cui, T.Y., Zhang, L., Hartman, L., Grahl, K., Guo-Yang, Z., Tarpey, J., and Damsky, C.H.: Adhesive and degradative properties of human placental cytotrophoblast cells in vitro. J. Cell Biol. 109:891–902, 1989.

Fisher, S.J., Librach, C., Zhou, Y., Dao, D., Kosten, K., Roth, I., Bass, K., and Damsky, C.H.: Regulation of human cytotrophoblast invasion. Placenta 13:A.17, 1992.

Fox, H.: White infarcts of the placenta. J. Obstet. Gynaecol. Br. Commonw. 70:980–991, 1963.

Fox, H.: Calcification of the placenta. J. Obstet. Gynaecol. Br. Commonw. 71:759–765, 1964.

Fox, H.: Perivillous fibrin deposition in the human placenta. Am. J. Obstet. Gynecol. 98:245–251, 1967a.

Fox, H.: The significance of placental infarction in perinatal morbidity and mortality. Biol. Neonate 11:87–105, 1967b.

Fox, H.: Fibrinoid necrosis of placental villi. J. Obstet. Gynaecol. Br. Commonw. 75:448–452, 1968.

Fox, H.: Effect of hypoxia on trophoblast in organ culture. Am. J. Obstet. Gynecol. 107:1058–1064, 1970.

Fox, H.: Pathology of the Placenta. Saunders, London, 1978.

Frame, L.T., Wiley, L., and Rogol, A.D.: Indirect immunofluorescent localization of prolactin to the cytoplasm of decidua and trophoblast cells in human placental membranes at term. J. Clin. Endocrinol. Metab. 49:435–437, 1979.

Frank, H.G., Malekzadeh, F., Kertschanska, S., Crescimanno, C., Castellucci, M., Lang, I., Desoye, G., and Kaufmann, P.: Immunohistochemistry of two different types of placental fibrinoid. Acta Anat. (Basel) 150:55–68, 1994.

Franken, H.: Beitrag zur Veranschaulichung von Struktur und Funktion der Plazenta. Zentralbl. Gynäkol. 76:729–745, 1954.

Freese, U.E.: The uteroplacental vascular relationship in the human. Am. J. Obstet. Gynecol. 101:8–16, 1968.

Freese, U.E., and Maciolek, B.J.: Plastoid injection studies of the uteroplacental vascular relationship in the human. Obstet. Gynecol. 33:160–169, 1969.

Fuchs, A.R., and Fuchs, F.: Endocrinology of human parturition: a review. Br. J. Obstet. Gynaecol. 91:948–967, 1984.

Fujikura, T.: Placental calcification and maternal age. Am. J. Obstet. Gynecol. 87:41–45, 1963a.

Fujikura, T.: Placental calcification and seasonal difference. Am. J. Obstet. Gynecol. 87:46–47, 1963b.

Fukamatsu, Y., Tomita, K., and Fukuta, T.: Further evidence of prolactin production from human decidua and its transport across fetal membrane. Gynecol. Obstet. Invest. 17:309–316, 1984.

Garel, J.-M., and Barlet, J.-P.: Calcitonin in the mother, fetus and newborn. Ann. Biol. Anim. Biochem. Biophys. 18:53–68, 1978.

Geller, H.F.: Über die Bedeutung des subchorialen Fibrinstreifens in der menschlichen Plazenta. Arch. Gynecol. 192:1–6, 1959.

Genbacev, O., Papic, N., Cuperlovic, M., Vicovac, L., Vuckovic, M., and Miller, R.K.: First trimester chorionic villous explants in culture as a model to study the origin and characteristics of extravillous cytotrophoblast [abstract]. Placenta 12:389, 1991.

Genbacev, O., Schubach, S.A., and Miller, R.K.: Villous culture of first trimester human placenta—model to study extravillous trophoblast (EVT) differentiation. Placenta 13:439–461, 1992.

Genbacev, O., DeMesey Jensen, K., Schubach Powlin, S., and Miller, R.K.: In vitro differentiation and ultrastructure of human extravillous trophoblast (EVT) cells. Placenta 14:463–475, 1993a.

Genbacev, O., Gerdner, K., and Miller, R.K.: Human cytotrophoblastic cell islands from first trimester placentae—proliferative and functional activity in vitro. Placenta 14:A.25, 1993b.

Genbacev, O., White, T.E.K., Gavin, C.E., and Miller, R.K.: Human trophoblast cultures: models for implantation and peri-implantation toxicology. Reprod. Toxicol. 7:75–94, 1993c.

Gille, J., Börner, P., Reinecke, J., Krause, P.-H., and Deicher, H.: Über die Fibrinoidablagerungen in den Endzotten der menschlichen Placenta. Arch. Gynecol. 217:263–271, 1974.

Gladwell, P., Duncan, P., Barham, K., and Kenny, J.: Amnioscopy of late pregnancy with fetal membrane and decidual cytology. Acta Cytol. (Baltimore) 18:333–337, 1974.

Gleich, G.J., and Adolphson, C.R.: The eosinophilic leukocyte: structure and function. Adv. Immunol. 39:177–253, 1986.

Glienke, W.: Zur Ultrastruktur der Septen der menschlichen Plazenta. Z. Mikrosk. Anat. Forsch. 88:111–147, 1974.

Globerson, A., Bauminger, S., Abel, L., and Peleg, S.: Decidual extracts suppress antibody response in vitro. Eur. J. Immunol. 6:120–122, 1976.

Golander, A., Hurley, T., Barrett, J., Handwerger, S.: Synthesis of prolactin by human decidua in vitro. J. Endocrinol. 82:263–267, 1979.

Gosseye, S., and Fox, H.: An immunohistological comparison of the secretory capacity of villous and extravillous trophoblast in the human placenta. Placenta 5:329–348, 1984.

Gossrau, R., Graf, R., Ruhnke, M., and Hanski, C.: Proteases in the human full-term placenta. Histochemistry 86:405–413, 1987.

Grannum, P.A.T., Berkowitz, R.L., and Hobbins, J.C.: The ultrasonic changes in the maturing placenta and their relation to fetal pulmonic maturity. Am. J. Obstet. Gynecol. 133:915–922, 1979.

Grosser, O.: Über Fibrin und Fibrinoid in der Placenta. Z. Anat. Entwicklungsgesch. 76:304–314, 1925.

Grosser, O.: Frühentwicklung, Eihautbildung und Placentation des Menschen und der Säugetiere. Bergmann, Munich, 1927.

Grünwald, P.: The lobular architecture of the human placenta. Bull. John Hopkins Hosp. 119:172–190, 1966.

Grünwald, P.: Fetal deprivation and placental insufficiency. Obstet. Gynecol. 37:906–908, 1971.

Grünwald, P.: Lobular structure of hemochorial primate placentas and its relation to maternal vessels. Am. J. Anat. 136:133–151, 1973.

Gu, Y., Jayatilak, P.G., Parmer, T.G., Gauldie, J., Fey, G.H., and Gibori, G.: Alpha 2-macroglobulin expression in the mesometrial decidua and its regulation by decidual luteotropin and prolactin. Endocrinology 131:1321–1328, 1992.

Gustavii, B.: Release of lysosomal acid phosphatase into the cytoplasm of decidual cells before the onset of labour in humans. Br. J. Obstet. Gynaecol. 82:177–181, 1975.

Haig, D.: Genetic conflicts in human pregnancy. Q. Rev. Biol. 68:495–532, 1993.

Haller, H., Radillo, O., Rukavina, D., Tedesco, F., Candussi, G., Petrovic, O., and Randic, L.: An immunohistochemical study of leucocytes in human endometrium, first and third

trimester basal decidua. J. Reprod. Immunol. 23:41–49, 1993.

Haller, U.: Beitrag zur Morphologie der Utero-Placentargefäße. Arch. Gynecol. 205:185–202, 1968.

Hamaguchi, M., Yamamoto, T., and Sugiyama, Y.: Production of prolactin by cultures of isolated cells from human first-trimester decidua. Obstet. Gynecol. 76:783–787, 1990.

Hamilton, W.J., and Boyd, J.D.: Trophoblast in human uteroplacental arteries. Nature 212:906–908, 1966.

Hamperl, H.: Über die endometrialen Granulozyten (endometriale Körnchenzellen). Klin. Wochenschr. 32:665–668, 1954.

Hansell, D.J., Bryant Greenwood, G.D., and Greenwood, F.C.: Expression of the human relaxin H1 gene in the decidua, trophoblast, and prostate. J. Clin. Endocrinol. Metab. 72:899–904, 1991.

Harman, C.R., Manning, F.A., Stearms, E., and Morrison, I.: The correlation of ultrasonic placental grading and fetal pulmonary maturation in five hundred sixty-three pregnancies. Am. J. Obstet. Gynecol. 143:941–943, 1982.

Harris, J.W.S., and Ramsey, E.M.: The morphology of human uteroplacental vasculature. Carnegie Inst. Contrib. Embryol. 38:43–58, 1966.

Hassler, O.: Placental calcifications. Am. J. Obstet. Gynecol. 103:348–353, 1969.

Healy, D.L., Muller, H.K., and Burger, H.G.: Immunofluorescence shows localisation of prolactin to human amnion. Nature 265:642–643, 1977.

Hearn, S., Walton, J., and Chapman, W.: Evidence that fibronectin in human placenta is derived from intermediate trophoblasts. Mod. Pathol. 5:64A, 1992.

Hein, K.: Licht- und elektronenmikroskopische Untersuchungen an der Basalplatte der reifen menschlichen Plazenta. Z. Zellforsch. 122:323–349, 1971.

Hellweg, G.: Über Auftreten und Verhalten der endometrialen Körnchenzellen im Verlauf der Schwangerschaft, im krankhaft veränderten Endometrium und außerhalb des Corpus Uteri. Virchows Arch. [Pathol. Anat.] 330:658–680, 1957.

Hertig, A.T.: Angiogenesis in the early human chorion and in the primary placenta of the macaque monkey. Contrib. Embryol. Carnegie Inst. 25:37–81, 1935.

Hertig, A.T.: La nidation des oeufs humains fécondes normaux et anormaux. In, Les Fonctions de Nidation Uterine et Leurs Troubles. J. Ferin and M. Gaudefroy, eds., pp. 169–213. Masson, Paris, 1960.

Hill, L.M., Breckle, R., Ragozzino, M.W., Wolfgram, K.R., and O'Brien, P.C.: Grade 3 placentation: incidence and neonatal outcome. Obstet. Gynecol. 61:728–732, 1983.

Hitschmann, J., and Lindenthal, O.T.: Der weisse Infarkt der Placenta. Arch. Gynäkol. 69:587–628, 1903.

Hobbins, J.C., and Winsberg, F.: Ultrasonography in Obstetrics and Gynecology. Williams & Wilkins, Baltimore, 1977.

Hofmann, G.E., Scott, R.T., Jr., Bergh, P.A., and Deligdisch, L.: Immunohistochemical localization of epidermal growth factor in human endometrium, decidua, and placenta. J. Clin. Endocrinol. Metab. 73:882–887, 1991.

Hofmann, G.E., Drews, M.R., Scott, R.T., Jr., Navot, D., Heller, D., and Deligdisch, L.: Epidermal growth factor and its receptor in human implantation trophoblast: immunohistochemical evidence for autocrine/paracrine function. J. Clin. Endocrinol. Metab. 74:981–988, 1992.

Hofmann, G.E., Glatstein, I., Schatz, F., Heller, D., and Deligdisch, L.: Immunohistochemical localization of urokinase-type plasminogen activator and the plasminogen activator inhibitors 1 and 2 in early human implantation sites. Am. J. Obstet. Gynecol. 170:671–676, 1994.

Hohn H.P., Boots, L.R., Denker, H.W., and Höök, M.: Differentiation of human trophoblast cells in vitro stimulated by extracellular matrix. Trophoblast Res. 7:181–201, 1993.

Hörmann, G.: Die Fibrinoidisierung des Chorionepithels als Konstruktionsprinzip der menschlichen Plazenta. Z. Geburtshilfe Gynäkol. 164:263–269, 1965.

Hörmann, G.: Über die sogenannten Septen, Inseln, Zysten, Furchen und die Randzone der menschlichen Plazenta. Z. Geburtshilfe Gynäkol. 165:125–134, 1966.

Hoshina, M., Boothby, M., Hussa, R., Pattillo, R., Camel, H.M., and Boime, I.: Linkage of human chorionic gonadotrophin and placental lactogen biosynthesis to trophoblast differentiation and tumorigenesis. Placenta 6:163–172, 1983.

Hoshina, M., Hussa, R., Pattillo, R., and Boime, I.: Cytologic distribution of chorionic gonadotropin subunit and placental lactogen messenger RNA in neoplasms derived from human placenta. J. Cell Biol. 97:1200–1206, 1985.

Howorka, E., and Kapczynski, W.: Marginal circular haematoma disrupting the chorionic plate of the placenta. J. Obstet. Gynaecol. Br. Commonw. 78:280–282, 1971.

Hsi, B.L., and Yeh, C.J.: Monoclonal antibody GB25 recognizes human villous trophoblasts. Am. J. Reprod. Immunol. Microbiol. 12:1–3, 1986.

Hsi, B.L., Yeh, C.J., Samson, M., and Fehlmann, M.: Monoclonal antibody GB36 raised against human trophoblast recognizes a novel epithelial antigen. Placenta 8:209–217, 1987.

Huber, C.P., Carter, J.E., and Vellios, F.: Lesions of the circulatory system of the placenta: a study of 243 placentas with special reference to the developments of infarcts. Am. J. Obstet. Gynecol. 81:560–572, 1961.

Hui, K.Y., Haber, E., and Matsueda, G.R.: Monoclonal antibodies to a synthetic fibrin-like peptide bind to human fibrin but not to fibrinogen. Science 222:1129–1132, 1983.

Hunt, J.S.: Current topic: The role of macrophages in the uterine response to pregnancy. Placenta 11:467–475, 1990.

Hunt, J.S., Fishback, J.L., Chumbley, G., and Loke, Y.W.: Identification of class I MHC mRNA in human first trimester trophoblast cells by in situ hybridization. J. Immunol. 144:4420–4425, 1990.

Hunt, J.S., Hsi, B.L., King, C.R., and Fishback, J.L.: Detection of class I MHC mRNA in subpopulations of first trimester cytotrophoblast cells by in situ hybridization. J. Reprod. Immunol. 19:315–323, 1991.

Hunziker, R.D., and Wegmann, T.G.: Placental Immunoregulation. Crit. Rev. Immunol. 613:245–285, 1987.

Hustin, J., and Schaaps, J.-P.: Echocardiographic and anatomic studies of the maternotrophoblastic border during the first trimester of pregnancy. Am. J. Obstet. Gynecol. 157: 162–168, 1987.

Hustin, J., and Schaaps, J.-P.: Anatomical studies of the utero-placental vascularization in the first trimester of pregnancy. Trophoblast Res. 3:49–60, 1988.

Ikkala, E., Myllylae, G., and Nevanlinna, H.R.: Transfusion therapy in factor XII (FSF) deficiency. Scand. J. Haematol. 1:308–312, 1964.

Iklé, F.A.: Dissemination von Syncytiotrophoblastzellen im mütterlichen Blut während der Gravidität. Bull. Schweiz. Akad. Med. Wiss. 20:63–72, 1964.

Ikonicoff, L.K.: Histologie et histochimie de la substance fibrinoide au niveau des villositis placentaires humaines. Rev. Fr. Gynecol. 66:139–146, 1971.

Ishizaki, Y., and Belter, L.F.: Melanin deposition in the placenta as a result of skin lesions (dermatopathic melanosis of placenta). Am. J. Obstet. Gynecol. 79:1074–1077, 1960.

Iwanaga, S.: Ultrastructural observations on human endometrial stromal cells during the normal menstrual cycle—with special reference to so-called "predecidual cells." Nippon Sanka Fujinka Gakkai Zasshi 35:177–182, 1983.

Jackson, G.M., Edwin, S.S., Varer, M.W., Casal, D., and Mitchell, M.D.: Regulation of fetal fibronectin production in human chorion cells. Am. J. Obstet. Gynecol. 169:1431–1435, 1993.

Javert, C.T.: Decidual bleeding in pregnancy. Ann. N.Y. Acad. Sci. 61:700–712, 1955.

Jeacock, M.K., Scott, J., and Plester, J.A.: Calcium content of the human placenta. Am. J. Obstet. Gynecol. 87:34–40, 1963.

Johnson, P.M., and Faulk, W.P.: Immunological studies of human placenta: identification and distribution of proteins in immature chorionic villi. Immunology 34:1027–1036, 1978.

Kaiser, R.: Über Rückbildungsvorgaenge in der Dezidua während der Schwangerschaft. Arch. Gynecol. 192:209–220, 1960.

Kanzaki, H., Crainie, M., Lin, H., Yui, J., Guilbert, L.J., Mori, T., and Wegmann, T.G.: The in situ expression of granulocyte-macrophage colony-stimulating factor (GM-CSF) mRNA at the maternal-fetal interface. Growth Factors 5:69–74, 1991.

Katz, V.L., Bowes, W.A., and Sierkh, A.E.: Maternal floor infarction of the placenta associated with elevated second trimester serum alpha-fetoprotein. Ám. J. Perinatol. 4:225–228, 1987.

Kaufman, H., and Adams, E.: Murexide, another approach to the histochemical staining of calcium. Lab. Invest. 6:275–280, 1957.

Kaufmann, P.: Entwicklung der Plazenta. In, Die Plazenta des Menschen. V. Becker, T.H. Schiebler, and F. Kubli, eds. Thieme, Stuttgart, 1981a.

Kaufmann, P.: Fibrinoid. In, Die Plazenta des Menschen. V. Becker, T.H. Schiebler, and F. Kubli, eds. Thieme, Stuttgart, 1981b.

Kaufmann, P.: Basic morphology of the fetal and maternal circuits in the human placenta. Contrib. Gynecol. Obstet. 13:5–17, 1985.

Kaufmann, P., and Stark, J.: Die Basalplatte der reifen menschlichen Placenta. I. Semidünnschnitt-Histologie. Z. Anat. Entwicklungsgesch. 135:1–19, 1971.

Kaufmann, P., and Stark, J.: Semidünnschnitt-zytochemische und immunautoradiographische Befunde zum Hormonstoffwechsel der reifen menschlichen Plazenta. Verh. Anat. Ges. 67:245–249, 1973.

Kaufmann, P., Schröder, H., and Leichtweiss, H.-P.: Fluid shift across the placenta. II. Fetomaternal transfer of horseradish peroxidase in the guinea pig. Placenta 3:339–348, 1982.

Kaufmann, P., Luckhardt, T.M., and Elger, W.: The structure of the tupaia placenta. II. Ultrastructure. Anat. Embryol. (Berl.) 171:211–221, 1985.

Kawagoe, K.: Immune reaction between maternal and fetal tissue at the nidatory site of tubal pregnancy. Nippon Sanka Fujinka Gakkai Zasshi 37:2691–2696, 1985.

Kawagoe, K., Kawana, T., and Sakamoto, S.: Ultrastructure of the nidatory site in tubal pregnancy. Acta Obstet. Gynaecol. Jpn. 33:403–410, 1981.

Kawano, T., Morimoto, K., and Uemura, Y.: Urokinase inhibitor in human placenta. Nature 217:253–254, 1968.

Kazzi, G.M., Gross, T.L., and Sokol, R.J.: Fetal biparietal diameter and placental grade: predictors of intrauterine growth retardation. Obstet. Gynecol. 62:755–759, 1983.

Kearns, M., and Lala, P.K.: Life history of decidual cells: a review. Am. J. Reprod. Immunol. 3:78–82, 1983.

Keiffer, H.: Le placenta myometrial humain; le mechanisme de sa secretion, excretion et absorption. Arch. Biol. 38:93–108, 1928.

Kephart, G.M., Andrade, Z.A., and Gleich, G.J.: Localization of eosinophil major basic protein onto eggs of Schistosoma mansoni in human pathologic tissue. Am. J. Pathol. 133:389–396, 1988.

Khan, H., Ishihara, O., Elder, M.G., and Sullivan, M.H.: A comparison of two populations of decidual cells by immunocytochemistry and prostaglandin production. Histochemistry 96:149–152, 1991.

Khan, H., Ishihara, O., Sullivan, M.H., and Elder, M.G.: Changes in decidual stromal cell function associated with labour. Br. J. Obstet. Gynaecol. 99:10–12, 1992.

Khong, T.Y., DeWolf, F., Robertson, W.B., and Brosens, I.: Inadequate maternal vascular response to placentation in preeclampsia and intrauterine fetal growth retardation. Br. J. Obstet. Gynaecol. 93:1049–1059, 1986a.

Khong, T.Y., Lane, E.B., and Robertson, W.B.: An immunocytochemical study of fetal cells at the maternal-placental interface using monoclonal antibodies to keratins, vimentin and desmin. Cell Tissue Res. 246:189–195, 1986b.

Khudr, G., Soma, H., and Benirschke, K.: Trophoblastic origin of the X-cell and the placental giant cell. Am. J. Obstet. Gynecol. 115:530–533, 1973.

Kim, C.K., and Benirschke, K.: Autoradiographic study of the "X-cells" in the human placenta. Am. J. Obstet. Gynecol. 109:96–102, 1971.

Kim, C.K., Altshuler, G.P., and Benirschke, K.: Karyotypic analysis of the X-cell in the human placenta. Obstet. Gynecol. 37:72–82, 1971a.

Kim, C.K., Naftolin, F., and Benirschke, K.: Immunohistochemical studies of the "X-cell" in the human placenta with anti-human chorionic gonadotropin and anti-human placental lactogen. Am. J. Obstet. Gynecol. 111:672–676, 1971b.

King, A., and Loke, Y.W.: Differential expression of blood-group-related carbohydrate antigens by trophoblast subpopulations. Placenta 9:513–521, 1988.

King, A., and Loke, Y.W.: Uterine large granular lymphocytes: a possible role in embryo implantation? Am. J. Obstet. Gynecol. 162:308–310, 1990.

King, A., and Loke, Y.W.: On the nature and function of human uterine granular lymphocytes. Immunol. Today 12:432–435, 1991.

King, A., Birkby, C., and Loke, Y.W.: Early human decidual cells exhibit NK activity against the K562 cell line but not against first trimester trophoblast. Cell. Immunol. 118:337–344, 1989.

King, A., Kalra, P., and Loke, Y.W.: Human trophoblast cell resistance to decidual NK lysis is due to lack of NK target structure. Cell. Immunol. 127:230–237, 1990.

King, B.F., and Blankenship, T.N.: Expression of proliferating cell nuclear antigen (PCNA) in developing macaque placentas. Placenta 14:A.36, 1993.

Kirby, D.R.S., Billington, W.D., Bradbury, S., and Goldstein, D.J.: Antigen barrier of mouse placenta. Nature 204:548–549, 1964.

Kirkinen, P., and Jouppila, P.: Intrauterine membranous cyst: a report of antenatal diagnosis and obstetric aspects in two cases. Obstet. Gynecol. 67:26S–30S, 1986.

Kisalus, L.L., and Herr, J.C.: Immunocytochemical localization of heparan sulfate proteoglycan in human decidual cell secretory bodies and placental fibrinoid. Biol. Reprod. 39:419–430, 1988.

Kisalus, L.L., Herr, J.C., and Little, C.D.: Immunolocalization of extracellular matrix proteins and collagen synthesis in first trimester human decidua. Anat. Rec. 218:402–415, 1987.

Klein, G.: Makroskopisches Verhalten der Utero-Placentargefässe. In, Die menschliche Placenta. Beiträge zur normalen und pathologischen Anatomie derselben. Hofmeier, ed., pp. 72–87. Bergmann, Wiesbaden, 1890.

Kliman, H.J., and Feinberg, R.F.: Human trophoblast-extracellular matrix (ECM) interactions in vitro: ECM thickness modulates morphology and proteolytic activity. Proc. Natl. Acad. Sci. U.S.A. 87:3057–3061, 1990.

Kliman, H.J., Nestler, J.E., Sermasi, E., Sanger, J.M., and Strauss, J.F., III: Purification, characterization, and in vitro differentiation of cytotrophoblasts from human term placentae. Endocrinology 118:1567–1582, 1985.

Kliman, H.J., Feinman, M.A., and Strauss, J.F., III: Differentiation of human cytotrophoblasts into syncytiotrophoblasts in culture. Trophoblast Res. 2:407–421, 1987.

Kliman, H.J., Feinberg, R.F., and Haimowitz, J.E.: Human trophoblast-endometrial interactions in an in vitro suspension culture system. Placenta 11:349–367, 1990.

Klinger, H.P.: The sex chromatin in fetal and maternal portions of the human placenta. Acta Anat. (Basel) 30:371–397, 1957.

Klinger, H.P., and Ludwig, K.S.: Sind die Septen und die grosszelligen Inseln der Placenta aus mütterlichem oder kindlichem Gewebe aufgebaut? Z. Anat. Entwicklungsgesch. 120:95–100, 1957.

Klopper, H.: The new placental proteins. Placenta 1:77–89, 1980.

Kölliker, A.: Entwicklungsgeschichte des Menschen und der höheren Thiere. 1st Ed. Engelmann, Leipzig, 1861.

Kölliker, A.: Entwicklungsgeschichte des Menschen und der höheren Thiere. 2nd Ed. Engelmann, Leipzig, 1879.

Kohnen, G., Kosanke, G., Korr, H., and Kaufmann, P.: Comparison of various proliferation markers applied to human placental tissue. Placenta 14:A38, 1993.

Korhonen, M., Ylanne, J., Laitinen, L., Cooper, H.M., Quaranta, V., and Virtanen, I.: Distribution of the alpha 1-alpha 6 integrin subunits in human developing and term placenta. Lab. Invest. 65:347–356, 1991.

Kosanke, G.: Methodological studies of proliferation markers applied to human placental villi. Biology doctoral thesis, Sciences Faculty, Technical University of Aachen, 1994.

Kottsova, N.A., Bystrova, O.A., Susloparov, L.A., and Mikhailov, V.M.: Changes in the cellular composition of the deciduous membrane in physiologic pregnancy and late toxicosis. Arkh. Anat. Gistol. Embriol. 97:76–82, 1989.

Krafft, M.-L.: Über den Halte- und Verspannungsapparat der plazentaren Randzone und der Eihäute. (Nach graphischen Rekonstruktionen.) Inaugural dissertation, Berlin, 1973.

Kratzsch, E., and Grygiel, I.-H.: Über das Vorkommen eines spezifischen Enzyms der Glucuronsäurebildung im menschlichen Amnion. Z. Zellforsch. 123:566–571, 1972.

Kretschmann, H.-J.: Über Feinstruktur des subchorialen Placentarfibrins im Vergleich mit der des Blutfibrins. I. Orthoskopische Analyse. Acta Anat. (Basel) 66:339–364, 1967a.

Kretschmann, H.-J.: Über die Feinstruktur des subchorialen Placentarfibrins im Vergleich mit der des Blutfibrins. II. Experimentelle Studie über Veränderungen der Feinstruktur des Blutfibrins. Acta Anat. (Basel) 66:494–503, 1967b.

Krönicher, W.D.: Ein Beitrag zur Genese der Inseln in der menschlichen Placenta. Z. Mikrosk. Anat. Forsch. 89:777–803, 1975.

Krohn, K., Ljungqvist, A., and Robertson, B.: Trophoblastic and subtrophoblastic mineral salt deposition in hydramnios. Acta Pathol. Microbiol. Scand. 69:514–520. 1967.

Kubli, F.: Die chronische Placentarinsuffizienz. Gynakologe 1:53–60, 1968.

Kubota, T., Kamada, S., Hirata, Y., Eguchi, S., Imai, T., Marumo, F., and Aso, T.: Synthesis and release of endothelin-1 by human decidual cells. J. Clin. Endocrinol. Metab. 75:1230–1234, 1992.

Kühler, W.: Die Deciduaverteilung in der menschlichen Placenta. Inaugural dissertation, Wesel, pp. 1–38, 1890.

Kunicki, T.J., Nugent, D.J., Staats, S.J., Orchekowski, R.P., Wayner E.A., and Carter W.G.: The human fibroblast class II extracellular matrix receptor mediates platelet adhesion to collagen and is identical to the platelet Ia-IIa complex. J. Biol. Chem. 263:4516–4519, 1988.

Kurman, R.J., Main, C.S., and Chen, H.C.: Intermediate trophoblast: a distinctive form of trophoblast with specific morphological, biochemical and functional features. Placenta 5:349–369, 1984a.

Kurman, R.J., Young, R.H., Norris, H.J., Main, C.S., Lawrence, W.D., and Sculley, R.E.: Immunocytochemical localization of placental lactogen and chorionic gonadotropin in the normal placenta and trophoblastic tumors, with emphasis on intermediate trophoblast and the placental site trophoblastic tumor. Int. J. Gynecol. Pathol. 3:101–121, 1984b.

Kyodo, Y., Kobayashi, T., and Terao, T.: Studies on the immunohistochemical localization of coagulation fibrinolysis factors in the placenta, especially of placental plasminogen activator (PPA). Nippon Sanka Fujinka Gakkai Zasshi 38: 10–16, 1986.

Ladines Llave, C.A., Maruo, T., Manalo, A.M., and Mochizuki, M.: Decreased expression of epidermal growth factor and its receptor in the malignant transformation of trophoblasts. Cancer 71:4118–4123, 1993.

Lala, P.K., Kearns, M., and Colavincenzo, V.: Cells of the fetomaternal interface: their role in the maintenance of viviparous pregnancy. Am. J. Anat. 170:501–517, 1984.

Lala, P.K., Kearns, M., and Pahar, R.S.: Immunobiology of the decidual tissue: the maternal component of the fetomaternal interface. In, Immunoregulation and Fetal Survival. T. Gill and T.G. Wegmann, eds. Oxford University Press, New York, 1985.

Lang, I., Hartmann, M., Blaschitz, A., Dohr, G., Skofitsch, G., and Desoye, G.: Immunohistochemical evidence for the heterogeneity of maternal and fetal vascular endothelial cells in human full-term placenta. Cell Tissue Res. 274:211–218, 1993.

Lang, I., Hartmann, M., Blaschitz, A., Dohr, G., Kaufmann, P., Frank, H.G., Hahn, T., Skofitsch, G., and Desoye, G.: Differential lectin binding to the fibrinoid of human full term placenta: correlation with a fibrin antibody and the PAF-Halmi method. Acta Anat. (Basel) 1994 (in press).

Langhans, T.: Untersuchungen über die menschliche Placenta. Arch. Anat. Physiol., Anat. Abt. 188–267, 1877.

Lapan, B., and Friedman, M.M.: Tissue enzymes in gestation: comparative activities in the placenta and fetal membranes. Am. J. Obstet. Gynecol. 93:1157–1163, 1965.

Larsen, J.F., and Knoth, M.: Ultrastructure of the anchoring villi and trophoblastic shell in the second week of placentation. Acta Obstet. Gynecol. Scand. 50:117–128, 1971.

Larsen, L.G., Theilade, K., Skibsted, L., and Jacobsen, G.K.: Malignant placental site trophoblastic tumor: a case report and a review of the literature. APMIS Suppl. 23: 138–145, 1991.

Latta, J.S., and Beber, C.R.: The differentiation of a special form of trophoblast in the human placenta. Am. J. Obstet. Gynecol. 74:105–110, 1957.

Lawn, A.M., Wilson, E.W., and Finn, C.A.: The ultrastructure of human decidual and predecidual cells. J. Reprod. Fertil. 26:85–90, 1971.

Leivo, I., Laurila, P., Wahlstrom, T., and Engvall, E.: Expression of merosin, a tissue-specific basement membrane protein, in the intermediate trophoblast cells of choriocarcinoma and placenta. Lab. Invest. 60:783–790, 1989.

Librach, C.L., Werb, Z., Fitzgerald, M.L., Chiu, K., Corwin, N.M., Esteves, R.A., Grobelny, D., Galardy, R., Damsky, C.H., and Fisher, S.J.: 92-kD Type IV collagenase mediates invasion of human cytotrophoblasts. J. Cell Biol. 113:437–449, 1991.

Liotta, L.A., Steeg, P.S., and Stetler-Stevenson, W.G.: Cancer metastasis and angiogenesis: an imbalance of positive and negative regulation. Cell 64:327–336, 1991.

Linthwaite, R. F.: Subchorial hematoma mole (Breus' mole). J.A.M.A. 186:867–870, 1963.

Logothetou Rella, H., Kotoulas, I.G., Nesland, J.M., Kipiotis, D., and Abazis, D.: Early human trophoblast cell cultures: a morphological and immunocytochemical study. Histol. Histopathol. 4:367–374, 1989.

Loke, Y.W.: Trophoblast antigen expression. Curr. Opin. Immunol. 1:1131–1134, 1989.

Loke, Y.W.: Experimenting with human extravillous trophoblast: a personal view. Am. J. Reprod. Immunol. 24:22–28, 1990.

Loke, Y.W., and Day, S.: Monoclonal antibody to human cytotrophoblast. Am. J. Reprod. Immunol. 5:106–108, 1984.

Loke, Y.W., and King, A.: Recent developments in the human maternal-fetal immune interaction. Curr. Opin. Immunol. 3:762–766, 1991.

Loke, Y.W., Butterworth, B.H., Margetts, J.J., and Burland, K.: Identification of cytotrophoblast colonies in cultures of human placental cells using monoclonal antibodies. Placenta 7:221–231, 1986.

Loke, Y.W., and Burland, K.: Human trophoblast cells cultured in modified medium and supported by extracellular matrix. Placenta 9:173–182, 1988.

Loke, Y.W., Gardner, L., and Grabowska, A.: Isolation of human extravillous trophoblast cells by attachment to laminin-coated magnetic beads. Placenta 10:407–415, 1989a.

Loke, Y.W., Gardner, L., Burland, K., and King, A.: Laminin in human trophoblast—decidua interaction. Hum. Reprod. 4:457–463, 1989b.

Loke, Y.W., Hsi, B.L., Bulmer, J.N., Grivaux, C., Hawley, S., Gardner, L., King, A., and Carter, N.P.: Evaluation of a monoclonal antibody, BC-1, which identifies an antigen expressed on the surface membrane of human extravillous trophoblast. Am. J. Reprod. Immunol. 27:77–81, 1992a.

Loke, Y.W., King, A., Gardner, L., and Carter, N.P.: Evidence for the expression of granulocyte-macrophage colony-stimulating factor receptors by human first trimester extravillous trophoblast and its response to this cytokine. J. Reprod. Immunol. 22:33–45, 1992b.

Luckett, W.P.: Origin and differentiation of the yolk sac and extraembryonic mesoderm in presomite human and rhesus monkey embryos. Am. J. Anat. 152:59–97, 1978.

Ludwig, K.S.: Die Rolle des Fibrins bei der Bildung der menschlichen Placenta. Acta Anat. (Basel) 38:323–331, 1959.

Ludwig, K.S.: Zur Feinstruktur der materno-fetalen Verbindung im Plazentom des Schafes (Ovis aries L.). Experientia 18:212, 1962.

Ludwig, H., and Metzger, H.: Das uterine Placentarbett post partum im Rasterelektronenmikroskop, zugleich ein Beitrag zur Frage der extravasalen Fibrinbildung. Arch. Gynecol. 210:251–266, 1971.

Lysiak, J., Khoo, N., Conelly, I., Stettler-Stevenson, W., and Peeyush, L.: Role of transforming growth factor (TGF) α and epidermal growth factor (EGF) on proliferation, invasion, and hCG production by normal and malignant trophoblast. Placenta 13:A41, 1992.

Maddox, D.E., Butterfield, J.H., Ackerman, S.J., Coulam, C.B., and Gleich, G.J.: Elevated serum levels in human pregnancy of a molecule immunochemically similar to eosinophil granule major basic protein. J. Exp. Med. 158:1211–1226, 1983.

Maddox, D.E., Kephart, G.M., Coulam, C.B., Butterfield, J.H., Benirschke, K., and Gleich, G.J.: Localization of a molecule immunochemically similar to eosinophil major basic protein in human placenta. J. Exp. Med. 160:29–41, 1984.

Maidman, J.E., Thorpe, L.W., Harris, J.A., and Wynn, R.M.: Fetal origin of X-cells in human placental septa and basal plate. Obstet. Gynecol. 41:547–552, 1973.

Malak, T.M., Ockleford, C.D., Bell, S.C., Dalgleish, R., Bright, N., and MacVicar, J.: Confocal immunofluorescence localization of collagen type-I, type-III, type-IV, type-V and type-VI and their ultrastructural organization in term human fetal membranes. Placenta 14:385–406, 1993.

Manaseki, S., and Searle, R.F.: Natural killer (NK) cell activity of first trimester human decidua. Cell. Immunol. 121:166–173, 1989.

Manivel, J.C., Niehans, G., Wick, M.R., and Dehner, L.P.: Intermediate trophoblast in germ cell neoplasms. Am. J. Surg. Pathol. 11:693–701, 1987.

Mansager, N., Bendon, R., Rosenn, B., Miodovnik, M., Mostello, D., and Siddiqi, T.A.: Maternal floor infarction: prenatal diagnosis and clinical significance [abstract 170]. Am. J. Obstet. Gynecol. 168:347, 1993.

Marais, W.D.: Human decidual spiral artery studies. I. Anatomy, circulation and pathology of the placenta. observations with a colposcope. J. Obstet. Gynaecol. Br. Commonw. 69:1–122, 1962.

Martinek, J.J.: Fibrinoid and the fetal-maternal interface of the rat placenta. Anat. Rec. 166:587–604, 1970.

Martinek, J.J.: Ultrastructure of the deciduotrophoblastic interface of the mouse placenta. Am. J. Obstet. Gynecol. 109:424–431, 1971.

Matsuo, H., Maruo, T., Murata, K., and Mochizuki, M.: Human early placental trophoblasts produce an epidermal growth factor-like substance in synergy with thyroid hormone. Acta Endocrinol. (Copenh.) 128:225–229, 1993.

Mau, G., and Netter, P.: Blutungen in der Frühschwangerschaft: ein Hinweis auf kindliche Mißbildungen? Z. Kinderheilk. 117:79–88, 1974.

McCombs, H.L., and Craig, J.M.: Decidual necrosis in normal pregnancy. Obstet. Gynecol. 24:436–442, 1964.

McCormick, J.N., Faulk, W.P., Fox, H., and Fudenberg, H.H.: Immunohistological and elution studies of the human placenta. J. Exp. Med. 91:1–13, 1971.

McKay, D.G., Hertig, A.T., Adams, E.C., and Richardson, M.V.: Histochemical observations on the human placenta. Obstet. Gynecol. 12:1–36, 1958.

McWey, L.A., Singhas, C.A., and Rogol, A.D.: Prolactin binding sites on human chorion-decidua tissue. Am. J. Obstet. Gynecol. 144:283–288, 1982.

Moe, N.: Deposits of fibrin and plasma proteins in the normal human placenta. Acta Pathol. Microbiol. Scand. 76:74–88, 1969a.

Moe, N.: Histological and histochemical study of the extracellular deposits in the normal human placenta. Acta Pathol. Microbiol. Scand. 76:419–431, 1969b.

Moe, N.: The cytotrophoblastic cell columns and the cell islands of the normal human placenta. Acta Pathol. Microbiol. Scand. 76:401–418, 1969c.

Moe, N.: The deposits of fibrin and fibrin-like materials in the basal plate of the normal human placenta. Acta Pathol. Microbiol. Scand. 75:1–17, 1969d.

Moll, U.M., and Lane, B.L.: Proteolytic activity of first trimester human placenta: localization of interstitial collagenase in villous and extravillous trophoblast. Histochemistry 94:555–560, 1990.

Moll, W., Nienartowicz, A., Hees, H., Wrobel, K.-H., and Lenz, A.: Blood flow regulation in the uteroplacental arteries. Trophoblast Res. 3:83–96, 1988.

Monaghan, J., O'Herlihy, C., and Boylan, P.: Ultrasound placental grading and amniotic fluid quantitation in prolonged pregnancy. Obstet. Gynecol. 70:349–352, 1987.

Montemagno, U.: La sostanza fibrinoide placentare. Arch. Ostetr. Ginecol. (Napoli) 72:585–596, 1967.

Morris, N.H., Eaton, B.M., Sooranna, S.R., and Steer, P.J.: NO synthase activity in placental bed and tissues from normotensive pregnant women. Lancet 342:679–680, 1993.

Mortimer, G., Mackay, M.M., and Stimson, W.H.: The distribution of pregnancy-associated prostaglandin synthetase inhibitor in the human placenta. J. Pathol. 159:239–243, 1989.

Mossman, H.W.: Comparative morphogenesis of the foetal membranes and accessory uterine structures. Contrib. Embryol. Carnegie Inst. 26:129–246, 1937.

Mossman, H.W.: Vertebrate Fetal Membranes: Comparative Ontogeny and Morphology; Evolution; Phylogenetic Significance; Basic Functions; Research Opportunities. Macmillan, London, 1987.

Mühlhauser, J., Crescimanno, C., Kaufmann, P., Höfler, H., Zaccheo, D., and Castellucci, M.: Differentiation and proliferation patterns in human trophoblast revealed by c-erbB-2 oncogene product and EGF-R. J. Histochem. Cytochem. 41:165–173, 1993.

Naeye, R.L.: Maternal floor infarction. Hum. Pathol. 16:823–828, 1985.

Nanaev, A.K., Milovanov, A.P., and Domogatsky, S.P.: Immunohistochemical localization of extracellular matrix in perivillous fibrinoid of normal human term placenta. Histochemistry 100:341–346, 1993a.

Nanaev, A.K., Milovanov, A.P., and Domogatsky, S.P.; Immunohistochemical localization of extracellular matrix in various types of fibrinoid of the normal human term placenta. Placenta 14:A.55, 1993b.

Nelson, D.M., Crouch, E.C., Curran, E.M., and Farmer, D.R.: Trophoblast interaction with fibrin matrix. Epithelialization of perivillous fibrin deposits as a mechanism for villous repair in the human placenta. Am. J. Pathol. 136:855–865, 1990.

Neuberg, M.: Decidual prolactin. Wiad. Lek. 45:376–380, 1992.

Neumann, E.: Die Picrocarminfärbung und ihre Anwendung auf die Entzündungslehre. Arch. Mikrosk. Anat. 18:130–150, 1880.

Nickel, R.E.: Maternal floor infarction: an unusual cause of intrauterine growth retardation. Am. J. Dis. Child. 142: 1270–1271, 1988.

Nikolov, S.D., and Schiebler, T.H.: Über die Gefässe der Basalplatte der reifen menschlichen Placenta. Licht- und elektronenmikroskopische Untersuchungen. Z. Zellforsch. 139:319–332, 1973.

Nitabuch, R.: Beiträge zur Kenntnis der menschlichen Plazenta. Inaugural dissertation, Stämpfli, Bern, 1887.

Ockleford, C.D., Malak, T., Hubbard, A., Bracken, K., Burton, S.A., Bright, N., Blakey, G., Goodliffe, J., Garrod, D., and d'Lacey, C.: Human amniochorion cytoskeletons at term. Placenta 14:A56, 1993.

Ockleford, C., Bright, N., Hubbard, A., d'Lacey, C., Smith, J., Gardiner, L., Sheikh, T., Albentosa, M., and Turtle, K.: Micro-trabeculae, macro-plaques or mini-basement membranes in human term fetal membranes. Philos. Trans. R. Soc. Lond. [Biol.] 342:121–136, 1994.

O'Connor, D.M., and Kurman, R.J.: Intermediate trophoblast in uterine curettings in the diagnosis of ectopic pregnancy. Obstet. Gynecol. 72:665–670, 1988a.

O'Connor, D.M., and Kurman, R.J.: Utilization of intermediate trophoblast in the diagnosis of an in utero gestation in endometrial curettings without chorionic villi. Mod. Pathol. 1:68A, 1988b.

Okudaira, Y., Hashimoto, T., Hamanaka, N., and Yoshinare, S.: Electron microscopic study on the trophoblastic cell column of human placenta. J. Electron Microsc. 20:93–106, 1971.

Okudaira, Y., Matsui, Y., and Kanoh, H.: Morphological variability of human trophoblasts in normal and neoplastic conditions—an ultrastructural reappraisal. In, Placenta: Basic Research for Clinical Application. H. Soma, ed. Karger, Basel, 1991.

Oláh, C.S., Gee, H., Rushton, I., and Fowlie, A.: Massive subchorionic thrombohaematoma presenting as a placental tumour: case report. Br. J. Obstet. Gynaecol. 94:995–997, 1987.

Ono, H., Ide, C., and Nishiya, I.: Electron microscopic study on early decidualization of the endometrium of pregnant mice, with special reference to gap junctions. Placenta 10: 247–261, 1989.

Ornoy, A., Benady, S., Kohen-Raz, R., and Russell, A.: Association between maternal bleeding during gestation and congenital anomalies in the offspring. Am. J. Obstet. Gynecol. 124:474–478, 1976.

Ortmann, R.: Histochemische Untersuchungen an menschlicher Plazenta mit besonderer Berücksichtigung der Kernkugeln (Kerneinschlüsse) und der Plasmalipoideinschlüsse. Z. Anat. Entwicklungsgesch. 119:28–55, 1955.

Ortmann, R.: Morphologie der menschlichen Placenta. Anat. Anz. 106/107:27–56, 1960.

Oswald, B., and Gerl, D.: Die Mikrofibrinoidablagerungen in der menschlichen Placenta. Acta Histochem. 42:356–359, 1972.

Pace, D., Morrison, L., and Bulmer, J.N.: Proliferative activity in endometrial stromal granulocytes throughout menstrual cycle and early pregnancy. J. Clin. Pathol. 42: 35–39, 1989.

Paddock, R., and Greer, E.D.: Origin of common cystic structure of human placenta. Am. J. Obstet. Gynecol. 13: 164–173, 1927.

Padykula, H.A., and Driscoll, S.G.: Decidual cell differentiation in the normal early gestational uterus includes lymphoid infiltration. Anat. Rec. 190:500–501, 1978.

Pampfer, S., Daiter, E., Barad, D., and Pollard, J.W.: Expression of the colony-stimulating factor-1 receptor (c-fms proto-oncogene product) in the human uterus and placenta. Biol. Reprod. 46:48–57, 1992.

Panigel, M., and Pascaud, M.: Les orifices artériels d'entrée du sang maternel dans la chambre intervilleuse du placenta humain. Bull. Assoc. Anat. 53rd Congres (Tours. No. 142), pp. 1287–1298, 1968.

Parhar, R.S., Yagel, S., and Lala, P.K.: PGE₂–mediated immunosuppression by first trimester human decidual cells blocks activation of maternal leukocytes in the decidua with potential anti-trophoblast activity. Cell Immunol. 120:61–74, 1989.

Park, W.W.: Disorders arising from the human trophoblast. In, Modern Trends in Pathology. D.H. Collins, ed., pp. 180–211. Butterworth, London, 1959.

Parmley, T.H., Gupta, P.K., and Walker, M.A.: "Aging" pigments in term human placenta. Am. J. Obstet. Gynecol. 139:760–766, 1981.

Peel, S., and Bulmer, D.: The fine structure of the rat metrial gland in relation to the origin of the granulated cells. J. Anat. 123:687–969, 1977.

Perrin, E.V.D.K.: Placenta as a reflection of fetal disease: a brief overview. In, Pathology of the Placenta. E.V.D.K. Perrin, ed. Churchill Livingstone, New York, 1984.

Petraglia, F., Sawchenko, P., Lim, A.T.W., Rivier, J., and Vale, W.: Localization, secretion, and action of inhibin in human placenta. Science 237:187–189, 1987.

Petrucha, R.A., and Platt, L.D.: Relationship of placental grade to gestational age. Am. J. Obstet. Gynecol. 144:733–735, 1982.

Petry, G.: Der Bau der menschlichen Eihaut und seine funktionelle Bedeutung. Klin. Wochenschr. 32:1020, 1954a.

Petry, G.: Studien über die morphologischen Grundlagen des Blasensprungs. Zentralbl. Gynäkol. 76:655–675, 1954b.

Pfeiffer, R.A.: Nanisme microcephalique letal: exemple de pathologie placentaire d'origine genetique? J. Genet. Hum. 22:259–261, 1974.

Pijnenborg, R., Dixon, G., Robertson, W.B., and Brosens, I.: Trophoblastic invasion of human decidua from 8 to 18 weeks of pregnancy. Placenta 1:3–19, 1980.

Pijnenborg, R., Robertson, W.B., Brosens, I., and Dixon, G.: Trophoblast invasion and the establishment of haemochorial placentation in man and laboratory animals. Placenta 2:71–92, 1981.

Piotrowicz, R.S., Orchekowski, D.J., Nugent, D.J., Yamada, K.Y., and Kunicki T.J.: Glycoprotein Ic-IIa functions as an activation-independent fibronectin receptor on human platelets. J. Cell Biol. 106:1359–1364, 1988.

Pitkin, R.M.: Calcium metabolism in pregnancy: a review. Am. J. Obstet. Gynecol. 121:724–737, 1975.

Pitkin, R.M., Reeynolds, W.A., Williams, G.A., and Hargis, G.K.: Calcium metabolism in normal pregnancy: a longitudinal study. Am. J. Obstet. Gynecol. 133:781–790, 1979.

Powell, H.C., Benirschke, K., Favara, B.E., and Pflueger, O.H.: Foamy changes of placental cells in fetal storage disorders. Virchows Arch. [A] 369:191–196, 1976.

Pozniak, M.A., Cullenward, M.J., Zickuhr, D., and Curet, L.B.: Venous lake bleeding: a complication of chorionic villus sampling. J. Ultrasound Med. 7:297–299, 1988.

Raghupathy, R., Singh, B., Barrington-Leigh, J., and Wegmann, T.G.: The ontogeny and turnover kinetics of paternal H-2 K antigenic determinants on the allogenic murine placenta. J. Immunol. 127:2074, 1981.

Raghupathy, R., Singh, B., and Wegmann, T.G.: Fate of antipaternal H-2 antibodies bound to the placenta in vivo. Transplantation 37:296, 1984.

Ramsey, E.M.: Circulation in the maternal placenta of the rhesus monkey and man, with observations on the marginal lakes. Am. J. Anat. 98:159–190, 1956.

Ramsey, E.M.: Circulation in the intervillous space of the primate placenta. Am. J. Obstet. Gynecol. 84:1649–1663, 1962.

Ramsey, E.M.: The story of the spiral arteries. J. Reprod. Med. 26:393–399, 1981.

Ramsey, E.M., and Donner, M.W.: Placental Vasculature and Circulation. Thieme, Stuttgart, 1980.

Ramsey, E.M., and Harris, J.W.S.: Comparison of uteroplacental vasculature and circulation in the rhesus monkey and man. Contrib. Embryol. Carnegie Inst. 38:59–70, 1966.

Ramsey, E.M., Corner, G.W., Jr., and Donner, M.W.: Serial and cineradioangiographic visualization of maternal circulation in the primate (hemochorial) placenta. Am. J. Obstet. Gynecol. 86:213–225, 1963.

Ramsey, E.M., Martin, C.B., Jr., McGaughey, H.S., Jr., Kaiser, I.H., and Donner, M.W.: Venous drainage of the placenta in rhesus monkeys: radiographic studies. Am. J. Obstet. Gynecol. 95:948–955, 1966.

Reddy, G.S., Norman, A.W., Willis, D.M., Goltzman, D., Guyda, H., Solomon, S., Philips, D.R., Bishop, J.E., and Mayer, E.: Regulation of vitamin D metabolism in normal human pregnancy. J. Clin. Endocrinol. Metab. 56:363–370, 1983.

Redline, R.W., and Lu, C.Y.: Specific defects in the anti-listerial immune response in discrete regions of the murine uterus and placenta account for susceptibility to infection. J. Immunol. 140:3947–3955, 1988.

Ren, S.G., and Braunstein, G.D.: Decidua produces a protein that inhibits choriogonadotrophin release from human trophoblasts. J. Clin. Invest. 87:326–330, 1991.

Reshef, E., Lei, Z.M., Rao, C.V., Pridham, D.D., Chegini, N., and Luborsky, J.L.: The presence of gonadotropin receptors in nonpregnant human uterus, human placenta, fetal membranes, and decidua. J. Clin. Endocrinol. Metab. 70:421–430, 1990.

Reynolds, S.R.M.: Formation of fetal cotyledons in the hemochorial placenta: a theoretical consideration of the functional implication of such an arrangements. Am. J. Obstet. Gynecol. 94:425–439, 1966.

Riley, S.C., Walton, J.C., Herlick, J.M., and Challis, J.R.: The localization and distribution of corticotropin-releasing hormone in the human placenta and fetal membranes throughout gestation. J. Clin. Endocrinol. Metab. 72:1001–1007, 1991.

Riddick, D.H., and Daly, D.C.: Decidual prolactin in human gestation. Semin. Perinatol. 6:L229–237, 1982.

Riley, S.C., Dupont, E., Walton, J.C., Luuthe, V., Labrie, F., Pelletier, G., and Challis, J.R.G.: Immunohistochemical localization of 3β-hydroxy-5-ene-steroid dehydrogenase delta5 → delta4 isomerase in human placenta and fetal membranes throughout gestation. J. Clin. Endocrinol. Metab. 75:956–961, 1992.

Ritson, A., and Bulmer, J.N.: Isolation and functional studies of granulated lymphocytes in first trimester human decidua. Clin. Exp. Immunol. 77:263–268, 1989.

Robb, J.A., Benirschke, K., and Barmeyer, R.: Intrauterine latent herpes simplex virus infection. I. Spontaneous abortion. Hum. Pathol. 17:1196–1209, 1986a.

Robb, J.A., Benirschke, K., Mannino, F., and Voland, J.: Intrauterine latent herpes simplex virus infection. II. Latent neonatal infection. Hum. Pathol. 17:1210–1217, 1986b.

Robertson, W.B.: Uteroplacental vasculature. J. Clin. Pathol. 29(Suppl.):9–17, 1976; R. Coll. Pathol. 10:9–17, 1976.

Robertson, W.B., and Manning, P.J.: Elastic tissue in uterine blood vessels. J. Pathol. 112:237–243, 1974.

Robertson, W.B., and Warner, B.: The ultrastructure of the human placental bed. J. Pathol. 112:203–211, 1974.

Robinson, L., Grau, P., and Crandall, B.F.: Pregnancy outcomes after increasing maternal serum alpha-fetoprotein levels. Obstet. Gynecol. 74:17–20, 1989.

Rohr, K.: Die Beziehungen der mütterlichen Gefäße zu den intervillösen Räumen der reifen Plazenta speziell zur Thrombose derselben ("weisser Infarkt"). Virchows Arch. [Pathol. Anat.] 115:505–534, 1889.

Romano, W.M., Lukash, L.A., Challis, J.R.G., and Mitchell, B.F.: Substrate utilization for estrogen synthesis by human fetal membranes and decidua. Am. J. Obstet. Gynecol. 155:1170–1175, 1986.

Rosen, J.F., Roginsky, M., Nathenson, G., and Finberg, L.: 25-Hydroxyvitamin D: plasma levels in mothers and their premature infants with neonatal hypocalcemia. Am. J. Dis. Child. 127:220–223, 1974.

Rosenberg, S.M., and Bhatnagar, A.S.: Sex steroid and human chorionic gonadotropin modulation of in vitro prolactin production by human term decidua. Am. J. Obstet. Gynecol. 148:461–465, 1984.

Rosenberg, S.M., Maslar, I.A., and Riddick, D.H.: Decidual production of prolactin in late gestation: further evidence for a decidual source of amniotic fluid prolactin. Am. J. Obstet. Gynecol. 138:681–685, 1980.

Rossant, J., and Croy, B.A.: Genetic identification of tissue of origin of cellular populations within the mouse placenta. J. Embryol. Exp. Morphol. 86:177–189, 1985.

Ruffolo, R., Benirschke, K., Covington, H.I., and Munro, A.B.: Electron microscopic study of the "X-cells" in septal cysts of the human placenta. Am. J. Obstet. Gynecol. 99:1147–1159, 1967.

Rukosuev, V.S., Nanaev, A.K., and Milovanov, A.P.: Participation of collagen types I, III, IV, V, and fibronectin in the formation of villi fibrosis in human term placenta. Acta Histochem. 89:11–16, 1990.

Ruoslahti, E., and Pierschbacher, M.D.: New perspectives in cell adhesion: RGD and integrins. Science 238:491–497, 1987.

Russell, J.G.B.: Antenatal diagnosis of placental calcification. J. Obstet. Gynaecol. Br. Commonw. 76:813–126, 1969.

Rutanen, E.M., Partanen, S., and Pekonen, F.: Decidual transformation of human extrauterine mesenchymal cells is associated with the appearance of insulin-like growth factor-binding protein-1. J. Clin. Endocrinol. Metab. 72:27–31, 1991.

Rutherford, R.N.: The significance of bleeding in early pregnancy as evidenced by decidual biopsy. Surg. Gynecol. Obstet. 74:1139–1153, 1942.

Sachs, H.: Quantitativ histochemische Untersuchung des Endometrium in der Schwangerschaft und der Placenta (Cytophotometrische Messungen). Arch. Gynecol. 205:93–104, 1968.

Saijonmaa, O., Laatikainen, T., and Wahlström, T.: Corticotrophin-releasing factor in human placenta: localization, concentration and release in vitro. Placenta 9:373–385, 1988.

Saito, S., Nishikawa, K., Morii, T., Enomoto, M., Narita, N., Motoyoshi, K., and Ichijo, M.: Cytokine production by CD16-CD56(bright) natural killer cells in the human early pregnancy decidua. Int. Immunol. 5:559–563, 1993.

Saji, M., Taga, M., and Minaguchi, H.: Epidermal growth factor stimulate cell proliferation and inhibits prolactin secretion of the human decidual cells in culture. Endocrinol. Jpn. 37:177–182, 1990.

Sakbun, V., Ali, S.M., Greenwood, F.C., and Bryant Greenwood, G.D.: Human relaxin in the amnion, chorion, decidua parietalis, basal plate, and placental trophoblast by immunocytochemistry and Northern analysis. J. Clin. Endocrinol. Metab. 70:508–514, 1990a.

Sakbun, V., Ali, S.M., Lee, Y.A., Jara, C.S., and Bryant Greenwood, G.D.: Immunocytochemical localization and messenger ribonucleic acid concentrations for human placental lactogen in amnion, chorion, decidua, and placenta. Am. J. Obstet. Gynecol. 162:1310–1317, 1990b.

Sala, M.A., Matheus, M., and Valeri, V.: Regional variation in the frequency of fibrinoid degeneration in the human term placenta. Z. Geburtshilfe Perinatol. 186:80–81, 1982a.

Sala, M.A., Valeri, V., and Matheus, M.: Michaelis-Gutmann bodies in human placental fibrinoid. Arch. Biol. (Bruxelles) 93:363–367, 1982b.

Sasagawa, M., Yamazaki, T., Sudo, Y., Kanazawa, K., and Takeuchi, S.: Immunohistochemical localization of hCG α, hCG β, CTP, hPL and SP1 on villous and extravillous trophoblasts in normal human pregnancy. Nippon Sanka Fujinka Gakkai Zasshi 39:1073–1079, 1987.

Sauramo, H.: Cytotrophoblast of the placenta and foetal membranes in normal and pathological obstetrics. Ann. Med. Exp. Fenn. 39:7–12, 1961.

Schaaps, J.P., and Hustin, J.: In vivo aspect of the maternal-trophoblastic border during the first trimester of gestation. Trophoblast Res. 3:39–48, 1988.

Scheuner, G.: Über die Verankerung der Nabelschnur an der Plazenta. Morphol. Jahrb. 106:73–89, 1964.

Schiebler, T.H., and Kaufmann, P.: Reife Plazenta. In, Die Plazenta des Menschen. V. Becker, T.H. Schiebler, and F. Kubli, eds. Thieme, Stuttgart, 1981.

Schiebler, T.H., and Knoop, A.: Histochemische und elektronenmikroskopische Untersuchungen an der Rattenplacenta. Z. Zellforsch. 50:494–552, 1959.

Schindler, A.M., Bordignon, P., and Bischof, P.: Immunohistochemical localization of pregnancy-associated plasma protein A in decidua and trophoblast: comparison with human chorionic gonadotrophin and fibrin. Placenta 5:227–235, 1984.

Schmidt-Matthiesen, H.: Das normale menschliche Endometrium. Thieme, Stuttgart, 1963.

Schuhmann, R.: Plazenton. Begriff, Entstehung, funktionelle Anatomie. In, Die Plazenta des Menschen. V. Becker, T.H. Schiebler, and F. Kubli, eds., pp. 192–207. Thieme, Stuttgart, 1981.

Schuhmann, R., and Wehler, V.: Histologische Unterschiede an Plazentazotten innerhalb der maternofetalen Strömungseinheit: ein Beitrag zur funktionellen Morphologie der Plazenta. Arch. Gynecol. 210:425–439, 1971.

Schultze, K.W.: Über Randsinusblutungen aus der Plazenta in der Schwangerschaft und unter der Geburt. Geburtshilfe Frauenheilkd. 13:708–715, 1953.

Schultze, K.W.: Über sog. Plazenta-Randsinusblutungen. Dtsch. Hebammen. Z. 20:1–4, 1968.

Schwartz, A., Sauer, J., Hradeckky, L., and Pavlik, V.: Die Zysten der menschlichen Plazenta. Zentralbl. Allg. Pathol. 117:185–190, 1973.

Scipiades, E., and Burg, E.: Über die Morphologie der menschlichen Placenta mit besonderer Rücksicht auf unsere eigenen Studien. Arch. Gynecol. 141:577–619, 1930.

Sengel, A., and Stöbner, P: Ultrastructure de l'endometre humain normal. III. Les cellules K. Z. Zellforsch. 133:47–57, 1972.

Sengupta, J., Given, R.L., Talwar, D., and Ghosh, D.: Endometrial response to deciduogenic stimulus in ovariectomized rhesus monkeys treated with oestrogen and progesterone: an ultrastructural study. J. Endocrinol. 124:53–57, 1990.

Serr, D.M., Sadowski, A.D., and Kohn, G.: The placental septa; a study based upon nuclear morphological sex difference. J. Obstet. Gynaecol. Br. Commonw. 65:747–777, 1958.

Shanklin, D.R., and Scott, J.S.: Massive subchorial thrombohaematoma (Breus' mole). Br. J. Obstet. Gynaecol. 82:476–487, 1975.

Sheppard, B.L., and Bonnar, J.: Scanning electron microscopy of the human placenta and decidual spiral arteries in normal pregnancy. J. Obstet. Gynaecol. Br. Commonw. 81:17–20, 1974a.

Sheppard, B.L., and Bonnar, J.: The ultrastructure of the arterial supply of the human placenta in early and late pregnancy. J. Obstet. Gynaecol. Br. Commonw. 81:497–511, 1974b.

Sheppard, B.L., and Bonnar, J.: The ultrastructure of the arterial supply of the human placenta in pregnancy complicated by fetal growth retardation. Br. J. Obstet. Gynaecol. 83:948–959, 1976.

Sheppard, B.L., and Bonnar, J.: The maternal blood supply to the placenta in pregnancy complicated by intrauterine fetal growth retardation. Trophoblast Res. 3:69–82, 1988.

Shipley, C.F., and Nelson, G.H.: Prenatal diagnosis of a placental cyst: comparison of postnatal biochemical analyses of cyst fluid, amniotic fluid, cord serum, and maternal serum. Am. J. Obstet. Gynecol. 168:211–213, 1993.

Shorter, S.C., Jackson, M.C., Sargent, I.L., Redman, C.W., and Starkey, P.M.: Purification of human cytotrophoblast from term amniochorion by flow cytometry. Placenta 11:505–513, 1990.

Shorter, S.C., Vince, G.S., and Starkey, P.M.: Production of granulocyte colony-stimulating factor at the maternofoetal interface in human pregnancy. Immunology 75:468–474, 1992.

Shorter, S.C., Starkey, P.M., Ferry, B.L., Clover, L.M., Sargent, I.L., and Redman, C.W.G.: Antigenic heterogeneity of human cytotrophoblast and evidence for the transient expression of MHC class I antigens distinct from HLA-G. Placenta 14:571–582, 1993.

Simmen, R.C.M., Ko, Y., Liu, X.H., Wilde, M.H., Pope, W.F., and Simmen, F.A.: A uterine cell mitogen distinct from epidermal growth factor in porcine uterine luminal fluids: characterization and partial purification. Biol. Reprod. 38:551–561, 1988.

Singer, M., and Wislocki, G.B.: The affinity of syncytium, fibrin and fibrinoid of the human placenta for acid and basic dyes under controlled conditions of staining. Anat. Rec. 102:175–194, 1948.

Sinha, A.A.: Ultrastructure of human amnion and amniotic plaques of normal pregnancy. Z. Zellforsch. 122:1–14, 1971.

Sohval, A.R., Gaines, J.A., and Strauss, L.: Chromosomal sex determination in the human newborn and fetus from examination of the umbilical cord, placental tissue, and fetal membranes. Ann. N.Y. Acad. Sci. 75:905–922, 1959.

Soma, H., Satoh, M., Higashi, S., Horikiri, H., Hata, T., Isaka, K., and Malla, D.: Fine structure and biological properties of chorionic cysts. In: Placenta: Basic Research for Clinical Application. H. Soma, ed., pp. 200–208, Karger, Basel, 1991.

Sonnenberg, A., Modderman, P.W., and Hogervorst, F.: Laminin receptor on platelets is the integrin VLA-6. Nature 336:487–489, 1988.

Sorensen, F.B., Marcussen, N., Daugaard, H.O., Kristiansen, J.D., Moller, J., and Ingerslev, H.J.: Immunohistological demonstration of intermediate trophoblast in the diagnosis of uterine versus ectopic pregnancy: a retrospective survey and results of a prospective trial. Br. J. Obstet. Gynaecol. 98:463–469, 1991.

Spanner, R.: Der Kreislauf im intervillösen Raum des Menschen: Untersuchungen an den Uteroplacentargefässen schwangerer Uteri. Anat. Anz. 78:127–129, 1934.

Spanner, R.: Mütterlicher und kindlicher Kreislauf der menschlichen Placenta und seine Strombahnen. Z. Ges. Anat. 105:163–242, 1935.

Spanner, R.: Zellinseln und Zottenepithel in der zweiten Hälfte der Schwangerschaft. Morphol. Jahrb. 86:407–461, 1941.

Spornitz, U.M.: The functional morphology of the human endometrium and decidua. Adv. Anat. Embryol. Cell Biol. 124:1–99, 1992.

Spornitz, U.M., and Ludwig, K.S.: Die Ultrastruktur der menschlichen Deziduazelle. Acta Anat. (Basel) 120:245, 1984.

Stark, J., and Kaufmann, P.: Die Basalplatte der reifen menschlichen Placenta. II. Gefrierschnitt-Histochemie. Z. Anat. Entwicklungsgesch. 135:185–201, 1971.

Stark, J., and Kaufmann, P.: Die Basalplatte der reifen menschlichen Placenta. III. Bindegewebs- und Deciduazellen. Arch. Gynecol. 213:399–417, 1973.

Stark, J., and Kaufmann, P.: Infarktgenese in der Placenta. Arch. Gynecol. 217:189–208, 1974.

Stegner, H.E., Sachs, H., and Uthmöller, E.: Elektronenmikroskopische Untersuchungen am experimentellen Deziduom der Ratte. Z. Geburtshilfe Gynäkol. 174:241–251, 1971.

Steininger, H.: Über die Herkunft von Septen und Inseln der menschlichen Plazenta. Arch. Gynecol. 226:261–275, 1978.

Stieve, H.: Neue Untersuchungen über die Placenta, besonders über die Entstehung der Placentasepten. Arch. Gynecol. 161:160–167, 1936.

Stieve, H.: Die Entwicklung und der Bau der menschlichen Placenta. I. Zotten, Trophoblastinseln und Scheidewaende in der ersten Hälfte der Schwangerschaft. Z. Mikrosk. Anat. Forsch. 48:287–358, 1940.

Stieve, H., and von der Heide, I.: Über die Entwicklung der Septen in der menschlichen Plazenta. Anat. Anz. 92:1–16, 1941.

Straatsburg, I.H., and Gossrau, R.: Enzyme histochemistry of the regressing rat decidua and metrial gland. Acta Histochem. 94:202–219, 1993.

Sunderland, C.A., Bulmer, J.N., Luscombe, M., Redman, C.W.G., and Stirrat, G.M.: Immunohistological and biochemical evidence for a role for hyaluronic acid in the growth and development of the placenta. J. Reprod. Immunol. 8:197–212, 1985.

Sutcliffe, R.G., Davies, M., Hunter, J.B., Waters, J.J., and Parry, J.E.: The protein composition of the fibrinoid material at the human uteroplacental interface. Placenta 3:297–308, 1982.

Sutherland, A.E., Calarco, P.G., and Damsky, C.H.: Expression and function of cell surface extracellular matrix receptors in mouse blastocyst attachment and outgrowth. J.Cell Biol. 106:1331–1348, 1988.

Swinburne, L.M.: Leucocyte antigens and placental sponge. Lancet 2:592–593, 1970.

Takayama, M., Isaka, K., Suzuki, Y., Funayama, H., Akiya, K., and Bohn, H.: Comparative study of placental protein 19, human chorionic gonadotrophin and pregnancy-specific β1-glycoprotein as immunohistochemical markers for extravillous trophoblast in pregnancy and trophoblastic disease. Histochemistry 93:167–173, 1989.

Tarachand, U.: Morphogenesis and postulated functions of decidual cells. Biol. Res. Pregnancy Perinatol. 6:187–190, 1985.

Tarachand, U.: Decidualisation: origin and role of associated cells. Biol. Cell 57:9–16, 1986.

Tavare, J.M., and Holmes, C.H.: Differential expression of the receptors for epidermal growth factor and insulin in the developing human placenta. Cell Signal 1:55–64, 1989.

Tekelioglu-Uysal, M., Edwards, R.J., and Kisnisci, H.A.: Ultrastructural relationships between decidua, trophoblast and lymphocytes at the beginning of human pregnancy. J. Reprod. Fertil. 42:431–438, 1975.

Thiede, H.A., and Choate, J.W.: Chorionic localization in the human placenta by immunofluorescent staining. II. Demonstration of hCG in the trophoblast and amnion epithelium of immature and mature placentas. Obstet. Gynecol. 22:433–443, 1963.

Thliveris, J.A., and Speroff, L.: Ultrastructure of the placental villi, chorion laeve, and decidua parietalis in normal and hypertensive pregnant women. Am. J. Obstet. Gynecol. 129:492–498, 1977.

Thomas, J.B.: Breus' mole. Obstet. Gynecol. 24:794–797, 1964.

Thomsen, K., and Willemsen, R.: Histochemische Untersuchungen über die Produktionsorte der Choriongonadotropine. Acta Endocrinol. (Copenh.) 30:161–174, 1959.

Thrailkill, K.M., Golander, A., Underwood, L.E., Richards, R.G., and Handwerger, S.: Insulin stimulates the synthesis and release of prolactin from human decidual cells. Endocrinology 124:3010–3014, 1989.

Thrower, S., Bulmer, J.N., Griffin, N.R., and Wells, M.: Further studies of lectin binding by villous and extravillous trophoblast in normal and pathological pregnancy. Int. J. Gynecol. Pathol. 10:238–251, 1991.

Tighe, J.R., Garrod, P.R., and Curran, R.C.: The trophoblast of the human chorionic villus. J. Pathol. Bacteriol. 93:559–567, 1967.

Tindall, V.R., and Scott, J.S.: Placental calcification: a study of 3,025 singleton and multiple pregnancies. J. Obstet. Gynaecol. Br. Commonw. 72:356–373, 1965.

Torpin, R.: Subchorial haematoma mole: hypothetical aetiology. J. Obstet. Gynaecol. Br. Emp. 67:990, 1960.

Torpin, R.: Breus subchorial hematoma mole at three or four months of pregnancy. Pacific Med. Surg. 74:226–227, 1966.

Tsang, R.C., Donavan, E.F., and Steichen, J.J.: Calcium physiology and pathology in the neonate. Pediatr. Clin. North Am. 23:611–626, 1976.

Tuttle, S.E., O'Toole, R.V., O'Shaughnessy, R.W., and Zuspan, F.P.: Immunohistochemical evaluation of human placental implantation: an initial study. Am. J. Obstet. Gynecol. 153:239–244, 1985.

Uhlendorf, B., and Kaufmann, P.: Die Entwicklung des Plazentastieles beim Meerschweinchen. Zentralbl. Veterinarmed. [C] 8:233–247, 1979.

Vernof, K.K., Benirschke, K., Kephart, G.M., Wasmoen, T.L., and Gleich, G.J.: Maternal floor infarction: relationship to X cells, major basic protein, and adverse perinatal outcome. Am. J. Obstet. Gynecol. 167:1355–1963, 1992.

Vicovac, L., Jones, C.J.P., and Aplin, J.D.: Morphogenesis of human placental anchoring villi in culture. Placenta 14: A.80, 1993.

Wachstein, M., Meagher, J.G., and Ortiz, J.: Enzymatic histochemistry of the term human placenta. Am. J. Obstet. Gynecol. 87:13–26, 1963.

Wadsworth, P.F., Lewis, D.J., and Heywood, R.: The ultrastructural features of progestagen-induced decidual cells in the rhesus monkey (Macaca mulatta). Contraception 22: 189–198, 1980.

Waidl, E.: Die Entstehung der Septen und Furchen der menschlichen Plazenta. Geburtshilfe Frauenheilkd. 23:757–766, 1963.

Wakuda, K., and Yoshida, Y.: Cytofluorometric nuclear DNA analysis and immunohistochemical study on the proliferative activity of the trophoblasts in human early gestation. Nippon Sanka Fujinka Gakkai Zasshi 42:1182–1188, 1990.

Wakuda, K., and Yoshida, Y.: DNA ploidy and proliferative characteristics of human trophoblasts. Acta Obstet. Gynecol. Ocand. 71.12–16, 1992.

Wang, D., Fujii, S., Konishi, I., Nanbu, Y., Iwai, T., Nonogaki, H., and Mori, T.: Expression of c-erbB-2 protein and epidermal growth factor receptor in normal tissues of the female genital tract and in the placenta. Virchows Arch. [A] 420:385–393, 1992.

Wanner, A.: Wird bei der Geburtsplacenta des Menschen die Basalplatte von Trophoblastzellen oder Zellen mütterlicher Herkunft überzogen? Acta Anat. (Basel) 63:545–558, 1966.

Wasmoen, T.L., Loegering, D.A., Coulam, C.B., Gleich, G.J., and Benirschke, K.: Characterization of a pregnancy-associated protein immunochemically similar to the major basic protein of eosinophils. Fed. Proc. 44:420, 1985.

Wasmoen, T.L., Benirschke, K., and Gleich, G.J.: Demonstration of immunoreactive eosinophil granule major basic protein in the plasma and placentae of non-human primates. Placenta 8:283–292, 1987a.

Wasmoen, T.L., Coulam, C.B., Leiferman, K.M., and Gleich, G.J.: Increase of plasma eosinophil major basic protein levels late in pregnancy predicts onset of labor. Proc. Natl. Acad. Sci. U.S.A. 84:3029–3032, 1987b.

Wasmoen, T.L., Bell, M.P., Loegering, D.A., Gleich, G.J., Prendergast, F.G., and McKean, D.J.: Biochemical and amino acid sequence analysis of human eosinophil granule major basic protein. J. Biol. Chem. 263:12559–12563, 1988.

Wasmoen, T.I., McKean, D.J., Benirschke, K., Coulam, C.B., and Gleich, G.J: Evidence of eosinophil granule major basic protein in human placenta. J. Exp. Med. 170:2051–2063, 1989.

Wasmoen, T.L., Coulam, C.B., Benirschke, K., and Gleich, G.J.: Association of immunoreactive eosinophil major basic

protein with placental septa and cysts. Am. J. Obstet. Gynecol. 165:416–420, 1991.

Watanabe, S.: Studies of endometrial granulocytes in early pregnant decidual tissue by means of double immunofluorescent staining and flow cytometry. Nippon Sanka Fujinka Gakkai Zasshi 39:972–979, 1987.

Weber, J.: The site of production of gonadotrophin in the placenta at term. Acta Obstet. Gynecol. Scand. 40:139–151, 1961.

Weller, P.F., and Götzl, E.J.: The human eosinophil: roles in host defense and tissue injury. Am. J. Pathol. 100:793–820, 1980.

Wells, M., Hsi, B.-L., Yeh, C.-J., and Faulk, W.P.: Spiral (uteroplacental) arteries of the human placental bed show the presence of amniotic basement membrane antigens. Am. J. Obstet. Gynecol. 150:973–977, 1984.

Welsh, A.O., and Enders, A.C.: Light and electron microscopic examination of the mature decidual cells of the rat with emphasis on the antimesometrial decidua and its degeneration. Am. J. Anat. 172:1–29, 1985.

Welsh, A.O., and Enders, A.C.: Chorioallantoic placenta formation in the rat. III. Granulated cells invade the uterine luminal epithelium at the time of epithelial cell death. Biol. Reprod. 49:38–57, 1993.

Weser, H., and Kaufmann, P.: Lichtmikroskopische und histochemische Untersuchungen an der Chorionplatte der reifen menschlichen Placenta. Arch. Gynecol. 225:15–30, 1978.

Wewer, U.M., Faber, M., Liotta, L.A., and Albrechtsen, R.: Immunochemical and ultrastructural assessment of the nature of pericellular basement membrane of human decidual cells. Lab. Invest. 53:624–633, 1985.

Wewer, U.M., Faber, M., Liotta, L.A., and Albrechtsen, R.: Correspondence: decidual cells. Lab. Invest. 55:120–121, 1986.

Wewer, U.M., Albrechtsen, R., Fisher, L.W., Young, M.F., and Termine, J.D.: Osteonectin/SPARC/BM-40 in human decidua and carcinoma, tissues characterized by de novo formation of basement membrane. Am. J. Pathol. 132:345–355, 1988.

Wieloch, J.: Beitrag zur Kenntnis des Baues der Placenta. Arch. Gynäkol. 118:112–119, 1923.

Wiese, K.-H.: Licht- und elektronenmikroskopische Untersuchungen an der Chorionplatte der reifen menschlichen Plazenta. Arch. Gynecol. 218:243–259, 1975.

Wigger, H.J.: Villous fibrinoid of the placenta: result of holocrine secretion of the cytotrophoblast. Am. J. Pathol. 86: 8a, 1977.

Wigglesworth, J.S.: Morphological variations in the insufficient placenta. J. Obstet. Gynaecol. Br. Commonw. 71: 871–884, 1964.

Wigglesworth, J.S.: Vascular anatomy of the human placenta and its significance for placental pathology. J. Obstet. Gynäkol. Br. Commonw. 76:979–989, 1969.

Wilkin, P.: Morphogenese. In, Le Placenta Humain. J. Snoeck, ed., pp. 23–70. Masson, Paris, 1958.

Winkler, F.N.: Zur Kenntnis der menschlichen Plazenta. Arch. Gynecol. 4:238–265, 1872.

Wislocki, G.B.: The histology and cytochemistry of the basal plate and septa placentae of the normal human placenta delivered at full term. Anat. Rec. 109:359, 1951.

Wislocki, G.B., and Streeter, G.L.: On the placentation of the macaque (Macaca mulatta) from the time of implantation until the formation of the definitive placenta. Contrib. Embryol. Carnegie Instit. 27:1–66, 1938.

Witter, F.R., and Sanders, R.C.: Maternal hemorrhage into the amniotic sac producing an apparent umbilical cord mass on sonogram. Am. J. Obstet. Gynecol. 155:649–651, 1986.

Wolf, H.K., and Michalopoulos, G.K.: Proliferating cell nuclear antigen in human placenta and trophoblastic disease. Pediatr. Pathol. 12:147–154, 1992.

Wolska, W.: Über die von Ruge beschriebene Vaskularisation der Serotina. Thesis, Bern, 1888.

Wu, W.X., Brooks, J., Millar, M.R., Ledger, W.L., Saunders, P.T., Glasier, A.F., and McNeilly, A.S.: Localization of the sites of synthesis and action of prolactin by immunocytochemistry and in-situ hybridization within the human uteroplacental unit. J. Mol. Endocrinol. 7:241–247, 1991.

Wynn, R.M.: Electron microscopy of the developing decidua. Fertil. Steril. 16:16–26, 1965.

Wynn, R.M.: Fetomaternal cellular relations in the human basal plate: an ultrastructural study of the placenta. Am. J. Obstet. Gynecol. 97:832–850, 1967a.

Wynn, R.M.: Intra-uterine devices: effects on ultrastructure of human endometrium. Science 156:1508–1510, 1967b.

Wynn, R.: Ultrastructural development of the human decidua. Am. J. Obstet. Gynecol. 118:652–670, 1974.

Wynn, R.M.: Fine structure of the placenta. In, The Placenta and its Maternal Supply Line. P. Gruenwald, ed., pp. 56–79. Medical Technical Publications, Lancaster, 1975.

Yeh, I., O'Connor, D.M., and Kurman, R.J.: Further immunocytochemical characterization of intermediate trophoblast. Mod. Pathol. 1:106A, 1988.

Yeh, I., O'Connor, D.M., and Kurman, R.J.: Vacuolated cytotrophoblast: a sub-population of trophoblast in the chorion laeve. Placenta 10:429–438, 1989.

Yeh, I.T., O'Connor, D.M., and Kurman, R.J.: Intermediate trophoblast: further immunocytochemical characterization. Mod. Pathol. 3:282–287, 1990.

Young, R.H., Kurman, R.J., and Scully, R.E.: Proliferations and tumors of intermediate trophoblast of the placental site. Semin. Diagn. Pathol. 5:223–237, 1988.

Yuen, B.H., Moon, Y.S., and Shin, D.H.: Inhibition of human chorionic gonadotropin production by prolactin from term human trophoblast. Am. J. Obstet. Gynecol. 154:336–340, 1986.

Zeng, C.X., and Fu, X.S.: Immunocytochemical localization of human chorionic gonadotropin and placental lactogen in normal placentae. Chung Hua Fu Chan Ko Tsa Chih 26: 155–157, 188, 1991.

Zhemkova, Z.P.: Sex chromatin in human placenta. Arkh. Anat. Histol. Embriol. 39:24–32, 1960.

Zhou, Y., Damsky, C.H., Chiu, K., Roberts, J.M., and Fisher, S.J.: Preeclampsia is associated with abnormal expression of adhesion molecules by invasive cytotrophoblasts. J. Clin. Invest. 91:950–960, 1993.

12
Anatomy and Pathology of the Placental Membranes

The term membranes is usually taken to be synonymous with the amnion and the chorion laeve. The membranes represent the "bag of waters" that encloses the fetus. They are distinct from the chorion frondosum, which is the actual placental tissue and forms a specialized, thickened part of the membranes. The membranes normally insert at the edge of the placenta and contain the amnionic fluid and the fetus. Membranes rupture during delivery owing to stretching or the mechanical force of the accoucheur. Several distinct layers are present in the membranes, and the structure and function of the membranes have received considerable attention primarily because of an interest in the turnover of the water they contain. Enzymatic activity of the membranes during the initiation of labor has been of additional interest. Most recently, the composition of the various extracellular connective tissue components has come under scrutiny. Comprehensive surveys of many of these aspects, particularly the structural nature of the membranes, are found in Bourne's (1962) and Schmidt's (1992) books on the topic. Amnionic fluid mechanics are reviewed comprehensively by Barnes and Seeds (1972).

There are three distinct layers of the membranes. Their origin and interdependence must be understood if one wishes to comprehend their complexity (Figure 169). The inner layer is the *amnion*. A thin, avascular layer of epithelial cells and connective tissue, it is derived from the fetal ectoderm by cavitation within the embryonic knot (Luckett, 1973) and is contiguous, over the umbilical cord, with the fetal skin. Confirmation of epidermal origin has come from the studies of Nanbu et al. (1989), who demonstrated the fetal differentiation antigen CA 125 in the fetal periderm (outer layer of epidermis) and the amnionic epithelium.

The amnion is passively attached to the next layer, the *chorion laeve*, by the internal pressures of amnionic fluid. The chorion laeve, a much more complex tissue, is comprised of connective tissue within which there are the fetal (chorioallantoic) blood vessels. The villi of the chorion frondosum originate from the chorion. At the parietal, free surface of the membranes one finds their atrophied remains, even in term pregnancy specimens. These former villi then are round "balls" of connective tissue, usually lack trophoblastic cover, and possess no vessels. On the outer surface of the chorion rest also the remains of the cytotrophoblastic cells of the trophoblastic shell. They undergo much change with advancing gestation; they are somewhat vesicular and often atrophy.

These cells, as the remaining villi, are intimately intermingled with the outermost layer, the *decidua* capsularis. The decidua, representing modified endometrium, is the only maternal component of the membranes. A variety of trophoblastic cells are present within this area, and it is essentially impossible to obtain "clean" decidual cells from this tissue for experimental work. The decidua capsularis also normally contains a few maternal blood vessels, some phagocytes, and other inflammatory cells. At the placental margin, this decidua capsularis is contiguous with the decidua basalis, where it delimits the marginal sinus. The tissue at the base of the actual placenta, to which the normal villous tissue is anchored, is the maternal floor. One often finds degenerative processes and inflammation at this location, and hemorrhages are frequent at this site. They have been referred to as being the result of a marginal sinus thrombosis, a term that is no longer defensible. When one stretches the edge of the membranes away from the placenta, one can see the friable tissue that constitutes this marginal decidua. When it is disrupted, one enters the intervillous blood space, the marginal sinus. In Figures 170 and 171, the margin of the placental membrane attachment is seen in situ. The uterus depicted also clearly shows a lack of fusion between the decidua capsularis and the decidua vera (or parietal decidua), as is similarly shown in Figure 172.

FIGURE 169. Microscopic appearance of normal "membranes." Amnion epithelium (A) sits on a thin layer of connective tissue that is separable from chorion in an ill-defined plane (P). Dense chorionic connective tissue (C) is irregularly studded with atrophic former villi (V) and has at its outer surface a layer of trophoblastic cells (next to V). At the periphery one finds the decidua capsularis (D) with maternal vessels (M) and frequent fibrin (F) deposits. H&E. ×16.

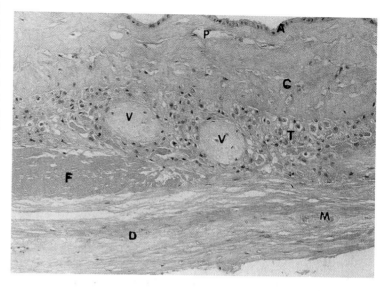

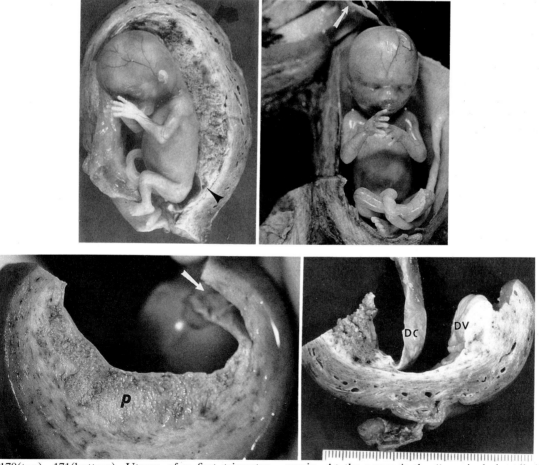

FIGURES 170(top), 171(bottom). Uterus of a first trimester pregnancy with a 7.5 cm fetus in situ. It was removed because of carcinoma of the cervix. Note the large myometrial vessels and the distance of the implanted placenta from the endo-cervix. At the arrow is the "marginal sinus." At right, the membranes have been elevated from the decidua vera (DV) to show the fact that the decidua vera and decidua capsularis (DC) do not "grow together." The cervix has been removed.

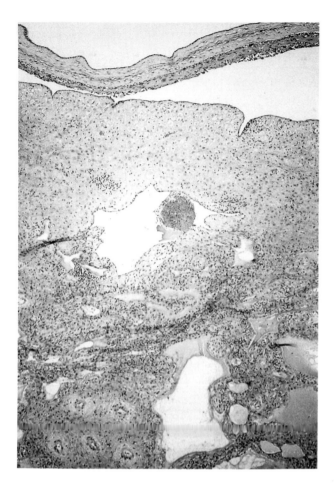

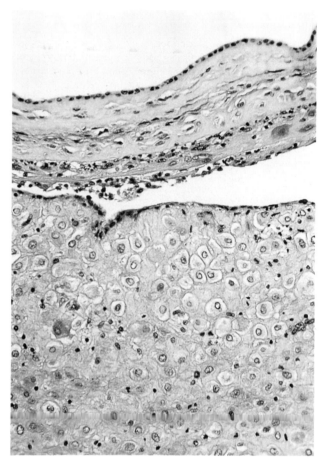

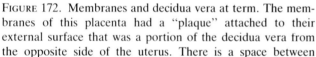

FIGURE 172. Membranes and decidua vera at term. The membranes of this placenta had a "plaque" attached to their external surface that was a portion of the decidua vera from the opposite side of the uterus. There is a space between decidua capsularis and decidua vera; the latter is covered by well preserved uterine epithelium. True "fusion" between the two deciduas has not occurred. H&E. A ×10; B ×240.

For the purposes of this presentation, we start with a brief summary of the development of the membranes. In the following segments we discuss each layer separately and identify the associated pathological processes. This organization of material is not to say, however, that these structures are independent; often they have substantial interactions. There is, however, much misunderstanding of the perceived unity of the membranes, particularly in biochemical studies. It is thus important that one clearly distinguishes between these structures.

DEVELOPMENT

The trophoblast of the implanting blastocyst can be subdivided into one early implanting half (the cells surrounding the implantation pole or the basal chorion) and one later implanting half (that surrounding the antiimplantation pole or the capsular chorion) (Figures 24b,c, 208). The developmental processes, described in Chapter 6, are valid for the basal chorion. With the appearance of the first villi, the basal chorion becomes the chorion frondosum, the forerunner of the later placenta. The capsular chorion, which implants a few days later (Figure is 24b,c) initially undergoes a corresponding, though delayed, development. It proceeds with the processes of lacuna formation and consecutive transformation of the trabeculae into small villous trees, identical to those that take place at the implantation pole. At this stage it is called the *capsular chorion frondosum*. Within a few days, however, beginning at the end of the 3rd week p.c., the first degenerative changes at the antiimplantation pole can be observed. They result in the regression of newly formed villi, a process that slowly spreads laterally over the blastocyst surface (Hamilton & Boyd, 1960). As soon as the villi degenerate, the surrounding intervillous space obliterates. Finally, the primary chorionic plate of the respective region, the obliterated intervillous space together with its villous remnants, and the trophoblastic shell fuse (Figure 208), forming a multilayered compact lamella, the *smooth chorion (chorion laeve)* (Figure 173). The first patches of the smooth chorion are formed roughly opposite the implantation pole. From there they gradually spread over about 70% of the surface of the chorionic sac. This process continues until the fourth

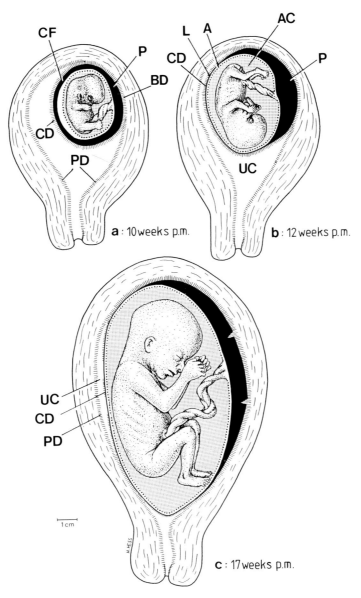

FIGURE 173. Late stages of the development of the fetal membranes. (a) Until 10 weeks p.m. the embryo is surrounded by a unit of chorion frondosum (CF); its later specialization into chorion laeve and the placenta is indicated by a slight increase in thickness (P) only. The chorion frondosum is covered by the capsular decidua (CD), which is continuous with basal decidua (BD) at the placental site and with the parietal decidua (PD), which lines the uterine cavity. The amnion (dotted line) is not fused in most places with the chorion frondosum. (b) Two weeks later (12th week p.m.), the original chorion frondosum has differentiated into the thick placenta (P) and the thinner fetal membranes that surround the inner amnionic cavity (AC). At this stage, the membranes are composed of inner amnion (A), intermediate chorion laeve (L), and outer capsular decidua (CD). Because of the embryo's small size, the uterine cavity (UC) is largely open. (c) From 17 weeks on, the membranes come into close contact with the uterine wall. The remainder of the capsular decidua (CD) fuses with the parietal decidua (PD) and largely closes the uterine cavity (UC). From then on, the chorion laeve contacts the parietal decidua. (Modified from Kaufmann, 1981.)

lunar month, when it slowly comes to a halt (Wynn, 1968; Boyd & Hamilton, 1970).

The differentiation process into chorion frondosum and chorion laeve is paralleled by changes in the surrounding maternal tissues. The superficial layer of the endometrium, which is characterized throughout implantation by the transformation of endometrial stromal cells into decidual cells, is henceforth called the decidua. Depending on its spatial relation to the implanting chorionic sac, it is subdivided into several segments (Figure 174). The decidua below and lateral to the blastocyst, or later that below the placenta, is called the *basal decidua* (decidua basalis). With complete interstitial implantation, the decidua closes over the blastocyst. This protruding layer is called the *capsular decidua* (decidua capsularis). All those parts of the decidua that line the

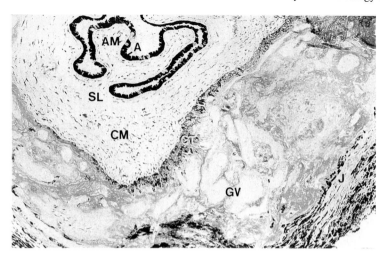

FIGURE 174. Membranes near their lateral placental attachment, showing lactate dehydrogenase activity. A = amnion epithelium; AM = amnionic mesenchyme; SL = spongy (intermediate) layer; CM = chorionic mesenchyme; CT = cytotrophoblast; GV = degenerative ghost villi; J = junctional zone, consisting of basal trophoblast and decidua. Ghost villi are frequent at the placental margin; more peripherally, the trophoblastic layers will fuse. Cryostat section. ×75.

uterine cavity without being in contact with the blastocyst (i.e., at the opposing uterine wall) are called the *parietal decidua* (decidua vera). With increasing diameter of the chorionic sac, the capsular decidua focally degenerates, so that in such places the external surface of the smooth chorion (trophoblast cells) borders the uterine cavity (Figure 173c). This surface finally touches the parietal decidua (Figures 173b,c). Between the 15th and 20th weeks p.c., the smooth chorion, together with its attached residual capsular decidua, locally fuses with the parietal decidua, thereby largely obliterating the uterine cavity (Figure 173c). From this date onward, the smooth chorion has contact with the decidual surface of the uterine wall over nearly its entire surface and may function as a paraplacental exchange organ. The efficiency of this exchange, however, is limited by the absence of fetal vessels within the smooth chorion.

A third tissue, the amnion, contributes to the development of the membranes. During the first steps of implantation an enlarged intercellular space between embryoblast and neighboring trophoblastic cells can be observed. Some small cells, lining the inner surface of the trophoblast in this particular region, have been named the amniogenic cells. They are the forerunners of the *amnionic epithelium*; the cleft separating them from the embryoblast is the early *amnionic cavity* (Hertig & Rock, 1941; Starck, 1975; Hinrichsen, 1990) (Figure 208). Because of its continuous expansion, the amnionic cavity slowly surrounds the embryo from all sides and finally covers the umbilical cord. In addition, through fetal growth and production of *amnionic fluid*, the amnionic cavity is expanded.

Extraembryonic mesoblast, formed during the lacunar stage (see Chapter 6, Figure 24d), not only lines the inner surface of the blastocyst cavity but also covers the external surface of the amnionic epithelium, thus giving rise to the *amnionic mesoderm*. Amnionic mesoderm and the extraembryonic mesoblast covering the trophoblast (*chorionic mesoderm*) are separated by a cavity called the exocoel (Figure 208) (Hertig, 1945, 1968). Those mesoblast cells that line the cavity are transformed into a mesothelium (Heuser's membrane). Fluid accumulation within the amnionic cavity causes its expansion, so it slowly compresses the exocoel. During the 6th to 7th week p.c., the amnionic vesicle has become so large its mesoderm locally fuses with the chorionic mesoderm (Figure 208). This process starts in the areas surrounding the cord insertion at the chorionic plate and is largely completed after another 5 weeks (until the 12th week p.c.). The amnionic vesicle then completely occupies the exocoel (Figure 173) (Boyd & Hamilton, 1970). Only cleft-like remnants of the latter may be detectable during later stages of pregnancy, although one can always detach the amnion from the chorion. According to Grosser (1927), the mesothelium of both mesoderm layers disappears as soon as they come into contact with each other or even fuse. Fusion never is perfect, however, and amnion and chorion can always easily slide against each other. Histologically, they even seem to be separated by a system of slender, fluid-filled clefts (see below, intermediate layer of chorion). Bundles of connective tissue fibers exist, crossing from one to the other layer; however, they are locally restricted and are laterally surrounded by the above clefts. Different from the situation in the membranes, the expanding amnion not only becomes closely attached to the surface of the cord but firmly fuses with it. It cannot be dislodged from the cord.

As soon as the amnion is attached to the surfaces of the placenta, umbilical cord, and chorion laeve, its nomenclature becomes specified. The names *placental amnion*, *umbilical amnion*, and *reflected amnion* are widely used. Although histologically the reflected amnion and chorion laeve are evidently separate structures, macroscopically they are summarized under the name "membranes."

The structure of the membranes generally remains constant from the 4th month until term (Petry, 1962; Schmidt, 1992). Their mean thickness after separation from the uterine wall during labor is about 200 to 300 μm, with a slight tendency to increase as one gets closer to the placenta. Because of local edematous swelling of the amnionic mesoderm, considerably thicker membranes are sometimes observed (Bourne, 1962). After birth, the following layers can be seen histologically.

1. Amnionic epithelium and basal lamina (20–30 μm thickness)

2. Amnionic mesoderm (about 15–30 μm thickness)
3. Intermediate zone (highly variable thickness)
4. Chorionic mesoderm (15–20 μm thickness)
5. Trophoblast (10–50 μm thickness)
6. Decidua (up to 50 μm thickness)

Amnion

The amnion is composed of an inner layer of epithelial cells, planted on a basement membrane that, in turn, is connected to a thin connective tissue membrane by filamentous strands (Danforth & Hull, 1958). When the membrane is allowed to fix while stretched, the surface appears flat; when it is allowed to contract, many folds appear. It is a translucent structure that is frequently detached from the rest of the membranes by the forces of labor. It can almost always be easily separated from the underlying chorion, with which it never truly fuses, cellularly speaking.

As mentioned, this "fusion" of amnion and chorion completes around the 12th week of development (Boyd & Hamilton, 1970). Before that time, the amnion forms a separate bubble within the chorionic sac; it is surrounded and separated from the chorion by chorionic fluid, the magma reticulare, a viscous, thixotropic gel within which some stellate cells are dispersed (Figure 175). It is important to recognize that the amnion does not possess its own blood vessels, in contrast to the opinion expressed by Donskikh (1957), who believed them to be present in early embryos. His drawings, however, are not convincing.

The amnion obtains its nutrition and oxygen from the surrounding chorionic fluid, the amnionic fluid, the fetal surface vessels, and during early gestation the magma reticulare. It is of parenthetical interest here to note that magma reticulare-like differentiation has been described in yolk sac tumors, and that these elements stain positively with antibodies to vimentin and cytokeratin, thus displaying both mesenchymal and epithelial characteristics (Michael et al., 1988). The latter is valid also for the amnionic epithelium. Despite its clearly epidermal origin, the cells not only express epidermal markers such as CA 125 (Nanbu et al., 1989) and general epithelial markers such as cytokeratins (Beham et al., 1988), they also express vimentin (Beham et al., 1988; Wolf et al., 1991). The latter is thought to be a marker for mesenchymally derived cells.

It is of historical interest also to note that Cane (1888) considered the amnion to secrete the amnionic fluid, which then was said to mold the early amnionic membrane. He also considered that it was responsible for the supply of oxygen by its rhythmic contractions, deemed to be analogous to the condition prevailing in birds. These hypotheses can now be laid aside.

Amnionic Epithelium: Different Cell Types or Cell Degeneration

The amnionic epithelium is a highly variable tissue, composed of a single layer of flat, cuboidal to columnar cells (Bautzmann & Schröder, 1955; Hempel, 1972; Schmidt, 1992). Columnar cells normally have been observed near the insertion of the membranes at the placental margin (Bou-Resli et al., 1981), whereas the cells generally flatten further in the periphery. Despite the diversity in shape, there appears to be only a single, uniform cell type (Sinha, 1971; Hempel, 1972; King, 1980). Previous findings by Thomas (1965), Armstrong et al. (1968), and Wynn and French (1968) resulted in

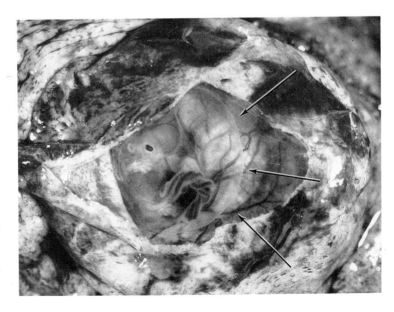

FIGURE 175. Intact placenta and fetus at 8 weeks of pregnancy, the chorion laeve having been opened. Arrows point to the amnionic bubble within the magma reticulare. Note also the early spiraling of the umbilical cord. ×3.

the suggestions of the existence of different cell types, such as Golgi and fibrillar cells, or light and dark cells. These types could not be verified, however, in later studies.

According to Hoyes (1972), an artifactual genesis of the previous findings (due to inappropriate fixation and inappropriate osmolarity of the fixative) may be the explanation. The differences in nomenclature may also result from different amounts of fluid content. Thus Hebertson et al. (1986) noted in their electron microscopic study of the epithelium that the normal thickness was much increased (to 18–56 μm) in diabetic pregnancies, canals were reduced in the presence of hydramnios, and other changes could be correlated with oligo- and polyhydramnios. Moreover, as discussed by Wynn and French (1968), a certain structural diversity of the cells may result from degenerative processes. These authors considered that the often present vesicles may reflect pinocytotic events. Histological examination of the amnionic epithelium shows it to exhibit many different appearances. Often it is tall and columnar, whereas at other times it is flat and more squamous (Figure 176). The varied appearance of the epithelial cells may be the result of different manners of fixation during preparation for microscopy, and it may also result from different amounts of fluid content. Numerous gaps in the amnionic epithelium may be signs of such an expulsion of dying cells from the epithelium

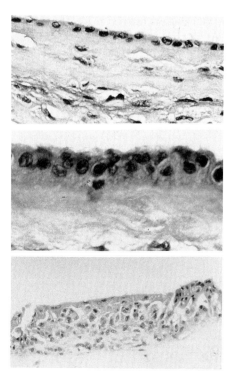

FIGURE 176. Different thicknesses of amnionic epithelium from three normal pregnancies. H&E. ×160.

into the amnionic fluid, resulting in frequent defects of the epithelial layer. The remains may be the channels that Bourne and Lacy (1960) interpreted to be channels for preferred fluid exchange. Similar channels and complex cellular arrangements of the amnionic epithelium have been identified in the surface by the electron microscopic studies of King (1982). This investigator also drew attention to the significant differences in the epithelial structure of the amnion when it is obtained from the free membranes or represents that of the cord. The development of micro-"blebs," frequent cell shedding, and the importance of the basal membrane for the maintenance of the integrity of the sac were emphasized in the studies of Herendael et al. (1978). The influence of labor on the structure of the amnionic epithelium has been studied by Sonek et al. (1991).

Cytological and Functional Aspects of the Amnionic Epithelium

During early pregnancy the bulging apical surfaces of the cells are covered by loosely scattered microvilli (Hoyes, 1968a,b; Lister, 1968; Ludwig et al., 1974). The number of microvilli increases later in the pregnancy. The microvillous surface is characterized by a densely packed glycocalyx with a high concentration of anionic binding sites (King, 1982). Intracellularly, a pronounced rough endoplasmic reticulum, numerous lipid droplets, and glycogen stores are evident. The ultrastructural findings are thought to favor intra-amnionic lipid synthesis, rather than a degenerative origin of the droplets (Armstrong et al., 1968; van Bogaert et al., 1978; King, 1980). So far, however, there is no explanation for such a possible secretion. According to Benedetti et al. (1973), the lipids cannot be explained as the result of absorption from the amnionic fluid, because the respective hydrolytic enzymes are absent. Most authors favor the view that the lipids are derived from the maternal circulation and, after some chemical changes, are secreted into the amnionic fluid (Polano, 1922; Szendi, 1940; Schmidt, 1965a,b, 1967; Armstrong et al., 1968; Pomerance et al., 1971; Schmidt et al., 1971). Not all findings, however, are in agreement with this concept. Some point to a fetal origin of the lipids and thus to their resorption from the amnionic fluid. According to Polishuk et al. (1965) and Pritchard et al. (1968) the intraamnionic lipids are chemically similar to those of the vernix. Vernix caseosa is derived from fetal sources (i.e., secretory ducts of the fetal skin mixed with desquamated skin cells) (Brusis et al., 1975). Even the degenerative character of the lipid droplets is still under discussion, although there is no ultrastructural evidence to support degeneration. The amount of lipid droplets increases throughout pregnancy (Yoshimura et al., 1980); maximum amounts have been reported following fetal hypoxia (Bourne, 1962; Bartman & Blanc, 1970) and fetal death (Yoshimura et al., 1980).

Substantial evidence exists to suggest a significant role for prostaglandins in the initiation and maintenance of uterine contractions (Olson et al., 1983; Smieja et al., 1993). Among the sources of prostaglandins for parturition, the amnionic epithelium seems to play a pivotal role because of its strategic anatomical location, with its close relation to amnionic fluid, myometrium, and uterine cervix. With the onset of labor, the production of prostaglandins increases (Olson et al., 1983; Kinoshita et al., 1984; Skinner & Challis, 1985; Mitchell, 1988; Lopez Bernal et al., 1989). Moreover, it is the nearly exclusive source for prostaglandin E_2 (PGE_2) (Okazaki et al., 1981a). The release of the latter hormone is regulated by intrinsic stimulatory properties of the membranes but not of the villous chorion (McCoshen et al., 1986).

In this context several questions arise: Do the membranes have the lipid precursors (arachidonic acid) for the synthesis of prostaglandins, and where are these metabolites manufactured and located? Foster and Das (1984) have contributed relevant studies. They separated amnion from chorion of normal membranes that they obtained following the normal onset of labor and analyzed the lipid content. This investigation contrasts with earlier studies that used combined membranes. It must be mentioned that the chorion was not freed from its decidual investment, and that inferences drawn with respect to the precise localization of prostaglandin precursors cannot be made from this study alone. Nevertheless, the chorion had considerably more lipid (in milligram per deciliter) than the amnion, as can be seen in the following summary of their findings.

Lipid Components	Amnion (mg/dl)	Chorion (mg/dl)
Total lipid	470	1,530
Nonpolar lipids	319	1,042
Cholesterol esters	44	263
Cholesterol	71	210
Triglycerides	160	416
Free fatty acids	44	153
Phospholipids	150	488

Olson and Smieja (1988) studied the incorporation of arachidonic acid into amnion and found that there was no difference, regardless of whether labor had preceded.

Enzymes involved in prostaglandin biosynthesis include phospholipases, prostaglandin synthase, and prostaglandin endoperoxide synthase (or cyclooxygenase). They have been found in human amnion (Okazaki et al., 1981b; Bryant-Greenwood et al., 1987;

Toth & Rao, 1992; Smieja, 1993; Toth et al., 1993). It is interesting that the enzymes are regulated by human chorionic gonadotropin (hCG) (Toth & Rao, 1992), the receptors of which are found on the amnionic epithelium (Rao & Lei, 1989; Reshef et al., 1990; Toth et al., 1993). The complexity of the intraamnionic regulatory mechanisms is increased by some additional findings: Corticotropin-releasing hormone (CRH) (Jones & Challis, 1989) and glucocorticoids (Gibb & Lavoie, 1990) themselves modulate prostaglandin production; CRH mRNA was demonstrated in amnionic membrane of term pregnancies (Okamoto et al., 1990). Its production is modulated by glucocorticoids and progesterone (Jones et al., 1989).

Interleukins also are well known to regulate prostaglandin biosynthesis. According to the in situ hybridization and polymerase chain reaction studies by Rote et al. (1993), normal amnionic and chorionic cells of the membranes produce interleukin-1β in vitro; the application of endotoxin induced additional expression of interleukin-6. In conclusion, the authors speculated that intraamnionic infections induce production of interleukins, which increase prostaglandin production. Much additional investigation relates to prostaglandin initiation during the process of chorioamnionitis and is covered in Chapter 20. 15-Hydoxyprostaglandin dehydrogenase as a prostaglandin metabolizing and inactivating enzyme was found in membranes and villous trophoblast (Cheung et al., 1990). Casey et al. (1989) found prostaglandin dehydrogenase in the decidua capsularis and proposed that it regulates levels of prostaglandin therein as well as in the amnionic fluid, uterus, and blood.

The interactions between prostaglandins and oxytocin in the regulation of uterine contractions are only poorly understood. In humans, oxytocin acts as the myometrial contraction stimulator, but only when it is combined with increased levels of $PGF_{2\alpha}$ (Fuchs et al., 1983). Production of the latter is stimulated by oxytocin through a receptor-mediated process (Roberts et al., 1976). Benedetto et al. (1990) were able to demonstrate the oxytocin receptors in the amnion as well as in the chorion laeve.

Finally, leukotrienes, another cytokine group derived from arachidonic acid, are produced by the amnion (Rees et al., 1988). The authors discussed that these cytokines may effect uterine contractility in addition to their function as mediators of immune reaction and vasodilation.

From a functional perspective, perhaps more interesting are some findings concerning the intercellular junctions and the basal lamina of the amnion. The amnionic cells are connected to each other by numerous desmosomes, which focally bridge the long, winding lateral intercellular spaces; some additional gap junctions have been observed in the laterobasal region (King, 1982; Bartels & Wang, 1983; Wang, 1984). Tight junctions occluding the lateral intercellular spaces, and thus limiting paracellular transport, could not be observed between the cells, with the exception of a few during the first months of pregnancy (King, 1982; Bartels & Wang, 1983). Consequently, the intercellular clefts may represent an effective route for paracellular transfer, as has been demonstrated by tracer studies (King, 1982; Matsubara & Tamada, 1991). This point is of particular importance, as there are no hints for an effective transcellular pathway for macromolecules.

There are, however, some findings concerning the basal lamina that restrict the relevance of the above interpretations. The amnionic cells have a highly folded basal surface that interdigitates intensely with the basal lamina to which they are fixed by numerous hemidesmosomes (Danforth & Hull, 1958; Verbeek et al., 1967; King, 1980, 1982; Bartels & Wang, 1983; Wang, 1984). According to the histochemical studies of King (1985), the basal lamina contains large quantities of proteoglycans, rich in heparan sulfate. The latter substance may serve as a permeability barrier to anionic macromolecules. Also Klima et al. (1991), Wolf and Schmidt (1991), and Singhas (1992) have described by means of lectin-binding studies the presence of glyco-conjugates in the amnion and discussed the influence of these substances on amnionic fluid transfer. These findings are in agreement with two others. Liotta et al. (1980) observed restricted permeability of an isolated basal lamina preparation of human amnion to a 60,000 dalton protein; and Sutcliffe (1975) reported that the amnionic fluid contains a much smaller amount of protein than is found in fetal and maternal serum. Thus the amnionic basal lamina must also be considered to participate in the barrier function (King, 1985).

Concerning the regulation of transamnionic fluid transfer, Beham et al. (1988), Wolf et al. (1991), and Ockleford et al. (1993) have studied the distribution of cytoskeletal filaments within the amnionic epithelium. Actin, α-actinin, spectrin, ezrin, cytokeratins, vimentin, and desmoplakin have been found. The specialized arrangement of this intracellular filament system indicates a role in the structural integrity and modulation of cell shape as well as in junctional permeability (Wolf et al., 1991). Casey et al. (1991) demonstrated that amnionic epithelial cells produce endothelin-1 and thus are one of the potential sources for endothelin in the amnionic fluid, where it appears in concentrations exceeding those of the blood plasma by 10- to 100-fold. Epidermal growth factor, interleukin-1, and tumor necrosis factor α increased amnionic endothelin production. Amnionic endothelin may be involved in the regulation of amnionic fluid homeostasis, as it is known

to promote water transfer across the epithelia of other organs.

The amnion is involved in the turnover of the amnionic fluid. There is great immunohistochemical activity of carbonic anhydrase isoenzymes CA-1 and CA-2 (Crescimanno et al., 1993; Mühlhauser et al., 1994); this enzyme is involved in bicarbonate/carbon dioxide exchange. This fact makes it likely that the epithelium is responsible for regulating the pH of the amnionic fluid, keeping it constant at about 7.10. In doing so, the amnionic epithelium is at least partly involved in fetal pH regulation, as the fetus delivers considerable amounts of protons and bicarbonate via his or her kidneys into the amnionic fluid.

Amnionic epithelium not only participates in fetal CO_2 clearance but also in the clearance of fetal vasopressin, for instance, which is excreted via the fetal urine. It is removed from the amnionic fluid by diffusion- and swallowing-independent mechanisms (Uyehara & Claybaugh, 1988). It is likely that the degrading peptidases are active in the amnionic epithelium as well as in the amnionic fluid. In this context it may be of interest that Gossrau et al. (1987) described dipeptidylpeptidase IV activities in the amnionic epithelium and speculated about its hydrolytic action both intracellularly and in the amnionic fluid.

Epithelial participation in the secretion of amnionic fluid and in its resorption have long been under discussion (Bourne, 1962; Armstrong et al., 1968; Kratzsch & Grygiel, 1972; Smadja et al., 1974; Weser & Kaufmann, 1978), but until now this secretory activity has been speculative. It is generally accepted that the sources of the amnionic fluid are multiple and that the role of the amnion in maintaining its composition is still uncertain. The general functional description of the amnion as an epithelial lining that is contributing to the homeostasis of the amnionic fluid is supported by many clinical findings (see below), but they add little to the resolution of the precise interactions. Several groups of investigators have used immunohistochemical means to detect hormones such as hCG and human chorionic somatotropin (hCS) in the amnionic cells (Thiede & Choate, 1963; Kim et al., 1971; de Ikonicoff & Cedard, 1973). It is likely, however, that these hormones are the result of resorption from the amnionic fluid with subsequent degradation, rather than reflecting any local hormone synthesis.

The structural studies support the view that the amnionic epithelium is metabolically highly active throughout gestation. This point is also supported by the histochemical proof of high activity of various enzymes (Weser & Kaufmann, 1978). The histochemical study of enzymes related to energy metabolism suggested a predominating anaerobic glycolysis due to restricted oxygen supply (Benedetti et al., 1973). The absence of vessels in the mesenchymal layers of the amnion raises the question of the source of its nutrients and oxygen. They may be supplied by diffusion from the deeper layers of the uterine wall or via the amnionic fluid from the fetus. Wolf and Desoye (1993) have described the presence of glucose transporter proteins 1 and 3 predominantly at the apical surface of amnionic epithelial cells, whereas glucose transporter protein 4 and insulin receptor could not be detected. Thus it is likely that these cells cover their glucose requirements from the amnionic fluid with an insulin-independent mechanism. Furthermore, Bourne (1962) reported a monochorionic, diamnionic twin pregnancy in which the ipsilateral amnion in the "dividing membrane" degenerated following the death of one fetus. This finding can be explained in different ways; it simply may be an indicator that the fetus is important for supplying the amnion with nutrients and gases; alternatively, the degenerating fetal tissues may affect adversely the epithelium.

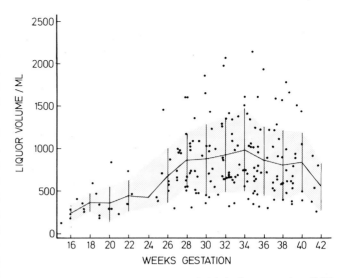

FIGURE 177. Volume of amnionic fluid during gestation (187 determinations). Mean values ± 1 SD. There is a wide range, with a final decrease during the last 4 weeks of gestation. (Modified from Queenan et al., 1972.)

Amnionic Fluid

It is commonly accepted that the amnionic fluid is derived from multiple sources: (1) possible secretory processes of the amnionic epithelium; (2) filtration of fluid from maternal vessels via the parietal decidua and the chorion laeve; (3) filtration from the fetal vessels via the chorionic plate and via the umbilical cord; (4) urination by the fetus; and (5) during early stages of pregnancy, by filtration from intracorporeal fetal vessels via the fetal skin. Its composition is influenced by continuous resorptive processes by the fetal digestive tract and the amnion and by pressure-dependent fetomaternal filtration across the membranes. The volume of the fluid is not static, varying among the stages of pregnancy as well as among individuals. A careful determination of the development of amnionic fluid volumes throughout pregnancy by a dilution method during amniocentesis has been presented by Queenan et al. (1972) (Figure 177). The results showed a wide range of volumes, with a mean of 239 ml at 15 to 16 weeks p.m., a maximum mean of 984 ml at 33 to 34 weeks p.m., and a slight final decrease to term (836 ml). After term (41–42 weeks p.m.), the mean volume was reduced to 544 ml.

The composition of the amnionic fluid has been described in detail by Schmidt (1992) and is reviewed only briefly here. The pH is usually 7.10, with a maximum value of 7.40; the osmotic pressure is about 255 mosm.

Further constituents are the following,

Glucose (5–20 mg/dl)
Amino acids
Proteins (280–780 mg/dl) (α_1-albumin; α_2-albumin; β-globulin; γ-globulins: IgA, IgG, IgM; α_1-fetoprotein; lipoproteins)
Lipids (40 mg/dl), largely as lipid droplets measuring 1 to 30 μm in diameter, composed of cholesterol, triglycerides, diglycerides, free fatty acids, phospholipids (Among the latter the ratio of lecithin to sphingomyelin (L/S ratio) as performed during prenatal diagnosis is thought to be a reliable parameter in determining pulmonary maturity; it has also been suggested that surfactant may stabilize the amnionic sac.) (Hills, 1994)

Urea (20–40 mg/dl)
Uric acid
Creatinine
Bilirubin

In addition, a broad variety of hormones has been found in the amnionic fluid (Schindler, 1982).

Progesterone, estradiol, estriol, testosterone, aldosterone, cortisol
Luteinizing hormone (LH), follicle stimulating hormone (FSH), hCG, human placental lactogen (hPL), prolactin, adrenocorticotropic hormone (ACTH), growth hormone (hGH), somatomedin, thyrotropin (TSH)
Thyroid hormones, parathyroid hormone, oxytocin, glucagon, insulin, hypothalamic-releasing hormones, neurophysin

Moreover, numerous enzymes have been found, most of which are, according to Schmidt (1992), thought to be derived from the membranes by secretion or by cell shedding. Among the regulating factors of enzymes (proteases) are tissue-type plasminogen activator (t-PA) and urokinase-type plasminogen activator (u-PA) as well as their respective inhibitors PAI-1 and PAI-2 (Kjaeldgaard et al., 1989). These activators and inhibitors regulate the fibrinolytic/proteolytic activities of amnionic fluid plasminogen, which is possibly involved in the etiology of membrane rupture (Jenkins et al., 1983).

After staining with Nile blue, hematoxylin and eosin, Giemsa or Papanicolaou stains, a variety of amnionic fluid cells can be observed, their number steadily increasing throughout pregnancy and reaching values at term of up to 80 cells/mm³. Their origin has not been satisfactorily determined in every case because after exfoliation from their tissue of origin they usually undergo structural changes (Schmidt, 1992). The following cells types have been classified by Schmidt (1992).

1. Large anuclear flat cells (diameter 40–50 mm), probably exfoliated keratinocytes
2. Nucleated squamous epithelial cells (diameter 30–50 μm): type b originating from the oral mucous membrane, type c possibly

originating from the amnionic epithelium of the cord, type d derived from the fetal vulva and vagina
3. Small round to oval cells (diameter 18–25 μm) originating from the fetal urinary tract
4. Variety of special cell forms such as polynuclear cells from the urinary tract (transitional epithelium) and others

Chromosomal Determinations

Bautzmann et al. (1960) and other students of the amnionic membrane have often made flat membrane preparations for investigation. These preparations allow one to see more clearly the squamous nature of the epithelium and to demonstrate its occasional defects. These preparations also lend themselves to observing the lipid droplets in the epithelium whose numbers increase with maturation (Bautzmann & Hertenstein, 1957; Danforth & Hull, 1958; Schmidt, 1963). Occasional giant cells ("colossal cells") with large vacuoles are seen to include large vacuoles. Such preparations also show relatively frequent polyploid nuclei. The epithelial cells, however, divide under normal conditions by regular mitosis (Schwarzacher & Klinger, 1963). Multinucleated cells, particularly binucleated cells, are most commonly found in newborns. Mitoses become rare after the sixth gestational month. In cytophotometric measurements, Schindler (1961) showed, in specimens from early gestation, that the polyploid cells are tetraploid and octoploid, with a concomitant increase in their cytoplasm. These observations have assumed greater significance as the use of amniocentesis for chromosomal determination of the fetus has been more widely practiced. The finding of mixed cell populations (mosaicism) is here of concern; it demands an explanation (Kalousek & Dill, 1983). These authors studied 117 specimens and concluded that the mosaic (aneuploid) cell populations they found invariably came from the membranes. The cells were not found in fetal lymphocytes when they were studied after birth. They had only 47 completely successful cultures with two aneuploid admixtures, but it is not clear that they grew amnion epithelium, as opposed to chorionic fibroblasts. Nevertheless, they reviewed other reports of mosaicism of cell lines from amnionic fluid culture (origin of these cells also unknown), where the fetus was eventually found to be normal. Similarly perplexing mosaicism has been detected in chorionic villus biopsy (CVS) specimens by a number of investigators. Linton and Lilford (1986), for instance, found complex XY/XYY mosaicism; and all 14 metaphases contained an extra chromosome 16q-. It was associated with a karyotypically normal fetus in a case described by Breed et al. (1986). In parallel cultures of amnionic fluid cells and samples from CVS, Verjaal et al. (1987) also found discrepancies and warned that great care must be taken when interpreting such abnormalities. Their findings supported the view of Hogge et al. (1985) that such errors occur as often as in 2% of CVS. Schulze et al. (1987) had experience with two aneuploid mosaics (46,XX/47,XX+3 and 46,XX/47,XX+15) and normal 46,XX newborns. Crane and Cheung (1988) suggested that postzygotic nondisjunction of chromosomes in the cytotrophoblast is the most likely cause of such mosaicism. They described 15 cases of mosaicism after CVS, identified in direct preparations from the biopsy specimen, thus ruling out an artifact of tissue culture. They suggested that the processing of multiple individual fragments of tissue might avoid mistaken diagnosis. The most recent methodology for evaluating the fetal genotype and studying differences in the genetic contributions of fetus versus placenta involves a molecular analysis of the DNA extracted from both tissues. Butler et al. (1988) studied 50 paired samples from these sources and found differences in the hypervariable regions of repetitive DNA in four pairs, whereas they were alike in the others. This finding may indicate that mitotic

crossing-over or other mechanisms of chromosomal segregation occur. These points must be considered for a meaningful interpretation of cytogenetic studies from placenta and amniotic fluid. Furthermore, mitotic errors in the delicate amnionic membrane of early gestation might be one mechanism that leads to defects in its structure and thus to the future amnionic band development. Additional discussion of this important topic is found in Chapter 21.

Another still poorly understood feature of the developing membranes is that the X inactivation ("lyonization") of its cells appears to be nonrandom. Ropers et al. (1978) reviewed the studies on this topic and analyzed the glucose-6-phosphate dehydrogenase (G-6-PD) activity of heterozygotic females. Preferential activity of the maternal X chromosome-derived isozyme activity was found in the membranes of the placenta, analogous to earlier observations in rodents (Frels et al., 1979; Rastan et al., 1980). Confirmation of these results has come from the study by Harrison and Warburton (1986). They also used the variants of G-6-PD as markers for "lyonization," but the mechanism leading to this preferential expression of the maternal allele and the possible reasons for it are unknown at present.

Cellular Metaplasia and Glycogen

Metaplastic processes are frequent in the amnionic epithelium. They are present in at least one-fourth of mature placentas, most prominently around the umbilical cord; they must not be confused with amnion nodosum. We refer to them as "squamous metaplasia," a misnomer, as Bourne (1960) noted. The amnion is squamous, and these areas of metaplasia do not form in response to some chronic irritation or inflammation (e.g., in the bronchus of smokers). They merely betray maturity and are not found in immature placentas. This so-called squamous metaplasia of the amnion is actually focal keratinization of the epithelium (Figures 178, 179). It is a regular feature of the amnion in many other species, such as whales, sheep, and others, in which nodules of keratin stud the cord and amnion. Some species even have melanin pigment in these structures. In the term human placenta these areas of squamous metaplasia are visible as hydrophobic foci of tiny, concentric elevations. They are most commonly found in the vicinity of the cord insertion. Squamous metaplasia occurs in up to 60% of term placentas. Sinha (1971) provided a detailed electron microscopic study of squamous metaplasia. In animals, these plaques (occasionally referred to as pustules) may be 15 cells thick. They may have no similarity to amnion cells but more resemble the epidermis and usually include keratohyaline granules and melanin. In this context, one must recall the developmental and structural continuity (Figure 208) of amnionic epithelium and the squamous fetal skin.

An interesting consideration is whether, in cases of ichthyosis congenita, the amnion participates in the excessive keratinization that is seen in the epidermis. One report of marked plaque formation in ichthyosis has come from Coston (1908). He observed a large placenta whose cord and amnion were covered with ichthyotic patches. This finding has not been our experience. The placenta of the X-linked type of ichthyosis (the commonest form of this disease) is structurally normal. A biochemical study by Bedin et al. (1981) of the steroid sulfatase in placentas from women has shown that the locus determining this critical enzyme for the disease is not inactivated. Garcia et al. (1977) observed the concurrence of amnion nodosum and congenital ichthyosis in four cases. Amnionic plaques of the membranes were correctly interpreted to result from oligohydramnios, rather than from excessive squamous metaplasia. Our conclusion is that, although ectodermal in origin, the amnion does not have the capacity to exhibit the lesion of ichthyosis congenita. In a case of severe, fatal lamellar ichthyosis seen by us, the amnion was attached to the fetal skin because of oligohydramnios, but its remnants, located around the cord insertion, were free from keratinization. There was some excessive squamous metaplasia on the cord surface,. with prominent desmosomes but lacking keratohyaline granules and true keratin. Moreover, no macroscopic plaques were present despite severe fetal skin involvement. An unresolved question is the cause of the common oligohydramnios in these pregnancies and the concomitant fetal deformities. The latter are frequently much in excess of those found with Potter's

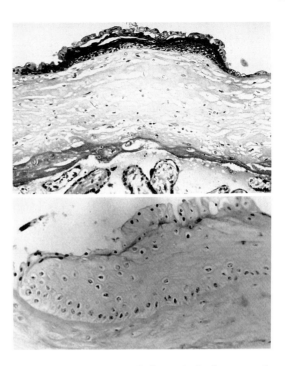

FIGURE 179. Squamous metaplasia, typical of mature placenta (top), and amnion epithelium (bottom). H&E. Top ×160; bottom ×250.

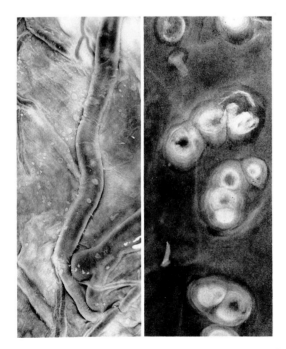

FIGURE 178. Squamous metaplasia of the amnion. At left is a surface view showing the concentric layers of keratin. At right one sees the tiny nodules of keratin irregularly present over vessels and chorion, different from amnion nodosum.

syndrome and are presumably a part of the genetic abnormality ichthyosis. Keratinization was also found to be absent in the rare harlequin fetuses of the Neu-Laxova syndrome (Karimi-Nejad et al., 1987), in which hyperkeratosis is a prominent feature of the infant's skin.

During early pregnancy the amnionic epithelium contains cytoplasmic glycogen, and it is not significantly increased in the placentas of women with diabetes. Increased amounts of glycogen in the placentas of diabetics have been found to occur only around the major fetal vessels (Robb & Hytten, 1976). Other vacuoles are frequently present in the epithelial cells; and they may be engaged in transport activity (Figure 180). In cases of fetal death, the epithelium shows extensive degeneration, particularly when studied electron microscopically (Mukaida et al., 1977).

Amnionic Mesoderm

The amnionic epithelium rests on a basal lamina that is composed mainly of collagen IV fibrils (Yurchenco & Ruben, 1994), laminin (Aplin and Allen, 1985), and heparan sulfate proteoglycan (Foltz et al., 1982). It is associated with the basal cell surface by means of fibronectins. Its functional influence on transamnionic transfer has been dealt with earlier. The lamina is fixed to the neighboring stroma by anchoring plaques con-

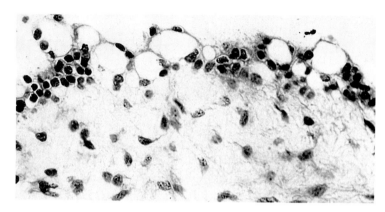

FIGURE 180. Ballooning degeneration of amnionic epithelium in a 20 week abortus after 3 weeks of bleeding. H&E. ×400.

taining collagen IV, which are attached to anchoring fibrils in the surrounding tissue that contain collagen VII (Keene et al., 1987). In addition, collagen V appears in the immediate area of the basal lamina (Modesti et al., 1984).

The following compact stromal layer has a varying thickness. It contains collagen types I and III (Madri et al., 1983) and fibronectins (Linnala et al., 1993) that are largely secreted by the amnionic epithelial cells. The distribution of the various collagen types in the various mesenchymal layers of the amnion has been described in detail by Malak et al. (1993). The compact stroma is composed of bundles of 30 nm collagen fibrils that are intermingled with 18 nm fibrils (Aplin & Allen, 1985). The three-dimensional structure of these fibrils and their association with the basal lamina as well as with the basal surface of amnionic epithelium has been beautifully illustrated by Campbell et al. (1989). The two types of fibers together form a coarse meshwork of bundles, in which, according to Bourne (1962), some elastic fibers can also be integrated. The latter finding has been contested by Aplin and Allen (1985), so it remains open whether the well known elasticity of the amnion is due to the presence of elastic material or to the arrangement of the collagenous bundles. Composition and fiber arrangement are important factors for the tensile strength of the amnion and thus may be discussed in context with causes for preterm rupture of the membranes. A characteristic layering of the amnionic mesoderm, as it has been described for the amnion of the chorionic plate (Bourne, 1962), is less pronounced in the amnionic membrane. The ability to identify several distinct layers of connective tissue probably depends to some degree on the state of its contraction and fixation, as well as on one's imagination. It is evident, however, that the compact collagenous layer near the epithelium is largely devoid of connective tissue cells. Ockleford et al. (1994), based on immuno-histochemical studies, have suggested that it represents a giant lamina reticularis representing the inner part of a basal membrane and thus belonging to the amnionic

basal lamina. The deeper part of the amnionic mesenchyme, also called the fibroblast layer (Bou-Resli et al., 1981), contains a more or less dense network of branched fibroblasts.

Bartels and Wang (1983) failed to observe intercellular junctions connecting these cells. Additionally, some macrophages can be observed as early as the 7th week of gestation (5- to 6-mm embryo). Schwarzacher (1960) likened them to Hofbauer cells. In electron microscopic studies of the amnion, Hoyes (1968a,b) suggested that these macrophages derive from the epithelium, and that they decrease in number toward term. In light of the modern findings regarding the biology of placental macrophages (see Chapter 7), however, there are no longer arguments regarding an epithelial derivation. The bundles of collagen fibers are arranged in clearly separated layers of varying fiber orientation (Bou-Resli et al., 1981). Aplin and Allen (1985) described the synthesis of collagens I, III, and IV, as well as of laminin and fibronectin, by amnionic epithelial cells in culture. From these findings they concluded that the epithelium not only produces the basal lamina; it is also involved in the synthesis of the stromal fibers, at least of the compact layer, which is largely devoid of fibroblasts.

Medley of Themes

The sex chromatin (Barr body) of amnionic epithelial cells and of the underlying connective tissue is easily observed. Using this marker, Klinger and Schwarzacher (1962) demonstrated in a fetus with XY/XXY mosaicism that the amnion was also mosaic. Some areas were sex chromatin-positive and others were sex chromatin-negative. Moreover, they showed clearly that the connective tissue underlying one type of epithelium occasionally had a different karyotype. This observation proved, once and for all, that these tissues have different embryological origins. We indicated earlier that we believe the peripheral connective tissue of the amnion is a condensation of the cellular elements that are dispersed in the magma reticulare of the primitive chorionic sac. Parenthetically, it may be noted that an improved method for the histological detection of sex chromatin in formalin-fixed tissues has been described (Davis & Penny, 1981). It employs pronase and acid hydrolysis prior

FIGURE 181. Two sets of "dividing membranes" (A,B) of diamnionic, monochorionic twins, with one twin having died days before birth. Note the necrosis of the epithelium on the right sides at various stages of degeneration. H&E. A ×160; B ×250.

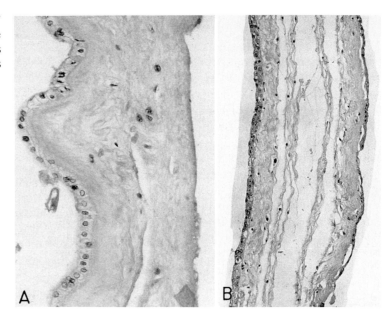

to quinacrine staining. Perhaps the earliest time sex chromatin can be observed in human embryos is on day 13. Thorburn (1964) identified the Barr bodies readily in trophoblast. Other authors who have described the sex chromatin in membranes and trophoblast are Bohle and Hienz (1956) and Verma and Ghai (1971).

Efforts to study the possible existence of smooth musculature in human amnions have usually employed flat, surface preparations of membranes. From studies in chickens and reptiles it is known that an orderly arrangement of a smooth muscle plexus in the amnion produces regular contractions, possibly to ensure mixing of fluid and rocking of the embryo (Bautzmann & Schöder, 1953; Bautzmann, 1956). Such structures have not been found in mammals. In early human amnions, only net-like fibrocytic cell arrangements are identifiable in the connective tissue of the amnion; muscle is absent.

There are also no nerves, lymphatics, or blood vessels in the amnion. Because the amnion is avascular, it must subsist on the nutrients and gaseous exchange of surrounding fluids and structures. This point is particularly well demonstrated by the large portions of amnion that are apposed as the "dividing membranes" in diamnionic monochorionic twins. Here the large stretches of amnion are kept alive by the amnionic fluid surrounding them. Consequently, when one fetus dies, that portion of its amnionic surface dies as well. The epithelial cells undergo necrosis, as is shown in Figure 181A (see also Bourne, 1962). It is surprising that the living amnion from the opposing twin's side is not able to sustain this portion of membrane, as the dividing membranes are so thin and delicate. Although it is also possible that the death of the amnionic epithelium in these circumstances comes about by the liberation of noxious substances from a macerating fetus, it is unlikely. The amnion overlying the placenta proper takes much longer to die. It is obviously being kept alive by the oxygen gradients from the persisting intervillous circulation.

Clinical and Research Applications

Because the amnion can be so readily separated from the chorion, and because it is so widely available, it has often been used as dressing for burns and other wounds (Editorial, 1984; Redmond, 1984). This practice appears to have special merits in that the

epithelium does not possess HLA-type antigens and even fails to elicit an immunological reaction when transplanted (Akle et al., 1981). Moreover, antibacterial properties of the amnion are well documented. The antimicrobial effect is thought to be related to the close adherence of the membrane to the wound surface (Talmi et al., 1991).

Of course, amnion has also been a favorite cellular material for virologists in that it can readily be established in culture, particularly when it is obtained from young pregnancies and from patients with toxemia of pregnancy (Jonas & Caunt, 1965). When such cultures are treated with cortisone, profound changes occur in the membranous surface of the amnionic epithelial cells (Polet, 1966). It is also worthy of note that the injection of transformed human amnion cells into cortisone-treated mice induces tumor growth with cartilage and bone formation, presumably by stimulating host cells to undergo this differentiation (Anderson et al., 1964). In other studies, the amnion has been used to serve as a substratum for axons in tissue culture (Davis et al., 1987) and for the cultivation of trophoblast; after removal of the epithelial cells the remaining connective tissue matrix, together with the epithelial basal lamina, serves as an excellent substratum for the monolayer culture of cytotrophoblast, even allowing syncytial fusion of the latter (Bullen et al., 1990).

Chorion Laeve

The chorionic membrane is a tough fibrous tissue layer that carries the fetal blood vessels. The villi arise from its outer surface; and on the inside of the chorion is the amnion, which is only loosely attached. It has been convenient for many authors to speak of the "placental chorion"—the membrane that covers the placental disk proper. In agreement with the anatomical literature, we call it the chorionic plate. On the other hand, the "reflected chorion" is the chorion laeve or extraplacental membrane (Bourne, 1962), which is the tissue that we discuss in greater detail in this chapter.

Intermediate (Spongy) Layer

When studying the membranes after birth, one realizes that the reflected amnion and chorion can easily slide, separating the two membranes from each other. This phenomenon is due to the existence of the spongy layer, which results from incomplete fusion of amnionic and chorionic mesoderm during early pregnancy. This intermediate layer is composed of loosely arranged bundles of collagen fibers with a few scattered fibroblasts, separated by a communicating system of clefts (Schmidt, 1956; Petry, 1962; Bou-Resli et al., 1981). The clefts are remainders of the formerly existing now largely obstructed exocoel (Figure 208). This view has been corroborated by immunohistochemical/confocal laser studies by Ockleford et al. (1993).

It is difficult to decide whether accidental cells lining these clefts are also fibroblasts or are the remainder of the original amnionic and chorionic mesothelium. The presence of collagen type IV in this zone (Malak et al., 1993; Ockleford et al., 1993), which is a typical basal lamina molecule, makes a mesothelial origin of these cells likely (Ockleford et al., 1993). In addition, macrophages have been observed (Schmidt, 1956).

Chorionic Mesoderm

The spongy layer continues without sharp demarcation into the next connective tissue layer, already belonging to the chorion laeve.

This connective tissue is derived from the embryo (Luckett, 1971). When restudying human and rhesus monkey embryonic material, Luckett found that the extraembryonic mesoderm comes from the primitive streak. It develops on day 12 from the caudal pole of the embryonic shield and differentiates in human embryos on about day 14. The cells of the primitive streak move peripherally; there they form the cores of the primitive villi. Luckett did not totally exclude the idea that there may be some minor contribution derived from trophoblast, but in our view it is unlikely. For example, even well differentiated choriocarcinomas never produce connective tissue, which would be expected at least occasionally, as such behavior is seen with virtually all other neoplasms.

Another reason for asserting that chorionic connective tissue has an embryonic origin comes from the embryological studies on reconstituted mouse embryos (Rossant & Croy, 1985). Rossant and Croy took inner cell masses of mice with distinct isoenzymes and in situ genetic markers and placed them into different trophoblastic shells. They then followed the placental development and deduced that only 4% of the mouse placenta was derived from the embryo. This portion was composed primarily of fetal capillaries. Mouse placental tissue has generally little connective tissue.

The formation of the extraembryonic mesenchyme has been studied in exquisitely prepared electron micrographs of early rhesus monkey ova from days 19 to 60 (Enders & King, 1988). The first evidence of mesenchyme was peripheral to the primitive endoderm, the "hypoblast." These authors showed convincing evidence that the rough endoplasmic reticulum of this mesenchyme has intracisternal densities that are not shared by other connective tissue. This feature allows one also to determine its origin. It

could be followed into the early villous structures on day 13. Also arguing against a trophoblastic origin of villous mesenchyme is the finding that there is always a complete basal lamina underlying the trophoblast. Enders and King's meticulous study showed that the earliest blood vessel formation comes from this villous mesenchyme, which differentiates focally into endothelium as early as day 13 but more actively later.

The composition of the chorionic mesoderm is similar to that of the fibroblast layer of the amnion, consisting of a coarse network of collagen bundles intermingled with finer argyrophilic fibrils. The distribution of the various collagen types I, III, IV, V, and VI has been detailed by Malak et al. (1993). Hessle and Engvall (1984) and Hessle et al. (1984) focused on the distribution of collagen VI. Fibroblasts and macrophages are regular findings. According to Wang and Schneider (1982) and Bartels and Wang (1983), many of the fibroblasts are likely to represent myofibroblasts. They are connected to each other by gap junctions, which allow intercellular coupling. Most of the studies that concern collagen composition and tensile properties of the membranes (e.g., Aplin et al., 1986; Teodoro et al., 1990; Malak et al., 1993) deal with the mesenchyme of the amnion and that of the chorion. For details we refer to these papers. It is likely that both layers equally contribute to the mechanical stability of the membranes.

The structure of the chorion laeve has been extensively studied by Hoyes (1970, 1971). His earlier contribution, although specifically dealing with the mesenchyme of the amnion, has two important features. Hoyes noted that prior to the attachment of amnion to chorion the mesenchymal cells have a continuous configuration with highly developed endoplasmic reticulum. Later, they disintegrate into dispersed elements. Hoyes believed that the Hofbauer cells found during later development resulted from degenerating connective tissue elements, a notion that is no longer in agreement with the modern views regarding the derivation of the placental macrophages (see Chapter 7). It appears to us more likely that these cells take their origin from the fetal vascular compartment. Santiago-Schwarz and Fleit (1988) described a population of cells in cord blood that, upon culturing, developed into macrophages. In a later paper, Hoyes (1971) described the mesenchymal elements. He considered them to be similar to those of the amnion.

The connective tissue is followed by a basal lamina that is highly variable in terms of thickness and structure. It is composed of laminin and collagen IV and shows accumulations of fibronectin and collagen III in its immediate surrounding area (Aplin & Campbell, 1985). Increased amounts of extracellular debris can be observed near the basal lamina (Lister, 1968). Fetal vessels exist up to the 6th month; they are branches of the umbilical vessels, extending via the chorionic plate into the mesoderm of the former chorion frondosum; during the last trimester these vessels are usually absent (Hoyes, 1971). Band-like groups of cells that are rich in lipid droplets and glycogen stores (found between the collagen bundles) have been discussed to be residues of the former capillary endothelium (Hoyes, 1971). This author traced the development of those capillaries that are present up to the third month; they then thrombose and gradually disappear. Lister (1968) claimed to have found some capillaries in abnormal placentas near term, but this observation was shared by neither Hoyes (1971) nor us.

From histochemical studies of fetal membranes—largely periodic acid-Schiff (PAS) and similar reactions—Sala and Matheus (1984) concluded that the membranes are not merely a container for the fetus, but that because of their polysaccharide content they participate in the exchange of water and electrolytes. They found that more neutral polysaccharides were present in the trophoblastic shell of term placental membranes and decidua than elsewhere; the acid mucopolysaccharides were most prominent in the connective tissue layers and decidua.

Trophoblast Layer

A highly variable layer of trophoblast cells persists until term. These cells are the only residues of the former villi of the chorion frondosum, intermingled with the trophoblastic residues of the primary chorionic plate and the trophoblastic shell.

The trophoblast is separated from the chorionic mesoderm by the above-mentioned basal lamina, on which it rests as a more or less uninterrupted, mostly even, multilayered stratum. Toward the uterine wall, the trophoblast interdigitates intensely with the decidua. Near the placental margin the trophoblast splits into two layers, flanking an intermediate fibrinoid lamella of increasing thickness. Ghost villi may be encased in the latter, which consist of clearly identifiable villous stroma surrounded by fibrinoid with some scattered trophoblast cells (Figure 169). At the placental margin, transition of the ghost villi into intact villi, surrounded by maternal blood, may lead smoothly to the placenta (Bühler, 1964). In other cases, abrupt changes from the placental margin into a uniform trophoblast layer of the chorion laeve are observed (Figure 173).

The trophoblast cells of the membranes, together with all the other cytotrophoblast residing outside the placental villi, is now subsumed under the heading extravillous cytotrophoblast. This summarizing term is justified, as all of these cells show the same behavior despite their different locations (chorionic plate, basal plate, cell columns, cell islands, septa, membranes).

The structure of the trophoblast cells of the membranes is variable (Bou-Resli et al., 1981), as it is in all other extravillous trophoblast populations. Several stages of differentiation can be found, including proliferating, undifferentiated rounded cells with large, oval nuclei and scarce organelles resting on the basal lamina that incorporate ^{3}H-thymidine (Kaltenbach & Sachs, 1979) and nonproliferating, differentiated, large polygonal cells with highly irregular, invaginated nuclei and condensed cytoplasm, with ample rough endoplasmic reticulum, lipid droplets, and glycogen. These cells have a highly active energy metabolism and express alkaline phosphatase (Petry, 1962). Some of the latter cells that are located nearer the decidua are obviously degenerative in nature. As the result of degeneration, foci of fibrinoid can be observed between the cells. It is probably identical with the amorphous material described by Bou-Resli et al. (1981). During earlier stages of pregnancy, a complete layer of syncytiotrophoblast marks the border to the decidua. It becomes interrupted as pregnancy advances. In the term placenta its complete continuity is no longer observed (Lister, 1968).

The trophoblast cells are separated from each other by a system of partly dilated intercellular clefts, bordered by a few microvilli and irregular cytoplasmic processes. The clefts are filled with a largely amorphous material (Bou-Resli et al., 1981) with some loosely arranged collagen fibers and bundles of a fine fibrillar material that resembles fibrin or fibrinoid. Immunohistochemically this material contains laminin, collagen IV, heparan sulfate proteoglycan, all three known to be usual basal lamina constituents; in addition, oncofetal fibronectin but no fibrin is present. Thus the area corresponds to the matrix-type fibrinoid described by Frank et al. (1994) which is a secretory product of trophoblast rather than a blood clotting product as postulated for fibrin. The presence of fibronectin in this trophoblastic layer has also been described by Yamaguchi et al. (1985) and that of collagen IV and laminin by Aplin and Campbell (1985), Malak et al. (1993), and Ockleford et al. (1993); the latter authors pointed to the similarity with basal lamina material.

The trophoblast cells are connected to each other by desmosomes (Bourne, 1962; Lister, 1968; Bou-Resli et al., 1981; Bartels & Wang, 1983; Wang & Schneider, 1987). In addition, occluding junctions and gap junctions have been described (Bartels & Wang, 1983). The function of the occluding junctions is still open to question. As concluded from their focal arrangement and from physiological studies (Battaglia et al., 1968; Lloyd et al., 1969; Chez et al., 1970; Seeds et al., 1977) the junctions cannot limit the permeability of the chorion laeve; physiologically, this layer must be regarded as a leaky membrane. The extracellular matrix may be involved in the permeability properties (Bartels & Wang, 1983), as discussed for the amnionic epithelium. This assumption, however, also cannot explain why the layer seems to be permeable for placental lactogen (hPL) with a molecular weight of about 22,000 daltons (Chez et al., 1970), whereas it was found to be impermeable to the much smaller inulin molecule (5,500 daltons) (Battaglia et al., 1962).

Another interesting view has been stressed by Bartels and Wang (1983). The existence of gap junctions between the trophoblast cells suggests that these cells are coupled metabolically. Gap junctions could not be detected between the individual cells of the villous cytotrophoblast or between villous cytotrophoblast and syncytiotrophoblast (Metz et al., 1979; Reale et al., 1980). Large amounts of renin have been detected immunohistochemically within the cytotrophoblast of the chorion laeve (Symonds et al., 1970; Poisner et al., 1981), and it has been demonstrated in other tissues that renin-producing cells are coupled by gap junctions (Boll et al., 1975; Forssmann & Taugner, 1977). The probable renin synthesis attributed to these cells is the only concrete functional finding, although there are some vague histochemical hints that the trophoblast of the smooth chorion is also involved in steroid biosynthesis (Benedetti et al., 1973) and that some cells at the trophoblastic decidual interface express hPL (Sakbun et al., 1990b). Another finding makes it likely that the trophoblast cells of this site are more than mere residual or even degenerating elements, as they bind epidermal growth factor to such an extent that they must be designated a real target tissue of this growth-stimulating and growth-regulating molecule (Rao et al., 1984).

Immunological Considerations of the Trophoblast

Because embryonic cells such as the membranous trophoblast contain both maternally and paternally derived chromosomes, a maternal immune reaction should be expected as soon as the embryonic cells are in contact with maternal tissues such as decidua. In the membranes trophoblastic and decidual cells often come into close contact without fibrinoid being interposed. However, neither inflammatory cells (granulocytes) nor immune-mediating cells (lymphocytes) can be found in unusual numbers in this maternofetal junctional zone.

The explanation may be that the membranous extravillous trophoblast expresses class I major histocompatibility complex (MHC) antigens differently from other embryoblast-derived cells (Hunt & Fishback, 1989). They do not express allotypic determinants associated with maternal or paternal class I antigens, and their antigens have lower-than-usual molecular weights (Ellis et al., 1986). How these special class I MHC antigens might function to suppress immunological problems and enhance pregnancy success is a critical and still open question. Interestingly, some tumor cells exhibit similar class I MHC patterns, which help to establish residency in host tissues (Hunt & Fishback, 1989).

Decidua

The decidual layer that is attached to the membranes after birth is largely derived from the parietal decidua (Figure 173), with some additional residual elements of the capsular decidua. Whether the individual cells are derived from one or the other layer cannot be distinguished. Because the capsular decidua undergoes degeneration early and becomes discontinuous (Figure 173c), it is likely that the remaining cells are mostly of parietal origin.

In most morphological descriptions of the membranes, the decidua is only peripherally discussed or not mentioned at all. Therefore it is difficult to decide if it is structurally different from the basal decidua, which has been the subject of numerous studies. The only modern description of the parietal decidua is based on rhesus monkey membranes (King, 1981). As far as can be determined from the early descriptions by Petry (1962) and Bourne (1962), the results can be extrapolated to humans. The cells of this layer obviously do not comprise a uniform population. They all have elongated cell bodies surrounded by more or less prominent and partly condensed meshworks of fine fibrils. Most of the cells have well developed granular endoplasmic reticulum, numerous mitochondria, and a prominent Golgi apparatus. The cell surfaces of many cells are characterized by stalk-like cytoplasmic processes that contain secretory granules, which are also well known in the decidua basalis (Wynn, 1974; Kisalus & Herr, 1988).

The cells are surrounded by a basal membrane-like material that contains typical basal laminas of various collagens (Wewer et al., 1985), heparan sulfate proteoglycan (Kisalus et al., 1987; Kisalus & Herr, 1988), and laminin. Charpin et al. (1985) studied laminin distribution. They considered laminin to be the protein that had been demonstrated around decidual cells by Wynn (1974). Because laminin has never been found in nondecidualized endometrium, they suggested that it is deposited under hormonal control. The same is probably valid for the other basal lamina molecules. Because laminin has an adhesive quality, they proposed that it may be involved in the attachment and nesting of the blastocyst.

In their delineation of placental villi with immunofluorescent antibodies directed against complement C3 breakdown products (C3d), Leivo and Engvall (1986) observed a strong localization in the trophoblastic basement membrane and decidua but none in the basement membranes of villous capillaries. They considered it possible that the complement originates from *maternal* plasma, as none was found in fetal capillaries, and it was also not produced by trophoblast. Because C3d has been found in glomeruli, its immunological relation to placenta, amply demonstrated by early studies, may have a new explanation. Laminin has a strong affinity for C3d, and it may be for this reason that it is bound at these sites.

Some of the decidual cells have been shown to express relaxin, a hormone that, however, is secreted also by cyto- and syncytiotrophoblast of different origin (Sakbun et al., 1990a).

The deeper layers of the parietal decidua, which remain in utero, are richly supplied with maternal blood vessels (Arts, 1961). In the superficial parts of the decidua that are attached to the membranes after birth, maternal vessels are the exception; if there are any vessels here, only some capillaries, smaller arterioles, and venules can be identified.

Tensile Properties of the Membranes

Some investigators have wondered why the relatively thin amnion withstands pressures so readily, and many have conducted measurements of its tensile strength. Independently, Polishuk et al. (1962, 1964), Laufer et al. (1966), and MacLachlan (1965) developed an apparatus to measure the tensile strengths of amnion and whole membranes. The tensile strength of amnion is greater than that of chorion. According to Klima et al. (1989), the amount and arrangement of fibers of the compact layer of amnionic mesenchyme is primarily responsible for the tensile properties. The tensile strength of the amnion was estimated to be even greater than would be needed for a successful gestation, and they found that the strength is greater during early gestation than near term.

The average thickness of the membranes is 0.56 mm, the amnion making up one-third. The average tensile strength is 205 g/cm (50–500 g/cm) (Lavery et al., 1980). Studies of details in membrane strength in prematurely ruptured sacs have supported earlier findings (Danforth et al., 1953). They pointed out that the membranes thin out appreciably at the site of rupture, but that their possibly reduced strength is not the explanation for rupture (Artal et al., 1976).

More recent studies have pointed out that the membranes have a great ability to withstand trauma. They can expand to twice normal size during pregnancy and labor. Physically they display both viscosity and elasticity, properties that are believed to explain the various unusual physical features (Lavery & Miller, 1977).

Kanayama and colleagues (1985) analyzed the collagen of normal and prematurely ruptured membranes. They recognized types I, III, and V in these extracts and found altered ratios between the types in specimens from prematurely ruptured membrane cases. There was a particular reduction in collagen type III, and they deduced from their analysis that it related to an increase in trypsin content and a decrease in α_1-antitrypsin.

Amnionic epithelium and the few neighboring fibroblasts continue to synthesize and to depose collagens and other matrix molecules until term, depending on the presence of vitamin C (Aplin et al., 1986). As was shown by Teodoro et al. (1990), the membranes of patients with premature rupture have 44% less collagen than is normal. Future studies in this area are particularly important, especially taking into consideration the local area of the membrane involved.

Kanayama et al. (1985) were unable to demonstrate the presence of elastins in any membranes, a finding that was somewhat contradicted by the results of Evaldson et al. (1987), who found no decrease in overall collagen content in prematurely ruptured membranes. Perhaps it is the relative proportion of collagen types that is significant.

Lower collagen/hexosamine ratios reduce tensile strength. Meudt (1966) found that meconium exposure had the same effect but offered no quantitative data. Lavery et al. (1980) provided such data and noted that although tensile strength is reduced the presence of meconium does not correlate with premature rupture of membranes. Surprisingly, amnions from pregnancies with premature rupture of membranes had higher tensile strengths than those with timely membrane rupture. Intrauterine pressures were not held to be responsible for membrane rupture. Other studies showed that proteases, presumably released from bacteria, reduce the strength and elasticity of membranes (McGregor et al., 1987). Premature rupture occurs also with chorioamnionitis (Naeye, 1982). Fibronectins are also involved in the tensile properties of the membranes: smoking inhibits fibronectin production and is associated with preterm rupture (Shimizu et al., 1992).

When collagen content of amnionic membranes was studied, it was found to decrease significantly during the last 8 weeks of pregnancy; it may be reduced in membranes from prematurely ruptured sacs (Skinner et al., 1981). Al-Zaid and colleagues (1980) found no decrease but, rather, a dissolution of fibers near the site of membrane rupture. It was examined electron microscopically by Ibrahim et al. (1983). From samples obtained at cesarean section from the cervical and opposite sides of membranes, they showed that a disruption of the collagen fibrils occurs near the site of membrane rupture. High in the uterus the amnionic epithelium had a flattened, stretched appearance, and gaps separated the cells.

It is not logical to deduce from a study of the membranes in general what the nature of the membranes at the site of rupture may be. It seems that it is not so much the general membrane strength that is important but, rather, that a local alteration occurs near the site of the membranes overlying the endocervix during the process that leads to their rupture. Studies of active and latent collagenase have shown that during labor the placenta, cervix, and maternal serum contain high levels of the active enzyme (Rajabi et al., 1990). Collagenase is produced by "stromal cells" and is possibly related to onset of labor. The levels in umbilical cord were markedly lower. By incubating membranes in "pseudoamnionic fluid" and studying the biomechanical properties with and without the addition of enzyme inhibitors, Artal et al. (1979) suggested that membrane rupture is perhaps regulated by enzymes.

In an attempt to explain why membrane rupture frequently occurs distal from the internal uterine os, Lavery et al. (1982) constructed a complex rheological model. From it they suggested that local flaws develop under the stress of Braxton-Hicks contractions and with labor. Opitz and Bernoth (1962) examined the site of rupture with polarizing optics; they observed the development of parallel "rupture lines" of collagen. The ability of the amnion to slide over the chorion is probably partly responsible for the variations in membrane rupture. This ability is enhanced, as Schwarzacher (1960) pointed out, by residues of magma reticulare (see above, spongy layer) between amnion and chorion that exist to term. This remnant of extraamnionic fluid presumably is also responsible for the sonographic "tenting" seen of some amnions after failed amniocentesis (Platt et al., 1982). It is possibly also the reason that, with repeated amniocentesis, the amnion often detaches from the chorion and thus allows the collection of amnionic fluid underneath. This mechanism probably led to the retained chorion of the patient reported by Stempel and Nelson (1982).

The studies by Wynn et al. (1967) with pig amnion suggested that "healing" of earlier defects may result from the regenerative processes in the amnion. They may also explain cessation of fluid leakage in such pregnancies. These authors are the only ones who clearly stated an opinion that the amnion is nourished by amnionic fluid.

Cysts, Tumors, Hemorrhage

Localized edema with resultant cyst formation is occasionally seen on the amnionic surface. It is not usually associated with clinical problems (Figure 182). Occasionally, such cysts are amnionic epithelial inclusions. No real tumors have been noted to develop in the amnion. To be sure, rare rests of cartilage, skin, or bone may be found underneath the amnionic epithelium (Figure 183), but they are not generally neoplastic. Some of these structures may represent the remains of aborted ("vanished") twins. This possibility is unlikely because "vanished twins" (discussed in Chapter 25) have usually a different microscopic appearance. An unusual case of an "epidermoid cyst" is seen in Figure 184. Other investigators have described teratomas in the membranes (e.g., Fox & Butler-Manuel, 1964; Joseph & Vogt, 1973; Nickell & Stocker, 1987). These "tumors" have usually had the appearance of acardiac twins, also discussed in greater detail in Chapter 25. Although these authors stated emphatically that no umbilical cord attached them to the membranes, a feature that is usually held to be a sine qua non for acardiac twins, the appearance of the lesions described is that of acardiacs. Smith and Pounder (1982) came to the same conclusion. They described a 3.0 × 2.0 × 1.5 cm mass at the edge of a placenta, covered with skin and broadly attached to the chorion (not decidua, as they stated). It also contained glia, intestine, cartilage, and fat. They referred to other, similar cases, especially that originally described by Küster (1928), and suggested that the lesion was most similar to an amorphous acardiac twin, under which heading this topic is further developed. Despite the lack of organization of such "teratomas," a

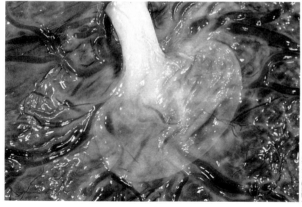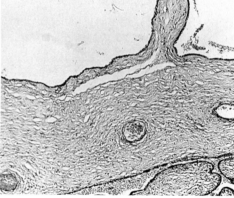

FIGURE 182. Amnionic cyst surrounding the umbilical cord. The cyst (left) contained 5 ml of clear fluid. There was no evidence of a vanished twin. H&E. ×160.

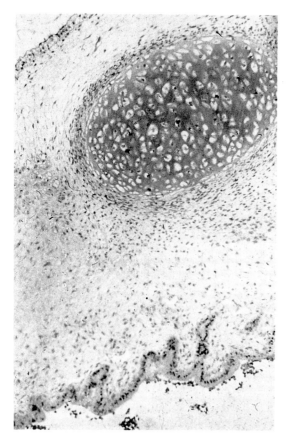

FIGURE 183. Subamnionic mature cartilage in normal placenta. H&E. ×100.

feature that is also found in some bona fide acardiacs, some recognizable structures are depicted in most of the above descriptions. The difficult decision as to whether such a lesion represents a teratoma or an acardiac twin has been pursued since Küster (1928) described a

walnut-sized lesion composed of external skin, bone, cartilage, connective tissue, nerves, fat, glands, and smooth muscle. She leaned toward a teratoma. Unger (1989) has reconsidered this problem, but there is no resolution. To invoke their origin from aberrant germ cells seems unwarranted without further supportive evidence. Other teratomas of the placenta fall into the same category. See further details under acardiacs in Chapter 25.

Hemorrhage into areas underneath the amnion most commonly originates from chorionic vessels. It is seen in many placentas when they are examined by the pathologist because the attendants in the delivery room have collected blood for the determination of fetal pH and blood groups and to undertake other laboratory tests. Rarely is such subamnionic blood of prenatal origin; and the age-old question of whether the placental surface can be damaged by the fetus (? scratching) has remained unresolved. Shanklin and Scott (1975) found subamnionic hemorrhages in 1 of 400 placentas. They preferred to call them hematomas and indicated that inappropriate traction on the umbilical cord by the accoucheur was the common cause of this hemorrhage. There are, however, ultrasonographic observations that suggest the occurrence of subamnionic and, certainly more frequently, subchorionic hematomas, representing intervillous thromboses. It is normal to find small laminated fibrin deposits underneath the chorionic plate at term, presumably accumulating from eddying in the intervillous circulation. These deposits may acquire major proportions, however, and they then represent a pathological feature. Sonographers have been much interested in this topic, as it is demonstrable with their equipment. Nyberg et al. (1990) found that marginal abruptios "tend to dissect beneath the placental membranes" resulting in subchorionic hematomas. This site

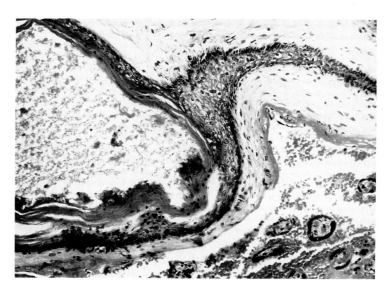

FIGURE 184. Subamnionic squamous epithelium-lined cyst with keratinization in normal placenta. H&E. ×160.

is by far the most common type of abruptio seen by sonography (91% before 20 weeks) and may mimic other placental sonographic masses, such as angiomas. In addition, these authors recognized what they termed "preplacental hematomas"—deposits between placenta and amniotic fluid. They are considered to be subchorial or subamnionic in location; some authors believed that they may originate from ruptured vessels (DeSa, 1971), and large ones possibly correspond to the Breus' mole (Shanklin & Scott, 1975). Anechoic placental "lakes" underneath the chorionic plate are common and probably of no significance, as most disappear with delivery. It was found that 80% of subchorial hematomas recognized before 20 weeks result in normal term delivery, and that their size is the most important prognostic determinant. Thus Abu-Yousef et al. (1987) found that significant, large hematomas are associated with a grave prognosis and that they always extend to the margin. Pearlstone and Baxi (1993) reviewed 14 studies and found that these lesions are common (occurring as often as in 4–48% of pregnancies), that their etiology was still undetermined, and that a risk for premature delivery exists with large thrombi. One such large thrombus was reported in an early publication by Cooperberg et al. (1979). Oláh et al. (1987) delivered a normally grown fetus who later died at 28 weeks with a huge subchorionic "thrombohematoma." It appeared as a placental tumor sonographically. The placenta weighed 700 g (!) and was circumvallate; the hematoma was 15 × 5 cm. Conversely, Pedersen and Mantoni (1990), although also finding subchorionic hematomas with great frequency among threatened abortions that exhibited vaginal bleeding (18%), stated that their presence did not enhance the frequency of abortion. Large preplacental hematomas (Pedersen and Mantoni observed hematomas of 2–150 ml) may produce clinical symptomatology similar to abruptios, and fetal demise can occur when the hematoma is large enough. Some authors believe such hematomas can compress the umbilical cord. The various controversies about the entity were discussed by Spirt et al. (1993). Dickey et al. (1992) also found these hematomas commonly by sonography and related adverse outcomes only to cases with vaginal bleeding. Fleischer et al. (1988) found a correlation with elevated α-fetoprotein levels, as did Bernstein et al. (1992). Because of the presence of antinuclear antibodies in three of five patients with subchorionic hematomas, Baxi and Pearlstone (1991) recommended that these patients be screened for such antibodies, irrespective of their obstetrical history. We have seen a number of such hematomas among midtrimester losses. They differ from Breus' moles in that they are not focal and the chorionic plate is uniformly elevated rather than, as in Breus' moles, in pockets.

When fetuses survive, they often become growth-retarded.

True amnionic cysts are rarely present on the placental surface. The commonest cysts found here are located underneath the chorion; they take their origin from X cell deposits in which central liquefaction has occurred. Bleeding into such cysts may occur, and the cysts may also be large and multiple. The associated fetus or newborn may be normal or small for gestational age; growth retardation occurs occasionally because X cells are especially prevalent in placentas with severe, extensive ischemic degeneration. These features are discussed further in Chapter 11.

Amniotic Fluid Embolism

Vernix caseosa often dissects underneath the amnion. Indeed, such rupture of only the amnionic sac leads to "double sacs," and it is seen also in patients with "high leaks." Patients who have had clinical fluid discharge and in whom later intact membranes are observed have similar membrane ruptures. Reisfield (1958) considered it to result from a congenital defect, but this conclusion is probably not valid. This rupture may occur before delivery, presumably when the amnion breaks before the chorion does. Amnionic fluid with cellular debris (squames, fat, hair) can then be pushed underneath the amnion (Figure 185), at times in impressive amounts. The material may appear as white flakes that can be moved back and forth under the amnion. In general, this finding has no significance whatsoever; earlier students of the matter, however (Leary & Hertig, 1950), considered that such subamnionic vernix may gain access to the maternal vascular space and thus initiate the clinical spectrum of amnionic fluid embolism. Indeed, some of their pictures showed squamous cells in the intervillous space and within the "decidual sinusoids." Whether they got there by dissection from the subamnionic space is a matter of conjecture. This separation between amnion and chorion can also occur spontaneously before birth, and amnionic fluid may then enter this space, a feature that is sometimes recognized sonographically (Borlum, 1989). Borlum emphasized that such "chorioamniotic separation" is not a contraindication to amniocentesis.

Amnionic fluid embolism has been recognized as an important cause of maternal death; it occurs most commonly after tumultuous labor and occasionally during cesarean section. Steiner and Lushbaugh (1941) first reported the entity. Clinical features include severe dyspnea, shock, and afibrinogenemia. Amnionic fluid embolism may lead to death. At autopsy one finds fragments of vernix caseosa, fat, squames, and fetal hair, as

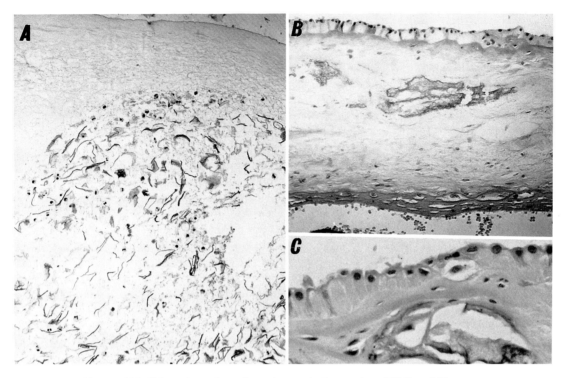

FIGURE 185. Dissection of vernix underneath the amnion. H&E. ×160.

well as thrombotic material in the pulmonary capillaries (Figure 186). The problem is well illustrated in an authoritative study by Landing (1950b). Although the diagnosis of amniotic fluid embolism is often suspected, it is only occasionally diagnosed with accuracy during life (Resnik et al., 1976; Haddad, 1985). The pathological interpretation of vernix in pulmonary capillaries is frequently difficult, particularly when it is attempted from blood smears of living patients. It must be realized that the embolization is probably a relatively brief event, wherein circulating vernix is quickly filtered out in the periphery and lung. Contamination of specimens by dandruff simulates the microscopic appearance closely. Squames are also often contained in staining solutions and so simulate the true vernix that one must make a positive interpretation with great circumspection. Finding vernix in blood smears is absolutely diagnostic. It seems unlikely that vernix enters maternal vessels by dissection of the amnion. It probably enters large veins that are opened during cesarean section or tumultuous labor, and in patients with placenta previa accreta. Similarly opened uterine vessels have been considered

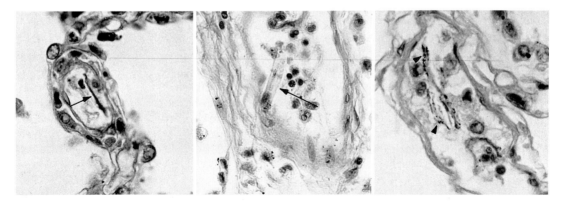

FIGURE 186. Pulmonary blood vessels containing various elements of vernix in a fatal amniotic fluid embolism. On the left is a squame, in the middle a hair, and on the right squames with meconium pigment. H&E. ×240.

by Landing (1950b) to be sites of entry. Bendon and Ray (1986) reported five cases of prolonged amnionic fluid leakage; they believed that the squames they found in and underneath the chorion represented vernix. In one it had elicited a foreign-body giant cell reaction. Although it was certainly not the cause of the chorioamnionitis in that case, their Figure 2 clearly showed that the squames had access to the maternal intervillous space.

Amnionic fluid embolism is fatal in more than 80% of cases. The clinical diagnosis is thus of considerable importance (Tuller, 1957; Philippe et al., 1961; Guidotti et al., 1981). Cases have been reported after repeated amniocentesis (Paterson et al., 1977) and even in undelivered patients with cord entanglement that led to abruption of the placental margin (Corridan et al., 1980). Amnionic fluid embolism causes not only pulmonary hypertension when the lung capillaries are plugged but also shock, hypotension, and uncontrolled bleeding. The "consumption coagulopathy" that follows the disseminated intravascular coagulation has been thought to result from the thromboplastin-containing liquor. Many coagulation studies on amnionic fluid have been reported (Beller et al., 1963), and the principal coagulative protein in amnionic fluid appears to be tissue factor (Lockwood et al., 1991). It must be cautioned, however, that the accurate diagnosis of embolism is difficult during life; afibrinogenemia more often results from abruption, the dead fetus syndrome, and other complications of pregnancy than from embolism with liquor. Moreover, it must be appreciated that several studies have supported earlier notions of the possible involvement of arachidic acid and leukotrienes during the catastrophic process that follows amniotic fluid embolism (Clark, 1985, 1988; Azegami & Mori, 1986). Although a central focus of past considerations has been the presumed pulmonary hypertension in this condition, Clark et al. (1988) have shown convincingly that left-sided heart failure is the principal cause of death in this devastating disorder.

Even greater care must be exercised in the diagnosis of amniotic fluid embolism during early pregnancy. The overwhelming evidence suggests that the fluid before 20 weeks is unable to cause coagulation. Vernix is not found in any quantity before the third trimester, certainly not at times of genetic amniocentesis. Clark et al. (1986) made the point that blood obtained from pulmonary arteries of pregnant and nonpregnant patients often contain squamous cells. They assumed that this cellular material originates from venous puncture, rather than from amniotic fluid. Although this statement may be true, it is our opinion that these cells usually derive from contamination with debris contained in fixing or staining solutions and, most commonly, from dandruff of technicians.

Meconium

Meconium is the bile-stained intestinal content of the fetus. It is often admixed with mucus. Meconium is present in the small bowel of fetuses long before midgestation but is usually not eliminated until after birth. When meconium is discharged before parturition, the baby and placenta may be meconium-stained and deeply green. It is a common event. With consecutive placental examinations, we have found in San Diego that macroscopic meconium staining occurred in 17.81% of 12,951 placentas, and Nathan et al. (1994) found it in 19%. In addition, in our material there were 130 hemosiderin-stained placentas (1%), a total of 5% of the stained placentas overall. Fujikura and Klionsky (1975) reviewed the 42,000 placenta examinations of liveborn infants enrolled in the oft-cited large, prospective Collaborative Perinatal Study that was conducted during the 1960s. These authors identified staining in 10.3%; and 18.1% of neonatal deaths had meconium-stained placentas. However, their case material contained many instances of erythroblastosis, a condition now rarely encountered. Therefore many of the placentas may well have been stained with hemolyzed blood pigments rather than with meconium. Most recently, Kallakury et al. (1993) found that 19 of 23 discolored placentas (of 100 consecutive organs examined) contained meconium and even more contained iron pigment. They concluded that no relation to fetal well-being could be identified.

The reason for the discharge of meconium is complex. When it occurs it usually takes place during the last month of pregnancy and with an even greater frequency in postterm pregnancies. It may be of some importance to differentiate various types of meconium staining of the fetal surface of the placenta. Such differentiation is represented in a simplified fashion as follows:

Gross features	Clinical outcome
Acute meconium staining: blue-green, glistening placenta, covered with green, slimy meconium	Typically normal.
Subacute meconium staining: slippery, edematous, membranes with dark discoloration	High risk of association with asphyxia and cerebral palsy; meconium aspiration syndrome.
Chronic meconium staining: dull and diffuse, muddy, cord sometimes stained throughout	Some of the infants with brown-green discoloration later manifest placental and membranes damage, assumed to be secondary to prenatal hypoxia.

In a study conducted by Usher et al. (1988) of 5,915 pregnancies 1 week before term, 1,408 pregnancies prolonged 1 to 2 weeks past term, and 340 pregnancies longer than 42 weeks (15.3%, 27.0%, and 31.5%, respectively) had meconium staining. Although meconium discharge was positively correlated with fetal distress, meconium staining occurred without fetal distress in 10.9%, 18.8%, and 16.2% in the respective groups. Similarly, Rogers et al. (1990) found no good correlation between meconium discharge and neonatal blood pH determinations. Trimmer and Gilstrap (1991) unsuccessfully attempted to correlate the thickness (the "meconiumcrit" of Weitzner et al., 1990) of meconium-stained fluid with outcome. Despite these findings, meconium has assumed great importance in medicolegal pursuits (see Chapter 27 and below).

Meconium is moved in the intestinal lumen by contractions of the intestine's muscular wall. This movement is regulated by a variety of hormones, one of which is motilin, a 22-amino-acid polypeptide. Motilin is released during the fasting period and induces movement of the "activity front" of the small intestine. In a variety of experimental animals and in human volunteers, the infusion of this polypeptide caused intestinal motor activity that can be interrupted by high doses of gastrin and insulin (Vantrappen et al., 1979). When motilin was measured in the umbilical cord blood of neonates, it was found that those with fetal distress had levels elevated above the normal 32 to 127 pmol/L (Lucas et al., 1979b). Lucas et al. (1979a) suggested that meconium discharge was the result of elevated motilin levels, which in turn were induced by fetal distress. In subsequent studies by Lucas et al. (1979a), it was found that six of eight gastrointestinal hormones were also elevated in cases complicated by fetal distress. This finding suggested to these investigators that these hormones may be powerful mediators in the many complications that follow fetal distress.

Immature fetuses had significantly lower levels of motilin than did mature infants. Our own studies of motilin levels in mature infants with and without meconium discharge are somewhat different (Mahmoud et al., 1988). In part, the different findings may be the result of our using different antibodies. We found that motilin levels of infants who had passed meconium were 177 fmol/ml of cord blood, whereas those who did not pass meconium had only 111 fmol/ml. No relation to fetal distress was found in this study. Because of the underdeveloped production of motilin in immature fetuses, it may be easily understood that meconium discharge is rare in premature infants, whereas it is common in postmature infants. Whether fetal distress is a primary signal for an increase in motilin and for meconium discharge is still uncertain. It is certainly true that many term stillbirths never have discharged meconium despite prolonged periods of distress that eventually lead to their demise.

Putative meconium presence in greenish amniotic fluid of very premature infants often results from hematoidin and other blood-derived pigments that have the same spectral absorbance. It must be said that it may be difficult to properly define meconium staining of amnionic fluid. For instance, Falciglia et al. (1993) described a 610 g infant with intrauterine meconium aspiration syndrome and pigmented material in the lung at autopsy. It is not clear to us that this green-stained fluid and the yellow pigment of the lung truly represented discharged meconium, as other pigments have similar spectral characteristics. In fact, we have never seen meconium discharge at that young gestational age. We may need to have a better definition for the material in the amnionic fluid and lungs. For each of the cases of midtrimester amniocenteses with meconium-stained liquor, Karp and Schiller (1977) suggested that a reason for fetal distress could be envisaged. Three times it had been due to significant prenatal bleeding, once there was marked hypertensive disease in the mother, and twice unsuccessful amniocenteses had preceded it. These investigators did spectrophotometric studies and found absorbance peaks at 405 μm, which is usually considered to be diagnostic of meconium but can be mimicked by other bile pigments. Their fetuses did well.

Golbus and Stephens (1979) performed similar spectrophotometric studies on fluid obtained from genetic amniocentesis. Discolored fluid had a large 405 to 415 nm peak, shared with meconium and oxyhemoglobin, as well as peaks at 540 and 575 nm. The latter peaks were due to blood pigments, believed to derive from disintegrating old blood. Allen (1985) found a 1.67% incidence of "meconium"-stained fluid among 4,709 midtrimester amniocenteses, with a 5.06% fetal mortality. He excluded fetuses with brownish amnionic fluid from the analysis. In the discussion that followed his paper, various data were summarized and the difficulty of using spectrophotometry as a sole determinant of meconium was considered. In studies of brown and green fluids from amniocenteses, Hankins et al. (1984) found that brown and green fluids had similar absorption spectra; the authors concluded that the staining at midgestation is more likely secondary to hemolysis than to meconium discharge. We concur with that assessment. Legge (1981) detected the presence of hemoglobin in brownish fluids by chemical means. Alger et al. (1984) made a determined effort to differentiate among the pigments of second trimester "meconium-like" substances. They studied 123 fluids, irrespective of their gross discoloration. They found that 91% of the clear fluids had an absorption peak at 405 μm, representing a pigment generally absent at term. Its presence was not correlated with fetal outcome, but it had a higher frequency in the presence of circumvallate placentas and in those with abruptio placentae. The substance was identified as methemoglobin. The authors emphatically denied the ability of a fetus to discharge meconium before 20 weeks. They reviewed what is known of early fetal intestinal motility and anal innervation. Abramovich and Gray (1982), on the other hand, went so far as to suggest that the fetus routinely defecates until 16 weeks but ceases to do so by 18 to 20 weeks. Boué et al. (1988) found the appearance of intestinal "microvillar enzymes" in amnionic fluid as early as at 12 to 13 weeks' gestation and suggested that it appeared as the anal membrane ruptured. When fetal anal sphincter control is established (18 weeks), however, the enzyme disappears quickly. Whether this evidence should be considered "defecation" is moot. Ostrea and Naqvi (1982) found that the passage of meconium was strongly dependent on gestational age. Eighty percent of their premature infants with meconium staining were older than 34 weeks' gestation, even when they had presented as breeches. Their overall incidence was only 6.5%. Recall that although the tensile strength of meconium-stained membranes is reduced the frequency of premature rupture of membranes is not increased with meconium staining (Lavery et al., 1980). Franqoual et al. (1986) identified coproporphyrin and hemoglobin chemically in stained fluids. Zorn et al. (1986) also studied midtrimester staining to rule out the presence of true meconium. Bilirubin staining of amniotic fluid has been associated with intestinal obstruction and hydramnios (Grimes & Cassady, 1970); these authors suggested that the pigment may derive from disturbed placental exchange. Could it not equally well derive from prenatal vomiting of bile-stained gastrointestinal content? This situation certainly occurred in one of our cases with jejunal obstruction, which was complicated by hydramnios. Griffiths and Burge (1988) found three similar cases with intestinal obstruction and bile vomiting in utero.

The conclusion that can be reached from all of these investigations is that meconium discharge of immature pregnancies is rare and that it is unreliably assessed by current technology. The reason, of course, is that hemoglobin is the common precursor of all these pigments. It may be more useful to determine if there is hemosiderin as iron-containing crystals in histological preparations of the discolored placental surface. This test would be a more reliable indicator of decomposed blood. The formation of pigments in vivo has been a long-standing investigative challenge for pathologists. In particular, it has been questioned whether extracellular formation of hemosiderin and hematoidin is possible. This topic was fully reviewed by Muir and Niven (1935), who experimented with the injection of red blood cells and hemolyzed blood into rodents and rabbits. Generally speaking, hemosiderin was formed within cells only after about 24 hours; hematoidin, in crystal form, followed in about 7 days. Muir and Niven (1935) did not find it in extracellular sites. They assumed that it derives intracellularly from hemosiderin after removal of the iron. This moiety is the same as the bilirubin of meconium. We believe that hematoidin and bilirubin cannot be reliably distinguished from each other at present by either light microscopy or spectrophotometry.

For some reason, meconium has become the "red flag" for obstetricians and for the law profession as well (Sepkowitz, 1987). Meconium, as it is often portrayed, is the result of preceding fetal distress and hypoxia (Mitchell et al., 1985; Zorn et al., 1986). Numerous studies, on the other hand, indicate that correlations between meconium discharge and fetal pH or with tocograms are poor (Steer et al., 1989). The finding of meconium during labor is in fact a complex topic. The amount of gastrointestinal hormone accumulating in the fetus may reach an optimal quantity at the normal 40 weeks' gestation; and when gestation goes beyond that time, meconium discharge becomes increasingly likely. Meconium is thus perhaps correlated with postmaturity (or "postdatism") more closely than with distress (Ostrea & Naqvi, 1982). It is not to say that postmature babies infrequently suffer some distress. Their discharge of meconium, however, may merely reflect the maturation of the system (see also Usher et al., 1988). As mentioned earlier, many term stillbirths never have discharged meconium, despite prolonged periods of distress that eventually lead to their demise. Yeomans and colleagues (1989) correlated meconium in amnionic fluid with fetal acid-base status. They concluded that "meconium-stained amniotic fluid correlates poorly with infant condition at birth as reflected by umbilical cord acid-base measurements." Their report also provided a valuable review of the views, pro and con, that meconium relates to fetal hypoxia.

Meconium has deleterious sequelae when it is aspirated by the fetus (Byrne & Gau, 1987) and on the amnion and umbilical cord as well. At times the meconium is quickly expectorated when aspirated, and it then has no untoward consequence, whereas at other times it leads to fatal pulmonary complications despite proper airway management (Davis et al., 1985). Dooley et al. (1985) studied outcome in infants who had meconium present below the vocal cords and related its discharge to intrapartum events; they found that no change in therapeutic maneuvers would have saved the infants (see, however, Falciglia, 1988). The quality of meconium differs from case to case. In some infants mucinous material may be present that the newborn's respiratory tract finds more difficult to eliminate. Likewise, it must be appreciated that not all babies born

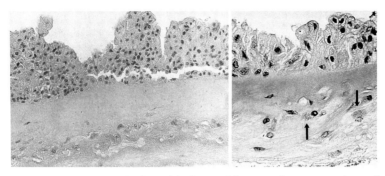

FIGURE 187. Heaping and degeneration of amnionic epithelium with meconium macrophage (arrows) after 20 hours of exposure (right) to meconium. H&E. Left ×160; right ×400.

from a meconium-containing amnionic environment suffer meconium aspiration. They may have ceased to breathe in utero as a result of chronic distress (Kaplan, 1983). Thus the problem is complicated and must be evaluated on individual merits. One must also consider the possibility that aspirated meconium causes degenerative changes in the alveolar epithelium similar to those seen in the amnion. Thus the meconium aspiration syndrome may represent a form of chemical pneumonitis with acute respiratory distress syndrome. Others (Katz & Bowes, 1992) have suggested that the deleterious pulmonary effect of meconium aspiration may be initiated by asphyxia. Many experimental studies have been conducted with meconium inhalation before and after birth; some have yielded conflicting results. Goodlin (1968), for instance, found that there was little difference of saline and meconium in his rabbit experiments. Wiswell et al. (1992) observed the changes in piglets, and Goetzman (1992) summarized all aspects of the meconium aspiration syndrome. Yoder (1994) reviewed treatment regimens and reemphasized that not all meconium is equal.

Meconium is noxious in other ways (Rubovits et al., 1938). When meconium has been present in the amnionic cavity for many hours, the amnionic epithelium begins to show degenerative changes. There is vacuolation, heaping up, loss of cells, and eventually necrosis (Figure 187). Moreover, muscle cells of the umbilical vessels of the umbilical cord and their ramifications on the placental surface may degenerate when the meconium presence has been long-standing (Figure 188). This change was first described by Altshuler and Hyde (1989), who also provided evidence that damage to the fetal vascular tissue may exacerbate fetal cerebral hypoperfusion and thereby augment possibly existing fetal hypoxia. When they experimentally exposed segments of umbilical veins obtained from cesarean sections and exposed them to meconium solutions, the muscular wall contracted markedly and rapidly. In addition, necrosis of vascular walls was believed to be a consequence of meconium exposure. Exactly how long this exposure must have existed before visual vascular alterations occur is not known, but we estimate that it is many hours. In subsequent studies, Altshuler et al.

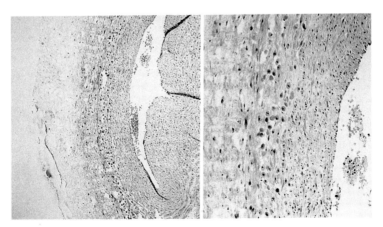

FIGURE 188. Degenerating muscle of umbilical cord blood vessel after chronic meconium exposure. H&E. Left ×64; right ×160. (Courtesy Dr. G. Altshuler.)

(1992) examined 1,100 meconium-stained placentas among which they found 10 with vascular necrosis; two placentas had ulcerated cords. This topic is further discussed in Chapter 13.

It is incorrect to assert, however, that meconium *causes* chorioamnionitis (Dominguez et al., 1960; see also Lauweryns et al., 1973). To be sure, when degenerative changes in the surface do occur, they are sometimes followed by inflammation, but the "amnionic sac infection syndrome" is not caused by meconium. In the retrospective study undertaken by Burgess and Hutchins (1994), the authors believed not only that meconium induces typical arterial necrosis of the cord but that inflammation of membranes and fetal lung may result. Their inflammation of the membranes was less severe than that usually seen in chorioamnionitis. We often see deeply meconium-stained placentas, obviously having been exposed to meconium for many hours, that do not have inflammation. A study by Novak and Kokomoor (1988) found meconium in about 13% of 1,024 consecutive placentas, 30 of which came from premature infants. The latter had 53% "chronic staining" in contrast to 17% in the term placentas. Also, 60% of the premature placentas, had inflammation with the staining, whereas it was seen in only 26% of the mature placentas. Villous edema was also more common in the premature placentas, and the authors concluded that meconium-stained placentas come from populations with different characteristics. It is likely that the more immature babies had chorioamnionitis independent of the meconium discharge, as inflammation is much commoner in premature infants anyway.

The pigment of meconium can be seen in cells of the membranes. It is not only the pigment that is found, phagolysosomes are full of debris when examined ultrastructurally (Figure 189). For routine purposes, it suffices to make light microscopic observations. When hemosiderin is to be ruled out, a Prussian blue stain quickly differentiates between these two pigments. Meconium-laden macrophages are large, ovoid or round cells in amnion and later in the chorion that have a yellow-brown-green content. They are often vacuolated (Figure 190). It is our opinion that these macrophages usually "lie in waiting" in amnion and chorion, and that they are normally inactive and unoccupied. When meconium or other substances come by, they spring into functional activity. Bourne (1962) offered some photographs suggesting that meconium may stream through passageways of the epithelium, but it is more likely that these areas represent already damaged epithelium. In detailed studies of the ultrastructure of placenta and membranes, Lister (1968) concluded that the meconium appears as electron-dense granules that are associated with debris and frequent cellular degeneration. There are, however, also rare circumstances where the membranes definitely do not have green meconium staining and histologically have pigmented macrophages that do not stain with iron stains. This finding was prominent in a placenta of a case of characteristic α-thalassemia that we saw. Hemolysis was not clinically

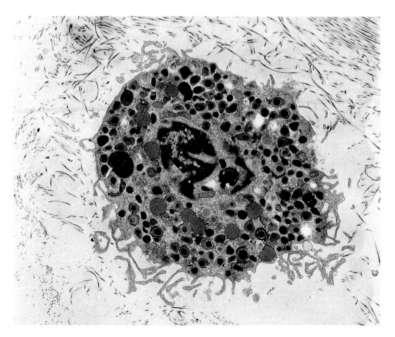

FIGURE 189. Meconium macrophage filled with lipid and lysosomes in a patient also having gastroschisis. Some lysosomes contain membranous debris and other heterogeneous material. Transmission electron micrograph. ×15,200. (Courtesy Dr. M. Grafe.)

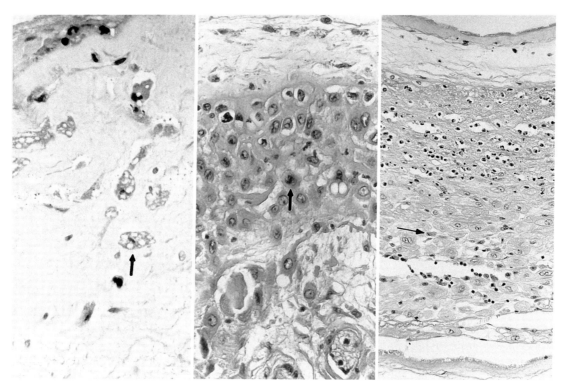

FIGURE 190. Different types of meconium macrophage in membranes after prolonged exposure. Note that the amnion is degenerated in all, and only the right membranes show minimal inflammation. (Left) Vacuolated cells with pigment. (Middle) Finely pigmented cells penetrating into trophoblast layer. (Right) Degenerating decidua with macrophages at arrows. H&E. Left, middle ×400; right ×200.

observed, and the nature of the pigment was not determined. One can always speculate of course that meconium had been discharged days earlier, but there was no such evidence. Furthermore, in a child with anal atresia and a rectourinary fistula we saw meconium staining because of meconuria. In other cases, bile vomiting may be the cause of such pigmented macrophages.

When meconium is discharged a short time before birth, it may be wiped or washed off the surface without leaving a stain. Later, it stains the amnion, and thereafter the chorion stains permanently. When studies were done to estimate the time interval for the staining to become permanent, it was determined histologically that meconium-stained macrophages could be found in the amnion within 1 hour of exposure, and staining of the chorion occurred after 3 hours (Miller et al., 1985). When it has been present for longer times, it cannot be dated reliably. From their review of the literature, Fujikura and Klionsky (1975) estimated that 4 to 6 hours transpires before meconium reaches the chorion. These figures are estimates only, because it is difficult to undertake such observations prospectively in vivo. Similar time tables have been established for the staining of fingernails and vernix. Desmond et al. (1956) found that it took 4 to 6 hours of bathing the toes of

neonates in meconium-containing fluid before the nails were stained and 12 to 14 hours for the vernix to be stained. The further progression of meconium staining of the membranes is as follows: Bile pigment stains the center of the umbilical cord, usually without being taken up in many macrophages, and the amnionic epithelium degenerates. The meconium is then transferred to macrophages that reside within the decidua. With long-standing meconium exposure and when the rare uterus with attached placenta becomes available for study, one may even observe meconium-stained macrophages within the myometrium. It is possible that some meconium is ultimately completely removed by this exchange, by swallowing, and by in utero inhalation of the material. It is also conceivable that in some instances fetuses discharge meconium repeatedly. This fact further complicates our ability to assign firm time sequences of placental meconium staining. The frequent meconium discharge in postterm fetuses and its effect on the fetus is complicated by the increasing incidence of oligohydramnios after term. The volume of amnionic fluid decreases significantly near term and thereafter (Clement et al., 1987). Suggestions that indomethacin induces both meconium discharge and oligohydramnios (Itskovitz et al., 1980) have not yet been confirmed. Prophylactic amnioinfusion with saline in thick meconium

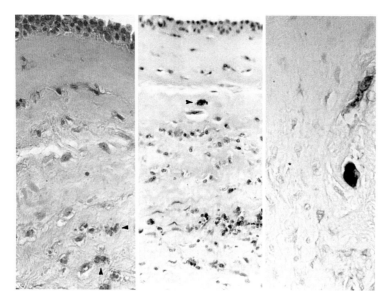

FIGURE 191. Hemosiderin macrophages (arrow-heads) in circumvallate placentas of the second trimester. Left: H&E. ×160. Middle: and H&E. ×100. Right: Prussian blue. ×400.

discharge has sometimes been beneficial in the ultimate outcome (Macri et al., 1992; Uhing et al., 1993). Many of the outstanding questions regarding meconium have been addressed in a searching contemporary contribution by Benirschke (1994).

It is essential that hemosiderin be differentiated from meconium. It derives from hemolyzed red blood cells and is commonly found in association with circumvallate placentas, in the placentas of erythroblastotic infants, with abruptio placentae, and with thromboses and other circumstances wherein bleeding has occurred. Although such placentas often have a brownish tint, they may be green and simulate meconium macroscopically. Clayton et al. (1969) spectrophotometrically studied the fluid pigments of hydropic fetuses and those with hemolyzed blood. They emphasized the difficulties of differentiating these moieties. Hemosiderin is comprised of granular particles, and it has a characteristic sheen (refringence) when the focus of the light microscope, or its substage, is changed (Figure 191). Hemosiderin is strongly positive with iron stains, but as mentioned earlier in the chapter hematoidin cannot be reliably distinguished from the bilirubin of meconium.

GASTROSCHISIS

The amnionic epithelial cells seen with gastroschisis have a characteristic fine, uniform, extensive vacuolation (Ariel & Landing, 1985) (Figure 192). Although this association was startling when first found, it is now known to be regularly present, is virtually diagnostic of gastroschisis, and is not found in fetuses with omphalocele. The fine vacuoles of amnion seen with gastroschisis contain lipid when examined electron microscopically (Grafe & Benirschke, 1990), but the origin of the lipid is still obscure. It is possible that it comes from the opened abdominal cavity of the fetus, but that possibility must be ascertained by future studies. The assumption is somewhat contradicted by the finding that the fibrin/

fibrous coating of intestines in this condition apparently contains no lipid (Tibboel et al., 1986). As was summarized earlier in the chapter, lipid has been found in small quantities by histochemical staining of the amnionic epithelium during early pregnancy and particularly in specimens from term pregnancies. Moreover, the quantity of cellular lipid content in amnionic fluid cells was formerly used reasonably successfully to estimate the length of gestation (van Bogaert et al., 1978). Schmidt (1963) studied lipid removal from the amnionic sac in the chick embryo and concluded that lipid injected into the extraembryonic coelom of the chick is absorbed by amnionic epithelium. Later, lipid in amnionic cells again becomes a component of the amnionic fluid, from where it reaches the fetal intestine. Schmidt considered similar pathways for the human embryo. Pritchard et al. (1968) found the composition of the lipid in amnionic cells to be similar to that of the

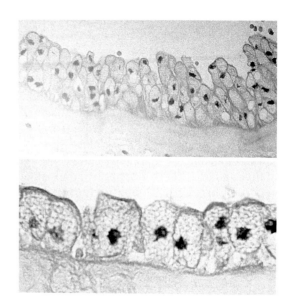

FIGURE 192. Characteristically vacuolated amnionic epithelium in two cases of gastroschisis. H&E. Top ×400; bottom ×640.

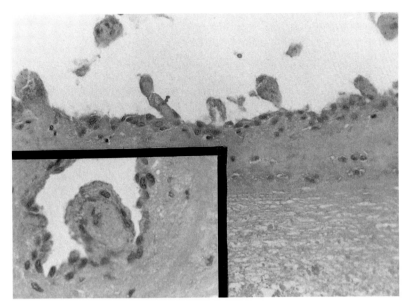

FIGURE 193. Amnion in a case of congenital epidermolysis bullosa and duodenal atresia. The child was delivered at 26 weeks' gestation and had numerous bullae. The amnion has polypoid expansions that were produced by apparent "hernia- tion" of connective tissue through superficial defects. These protrusions were covered by degenerating amnionic epi- thelium. H&E. ×256; inset ×400.

amnionic fluid and to vernix; they suggested that most of the lipid in vernix is produced by amnionic epithelium. We believe that the reverse occurs, and that vernix is derived from fetal sebum, which becomes incorporated into amnionic epithelium.

EPIDERMOLYSIS BULLOSA

Epidermolysis bullosa, a rare condition, has been associated with amnionic lesions. Faulk et al. (1988) reported that a term newborn with this disease had an amnionic surface with multiple polypoid protrusions covered by epithelial cells. We saw a 26-week pre- mature infant with this disease and duodenal atresia. Its amnion also had lesions similar to those described by Faulk et al. (1988). There were apparent protrusions of the connective tissue through epithelial defects. Thus polyp-like excrescences were produced that were partially covered by amnionic epithelium (Figure 193). There was no inflammation but many pigmented macrophages existed in the connective tissue of the membranes. Thus it appears that the amnion shares the immunological features of this disease with the skin.

Amnion Nodosum

Amnion nodosum, a relatively common condition, was first so named by Landing (1950a) when he observed small granules on the placental surfaces from preg- nancies complicated by severe oligohydramnios. The lesion had been known since Pilgram (1889) and was described in the German literature as *Amnionknötchen*, so termed by v. Franqué (1897). Blanc (1961) assigned the name vernix granulomas to it and expanded on the pathology of associated fetal lesions in a later contri- bution (Blanc et al., 1962). The term vernix granuloma, although denoting its relation to vernix, was not adopted because the lesions are clearly not granulomas.

Amnion nodosum is most commonly found in the placentas of fetuses with renal agenesis or following premature and prolonged amniorrhea, in the placenta of the donor twin of the twin transfusion syndrome (the "stuck twin"), in diamnionic acardiac twins, character- istically in sirenomelia, and with some other distur- bances that lead to prolonged oligohydramnios. It is clearly the result of deficient amnionic fluid over a prolonged period. The nodules are most pronounced on the placental surface, but they may rarely extend onto the membranes as well. They are only rarely found on the umbilical cord surface. Most cases of amnion nodosum show fine granules that are best seen in oblique light (Figure 194). They are different from the granules of squamous metaplasia, which is typically more plaque-like, patchy, and hydrophobic. Amnion nodosum is frequently brown-yellow and not shiny. The nodules are composed of squames and hair intermixed with sebum. They are from vernix that has been "rubbed" into defects of the amnionic surface. Probably the first event is that the amnionic epithelium becomes defective because of absent fluid, which then allows vernix to attach to the defect (Figures 195, 196). There is no inflammatory or other tissue reaction of the amnion to the presence of the vernix. At times the edges of the granules become covered with regenerating

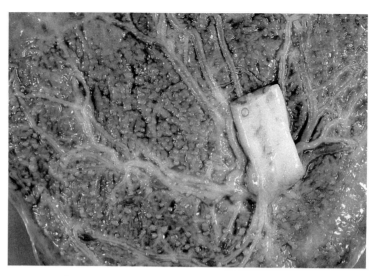

FIGURE 194. Macroscopic appearance of amnion nodosum in a child with renal agenesis. Note the uniform presence of fine granules, mostly sparing the vessel surfaces and not present on the cord.

amnionic epithelial cells. The finding that the cord surface is so rarely involved and that the free membranes are also usually less markedly affected is probably due to the fact that their epithelium is better nourished by underlying umbilical and chorionic blood flow.

Electron microscopic studies have shown that most of the nodules are composed of acellular debris, degenerating cellular walls, hair fragments, and squamous cells. Bartman and Driscoll (1968) discussed the possibility, originally suggested by Bourne (1960), that the nodules originate from the amnionic epithelium; but Salazar et al. (1974) clearly demonstrated their origin from vernix. The latter authors described many cell types present within the nodules; they also contain remnants of cells, old cell walls, and fibrillar material. The centers of amnion nodosum are positive with PAS and alcian blue stains. Salazar et al. (1974) laid to rest the notion of the cellular origin from squamous hyperplasia and metaplasia. Surprisingly, they saw some nodules covered by thin, symplastic amnionic epithelium that they considered as possibly having regenerated.

Amnion nodosum develops during late fetal life. There is not enough vernix during early pregnancy to produce this lesion. Although oligohydramnios has been verified as early as at 16 weeks in the case of urethral obstruction reported by Wagner and Tygstrup (1963), the amnion was still normal. Alternatively, as shown in Figure 195, with such gestations the amnion shows only minute foci of cellular degeneration. When renal anomalies exist in only one of monoamnionic twins, as in the sirenomelia described by Kohler (1972) and substantiated by many subsequent cases, there is no

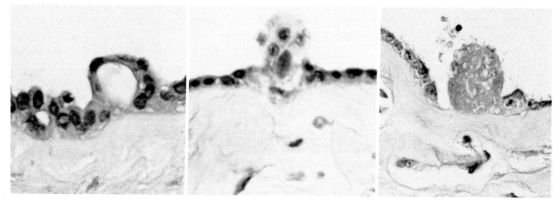

FIGURE 195. Early stages in the development of amnion nodosum. Focal ballooning, necrosis, and apposition of debris are present in therapeutic abortions performed because of recognized oligohydramnios due to renal agenesis or renal cystic disease. H&E. ×400.

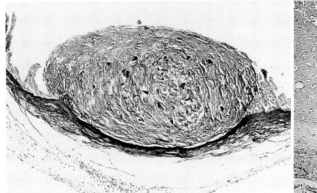 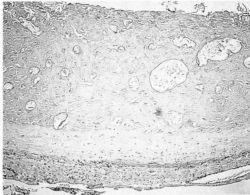

FIGURE 196. Late stages of amnion nodosum. (Left) One nodule. (Right) A larger plaque. Both contain squames, fat, and hair. Left: PTAH. ×1,160. Right: H&E. ×200.

amnion nodosum. Not only does amnion nodosum not develop in such monoamnionic twins, but the pulmonary hypoplasia that is so characteristic of newborns associated with severe oligohydramnios is also prevented. Brown et al. (1978) described two cases of oligohydramnios secondary to amniorrhea, similar to that originally delineated by Bain et al. (1964). In Brown's two cases, amnion nodosum was present in only one, a fetus of 1,000 g; the other, weighing 600 g at 27 weeks, lacked amnion nodosum. The explanation for such apparent discrepancies is that at that early age little vernix exists to allow amnion nodules to develop. It need not be hypothesized, as did Bain and colleagues, that the vernix had drained out with the amniorrhea, or that "trauma" or close contact with the fetal surface is necessary to produce the nodules, as has often been suggested. The nodules are much too finely distributed to have derived from the trauma of scratching or from close fetal contact with the amnion. We believe that it forms by apposition of vernix debris to foci of dying amnion epithelium—areas of epithelium that are no longer supported by the nutrition and oxygen normally contained in amnionic fluid.

There are numerous other reports of amnion nodosum, itemized in the contributions of Thompson (1960), Masson et al. (1966), Fitch and Lachance (1972), and Wentworth and Turnbull (1969). A comprehensive study of 100 cases of oligohydramnios may be found in the poorly accessible thesis of Déglon (1978). These studies also considered the pathogenesis of pulmonary hypoplasia and the fetal deformities associated with oligohydramnios. The dispute here is whether pulmonary hypoplasia follows the inability of the lung to inhale normal amounts of liquor, or it is a phenomenon due to compression in a too tight uterus. Breathing motions alone do not determine the future of lung development; it is the availability of amnionic fluid that is a prerequisite for useful breathing expansion of the

lung (Wigglesworth & Desai, 1982; Kilbride et al., 1988). This claim is supported by experimental studies of fluid withdrawal from the amnion of rats (Symchych & Winchester, 1978). Lung fluid production may be another important facet, as derives from rare and complex anomalies.

The poor prognosis of fetuses associated with oligohydramnios and identified sonographically during the second trimester has been the topic of articles by Barss et al. (1984) and Mercer and Brown (1986). Wong and colleagues (1985) criticized this mode of detection if it is not followed up by confirmation through amnioscopy or amniocentesis. An additional consideration regarding pulmonary development is the secretion of fluid by the respiratory tract. When laryngeal atresia exists, the fetal lung may overexpand owing to this secretion, with hydramnios ensuing from obstruction to venous return (Silver et al., 1988).

Amnionic Bands

The existence of amnionic bands as a cause of amputations and other fetal debilities can hardly be disputed, although such doubts are expressed in the literature with regularity. These doubts began with Streeter (1930), who believed the defects to be of "germ plasm" origin. Others have shared this doubt in the primacy of amnion disruption (Patterson, 1962; Woolnough, 1987; Lockwood et al., 1989). Doubt has been expressed particularly with cases involving major congenital anomalies, such as exencephaly, ectopia cordis, and spinal disruptions (Chaurasia, 1978). These cases are frequently associated with broad amnionic adhesions. Several reviews of these cases have suggested that we may deal with two or three distinct entities: (1) amnionic bands (with constriction possible of fingers, extremities, umbilical cord but generally normal fetus); (2) amnionic sheets (usually attached broadly to the skull and often the facies); (3) the limb–body wall complex (with amnionic sheets and gross disruptions). The last word has not been spoken on this complicated issue, especially as to etiology and pathogenesis. It is clear, however, that the amnionic sheets are frequently associated with many other fetal anomalies (e.g., exencephaly, meningocele, bony defects, single umbilical artery [SUA]), which is not the case with the typical bands that entangle the fingers. There may be overlaps, as suggested by Moerman et al. (1992). These authors provided a useful differentiation between these features and suggested that the latter two categories are associated with disturbances of early embryogenesis, thus leaving the amnion attached to the forehead in a broad sheet. Numerous cases of constriction of umbilical cord, limbs, and fingers have been presented that leave little doubt, however, that true bands from disruption of the amnionic sac do occur, that they can cause amputations, even fusion of fingers and toes, and that they may cause fetal death by encircling the cord (Hong & Simon, 1963; Ashkenazy et al., 1982). Baker and Rudolph (1971), who reported on 13 cases, thought that bands occurred only rarely (1 per 10,000 births). Bands can be a cause of spontaneous abortion with macerated fetuses, which must be carefully inspected to arrive at the correct diagnosis (Figures 197–199). Thus Kalousek (1987; Kalousek & Bamforth, 1988) found bands much more frequently, as often as 1 per 53 previable fetuses, when compared to 1 per 2,500 to 1 per 10,000 liveborns. At times it has even been witnessed that a smaller limb is delivered with a fetus. We have seen a newborn with

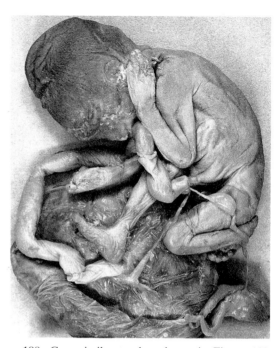

FIGURE 198. Case similar to that shown in Figure 199, with encircling of extremities and cord. Aborted fetus. (Courtesy Dr. G. Altshuler; Reprinted with permission of Altshuler, G. and McAdams, A.J.: The role of the placenta in fetal and perinatal pathology. Am. J. Obstet. Gynecol. 113:616–626, 1972.)

a foot amputation whose placenta was accompanied by one small macerated foot. The gestational age of the foot was estimated (from its length) to be 20 weeks. The term neonate suffered osteomyelitis later in the amputated stump. These findings indicated to us that amputation had occurred at an earlier fetal age. Such was also the case in the patient reported by Torpin and Faulkner (1966). Doubtlessly, the fetus moves and becomes entangled in these remnants of amnion; and because the fingers move most actively it is probable that amputation of fingertips is the most common sequela of amnionic bands. Most fetuses with amputations due to amnionic bands are otherwise normal, and the placental surface is usually completely devoid of amnion. In such cases, one usually finds remnants of amnion only around the umbilical cord. A small sac is often found at the placental end of the cord, where the bands originate (Figures 199 and 200) (Patterson, 1962). The amnion is so firmly attached to the cord surface that it does not detach from it and is not capable of disruption with band formation. The placental surface is usually somewhat opaque owing to infiltration with enlarged macrophages. This situation is particularly true when the amnion has been missing for long periods (Figure 199). The entire topic of amnionic disruption and bands has been exhaustively treated by Torpin (1968) in a book that has innumerable references and

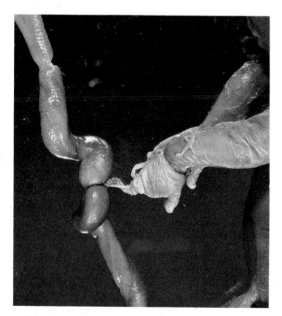

FIGURE 197. Spontaneous abortion at 15 weeks with amnionic bands encircling a constricting umbilical cord and tips of fingers.

FIGURE 199. Surface of the placenta of a term fetus with an amnionic remnant issuing from the base of the cord. The band had encircled the leg and nearly amputated it (Figure 201). Note the opacity of the membranes.

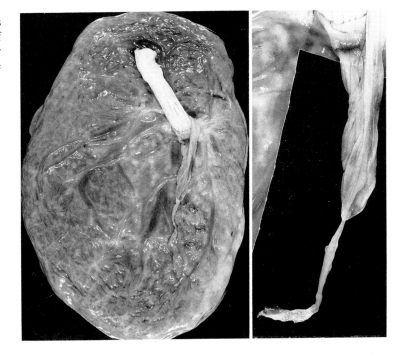

illustrations. Not only did he collect more than 400 cases from the literature, he also gave a detailed account of the many cases he had himself encountered. This volume should be consulted with respect to the history and other aspects of this relatively common cause of fetal anomalies. Moreover, it was Torpin who first contradicted the theories of Streeter and assigned a later amnion rupture as the etiological event. Constriction of extremities is perhaps the commonest or best known feature (Figure 201). We believe that the mobility of hands and feet is responsible. It should be cautioned, however, that not every case of amnionic rupture necessarily leads to entangling and constriction.

Another comprehensive review of most aspects of amnionic bands is that of Seidman et al. (1989). These authors bemoan the fact that the syndrome is surely underdiagnosed and emphasize that no two cases are alike, especially when one includes the limb–body wall complex. Single umbilical artery and short umbilical cords were found to be common associations. The karyotype of associated fetuses has almost always been normal, and the etiology is still disputed. This other type of amnionic disruption leads to different fetal deformities. They have been assumed to be associated with *early* amnion rupture, although different interpretations exist. Indeed the sheets are so large and

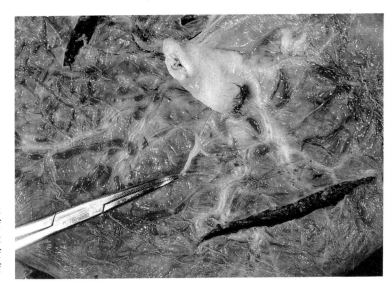

FIGURE 200. Placental surface of an infant with an amputated arm. The tiny remnants (clamp) of amnionic bands were initially not recognized at inspection after delivery. The importance of recognizing bands cannot be overemphasized if proper clinical counseling is to occur.

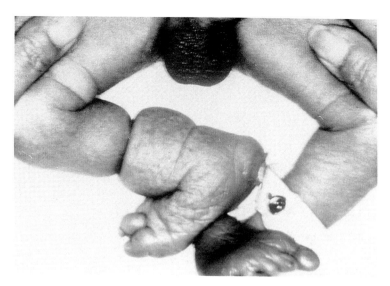

FIGURE 201. Note the extreme constriction of the right foreleg due to the amnionic bands shown in Figure 199. The infant also had several amputated toes.

often so well shown by sonography (they are contiguous with the ectoderm of the face and other parts of the body) that one should question the association with amnionic disruption. The anomalies are characterized by more profound defects commonly involving the face, skull, and abdomen. Often exencephaly, clubbed feet, and a variety of other features are observed. Although these disruptive events were once also held to be sequelae of amnion rupture, the mechanism that produces them is surely different from the typical bands. Shephard et al. (1988) conjectured that the frequent facial disruption of these fetuses may result from the "stickiness" of these areas in early embryos. This explanation is highly unlikely. Stickiness would not produce the large variety of other anomalies, nor would it be associated with a sheet of amnion whose epithelium is contiguous with the facial ectoderm. Incomplete embryonic folding and neural tube closure are more likely the mechanism. Because of fetal growth retardation and hydramnios, these "limb–body wall complexes" (Patten et al., 1986) are often recognized antenatally. Pysher (1980) described such a case that affected only one of monozygotic twins, and Woolnough (1987) described it in a dizygotic twin. We have seen it in one of presumably monozygotic but dichorionic twins. It had broad amnionic adhesions and many other anomalies (truncus, short bowel, ureteromegaly). In observations of amnionic bands described by Lockwood et al. (1989) and their review of the literature, emphasis was laid on the fact that only one of monozygotic (rarely a dizygotic) twins may be affected, making an external cause unlikely. Hartwig et al. (1989) reviewed this limb–body wall malformation complex more completely and concluded that only some cases have broad amnionic adhesions, and that others cannot be explained by this mechanism. They favored other, more complex disturbances of early em-

bryogenesis in their etiology. It was especially deemed to be so because apparently unrelated anomalies (e.g., truncus arteriosus) were sometimes encountered in such fetuses. It must be cautioned, however, that delivery often disrupts the areas of amnionic adhesion, and reconstruction may be difficult. Characteristic of the limb –body wall complex is that the amnion is contiguous with some portion of the body wall, often either the abdomen or the skull (Figure 202). This interesting spectrum of anomalies has therefore received attention since the beginning of the century (e.g., Ballantyne, 1904; Woyton, 1961; Torpin, 1968; Chaurasia, 1978; Higginbottom et al., 1979; Bieber et al., 1984; Seidman et al., 1989). Most commonly it has been assumed that these gross malformations result from an "early amnion rupture," but truthfully the exact differences of etiology between it and the more classical amnionic band syndrome are not known. We prefer to see them as a different entity and consider amnionic sheets separately from true bands.

For these reasons and because "amnionic intrusion" (Fort, 1971) (i.e., the prenatal intraamnionic invasion by perinatologists) is now so common, many investigators have attempted to understand these features by experimental reduction of amnionic fluid and disruption of the fetal sacs. After doing it in mice, Trasler et al. (1956) found a high incidence of cleft palate, which is also a common feature of this syndrome in humans. DeMyer and Baird (1969) found similar defects and skeletal abnormalities in rat fetuses when amniocentesis was performed between days 14 and 16; and Kino (1972), Singh and Singh (1978), and Houben and Huygens (1987) observed that limb defects follow focal hemorrhages in the limbs after amniocentesis in rats. None of these experiments, however, produced adhesions. Whether they bear any relation to the massive

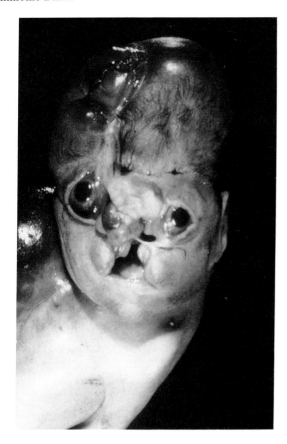

FIGURE 202. Abnormal skull and partial exencephaly secondary to broad amnionic adhesions. (Courtesy Dr. Cynthia Kaplan; from Kaplan, 1980, with permission.)

anomalies seen in the limb–body wall complex, is doubtful. Lockwood et al. (1989) suggested that these hemorrhages are a primary agency in the formation of amputations and the band syndrome in general. Among the 2,300 amniocenteses reported by Porreco et al. (1982), adverse outcomes usually related to complica-tions from anterior placentas; amnionic adhesions were not recorded (see below).

It has been noted that pregnancies complicated by apparent bands, identified with ultrasonographic techniques, often have a benign outcome, without fetal adhesions present; at birth, no amnionic bands can be found (Wehbeh et al., 1993). The discrepancy was first noted by Mahony et al. (1985) and further elaborated on by Randel et al. (1988) in their sonographic study of 17 patients. In the patients with this condition, the membranes were intact, and the apparent bands repre-sented indentations of the free membranes by endo-metrial synechiae or were the sequelae of former endo-metrial trauma. In most patients there is a history of repeated therapeutic abortion, myomectomy, or infec-tion. Presumably, it has led to the formation of endo-metrial synechiae, around which the amnion expands; sonographically it appears as bands. In two cesarean sections of patients with amnionic sheets, however, no uterine anomalies were identified. Such a case is shown in Figure 203. During sonography, a peculiar "stalk" was seen near term. This 36-year-old patient had a transverse lie with primary cesarean section. Although she was multiparous, no other risk factors were ascer-tained. The decidual adhesive band is clearly visible. There were no other pathological findings or complica-tions. Future studies are needed to clarify this condition. For clinical purposes it is important to distinguish it from true amnionic bands. These uterine adhesions have also been termed amniotic sheets, but they are different from the sheets discussed above in the limb–body wall complex. It is unfortunate that the two names have been used for different conditions.

When sections are made of amnionic bands, the bands are found to consist of normal-appearing amnionic epi-thelium with its connective tissue. There are few signs of degeneration, and inflammation is absent; there is also no evidence that bands may derive by a mechanism

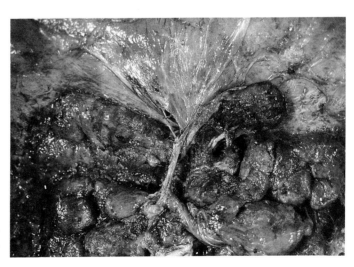

FIGURE 203. "Amnionic sheet." This stalk was identified sonographically as a stalk. It represents an adhesion in the uterine cavity.

of "adhesions," as suggested by Lockwood et al. (1989). Because the amnion does not completely attach itself to the chorion until the 12th week (Boyd & Hamilton, 1970), we assume that in the typical amnionic band syndrome cases the rupture of the amnion occurred prior to the 3rd month. It would then allow the fetus to escape into the chorionic sac and to become entangled in the amnionic remains when moving. The amnion, whose growth it appears is mediated by stretching of an enlarging sac, shrivels when ruptured; its remains then produce the amnionic adhesions. The fetus may not always entangle, but one finds spontaneously denuded placentas without fetal amputations only rarely. They then usually relate to the disruptions that occur during the process of labor, and the entire amnion is present—not, as in the band syndrome, only small portions thereof. Torpin (1968, 1969) made the point that it is at times difficult to identify band formation on the placental surface. He advocated that the placenta be studied under water, which enhances the detection of placental structural abnormalities. He also described the case of a fetus from whose mouth a 94 cm long piece of amnionic band was extracted (Torpin et al., 1964).

The etiology of these bands has stimulated the interest of obstetricians and dysmorphologists. We and others have questioned patients extensively as to possible traumatic or other significant events of early pregnancy, always with negative results. We have seen a set of twins who may shed some light on this question. A woman with previous salpingectomy had in vitro fertilization with transfer of five ova. Three of the ova "took," and the pregnancy was followed closely by sonography. At 6 weeks an abdominal catastrophe was diagnosed as uterine rupture from placenta percreta of one triplet that had nested near the tubal stump. It was resected, and the pregnancy went to term. One placenta was normal the other had an opaque surface and the remnants of a shriveled amnion around the cord with a small extension of band. The newborn had a single finger constriction. It was speculated that the amnion disruption occurred at the time of uterine rupture or during its repair. Many of these aspects were well discussed in Torpin's book (1968) and by Street and Cunningham (1964). Rarely have toxins such as lysergic acid diethylamide (LSD) been implicated (Blanc et al., 1971). As a rule, the mothers do not recall anything unusual about their pregnancy. The few exceptions of antenatal trauma have been well documented in Torpin's classical book (1968). It must be emphasized that the event typically occurs spontaneously. It is an open question whether excessive fetal activity or defective amnion development are causes of such rupture. Garza and colleagues (1988) concluded that amnionic bands are not hereditary. Only one study suggested that it may rarely occur in families repetitively (Lubinsky

et al., 1983). These authors described two families with possible band-related amputations and reviewed the sparse literature. Hereditary collagen defects (Ehlers-Danlos syndrome and osteogenesis imperfecta) were implicated by Young et al. (1985), but we have seen several cases of both conditions with entirely normal membranes; moreover, in one reported case of Ehlers-Danlos type III, no untoward membrane complication was reported (Atalla & Page, 1988). It must be cautioned, however, that it is of course the *fetus* who must be affected with this collagen defect to exhibit possible ill-effects from this condition. There is thus the report by Barabas (1966) that reviewed the gestational history of 18 patients with this syndrome. In his series, 14 of 18 patients (78%) were born prematurely secondary to premature rupture of the membranes. This large number suggests strongly, as did the author, that membrane integrity in this genotype may be adversely affected. Likewise, Levick (1989) found an increased number of miscarriages and intrauterine fetal deaths in families, even in those where the father had the disease. She studied three families with this defect and attributed miscarriage to "cervical laxity or premature rupture of fetal membranes." In neither report were bands described. Most authors consider that amnionic bands represent a sporadic event without recurrence risk; the usual discordance in monozygotic twins is further support. Some authors have described occasional families with possible band-related recurrent amputations, but it is exceptional (see also Lockwood et al., 1989). The notion that once the amnion has ruptured during early life the chorion allows fluid transfer and oligohydramnios, as suggested by Lockwood et al. (1989), has no merit. Nor has their suggestion that possible ensuing oligohydramnios leads to fetal skin abrasions. Amnionic bands have been described in monkeys at least twice (Tarantal & Hendrickx, 1987), and we have been shown a chimpanzee with typical finger amputations.

The nomenclature of modern dysmorphologists refers to these anomalies as the ADAM complex (amniotic deformities, adhesions, mutilation). The incidence of amnionic bands is difficult to assess. An epidemiological study was undertaken in Atlanta to identify the prevalence of TEARS (the early amnion rupture sequence). It was found to be 1.16 per 10,000 births among 388,325 live births assessed (Garza et al., 1988). These authors identified 45 cases of such severe, disruptive injuries. The incidence was higher in Blacks and correlated with low maternal age. There was a 30% mortality rate. On occasion, amnionic bands have been recognized by sonography; more commonly though the amnionic sheets are seen sonographically. It has also been suggested that amniocentesis might be the cause of early amnion disruption and of bands (Rehder & Weitzel, 1978; Moessinger et al., 1981), but this cause must be uncom-

FIGURE 204. Extramembranous pregnancy. A = Amnion; C = Chorion; AS = Amnionic SAC. (Reprinted with permission from the American College of Obstetricians and Gynecologists [Perlman, M. et al., Extramembranous pregnancy: maternal, placental, and perinatal implications. Obstetrics and Gynecology 55:345–375, 1980].)

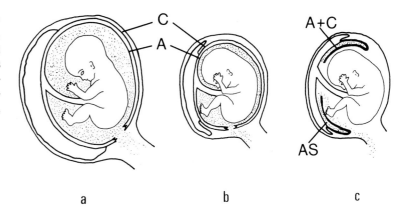

a   b   c

mon. Amniocentesis is done too late during gestation to detach the amnion from the chorion. Christiaens and colleagues (1989) provided evidence that chorionic villous sampling (CVS) may occasionally be held responsible for such injury. Although this point has been debated in recent literature it is the sense that only very early CVS may be related to this anomaly (see Chapter 21). Seeds et al. (1982) also described such an occurrence. Moessinger et al. (1981) found an arm constriction in an aborted fetus after complicated CVS with chorioamnionitis ensuing. Lage et al. (1988) have also been skeptical of the role of amniocentesis in the causation of amnionic bands. Moreover, the experimental studies cited above suggest that the sequelae of early fluid withdrawal differ from what is observed clinically in this syndrome, which is frequently referred to as Streeter's bands, after his early description (Streeter, 1930). There are also bands that completely encircle the abdomen or an extremity (Figure 201) and that have caused deep furrows and produced sloughing of skin. Finally, there are cases in which the circulation of the umbilical cord has been interrupted by bands composed of amnion (Figures 197, 198) (Kohler & Collins, 1972; Ashkenazy et al., 1982). Furthermore, in some cases bands have caused fusion of fingertips, with a space remaining at their base. All these varieties cannot be rationally explained by "germ plasm defects"; the primacy of the simple bands from sac disruption makes much more sense. We admit that the limb–body wall complexes do not have similar amputations, and as a rule they lack amputations. Their pathogenesis is different, and the broad amnionic sheet adhesions are surely the reason for their short umbilical cords. Some authors have suggested that short cords are not a related feature, but that has not been our experience and it is certainly not the case in Moerman's review (1992). The complete review of pathogenesis and associated features provided in the report of two cases by Seidman et al. (1989) should be consulted. Lockwood and his colleagues (1988, 1989) provided suggestions on how to

diagnose amnionic bands in twins, and they considered their pathogenesis. They reviewed 15 cases of amnionic bands in twin gestations, all of them in monochorionic (identical) twins. The absence of this syndrome in dizygotic (dichorionic twins), and other considerations led these authors to reject an "exogenous" etiology. The spectrum of anomalies in these twins, however, makes it clear that no single entity is being discussed.

Extramembranous Pregnancy

Not only may the amnion rupture, with the fetus developing outside the amnion although still contained within the chorion, but the entire chorion (laeve) may rupture as well. The fetus then lies in the endometrial cavity, and the pregnancy is referred to as "extramembranous." Although several previous cases were well described, the first observation made in situ was by Hofbauer

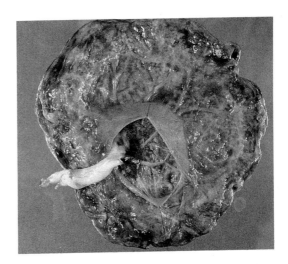

FIGURE 205. Extramembranous pregnancy. Note the circumvallate nature of the surface and the diminutive opening through which the cord emerges. Infant died from pulmonary hypoplasia.

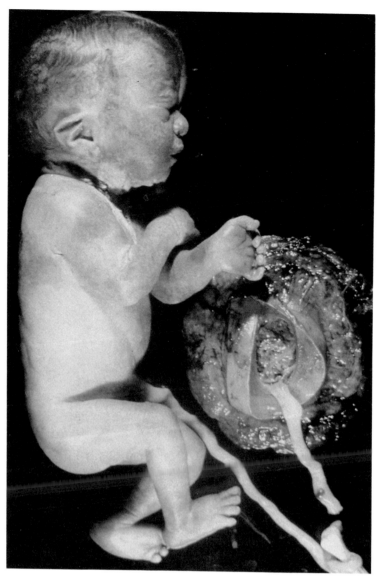

FIGURE 206. Extramembranous pregnancy with fetus. Note the size of the fetus and the membrane opening. There is a circumvallate placenta; and marked pulmonary hypoplasia is present.

(1929), who provided an excellent picture: The patient underwent a hysterectomy for mistaken diagnosis and gave a history of repeated prenatal hemorrhage that had been a major problem. Torpin (1968) collected 100 such cases and illustrated them well. These cases are rare circumstances and they are usually associated with prolonged "amniorrhea" (actually representing periodic fetal urination). Commonly there are severe positional deformities of the fetus associated with extramembranous gestation, and pulmonary hypoplasia is a characteristic sequela (Benirschke, 1977). Occasionally, such fetuses have survived, as in the cases reported by Perlman et al. (1980) (Figure 204). These authors collected the few cases reported since Torpin's 1968 review. We also witnessed three cases during the 1980s

and have seen others since then. We are impressed with the uniformity of the placental findings. The placenta is typically circumvallate, the cords are short, and in the membranes one finds substantial quantities of post-hemorrhagic hemosiderin (Figure 205). There may be sparse amnion nodosum over the placental tissue, but it is not striking. The remaining edge of the membranes is relatively normal, as was depicted by Perlman and his colleagues (1980). Most of these pregnancies abort or terminate prematurely. They are occasionally associated with infection. Evidence that the fetus must have escaped from the membranes much earlier is manifested by the diminutive hole that usually remains in the membranes. The hole may barely admit the umbilical cord, let alone fetal parts (Figure 206). As in the other cases

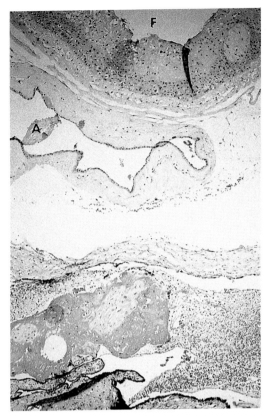

FIGURE 207. Membrane insertion in the extramembranous pregnancy shown in Figure 206. Below is villous tissue; membranes are folded at the right, and the fetus lay in space F. Much necrotic debris and inflammatory exudate are present at the margin. A = Focal amnion nodosum. H&E. ×64.

of bands and membrane rupture, the etiology remains obscure. It is nevertheless interesting to reflect on fetal life within the endometrium and to ponder the pathogenesis of circumvallate placentation. The placental membranes that have folded over appear essentially normal (Figure 207), with the exception of some minor degree of amnion nodosum and hemosiderin. Panayiotis and Grunstein (1979) have reported that one of dichorionic twins suffered prolonged amniorrhea and was born with severe growth retardation (1,600 g) and typical Potter syndrome-like features. The placenta was characteristically circumvallate, and the co-twin (2,150 g) survived. Extramembranous development was reported by Vago and Chavkin (1980) as having occurred after amniocentesis that led to amniorrhea. Despite deformities and some pulmonary hypoplasia, the 1,520 g neonate survived. The placenta was typical.

References

Abramovich, D.R., and Gray, E.S.: Physiologic fetal defecation in midpregnancy. Obstet. Gynecol. 60:294–296, 1982.

Abu-Yousef, M.M., Bleicher, J.J., Williamson, R.A., and

Weiner, C.P.: Subchorionic hemorrhage: sonographic diagnosis and clinical significance. Am. J. Roentgenol. 149: 737–740, 1987.

Akle, C.A., Adinolfi, M., Welsh, K.I., Leibowitz, S., and McColl, I.: Immunogenicity of human amniotic epithelial cells after transplantation into volunteers. Lancet 2:1003–1005, 1981.

Alger, L.S., Kisner, H.J., and Nagey, D.A.: The presence of a meconium-like substance in second-trimester amniotic fluid. Am. J. Obstet. Gynecol. 150:380–385, 1984.

Allen, R.: The significance of meconium in midtrimester genetic amniocentesis. Am. J. Obstet. Gynecol. 152:413–417, 1985.

Altshuler, G., and Hyde, S.: Meconium induced vasoconstriction: a potential cause of cerebral and other fetal hypoperfusion and of poor pregnancy outcome. J. Child Neurol. 4:137–142, 1989.

Altshuler, G., and McAdams, A.J.: The role of the placenta in fetal and perinatal pathology. Am. J. Obstet. Gynecol. 113:616–626, 1972.

Altshuler, G., Arizawa, M., and Molnar-Nadasdy, G.: Meconium-induced umbilical cord vascular necrosis and ulceration: a potential link between the placenta and poor pregnancy outcome. Obstet. Gynecol. 79:760–766, 1992.

Al-Zaid, N.S., Bou-Resli, M.N., and Goldspink, G.: Bursting pressure and collagen content of fetal membranes. Br. J. Obstet. Gynaecol. 87:227–229, 1980.

Anderson, H.C., Merker, P.C., and Fogh, J.: Formation of tumors containing bone after intramuscular injection of transformed human amnion cells (FL) into cortisone treated mice. Am. J. Pathol. 44:507–519, 1964.

Aplin, J.D., and Allen, T.D.: The extracellular matrix of human amniotic epithelium: ultrastructure, composition and deposition. J. Cell Sci. 79:119–136, 1985.

Aplin, J.D., and Campbell, S.: An immunofluorescence study of extracellular matrix associated with cytotrophoblast of the chorion laeve. Placenta 6:469–479, 1985.

Aplin, J.D., Campbell, S., Donnai, P., Bard, J.B.L., and Allen, T.D.: Importance of vitamin C in maintenance of the normal amnion: an experimental study. Placenta 7:377–389, 1986.

Ariel, I.B., and Landing, B.H.: A possible distinctive vacuolar change of the amniotic epithelium associated with gastroschisis. Pediatr. Pathol. 2:283–289, 1985.

Armstrong, W.D., Wilt, J.C., and Pritchard, E.T.: Vacuolation in the human amnion cell studied by time-lapse photography and electron microscopy. Am. J. Obstet. Gynecol. 102:932–948, 1968.

Artal, R., Sokol, R.J., Neuman, M., Burstein, A.H., and Stojkov, J.: The mechanical properties of prematurely and non-prematurely ruptured membranes: methods and preliminary results. Am. J. Obstet. Gynecol. 125:655–659, 1976.

Artal, R., Burgeson, R.E., Hobel, C.J., and Hollister, D.: An in vitro model for the study of enzymatically mediated biomechanical changes in the chorioamniotic membranes. Am. J. Obstet. Gynecol. 133:656–659, 1979.

Arts, N.F.T.: Investigations on the vascular system of the placenta. II. The maternal vascular system. Am. J. Obstet. Gynecol. 82:159–166, 1961.

Ashkenazy, M., Borenstein, R., Katz, Z., and Segal, M.: Constriction of the umbilical cord by an amniotic band after midtrimester amniocentesis. Acta Obstet. Gynecol. Scand. 61:89–91, 1982.

Atalla, A., and Page, I.: Ehlers-Danlos syndrome type III in pregnancy. Obstet. Gynecol. 71:508–509, 1988.

Azegami, M., and Mori, N.: Amniotic fluid embolism and leukotrienes. Am. J. Obstet. Gynecol. 155:1119–1124, 1986.

Bain, A.D., Smith, I.I., and Gauld, I.K.: Newborn after prolonged leakage of liquor amnii. B.M.J. 2:598–599, 1964.

Baker, C.J., and Rudolph, A.J.: Congenital ring constriction and intrauterine amputations. Am. J. Dis. Child. 121:393–400, 1971.

Ballantyne, J.W.: Manual of Antenatal Pathology and Hygiene. The Embryo. William Greene & Sons, Edinburgh, 1904.

Barabas, A.P.: Ehlers-Danlos syndrome: associated with prematurity and premature rupture of foetal membranes; possible increase in incidence. B.M.J. 2:682–684, 1966.

Barnes, A.C., and Seeds, A.E.: The Water Metabolism of the Fetus. Charles C Thomas, Springfield, IL, 1972.

Barss, V.A., Benacerraf, B.R., and Frigoletto, F.D.: Second trimester oligohydramnios, a predictor of poor fetal outcome. Obstet. Gynecol. 64:608–610, 1984.

Bartels, H., and Wang, T.: Intercellular junctions in the human fetal membranes. Anat. Embryol. (Berl.) 166:103–120, 1983.

Bartman, J., and Blanc, W.A.: Ultrastructure of human fetal placental membranes in chorio-amnionitis and meconium exposure. Obstet. Gynecol. 35:554–561, 1970.

Bartman, J., and Driscoll, S.G.: Amnion nodosum and hypoplastic cystic kidneys; an electron microscopic and microdissection study. Obstet. Gynecol. 32:700–705, 1968.

Battaglia, F.C., Hellegers, A.E., Meschia, G., and Barron, D.H.: In vitro investigations of the human chorion as a membrane system. Nature 196:1061–1063, 1962.

Battaglia, F.C., Behrman, R.E., Meschia, G., Seeds, A.E., and Bruns, P.D.: Clearance of inert molecules, Na, and Cl ions across the primate placenta. Am. J. Obstet. Gynecol. 102:1135–1143, 1968.

Bautzmann, H.: Fruchthüllenmotorik und Embryokinese: Ihre Natur und ihre Bedeutung für eine physiologische Embryonalentwicklung bei Tier und Mensch. Arch. Gynecol. 187:519–545, 1956.

Bautzmann, H., and Hertenstein, C.: Zur Histogenese und Histologie des menschlichen fetalen und Neugeborenen-Amnion. Z. Zellforsch. 45:589–611, 1957.

Bautzmann, H., and Schröder, R.: Studien zur funktionellen Histologie und Histogenese des Amnions beim Hühnchen und beim Menschen. Z. Anat. Entwicklungsgesch. 117:166–214, 1953.

Bautzmann, H., and Schröder, R.: Vergleichende Studien über Bau und Funktion des Amnions: neue Befunde am menschlichen Amnion mit Einschluß seiner freien Bindegewebs- oder sog. Hofbauerzellen. Z. Anat. 119:7–22, 1955.

Bautzmann, H., Schmidt, W., and Lemburg, P.: Experimental electron- and light-microscopic studies on the function of the amnion-apparatus of the chick, the cat and man. Anat. Anz. 108:305–310, 1960.

Baxi, L.V., and Pearlstone, M.M.: Subchorionic hematomas and the presence of autoantibodies. Am. J. Obstet. Gynecol. 165:1423–1424, 1991.

Bedin, M., Weil, D., Fournier, T., Cedard, L., and Frezal, J.: Biochemical evidence for non-inactivation of the steroid sulfatase locus in human placenta and fibroblasts. Hum. Genet. 59:256–258, 1981.

Beham, A., Denk, H., and Desoye, G.: The distribution of intermediate filament proteins, actin and desmoplakins in human placental tissue as revealed by polyclonal and monoclonal antibodies. Placenta 9:479–492, 1988.

Beller, F.K., Douglas, G.W., Debrovner, C.H., and Robinson, R.: The fibrinolytic system in amniotic fluid embolism. Am. J. Obstet. Gynecol. 87:48–55, 1963.

Bendon, R.W., and Ray, M.B.: The pathologic findings of the fetal membranes in very prolonged amniotic fluid leakage. Arch. Pathol. Lab. Med. 110:47–50, 1986.

Benedetti, W.L., Sala, M.A., and Alvarez, H.: Histochemical demonstration of enzymes in the umbilical cord and membranes of human term pregnancy. Eur. J. Obstet. Gynecol. Reprod. Biol. 3:185–189, 1973.

Benedetto, M.T., de Cicco, F., Rossielli, F., Nicosia, A.L., Lupi, G., and Dell'Acqua, S.: Oxytocin receptor in human fetal membranes at term and during labor. J. Steroid Biochem. 35:205–208, 1990.

Benirschke, K.: Effects of placental pathology on the embryo and the fetus. In, Handbook of Teratology. Vol. 3. J.G. Wilson and F.C. Fraser, eds., pp. 79–115. Plenum Press, New York, 1977.

Benirschke, K.: Placenta pathology: questions to the perinatologist. J. Perinatol. (in press, 1994).

Bernstein, I.M., Barth, R.A., Miller, R., and Capeless, E.L.: Elevated maternal serum alpha-fetoprotein: association with placental sonolucencies, fetomaternal hemorrhage, vaginal bleeding, and pregnancy outcome in the absence of fetal anomalies. Obstet. Gynecol. 79:71–74, 1992.

Bieber, F.R., Mostoufi-Zadeh, M., Birnholz, J.C., and Driscoll S.G.: Amniotic band sequence associated with ectopia cordis in one twin. J. Pediatr. 105:817–819, 1984.

Blanc, W.A.: Vernix granulomatosis of amnion ("amnion nodosum") in oligohydramnios: lesion associated with urinary anomalies, retention of dead fetuses, and prolonged leakage of amniotic fluid. N.Y. J. Med. 61:1492–1496, 1961.

Blanc, W.A., Apperson, J.W., and McNally, J.: Pathology of the newborn and of the placenta in oligohydramnios. Bull. Sloane Hosp. Women 7:51–64, 1962.

Blanc, W.A., Mattison, D.R., Kane, R., and Chauhan, P.: L.S.D., intrauterine amputations, and amniotic-band syndrome. Lancet 2:158–159, 1971.

Bohle, A., and Hienz, H.A.: Zellkernmorphologische Geschlechtsbestimmung an der Placenta. Klin. Wochenschr. 34:981–985, 1956.

Boll, H.U., Forssmann, W.G., and Taugner, R.: Studies on the juxtaglomerular apparatus. IV. Freeze-fracturing of membrane surfaces. Cell Tissue Res. 161:459–469, 1975.

Borlum, K.-G.: Second-trimester chorioamniotic separation and amniocentesis. Eur. J. Obstet. Gynecol. Reprod. Biol. 30:35–38, 1989.

Boué, A., Muller, F., Briard, M.L., and Boué, J.: Interest of biology in the management of pregnancies where a fetal malformation has been detected by ultrasonography. Fetal Ther. 3:14–23, 1988.

Bou-Resli, M.N., Al-Zaid, N.S., and Ibrahim, M.E.A.: Full-term and prematurely ruptured fetal membranes. Cell Tissue Res. 220:263–278, 1981.

Bourne, G.L.: The microscopic anatomy of the human amnion and chorion. Am. J. Obstet. Gynecol. 79:1070–1073, 1960.

Bourne, G.L.: The Human Amnion and Chorion. Lloyd-Luke, London, 1962.

Bourne, G.L., and Lacy, D.: Ultra-structure of human amnion and its possible relation to the circulation of amniotic fluid. Nature 168:952–954, 1960.

Boyd, J.D., and Hamilton, W.J.: The Human Placenta. Heffer & Sons, Cambridge, 1970.

Breed, A., Mantingh, A., Govaerts, L., Booger, A., Anders, G., and Laurini, R.: Abnormal karyotype in the chorion, not confirmed in a subsequently aborted fetus. Prenat. Diagn. 6:375–377, 1986.

Brown, D.R., Doshi, N., and Taylor, P.M.: Oligohydramnios and fatal pulmonary hypoplasia without amnion nodosum. J. Reprod. Med. 20:293–296, 1978.

Brusis, E., Nitsch, B., and Wengeler, H.: Fruchtwasser und Amnion. In, Klinik der Frauenheilkunde und Geburtshilfe. Vol. 4. G. Döderlein and K.H. Wulf, eds., pp. 667–750. Urban & Schwarzenberg, Munich, 1975.

Bryant-Greenwood, G.D., Rees, M.C.P., and Turnbull, A.C. Immunohistochemical localization of relaxin, prolactin and prostaglandin synthase in human amnion, chorion and decidua. J. Endocrinol. 114:491–496, 1987.

Bühler, F.R.: Randbildungen der menschlichen Placenta. Acta Anat. (Basel) 59:47–76, 1964.

Bullen, B., Bloxam, D., Ryder, T.A., Mobberley, M.A., and Bax, C.M.: Two-sided culture of human placental trophoblast: morphology, immunohistochemistry and permeability properties. Placenta 11:431–450, 1990.

Burgess, A.M., and Hutchins, G.M.: Inflammation of the lungs, umbilical cord, and placenta associated with meconium passage in utero: review of 123 autopsied cases [abstract 4]. Mod. Pathol. 7(1):1P, 1994.

Butler, W.J., Schwartz, C.E., Sauer, S.M., Wilson, J.T., and McDonough, P.G.: Discordance in deoxyribonucleic acid analysis of fetus and trophoblast. Am. J. Obstet. Gynecol. 158:642–645, 1988.

Byrne, D.L., and Gau, G.: In utero meconium aspiration: an unpreventable cause of neonatal death. Br. J. Obstet. Gynaecol. 94:813–814, 1987.

Campbell, S., Allen, T.D., Moser, B.B., and Aplin, J.D.: The translaminal fibrils of the human amnion basement membrane. J. Cell Sci. 94:307–318, 1989.

Cane, F.E.: The functions of the amnion. Lancet 2:1274, 1888.

Casey, M.L., Delgadillo, M., Cox, K.A., Niesert, S., and MacDonald, P.C.: Inactivation of prostaglandins in human decidua vera (parietalis) tissue: substrate specificity of prostaglandin dehydrogenase. Am. J. Obstet. Gynecol. 160:3–7, 1989.

Casey, M.L., Word, R.A., and MacDonald, P.C.: Endothelin-1 gene expression and regulation of endothelin mRNA and protein biosynthesis in avascular human amnion. J. Biol. Chem. 266:5762–5768, 1991.

Charpin, C., Kopp, F., Pourreau-Schneider, N., Lissitzky, J.C., Lavaut, M.N., Martin, P.M., and Toga, M.: Laminin distribution in human decidua and immature placenta: an immunoelectronmicroscopic study (avidin-biotin-peroxidase complex method). Am. J. Obstet. Gynecol. 151:822–826, 1985.

Chaurasia, B.D.: Amniochorionic bands and adhesions with fetal deformities. Anat. Anz. 144:158–162, 1978.

Cheung, P.Y., Walton, J.C., Tai, H.H., Riley, S.C., and Challis, J.R.: Immunocytochemical distribution and localization of 15-hydroxyprostaglandin dehydrogenase in human fetal membranes, decidua, and placenta. Am. J. Obstet. Gynecol. 163:1445–1449, 1990.

Chez, R.A., Josimovich, J.B., and Schultz, S.G.: The transfer of human placental lactogen across isolated amnion-chorion. Gynecol. Invest. 1:312–318, 1970.

Christiaens, G.C.M.L., van Baarlen, J., Huber, J., and Leschot, N.J.: Fetal limb constriction: a possible complication of CVS. Prenat. Diagn. 9:67–71, 1989.

Clark, S.L.: Arachidic acid metabolites and the pathophysiology of amniotic fluid embolism. Semin. Reprod. Endocrinol. 3:253–257, 1985.

Clark, S.L.: Amniotic fluid embolism and leukotrienes. Am. J. Obstet. Gynecol. 158:681, 1988.

Clark, S.L., Pavlova, Z., Greenspoon, J., Horenstein, J., and Phelan, J.P.: Squamous cells in the maternal pulmonary circulation. Am. J. Obstet. Gynecol. 154:104–106, 1986.

Clark, S.L., Cotton, D.B., Gonik, B., Greenspoon, J., and Phelan, J.P.: Central hemodynamic alterations in amniotic fluid embolism. Am. J. Obstet. Gynecol. 158:1124–1126, 1988.

Clayton, E.M., Waller, D.H., and Foster, E.B.: The significance of heme pigments in amniotic fluid. Obstet. Gynecol. 34:641–647, 1969.

Clement, D., Schifrin, B.S., and Kates, R.B.: Acute oligohydramnios in postdate pregnancy. Am. J. Obstet. Gynecol. 157:884–886, 1987.

Cooperberg, P.L., Wright, V.J., and Carpenter, C.W.: Ultrasonographic demonstration of a placental maternal lake. J. Clin. Ultrasound 7:62–64, 1979.

Corridan, M., Kendall, E.D., and Begg, J.D.: Cord entanglement causing premature placental separation and amniotic fluid embolism: case report. Br. J. Obstet. Gynaecol. 87:935–940, 1980.

Coston, H.R.: Report of a case of ichthyosis fetalis; placenta and membranes involved. Am. J. Obstet. Dis. Women Child. 58:650–654, 1908.

Crane, J.P., and Cheung, S.W.: An embryonic model to explain cytogenetic inconsistencies observed in chorionic villus versus fetal tissue. Prenat. Diagn. 8:119–129, 1988.

Crescimanno, C., Mühlhauser, J., Castellucci, M., Rajaniemi, H., Parkkila, S., and Kaufmann, P.: Immunocytochemical expression patterns of carbonic anhydrase isoenzymes in human placenta, cord and membranes. Placenta 14:A11, 1993.

Danforth, D.N., and Hull, R.W.: The microscopic anatomy of the fetal membranes with particular reference to the detailed structure of the amnion. Am. J. Obstet. Gynecol. 75:536–550, 1958.

Danforth, D.N., Elin, T.W., and Stanes, M.N.: Studies on fetal membranes. I. Bursting tension. Am. J. Obstet. Gynecol. 65:480–490, 1953.

Davis, J.R., and Penny, R.J.: Improved fluorescence method for identifying sex chromatin in formalin-fixed tissue. Am. J. Clin. Pathol. 75:731–733, 1981.

Davis, R.O., Philips, J.B., III, Harris, B.A., Wilson, E.R., and Huddleston, J.F.: Fatal meconium aspiration syndrome occurring despite airway management considered appropriate. Am. J. Obstet. Gynecol. 151:731–736, 1985.

Davis, G.E., Blaker, S.N., Engvall, E., Varon, S., Manthorpe, M., and Gage, F.H.: Human amnion membrane serves as a substratum for growing axons in vitro and in vivo. Science 236:1106–1109, 1987.

Déglon, P.: Lésions placentaires et foetales dans 100 cas d'oligohydramnios. Thesis, University of Lausanne, 1978.

De Ikonicoff, L.K., and Cedard, L.: Localization of human chorionic gonadotropic and somatomammotropic hormones by the peroxidase immuno-enzymologic method in villi and amniotic epithelium of human placenta (from six weeks to term). Am. J. Obstet. Gynecol. 116:1124–1132, 1973.

DeMyer, W., and Baird, I.: Mortality and skeletal malformations from amniocentesis and oligohydramnios in rats: cleft palate, clubfoot, microstomia, and adactyly. Teratology 2:33–38, 1969.

DeSa, D.J.: Rupture of fetal vessels on placental surface. Arch. Dis. Child. 46:495–501, 1971.

Desmond, M.M., Lindley, J.E., Moore, J., and Brown, C.A.: Meconium staining of newborn infants. J. Pediatr. 49:540–549, 1956.

Dickey, R.P., Olar, T.T., Curole, D.N., Taylor, S.N., and Matulich, E.M.: Relationship of first-trimester subchorionic bleeding detected by color Doppler ultrasound to subchorionic fluid, clinical bleeding, and pregnancy outcome. Obstet. Gynecol. 80:415–420, 1992.

Dominguez, R., Segal, A.J., and O'Sullivan, J.A.: Leukocytic infiltration of the umbilical cord: manifestation of fetal hypoxia due to reduction of blood flow in the cord. J.A.M.A. 173:346–349, 1960.

Donskikh, N.V.: New views on vascularity of the human amnion. Akush. Ginekol. (Mosk.) 33:93–94, 1957 (Russian).

Dooley, S.L., Pesavento, D.J., Depp, R., Socol, M.L., Tamura, R.K., and Wiringa, K.S.: Meconium below the vocal cords at delivery: correlation with intrapartum events. Am. J. Obstet. Gynecol. 153:767–770, 1985.

Editorial: Anyone for amnion? Lancet 1:719, 1984.

Ellis, S.A., Sargent, I.L., Redman, C.W., and McMichael, A.J.: Evidence for a novel HLA antigen found on human extravillous trophoblast and a choriocarcinoma cell line. Immunology 59:595–601, 1986.

Enders, A.C., and King, B.F.: Formation and differentiation of extraembryonic mesoderm in the rhesus monkey. Am. J. Anat. 181:327–340, 1988.

Evaldson, G.R., Larsson, B., and Jiborn, H.: Is collagen content reduced when the fetal membranes rupture? A clinical study of term and prematurely ruptured membranes. Gynecol. Obstet. Invest. 24:92–94, 1987.

Falciglia, H.S.: Failure to prevent meconium aspiration syndrome. Obstet. Gynecol. 71:349–353, 1988.

Falciglia, H.S., Kosmetatos, N., Brady, K., and Wesseler, T.A.: Intrauterine meconium aspiration in an extremely premature infant. Am. J. Dis. Child. 147:1035–1037, 1993.

Faulk, W.P., Hsi, B.-L., Yeh, C.-J.G., McIntyre, J.A., and Stevens, P.J.: Epidermolysis bullosa fetalis: an immunogenetic disease of extraembryonic exoderm? Am. J. Obstet. Gynecol. 158:150–157, 1988.

Fitch, N., and Lachance, R.C.: The pathogenesis of Potter's syndrome of renal agenesis. Can. Med. Assoc. J. 107:653–656, 1972.

Fleischer, A.C., Kurtz, A.B., Wapner, R.J., Ruch, D., Sacks, G.A., Jeanty, P., Shah, D.M., and Boehm, F.H.: Elevated alpha-fetoprotein and a normal fetal sonogram: association with placental abnormalities. Am. J. Roentgenol. 150:881–883, 1988.

Foltz, C.M., Russo, R.G., Terranova, V.P., and Liotta, L.A.: Interactions of tumous cells with whole basement membrane in the presence or absence of endothelium. In, Interaction of Platelets and Tumour Cells. G.A. Jamieson and A.R. Scipio, eds., pp. 353–371. Alan R. Liss, New York, 1982.

Forssmann, W.G., and Taugner, R.: Studies on the juxtaglomerular apparatus. V. The juxtaglomerular apparatus in Tupaia with special reference to intercellular contacts. Cell Tissue Res. 177:291–305, 1977.

Fort, A.T.: Prenatal intrusion into the amnion. Am. J. Obstet. Gynecol. 110:432–455, 1971.

Foster, H.W., and Das, S.K.: Study of lipids in human amnion and chorion. Am. J. Obstet. Gynecol. 149:670–673, 1984.

Fox, H., and Butler-Manuel, R.: A teratoma of the placenta. J. Pathol. Bacteriol. 88:137–140, 1964.

Frank, H.G., Malekzadeh, F., Kertschanska, S., Crescimanno, C., Castellucci, M., Lang, I., Desoye, G., and Kaufmann, P.: Immunohistochemistry of two different types of placental fibrinoid. Acta Anat. 150:55–68, 1994.

Franqoual, J., Lindenbaum, A., Benattar, C., Dehan, M., Cohen, H., and Leluc, R.: Importance of simultaneous determination of coproporphyrin and hemoglobin in contaminated amniotic fluid. Clin. Chem. 32:877–878, 1986.

Franqué, O.v.: Zur Kenntnis der Amnionanomalien. Monatsschr. Geburtshilfe Gynäkol. 6:36–41, 1897.

Frels, W.I., Rossant, J., and Chapman, V.M.: Maternal X chromosome expression in mouse chorionic ectoderm. Dev. Genet. 1:123–132, 1979.

Fuchs, A.R., Periysamy, S., Alexandrova, M., and Soloff, M.: Correlation between oxytocin receptor concentration and responsiveness to oxytocin in pregnant myometrium: effects of ovarian steroids. Endocrinology 113:742–749, 1983.

Fujikura, T., and Klionsky, B.: The significance of meconium staining. Am. J. Obstet. Gynecol. 121:45–50, 1975.

Garcia, A.G.P., Consorte, S.M., Lana, A.M.A., and Friede, R.: Amnion nodosum and congenital ichthyosis. Am. J. Clin. Pathol. 67:567–572, 1977.

Garza, A., Cordero, J.F., and Mulinare, J.: Epidemiology of the early amnion rupture spectrum of defects. Am. J. Dis. Child. 142:541–544, 1988.

Gibb, W., and Lavoie, J.C.: Effects of glucocorticoids on prostaglandin formation by human amnion. Can. J. Physiol. Pharmacol. 68:671–676, 1990.

Goetzman, B.W.: Meconium aspiration. Am. J. Dis. Child. 146:1282–1283, 1992.

Golbus, M.S., and Stephens, J.D.: Prenatal diagnosis, chromosomal abnormalities and neural tube defects. Clin. Perinatol. 6:245–254, 1979.

Goodlin, R.C.: Meconium aspiration. Obstet. Gynecol. 32: 94–95, 1968.

Gossrau, R., Graf, R., Ruhnke, M., and Hanski, C.: Proteases in the human full-term placenta. Histochemistry. 86: 405–413, 1987.

Grafe, M.J., and Benirschke, K.: Ultrastructural study of the amniotic epithelium in a case of gastroschisis. Pediatr. Pathol. 10:95–101, 1990.

Griffiths, D.M., and Burge, D.M.: When is meconium stained liquor actually bile stained vomitus? Arch. Dis. Child. 63: 201–202, 1988.

Grimes, L.D., and Cassady, G.: Fetal gastrointestinal obstruction. Am. J. Obstet. Gynecol. 106:1196–1200, 1970.

Grosser, O.: Frühentwicklung, Eihautbildung und Placentation des Menschen und der Säugetiere. J.F. Bergmann, Munich, 1927.

Guidotti, R.J., Grimes, D.A., and Cates, W.: Fatal amniotic fluid embolism during legally induced abortion, United States, 1972 to 1978. Am. J. Obstet. Gynecol. 141:257–261, 1981.

Haddad, F.S.: Amniotic fluid embolism: a review of the literature and a case report with recovery. J. Indian Med. Assoc. 17:76–79, 1985.

Hamilton, W.J., and Boyd, J.D.: Development of the human placenta in the first three months of gestation. J. Anat. 94:297–328, 1960.

Hankins, G.D.V., Rowe, J., Quirk, J.G., Trubey, R., and Strickland, D.M.: Significance of brown and/or green amniotic fluid at the time of second trimester genetic amniocentesis. Obstet. Gynecol. 64:353–358, 1984.

Harrison, K.B., and Warburton, D.: Preferential X-chromosome activity in human female placental tissue. Cytogenet. Cell Genet. 41:163–168, 1986.

Hartwig, N.G., Vermej-Keers, C.H.R., de Vries, H.E., Kagie, M., and Kragt, H.: Limb body wall malformation complex: an embryologic etiology? Hum. Pathol. 20:1071–1077, 1989.

Hebertson, R.M., Hammond, M.E., and Bryson, M.J.: Amniotic epithelial ultrastructure in normal, polyhydramnic, and oligohydramnic pregnancies. Obstet. Gynecol. 68:74–79, 1986.

Hempel, E.: Die ultrastrukturelle Differenzierung des menschlichen Amnionepithels unter besonderer Berücksichtigung des Nabelstranges. Anat. Anz. 132:356–370, 1972.

Herendael, B.J.v., Oberti, C., and Brosens, I.: Microanatomy of the human amniotic membranes: a light microscopic, transmission, and scanning electron microscopic study. Am. J. Obstet. Gynecol. 131:872–880, 1978.

Hertig, A.T.: On the development of the amnion and exocoelomic membrane in the previllous human ovum. Yale J. Biol. Med. 18:107–115, 1945.

Hertig, A.T.: Human Trophoblast. Charles C Thomas. Springfield, IL, 1968.

Hertig, A.T., and Rock, J.: Two human ova of the previllous stage having an ovulation age of about eleven and twelve days respectively. Contrib. Embryol. Carnegie Inst. 29: 127–156, 1941.

Hessle, H., and Engvall, E.: Type VI collagen. J. Biol. Chem. 259:3955–3961, 1984.

Hessle, H., Sakai, L.Y., Hollister, D.W., Burgeson, R.E., and Engvall, E.: Basement membrane diversity detected by monoclonal antibodies. Differentiation 26:49–54, 1984.

Higginbottom, M.C., Jones, K.L., Hall, B.D., and Smith, D.W.: The amniotic band disruption complex: timing of amnion rupture and variable spectra of consequent defects. J. Pediatr. 95:544–549, 1979.

Hills, B.A.: Further studies of the role of surfactant in premature rupture of the membranes. Am. J. Obstet. Gynecol. 170:195–201, 1994.

Hinrichsen, K.: Embryogenese, äußere Körperform und Nabelbildung. In, Humanembryologie. K. Hinrichsen, ed. Springer, Heidelberg, 1990.

Hofbauer, J.: Extrachoriale Fruchtentwicklung, in situ beobachtet. Arch. Gynecol. 135:332–333, 1929.

Hogge, W.A., Schonberg, S.A., and Golbus, M.S.: Prenatal diagnosis by chorionic villus sampling: lessons of the first 600 cases. Prenat. Diagn. 5:393–400, 1985.

Hong, C.Y., and Simon, M.A.: Amniotic bands knotted about umbilical cord: a rare cause of fetal death. Obstet. Gynecol. 22:667–670, 1963.

Houben, J.J., and Huygens, R.: Subcellular effects of experimental oligohydramnios on the developing rat limb. Teratology 36:107–116, 1987.

Hoyes, A.D.: Fine structure of human amniotic epithelium in early pregnancy. J. Obstet. Gynaecol. Br. Commonw. 75: 949–962, 1968a.

Hoyes, A.D.: Ultrastructure of the epithelium of human umbilical cord. J. Anat. 103:388–389, 1968b.

Hoyes, A.D.: Ultrastructure of the human mesenchymal layers of the human chorion in early pregnancy. Am. J. Obstet. Gynecol. 106:557–566, 1970.

Hoyes, A.D.: Ultrastructure of the mesenchymal layers of the human chorion laeve. J. Anat. 109:17–30, 1971.

Hoyes, A.D.: Fine structure of human amnionic epithelium following short term preservations in vitro. J. Anat. 111: 43–54, 1972.

Hunt, J.S., and Fishback, J.L.: Amniochorion: immunologic aspects—a review. Am. J. Reprod. Immunol. 21:114–118, 1989.

Ibrahim, M.E.A., Bou-Resli, M.N., Al-Zaid, N.S., and Bishay, L.F.: Intact fetal membranes: morphological predisposal to rupture. Acta Obstet. Gynecol. Scand. 62:481–485, 1983.

Itskovitz, J., Abramovici, H., and Brandes, J.M.: Oligohydramnion, meconium and perinatal death concurrent with indomethacin treatment in human pregnancy. J. Reprod. Med. 24:137–140, 1980.

Jenkins, D.M., O'Neill, M., Matter, M., France, V.W., Hsi, B.L., and Faulk, W.P.: Degenerative changes and detection of plasminogen in fetal membranes that rupture prematurely. Br. J. Obstet. Gynaecol. 90:841–846, 1983.

Jonas, E.G., and Caunt, A.E.: Clinical evaluation of human amnion tissue culture. B.M.J. 1:898–901, 1965.

Jones, S.A., and Challis, J.R. Local stimulation of prostaglandin production by corticotropin-releasing hormone in human fetal membranes and placenta. Biochem. Biophys. Res. Commun. 159:192–199, 1989.

Jones, S.A., Brooks, A.N., and Challis, J.R.: Steroids modulate corticotropin-releasing hormone production in human fetal membranes and placenta. J. Clin. Endocrinol. Metab. 68:825–830, 1989.

Joseph, T.J., and Vogt, P.J.: Placental teratomas. Obstet. Gynecol. 41:574–578, 1973.

Kallakury, B., Kelty, R., Ross, J.S., and Amyot, K.: Prevalence, histological characteristics and clinical significance of meconium in placentas [abstract 26]. Mod. Pathol. 6:5P, 1993.

Kalousek, D.: Amniotic band syndrome in previable fetuses. Pediatr. Pathol. 7:488, 1987.

Kalousek, D.K., and Bamforth, S.: Amnion rupture sequence in previable fetuses. Am. J. Med. Genet. 31:63–73, 1988.

Kalousek, D.K., and Dill, F.J.: Chromosomal mosaicism confined to the placenta in human conceptions. Science 221:665–667, 1983.

Kaltenbach, F.J., and Sachs, W.: The uptake of tritiated thymidine in human fetal membranes during the last third of pregnancy. Z. Geburtshilfe Perinatol. 183:285–295, 1979.

Kanayama, N., Terao, T., Kawashima, Y., Horiuchi, K., and Fujimoto, D.: Collagen types in normal and prematurely ruptured amniotic membranes. Am. J. Obstet. Gynecol. 153:899–903, 1985.

Kaplan, C.: Placental pathology in perinatal disease. In, Gynecology and Obstetrics. Vol 3 J.J. Sciarra, ed., Chapter 106, pp. 1–21. Harper & Row, Hagerstown, MD, 1980.

Kaplan, M.: Fetal breathing movements: an update for the pediatrician. Am. J. Dis. Child. 137:177–181, 1983.

Karimi-Nejad, M.H., Khajavi, H., Gharavi, M.J., and Karimi-Nejad, R.: Neu-Laxova syndrome: report of a case and comments. Am. J. Med. Genet. 28:17–23, 1987.

Karp, L.E., and Schiller, H.S.: Meconium staining of amniotic fluid at midtrimester amniocentesis. Obstet. Gynecol. 50: 47s–49s, 1977.

Katz, V.L., and Bowes, W.A.: Meconium aspiration syndrome: reflections on a murky subject. Am. J. Obstet. Gynecol. 166:171–183, 1992.

Kaufmann, P.: Entwicklung der Plazenta. In, Die Plazenta des Menschen. V. Becker, T.H. Schiebler, and F. Kubli, eds. Thieme, Stuttgart, 1981.

Keene, D.R., Sakai, L.Y., Lunstrum, G.P., Morris, N.P., and Burgeson, R.E.: Type VII collagen forms an extended network of anchoring fibrils. J. Cell Biol. 104:611–621, 1987.

Kilbride, H.W., Thibeault, D.W., Yeast, J., Maulik, D., and Grundy, H.O.: Fetal breathing is not a predictor of pulmonary hypoplasia in pregnancies complicated by oligohydramnios. Lancet 1:305–306, 1988.

Kim, C.K., Naftolin, F., and Benirschke, K.: Immunohistochemical studies of the "X cell" in the human placenta with anti-human chorionic gonadotropin and anti-human placental lactogen. Am. J. Obstet. Gynecol. 111:672–676, 1971.

King, B.F.: Developmental changes in the fine structure of rhesus monkey amnion. Am. J. Anat. 157:285–307, 1980.

King, B.F.: Developmental changes in the fine structure of the chorion laeve (smooth chorion) of the rhesus monkey placenta. Anat. Rec. 200:163–175, 1981.

King, B.F.: Cell surface specializations and intercellular junctions in human amnionic epithelium: an electron microscopic and freeze-fracture study. Anat. Rec. 203:73–82, 1982.

King, B.F.: Distribution and characterization of anionic sites in the basal lamina of developing human amniotic epithelium. Anat. Rec. 212:57–62, 1985.

Kino, Y.: Reductive malformations of the limbs in the rat fetus following amniocentesis. Congen. Anom. (Japan) 12: 35–44, 1972.

Kinoshita, K., Satoh, K., and Sakamoto, S.: Human amniotic membrane and prostaglandin biosynthesis. Biol. Res. Pregnancy Perinatol. 5:61–67, 1984.

Kisalus, L.L., and Herr, J.C.: Immunocytochemical localization of heparan sulfate proteoglycan in human decidual cell secretory bodies and placental fibrinoid. Biol. Reprod. 39: 419–430, 1988.

Kisalus, L.L., Herr, J.C., and Little, C.D.: Immunolocalization of extracellular matrix proteins and collagen synthesis in first-trimester human decidua. Anat. Rec. 218:402–415, 1987.

Kjaeldgaard, A., Pschera, H., Larsson, B., Gaffney, P., and Astedt, B.: Plasminogen activators and inhibitors in amniotic fluid. Fibrinolysis 3:203–206, 1989.

Klima, G., Zerlauth, D., Richter, J., and Schmidt, W.: Die Mikrotextur von Amnion- und Chorionbindegewebe. Anat. Anz. 168:395–400, 1989.

Klima, G., Zerlauth, B., Wolf, H.J., and Schellnast, R.: A study of lectin bindings to the fetal membranes. Anat. Anz. 173:87–91, 1991.

Klinger, H.P., and Schwarzacher, H.G.: XY/XXY and sex chromatin positive cell distribution in a 60 mm human fetus. Cytogenetics 1:266–290, 1962.

Kohler, H.G.: An unusual case of sirenomelia. Teratology 6:295–302, 1972.

Kohler, H.G., and Collins, M.L.: Ligation of the umbilical cord by torn amniotic membrane. J. Obstet. Gynaecol. Br. Commonw. 79:183–184, 1972.

Kratzsch, E., and Grygiel, I.-H.: Über das Vorkommen eines spezifischen Enzyms der Glucuronsäurebildung im menschlichen Amnion. Z. Zellforsch. 123:566–571, 1972.

Küster, J.: Adultes Teratom ("Dermoid") der Placenta. Arch. Gynecol. 133:93–99, 1928.

Lage, J.M., Van Marter, L.J., and Bieber, F.R.: Questionable role of amniocentesis in the formation of amniotic bands. J. Reprod. Med. 33:71–73, 1988.

Landing, B.H.: Amnion nodosum: a lesion of the placenta apparently associated with deficient secretion of fetal urine. Am. J. Obstet. Gynecol. 60:1339–1342, 1950a.

Landing, B.H.: The pathogenesis of amniotic-fluid embolism. N. Engl. J. Med. 243:590–596, 1950b.

Laufer, A., Polishuk, W.Z., Boxer, J., and Ganzfried, R.: Studies of amniotic membranes. J. Reprod. Fertil. 12:99–105, 1966.

Lauweryns, J., Bernat, R., Lerut, A., and Detournay, G.: Intrauterine pneumonia: an experimental study. Biol. Neonate 22:215–231, 1973.

Lavery, J.P., and Miller, C.E: The viscoelastic nature of chorioamniotic membranes. Obstet. Gynecol. 50:467–472, 1977.

Lavery, J.P., Miller, C.E., and Johns, P.: Effect of meconium on the strength of chorioamniotic membranes. Obstet. Gynecol. 56:711–715, 1980.

Lavery, J.P., Miller, E., and Knight, R.D.: The effect of labor on the rheologic response of chorioamniotic membranes. Obstet. Gynecol. 60:87–92, 1982.

Leary, O.C., and Hertig, A.T.: Pathogenesis of amniotic fluid embolism. I. Possible placental factors—aberrant squamous cells in placenta. N. Engl. J. Med. 243:588–590, 1950.

Legge, M.: Dark brown amniotic fluid—identification of contributing pigments. Br. J. Obstet. Gynaecol. 88:632–634, 1981.

Leivo, I., and Engvall, E.: C3d fragment of complement interacts with laminin and binds to basement membranes of glomerulus and trophoblast. J. Cell Biol. 103:1091–1100, 1986.

Levick, K.: Pregnancy loss and fathers with Ehlers-Danlos syndrome. Lancet 2:1151, 1989.

Linnala, A., Balza, E., Zardi, L., and Virtanen, I.: Human amnion epithelial cells assemble tenascins and three fibronectin isoforms in the extracellular matrix. FEBS Lett. 317: 74–78, 1993.

Linton, G., and Lilford, R.J.: False-negative finding on chorionic villus sampling. Lancet 2:630, 1986.

Liotta, L.A., Lee, C.W., and Morakis, D.J.: New method for preparing large surfaces of intact human basement membrane for tumor invasion studies. Cancer Lett. 11:141–152, 1980.

Lister, U.M.: Ultrastructure of the human amnion, chorion and fetal skin. J. Obstet. Gynaecol. Br. Commonw. 75: 327–341, 1968.

Lloyd, S.J., Garlid, K.D., Reba, R.C., and Seeds, A.E.: Permeability of different layers of the human placenta to isotopic water. J. Appl. Physiol. 26:274–276, 1969.

Lockwood, C., Ghidini, A., and Romero, R.: Amniotic band syndrome in monozygotic twins: prenatal diagnosis and pathogenesis. Obstet. Gynecol. 71:1012–1016, 1988.

Lockwood, C., Ghidini, A., Romero, R., and Hobbins, J.C.: Amniotic band syndrome: reevaluation of its pathogenesis. Am. J. Obstet. Gynecol. 160:1030–1033, 1989.

Lockwood, C.J., Bach, R., Guha, A., Zhou, X., Miller, W.A., and Nemerson, Y.: Amniotic fluid contains tissue factor, a potent initiator of coagulation. Am. J. Obstet. Gynecol. 165:1335–1341, 1991.

Lopez Bernal, A., Hansell, D.J., Khong, T.Y., Keeling, J.W., and Turnbull, A.C.: Prostaglandin E production by the fetal membranes in unexplained preterm labour and preterm labour associated with chorioamnionitis. Br. J. Obstet. Gynaecol. 96:1133–1139, 1989.

Lubinsky, M., Sujansky, E., Sanger, W., Salyards, P., and Severn, C.: Familial amniotic bands. Am. J. Med. Genet. 14:81–87, 1983.

Lucas, A., Adrian, T.E., Aynsley-Green, A., and Bloom, S.R.: Gut hormones in fetal distress. Lancet 2:968, 1979a.

Lucas, A., Christofides, N.D., Adrian, T.E., Bloom, S.R., and Aynsley-Green, A.: Fetal distress, meconium, and motilin. Lancet 1:718, 1979b.

Luckett, P.: The origin of extraembryonic mesoderm in the early human and rhesus monkey embryos. Anat. Rec. 169: 369–370, 1971.

Luckett, W.P.: Amniogenesis in the early human and rhesus monkey embryos. Anat. Rec. 175:375, 1973.

Ludwig, H., Metzger, H., Korte, M., and Wolf, H.: Die freie Oberfläche des Amnionepithels: rasterelektronenmikroskopische Studie. Arch. Gynecol. 217:141–154, 1974.

MacLachlan, T.B.: A method for the investigation of the strength of the fetal membranes. Am. J. Obstet. Gynecol. 91:309–313, 1965.

Macri, C.J., Schrimmer, D.B., Leung, A., Greenspoon, J.S., and Paul, R.H.: Prophylactic amnioinfusion improves outcome of pregnancy complicated by thick meconium and oligohydramnios. Am. J. Obstet. Gynecol. 167:117–121, 1992.

Madri, J.A., Williams, S.K., Wyatt, T., and Mezzio, C.: Capillary endothelial cell cultures: phenotypic modulation by matrix components. J. Cell Biol. 97:153–165, 1983.

Mahmoud, E.L., Benirschke, K., Vaucher, Y.E., and Poitras, P.: Motilin levels in term neonates who have passed meconium prior to birth. J. Pediatr. Gastroenterol. Nutr. 7:95–99, 1988.

Mahony, B.S., Filly, R.A., Callen, P.W., and Golbus, M.S.: The amniotic band syndrome: antenatal sonographic diagnosis and potential pitfalls. Am. J. Obstet. Gynecol. 152:63–68, 1985.

Malak, T.M., Ockleford, C.D., Bell, S.C., Dalgleish, R., Bight, N., and MacVicar, J.: Confocal immunofluorescence localization of collagen type-I, type-III, type-IV, type-V and type-VI and their ultrastructural organization in term human fetal membranes. Placenta 14:385–406, 1993.

Masson, J.C., Philippe, E., Korn, R., Irrmann, M., Dehalleux, J.M., and Gandar, R.: Amnion nodosum. Rev. Fr. Gynecol. Obstet. 61:701–707, 1966.

Matsubara, S., and Tamada, T.: Ultracytochemical study of the permeability of the human amniotic epithelium. Acta Obstet. Gynaecol. Jpn. 43:641–646, 1991.

McCoshen, J.A., Tulloch, H.V., Johnson, K., and Odowichuk, C.: Evidence of a differential chorionic influence on prostaglandin E_2 release by human amnion before and after term labour. Placenta 7:479, 1986.

McGregor, J.A., French, J.I., Lawellin, D., Franco-Buff, A., Smith, C., and Todd, J.K.: Bacterial protease-induced reduction of chorioamniotic membrane strength and elasticity. Obstet. Gynecol. 69:167–174, 1987.

Mercer, L.J., and Brown, L.G.: Fetal outcome with oligohydramnios in the second trimester. Obstet. Gynecol. 67:840–842, 1986.

Metz, J., Weihe, E., and Heinrich, D.: Intercellular junctions in the full term human placenta. I. Syncytiotrophoblastic layer. Anat. Embryol. (Basel) 158:41–50, 1979.

Meudt, R.: Beitrag zur Festigkeit der menschlichen Eihaut. Gynaecologia 162:430–434, 1966.

Michael, H., Ulbright, T.M., and Brodhecker, C.: Magma reticulare-like differentiation in yolk sac tumor and its pluripotential nature. Mod. Pathol. 1:63A, 1988.

Miller, P.W., Coen, R.W., and Benirschke, K.: Dating the time interval from meconium passage to birth. Obstet. Gynecol. 66:459–462, 1985.

Mitchell, J., Schulman, H., Fleischer, A., Farmakides, G., and Nadeau, D.: Meconium aspiration and fetal acidosis. Obstet. Gynecol. 65:352–355, 1985.

Mitchell, M.D.: Sources of eicosanoids within the uterus during pregnancy. In, The Onset of Labor: Cellular and Integrative Mechanisms. D. McNellis ed., pp. 165–181. Perinatology Press, Ithaca, NY, 1988.

Modesti, A., Kalebic, T., Scarpa, S., Togo, S., Grotendorst, G., Liotta, L.A., and Triche, T.J.: Type V collagen in human amnion is a 12nm fibrillar component of the pericellular interstitium. Eur. J. Cell Biol. 35:246–255, 1984.

Moerman, P., Fryns, J.-P., Vandenberghe, K., and Lauweryns, J.M.: Constrictive amniotic bands, amniotic adhesions, and limb-body wall complex: discrete disruption sequences with pathogenetic overlap. Am. J. Med. Genet. 42:470–479, 1992.

Moessinger, A.C., Blanc, W.A., Byrne, J., Andrews, D., Warburton, D., and Bloom, A.: Amniotic band syndrome associated with amniocentesis. Am. J. Obstet. Gynecol. 141:588–591, 1981.

Mühlhauser, J., Crescimanno, C., Rajaniemi, H., Parkkila, S., Castellucci, M., Milovanov, A.S., and Kaufmann, P.: Immunohistochemistry of carbonic anhydrase in the human placenta and fetal membranes. Histochemistry 101:91–98, 1994.

Muir, R., and Niven, J.S.F.: The local formation of blood pigments. J. Pathol. 41:183–197, 1935.

Mukaida, T., Yoshida, K., Kikyokawa, T., and Soma, H.: Surface structure of the placental membranes. J. Clin. Electron Microsc. 10:447–448, 1977.

Naeye, R.L.: Factors that predispose to premature rupture of the fetal membranes. Obstet. Gynecol. 60:93–98, 1982.

Nanbu, Y., Fujii, S., Konishi, I., Nonogaki, H., and Mori, T.: CA 125 in the epithelium closely related to the embryonic ectoderm: the periderm and the amnion. Am. J. Obstet. Gynecol. 161:462–467, 1989.

Nathan, L., Leveno, K.J., Carmody, T.J., Kelly, M.A., and Sherman, M.L.: Meconium: a 1990s perspective on an old obstetric hazard. Obstet. Gynecol. 83:329–332, 1994.

Nickell, K.A., and Stocker, J.T.: Placental teratoma: a case report. Pediatr. Pathol. 7:645–650, 1987.

Novak, R., and Kokomoor, F.: Placental pathology of meconium-stained premature infants [abstract 35]. Mod. Pathol. 1:7p, 1988.

Nyberg, D.A., Mahony, B.S., and Pretorius, D.H.: Diagnostic Ultrasound of Fetal Anomalies: Text and Atlas. Year Book, Chicago, 1990.

Ockleford, C., Bright, N., Hubbard, A., d'Lacey, C., Smith, J., Gardiner, L., Sheikh, T., Albentosa, M., and Turtle, K.: Micro-trabeculae, macro-plaques or mini-basement membranes in human term fetal membranes. Philos. Trans. R. Soc. Lond. [Biol] 342:121–136, 1994.

Ockleford, C.D., Malak, T., Hubbard, A., Bracken, K., Burton, S.A., Bright, N., Blakey, G., Goodliffe, J., Garrod, D., and d'Lacey, C.: Human amniochorion cytoskeletons at term. Placenta 14:A56, 1993.

Okamoto, E., Takagi, T., Azuma, C., Kimura, T., Tokugawa, Y., Mitsuda, N., Saji, F., and Tanizawa, O.: Expression of the corticotropin-releasing hormone (CRH) gene in human placenta and amniotic membrane. Horm. Metab. Res. 22: 394–397, 1990.

Okazaki, T., Casey, M.L., Okita, J.R., MacDonald, P.C., and Johnston, J.M.: Initiation of human parturition. XII. Biosynthesis and metabolism of prostaglandins in human fetal membranes and uterine decidua. Am. J. Obstet. Gynecol. 139:373–381, 1981a.

Okazaki, T., Sagawa, N., Bleasdale, J.E., Okita, J.R., MacDonald, P.C., and Johnston, J.M.: Initiation of human parturition. XIII. Phospholipase C, phospholipase A2, and diacylglycerol lipase activities in fetal membranes and decidua vera tissues from early and late gestation. Biol. Reprod. 25:103–109, 1981b.

Oláh, K.S., Gee, H., Rushton, I., and Fowlie, A.: Massive subchorionic thrombohaematoma presenting as a placental tumor: a case report. Br. J. Obstet. Gynaecol. 94:995–997, 1987.

Olson, D.M., and Smieja, Z.: Arachidonic acid incorporation into lipids of term human amnion. Am. J. Obstet. Gynecol. 159:995–1001, 1988.

Olson, D.M., Skinner, K., and Challis, J.R.: Prostaglandin output in relation to parturition by cells dispersed from human intrauterine tissues. J. Clin. Endocrinol. Metab. 57:694–699, 1983.

Opitz, H., and Bernoth, E.: Strukturuntersuchungen der menschlichen Eihaut nach vor- und rechtzeitigem Blasensprung. Arch. Gynecol. 196:435–446, 1962.

Ostrea, E.M., and Naqvi, M.: The influence of gestational age on the ability of the fetus to pass meconium in utero: clinical implications. Acta Obstet. Gynecol. Scand. 61:275–277, 1982.

Panayiotis, G., and Grunstein, S.: Extramembranous pregnancy in twin gestation. Obstet. Gynecol. 53:34S–35S, 1979.

Paterson, W.G., Grant, K.A., Grant, J.M., and McLean, N.: The pathogenesis of amniotic fluid embolism with particular reference to transabdominal amniocentesis. Eur. J. Obstet. Gynecol. Reprod. Biol. 7:319–324, 1977.

Patten, R.M., Allen, M.V., Mack, L.A., Wilson, D., Nyberg, D., Hirsch, J., and Viamont, T.: Limb-body wall complex: in utero sonographic diagnosis of a complicated fetal malformation. Am. J. Radiol. 146:1019–1024, 1986.

Patterson, T.J.S.: Amniotic bands. In, The Human Amnion and Chorion. G.L. Bourne, ed. Lloyd-Luke, London, 1962.

Pearlstone, M., and Baxi, L.: Subchorionic hematoma: a review. Obstet. Gynecol. Surv. 48:65–68, 1993.

Pedersen, J.F., and Mantoni, M.: Prevalence and significance of subchorionic hemorrhage in threatened abortion: a sonographic study. Am. J. Roentgenol. 154:535–537, 1990.

Perlman, M., Tennenbaum, A., Menash, M., and Ornoy, A.: Extramembranous pregnancy: maternal, placental, and perinatal implications. Obstet. Gynecol. 55:34S–37S, 1980.

Petry, G.: Die Bedeutung der Embryonalhüllen bei der Frage nach der Herkunft alkalischer Phosphatase im menschlichen Fruchtwasser. Z. Geburtshilfe Gynäkol. 158:171–180, 1962.

Philippe, E., Dourov, N., Muller, P., and Fruhling, L.: Le substratum morphologique de l'embolie amniotique: a propos de deux observations d'incoagulabilité sanguine par embolie amniotique. Ann. Anat. Pathol. 6:479–496, 1961.

Pilgram, H.: Die Zotten und Karunkeln des menschlichen Amnion. Marburg, 1889. Cited by Blanc et al. (1962).

Platt, L.D., DeVore, G.R., and Gimovsky, M.L.: Failed amniocentesis: the role of membrane tenting. Am. J. Obstet. Gynecol. 144:479–480, 1982.

Poisner, A.M., Wood, G.W., Poisner, R., and Inagami, T.: Localization of renin in trophoblasts in human chorion laeve at term pregnancy. Endocrinology 109:1150–1155, 1981.

Polano, O.: Beiträge zur Anatomie und Physiologie des menschlichen Amnions. Z. Anat. Entwicklungsgesch. 63: 539–553, 1922.

Polet, H.: The effect of hydrocortisone on the membranes of primary human amnion cells in vitro. Exp. Cell Res. 41: 316–323, 1966.

Polishuk, W.Z., Kohane, S., and Peranio, A.: The physical properties of fetal membranes. Obstet. Gynecol. 20:204–210, 1962.

Polishuk, W.Z., Kohane, S., and Hadar, A.: Fetal weight and membrane tensile strength. Am. J. Obstet. Gynecol. 20: 204–250, 1964.

Polishuk, W.Z., Boxer, J., and Granzfried, R.: Lipid in amniotic membranes. Am. J. Obstet. Gynecol. 91:61–64, 1965.

Pomerance, W., Biezenski, J.J., Moltz, A., and Goodman, J.: Origin of amniotic fluid lipids. II. Abnormal pregnancy. Obstet. Gynecol. 38:379–382, 1971.

Porreco, R.P., Young, P.E., Resnik, R., Cousins, L., Jones, O.W., Richards, T., Kernahan, C., and Matson, M.: Reproductive outcome following amniocentesis for genetic indications. Am. J. Obstet. Gynecol. 143:653–660, 1982.

Pritchard, E.T., Armstrong, W.D., and Wilt, J.C.: Examination of lipids from amnion, chorion, and vernix. Am. J. Obstet. Gynecol. 100:289–298, 1968.

Pysher, T.J.: Discordant congenital malformations in monozygous twins: the amniotic band disruption complex. Diagn. Gynecol. Obstet. 2:221–225, 1980.

Queenan, J.T., Thompson, W., Whitfield, C.R., and Shah, S.I.: Amniotic fluid volumes in normal pregnancies. Am. J. Obstet. Gynecol. 114:34–38, 1972.

Rajabi, M.R., Dean, D.D., and Woessner, J.F.: Changes in active and latent collagenase in human placenta around time of parturition. Am. J. Obstet. Gynecol. 163:499–505, 1990.

Randel, S.B., Filly, R.A., Callen, P.W., Anderson, R.L., and Golbus, M.S.: Amniotic sheets. Radiology 166:633–636, 1988.

Rao, C.V., and Lei, Z.M.: The presence of gonadotropin receptors in human placenta, amnion, chorion and decidua. Placenta 10:458, 1989.

Rao, C.V., Carman, F.R., Chegini, N., and Schultz, G.S.: Binding sites for epidermal growth factor in human fetal membranes. J. Clin. Endocrinol. Metab. 58:1034–1042, 1984.

Rastan, S., Kaufman, M.H., Handyside, A.H., and Lyon, M.F.: X-chromosome inactivation in extraembryonic membranes of diploid parthenogenetic mouse embryos

demonstrated by differential staining. Nature 288:172–173, 1980.

Reale, E., Wang, T., Zaccheo, D., Maganza, C., and Pescetto, G.: Junctions on the maternal blood surface of the human placental syncytium. Placenta 1:245–258, 1980.

Redmond, A.D.: Amnion dressing. Lancet 1:902, 1984.

Rees, M.C.P., di Marzo, V., Lopez Bernal, A., Tippins, J.R., Morris, H.R., and Turnbull, A.C.: Leukotriene release by human fetal membranes, placenta and decidua in relation to parturition. J. Endocrinol. 118:497–500, 1988.

Rehder, H., and Weitzel, H.: Intrauterine amputations after amniocentesis. Lancet 1:382, 1978.

Reisfield, D.R.: Congenital defect in the fetal membranes: a condition simulating spontaneous rupture. Bull. Sloane Hosp. Women 4:16–18, 1958.

Reshef, E., Lei, Z.M., Rao, C.V., Pridham, D.D., Chegini, N., and Luborsky, J.L.: The presence of gonadotropin receptors in nonpregnant human uterus, human placenta, fetal membranes, and decidua. J. Clin. Endocrinol. Metab. 70:421–430, 1990.

Resnik, R., Swartz, W.H., Plumer, M.H., Benirschke, K., and Stratthaus, M.E.: Amniotic fluid embolism with survival. Obstet. Gynecol. 47:295–298, 1976.

Robb, S.A., and Hytten, F.E.: Placental glycogen. Br. J. Obstet. Gynaecol. 83:43–53, 1976.

Roberts, J.S., McCraken, J.A., Gavagan, J.E., and Soloff, M.S.: Oxytocin-stimulated release of prostaglandin $F_{2\alpha}$ from ovine endometrium in vitro: correlation with estrous cycle and oxytocin-receptor binding. Endocrinology 99: 1107–1114, 1976.

Rogers, B.B., Widness, J.A., Coustan, D.R., and Singer, D.B.: Fetal acidosis and placental pathology [abstract 498]. Mod. Pathol. 3(1):85A, 1990.

Ropers, H.H., Wolff, G., and Hitzeroth, H.W.: Preferential X inactivation in human placenta membranes: is the paternal X inactive in early embryonic development of female mammals? Hum. Genet. 43:265–273, 1978.

Rossant, J., and Croy, B.A.: Genetic identification of tissue of origin of cellular populations within the mouse placenta. J. Embryol. Exp. Morphol. 86:177–189, 1985.

Rote, N.S., Menon, R., Swan, K.F., Lyden, T.W., and Fortunato, S.J.: Expression of IL-1β and IL-6 protein and mRNA in amniochorionic membrane. Placenta 14:A63, 1993.

Rubovits, W.H., Taft, E., and Neuwelt, F.: The pathologic properties of meconium. Am. J. Obstet. Gynecol. 36:501–505, 1938.

Sakbun, V., Ali, S.M., Greenwood, F.C., and Bryant-Greenwood, G.D.: Human relaxin in the amnion, chorion, decidua parietalis, basal plate, and placental trophoblast by immunocytochemistry and Northern analysis. J. Clin. Endocrinol. Metab. 70:508–514, 1990a.

Sakbun, V., Ali, S.M., Lee, Y.A., Jara, C.S., and Bryant-Greenwood, G.D.: Immunocytochemical localization and messenger ribonucleic acid concentrations for human placental lactogen in amnion, chorion, decidua, and placenta. Am. J. Obstet. Gynecol. 162:1310–1317, 1990b.

Sala, M.A., and Matheus, M.: Histochemical study of the fetal membranes in the human term pregnancy. Gegenbaurs Morphol. Jahrb. 130:699–705, 1984.

Salazar, H., Kanbour, A.I., and Pardo, M.: Amnion nodosum: ultrastructure and histopathogenesis. Arch. Pathol. 98:39–46, 1974.

Santiago-Schwarz, F., and Fleit, H.B.: Identification of non-adherent mononuclear cells in human cord blood that differentiate into macrophages. J. Leukocyte Biol. 43:51–59, 1988.

Schindler, A.E.: Hormones in human amniotic fluid. Monogr. Endocrinol. 21:1–158, 1982.

Schindler, P.D.: Nuclear deoxyribonucleic acid (DNA) content, nuclear size and cell size in the human amnion epithelium. Acta Anat. (Basel) 44:273–285, 1961.

Schmidt, W.: Der Feinbau der reifen menschlichen Eihäute. Z. Anat. Entwicklungsgesch. 119:203–222, 1956.

Schmidt, W.: Struktur und Funktion des Amnionepithels von Menschen und Huhn. Z. Zellforsch. 61:642–660, 1963.

Schmidt, W.: Über den paraplacentaren, fruchtwassergebundenen Stofftransport beim Menschen. I. Histochemische Untersuchung der in den Eihäuten angereicherten Stoffe. Z. Anat. Entwicklungsgesch. 124:321–334, 1965a.

Schmidt, W.: Untersuchungen zur Frage des paraplazentaren Stofftransportes beim Menschen. Anat. Anz. 115:161–163, 1965b.

Schmidt, W.: Über den paraplacentaren, fruchtwassergebundenen Stofftransport beim Menschen. II. Nachweis der vom Amnion abgegebenen Lipide im Fruchtwasser und im Dünndarm des Keimes. Z. Anat. Entwicklungsgesch. 126:276–288, 1967.

Schmidt, W.: The amniotic fluid compartment: the fetal habitat. Adv. Anat. Embryol. Cell Biol. 127:1–100, 1992.

Schmidt, W., Eberhagen, D., and Svejcar, J.: Über den paraplazentaren, fruchtwassergebundenen Stofftransport beim Menschen. III. Quantitative und qualitative Analyse der im Fruchtwasser enthaltenen Stoffe. Z. Anat. Entwicklungsgesch. 135:210–221, 1971.

Schulze, B., Schlesinger, C.H., and Miller, K.: Chromosomal mosaicism confined to chorionic tissue. Prenat. Diagn. 7:451–453, 1987.

Schwarzacher, H.G.: Beitrag zur Histogenese des menschlichen Amnion. Acta Anat. (Basel) 43:303–311, 1960.

Schwarzacher, H.G., and Klinger, H.P.: Die Entstehung mehrkerniger Zellen durch Amitose in Amnionepithel des Menschen und die Aufteilung des chromosomalen Materials auf deren einzelne Kerne. Z. Zellforsch. 60:741–754, 1963.

Seeds, A.E., Eichhorst, B.C., and Stolee, A.: Factors determining human chorion laeve permeability in vitro. Am. J. Obstet. Gynecol. 128:13–21, 1977.

Seeds, J.W., Cefalo, R.C., and Herbert, W.N.P.: Amniotic band syndrome. Am. J. Obstet. Gynecol. 144:243–248, 1982.

Seidman, J.D., Abbondanzo, S.L., Watkin, W.G., Ragsdale, B., and Manz, H.J.: Amniotic band syndrome: report of two cases and review of the literature. Arch. Pathol. Lab. Med. 113:891–897, 1989.

Sepkowitz, S.: Influence of the legal imperative and medical guidelines on the incidence and management of the meconium-stained newborn. Am. J. Dis. Child. 141:1124–1127, 1987.

Shanklin, D.R., and Scott, J.S.: Massive subchorial throm-

bohaematoma (Breus' mole). Br. J. Obstet. Gynaecol. 82:476–487, 1975.

Shephard, T.H., Fantel, A.G., Fujinaga, M., and Fitzsimmons, J.: Amniotic band disruption syndrome: why do their faces look alike? [abstract]. Congen. Anom. (Japan) 37:491–492, 1988.

Shimizu, T., Dudley, D.K.L., Borodchack, P., Belcher, J., Perkins, S.L., and Gibb, W.: Effect of smoking on fibronectin production by human amnion and placenta. Gynecol. Obstet. Invest. 34:142–145, 1992.

Silver, M.M., Thurston, W.A., and Patrick, J.E.: Perinatal pulmonary hyperplasia due to laryngeal atresia. Hum. Pathol. 19:110–113, 1988.

Singh, G., and Singh, S.: Hemorrhage induced by amniocentesis and vascular clamping in the limbs of rat fetuses. Congen. Anom. (Japan) 18:89–93, 1978.

Singhas, C.A.: Lectin histochemistry of the human amniochorionic membrane complex. Placenta 13:523–534, 1992.

Sinha, A.A.: Ultrastructure of human amnion and amniotic plaques of normal pregnancy. Z. Zellforsch. 122:1–14, 1971.

Skinner, K.A., and Challis, J.R.: Changes in the synthesis and metabolism of prostaglandins by human fetal membranes and decidua at labor. Am. J. Obstet. Gynecol. 151:519–523, 1985.

Skinner, S.J., Campos, G.A., and Liggins, G.C.: Collagen content of human amniotic membranes: effect of gestational length and premature rupture. Obstet. Gynecol. 57:487–489, 1981.

Smadja, A., Hoang Ngoc Minh, and Nguyen, T.L.: Conception nouvelle sur la physiologie de la circulation amniotique. Rev. Fr. Gynecol. 69:111–114, 1974.

Smieja, Z., Zakar, T., Walton, J.C., and Olson, D.M.: Prostaglandin endoperoxide synthase kinetics in human amnion before and after labor at term and following preterm labor. Placenta 14:163–175, 1993.

Smith, L.A., and Pounder, D.J.: A teratoma-like lesion of the placenta: a case report. Pathology 14:85–87, 1982.

Sonek, J., Gabbe, S.G., Iams, J.D., and Kniss, D.A.: Morphologic changes in the human amnion epithelium that accompany labor as seen with scanning and transmission electron microscopy. Am. J. Obstet. Gynecol. 164:1174–1180, 1991.

Spirt, B.A., Gordon, L.P., and Silverman, R.K.: Letter to the editor. J. Ultrasound Med. 3:167–168, 1993.

Starck, D.: Embryologie. Thieme, Stuttgart, 1975.

Steer, P.J., Eigbe, F., Lissauer, T.J., and Beard, R.W.: Interrelationships among abnormal cardiotocograms in labor, meconium staining of the amniotic fluid, arterial cord blood pH, and Apgar scores. Obstet. Gynecol. 74:715–720, 1989.

Steiner, P.E., and Lushbaugh, C.C.: Maternal pulmonary embolism by amniotic fluid as cause of obstetric shock and unexpected deaths in obstetrics. J.A.M.A. 117:1245–1254, 1340–1345, 1941.

Stempel, L.E., and Nelson, D.M.: Retained chorionic membrane following repeated amniocenteses. Am. J. Obstet. Gynecol. 142:242–243, 1982.

Street, D.M., and Cunningham, F.: Congenital anomalies

caused by intra-uterine bands. Clin. Orthop. 37:82–97, 1964.

Streeter, G.L.: Focal deficiencies in fetal tissues and their relation to intrauterine amputations. Contrib. Embryol. Carnegie Inst. 22:1–15, 1930.

Sutcliffe, R.G.: The nature and origin of the soluble protein in human amniotic fluid. Biol. Rev. 50:1–33, 1975.

Symchych, P.S., and Winchester, P.: Animal model: amniotic fluid deficiency and fetal lung growth in the rat. Am. J. Pathol. 90:779–782, 1978.

Symonds, E.M., Skinner, S.L., Stanley, M.A., Kirkland, J.A., and Ellis, R.C.: An investigation of the cellular source of renin in human chorion. J. Obstet. Gynaecol. Br. Commonw. 77:885–890, 1970.

Szendi, B.: Experimentelle Untersuchungen beim Menschen Über den Austausch und die intrauterine Rolle des Fruchtwassers. Arch. Gynecol. 170:205–227, 1940.

Talmi, Y.P., Sigler, L., Inge, E., Finkelstein, Y., and Zohar, Y.: Antibacterial properties of human amniotic membranes. Placenta 12:285–288, 1991.

Tarantal, A.F., and Hendrickx, A.G.: Amniotic band syndrome in a rhesus monkey: a case report. J. Med. Primatol. 16:291–299, 1987.

Teodoro, W.R., Andreucci, D., and Palma, J.A.: Short communication: placental collagen and premature rupture of fetal membranes. Placenta 11:549–551, 1990.

Thiede, H.A., and Choate, J.W.: Chorionic localization in the human placenta by immunofluorescent staining. II. Demonstration of hCG in the trophoblast and amnion epithelium of immature and mature placentas. Obstet. Gynecol. 22:433–443, 1963.

Thomas, C.E.: The ultrastructure of human amnion epithelium. J. Ultrastruct. Res. 13:65–84, 1965.

Thompson, V.M.: Amnion nodosum. J. Obstet. Gynaecol. Br. Emp. 67:611–614, 1960.

Thorburn, M.J.: Sex-chromatin in a 13-day embryo. Lancet 1:277–278, 1964.

Tibboel, D., Vermey-Keers, C., Klück, P., Gaillard, J.L.J., Kloppenberg, J., and Molenaar, J.C.: The natural history of gastroschisis during fetal life: development of the fibrous coating on the bowel loops. Teratology 33:267–272, 1986.

Torpin, R.: Fetal Malformations Caused by Amnion Rupture during Gestation. Charles C Thomas, Springfield, IL, 1968.

Torpin, R.: The Human Placenta. Its Shape, Form, Origin and Development. Charles C Thomas, Springfield, IL, 1969.

Torpin, R., and Faulkner, A.: Intrauterine amputation with the missing member found in the fetal membranes. J.A.M.A. 198:185–187, 1966.

Torpin, R., Goodman, L., and Gramling, Z.W.: Amnion string swallowed by fetus. Am. J. Obstet. Gynecol. 90:829–830, 1964.

Toth, P., and Rao, C.V.: Direct novel regulation of cyclooxygenase (COX) and prostacyclin synthase (PGI$_2$-S) by hCG in human amnion. Placenta 13:A63, 1992.

Toth, P., Li, X., and Rao, C.V.: Expression of hCG/LH receptor gene and its functional coupling to the regulation of cyclooxygenase-1 and -2 enzymes in human fetal membranes. Placenta 14:A78, 1993.

Trasler, D.G., Walker, B.E., and Fraser, F.C.: Congenital malformations produced by amniotic-sac puncture. Science 124:439, 1956.

Trimmer, K.J., and Gilstrap, L.C.: "Meconiumcrit" and birth asphyxia. Am. J. Obstet. Gynecol. 165:1010–1013, 1991.

Tuller, M.A.: Amniotic fluid embolism, afibrinogenemia, and disseminated fibrin thrombosis: Case report and review of the literature. Am. J. Obstet. Gynecol. 73:273–287, 1957.

Uhing, M.R., Bhat, R., Philobos, M., and Raju, T.N.K.: Value of amnioinfusion in reducing meconium aspiration syndrome. Am. J. Perinatol. 10:43–45, 1993.

Unger, J.: Placental teratoma. Am. J. Clin. Pathol. 92:371–373, 1989.

Usher, R.H., Boyd, M.E., McLean, F.H., and Kramer, M.S.: Assessment of fetal risk in postdate pregnancies. Am. J. Obstet. Gynecol. 158:259–264, 1988.

Uyehara, C.F.T., and Claybaugh, J.R.: Vasopressin metabolism in the amniotic sac of the fetal guinea pig. Endocrinology 123:2040–2047, 1988.

Vago, T., and Chavkin, J.: Extramembranous pregnancy: an unusual complication of amniocentesis. Am. J. Obstet. Gynecol. 137:511–512, 1980.

Van Bogaert, L.-J., Maldague, P., and Staquet, J.-P.: Morphologic changes in the amniotic epithelium in relation to placental weight and fetal maturity. Arch. Gynecol. 226: 241–245, 1978.

Vantrappen, G., Janssens, J., Peeters, T.L., Bloom, S.R., Christofides, N.D., and Hellemans, J.: Motilin and the interdigestive migrating motor complex in man. Am. J. Dig. Dis. 24:497–500, 1979.

Verbeek, J.H., Robertson, E.M., and Haust, M.D.: Basement membranes (amniotic, trophoblastic, capillary) and adjacent tissue in term placenta. Am. J. Obstet. Gynecol. 99:1136–1146, 1967.

Verjaal, M., Leschot, N.J., Wolf, N.J., and Treffers, P.E.: Karyotypic differences between cells from placenta and other fetal tissues. Prenat. Diagn. 7:343–348, 1987.

Verma, I.C., and Ghai, O.P.: Study of sex chromatin in amniotic membranes of newborns. Indian J. Med. Res. 59:1660–1665, 1971.

Wagner, G., and Tygstrup, I.: Oligohydramnios and urinary malformations in early human pregnancy. Acta Pathol. Microbiol. Scand. 59:273–278, 1963.

Wang, T.: Fetalmembranen des Menschen. Fortschr. Med. 46:1185–1188, 1984.

Wang, T., and Schneider, J.: Myofibroblasten im Bindegewebe des menschlichen Amnions. Z. Geburtshilfe Perinatol. 186:164–168, 1982.

Wang, T., and Schneider, J.: Cellular junctions on the free surface of human placental syncytium. Arch. Gynecol. 240: 211–216, 1987.

Wehbeh, H., Fleisher, J., Karimi, A., Mathony, A., and Minkoff, H.: The relationship between the ultrasonographic diagnosis of innocent amniotic band development and pregnancy outcomes. Obstet. Gynecol. 81:565–568, 1993.

Weitzner, J.S., Strassner, H.T., Rawlins, R.G., Mack, S.R., and Anderson, R.A.: Objective assessment of meconium content of amniotic fluid. Obstet. Gynecol. 76:1143–1144, 1990.

Wentworth, P., and Turnbull, I.: Bilateral renal agenesis (Potter's syndrome) J. Reprod. Med. 3:87–91, 1969.

Weser, H., and Kaufmann, P.: Lichtmikroskopische und histochemische Untersuchungen an der Chorionplatte der reifen menschlichen Placenta. Arch. Gynecol. 225:15–30, 1978.

Wewer, U.M., Faber, M., Liotta, L.A., and Albrechtsen, R.: Immunochemical and ultrastructural assessment of the nature of pericellular basement membrane of human decidual cells. Lab. Invest. 53:624–633, 1985.

Wigglesworth, J.S., and Desai, R.: Is fetal respiratory function a major determinant of perinatal survival? Lancet 1: 264–267, 1982.

Wiswell, T.E., Foster, N.H., Slayter, M.V., and Hachey, W.E.: Management of a piglet model of the meconium aspiration syndrome with high-frequency or conventional ventilation. Am. J. Dis. Child. 146:1287–1293, 1992.

Wolf, H.J., and Desoye, G.: Immunohistochemical localization of glucose transporters and insulin receptors in human fetal membranes at term. Histochemistry 100:379–385, 1993.

Wolf, H.J., and Schmidt, W.: Histochemical study of carbohydrate metabolism in fetal membranes. Acta Histochem. 91:3–11, 1991.

Wolf, H.J., Schmidt, W., and Drenckhahn, D.: Immunocytochemical analysis of the cytoskeleton of the human amniotic epithelium. Cell Tissue Res. 266:385–389, 1991.

Wong, F.W.S., Loong, E.P.L., and Chang, A.M.Z.: Ultrasound diagnosis of meconium-stained amniotic fluid. Am. J. Obstet. Gynecol. 150:359, 1985.

Woolnough, H.C.: Amniotic band syndrome. [abstract]. Teratology 36:150, 1987.

Woyton, J.: Encephalocele attached to the placenta. Am. J. Obstet. Gynecol. 81:1028–1032, 1961.

Wynn, R.M.: Morphology of the placenta. In, Biology of Gestation. N.S. Assali, ed. Academic Press, Orlands, FL, 1968.

Wynn, R.: Ultrastructural development of the human decidua. Am. J. Obstet. Gynecol. 118:652–670, 1974.

Wynn, R.M., and French, G.L.: Comparative ultrastructure of the mammalian amnion. Obstet. Gynecol. 31:759–774, 1968.

Wynn, R.M., Sever, P.S., and Hellman, L.M.: Morphologic studies of the ruptured amnion. Am. J. Obstet. Gynecol. 99:359–367, 1967.

Yamaguchi, Y., Isemura, M., Yosizawa, Z., Kurosawa, K., Yoshinaga, K., Sato, A., and Suzuki, M.: Changes in the distribution of fibronectin in the placenta during normal human pregnancy. Am. J. Obstet. Gynecol. 152:715–718, 1985.

Yeomans, E.R., Gilstrap, L.C., Leveno, K.J., and Burris, J.S.: Meconium in the amniotic fluid and fetal acid-base status. Obstet. Gynecol. 73:175–178, 1989.

Yoder, B.A.: Meconium-stained amniotic fluid and respiratory complications: impact of selective tracheal suction. Obstet. Gynecol. 83:77–84, 1994.

Yoshimura, S., Nishimura, T., and Yoshida, Y.: The morphometry of the sudan-III-positive granules in the cytoplasm of the human amniotic epithelium. Acta Cytol. (Baltimore) 224:44–48, 1980.

Young, I.D., Lindenbaum, R.H., Thompson, E.M., and Pembrey, M.E.: Amniotic bands in connective tissue disorders. Arch. Dis. Child. 60:1061–1063, 1985.

Yurchenco, P.D., and Ruben, G.C.: Basement membrane structure in situ: evidence for lateral associations in the type IV collagen network. J. Cell Biol. 105:2559–2568, 1994.

Zorn, E.M., Hanson, F.W., Greve, L.C., Phelps-Sandall, B., and Tennant, F.R.: Analysis of the significance and origin of the discolored amniotic fluid detected at midtrimester amniocentesis. Am. J. Obstet. Gynecol. 154:1234–1240, 1986.

13
Anatomy and Pathology of the Umbilical Cord and Major Fetal Vessels

DEVELOPMENT

The development of the umbilical cord is closely related to that of the amnion (see Chapter 12). Throughout the last days of the second week p.c. the blastocystic cavity is being filled by a loose meshwork of mesoderm cells, the extraembryonic mesoblast, which surrounds the embryoblast (Figure 208, day 13). The embryoblast at that time is composed of two vesicles: the amnionic vesicle and the primary yolk sac. When these two vesicles are in contact with each other, they form the double-layered embryonic disk. During the following days the extraembryonic mesoderm cells are rearranged in such a way that they line the inner surface of the trophoblastic shell, as chorionic mesoderm. They also cover the surface of the two embryonic vesicles (Figure 208, day 18). Between the two mesoderm layers the exocoelomic cavity forms. It largely separates the embryo and its mesodermal cover from the chorionic mesoderm. The exocoelom is bridged by the mesoderm in only one place, which lies basal to the amnionic vesicle. This mesenchymal connection is referred to as the connecting stalk (Figure 208, day 18). It fixes the early embryo to the membranes and is the early forerunner of the umbilical cord. During the same period (around day 18 p.c.) a duct-like extension of the yolk sac, originating from the future caudal region of the embryo, develops into the connecting stalk. This structure is the transitory allantois, the primitive extraembryonic urinary bladder.

The three subsequent weeks are characterized by three developmental processes.

1. The embryo rotates in such a way that the yolk sac vesicle, originally facing the region opposite the implantation site, is turned toward the implantation pole.
2. The amnionic vesicle enlarges considerably, extending around the embryo.
3. The originally flat embryonic disk is bent in the anteroposterior direction and rolled up in the lateral direction. It thus "herniates" into the amnionic vesicle. As the embryo bends it subdivides the yolk sac into an intraembryonic duct (the gut) and an extraembryonic part (the omphaloenteric or omphalomesenteric duct), which is dilated peripherally to form the extraembryonic yolk sac vesicle.

Both the allantois and the extraembryonic yolk sac extend into the mesenchyme of the connecting stalk (Figure 208, day 22). Between days 28 and 40 p.c. the expanding amnionic cavity has surrounded the embryo so far that the connecting stalk, the allantois, and the yolk sac are compressed to a slender cord, which is then covered by amnionic epithelium (Figure 208, day 28).

They thus form the umbilical cord. The cord lengthens as the embryo "prolapses" backward into the amnionic sac (Hertig, 1962). During the same process of expansion, the amnionic mesenchyme locally touches and finally fuses with the chorionic mesoderm, occluding the exocoelomic cavity. This process persists until the middle of pregnancy when, at approximately 12 weeks, the amnionic cavity completely occupies the exocoelom so that amnionic and chorionic mesenchyme have fused everywhere.

During the 3rd week p.c. the extraembryonic yolk sac, the omphalomesenteric duct that connects with the embryonic gut, and the allantois become supplied with fetal vessels. All mammals use either allantoic or yolk sac vessels for vascularization of the placenta. The human allantoic vessels, two allantoic arteries originating from the internal iliac arteries and one allantoic vein that enters the hepatic vein, invade the placenta and become connected to the villous vessels. The allantoic participation in placental vascularization is the reason for the name "chorioallantoic" placenta. In contrast, with choriovitelline or vitelline placentation (e.g., that of rodents and bats) the yolk sac vessels establish fetoplacental vascular connections.

The development of the cord has been treated in great detail in the classical text by Cullen (1916). Unfortunately, this book is so inaccessible that it is rarely cited, let alone read. Another major review with special reference to comparative anatomy is that by Arvy and Pilleri (1976a). This volume brings together an enormous amount of material and is of particular interest because so many features considered to be abnormal in human placentas are normal features in some other species. Thus many animals have pronounced squamous metaplasia on the cord's surface and nodules, not only near its abdominal end, which make the surface feel somewhat sandy.

Amnionic Epithelium

The cord is covered by amnionic epithelium. Near the umbilicus, a largely unkeratinized, stratified squamous epithelium provides the transition from the abdominal wall to the cord's surface. Farther away from the umbilicus, the epithelium transforms into a stratified columnar epithelium (two to eight layers) and finally into a simple columnar epithelium (Hoyes, 1969; Sinha, 1971; Hempel, 1972). The latter continues developing into the simple columnar to cuboidal epithelium of the

319

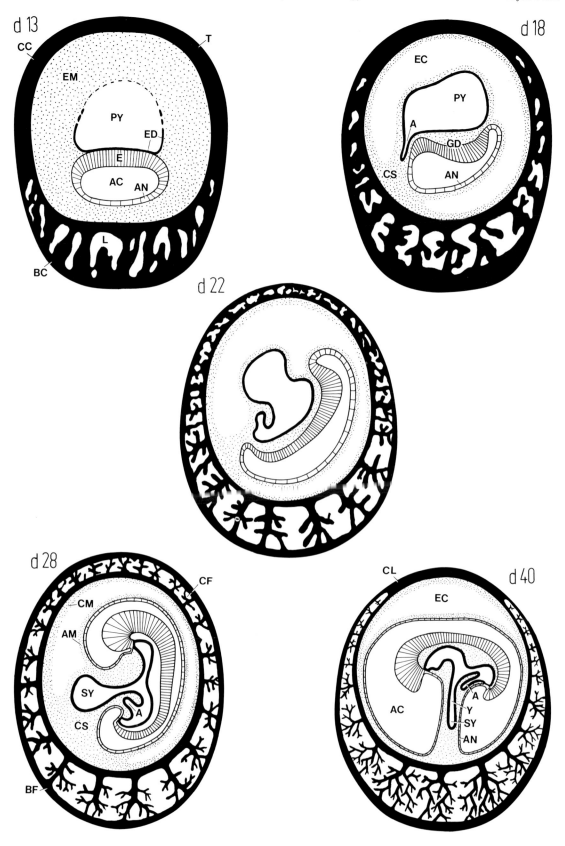

placental amnionic surface. The basal cells of the stratified parts of the amnion resemble the amnionic epithelium of the membranes, whereas the superficial cells sometimes are squamous, poor in organelles, and pyknotic (Bourne, 1962). Parry and Abramovich (1970) found two principal cell types, with intermediates. In contrast to earlier theories, they suggested that these cells do not have any water-regulatory function. Therefore if there is a larger water content in the proximal portion of the cord it must have other underlying causes. In this context it is interesting to note that Gebrane-Younes and coworkers (1986), based on the ultrastructure of the umbilical endothelium and other wall components, have suggested a considerable fluid transudation out of the umbilical vessels into the amnionic fluid.

In general, the amnion of the cord is structurally similar to that described in the membranes (see Chapter 12). Moreover, there are no indications that it is different in terms of its basic functions (see Chapter 12). In contrast to the amnion that covers the chorionic surface of the placenta, however, and that of the membranes where it is easily detached, the amnion of the cord grows firmly into the central connective tissue core. It cannot be dislodged.

Wharton's Jelly

The connective tissue of the cord, or Wharton's jelly, is derived from the extraembryonic mesoblast. McKay et al. (1955) referred to this jelly-like material as a "thixotropic gel" because it liquefies when touched (see also Bacsich & Riddell, 1945). The incorporation of this mesenchyme into the cord substance and the sub-amnionic layers probably accounts for their mucoid and compressible structures. The importance of this faculty

was stressed by Reynolds (1952). He likened the compressed (by distended fetal vessels) Wharton's jelly to erectile tissue. It is clearly true that a filled umbilical cord is a relatively firm, rigid structure, and that with expansion and contraction of the vasculature its thickness and turgidity vary. Wharton's jelly is composed of a ground substance of open-chain polysaccharides (hyaluronic acid: Graumann, 1964; carbohydrates with glycosyl and mannosyl groups: Yamada & Shimizu, 1976), distributed in a fine network of microfibrils and little collagen. It contains evenly distributed spindle-shaped fibroblasts with long extensions (Parry, 1970) and numerous mast cells. These cells can be stained selectively, surround the vessels densely, and are also found underneath the cord surface (Moore, 1956). There are surprisingly few macrophages in the umbilical cord. Even when the cord is deep green owing to meconium staining and when meconium-filled macrophages are readily seen in the membranes, only relatively few activated and pigmented macrophages are seen in the cord substance. Similarly, after intrafunicular bleeding hemosiderin is not formed in situ.

The tensile properties of the cord have been reported by Ghosh et al. (1984). No significant differences in the tensile parameters with respect to the sex of the baby have been found, but there was a significant positive correlation between the tensile breaking load and the birth weight of the infant. The average tensile breaking load is 2.49 times the weight of the baby at birth.

Structure of Umbilical Vessels

There are normally two arteries and one vein in the human umbilical cord (Figure 209). An originally developed second umbilical vein atrophies during the second month of pregnancy. In rare cases—1% accord-

---

FIGURE 208. Development of the umbilical cord and amnion. (a) Day 13 p.c. The embryonic disk consists of two epithelial layers: the ectoderm (E), which is contiguous with the amnionic epithelium (AN), and the entoderm (ED), which partially surrounds the primary yolk sac cavity (PY). Both vesicles are surrounded by the extraembryonic mesoderm (EM). T = trophoblast; CC = capsular chorion; L = lacuna; BC = basal chorion. (b) Day 18 p.c. At this stage the entoderm has become closely applied to the periphery of the yolk sac; and at the presumptive caudal end of the germinal disk (GD) the allantoic invagination (A) has occurred. In the extra-embryonic mesoderm, the exocoelom (EC) has cavitated. A mesenchymal bridge, the connecting stalk (CS), has developed and will ultimately form the umbilical cord. (c) Day 28 p.c. The embryo has begun to rotate and fold. The primary yolk sac is being subdivided into the intraembryonic intestinal tract and the secondary (extraembryonic) yolk sac (SY). The secondary yolk sac and allantois extrude from the future

embryonic intestinal tract into the connecting stalk. The amnionic sac largely surrounds the embryo because of its folding and rotation. Villous formation has occurred at the entire periphery of the chorionic vesicle, forming the chorion frondosum (CF). BF = basal chorion frondosum; CM = chorionic mesoderm; AM = amnionic mesoderm. (d) Day 40 p.c. The embryo has now fully rotated and folded. It is completely surrounded by the amnionic cavity and is attached to the umbilical cord. The latter has developed from the connecting stalk as it has become covered by amnionic membrane. The exocoelom has become largely compressed by the expansion of the amnionic cavity (AC). At the abembryonic pole of the chorionic vesicle, the recently formed placental villi gradually atrophy, forming the chorion laeve (CL). Only that portion that retains villous tissue, which has the insertion of the umbilical cord, develops into the placental disk. Y = yolk sac.

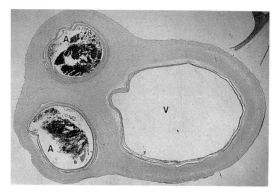

FIGURE 209. Cross section of mature umbilical cord near its placental insertion. Wharton's jelly is compressed by the expanded umbilical vein (V) and two arteries (A). H&E. ×10. (From Schiebler & Kaufmann, 1981, with permission.)

ing to Boyd and Hamilton (1970)—there is only one umbilical artery (see below), an anomaly that may be associated with multiple fetal malformations (Lemtis, 1966, 1968). Local fusion of the two arteries has also been reported (Kelber, 1976). The arrangement is different in many other species. For example, two arteries and two veins are found in the nine-banded armadillo, with many subtle variations (Benirschke et al., 1964); and, as indicated earlier, other animals may have an admixture of yolk sac (vitelline) vessels. Cats have four vessels of each type. The notion of a "double umbilicus" (Reeves, 1916) is based on a single observation of a somewhat displaced, doubled umbilical vein found in an adult, with puckering of the skin. In another case, described by Murdoch (1966), there were two umbilical veins, and a portion of the cord was separated, giving it a partially split appearance. The mean intravital

diameter of the arteries is around 3 mm, with a slight tendency to increase toward the placenta. The venous diameter is around twice this size (Figure 209).

Human umbilical vessels differ from the major vessels of the body in many ways. The endothelial cells of both the arteries and the veins are unusually rich in organelles (Parry & Abramovich, 1972; Las Heras & Haust, 1981) and thus structurally different from the endothelium of the villous vessels. Gebrane-Younes et al. (1986) have given a careful account of the ultrastructure of the endothelium. They described ultrastructural evidence that transudation of fluid through the umbilical vessel walls contributes to the formation of amnionic fluid.

Despite all differences among umbilical and villous endothelium, human umbilical vein-derived endothelial cells (HUVECs) are often used for cell culture as models for "placental endothelium." The findings by Lang et al. (1993) suggest that we should be careful with the interpretation of such experiments. These authors described considerable differences among umbilical and villous endothelium with respect to cell surface markers and receptors for transferrin and immunoglobulin G (IgG).

Slender endothelial extensions, penetrating the basal lamina, may interdigitate with the neighboring muscle cells and form an endotheliomuscular system (Nikolov & Schiebler, 1973). The arteries possess no internal elastic membrane and have much less elastica in general (Boyd & Hamilton, 1970; Nikolov & Schiebler, 1973). The vein, on the other hand, has an elastic subintimal layer (Figure 210). The muscular coat of the arteries consists of a system of crossing spiraled fibers (von Hayek, 1936; Goerttler, 1951; Scheuner, 1964). The venous muscular coats are thinner and composed of more separate layers of longitudinal or circular fibers.

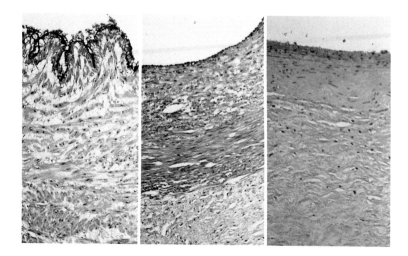

FIGURE 210. Umbilical cord sections of a stillborn with necrosis (due to thrombosis) of one umbilical artery (right) and a normal artery (middle) and vein (left). In these sections one may observe the presence of a delicate subendothelial elastica only in the vein at left. von Gieson. ×160.

Cardoso and colleagues (1992) have analyzed the extracellular matrix of isolated umbilical arteries. In general, hyaluronic acid was increased, whereas heparane sulfate and chondroitin-4-sulfate and chondroitin-6-sulfate were reduced in normal umbilical arteries compared to their levels in normal adult arteries. Following hypertension during pregnancy the total glycosaminoglycan and collagen content of the umbilical arteries were reduced; these changes were unlikely to impair the hemodynamic properties of the cord vessels. Each umbilical vessel is surrounded by crossing bundles of spiraled collagen fibers that form a kind of adventitia. Electron microscopic and immunohistochemical studies by Takechi et al. (1993) revealed that the stromal cells embedded in this collagen meshwork are myofibroblasts rather than typical fibroblasts. Myofibroblasts are fiber-producing cells that have contractile properties similar to those of smooth muscle cells. These results were supported by Nanaev and coworkers (1992), who found myofibroblasts lining fiber-free, jelly-filled spaces, possibly regulating the turgor of the cord and thus helping to avoid fatal bends of the vessels. The fiber-free spaces should not be misunderstood as lymphatic vessels. The latter are completely absent from the umbilical cord and the placenta. The umbilical vessels also lack vasa vasorum. Fetuses beyond 20 weeks' gestation, however, have vasa vasorum in the intraabdominal portions of their umbilical arteries (Clarke, 1965). In addition, extensions of Wharton's jelly pervade the strands of muscle.

INNERVATION

There is general agreement with the findings by Spivack (1943) that no nerves traverse the umbilical cord from fetus to placenta, and that the placenta has no neural supply. A number of investigators, however, have since investigated this apparent lack of nerves, and some have come to different conclusions. Kernbach (1963) studied the amnion with Cajal stains and considered the powdery Nissl substance of X cells (see Chapter 15) to represent sympathicoblasts with nerve fibers. He also believed that he had identified nerves in the amnion (Kernbach, 1969). Ten Berge (1963) reviewed the older literature on this topic and found only three authors who claimed to have demonstrated nerves by "persevering techniques." Ten Berge was unable to obtain convincing preparations with a variety of stains. He believed, however, that the responsiveness to oxygen perfusion and a variety of pharmacological agents argues in favor of innervation. Fox and Jacobson (1969) stained various segments of umbilical cords from abortuses and term placentas with methylene blue and observed fibers in all segments of all cords. The fibers were most easily seen in Wharton's jelly but surrounded and entered the vascular walls. Fox and Jacobson (1969) interpreted the fibers to be neural elements. It is possible that these structures relate to the vagal fibers described in embryos by Pearson and Sauter (1969), which are thought to be instrumental in closing the ductus venosus after birth. The same authors subsequently investigated the sacral portions of embryos and found convincing evidence for a neural supply of umbilical arteries (Pearson & Sauter, 1970). Some neural

elements terminate before entering the cord, whereas others penetrate it. This report was in contrast to the older literature, which was reviewed.

Ellison (1971) then took up the topic and studied the cords with a thiocholine technique. He demonstrated acetylcholinesterase-positive nerve endings in the proximal 20 cm of umbilical cord, but the placental side invariably gave negative results. The illustrations of tiny nerves present around the umbilical vessels appear convincing. Because they frequently showed degenerative changes, they were interpreted as having a primarily prenatal function. Ellison (1971) was unable to confirm the assertion by Fox and Jacobson (1969) of a subamnionic neural plexus and interpreted it as an artifact. Electron microscopic search for innervation of the human umbilical cord has generally been negative (Nadkarni, 1970). Fox (1978), who cited other studies, believed that the topic may be controversial because of the paucity of fibers. Lachenmayer (1971) examined guinea pig and human cords and the intrafetal portions of vessels for formaldehyde-induced fluorescence, which is considered to be specific for catecholamines. He found no evidence of nerve fibers in the cord vessels, but they were present within the fetus and the immediate vicinity of the umbilicus. He considered the cord to be a model of a nerve-free effector organ. Later studies (e.g., those by Nikolov & Schiebler, 1973, and Papaloucas et al., 1975) have corroborated this view. Moreover, immunohistochemical examination of cords obtained from first, second, and third trimester pregnancies, and using a panel of antibodies directed against neural and glial structures, failed to identify any nerve tissues in the middle and placental segment of the human umbilical cord (Fox & Khong, 1990).

Contractility of Umbilical Vessels

There has been much interest in the mechanisms of closure of umbilical vessels after birth (Editorial, 1966). Yao et al. (1977) observed umbilical cords after delivery and witnessed that irregular constrictions of arteries occurred at irregular intervals. Davignon et al. (1965) showed that increased transmural pressures exerted on the umbilical arteries led to vasoconstriction. This finding is usual in the guinea pig also. Throughout the last 2 weeks of pregnancy the cord vessels show increasing responsiveness to mechanical irritation, which is not present during the prior periods of pregnancy. This response and other mechanisms indirectly confirm the absence of a neural mechanism operating in cord vessels (Shepherd, 1968).

Electron microscopic observations led Röckelein and Scharl (1988) to the assumption that an endotheliomuscular interaction mediated by the endotheliomuscular interdigitations (Nikolov & Schiebler, 1973) may play an important role. As a consequence of muscular contraction, the authors describe a cytoplasmic prolapse of smooth muscle cells into the endothelial cells, causing a kind of "hydrops" of the latter. Seemingly hydropic endothelial cells of umbilical arteries deeply protruding into the arterial lumens and partly occluding them have been seen by many authors.

Sometimes they have been interpreted as a pathological finding, for example in the allantoic vessels obtained from human immunodeficiency virus (HIV)-positive mothers (Jimenez et al., 1988). According to Röckelein & Hey (1985) and Hey & Röckelein (1989), this phenomenon is more likely to be a result of postpartal muscle contraction or even an artifact due to delayed fixation. We agree.

It has been well recognized for many years that the vessels are exquisitely sensitive to various endocrine mediators (e.g., serotonin, angiotensin, and oxytocin) (LeDonne & McGowan, 1967; Dyer, 1970; Winters, 1970). Moreover, smooth muscle contractility of the vessel walls is influenced in paracrine loops by substances produced within the neighboring endothelial cells. Among these mediators, prostaglandins have been shown to be produced within the umbilical vascular endothelium. Despite earlier observations to the contrary, it is now known that the endothelium of the umbilical vein produces far more prostaglandins than does that of the arteries (Harold et al., 1988). However, there is little production of prostaglandins (PG) in placental surface vessels. Karbowski and coworkers (1991) have cultured umbilical vein endothelial cells from smoking mothers and diabetic mothers; and they found that the synthesis rates of PGI_2 and PGE_2 were significantly reduced compared to those from normal control mothers. Because both prostaglandins are potent vasodilators and platelet aggregation inhibitors, the authors conclude that impaired placental perfusion in smoking and diabetic mothers may be mediated by the altered umbilical endothelium. McCoshen et al. (1989) found by incubation experiments that the cord (presumably its amnionic surface) is the major source of PGE_2 in the gestational sac during labor.

Another vasodilator that has attracted much attention is nitrous oxide—identical with the endothelial-derived relaxing factor from the older literature (Pinto et al., 1991)—which is produced from the conversion of L-arginine to citrulline by nitric oxide synthase (NOS); the latter enzyme has been detected immunohistochemically not only in villous syncytiotrophoblast but also in fetal villous and umbilical endothelium (Myatt et al., 1993). Atrial natriuretic peptide (NAP) is another potent vasodilator that in addition seems to be involved in fetal fluid hemostasis. Its binding sites have been detected in umbilical smooth muscle cells (Salas et al., 1991). Immunoreactivity for the peptide itself and its messenger RNA have been found in the umbilical endothelium (Cai et al., 1993a,b) even though Inglis and colleagues (1993) have questioned local umbilical synthesis. They suggested an endocrine action of the peptide that is released from the fetal heart into the circulation (for review see Macara et al., 1993); messenger RNA for ANP is present in cardiomyocytes of fetuses as early as 19 weeks (Gardner et al., 1989).

Vasoconstrictor substances found in umbilical endothelium comprise angiotensin II, 5-hydroxytryptamine (5-HT), thromboxane (Macara et al., 1993), neuropeptide Y (NPY) (Cai et al., 1992, 1993a), and endothelin-1 (Hemsen et al., 1991). However, Gu and coworkers (1991) detected endothelin-1 and endothelin-2 only in fibroblasts and amnionic epithelium of human cords, not in endothelium. Bindings sites for endothelin-1 have been described in the media of umbilical vessels, the activity of the arteries exceeding that of the vein (Rath et al., 1993). The functions of these vasoconstrictors are still under discussion. NPY and angiotensin II, which are found most abundantly in the endothelial cells, cause relatively weak or no responses on the term umbilical artery in vitro (White, 1989). When White compared the effects of various vasoactive agents on the arteries in premature and term placentas, significant differences were found. Immature vessels were more sensitive to angiotensin II, arachidonic acid, and oxytocin; term vessels reacted more to vasopressin, norepinephrine, PGD_2 and PGE_2. In vitro 5-HT and endothelin-1 were found to be powerful vasoconstrictors on all levels of the fetoplacental circulation (Maclean et al., 1992). The latter substances are also under discussion as mediators of closure of placental circulation at birth (Hemsen et al., 1991).

These findings shed a new light on the highly complex mechanisms of autoregulation, not only of the umbilical circulation but also of the villous circulation, as most of these mediators have been described also in the walls of the larger chorionic and villous vessels (for review see Macara et al., 1993). Additional studies are needed to elucidate the complicated interactions of these substances, as they are likely to be involved in abnormal conditions, such as intrauterine growth retardation (IUGR) and a high Doppler resistance index.

The vessels of patients with preeclampsia, growth-retarded fetuses, and diabetes, as well as those of smoking mothers, show reduced prostacyclin production (Busacca et al., 1982; Dadak et al., 1982; Jogee et al., 1983; Mäkilä et al., 1983). Similar effects have been found in vitro by Karbowski et al. (1991). Degeneration of endothelium from umbilical vessels had earlier been shown to occur in smoking mothers (Asmussen & Kjeldsen, 1975). Other effects of smoking on the placenta have been discovered as well; most are discussed in Chapter 19. One example is that the steroid production is altered (Mochizuki et al., 1984); others are trophoblastic degeneration, microvascular changes, and several other effects (Wigger et al., 1984). Although it is attractive to consider that prostaglandins are the principal mediators of umbilical vascular responses, some evidence has been adduced that there may be considerable differences among species (Dyer, 1970). Alcohol leads to a dose-dependent contractile response in umbilical arteries in vitro (Yang et al., 1986). Estrogens dilate the vessels (De Sa & Meirelles, 1977).

Hyrtl Anastomosis, False Knots, and Hoboken Nodes

An important macroscopic feature of umbilical arteries is the presence of an anastomosis between the two arteries near the surface of the placenta. The older literature (Hyrtl, 1870) and more recent studies have shown that 96% of cords have some sort of anastomosis (Priman, 1959; Arts, 1961). Most were seen 1.5 cm from the placental insertion and were either truly anastomotic vessels or the two arteries had fused. On rare occasions, two such communicating vessels exist. Like Hyrtl (1870), who attached much importance to this communication, we believe it to be meaningful for an equalization of flow and pressures between the two arteries and for the uniform distribution of blood to the different lobes of the placenta. Its relevance to an understanding of single umbilical artery, the commonest macroscopic anomaly of the placenta, is discussed below. Young (1972), who provided an admirable review of the literature, studied this anastomosis in many primate species and prepared an elaborate classification scheme for the different types found. He found that "lower" primates (e.g., lemurs) lacked it; New World monkeys had it in some 30% of cords, and Old World monkeys showed an 80% incidence. It is apparently a recent evolutionary development.

Often the looping of umbilical vessels is the cause for false knots of the cord. In most cases, local loops of the arteries, or sometimes even the vein, cause knot-like dilation of the cord. Occasionally, focal varicosities of the veins or perivascular accumulations of connective tissue result in a similar external appearance. Finally, there are the valves (nodes) of Hoboken (Hoboken, 1669; Spivack, 1936), named after a seventeenth century Dutch anatomist. Malpas and Symonds (1966) concluded that these crescentic folds in the inner wall of umbilical arteries are present after delivery, but that they do not exist in vivo. Reynolds (1952) was not so sure and depicted some of these vascular indentations. He speculated that they resulted from muscular constriction, a view that has been corroborated by electron microscopic studies: Röckelein and Scharl (1988) and Röckelein et al. (1990), speculated on the occurrence of some interference with postnatal closure of the cord vessels. On the other hand, most other observers believe that the folds have no physiological significance, as was inferred by Spivack (1936). They cautioned that incisive observations must be made immediately after cesarean section because the folds form quickly. Ideally, they are studied with sonography before birth.

ALLANTOIS

The allantoic duct, a minute connection to the fetal bladder, is frequently found in the proximal portions of the umbilical cord. Remnants may exist discontinuously throughout the cord. Complete obliteration of the duct is normally achieved by 15 weeks' gestation (Janosco et al., 1977). In the fetus the rudiment is referred to as the median umbilical ligament. The remains of this connection in the umbilical cord are always located centrally between the two umbilical arteries, and usually they consist of a collection of epithelial cells without lumens (Figure 211). The epithelium, when present, is generally of the transitional, bladder type. However, mucin-producing epithelium is also found occasionally because of the proximity to the yolk sac during development. Rarely is the allantois tissue accompanied by muscle, and even more uncommonly is the duct patent. Nevertheless, urination from the clamped umbilical stump has been reported, and cysts may even persist into adult life (Kreibich, 1947). A patent duct (urachus) on the abdominal wall may complicate pregnancy. Nielsen et al. (1982) reviewed 12 such cases from the literature and reported on an additional case. Their patient had a discharge from the umbilicus during pregnancy. Her bladder became infected, and pyelonephritis ensued. Infection is a common complication of this rare condition. An abscess of the allantoic duct remnant was described by Baill et al. (1989). It was found in the placenta of a 22 weeks' gestation placenta that was involved with chorioamnionitis and funisitis.

The allantoic remnant may be symptomatic at birth, presenting as a "giant umbilical cord" (Ente et al., 1970). In one of the two patients of these authors, the cord was tense and swollen to a 5 cm diameter. Urine discharged from it. The second patient also had an enlarged cord but only after the cord had separated during the neonatal period did urine pass through the duct. The authors stressed the association with a tense, "giant" cord swelling and contrasted it to that found with omphalomesenteric remnants. That was also the finding in a case reported by Chantler and his colleagues (1969), where a single umbilical artery ("fusion") was an associated anomaly. Browne (1925) described a cyst in the umbilical cord originating from the allantois. De Sa (1984) described a small cyst and likened its appearance to the cell nests

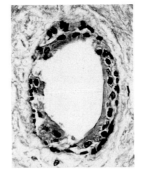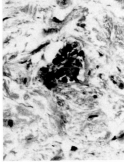

FIGURE 211. Two remnants of allantoic duct: the left is patent and the right obliterated. Note the absence of the muscular coat. H&E. ×525. (Courtesy G.L. Bourne.)

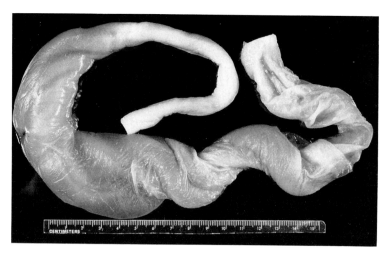

FIGURE 212. Edematous umbilical cord of a 32-week fetus with a large urachal extension into the cord. It was correctly diagnosed by sonography before birth. This cord weighed

180 g (compared with a normal weight of about 40 g). (Courtesy Dr. S. Kassel, Fresno, California.)

of von Brunn, which are characteristic for bladder epithelium. Such a case is shown in Figure 211. This stillborn had a prenatally diagnosed swelling at the abdomen. At delivery, the "giant," edematous cord (Figure 212) weighed 180 g (the average normal weight of the cord is 40–45 g). Sections showed that the urachus extended deep into the umbilical cord; it was accompanied by normal bladder musculature and was located in its usual place between the two arteries (Figure 213). The remarkable feature of this umbilical cord was that it had numerous vasa aberrantia. These vessels cannot be classified as vasa vasorum because they were similarly distributed around vessels and the urachus. Normally, vasa vasorum are confined to the intraabdominal portions of these structures. Furthermore, around all these small vessels were numerous islands of extramedullary hematopoiesis. The fetus presumably died because venous return was compressed by this large cyst in the cord.

Even if there is no macroscopic or clinical evidence of allantoic vestiges, careful histological examination may reveal their

presence. When studying the placental extremities of 1,000 cords, Jauniaux and coworkers (1989a) found such remnants in 14.6% of the cases.

Omphalomesenteric Duct

The omphalomesenteric duct arises through the lengthening of the umbilical stalk when the embryo retracts (herniates or prolapses) into the amnionic cavity. While the embryo is folding and the cord becomes established, the connection between the gut and the yolk sac lengthens. From the primary yolk sac develops the secondary structure that is connected to the fetal intestines. Detailed morphological descriptions of the

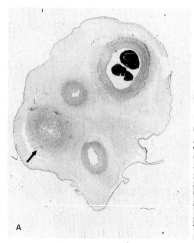
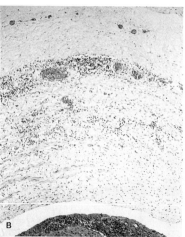

FIGURE 213. (A) Histological appearance of the umbilical cord shown in Figure 212. The arrow indicates the urachus. Note the presence of small vessels and vasa aberrantia around the

vein and one artery. (B) Vasa aberrantia around the umbilical vein in the same case. H&E. A ×6; B ×64.

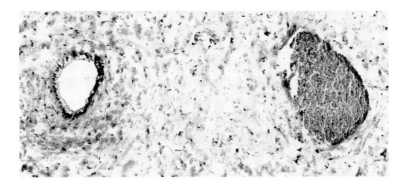

FIGURE 214. Omphalomesenteric duct remnant at left with mucus-producing epithelium and a small amount of musculature in the wall. At right are the remains of the vitelline vein. H&E. ×100.

intact, nonregressive yolk sac during the early stages of pregnancy have been provided by Gonzales-Crussi and Roth (1976), and Ukeshima et al. (1986). The yolk sac has a three-layered wall, consisting of an inner resorptive endodermal epithelium and an outer mesothelium, which are joined by some mesenchyme. Erythropoiesis was found in the mesenchyme from 6 to 8 weeks' gestation (Jones et al., 1993).

When the gut rotates and withdraws to its original cavity, this duct atrophies. Atrophy is usually complete by the 7th to 16th weeks (Janosco et al., 1977). Jones et al. (1993) described generalized degenerative changes for the 10th week. Meckel's diverticulum, a small outgrowth of the ileum, is a frequent remnant of this connection in the fetus. Only in exceptional cases can a larger duct be found. It then connects the ileum with the proximal part of the cord. Having thus an endodermal origin, it is not surprising that in remnants of this duct one may find liver, pancreas, stomach, and intestinal remains.

Minute vitelline ducts are frequently found on histological study in the umbilical cord. At the placental

extremities, the incidence seems to be lower; of 1,000 mature cords studied, only 1.5% showed remnants of the omphalomesenteric (vitelline) duct, whereas vitelline vessels were present in about 7% (Jauniaux et al., 1989a). Clinically, these vestiges are unimportant. The blood vessels that may accompany the vitelline duct are always tiny and may even contain red blood cells. It is noteworthy, however, that these vessels always lack a muscular coat, which, we believe, develops only under the influence of blood pressure. Thus when in sirenomelia the omphalomesenteric artery is probably converted to the sole umbilical artery (because the allantoic vessels failed to develop), this vessel acquires a "normal" muscular investment. Usually, vitelline vessels are composed only of endothelium. There are other points of view with respect to the single artery in sirens, and they are discussed at the end of this chapter.

Cysts of vitelline origin have been described many times. In contrast to the allantoic duct remnants, they often have muscular coats (Figure 214) and may occur in duplicate (Figure 215). True intestinal walls, including ganglion cells, may be present. Browne (1925)

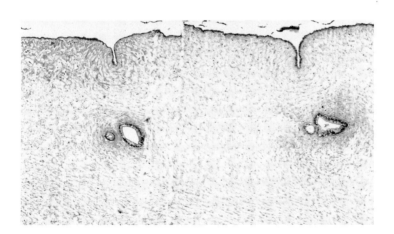

FIGURE 215. Microscopic section of a term pregnancy cord with four remnants of omphalomesenteric duct. The marginal position of such vestiges is typical. H&E. ×50.

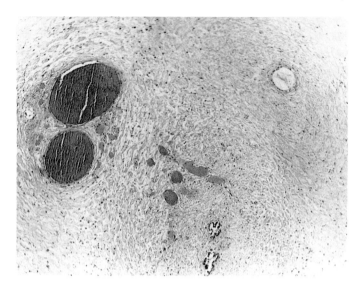

FIGURE 216. Plexus of small vitelline vessels accompanies the duct remnants (bottom center) in term cord. At top right is the dilated allantoic duct. H&E. ×64.

referred to a report of one such cyst as having caused fetal death, presumably due to compression of allantoic vessels. Three cases were reported by Heifetz and Rueda-Pedraza (1983b), one of which had many other anomalies. These authors reviewed six previously described cases and extensively discussed the embryology. Heifetz and Rueda-Pedraza made the point that the cysts (0.4–6.0 cm) are frequently surrounded by a plexus of small vessels (Figure 216) and that they usually lie in the proximal portion of the cord. Males outnumber females 4:1. Although these vitelline remnants are not particularly common and usually have no clinical significance, it is not always the case; and the question of what to do when such an anomaly is found is not always easy to answer. Heifetz and Rueda-Pedraza (1983b) thought that exploration of the neonate's abdomen is

not indicated. Schellong and Pfeiffer (1967), however, described a child with intestinal obstruction that developed after the umbilical stump had fallen off. A "wart-like" swelling had developed at the navel. Because it was later identified as the severed intestine that had entered the cord, they favored exploration when such structures are found.

Remnants of distended omphalomesenteric ducts can be associated with atresia of the small intestine and can be a rare cause of abdominal distension (Petrikovsky et al., 1988). One experienced obstetrician stated that he had severed the normal-appearing cord of a neonate who was later found to have nearly the entire length of small bowel within that cord. King (1968) described similar cases and referred to them as ileal "prolapse," a normal feature in early embryos (Figure 217). Such

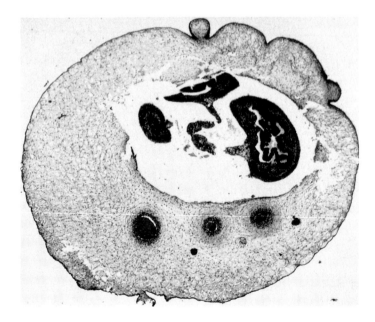

FIGURE 217. Cross section of an umbilical cord of an embryo with a crown-rump length of 4 cm from a tubal pregnancy. The large space (extraembryonic coelom) contains a loop of intestine; and below it are the two umbilical arteries (right) with tiny allantoic remnants below and between. At bottom left is the umbilical (allantoic) vein. H&E. ×25.

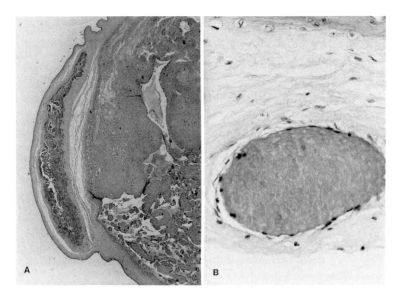

FIGURE 218. (A) Microscopic appearance of a yolk sac remnant in a term placenta. It consists of irregular fragments of phosphate deposits, underneath which are remains of omphalomesenteric vessels. The amnion is above and the chorion below. (B) Remains of a vitelline vessel in the proximal part of the cord. Note the squamous metaplasia on the cord surface. H&E. A × 50; B ×400.

remnants of intestine may be seen on the surface of the umbilical cord. Lee and Aterman (1968) reported an intestinal polyp arising 5 cm from the end of the cord. Dombrowski et al. (1987) described intestinal epithelium on the surface of the umbilical cord that was associated with a hemangioma of the cord. Harris and Wenzl (1963) described the only other similar case, in which they found pancreatic tissue within the anomaly. No islets of Langerhans, however, were present within that pancreatic remnant. In neither case was abdominal exploration necessary.

Fetal death occurred as a rather unusual complication of such an embryological remnant in the interesting case described by Blanc and Allan (1961). Prenatal exsanguinating hemorrhage had taken place into the amnionic sac from a "tear" in the umbilical cord, near the fetal surface. Because of the proximity of vitelline structures, including gastric mucosa, it was inferred that the umbilical vein had ulcerated owing to erosive activity within this location. Calcific masses accompanied this lesion.

The finding of liver tissue at the umbilicus (Shaw & Pierog, 1969) is rare and probably relates more to exomphalos (omphalocele) than to the vestiges herein described. Patel et al. (1989) reported a newborn with a markedly swollen umbilical cord (70 mm circumference) at its abdominal attachment that contained herniated bowel. Because of this case they determined the normal circumference of the umbilical cord in 191 neonates at different fetal ages and of various weights. The normal circumference was found to be 37.7 ± 7.3 mm. They cautioned that clamping large cords may cause bowel obstruction.

After regression of the omphalomesenteric duct, remainders of the detached yolk sac persist in many cases and can be found as 3 to 5 mm white-yellow disks in the chorionic plate. Meyer (1904) found them to be as large as 15 mm and wondered how such atrophic structures could become so large while degenerating. The yolk sac remnant is almost invariably located near the margin of the term placenta. It lies underneath the amnion and has a somewhat pasty consistency. This vestige must not be interpreted as being abnormal or perhaps as representing the site of former inflammation. Histologically, it stains deeply purple with hematoxylin. It appears to be calcified but is probably mostly a deposit of pasty phosphates (Figure 218). The calcareous nature of this material was discussed at length by Meyer (1904). Minute omphalomesenteric vessels may also accompany these yolk sac remnants. They can be seen coursing toward the umbilical cord (Figure 219). The yolk sac can be visualized as a small sac during early pregnancy (Reece et al., 1987). Ferrazzi et al. (1988) reported an overall success of 97% with this visualization at 7 weeks' gestation.

It is well recognized that the vessels are exquisitely sensitive to various mediators (e.g., serotonin, angiotensin, and oxytocin) (LeDonne & McGowan, 1967; Dyer, 1970; Winters, 1970). It is our impression that whatever alleged minute nerves may be demonstrated in the umbilical cord they are either artifacts of the preparative procedure or degenerating structures. The

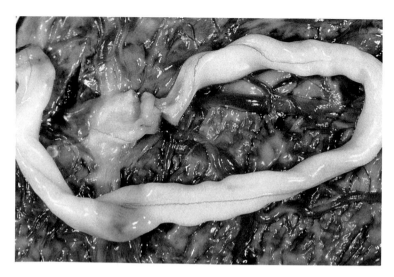

FIGURE 219. Vitelline vessels coursing from a yolk sac remnant (not seen) on the cord surface of a normal term placenta.

cord and certainly the placenta are here considered as having no functional neural investment, a conclusion that is shared by most authors (e.g., Lauweryns et al., 1969).

Spiral Turns of the Cord

The umbilical cord is usually spiraled, a quality referred to as chirality (Fletcher, 1993). A counterclockwise spiral (left) exceeds that of the opposite direction by a ratio of 7:1. The helices may be seen by ultrasonographic examination as early as during the first trimester of pregnancy (Figures 220, 221). Lacro et al. (1987) have studied this phenomenon in greater detail, efforts that evidently are not appreciated by everyone. For

instance, Eastman (1967) stated that, "as far as I am aware, knowledge about these helices is of no practical value whatsoever." Helices are readily seen by the 9th week of gestation. They usually number up to 40, but as many as 380 turns have been described. The number is already well established early in pregnancy, and it increases only insignificantly during the third trimester. It therefore follows that the cord length grows not by increased spiraling but by increasing the pitch between each turn of the spiral. It is uncommon to find an absence of spirals in the cord but when it occurs it has an ominous prognosis (Strong et al., 1993). Strong et al. found that 4.3% of newborn lacked cord twist, and that these infants had a significantly higher increase in perinatal mortality and other problems. Later these authors suggested that the umbilical coiling index

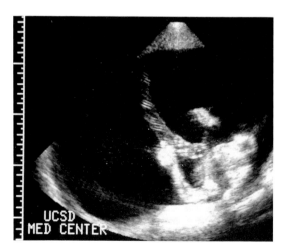

FIGURE 220. Sonographic appearance of a left umbilical helix in one monochorionic twin with the transfusion syndrome at 22 weeks' gestation. (Courtesy Dr. G.R. Leopold.)

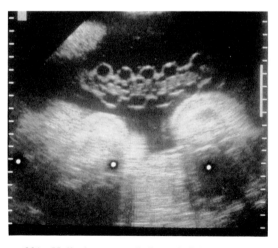

FIGURE 221. Helical nature of distended blood vessels in the umbilical cord is shown in this sonograph of a pregnancy at 38 weeks' gestation. (Courtesy Dr. G.R. Leopold.)

(number of coils divided by length of cord: average 0.21/cm) may identify the fetus at risk (Strong et al., 1994). When the index fell below the 10th percentile, more chromosomal errors, fetal distress, and meconium staining were identified. Animals with lengthwise fixation in their uterus and infants with fixation of their bodies to the placental surface (due to amnionic bands) have not only relatively short cords but also few or no umbilical helices (Spatz, 1968). The same is true for species with elongated embryos in elongated uterine horns (e.g., whales), a situation that hinders embryonic rotation (Slijper, 1960; Arvy & Pilleri, 1976b). This point thus infers that the turns must be induced by fetal rotations. Furthermore, because the left spirals outweigh the right spirals by approximately the same frequency as the distribution of handedness, Lacro et al. (1987) reasoned that the cerebral organization is the cause of the direction of spirals. The authors subsequently found that this hypothesis is incorrect, and that there was no correlation between the handedness of the fetus (or that of the mother) and the direction of spirals (Table 15). Furthermore, twins were found to have spirals in the same or opposite directions, although in general they had fewer twists than singletons and a different ratio. Monozygotic twins may have helices in different directions, an observation often made before. Only infants with single umbilical arteries had a significant reduction of spirals. No other anomalous development correlated, and one or the other twist was not more commonly associated with perinatal morbidity or mortality. It is interesting that an occasional cord may have helices in opposite directions (Figure 222). The spirals of the cord have been studied in 5,000 cords using morphometry and histology (Blackburn et al., 1988). A left twist was found in 79%, with a left/right ratio of 3.7:1.0; in twins the left direction was found in 61%, and mixed spiraling occurred in 26%. In contrast to the findings of Lacro et al. (1987), Blackburn et al. (1988) always found identical twins to spiral in the same

directions. Fetuses with single umbilical arteries had a 1.5:1.0 left/right ratio. These authors also gave figures for cord dry mass and weight/length ratios. Fletcher (1993) found a 76.5% left-handed spiral in patients at Abu Dhabi, a right-handed twist in 15.5%, and mixed in 6.5%. They found no sex difference.

Most authors have concluded that spiraling of the cord is the result of some fetal activity, and that the lack of spiraling may reflect fetal inactivity and possibly central nervous system (CNS) disturbances. Thus reduced coiling has poor prognosis (Strong et al., 1993). We have seen absent twists not only in many stillborns but also in the presence of various chromosomal errors and congenital syndromes, such as the Pena Shokeir syndrome and others. Another suggestion for the occurrence of spirals is that they are governed by the earth's rotational forces, and that like the familiar bathtub vortex (Sibulkin, 1983) there are differences in the chirality of cords between the hemispheres. This postulate has been disproved. Edmonds (1954) and Lacro et al. (1987) considered in detail the various theories that are the basis for umbilical cord spiraling. The causes remain unknown. In our experience, Schordania's (1929b) notion that long cords are more spiraled is correct, although it contradicts the findings of Chaurasia and Agarwal (1979), who studied a small number of specimens. The higher fetal mortality seen with intense spiraling (Figure 223) has been discussed.

The fact that frequently, but not always, the spirals represent distended umbilical arteries is well seen in Figure 224. This helical arrangement of vessels has been helpful in the diagnosis of fetal death, as in some such pregnancies gas can be visualized in an helical arrangement (Gruber, 1967). Several investigators have suggested that differential pressures of different-size umbilical arteries are the forces that produce the helices. The findings on single umbilical arteries (Lacro et al., 1987) tend to negate this notion. It may be that we are failing to differentiate true umbilical cord twists

TABLE 15. Distribution of the direction of the umbilical cord helix.

Source of cord	Direction of the cord helix			L/R ratio
	Left (%)	Right (%)	None (%)	
Live-born singletons	83	12	5	7.8
All twins (combined data for 290 sets)	66	18	11	3.7
Monochorionic twins	82	11	7	7.8
Dichorionic twins	77	16	8	4.8
Intrauterine deaths	73	8	18	8.7
Single umbilical artery (SUA)	63	22	15	2.8
SUA with problems	44	39	17	1.1
SUA without problems	72	14	14	5.2
Placental singletons ($n = 14,070$)	75	10	15	7.5

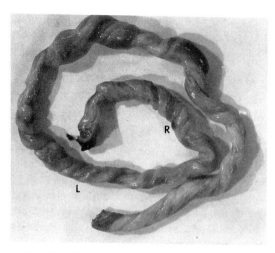

FIGURE 222. Umbilical cord with helices pointing in both right and left directions in a normal infant with a 52 cm cord and circumvallation.

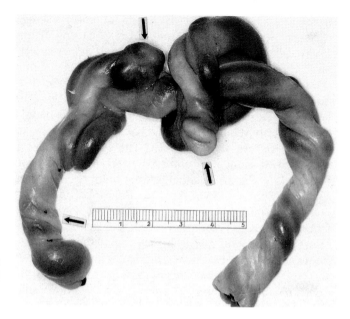

FIGURE 224. Umbilical cord with true and false knots in a live infant. Note that the arteries wind around the vein (left arrow), and in the knot the vein winds about the artery. False knots with vessels (top arrow) and with only Wharton's jelly (central arrow) are apparent as well.

from changes in which the umbilical arteries are merely wound around a less spiraled vein. Whether arteries are wound around the vein (Smart, 1962) or the vein winds around arteries (Potter, 1961) is irrelevant. Both arrangements can be seen in the same cord (Figure 224). The many arrangements that exist have been depicted by Hyrtl (1870) and Arvy and Pilleri (1976a), among others. These authors made numerous corrosion preparations of cords to investigate these features.

Length of the Cord

The length of the umbilical cord has been the topic of numerous studies. Most authors agree that excessively short and long cords correlate well with a variety of fetal problems. The normal length at term has been cited by Grosser (1927), who utilized data from various older studies but standards for measuring the length were supplied only more recently (e.g., Mills et al., 1983). These authors and Naeye (1985) used the large number of cord measurements from the Collaborative Perinatal Study and provided smoothed curves from 34 to 43 weeks' gestation. These data are not significantly different from ours. A mean length of 59.44 cm was determined by one of us (8,000 measurements, ranging from 24 to 146 cm); another author found it to be 66.54 cm (12,000 measured). When circled once about the neck the cord was 76.5 cm long, and when circled twice about the neck it was 93.5 cm. Thus wide variations were detected. As was suggested by Leonardo da Vinci, the umbilical cord has usually the same length as the baby. Figure 225 gives values for cord lengths as determined by a variety of authors. Manci et al. (1993) found that the length of the cord shrinks up to 7 cm during the first few hours after delivery, so accurate recording at birth is preferable.

There have been numerous other studies as well. Malpas (1964), stimulated by the birth of a baby with a

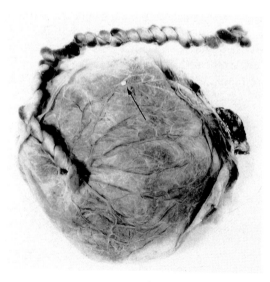

FIGURE 223. Term placenta of a stillborn infant with an intensely twisted umbilical cord. The cause of death was inferred to be the twisted cord, as there were no other findings. Note also the remains of the yolk sac (arrow).

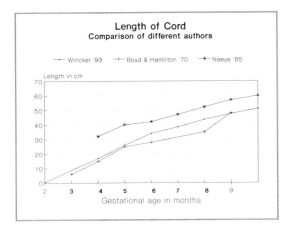

FIGURE 225. Length of umbilical cord as determined in three studies. (When exact numbers were not given, the approximate number was entered.)

129 cm long cord, measured 538 normal cords at term. He found a normal distribution, with an average length of 61 cm (30–129 cm). There was slight correlation with fetal and placental weights. Gardiner (1922) obtained an average length of 55 cm for normal cords. He considered less than 32 cm as "absolutely" short and more than 32 cm as "relatively" short. He also suggested what the length of the cord *should* be if it were to allow a normal delivery with cephalic or breech presentations with looping (he provided quantitative accounts of the frequency of coiling). He assumed that the length of the cord was determined by the amount of amnionic fluid and depended also on fetal movements. The complete findings of Malpas just cited supported the notion of Walker and Pye (1960) (average 54.1 cm, maximum values ranging from 17.8 to 121.9 cm) that most of the cord's length is achieved by the 28th week of pregnancy. During the 41st day p.c. the developing cord, the amnionic covering of which is still incomplete, has a mean length of about 0.5 cm. By the 4th lunar month it has grown to 16 to 18 cm and by the 6th month to 33 to 35 cm. It was also suggested that there may be a relation to umbilical arterial pressures, but this point was not well supported. In a series of 37 pairs of monozygotic twins studied, little difference was found from that of singletons. Naeye (1985) based his findings on the measurements of cords at birth from the Collaborative Perinatal Study (35,779 cases) and found that the cord grows progressively from 32 cm at 20 weeks to 60 cm at term. Although growth slowed progressively, it never ceased.

Abnormal Length, Nuchal Cord

Short cords (<40 cm) are correlated with neonatal problems and depressed intelligence quotient (IQ) values.

The essential question, however, remains whether the length of the cord is determined by prenatal CNS problems or the CNS problems that are so well correlated result from perinatal problems attending the delivery with a short cord. This question is of interest because it has been shown that short cords are not only more common with a variety of congenital anomalies but also that the length of the cord is usually determined by fetal movements during early fetal life. When the fetus is constrained, as occurs for instance with amnionic adhesions and in ectopic pregnancies, the cord is short (Miller et al., 1981). The possible relation between long cords and excessive fetal movements is more difficult to assess because of the deficiency of quantitative data on prenatal movements. It would also be of great interest to obtain more information as to whether children associated with long umbilical cords are "hyperactive" during later life.

Moessinger and his colleagues (1982) have investigated the question of the cord's length experimentally in rats. They injected curare (short cords), placed the rat fetuses in an extrauterine position (long cords), and produced oligohydramnios (short cords). It has also been learned that infants with Down syndrome (trisomy 21) have significantly shorter cords (45.1 cm versus 57.3 cm for controls), speculated to be due to the reduced fetal activity in utero (Moessinger et al., 1986). Likewise, with breech presentations, the cord is shorter by some 4.5 cm than with births from a vertex presentation (Soernes & Bakke, 1986). The latter authors also confirmed other investigators' findings that males have slightly longer cords than females (58.46 versus 56.90 cm in vertex; 53.78 versus 52.51 cm in breech). These correlations have led to further experiments in animals, where it was found that prenatal alcohol administration to rats shortens the cords (Barron et al., 1985), as does atenolol (a β-blocker) given to rabbits (Katz et al., 1987). In contrast, Fujinaga et al. (1990) have opined that the "stretch hypothesis" is faulty. Their findings verified that umbilical cords of humans and rats steadily increases with gestational age, although in some of their cases of oligohydramnios long cords were found. Moreover, their tenet was that the amount of amnionic fluid decreases with advancing gestational age and therefore "fetuses should be less active." This chapter is not the place to argue extensively over the merits of one or the other theory; suffice it to say that oligohydramneic fetuses may be just as active as those in normal environments and thus may be able to stretch their cords. It is also important to know how long the oligohydramnios had existed and how severe it was. Further data are definitely needed. Naeye and Tafari (1983) found that neonates with long cords were relatively hyperkinetic when compared with those who had shorter cords.

An interesting study of equine abortions was reported by Hong et al. (1993). They found that torsion of an excessively long umbilical cord is an important cause of fetal wastage in horses, making up some 4.5% of 1,211 cases. The normal cord length in horses was found to be 52 cm, whereas that of abortuses with torsion was 72 cm. Excellent photographs accompany this description.

There are rare cases of "achordia," which have mostly been associated with abdominal wall defects (Giacoia, 1992), as in Figure 226, or with acardiac fetuses (see Chapter 25). Most of these infants actually have a diminutive cord rather than no cord at all. Rupture of short cords and of cords with entanglement have been reported by Szécsi (1955). Several authors have delineated a "short cord syndrome" that includes a variety of associated anomalies (Grange et al., 1936; Arya & Gilbert, 1985; Gilbert, 1986). In the latter study, cords less than 15 cm were often associated with abdominal wall defects and evisceration, spinal and limb deformities, and other lesions. The authors thought of it as a "primary malformation."

An excessively long cord poses problems because the fetus may become entangled in it or the cord may prolapse, especially after the membranes rupture. The successful clinical management of gestations with long cords has been detailed by Katz et al. (1988). In general, long cords have more pronounced spiraling; and it may be inferred from this fact that the excessive length results from increased fetal movements. Umbilical cords measuring up to 300 cm have been reported (Arvy & Pilleri, 1976a). The greatest length we have measured was 165 cm. One would think that such excessively long, spiraled cords would also require greater perfusion pressure, but it has not been confirmed, and some studies suggest that it is not true.

Looping about the neck and extremities was found in 23% of overall obstetrical cases by Earn (1951), and it was more common with excessively long cords. He once found the cord to be wound eight times around the neck. The fetus in Figure 227 died because its cord was entwined around the neck three times; there was obstruction of venous return from the placenta. The constriction of the cord shown in Figure 228 led to its reduced size. It had been wound around the arm; and the depression of the arm, which was clearly discernible, bore testimony to this entwinement having caused the fetal death.

To find an entanglement of cords with extremities and bodies of young fetuses establishes that these abnormalities are not just features of labor and term pregnancy. Javert and Barton (1952) also made such observations. They studied 1,000 spontaneous abortions, of which 297 had sufficiently well preserved cords for study. Of these cases, 104 (35%) were abnormal, compared with a rate of 4.8% in a control group of "therapeutic" abortions; 13.4% were of excessive length and had looping. In those cases excessive fetal activity had often been observed before fetal death occurred. A case reported by Williams and colleagues (1981) is of considerable interest here. They had a patient with fetal growth retardation at 38 weeks' gestation in whom an emergency cesarean section was performed because of flat fetal heart rate tracings. The normally long umbilical cord was wound five times about the severely compressed and bruised neck. Various clinical findings, including oligohydramnios and

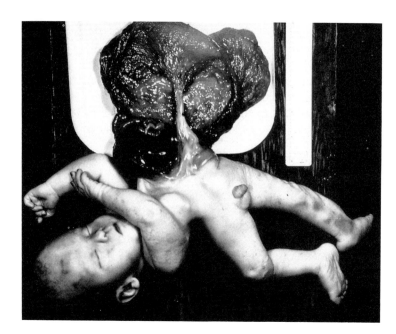

FIGURE 226. Excessively short umbilical cord at term with an abdominal wall defect (gastroschisis).

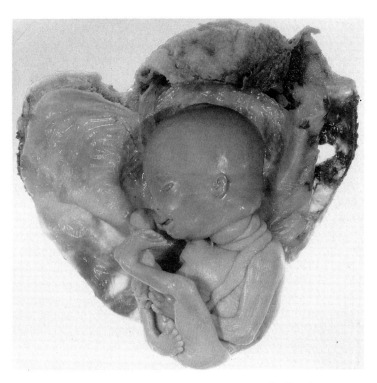

FIGURE 227. Stillborn fetus with the cord wrapped three times around its neck. Death was presumably due to obstruction to venous return from the placenta, not by obstruction to head vessels. Note the congestion of the head.

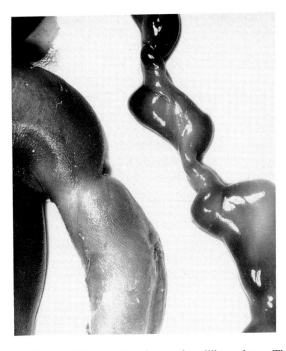

FIGURE 228. Umbilical cord and arm of a stillborn fetus. There is marked constriction of the arm and cord where the latter had wound firmly about the arm. The specimen was received with the amnion unruptured, so fetal motion alone must have caused the entanglement.

a lack of fetal movements, led them to suspect that this cord entanglement had been present for at least 2 months.

There have been numerous investigations of whether nuchal cords may cause fetal death or asphyxia during labor. Crawford (1962) found its incidence to be as high as 34% in vaginal vertex deliveries. He surmised that the significantly increased morbidity was related to deprivation of placental perfusion after expulsion of the fetus. At later analysis of his data, Crawford (1964) concluded that the incidence of nuchal cords rises steeply after 38 weeks' gestation, perhaps secondary to greater fetal activity or because of decreasing amniotic fluid volume. A somewhat similar incidence of nuchal cords and its complications was found by Kan and Eastman (1957) (one coil 20.6%, two coils 2.5%, three coils 0.5%), Reiss (1964), Horwitz et al. (1964), and others. McCurdy et al. (1994) were able to identify the presence of nuchal cords sonographically, confirming other radiologists' impressions. In their study, the presence of nuchal cords led to more admissions to the neonatal intensive case unit and to cesarean section.

There are some authors, however, who deny any relation of fetal distress and poor fetal outcome to problems of cord length. Sinnathuray (1966) and Kan and Eastman (1957) found no increase in perinatal mortality. Dippel (1964) wrote that nuchal cords are much "maligned" and observed a significant increase only in the frequency of irregular fetal heart rates and the need for resuscitation when they were present. He opined that a hasty delivery is rarely required. Spellacy and coauthors (1966) studied this phenomenon in 17,190 deliveries from the Collaborative Perinatal Study. They concluded that nuchal coils occurred in 20.4% of deliveries, that there was entwinement about the body in 2%, and that knots occurred in 1%. There were more complications with long cords, and with "tight" cords (i.e., cords that were short). Entanglement was the cause of depressed 1-minute Apgar scores but did not cause low 5-minute scores. Length of cord was also not correlated with the 1-year neurological status; stillbirths, though, were increased with true knots. McLennan et al. (1988) undertook a prospective study of 1,115 vaginal deliveries to ascertain the frequencies of knots and encirclement. Six knots (0.5%) and 158 cases with encirclement (14.2%) were found, with cords ranging from 27 to 122 cm in length. No warning of such knots or entanglements was identified in the gravidas, and the offspring had no problems, although the authors admitted that knots and entanglements are the cause of 10% of fetal deaths above 2,500 g. In their experience, the average cord length was 52 cm, the 10th percentile was 40 cm, and the 90th percentile was 69 cm. Giacomello (1988) reported the detection of nuchal cord in a large proportion of breech presentations by ultrasonography. He cautioned that assessment of the postdelivery incidence of nuchal cords is unreliable.

In recent years, obstetrical care has frequently involved extensive monitoring of fetal heart rates. Cord entanglement, cord prolapse, and other abnormalities during labor have thus become better correlated with compromised cord perfusion. Rayburn et al. (1981) reviewed some of these findings. They studied 536 term deliveries in an effort to correlate the findings of fetal heart rate monitoring with cord length. They defined "short cord" as all cords measuring less than 35 cm in length and a long cord as measuring more than 80 cm. Of the 32 cases with "cord accidents," 20 (62.5%) were found with long cords. The monitor tracings had "cord compression patterns." These authors advocated measuring cord length routinely after delivery, a recommendation since strongly repeated (Benirschke, 1991). Fribourg (1981) objected to this measurement as an idle enterprise because there are "no current means of performing measurements before the fact." This situation is changing, however, with improved sonographic techniques and with the development of velocimetry (Feinstein et al., 1985; Guidetti et al., 1987). A better understanding of the correlations just described is deemed especially important for infants whose poor outcome is otherwise unexplained. This consideration particularly concerns medical litigation.

It was mentioned earlier that infants born with nuchal cords are more often deprived of placental blood transfusion because their cords are severed by the obstetrician before extraction. Shepherd et al. (1985) noted that newborns with nuchal cords are significantly more anemic than controls, presumably because of reduced venous return from the placenta secondary to compression of the umbilical vein. More recently, Vanhaesebrouck et al. (1987) suggested that tight nuchal cords may be the cause of hypovolemic shock of the newly born. They observed two newborns with anemia and cord entanglement and suggested that entanglement occurs as often as in some 20% of births. Fetomaternal hemorrhage was ruled out to have caused the anemia by Kleihauer stains on maternal blood. These authors also suggested that problems of venous return from the placenta allowed pooling of blood in the placenta. Thus "fetoplacental" hemorrhage is the mode they used to explain the neonatal anemia in their cases. Anagnostakis and coauthors (1974) conjectured that the two neonatal deaths with pulmonary hemorrhages they saw may have resulted from increased pulmonary perfusion because of tight nuchal cords. This argument is difficult to accept, as nuchal cords are so common and lethal pulmonary hemorrhages are rare.

Premature separation of the cord with fetal bleeding may occur with short cords and when a "relative" short cord is induced by entangling. An interesting suggestion has been made by Akiyama et al. (1981), who were concerned with ascertaining clinically when the placenta had detached from the uterus so as to allow its delivery. When they clamped the cord immediately after delivery of the infant, pinched the placental end of the cord, and then squeezed the blood toward the placenta for 10 to 15 cm, they could assess the back-flow of blood in their fingers when slowly releasing the pressure. When back-flow was sensed, the placenta had not yet separated.

Eastman and Hellman (1961) emphasized that the "absolute" and "relative" lengths of cords are the important factors, not the actual measurement of the cord length. It is obvious that a long cord, wound about the neck five times, may in fact be a relatively short cord during fetal descent with delivery. Dislodgement of the placenta may then occur, which may cause bleeding. In the case described by Corridan and coauthors (1980), this complication was associated with fatal amnionic fluid embolism. The reader is also referred to Fox's (1978) book on the placenta for additional references. Fox (1978) and De Sa (1984) were not impressed with the opinion that mechanical factors such as traction play an important role in fetal compromise when short cords are present. Perhaps vascular spasm (Camilleri, 1964) is the important event. This hypothesis is supported by our finding a nuchal cord with fetal death in an otherwise well developed extrauterine (tubal) fetus. The umbilical cord of this fetus was occluded, yet it was clearly stationary.

Prolapse of the cord is associated more often with long cords than with those of normal length. At times this situation has grave prognostic significance for the fetus. Widholm and Nieminen (1963) recorded cord prolapse in 0.41% of 7,500 deliveries with a 13.4% perinatal mortality. This figure is similar to the results published by Brant and Lewis (1966), who urged that a prolapsed cord be kept warm so as to avoid spasm of vessels. A more recent review of the topic was provided by Levy et al. (1984), who found this complication more often in multiparous women. One-half of their study group had fetal malpresentations, one-third had premature onset of labor, and a variety of other abnormal factors were present. Good obstetrical management usually provided a good fetal outcome so long as the fetus was alive on admission. Dildy and Clark (1993) found that cord prolapse occurred in 1 of 275 deliveries, and that the risk was greatest with artificial rupture of membranes with high presenting fetal parts. It has been cautioned that many cases of fatal cord prolapse result from amniotomy, and that some occur after external fetal version (Lehman, 1983). It is now possible to make the diagnosis antenatally with ultrasonography, particularly when malposition and hydramnios suggest this possibility (Lange et al., 1985). A large study on causes of, or associations with, cord prolapse was undertaken by Critchlow et al. (1994). Their findings indicated a high cesarean section rate, 10% mortality, and high prematurity and breech rates; data on the length of the cord were not available. The hemodynamic response with fetal heart rate monitoring has been detailed by Lee and Hon (1963) and is of particular importance for cases with "occult" prolapse. These authors found prompt, marked bradycardia when the umbilical arteries were occluded and believed that it probably resulted from increased fetal blood pressure. This finding has come to be looked at as being pathognomonic for the detection of cord compression during monitored labor. The compressed umbilical cord may show profound pathological changes, such as hemorrhage, and even rupture at the site of compression. It leads occasionally to thrombosis, found when multiple sections are obtained but thrombi ensue more commonly in the surface chorionic vessels. That cord compression may have serious fetal neurological consequences is one of the reasons for taking the "cord compression pattern" of fetal heart monitoring seriously. Its effects on CNS damage has been amply studied in fetal sheep (Mallard et al., 1992). They detected that even short arterial occlusion may cause damage predominantly in the hippocampal area.

Site of Cord Insertion

The umbilical cord normally inserts on the placental tissue itself, more often near or at the center than elsewhere, as shown in Figure 229. In nearly 7% of term placentas it has a marginal insertion, which in the English literature is often referred to as a *Battledore placenta*. In about 1% of placentas the umbilical cord inserts on the membranes, referred to as *velamentous insertion*. Here the umbilical vessels course over the free membranes and, having lost their protection by Wharton's jelly, are more vulnerable to trauma and disruption.

Not only are the sites of insertion variable, the insertion itself may take an abnormal shape: The vessels may branch before the cord comes to the surface of the placenta with the *furcate cord insertion* (Ottow, 1923). At times the cord runs parallel to the placental surface or in the membranes before its vessels branch—the *interposition* (Ottow, 1922). The fetal end of the umbilical cord may also be anomalous, as is found primarily in infants with gastroschisis (short cords) (Figure 226) or with omphaloceles. These conditions can now be diagnosed prenatally and assume a greater importance in management than they did in the past (Didolkar et al., 1981). Some of these anomalies are associated with significant disturbances in fetal growth or during delivery and are thus of importance. Moreover, the formal genesis has interested students of the placenta so they may obtain a better insight into the factors that regulate placental growth. We have seen typical interposition in a case of trisomy 13 associated with a severely malformed fetus and extensive thrombosis of fetal vessels. The umbilical vein of the interposed segment had mural

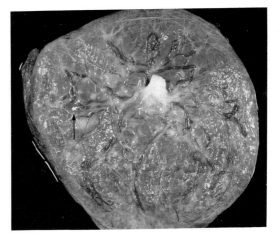

FIGURE 229. Normal term placenta with near-central insertion of the umbilical cord. Note the disperse distribution of the vessels, marginal membranes, and calcified yolk sac remnant (arrow).

thrombosis and old calcifications in the wall; the fetus had intestinal arterial thrombi.

Furcate Cord Insertion

Furcate cord insertion is a rare abnormality in which the umbilical vessels separate from the cord substance prior to reaching the surface of the placenta. They lose the protection afforded by Wharton's jelly and are prone to thrombosis and injury. The condition was first described in three patients by Hyrtl (1870) and received additional attention from Herberz (1938) (six cases) and Swanberg and Wiqvist (1951) (stillborn, hemorrhage). Four of Herberz' cases were associated with normal infants, and much discussion was devoted to its differentiation from velamentous insertion. Kessler (1960) also described fatal hemorrhage associated with this condition and supplied an extensive literature of intrapartum hemorrhage on request. The manner of insertion and the dissociation of vessels from the cord substance are well seen in Figure 230. This placenta was associated with normal outcome. The infant whose placenta is shown in Figure 231, however, was growth-retarded and had low Apgar scores. The furcate and velamentous cords had varices and numerous mural thrombi; many of the placental vessels had degenerations and calcifications in their walls. This case illustrates why the conditions "furcate" and "velamentous" have often posed semantic problems of classification.

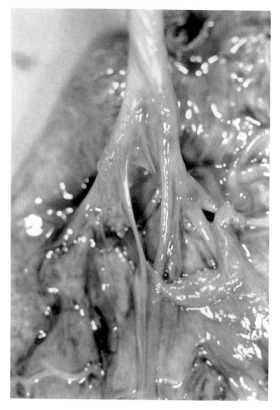

FIGURE 230. Furcate insertion of the umbilical cord. Note that the umbilical vessels leave the protection of Wharton's jelly several centimeters above the cord insertion on the placenta. (Courtesy Dr. W. Tench.)

Velamentous Cord Insertion

Because of its relative frequency and its importance to the course of pregnancy and delivery, membranous insertion of the umbilical cord has been studied by many investigators. Complications include rupture of membranous vessels and vasa previa. Moreover, vasa previa may be compressed during labor and cause fetal distress (Cordero et al., 1993). Velamentously inserted cords are associated with twinning and single umbilical artery (SUA). The incidence of various types of cord insertion varies among numerous reported series because the interpretation of what is truly a marginal or already a velamentous insertion or merely an excessively eccentric one differs in the eyes of the beholder. Nevertheless, Table 16 shows that most observers agree that the frequency of the velamentous insertion is around 1% of singleton term deliveries. The cord may insert reasonably close to the edge of the placenta. This insertion is much more common than the extreme situation, where the cord inserts at the apex of the membranous sac. In the latter configuration the long membranous course of the vessels makes them vulnerable to injury. It should be pointed out, though, that a membranous course of fetal blood vessels is not reserved to velamentous insertion of the cord. Often there are such membranous vessels issuing from marginally inserted cords, and they have the same serious prognosis. Also, membranous fetal vessels are not the same as vasa previa. The latter condition exists only when the membranous vessels course over the internal os uteri, previous (ahead of) to the fetal head during delivery.

Thrombosis of arteries (Figure 232) and veins (Figure 233) have both been seen, and thrombi may be associated with neonatal purpura and fetal death. Hemorrhages arise most commonly from the veins, and they are the most frequent complications of membranous vessels. Hemorrhages may even commence in utero before labor has begun (Bilek et al., 1962). More often they are found when the membranous vessels course over the internal os and are, as "vasa previa," broken by the exiting fetal head or by the obstetrical attendant who ruptures the membranes (Quek & Tan, 1972). Obolensky (1967) provided a description of the differential diagnosis of fetal (versus maternal) blood for such unsuspected vaginal bleeding. The manner by which fetal blood can be distinguished from maternal blood is discussed in greater detail in the discussion on hemorrhage due to placenta previa and in Chapter 17. Exsanguination from ruptured vasa previa can proceed within minutes. We have seen fatalities occur within 3 minutes of disruption through unrecognized velamentous vessels. Experience of successful immediate

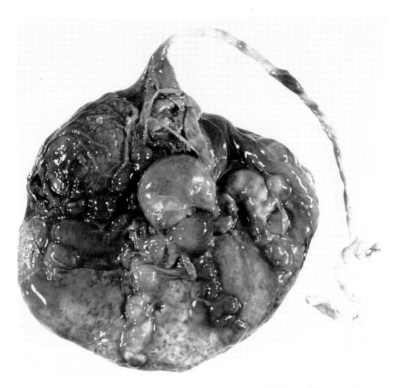

FIGURE 231. Velamentous, furcate insertion of the cord in a growth-retarded infant with low Apgar scores. There are numerous aneurysms, an extensive mural thrombosis, and vessel wall calcifications. (Courtesy Dr. M. Rockwell.)

blood transfusion has also been reported (Mitchell et al., 1957). The frequency of hemorrhages is difficult to assess but has been estimated by Quek and Tan (1972) to be 1 in 50 cases of velamentous insertions. The mortality rate from intrapartum rupture and hemorrhage was given as 58% by Rucker and Tureman (1945) in their report of three cases and in their comprehensive literature review. Remarkably, the mortality has been 73% when the hemorrhage occurred before delivery (Torrey, 1952). Pent (1979) went so far as to state that "an active obstetric service can expect to have one perinatal death each year due to vasa previa."

Hemorrhages have on occasion been recognized by palpation of vasa previa, by amnioscopy, and even

TABLE 16. Large series' frequencies of cord insertions in singletons.

Authors	Total	Cord insertion		
		Marginal (%)	Velamentous (%)	Normal (%)
Benirschke 1972–1975	4,601	8.5	1.5	90.0
Nöldeke (1934)	10,000	ng	1.1	
Grieco (1936)	23,469	?	0.41	
Earn (1951)	5,412	15	1.0	84.0
Di Terlizzi & Rossi (1955)	15,416	?	1.0	
Scott (1960)	3,161	2	1.5	96.5
Corkill (1961)	12,695	ng	0.024	
Eastman & Hellman (1961)	2,000	7	1.25	91.75
Thomas (1963)	18,316	5.2	1.3	93.5
Krone et al. (1965)	2,868	7.9	1.8	90.3
Scheffel & Langanke (1970)	37,963	ng	0.22	
Uyanwah-Akpom & Fox (1977)	1,000	5.6	1.6	92.8
Robinson et al. (1983)	44,677	8.5	1.5	90.0
This series (1984–1987)	12,787	9.17	1.27	89.56
Total	194,365	6.89	1.11	90.9

ng = not given.

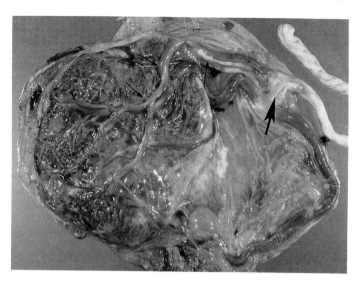

FIGURE 232. Velamentous (membranous) insertion of the umbilical cord (large arrow) with several calcified arterial thrombi (small arrows). Apgar scores were 1/9.

by sonography (Gianopoulos et al., 1987). Vasa previa have been diagnosed by ultrasonography (color Doppler) prior to hemorrhage, leading to elective section (Meyer et al., 1993). The aberrant vessels led to a succenturiate lobe. When velamentous vessels are compressed during labor, it may be recognized by a sinusoidal fetal heart rate pattern. An example is the twin pregnancy described by Antoine et al. (1982). These authors reviewed the dismal experience with vasa previa in twin pregnancies. Obstetricians have also occasionally made the diagnosis of bleeding due to vasa previa by examining vaginal blood during labor. Diagnostic methods have included Kleihauer stains and other techniques to detect fetal blood (Bergström, 1963; Carp et al., 1979; Vandriede & Kammeraad, 1981; Silva et al., 1985; Jones et al., 1987). Because of the ability to ascertain fetal blood in vaginal bleeding from vasa previa, it has become a topic for litigation, but Messer et al. (1987) surveyed 100 community

hospitals and concluded that such testing is currently not a "standard of care" in the United States.

As already stated, vasa previa are not confined to velamentous insertions. A marginally inserted cord may have aberrant branches that course over the membranes; even cords with more central position can have such vessels. Vasa previa may also occur with succenturiate lobes (Radcliffe et al., 1961) and in bilobed placentas (Waidl, 1960; Kouyoumdjian, 1980). Scheuner (1965) studied the histological characteristics of nine term velamentous insertions and discussed the rich literature of this condition in detail. He found that membranous vessels are firmly anchored to the chorion by collagenous fibers, which explains why it is that the vessels rupture so readily when the chorion breaks.

It has been of great interest to understand the pathogenesis of velamentous and marginal insertions of the umbilical cord. There are two mutually contradictory theories: (1) abnormal primary implantation ("polarity

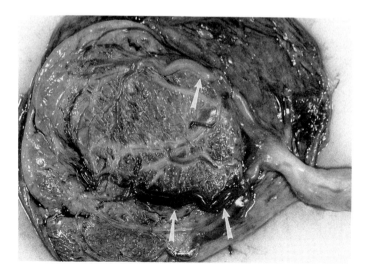

FIGURE 233. Velamentous insertion of the umbilical cord with sudden fetal death at 37 weeks. Note the large venous thrombi (arrows). The different ages of thrombi are seen in darker and lighter colors, indicating different degrees of hemolysis.

theory"); and (2) trophotropism. Arguments have been brought to bear for both of these points of view. We favor the second and believe that it derives stronger support from the various placental constellations one finds associated with this condition.

The primarily abnormal implantation theory postulates that at the nidation of the blastocyst the embryo does not face the endometrium; rather, it is located at the opposite side or is obliquely oriented. Thus when the vascular stalk develops, this trunk must seek its connection with the future area of placentation by extending its vessels from the embryo to the base of implantation. Eventually, the vessels must thereby become membranous in location. This view was championed by Hertig (1968), among others, despite the fact that in virtually all of the normal early embryos he discovered and described in meticulous detail the embryo had a "normal" (endometrial) position. Carnegie specimen 8671, however (his Figure 65), had a somewhat oblique orientation, which might have caused a marginal insertion of the cord. Beer (1954) suggested that the cord arises "from the most vascular portion of the decidua," an opinion that is difficult to comprehend. If that were the case, one would perhaps expect to find as high a frequency (or a higher one) of velamentous and marginal cords during the first trimester as that which occurs later in gestation—which is not the case.

Monie (1965) found 15.3% of velamentous cords and 14.7% of marginal cords among 183 specimens of 9- to 13-week abortuses. He confirmed that velamentous insertion was highly correlated with congenital anomalies (marginal cords were in between), and he provided a particularly good discussion and diagrams of the various notions published by earlier investigators. Monie acknowledged the frequency of velamentous cords in South American monkeys that have a superficial implantation. This finding negated earlier suggestions by Torpin (1953) that too deep an implantation may be the cause of velamentous cord insertion. Monie also reviewed the two types of velamentous insertion, normal and interpositional. Parenthetically, it may be mentioned that the umbilical cords of gorillas have

nearly always been found to be marginal and also relatively long, about 100 cm (Ludwig, 1961). Hathout (1964) searched for cord insertion sites in 131 abortions of up to 28 weeks' gestation. He found velamentous cords in 8.1% (three twins); 21.5% had marginal cords (one twin). It was central/eccentric in 70%. Because the abnormal cords were from midtrimester abortions, one might consider that the factors involved in trophotropism were also the cause of abortion. This contention is not supported by the extensive mathematical analysis of McLennan (1968), who sided with the theory of primarily disturbed placentation.

The case for trophotropism was first presented in detail by Strassmann (1902) in his large study of placenta previa and associated placental anomalies. The etiological role of trophotropism is supported by cogent considerations: Velamentous and marginal cords are much more common in twins and are almost invariably present in higher multiple births. They are common when intrauterine devices (IUDs) are found in the placental membranes. Some of these pregnancies have led to prenatal hemorrhages and abortion (Golden, 1973). Moreover, one can sonographically observe eccentric expansion of the placenta during the course of advancing pregnancy, which would leave the cord insertion site behind. The distribution of cord insertions of some consecutive twin placentas are recorded in Table 17. It can be seen that with the exception of diamnionic/dichorionic separate twin placentas there is an excessively high rate of abnormal cord insertions.

Finally, a series of successively undertaken ultrasonographs has shown that the placenta may "wander," called "dynamic placentation" (King, 1973). That is, when during early pregnancy a placenta previa was unmistakenly diagnosed (in 5.3% of patients), it converted to a "marginal" or higher-lying placenta with progressing pregnancy; a placenta previa was found at term in only 0.58% (Rizos et al., 1979). In the series published by Meyenburg (1976), which supports these observations, the point is made that an opposite migration never takes place. Regrettably, in none of these studies is the location of the umbilical cord mentioned—

TABLE 17. Distribution of cord insertion in twin placentas past 20 weeks.

Type of placenta	Pairs (no.)	Infants (no.)	Cord insertion (no.)					Marginal (%)	Velamentous (%)	Dead	
			Marginal		Velamentous		Eccentric or central				
			Twin A	Twin B	Twin A	Twin B				No.	%
MoMo	15	30	5	5	2	3	15	33	16	9	30.0
DiMo	247	494	69	77	36	29	283	30	13	110	22.0
DiDi fused	188	376	48	43	15	21	249	24	10	28	7.4
DiDi sep.	241	482	30	27	8	7	410	12	3	1	8.5
Total	691	1,382	152	152	61	60	957	21.9	8.7		

MoMo = monoamnionic/monochorionic; DiMo = diamnionic/monochorionic; DiDi = diamnionic/dichorionic.

neither at the time when the placenta was first localized nor after delivery. It would be desirable to collect this information in the future. The placental movement is not accomplished, of course, by the placenta unseating and relocating itself but, rather, through marginal atrophy on one side and expansion on the other, as well as through the development and thinning of the lower uterine segment. This mechanism is also the best one to explain the sickle-shaped, marginal placental atrophy that has been observed (Winter, 1978). Young (1978), who studied a large number of such early placentas previa, referred to the process as an "amoeba-like growth."

The most extensive writings on this topic come from Krone. In 1962 this author began studies showing that marginal and velamentous cords tend to correlate with fetal anomalies. In his early contributions, Krone (1960) presented data to show that 9% of normal infants had a markedly eccentric cord, as did 28% of malformed babies. Marginal and velamentous cord insertions were present in 6% and 26%, respectively. In a later study of 2,868 placental examinations, Krone et al. (1965) found that such cord insertional anomalies correlated with advanced maternal age and multiparity, and that they often followed abortions and curettage. He believed that the abnormal placentas could not be the cause of fetal anomalies because final placental shape occurs only *after* the "teratogenetic termination period" (Schwalbe, 1906).

These placentas, however, direct our attention to the existence of an abnormal nidation/placentation process (Krone, 1967). Our own studies of fetal anomalies and cord insertion clearly showed such a relation, and it has been noted by others as well (Robinson et al., 1983). The suggestion by Shanklin (1970) that abnormal cord insertion correlates with low birth weight was not supported by the study of Woods and Malan (1978), who evaluated 940 placentas with marginal or central cords. Nöldeke (1934) found that abnormally inserted cords occur more often in prematurely delivered infants. He noted increased difficulty of placental separation, as did Earn (1951). Their findings were not confirmed, however, by the study of Uyanwah-Akpom and Fox (1977). In all these considerations one must remember that twins must be excluded from any study so as to make the data truly comparable. This exclusion is often not done; so from many of the original papers it is impossible to discern the extent to which twins were present within the data sets and thereby increased the numbers of velamentous cords. Hence the numbers in Table 16 and in the reports must be interpreted with some caution.

Eddleman and colleagues (1992) reviewed the sonograms of the 82 cases of velamentous cord insertions seen in their 4-year experience (77 singletons). In none of them had the diagnosis been made before birth, including the three cases of vasa previa later identified. The infants born to these women had lower birth weights than controls and more intrapartum complications, but the mothers did not have higher parity or more frequently prior sections as is often assumed. Importantly, the study showed that sonographically this diagnosis cannot be expected to be made routinely.

Placental Surface Vessels

It is convenient to consider the placental vascular tree at this point, as future discussion of the thrombotic events of the cord often interrelate with those of the vasculature on the surface of the placenta. The distribution of the blood vessels across the placenta is not random, although we do not understand the mechanisms that govern their growth. Two principal patterns of vessel distribution have been described in the literature, and admixtures exist occasionally. The "disperse" pattern has a fine network of vessels that course from the cord insertion to the various placental cotyledons. The "magistral" pattern has arteries that course across the placental surface nearly to the edge without diminishing their diameters. The arteries have a fairly uniform diameter, and they have many branches. These two types are shown in Figure 234. They have been delineated by injection and corrosion techniques that employ a variety of materials, including lead salts and plastics (Hyrtl, 1870; Schordania, 1929a; Bacsich & Smout, 1938; Smart, 1962; Kishore & Sarkar, 1967; and others cited by these authors). Schordania (1929a), who is responsible for the aforementioned terminology, advanced the theory that the magistral type of vascularity leads to better-developed fetuses. This theory was not affirmed by the studies of Crawford (1959), however; and Bacsich and Smout (1938) failed to identify the arterial anastomoses in the periphery of the placenta that were delineated by Hyrtl (1870) and others. The same observation was made by Priman (1959). The superficial arteries are end-arteries, to which feature Bacsich and Smout (1938), incorrectly we believe, attributed the occurrence of white infarcts near term. The disperse type of vessel distribution is more commonly present (61.8%), with the magistral type occurring in 38.2% (Kishore & Sarkar, 1967). The latter authors found no association with placental size or anomalies but noted that the disperse type was more frequent in placentas with centrally inserted cords. There is no racial influence on these features (Andrade, 1968).

At the periphery, the arteries individually supply a single cotyledon, turning abruptly toward the maternal surface, then branch repeatedly, and finally become

FIGURE 234. Disperse and magistral distributions of placental arterial vessels.

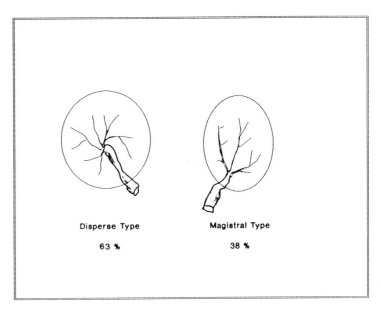

capillaries; the blood is then returned from the capillary loops of the cotyledon to the umbilical cord by veins that merge. It is crucial to recognize that in the overwhelming majority of cotyledons there is a 1:1 relation between artery and vein at the periphery. Otherwise, the transfusion syndrome of monochorial twins could not be understood. It is further remarkable that arteries always cross over veins, particularly nearer the cord insertion (Smart, 1962). Wentworth (1965) reported that only about 3% show the opposite condition. Bhargava, in a series of studies (Bhargava & Raja, 1969), suggested that veins may cross over arteries. They undertook a quantitative analysis of these features. In their material, this reversal of the normal pattern correlated significantly with abnormal fetal development and with hydramnios. However, according to Boyd and Hamilton (1970) the superficial position of one or few veins at points of arteriovenous crossing is not unusual even in normal placentas. They can thus be readily identified by macroscopic examination. Histologically, it is nearly impossible to make this distinction (Figure 235). Only Bhargava, in a series of studies (Bhargava & Raja, 1969), suggested that veins may cross over arteries. They undertook a quantitative analysis of these features. In their material, this reversal of the normal pattern correlated significantly with abnormal fetal development and with hydramnios. What makes these vessels assume this pattern so uniformly? Because we do not understand genetic influences on the placenta, it is our belief that when the earliest embryonic vessels grow into the placental surface, the subsequent perfusion, at first sluggish, determines the vascular pattern that ultimately results. It may well be subject to trophic or mechanical (pressure) forces. For a better comprehension of the complexities

of the vascularity in twin placentation, it would be helpful to have a better understanding of these vascular phenomena. It is further remarkable that the circumferential architecture of the placental surface vessels is

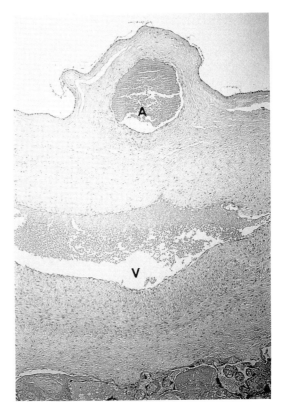

FIGURE 235. Microscopic appearance of the surface of the placenta, with the artery (A) above the vein (V). Note that the fetal side of both vessels has a much thinner muscular wall and that the artery lies on top of the vein. H&E. ×60.

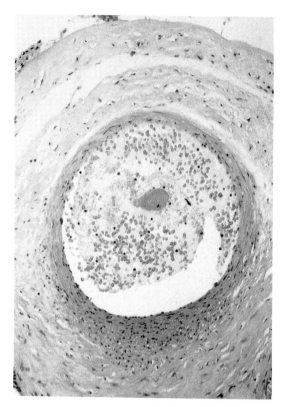

FIGURE 236. Differences in wall thickness of the umbilical vein branch at term. H&E. ×240.

asymmetrical (Figure 236). This area has been studied by Fujikura and Carleton (1968), who found that the thinning of the muscular wall of arteries (80%) commences after 12 weeks' gestation. Of the two theories they advanced (trophic growth of muscle and hemodynamic thinning), we favor the latter and believe that the pressure buckles and thins the superficial portions of the vessels, whereas the "fixed" portions resist this pressure. This phenomenon of thinning of the superficial aspect of chorionic vessels (also shared with cord vessels) may actually be a sequel of amnionic rupture and a change in intraamnionic pressure relation after the event of membrane rupture. Contrary to the observations of Fujikura and Carleton (1968), we believe this property to be shared by veins (Figure 235), a feature Fujikura and Hosoda (1990) have acknowledged. Unilateral thickening of the muscular walls of large chorionic veins (>1.0 mm diameter) on the chorionic side is a usual finding in all normal placentas after 17 weeks' gestation. The amnionic/chorionic wall thickness ratio may be 1:3 to 1:4. It is caused by muscular hyperplasia rather than by arteriosclerotic changes. Fujikura and Hosoda (1990) concluded differences in wall movement as etiological factors.

Surface arteries and veins are subject to spontaneous rhythmic contractions and to the influences of various mediators, such as serotonin, prostaglandins, atrial natriuretic peptide, nitric oxide, and endothelin-1 (Panigel, 1962; Panizza et al., 1981; Robaut et al., 1991; Salas et al., 1991; Omar et al., 1992; Myatt et al., 1993; Rath et al., 1993). Methyldopa, for instance, was found to decrease the placental vascular resistance in hypertensive disease when Doppler velocimetry was done (Rey, 1992). In general, the larger chorionic and stem vessels seem to behave like the umbilical vessels (see above) (Macara et al., 1993). Endothelin, on the other hand, is said to increase resistance in the arterial bed (Bodelsson et al., 1992).

Studies have also endeavored to correlate umbilical artery flow waveforms with abnormalities in the vascular beds of tertiary villi (McCowan et al., 1987). When the cord arterial pulsatility index is high, indicating peripheral vascular resistance, the peripheral arterial vessel count is low, a finding that is strongly correlated with growth-retarded fetuses (Hitschold et al., 1993). Similar studies by Doppler waveform analysis of umbilical cord flow showed that, during preterm labor, ritodrine (but not magnesium sulfate) affected umbilical vascular resistance (Brar et al., 1988). When different patterns of flow were thus determined with serial determinations, the placenta was subsequently found to have one large infarcted lobe supplied by one artery; and the authors believed that the infarction may have been the reason for the difference (Trudinger & Cook, 1988). The pattern of umbilical blood velocity waveforms changes abruptly at about 12 weeks' gestation. Prior to that time, there are no end-diastolic frequencies (EDFs), which in later life would be held to be an abnormal feature of fetal circulation. Fisk et al. (1988) and Loquet et al. (1988) simultaneously reported that no EDFs were observed before 12 weeks (as is normal in peripheral arteries), and that their appearance at the second trimester perhaps signals the development of vessels in the tertiary villi and the disappearance of the membranous circulation. It signals the sudden decrease of placental villous flow resistance.

A variety of disease processes affect placental surface vessels. The easiest to understand is hemorrhage after traumatic laceration. Disruption of chorionic vessels is commonest after amniocentesis and may lead to rapid fetal exsanguination (Goodlin & Clewell, 1974) and intraamnionic bleeding. It has been recognized by sonography during amniocentesis as a spurt. We have seen three such lacerations of surface vessels due to amniocentesis performed to assess fetal maturity in a patient with diabetes (Figure 237). The infant survived. In another case, where amniocentesis was performed at 12 weeks to obtain genetic information, the anterior

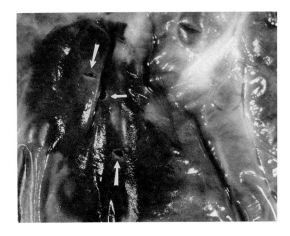

FIGURE 237. Three lacerations (arrows) due to amniocentesis performed to assess fetal maturity at 38 weeks' gestation in a patient with diabetes. A cesarean section was performed resulting in a live birth.

placenta had one surface vessel ruptured, and blood dissected underneath the amnion. When a stillborn fetus was eventually delivered, hemosiderin and nucleated red blood cells were found along the well defined needle track. Intraamnionic bleeding has been studied with sonographic surveillance and correlation with Kleihauer tests to determine the amount of RhoGam needed for Rh-negative patients (Lenke et al., 1985). It was found that bleeding occurred most commonly when, in anterior placentas, the placenta had to be traversed by the needle. No correlation with fetal-to-maternal hemorrhage has been found. A patient was referred to us with a posterior placenta that exsanguinated through a transverse laceration of a surface artery. The amniocentesis needle had produced this lesion after much amniotic fluid had been withdrawn, perhaps because the posterior placenta had then come closer. Considerable search may be required to identify such defects; the pallor of the placental tissue is the first sign of blood loss, the suspicion of which then leads to a detailed inspection for an explanation. Needle puncture of the fetus at amniocentesis has also been reported. When it occurs during early diagnostic procedures fetal scars may result (Broome et al., 1975, 1976); in later gestations, hemorrhage may ensue (Galle & Meis, 1982). The practice of cordocentesis may also cause hematoma and other injury to the umbilical cord. Jauniaux et al. (1989b) found, among 50 cases studied, one giant hematoma of the cord and four small hematomas that encircled the walls of the arteries. The needle puncture sites were readily visible in 37 cases. Thrombosis was not found, and these authors suspected that the injured vessel was repaired within 1 week. In a fortuitous section, De Sa (1984) depicted (his Figures 5–8) the disruption of an umbilical vein within a cord hematoma.

More frequent perhaps are hemorrhages that occur after laceration of velamentous vessels and vasa previa. This subject is discussed later in the chapter. A remarkable case was described by Tuggle and Cook (1978): An infant had experienced massive bleeding from a surface vein that led to cesarean section; no therapeutic intervention could be blamed for this spontaneous rupture. Because of the unusually long fingernails of the newborn, it was conjectured that the nails of the fetus may have caused the tear.

Nucleated Red Blood Cells

Another important observation is needed when examining the fetal blood within chorionic vessels (easiest done in the blood of the vessels on the fetal surface) or in the umbilical cord. That observation is to gain an appreciation of the presence of nucleated red blood cells (NRBCs) in the fetal circulation. In normal term pregnancies few red blood cells with nuclei are visible in the fetal blood during placental examination. There is, however, considerable controversy about the number of NRBCs in truly normal neonates. When many NRBCs are seen in the absence of anemia or erythroblastosis, it is a distinctly abnormal finding; and the pathologist should endeavor to ascertain the reason for their presence. There exists an extensive literature on this topic, and its findings are not always in agreement. One reason for discrepant results may be that, especially in older citations, the authors have not always excluded infants who suffered hypoxia or other causes for the presence of NRBCs. This aspect is fully discussed at the end of Chapter 9.

Cysts and Edema

Aside from the aforementioned cysts, we have seen a small amnionic epithelial inclusion cyst in a fetus with 47,XXX chromosome constitution. It was filled with clear fluid. On rare occasions cysts arise within Wharton's jelly. They are most obvious in the edematous umbilical cords that have been associated with respiratory distress syndrome of newborns (Coulter et al., 1975). Coulter and colleagues found 10% of babies to have edematous cords; the occurrence is more common in premature infants. These authors related the edema to reduced oncotic pressure. Edema is apparent in the markedly swollen, glistening umbilical cord shown in Figure 238. It resembles the condition of "mucoid degeneration" described by Bergman et al.

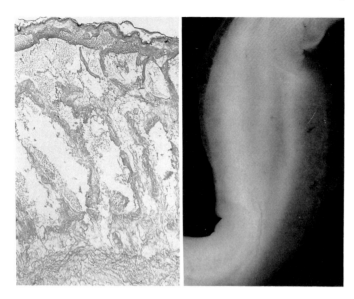

FIGURE 238. Marked edema in the umbilical cord of a normal newborn. Note the dissociation of fibrous tissue underneath the surface of the cord. H&E. ×160.

(1961). These investigators believed that one of their patients died as a result of this degeneration. Whether it is truly a degenerative event, however, remains to be ascertained. Rolschau (1978), on the other hand, found that edema of the cord had no influence on fetal development and well-being. The pathological change may be diffusely distributed or occur focally as cysts. Usually, the cysts in Wharton's jelly are not accompanied by fetal disease, and there is a normal fetal outcome. Severe distension, up to 5 cm diameter, occurs for unknown reasons occasionally and may then be accompanied by hydramnios and an excessive number of mast cells (Howorka & Kapczynski, 1971). Walz (1947) studied this phenomenon in more detail when he observed a growth-retarded infant with a normal placenta but an "arm-thick" umbilical cord that was difficult to ligate. It also had calcifications that are discussed shortly. The cord was 46 cm long and 7 cm thick. Histologically, it was edematous and had acute inflammatory cell infiltration, mural thrombi, and many areas of degeneration. Walz reviewed the older literature on this finding. Occasionally, the cord has a complete lack of Wharton's jelly, which is usually a sign of fetal growth retardation (Scott & Jordan, 1972). The association is not a strict one, however, and many infants with IUGR (e.g., renal agenesis) have normal cords. Nevertheless, experienced obstetricians regard lean cords as a sign of dysmaturity (Goodlin, 1987). Degeneration of cord substance, with an absence of Wharton's jelly, has also been reported by Labarrere et al. (1985). They found three cases of meconium-stained term neonates who died shortly after birth in whom the umbilical arteries were detached from the cord substance. Much of the amnionic epithelium of the cord was defective, as was Wharton's jelly. They speculated that there may have been incomplete fusion of amnion with cord and

likened the condition's etiology to that of furcate insertion. The pathological change may be diffusely distributed or occur focally as cysts. We have seen such degenerated cords with prolonged meconium staining on several occasions, not always associated with bad fetal outcome. The dissociated vessels, however, have usually been severely inflamed, and our opinion is that it is the result of meconium toxicity.

The water content of the umbilical cord has been studied in great detail by Scott and Wilkinson (1978). Edematous cords had a water content of 93.5%, and wrinkled cords had 89.2% water. The correlation with cystic spaces such as those of Figure 238 is then excellent. There is a tendency for the amount of Wharton's jelly or its water content to decrease with advancing gestation. Bender et al. (1978) provided a particularly useful review of the older literature on this topic and studied the relation of the amount of jelly to outcome. They found that infants with much jelly and more spiraling of vessels have better outcomes than those who do not. In the stillborn with a markedly spiraled, jelly-poor cord, it can be argued that the jelly has disappeared because of vascular compression. It is not proved that Wharton's jelly was primarily absent; in general, we are ignorant of the mechanisms that provide cord jelly and its water content. Realizing that the amnionic fluid decreases with advancing gestational age and that there may be a correlation with cord thickness, Silver et al. (1987a) sonographically studied the cord thickness, diameter, and circumference after birth. The cord diameter varied from 1.25 to 2.00 cm and its circumference from 2.4 to 4.4 cm. Fetal monitoring "compression patterns" increased in frequency with decreasing fluid content of the cord. It may also be mentioned that experimental evidence has indicated that in fetal lambs intermittent partial cord occlusion leads to cerebral necrosis (Clapp et al., 1988; Mallard et al., 1992). Gill and collaborators (1993) measured the quantity of jelly in umbilical cord; they found a positive relation to male fetuses, increased prepartum maternal weight, and heavier birth weight.

Excessively thin umbilical cords are abnormal and potential causes of fetal problems. This condition was referred to as the "thin cord syndrome" by Hall (1961). It may involve the entire cord or only portions of the umbilical cord. The latter is seen most often in cases in which the cord has become extremely thinned near the abdominal surface of the fetus due to torsion, so-called coarctation. It frequently leads to fetal death and abortion. In the prototype of abnormally thin cord there is a deficiency of Wharton's jelly, and compression of vessels is a greater possibility than when they are protected. Thin cords occur more often with growth-retarded fetuses and in preeclampsia, but unknown causes exist as well. Labarrere et al. (1985) presented three cases in which Wharton's jelly was deficient, with arteries free next to the umbilical cords and causing fetal demise. Meconium is often present and may be the cause of degenerative changes that are occasionally seen.

Single Umbilical Artery

Single umbilical artery (SUA) is the commonest true congenital anomaly of humans. An enormous literature has been created in efforts to explain its nature and significance. Our files contains more than 80 papers dealing with SUA, and many more are reviewed and critically analyzed in the review articles by Heifetz (1984) and Leung and Robson (1989). These reports can be consulted for all of the relevant literature.

Single umbilical artery was apparently first described by Vesalius. It did not attract further notice until the 40 cases listed by Otto (1830) and the later attention by Hyrtl (1870), who summarized 70 cases in an interesting monograph. Considering its incidence of about 1% in newborns (Heifetz compiled all data and reported there being a 0.63% frequency), it is surprising that its relation to anomalous fetal development was overlooked for so long—until we drew attention to it again (Benirschke & Brown, 1953; Benirschke & Bourne, 1960). Since then, there has been a veritable flood of information on SUA (Table 18). It can now be detected prenatally by ultrasonography (Tortora et al., 1984; Herrmann & Sidiropoulos, 1988), and Jones et al. (1993) made the point that it is unforgivable if it is not ascertained. Among the seven patients of Tortora et al. (1984), four had hydramnios, two were growth-retarded, two died, two survived with anomalies, and three were normal infants. Herrmann and Sidiropoulos (1988) found SUA

TABLE 18. Frequency of SUA in various populations.

Series of prospective deliveries	Total	SUA	
		No.	%
Review	332,067	2,099	0.63
Autopsies	18,614	357	1.92
Twin deliveries	1,323	51	3.85
Twin infants	2,399	56	2.33

Data from Heifetz (1984).

in four cases and drew attention to the growth retardation of the neonates. The relation of SUA to growth retardation has also been studied by Rolschau (1978). He found that SUA correlated with circumvallation of the placenta, and that marginal cord insertion was moderately well correlated with small placentas and fetuses. Velamentous insertion of the cord, however, had a strong negative effect on fetal and placental weights. Leung and Robson (1989) found SUA in 159 of 56,919 infants. Twins had an incidence of 8.8%, and it was usually the smaller twin who had the anomaly. SUA was associated with diabetes, epilepsy, preeclampsia, antepartum hemorrhage, hydramnios, and oligohydramnios. Anomalies were detected in 44.7% of the associated infants, and other placental abnormalities were found in 16.4%. Because of the frequency of renal anomalies (18.5%) these authors recommended that neonatal renal sonography be performed when SUA is found. Abuhamad et al. (1994) found sonographically that 70% of SUA locates to the left artery and that cytogenetic and complex anomalies were associated with that side. Theirs is the largest prospective series, and they found a 30% associated anomaly incidence.

Absence of one umbilical artery may occur as aplasia or as the consequence of atrophy of one artery. The latter mechanism is probably more frequent and can be seen to have occurred in many specimens when histological examination is undertaken (Figure 239). Degeneration of one artery occasionally occurs late in pregnancy, but when it took place some time before birth the arterial lumen gradually vanishes, and only a tiny muscular remnant then remains (Figure 240).

The question whether SUA due to "aplasia" has a prognosis different from that due to "atrophy" was examined in a large study by Altshuler et al. (1975). These authors found 19 placentas with SUA among 4,138 consecutive deliveries (0.46%). Altogether they analyzed 48 children with this anomaly and found no significant difference "in congenital malformations or neonatal mortality." The more frequent detection of SUA in term placentas than in placentas of early gestation further supports the view that the etiology involves arterial atrophy. On the other hand, early embryos with SUA have also been seen, and SUA has been observed

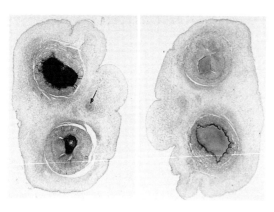

FIGURE 239. Umbilical cord from a placenta with marginal cord insertion. A degenerating second artery is seen (arrow). An elastic tissue stain (right) shows the internal elastica of the umbilical vein and its absence in both arteries. Left, H&E; right, von Gieson. ×10.

associated with many chromosomal anomalies and with exposure to such teratogens as thalidomide. It has even occurred in baboons so treated experimentally. SUA is also found almost regularly in association with sirenomelia and is present in the cords of most acardiac fetuses (malformed monozygotic twins; see Chapter 25) which also supports the notion of occasional "aplasia" as its origin.

It must be cautioned that SUA may be found at one end of the cord and not the other. We have therefore suggested that to verify its existence one must sample three areas of the umbilical cord. At times the arteries fuse far above the cord insertion on the placenta (Kelber, 1976) in a manner similar to their normal communication near the placenta. An interesting question is what happens when there is no communicating artery during early development, as is the case in some 4% of term umbilical cords (Priman, 1959). Because each artery supplies a portion of placental tissue, the area supplied by an atrophying artery would then presumably undergo atrophy. Such atrophic changes may explain the much higher frequency of SUA in multiple births. Trophotropic expansion and pressures from one twin placenta may then affect the placental expansion of the other placenta (Thomas, 1961). Such considerations may also relate to the finding that SUA is associated with lower birth weight, as the amount of some placental area would be reduced by the placental atrophy. This concept has been supported by the experimental ligation of one artery in sheep fetuses (Hobel et al., 1970). Bhargava et al. (1971) found a higher frequency of the magistral pattern of chorial blood vessels with SUA, and the vascular pattern of SUA differs from that of cords with fused arteries.

Much has been made of the significance of SUA with respect to other congenital anomalies in the fetus and how seriously one should look for such anomalies. It can now be said that there is no predilection for any specific type of fetal anomaly. Moreover, SUA is often found in perfectly healthy infants who eventually attain normal size and development. Therefore an extraordinary or invasive study of infants born with SUA is not warranted. To be sure, the pediatrician should be notified of its existence and then make certain by more detailed physical examination that the infant has no hidden anomalies. We do not perform radiographic or invasive study.

The SUA is commoner in European whites than in Orientals, in multiple births, in autopsy series (because of associated anomalies), in spontaneous abortions, with other placental anomalies [velamentous cord and chorangioma: 2.70% and 0.65%, respectively (Froehlich & Fujikura, 1966); perhaps circumvallates], and with chromosomal errors; it has no familial or genetic tendency. The suggested relation to the development of inguinal hernias has been disputed. Infants with SUA have lower birth weights and are more often born prematurely. When one considers all the details of the enormous study produced by Heifetz (1984), it is apparent that the diagnosis of SUA is made at birth; and when found one proceeds cautiously with additional studies in an attempt to find its possible cause and relevance. There is no reason, however, to change our view from that expressed earlier (Benirschke & Driscoll, 1967) that the "indiscriminate association of the absence of one umbilical artery with various and quite diverse chromosomal disorders indicates how limited the placenta is in expressing a variety of constitutional defects." Most likely, SUA is either part of a constellation of multiple anomalies, not its cause, or it develops during pregnancy due to atrophy; in the latter case it may be the reason for reduced fetal growth (small for gestational age, SGA). The importance of abnormal

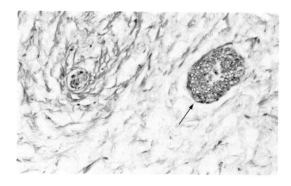

FIGURE 240. Muscular remnant of a "vanished" second umbilical artery (arrow); the other structure is a remnant of an allantoic duct. H&E. ×60.

cord insertion in SUA is borne out, for instance, in the study of Matheus and Sala (1980), who reported an incidence of 0.95%. Of their 42 SUA cases, 11.9% had velamentous insertion, and 33.3% were associated with abnormal fetuses. Kaplan et al. (1990) have suggested that SUA may be associated with cord accidents during labor. They reported on four infants with SUA who died suddenly in utero, presumably because of "cord accidents," but these infants were not growth-retarded because of SUA.

Perhaps a special case of SUA is that found nearly invariably with sireniform fetuses. The question posed by this finding is whether the SUA, arising usually directly from the aorta and immediately distal to the celiac artery, is of enteric ("omphalomesenteric," vitelline) nature or it is an allantoic vessel, as would be normal for the cord. This anomaly (sympus) has also been referred to as caudal regression syndrome, but this term is often inappropriately used; frequently there is no evidence for regression, particularly in the cases that are so descriptive of diabetic embryopathy (Benirschke, 1987). In any event, we have suggested that this vessel "steals" blood from the lower aortic blood flow and is thus responsible for the caudal maldevelopment (Stevenson et al., 1986). The older literature on this topic has been considered in this study of 11 sireniform fetuses. This review and the papers cited by Heifetz (1984) can be consulted when further insight into this phenomenon is desired. The dispute is not totally resolved, however, as studies in mice with this anomaly suggest the vessel to be allantoic in nature; it is thought only to take an abnormal course, with fusion of the two arteries (Schreiner & Hoornbeek, 1973). How complex these embryological considerations are can be seen in the study by Monie and Khemmani (1973). They induced SUA in rat fetuses with retinoic acid and described the vitelloumbilical anastomosis in the embryos. After due consideration they could not rule out the occasional existence of such anastomoses in human embryos; it is their opinion, however, that the SUA of symmelia represents a remaining allantoic vessel. These considerations are of interest only in that the view of persisting vitelline vessels would support the notion that when these vessels become dominant they can acquire muscular coats. This situation is not the case with the usual persistence of omphalomesenteric vessels; they are composed essentially only of endothelium.

More than three umbilical vessels are normal for many species (Benirschke et al., 1964), but it is rare in human umbilical cords. Painter and Russell (1977) described a stillborn with ectopia cordis and other anomalies; there were two umbilical veins, the right umbilical vein having persisted. Hathout (1964) mentioned that one of his cases had five vessels due to "division of both arteries" and one with four and a nodular embryo. One must take care, when assessing an increased number of vessels, not to be misled by the frequent looping that occurs in many cord vessels.

Placental Transfusion

When the fetus is delivered, the umbilical cord may break by the mechanisms discussed above, and bleeding may cease shortly thereafter. More commonly now, the attending obstetrician clamps the cord. With vaginal deliveries the amount of fetal blood remaining in the placenta is 2.5% of fetal body weight, even with prompt cord ligation. With cesarean section, that figure is 4.5% (Gruenwald, 1969). It has become customary to clamp both sides of the cord, even though the loss of placental fetal blood might be thought irrelevant. One reason for clamping has been the realization that, on occasion, an unrecognized twin may be present; that twin may exsanguinate quickly through intertwin arterial anastomoses of monochorial placentas. Moreover, the continuous blood issuing from the cut end of the cord is messy. On the other hand, a less turgid, "deflated" placenta may separate more readily when the uterus contracts.

Walsh (1968) found that postpartum hemorrhage and retained secundines are significantly more common when early clamping is practiced. The amount of fetal blood contained within the placenta varies. It is generally between 50 and 100 ml but is significantly greater in pregnancies of diabetic mothers (Kjeldsen & Pedersen, 1967; Klebe & Ingomar, 1974). Newton and Moody (1961) estimated that 9.4 ml of fetal blood per 100 g of placenta remained after delivery when the cord was ligated immediately, and there was 9.6 ml of maternal blood. The latter quantity did not change with delivery and clamping practices. When the cord was ligated after pulsations ceased, only 5 ml of fetal blood remained. They estimated that the term neonate may receive as much as 10% of his blood volume (26.6 ml) when cord ligation is delayed and the placental vessels allowed to empty. The presence of fetal blood is what imparts the red color to its tissue, not the maternal intervillous blood content, which has largely been squeezed out by uterine contractions.

Numerous studies have been conducted to ascertain whether it is best to allow as much blood to drain from the placenta into the fetus (under the influence of maternal uterine contractions) as possible before the cord is ligated and severed. Vardi (1965) reviewed the older literature and advocated that the delivered placenta be held above the infant but advised against "stripping" the cord. His studies showed that it is beneficial for the hematological and iron requirements of the infant to let as much blood drain into the fetus as possible. Yao et al. (1968) found marked hematological changes with different clamping times, studied up to 3 minutes. They thought that the maximum transfer had taken place by that time. Later these investigators studied the fetal/placental blood volume changes (Yao et al., 1969). When the cord was clamped within 5 seconds of birth the infant/placental volume distribution was 67%/33%; by 3 minutes it was 87%/13%. In later studies, which include a complete summary of their findings, Yao and Lind (1974, 1982) evaluated the consequences of cord clamping at various times after birth with respect to the development and behavior of the newborn infant. Special attention was paid to the occasional hypervolemia resulting from late clamping. Their recommendation was that for vaginal deliveries clamping be done within 30 seconds, providing the baby is not elevated. With cesarean section, elevation of the infant is to be avoided; and when there is no distress, the cord be handled as for vaginal births.

Fetal-to-maternal red blood cell transfer during labor is not influenced by the timing of cord ligation (Dunn et al., 1966; Moncrieff et al., 1986). An interesting study of residual placental fetal blood content and neonatal outcome was done by Philip et al. (1969). They found that, compared with normal newborns, asphyxiated neonates had already received more blood prenatally, irrespective of postnatal transfusions. There are other complex questions of cord clamping time (e.g., the increased frequency of neonatal bilirubinemia with draining of the placental blood into the fetus), but they are beyond the scope of this chapter (see Philip, 1973).

Detachment of the umbilicus from the infant is variable, occurring within a mean of 7.4 days (Oudesluys-Murphy et al., 1987) to 13.9 days (Novack et al., 1988). Numerous studies have endeavored to ascertain its causes, which remain unresolved. Cesarean section delays it by several days. Immature cords sepa-

rate later than mature ones, and infection can delay separation.

Knots

Excessively long umbilical cords are apt to become knotted. We have seen three knots in a 76 cm long cord with which the fetus suffered severe cerebral palsy. He was born without fibrinogen and had widespread petechiae. Much venous distension was evident behind the first knot. Collins (1993; Collins et al., 1993) also described triple knots associated with fetal demise and other cord abnormalities, such as torsion. Knots in the umbilical cord may not only cause fetal death (Figure 241), they may lead to significant prepartum hypoxia with lasting damage. There are some important questions: Does every knot cause some damage (Figure 242)? If not, when are umbilical cord knots clinically significant? Although knots are important clinical findings, with an associated fetal mortality of around 10% (Scheffel & Langanke, 1970), it is surprising how little has been written about them. Perhaps the topic is too obvious to demand the attention of many investigators.

Browne (1925) reported that true knots occur with a frequency of 0.4% to 0.5%. He performed perfusion experiments to ascertain the resultant perfusion pressure that presumably follows the presence of knots. The normal pressure in the umbilical vein (10 mmHg) was raised to 20 mmHg by one slack knot; two knots raised it to 60 mmHg. If a weight of 100 g was used to cause increased tension on the one knot, the perfusion pressure was raised to 100 mmHg. These findings were partially contradicted by the investigations of Chasnoff and Fletcher (1977), who did not find that elevated pressure for perfusion was required when a loose knot

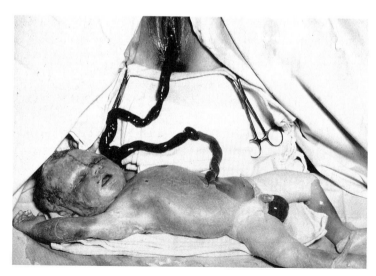

FIGURE 241. Macerated stillborn fetus. Death was due to a true knot with obstruction of venous return from the placenta 10 cm from the abdomen. Total length was 65 cm. Note the marked congestion of the cord distal to the knot.

FIGURE 242. Knot in the umbilical cord (actually two loops) that had no untoward sequelae.

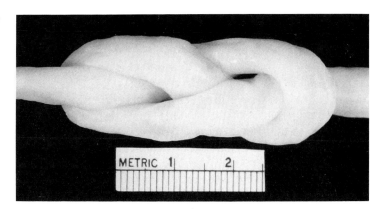

was laid; only when more than a 20 g weight was applied did the pressure requirements for perfusion rise markedly. They saw a 0.35% incidence of true knots among 2,000 consecutive deliveries: One infant was stillborn, one had low Apgar scores, five were normal.

Knots cause compression of Wharton's jelly at the site of knotting. When examined microscopically, one often finds mural thrombosis in the vein. Venous distension distal to the knot is a characteristic finding in knots with clinical significance, as is the tendency of the unknotted cord to curl if the knot had been present for some time. Parenthetically, it may be mentioned that stillbirth due to a cord knot has been recorded in an African green monkey (Brady, 1983). Its cord was unusually long, and there was congestion behind the knot. Chimpanzees and orangutans have also been reported to have true knots in some cords (Naaktgeboren & Wagtendonk, 1966).

False Knots

False knots should not be listed as knots at all. This term has become so customary, however, that it merits brief discussion. One such structure is shown in Figure 243. These anomalies are local redundancies of umbilical vessels, rather than knots, and they are often large. Their vasculature has been depicted by Hyrtl (1870), Arvy and Pilleri (1976a), and others. A rarely used term for these changes is nodus spurious vasculosus. When an excessive amount of Wharton's jelly is present, the term nodus spurious gelatinosus has been used. As far as can be determined, these structures have absolutely no clinical importance. Of course, there may be the occasional clot formed in this area, and it is conceivable that they might bleed. Despite their clinical irrelevance, questions persist just why these redundancies appear at all. What are the forces that regulate

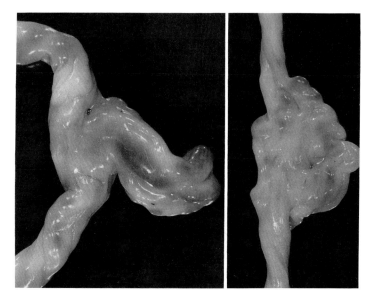

FIGURE 243. "False" knots, representing vascular redundancies.

the growth of fetal vessels in the first place, and do the false knots merely signify a temporal discrepancy of vascular growth with cord lengthening? Answers to these questions elude us at present.

A completely forgotten notion, the "angle of insertion" (*Insertionswinkel*) to which Hyrtl (1870) tried to draw attention, suggests that one may infer the position held in utero and reflect trophotropic departure of the placenta from its original site of implantation. This angle was between 0° and 90° in the original observations and is clearly variable when one examines placentas. Strassmann (1902) regretted that in his studies on placenta previa he failed to take note of this feature, which might have enhanced his conviction of the etiology.

Strictures

Significant reductions in the size of the umbilical cord are referred to as stricture, torsion, and coarctation. These abnormalities are often found on the abdominal surfaces of macerated fetuses with long, heavily spiraled cords. Javert and Barton (1952) have been depicted this problem in several of their illustrations. One must assume that the fetus has been so active as to have sheared off the blood supply at the site of torsion. In the previous edition of this book we were skeptical about the significance of this lesion and some of the case reports. Since then we have seen many additional cases that have convinced us it is a real phenomenon. One may even see much congestion on one side of the torsion and find thrombi. Because they are often macerated fetuses, the demonstration of thrombi is hampered.

A typical case of cord constriction is shown in Figure 244, and several authors have provided single case reports (King, 1926; Weber, 1963; Quinlan, 1965; Virgilio & Spangler, 1978; Robertson et al., 1981; Glanfield & Watson, 1986). These authors have shown that the phenomenon is not confined to abortions or to the fetal end of the cord. Glanfield and Watson (1986) reported a case with a fresh thrombus at the site of torsion at the twisted placental end of the cord that led to fetal death at 35 weeks' gestation. They also reviewed the sparse literature of this anomaly whose etiology is not known. Nevertheless, Weber (1963) stated that the constriction is rarely reported, although it is not uncommon, and described five cases.

Robertson et al. (1981) surmised that the cause of constriction is a primary deficiency of Wharton's jelly, a true coarctation. These investigators lost two fetuses with this lesion soon after amniocentesis. Hersh and Buchino (1988), who observed two successive deaths in one family due to torsion of the cord, also believed that primary absence of Wharton's jelly is the cause of this lesion. They had previously seen two similar cases in one family and hinted at the possibility that the recurrence risk is greater than what had been thought. There is, of course, normally a gradually diminishing amount of Wharton's jelly near the abdominal surface. It may be for this reason that the stricture is most commonly seen at that site. We have had such a case where with a 64 cm umbilical cord in a stillborn the two umbilical arteries exhibited significant, long-standing degenerative changes at this site. It was the cause of the fetal death.

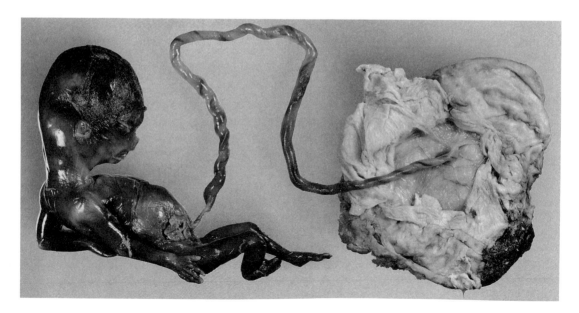

FIGURE 244. Spontaneous abortus at about 14 weeks' gestation. Note the markedly spiraled cord and severe constriction of the cord (coarctation, torsion) near the fetal surface that led to death.

Colgan and Luk (1982), who reported the death of one of monoamnionic/monochorionic twins from such a torsion, found thrombi in all three vessels at that site.

Rupture

It is not surprising that short cords may avulse from the placenta during descensus, particularly during a precipitous delivery. The cord may rupture completely or partially, and it may bleed or form hematomas. Bahary et al. (1965) reported a severely anemic newborn whose marginally inserted short cord (24 cm) had ruptured during descensus. They believed that velamentous cord insertion was the most frequent antecedent of this complication. Rhen and Kinnunen (1962) lost a fetus with a 50 cm cord before labor due to a ruptured umbilical vein. It occurred spontaneously after tumultuous movements by the fetus. Foldes (1957) reported a stillbirth after rupture in which the normally long cord was wound tightly around the neck. These authors reviewed the early literature of this rare event. Bleeding from the injured cord after amniocentesis has been recorded by ultrasonography (Romero et al., 1982); and the development of a cord hematoma following in utero transfusion, with bradycardia secondary to arterial spasm, was observed by Moise et al. (1987).

Such experiences and the question as to how much traction may be applied to the cord during delivery have stimulated systematic studies on the tensile strength of the umbilical cord (e.g., Crichton, 1973). Crichton tested 200 normal term umbilical cords without having their blood drained. He thus obtained a nearly normal distribution of breaking weights. Most cords ruptured when 12 pounds were applied, the extremes being 4 and 24 pounds. There was no correlation with fetal weight, length of cord, or placental weight. Although the cord ruptured most often (22.5%) at the site of its placental attachment, rupture could occur anywhere (Siddall, 1925). It must be said, however, that complete rupture is an uncommon event; most ruptures are partial and cause local hematomas or hemorrhage. Leinzinger (1972) reported such a case in association with hydramnios and reviewed the relevant literature, but the case reported by Golden (1973) must not be cited as one of umbilical cord rupture. In his patient the cord separated when traction was applied to it after the child was delivered; the hematoma was at the site of detachment, and there was an adjacent intrauterine device (IUD: Lippe's loop). The photograph he supplied suggests that the cord was either marginal or in a velamentous insertion, a finding that is frequently made when IUDs remain during pregnancy. The IUD was certainly not within the amnionic sac and had nothing directly to do with the traumatic postnatal

cord separation. More likely, the cord ruptured through velamentous vessels.

Hematoma

Hemorrhages into the cord substance are more common than complete rupture, and they may be similarly life-threatening. Figure 245 shows such an example, associated with a slightly shorter than average cord (42 cm). It has been conjectured in the past that such hemorrhages occur because of "fatty degeneration" of the cord (Browne, 1925), but we have not seen such changes. In our experience, cord hematomas are associated with short cords, trauma, and entangling. At times there are associated thrombi. Whichever event is the primary one is then unknown. Vu et al. (1984) reported on five cases; they stated that inflammation eventually occurs when the hemorrhage is not lethal. This finding is also contrary to our experience.

It is a common practice for the obstetrician to use a clamp to apply gentle traction to the cord after delivery. This practice may induce local hematoma formation, and such a history must be ascertained before the diagnosis of spontaneous hematoma is entertained. Hematomas due to cord clamping is often obvious because the serrations of a clamp remain visible. Traumatic injury to cord vessels during amniocentesis has often been reported (Gassner & Paul, 1976; James & Nickerson, 1976; Bobitt, 1979). This potential hazard, when it occurs, demands emergency attention.

Ruvinski et al. (1981), reviewing the entire literature (57 cases), found that hematomas of the cord are associated with a 50% fetal mortality. They described a

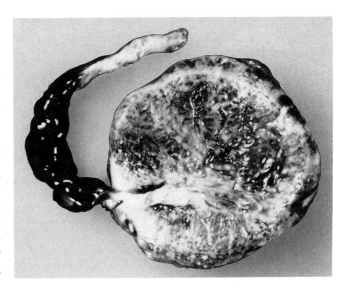

FIGURE 245. Stillbirth due to "rupture" (hematoma) of a 46 cm long umbilical cord.

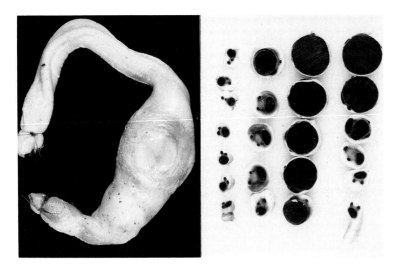

FIGURE 246. Aneurysmal dilatation of the umbilical vein with fatal compression of arteries resulting in a stillborn at term after a normal pregnancy and delivery. No cause was identified for this lesion. There were also no thrombi.

case diagnosed by ultrasonography prenatally, at 32 weeks. The hematoma measured 6 × 9 × 3 cm and was estimated to contain 100 ml of blood. The cord was 52 cm long and had a ruptured vein from which the sac-like extension of the hematoma took place. The fetus exsanguinated; it did not die from compression of vessels. In the cord shown in Figure 246, the aneurysmally distended vein was so huge that the arteries were compressed and the fetus stillborn. Remarkably, the external appearance was not one of hemorrhage. A similar case, but involving the umbilical artery, has been described by Fortune and Östör (1978). It was a 36-week spontaneous intrauterine death. The two umbilical arteries were looped, and one had an 8 × 3 cm aneurysmal dilatation that had obstructed the blood flow through the other vessels. There was no thrombosis, and no underlying pathology existed.

Gerlach (1968) had previously described a cherry-sized aneurysm of the umbilical artery in its abdominal portion of a child with anomalies. He concluded that it was part of a dysmorphic condition. The wall of that vessel was partially calcified. Two similar cases were described by Rissmann (1931); one was a stillborn, and the other lived. The classical report of cord hematoma is that of Dippel (1940), who found 36 cases. He believed that congenital thinning, fatty and mucoid degeneration of the vein wall, varices, and looping of a long cord are instrumental in the cause. Schreier and Brown (1962) depicted such a defect in the vein of a child who survived a large hematoma. When elastic stains are done on such cords it has been repeatedly found that the elastic fibers of the vein are focally deficient. Remarkably, the infant of the cord shown in Figure 247 survived, even though much clotted blood

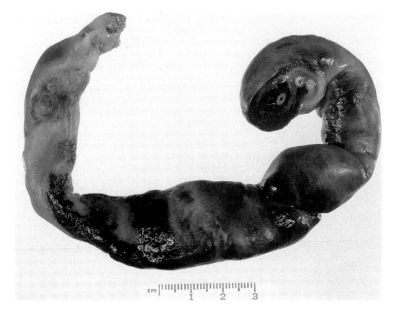

FIGURE 247. Large, 90 cm long umbilical cord with hematoma. The 5,300 g infant survived. Despite the large hematoma, the vascular lumens were patent and had no thrombus, as has been described by Bret and Bardiaux (1956).

was found in the distorted Wharton's jelly. Although the disruptive lesion is usually located in the vein (Dippel cited a 9:1 ratio), one of the cases described by Gardner and Trussell (1964) involved an artery in a patient who had a prolapsed cord. Other case reports have stressed that the overall mortality rate is around 50%, that hematomas may occur with long and short cords, with and without inflammation, and that their primary cause remains generally unknown (Irani, 1964; Ratten, 1969; Clare et al., 1979; Dillon & O'Leary, 1981). Although funisitis renders the cords generally slightly more friable, it was an infrequent finding. Syphilis, once thought to be a major cause, was specifically ruled out by Dippel (1940), and Fox (1978) agreed with the unimportant contribution of infection to hematomas. He lamented that the main etiology is unusually obscure but considered deficient Wharton's jelly as possibly important, particularly as hematomas are relatively more frequent in prolonged pregnancy. We have seen one case of cord hematoma with fatal prenatal myocardial infarct of the fetus. Aneurysms of cord and placental surface vessels are considered below.

Several investigators have attempted ultrastructural delineation of the vessels' unusual structure. We once saw an apparently normal umbilical artery that had two well defined lumens. Spiteri et al. (1966) were anxious to state that there was no sign of senescence in term arteries when they were compared with those of 7-week-old fetuses. This finding is in contrast, of course, to the expected degenerative changes seen in the aging intraabdominal portions of the umbilical arteries (Takagi et al., 1984). Vascular structure and changes induced in the umbilical vein by maternal smoking were investigated by Asmussen (1978). These studies showed damage to the intima, elastic subintimal membrane, and media. Also present are edema, deficiency of collagen, and myocyte proliferation. A peculiar feature of these large and thick umbilical vessels is that they allow penetration of many polymorphonuclear leukocytes in the usual inflammatory reaction of the amnionic sac infection syndrome. This trait is so striking and so different from other vessels that it is discussed in more detail in the consideration of chorioamnionitis. It may be related to the absence of a true adventitia, as seen in other bodily vessels. Moreover, in the umbilical cord, the extensions of Wharton's jelly penetrate the muscular walls of the arteries and vein, which may enhance transport of signals, such as leukotaxins.

Varices and Aneurysms

As happens with umbilical cords, surface vessels may have aneurysms that can bleed, thrombose, and rupture (Figure 248). Six such placentas with subamnionic hemorrhages from partially thrombosed chorionic vessels were described by De Sa (1971). He made the point that such thrombi are often associated with fetal growth retardation, diabetes, diffuse thromboses, and organized "cushions." These lesions must be differentiated from tears induced during delivery. It must also be cautioned that the obstetrician and neonatologist often draw blood from the chorionic vessels after birth, and the vessels may subsequently leak blood. Thus when a pathologist observes these surface hematomas, he or she must make sure that they are not artifacts of handling. Varices must not be confused with hemorrhagic subchorial cysts originating from degenerating trophoblastic cell islands. Note, however, that a number of cases have been described that are difficult to trace. They are instances where blood was found in the amniotic space and in which

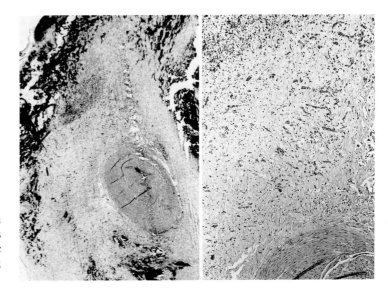

FIGURE 248. Umbilical cord of a patient with a palsied infant and hematoma. Numerous capillaries testify to probable early intrauterine traumatic hemorrhage with organization. H&E. Left ×40; right ×160.

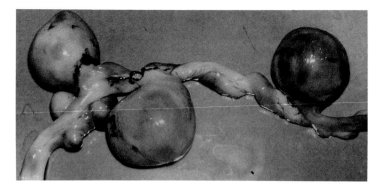

FIGURE 249. Multiple aneurysms of the umbilical cord associated with a single umbilical artery. The child was well at 3 years. (Courtesy R.E. Wybel, Bakersfield, California.)

subamnionic hemorrhages had occurred before birth. They originated from small lesions in vessels that could be demonstrated only by an injection study (Gad, 1968). Their etiology was often obscure. A similar case was reported by Leff (1931). The most detailed study of placental aneurysms derived from the examination of 1,000 consecutive placentas reported by Lemtis (1968), whose paper was accompanied by exemplary photographs. Lemtis found these lesions in 24 cases, one of which was a partial hydatidiform mole that had numerous aneurysms. Lemtis classified the anomalies into several types. The aneurysms were usually associated with atypical insertion of the cord, SUA, fetal growth retardation, or other placental anomalies; therefore Lemtis considered them to be true developmental abnormalities. In a set of dizygotic twins we saw, one twin's placenta had two chorionic venous aneurysms. This twin expired from completely spontaneous rupture during labor. Because rupture and exsanguination have been reported only during labor, it is our conviction that the aforementioned distension of the surface half of chorionic vessels after membrane rupture leads to this thinning and the vulnerability of potential aneurysms. Other large aneurysms we have seen have been described as "cirsoid." They were huge dilatations of surface vessels, often partially thrombosed and associated with thrombocytopenia of the neonate. In one such case, the subjacent main stem vessels had a mole-like myxoid distension. Siddiqi and colleagues (1992) described a classical umbilical arterial aneurysm in a two-vessel cord. It was noted to grow in repeated sonographic studies and had a partially calcified wall. It measured 13 × 5 cm and was 15 cm from the fetus; although it had no thrombus, the cardiac hypertrophy found in the stillborn infant suggested that it had circulatory consequences.

Varicosities in the umbilical cord are much more common than aneurysms. An example is illustrated in Figure 243. Real varix formations, such seen in Figures 249 and 250, are rare. A case was described by Leinzinger (1969), who also reviewed the sparse literature. Leinzinger observed during a normal delivery a

70 cm long umbilical cord that had a "peach-sized" varix of the umbilical vein that was largely thrombosed. He drew attention to the focally marked thinning of the wall of the umbilical vein, which has also been reported to be associated with necrosis of muscle wall and has attracted greater interest recently (Qureshi and Jacques, 1994). Altshuler and Hyde (1989) first depicted necrosis of umbilical vessel walls and suggested that it is the occasional result of chronic, severe meconium exposure. These authors also demonstrated in vitro that meconium may induce a significant contraction when strips of umbilical vein are exposed to solutions of meconium. Figure 251 shows a somewhat similar thinning of the vein wall in a child with cerebral palsy. Note that this thinning did not take place in a varix; there is no thrombus, nor is the thinned wall toward the cord surface, which might be expected if mechanical pressure had been the cause of this marked diminution in vessel wall thickness. Such areas of degeneration not only occur in the vein but may affect arteries for entirely

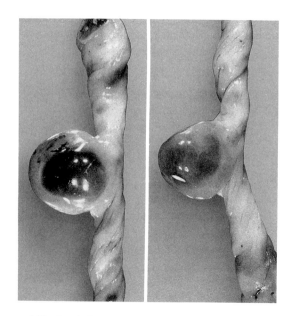

FIGURE 250. Partially thrombosed varix near the fetal end of the cord. A normal infant resulted with a 65 cm long cord.

FIGURE 251. Segmental thinning toward the middle of the cord in an umbilical vein (arrows). There was no apparent cause for this anomaly. The infant suffered cerebral palsy. H&E. Left ×60; right ×160.

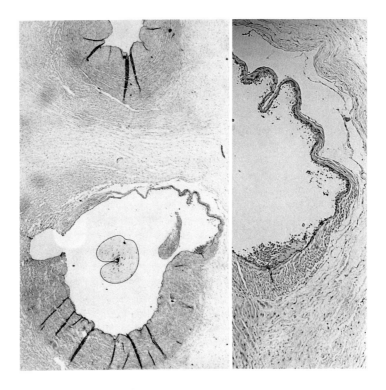

unknown reasons. To be sure, on occasion they are the sequelae of thrombosis, but they may occur without it. Within the stillborn whose umbilical artery is shown in Figure 252, a thin segment of artery had numerous rounded, degenerating myocytes. This process was confined to only one artery; it lay under the cord surface, and there was mild phlebitis. The short cord was loosely wound around the neck, but no reasonable cause of the lesion was identified. Similar "hypoplasia" of segments of umbilical vessels, usually veins, has been reported a few times in the literature. It is usually associated with rupture of the cord or hematomas (Bender et al., 1978).

Severe venous distension of the umbilical vein, detected sonographically, has been used as an indicator of severe hemolytic disease in the fetus (DeVore et al., 1981).

Thrombosis of the Umbilical Vessels

Thrombi of vessels in the umbilical cord are not uncommon. They may occur during early pregnancy and then lead to SUA, but this situation is not likely because of the difficulty of clotting during early pregnancy. More frequently, thrombi occur near term. The for-

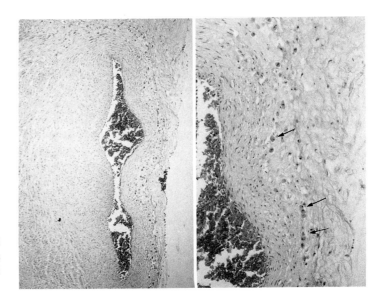

FIGURE 252. Segmental thinning of one umbilical arterial wall with degenerating, rounded myocytes (arrows) under the surface. A stillborn infant resulted with a short nuchal cord. H&E. Left ×60; right ×160.

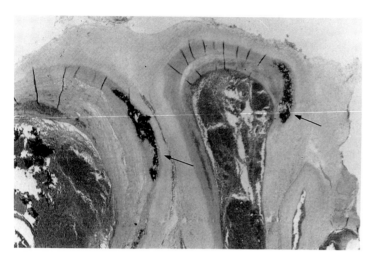

FIGURE 253. Partially calcified vessel walls (arrows) in the cord of a stillborn. The cord also had varices but no inflammation. H&E. ×60.

mation of thrombi with velamentous insertion of the cord is readily understandable. Here the membranous vessels course in the chorion, unprotected by Wharton's jelly; they are thus prone to injury from compression and are also subject to tears. Neonatal thrombocytopenia and bruising has been witnessed on several such occasions.

Severe inflammatory reactions of the cord often cause mural thrombi as well. Such a case with a surviving, bruised infant has been described by Wolfman et al. (1983). The umbilical vein of this premature infant of an otherwise uncomplicated pregnancy was inflamed and nearly completely thrombosed. In addition, there was one peculiar lesion of the cord with old inflammatory exudate surrounding the vessels. These lesions are often calcified and macroscopically resemble the precipitation ring in Ouchterlony plates. This unusual entity is further discussed in Chapter 20. Thrombi are frequent in this condition.

It is also easy to understand that thrombosis of cord vessels may occur in varices (Figures 250 and 253) and from looping and knotting of the umbilical cord. Likewise, the entangling of cords in monoamnionic twins, with vascular obstruction ensuing, and that from amnionic bands are mechanical reasons for thrombosis that can be readily envisaged. Thrombosis has also followed intravascular exchange transfusion and was there associated with an intrafunicular hematoma (Seeds et al., 1989). These situations can all compromise the circulation and lead to fetal death. The thrombi may break off and potentially embolize to the fetus or to the placenta, where they may cause infarction. Thrombosis may become so extensive as to compromise the circulation and lead to fetal death. Myocardial infarction with prenatal tamponade has been reported (Wolf et al., 1985).

Thrombi have been held responsible for amputations (Hoyme et al., 1982) and for a generalized bleeding tendency due to disseminated intravascular coagulation (DIC), or "consumption coagulopathy" (Williams & Benirschke, 1978). More remarkable are the thrombi that occur in the absence of all of these more readily understood complications, and they are perhaps the most common. We have seen many such cases that result in fetal death and others in children who developed cerebral palsy. In retrospect, there is often no good explanation for their genesis (Figure 254). There are numerous case reports on the subject; often the pathologist is unable to explain the origin of thrombi. Frequently thromboses of vessels in the cord are associated with similar events in the villous ramifications. Because of finding occasional deposits of calcium salts in such vessel walls and the apparent "organization" of these thrombosed vessels, it must be inferred that the clots have been present for days, if not weeks. Doshi and Klionsky (1979) also found it to be a frequent problem in severely ill newborns. They described 40 cases of DIC with thromboses in placental vessels, at least six of which had a prenatal onset. Coagulation problems caused by protein C or S deficiency are sometimes suspected, but they have rarely been proved to exist. Only the cases reported by Seligsohn et al. (1984) and Marcianiak et al. (1985) of familial protein C deficiency support this notion. The neonatal purpura fulminans of protein C deficiency was reviewed by Dreyfus et al. (1991) and depicted by Hartman et al. (1990). In these pedigrees prenatal thrombosis was not reported, although the condition at birth is summarized by the latter authors. One case of protein S deficiency during pregnancy has been reported (Tharakan et al., 1993). The pregnancy of this patient ended in a stillbirth with placental vascular thrombosis, and the patient had a pulmonary embolus. After anticoagulation she had a successful pregnancy. Unfortunately, the state of the placenta in each of these four newborns with massive venous thrombosis and fulminant purpura developing

FIGURE 254. Nearly occlusive venous thrombus with fetal death. The cord was long. H&E. ×40.

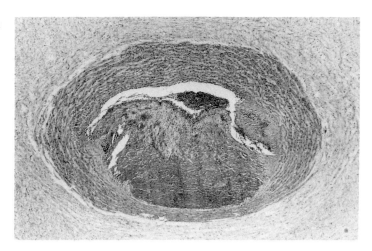

shortly after birth were not reported. Heifetz (1988) has reviewed three patient populations in addition to 68 cases gathered from the literature. The incidence of thrombosis was 1 in 1,300 deliveries, 1 in 1,000 perinatal autopsies, and 1 in 250 high risk gestations. Venous thromboses were more common than thromboses in one or both arteries, but the latter was more often lethal.

In two cases of arterial thrombosis we have witnessed, one umbilical artery had a completely necrotic wall, and many thrombi were found in the fetal chorionic vascular ramifications. One child died during the neonatal period with prenatal thrombosis of one pulmonary artery and an infarcted lung; the other survived but developed severe cerebral palsy. Maternal diabetes, which is occasionally associated with such thromboses, was not present, and no other morphological or clinical features helped to explain the cause of this fetal vascular coagulation.

Protein C deficiency was found to be associated with the 11 neonatal cases reported by Marco-Johnson et al. (1988). They established that the protein C levels are low in newborns, and that an inherited deficiency to explain neonatal thrombosis must be carefully documented. The relatives of their patients were not heterozygotes; and after successful therapy with heparin in four patients, their protein C levels gradually rose to normal. Five of their patients were one of twins; one of these twins developed the transfusion syndrome, and the co-twin had died at birth. One patient had a diabetic mother. Four infants had aortic thromboses (one also had renal thrombosis), and one had CNS thrombosis. The mechanism of this presumably acquired absence of protein C in these neonates remained unknown, and the placentas were not described.

It is often desirable to estimate the age of the thrombi. When calcification accompanies them, they are clearly old; for younger clots, the table derived from the detailed investigations on aging of thrombi by Leu and Leu (1989) is helpful.

There was such massive calcification in the walls of some vessels in a few cases (Rust, 1937; Walz, 1947; Perrin & Bel, 1965) that it became difficult to ligate the cord (Figure 253). Two of these infants survived. In others, the calcification affected fetal arteries with lethal consequences (Ivemark et al., 1962). Schiff et al. (1976) were the first to recognize a calcified cord antenatally. The three vessels were calcified virtually over the entire length of the cord and attended by much inflammation; the neonate died with pulmonary hypoplasia. There are some reports of venous thrombosis associated with severe fetal distress (Eggens & Bruins, 1984), cerebral palsy, massive fetomaternal hemorrhage (Hoag, 1986), and other complications. Occasionally, maternal smoking and diabetes have been implicated. Abrams et al. (1985) were able to make the diagnosis by sonography, and there are many other case reports, too numerous to list, that attest to thromboses as being an important problem in perinatology. It stands to reason that such occlusions, particularly when associated with villous vascular disease, raise fetal blood pressure; and like the experimental obliteration of placental vessels by microembolization (Trudinger et al., 1987), they may have abnormal sonographic consequences. Thrombi may also lead to fetal growth retardation. In an occasional case, one may observe strange phenomena that clearly betray long-standing prenatal problems, as shown in Figure 255. Here the cord of an infant with renal agenesis can be seen to be unusually long (77 cm) for an oligohydramneic pregnancy. The placenta had many thrombi in its surface vessels, and the partially calcified umbilical vein had ruptured. Squamous debris (vernix caseosa) had dissected underneath the cord surface. All of these findings suggest that the process had been ongoing for weeks prior to delivery. Parenthetically, it may be mentioned that fatal air embolization

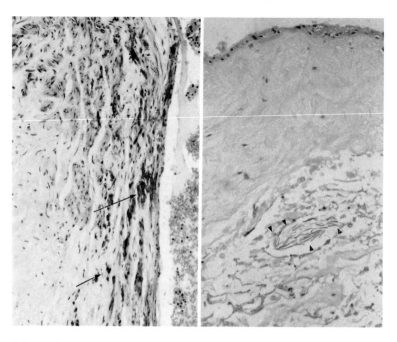

FIGURE 255. Umbilical cord (77 cm) in a case of renal agenesis with partial calcification of the vein wall (left, arrows) and vernix dissection (right, arrows). H&E. ×160.

has been reported when, during cesarean section, the placenta had to be incised (Allen et al., 1969). Also, the frequent amnion nodosum of the placental surface seen with renal agenesis or with other causes of severe oligohydramnios is rarely present on the cord's surface.

Khong and Dilly (1989) reviewed the topic of the rare calcifications in umbilical arteries and presented five new cases. These authors were of the opinion that the calcifications fall into two classes: (1) those with calcific thrombi; and (2) those with evidence of funisitis or inflammation of the amnionic sac (or both). They described two complete thromboses of one artery with calcification. In one the mother had a lupus-like disease, and there was 20% infarction of the placenta, with a liveborn at 35 weeks. In the other, a mother with a skin rash at 28 weeks' gestation gave birth to a severely growth-retarded (940 g), macerated fetus at 34 weeks' gestation with apparent amnionic bands with amputations and cord constriction. The other three cases (one living) had associated inflammation without recognized microorganisms.

Thrombosis of the Placental Vascular Tree

Mural and occlusive thrombi occur frequently in the superficial placental vessels and their villous ramifications. They are variably located across the fetal surface and within the placenta, and only occasionally are they accompanied by thrombi in the umbilical cord. Often these vascular occlusions have grave consequences. Surface thrombi are usually recognized during careful gross examination. When the vessel is hugely distended, as that shown in Figure 256A, the identification of thrombosis is easy. Much more frequently overlooked are such thrombi as seen in Figures 257 and 258. When thrombi are fresh, their gross appearance is that of a slightly enlarged vessel that may have an unusual color. It is not as shiny and blue as normal vessels. One is also unable to move the blood mechanically in thrombosed vessels; and of course histologically they are easily diagnosed (Figure 259). Older thrombi become white or yellow.

Mural thrombosis is much more frequent than complete obliteration of the vessel. Such thromboses may even calcify (Figure 260) but variations are frequent; and when thrombosis has occurred a long time before examination, the vessel may obliterate completely. It then appears as a fibrous strand that may be difficult to recognize as once having been a vessel. We have seen such thrombi in placentas of trisomy 18 and associated with cytomegalovirus infection, excessively long cords, cord knots, velamentous insertion, amputation necrosis in the fetus, severe chorioamnionitis, neonatal purpura, generalized fetal thrombosis, and many other conditions. They are not rare events and clearly bespeak a pathological prenatal environment. They may occur in arteries or veins, and the vascular wall may show various stages of degeneration or calcification. Thrombi are generally not a cause of local

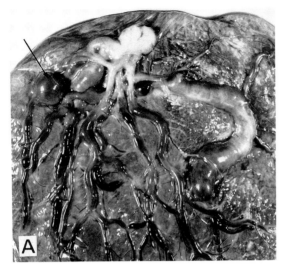
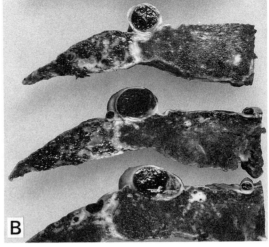

FIGURE 256. (A) Varix in a surface chorionic vein branch (arrow) and a hugely distended, thrombosed umbilical vein tributary (at right). Neonatal death occurred with umbilical vein thrombosis, renal necrosis, and possible maternal diabetes. (B) Layered thrombi are apparent in the cross sections.

inflammation. The topic has been discussed extensively in a study of cord lesions (Benirschke, 1994).

Similar thrombosis of the further ramifications of the vascular tree exist (Figure 261). If the thrombi have been occlusive for a prolonged time, the entire villous tree may become avascular and atrophy (Figure 262). It does not infarct; true infarction of villous tissue occurs only when the maternal blood supply is interrupted. The villous tissue merely atrophies over time. Localized thrombosis with early blanching of the affected villous district has been well illustrated by Fox (1966).

In the neonatal blood of neonates whose placental vessels had thrombi, one may detect schistocytes and find hematological derangements such as fibrinogen and platelet deficiencies. Kristiansen and Nielsen (1985) described three cases with fatal thromboses; they concluded that most often mechanical factors are the cause. The relation of thrombi to fetal deaths was evaluated by Cook et al. (1987). They found thrombi in 98% of fetal deaths, which is much in excess of our observations; moreover, we disagree with their interpretation of "organization" of the thrombotic material. In fact, true organization of dead tissues, as the pathologist knows it from renal or splenic infarcts, is rare in all placental degenerative lesions. That is, removal of debris by phagocytes and the ingrowth of granulation tissue with fibrous tissue substitution are phenomena not seen in true placental infarcts, nor do they occur in thrombosed placental vessels. Rather, these lesions shrink, and some phagocytes may appear; but eventually they

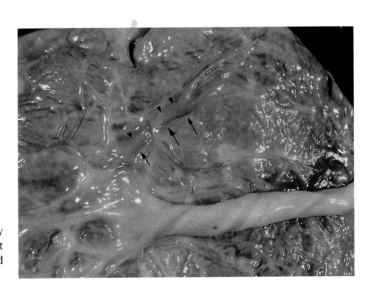

FIGURE 257. Thrombosis of an umbilical vein tributary (arrows). Note the discoloration (hemolysis). The infant had disseminated intravascular coagulation, exhibited schistocytes, and developed cerebral palsy.

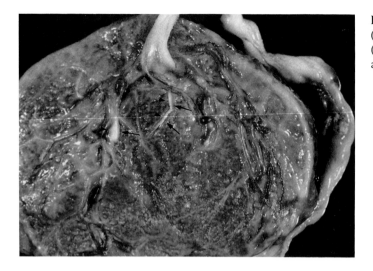

either become calcified, or the vessel atrophies. It may eventually disappear completely, becoming unrecognizable as having been a vessel.

As indicated, thromboses extend occasionally into the major ramifications of villous vessels. They may be occlusive; and their walls and the extensions of Wharton's jelly may calcify. When many placentas are examined histologically, one finds these lesions more often than they are suspected macroscopically. They are not always associated with recognizable surface thrombi (Figure 263), and often the etiology of the lesions remains unknown. They are frequently associated with fetal growth retardation and neonatal coagulation disorders. We have speculated that they may be the result of prenatal insults, such as virus infections or perhaps even trauma due to fetal motions, but the etiology remains often obscure. It is common to find

occlusions of placental vessels with stillborns but to differentiate thrombi from autolytic degeneration may be difficult. Caution must be exercised when these large stem villi are evaluated. Collagenous trabeculae therein have much the same appearance as old occlusive thrombi.

Obliterative vascular changes were probably first described by Merttens (1894). They have since been discussed at length by Becker and Dolling (1965), who

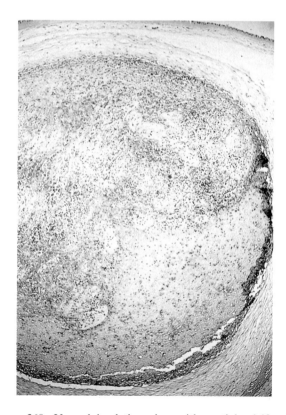

FIGURE 260. Unexplained thrombus with partial calcification (right margin) of a surface vein in a stillborn infant. H&E. ×26.

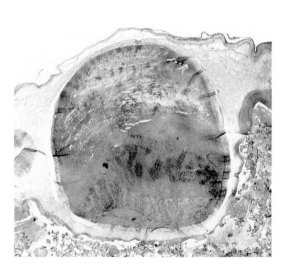

FIGURE 259. Layered thrombus in a dilated chorionic vein tributary. Stillbirth resulted, with a long cord. A sacrococcygeal teratoma was found. H&E. ×16.

FIGURE 261. Muscular hypertrophy and old occlusions in several of many stem vessels of a child with unexplained midforearm amputation. H&E. ×260.

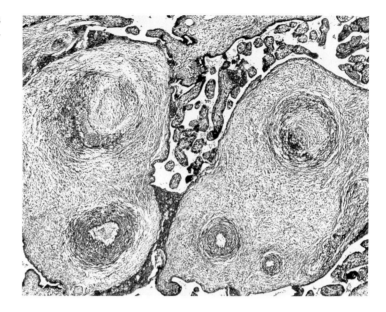

believed them to be the sequelae of infections during earlier fetal life. These authors found neovascularization and other phenomena, which they thought to be indications of organization. The former notion of syphilitic endovasculitis as the etiology was negated. Other authors cited by these investigators and by Fox (1966) found such vascular obliterations unduly commonly in diabetic pregnancies: 3.6% single arterial stem thrombi in live-born infants. Fox (1966) also observed them much more commonly in the placentas of stillborns.

Apparently dissatisfied with the varied literature of this topic, Fox studied fetal stem arteries from 682 placentas, 36 of which were from stillbirths (Fox, 1967). He observed three lesions: obliterative endarteritis, fibromuscular sclerosis, and thrombosis. These lesions were common in patients with diabetes (23%) and

hypertension (about 30%). From a comparison of material from live and dead infants he asserted that the "sclerosis" of vessel walls was a postmortem change. Similar vascular changes were held to be of postmortem nature by Theuring (1968) in his study of placentas from stillborns. He considered that the placenta continues to live after fetal death and that the vessels live in a tissue-culture-like environment to attain such occlusions. The longer the fetal death, the more extensive the occlusions. A similar position was taken by Altemani (1987), who concluded that because the placental perfusion after fetal death keeps the tissue alive many of the vascular occlusions seen in stillborns were of postmortem origin. He considered that true organization occurs in these vessels and alluded to the relation of vascular occlusions to hemorrhagic endovasculitis (HEV). The vascular changes found in dia-

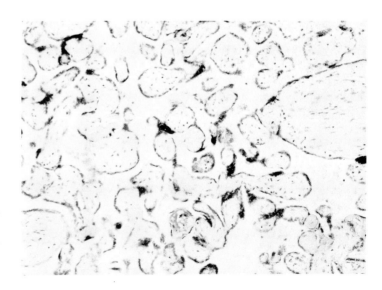

FIGURE 262. Diffuse atrophy (degeneration and disappearance) of villous vessels in a placenta with extensive surface thromboses. Fetal growth retardation was evident, and the infant had low Apgar scores. H&E. ×60.

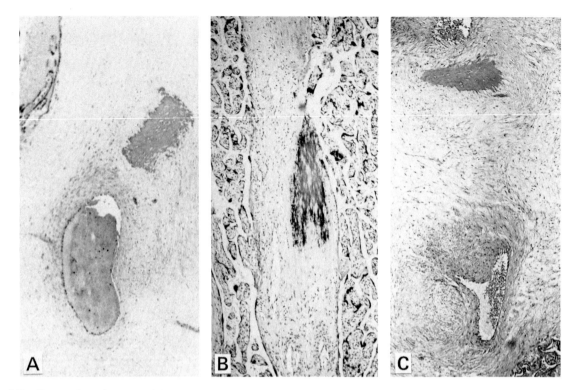

FIGURE 263. Composite of cases with villous stem vascular lesions. (A) Growth retardation, wavy ribs, 29 weeks' gestation. (B) Neonate with phocomelia. (C) Growth retardation, purpura, pulmonary hypoplasia, degeneration in several organs, neonatal death. All have calcified deposits in stem vessel walls, and some have thrombi or muscular lesions. H&E. ×60.

betics were considered by Fox (1967) to be true in vivo lesions, as had been suggested by Fujikura and Benson (1964) earlier, an observation that was supported by others. Dolff (1978) studied the phenomenon in serial sections, mostly in placentas of stillborn infants. Having duly considered the two principal theories (postnatal change versus prenatal endarteritis obliterans), Dolff came to the conclusion that (1) this lesion is an in vivo phenomenon of importance, and (2) the dynamics that lead to recanalization of the affected vessels is the function of the paravascular network of the placental stem vessels. Altemani and Lopes de Faria (1987) made a thorough study of the muscular and endothelial changes of main stem blood vessels in 50 stillborns and 50 controls. In their opinion, the occlusive changes seen were mostly a postmortem phenomenon that was not the cause of fetal demise. Becker and Röckelein (1989) saw in the "endarteritis obliterans" a common endstage of infections (syphilis, rubella) but also believed that diabetes and preeclampsia have pathogenic importance. In our view, this vascular lesion of main stem villous vessels is not a true inflammation but results most often from thrombosis of more proximal vessels or represents a postmortem phenomenon. In his study of postmortem changes of the placenta, Genest (1992) was able to time the vascular events and confirmed that most endothelial abnormalities occurred after fetal death. Karyorrhexis of villous capillaries occurred within 6 hours, stem villus vascular "septation" and complete obliteration took 2 days or more, and fibrosis of terminal villi took weeks to occur.

These considerations are important because the entity hemorrhagic endovasculitis (Sander, 1980) has aroused much controversy. Briefly stated, this concept evolved from the study of many formalin-fixed placentas seen in a registry of placentas collected from perinatal deaths and infants with perinatal problems. It was hypothesized that hemorrhagic endovasculitis (HEV) may play an important role in the etiology of these tragedies, and that it may be caused by a specific viral or other infectious agent. Hemosiderin was found in some cases to indicate the presumed antiquity of the lesion. HEV is not one lesion; it is a microangiopathy that etiologically and pathologically resembles the glomerulopathy of the hemolytic uremic syndrome. Proliferative, inflammatory vasculitis is not present. The pathological changes consist in endothelial degeneration, thrombosis, and diapedesis of red blood cells (Figure 264). Stevens and Sander (1984) found HEV to be present in 52% of stillborns and in 22% of liveborn infants. They found associations with preeclampsia, prolonged pregnancy, meconium staining,

FIGURE 264. Hemorrhagic endovasculitis (HEV) in a main stem villous vessel of a stillborn monozygotic twin. The other twin is well. H&E. ×160.

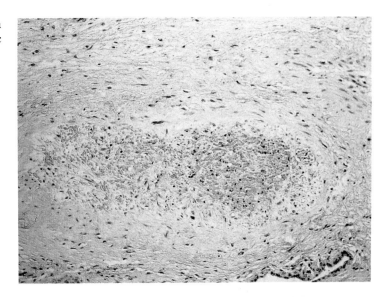

and growth retardation. Other investigators (Shen-Schwarz et al., 1986, 1988) found a much lower incidence of this lesion (0.67% after 20 weeks) and associated it with nuchal cords, meconium staining, and postmaturity. Many of these associations did not involve infection, and many infants survived; moreover, ultrastructural investigations have not shown organisms. The etiology must therefore be considered to include hypoxia, acidosis, and perhaps the DIC associated with the Shwartzman phenomenon.

Silver et al. (1987b, 1988) have done a complete analysis of HEV and confirmed the findings of Ornoy et al. (1976) that the fetal vascular occlusions are most frequently seen in the placentas of macerated stillborns. They presumed it to be a postmortem development. For that reason, they cultured villous tissue in vitro and sampled it at regular intervals for light and electron

microscopic study. They saw a similar lesion develop, in time, when organ explants were allowed to degenerate, confirming their original assumption. They believed that it is the sequela of focal or uniform postmortem autolysis of vessel walls. Our own assessment is that HEV is not a specific entity. Clearly, thrombotic lesions of villous stem vessels occur; and often they are associated with cord lesions and surface thrombi. They can be seen in a variety of clinical circumstances, as we have indicated. The occlusion of vessels after death, however, so much mimic degenerative lesions that they may be overinterpreted. Moreover, we now believe the "vascular anomaly" (proliferation of vessels in an abortus) shown in Figure 276 (Benirschke & Driscoll, 1967) to be a typical, albeit unusual postmortem phenomenon. In short, although HEV does exist, it does not represent a specific disease entity.

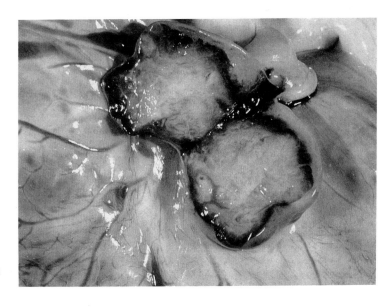

FIGURE 265. Angioma at the insertion of the cord in one twin.

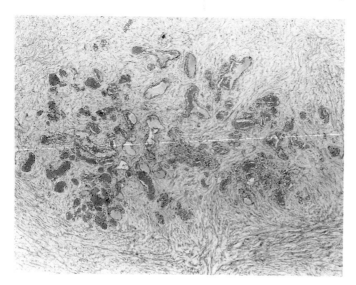

FIGURE 266. Histological appearance of a hemangioma of the umbilical cord. H&E. ×20. (From Benirschke & Dodds, 1967, with permission.)

TUMORS OF THE UMBILICAL CORD

Aside from the tumor-like swellings of aneurysms discussed above, only two true tumors occur in the umbilical cord: angiomas of great variety and significance and, much more rarely, teratomas.

As early as 1939 Marchetti was able to summarize 209 cases of placental angioma and added eight cases of his own, and Fortune and Östör (1980) summarized 58 cases. A cord angioma was not among this large group. Frequently, the fetus dies when large tumors exist in the cord; hemangiomas or other anomalies may coexist in the fetus (Barry et al., 1951; Corkill, 1961). Some authors have found myxoma-like Wharton's jelly in such tumors (Benirschke & Dodds, 1967; Fortune & Östör, 1980) or have interpreted them to be hamartomas. These neoplasms are never malignant and have a fairly uniform appearance (Figures 265, 266). Death often occurs because of obstruction of blood flow. Occasionally, an associated atrophic artery signifies their long existence before birth. Heifetz and Rueda-Pedreza (1983a), who have summarized much of the literature, noted that angiomas tend to occur at the placental end of the cord and arise from one or more umbilical vessels. Unlike chorangiomas, angiomas of the cord are also usually not associated with hydramnios. Thus the large angioma described by Barents (1953) was not associated with hydramnios and resulted in a normal infant. Mishriki et al. (1987) described an exception.

Resta et al. (1988) have described an angioma of the cord in association with extremely high (887–1,030 IU/ml) α-fetoprotein (AFP) levels in the maternal serum at 16 weeks' gestation. The lesion was unsuccessfully biopsied, and the fetus died 1 week later. A 3.2 × 1.8 × 2.0 cm angioma was found, in addition to severe narrowing of the cord at the fetal end. They found 22 cases of funicular angioma in the literature. Transplacental bleeding was excluded as possibly accounting for this 30-fold elevation. The neoplasms may attain rather large size, such as the 9 × 7 × 6 cm lesion found by Nieder and Link (1970) or that reported by Yavner and Redline (1989). The angiomyxoma of theirs was associated with a slightly elevated AFP level and was diagnosed sonographically at 19 weeks' gestation. The infant was delivered at 38 weeks and was normal. The large tumor (5.0 × 9.5 cm, 900 g) included a large cystic mass. Its location was typically near the fetal end of the cord. Other large tumors have been diagnosed prenatally. A cord angioma measuring 18 cm in length and associated with a cord that measured 9 cm in width was responsible for nonimmune hydrops of one of dichorionic twins successfully treated during the neonatal period and reported by Seifert et al. (1985). These authors postulated that the cause of the nonimmune hydrops was high-output cardiac failure. Dombrowski et al. (1987) reported a case of severe fetal hemorrhage from the angiomatous cord. Interestingly, this specimen also had intestinal epithelium on the cord's surface.

Teratomas are much less common than angiomas. Browne (1925) discussed the semantics of teratoma and dermoid. He reported one teratoma and one dermoid, with an anencephalic fetus. Smith and Majmudar (1985) presented the case of a term fetus with bladder exstrophy who also had a pendulous 1.8 × 0.6 cm tumor that was 30 cm from the placental surface. It was focally calcified and contained skin with appendages, colonic epithelium, smooth muscle, and connective tissue. The authors found four previously reported cases in the literature and six cases in which the lesions were located on the placental surface, the largest measuring 7.5 cm. All were benign.

One wonders if these teratomas represent variations of acardiac twins. The latter, however, usually have some longitudinal differentiation and should have their own, separate umbilical cords. Nevertheless, the possibility that "teratomas" of the cord may represent a form of acardiac fetus has been considered by several authors. Thus Kreyberg (1958) observed a stillborn premature infant with a 36-cm cord that had, 16 cm from its insertion, a bulky tumor with cystic cavities and a variety of tissues (?platysma, sebaceous glands, hair, myelinated nerves, glia). He cited other similar tumors, one the size of a child's head. Heckmann et al. (1972) illustrated their finding of a 9 × 7 cm tumor that was situated 25 cm from the fetal end of the cord and 45 cm from the placenta. It had an epidermoid surface and several chambers lined by skin and intestinal epithelium, as well as cartilage and lymphatic remnants. The child did well. The authors considered "displaced germ cells" as its origin.

References

Abrams, S.L., Callen, P.W., and Filly, R.A.: Umbilical vein thrombosis: sonographic detection in utero. J. Ultrasound Med. 4:283–285, 1985.

Abuhamad, A., Shaffer, W., Mari, G., Copel, J., Hobbins, J., and Evans, A.: Single umbilical artery: does it matter which artery is missing? [abstract 10]. Am. J. Obstet. Gynecol. 170:226, 1994.

Akiyama, H., Kohzu, H., and Matsuoka, M.: An approach to detection and expulsion with new clinical sign: a study based on hemodynamic method and ultrasonography. Am. J. Obstet. Gynecol. 140:505–511, 1981.

Allen, J.R., Carrera, G.M., and Weed, J.C.: Neonatal death due to embolism. J.A.M.A. 207:756–757, 1969.

Altemani, A.M.: Thrombosis of fetal placental vessels: a quantitative study in placentas of stillbirths. Pathol. Res. Pract. 182:685–689, 1987.

Altemani, A.M., and Lopes de Faria, J.: Non-thrombotic changes of fetal placental vessels: a qualitative and quantitative study. Pathol. Res. Pract. 182:676–683, 1987.

Altshuler, G., and Hyde, S.: Meconium induced vasoconstriction: a potential cause of cerebral and other fetal hypoperfusion and of poor pregnancy outcome. Child Neurol. 4:137–142, 1989.

Altshuler, G., Tsang, R., and Ermocilla, R.: Single umbilical artery: correlation of clinical status and umbilical cord histology. Am. J. Dis. Child. 129:697–700, 1975.

Anagnostakis, D., Kazlaris, E., Xanthou, M., and Maounis, F.: Umbilical cord entanglement: a cause of neonatal pulmonary hemorrhage? Helv. Paediatr. Acta 29:167–171, 1974.

Andrade, A.: Anatomical and radiographic study on the anastomosis and branching of the umbilical arteries in white and non-white Brazilians. Acta Anat. (Basel) 70:66–75, 1968.

Antoine, C., Young, B.K., Silverman, F., Greco, M.A., and Alvarez, S.P.: Sinusoidal fetal heart rate pattern with vasa previa in twin pregnancy. J. Reprod. Med. 27:295–300, 1982.

Arts, N.F.T.: Investigations on the vascular system of the placenta. I. General introduction and the fetal vascular system. Am. J. Obstet. Gynecol. 82:147–158, 1961.

Arvy, L., and Pilleri, G.: Le Cordon Ombilical. Funis Umbilicalis. Verlag Hirnanatomisches Institut, Ostermundigen (Bern), Switzerland, 1976a.

Arvy, L., and Pilleri, G.: The cetacean umbilical cord; studies of the umbilical cord of two Platanistoidea: Platanista gangetica and Pontoporia blainvillei. In, Investigations on Cetacea. Volume VII. G. Pilleri, ed., pp. 91–103. Brain Anatomy Institute, Berne, Switzerland, 1976b.

Arya, S., and Gilbert, E.F.: The short cord syndrome: pathogenetic considerations [abstract]. Lab. Invest. 52:1P, 1985.

Asmussen, I.: Ultrastructure of human umbilical veins. Acta Obstet. Gynecol. Scand. 57:253–255, 1978.

Asmussen, I., and Kjeldsen, K.: Intimal ultrastructure of human umbilical arteries: observations on arteries from newborn children of smoking and nonsmoking mothers. Circ. Res. 36:579–589, 1975.

Bacsich, P., and Riddell, W.J.B.: Structure and nutrition of the cornea, cartilage and Wharton's jelly. Nature 155:271, 1945.

Bacsich, P., and Smout, C.F.V.: Some observations on the foetal vessels of the human placenta with an account of the corrosion technique. J. Anat. 72:358–364, 1938.

Bahary, C.M., Gabbai, M., and Eckerling, B.: Rupture of the umbilical cord: report of a case. Obstet. Gynecol. 26:130–132, 1965.

Baill, I.C., Moore, G.W., and Hedrick, L.A.: Abscess of allantoic duct remnant. Am. J. Obstet. Gynecol. 161:334–336, 1989.

Barents, J.W.: Over tumoren van de navelstreng en de placenta. Nederl. Tijdschr. Verlosk. Gynaecol. 52:243–251, 1953.

Barron, S., Riley, E.P., Smotherman, W.P., and Kotch, L.E.: Umbilical cord length in rats is altered by prenatal alcohol exposure. Teratology 31:49A–50A, 1985.

Barry, F.E., McCoy, C.P., and Callahan, W.P.: Hemangioma of the umbilical cord. Am. J. Obstet. Gynecol. 62:675–680, 1951.

Becker, V., and Dolling, D.: Gefäßverschlüsse in der Placenta von Totgeborenen. Virchows Arch. [Pathol. Anat.] 338:305–314, 1965.

Becker, V., and Röckelein, G.: Pathologie der weiblichen Genitalorgane. I. Pathologie der Plazenta und des Abortes. Springer-Verlag, Heidelberg, 1989.

Beer, D.C.: Vasa previa: review of current concepts of management and report of a case. Obstet. Gynecol. 3:595–597, 1954.

Bender, H.G., Werner, C., and Karsten, C.: Zum Einfluß der Nabelschnurstruktur auf Schwangerschafts- und Geburtsverlauf. Arch. Gynecol. 225:347–362, 1978.

Benirschke, K.: You need a sympathetic pathologist! The borderline of embryology and pathology revisited. Teratology 36:389–393, 1987.

Benirschke, K.: College of American Pathologists conference XIX on examination of the placenta: summary. Arch. Pathol. Lab. Med. 115:720–721, 1991.

Benirschke, K.: Obstetrically important lesions of the umbilical cord. J. Reprod. Med. 39:262–272, 1994.

Benirschke, K., and Bourne, G.L.: The incidence and prognostic implication of congenital absence of one umbilical artery. Am. J. Obstet. Gynecol. 79:251–254, 1960.

Benirschke, K., and Brown, W.H.: A vascular anomaly of the umbilical cord: the absence of one umbilical artery in the umbilical cords of normal and abnormal fetuses. Obstet. Gynecol. 6:399–404, 1953.

Benirschke, K., and Dodds, J.P.: Angiomyxoma of the umbilical cord with atrophy of an umbilical artery. Obstet. Gynecol. 30:99–102, 1967.

Benirschke, K., and Driscoll, S.G.: The Pathology of the Human Placenta. Springer-Verlag, New York, 1967.

Benirschke, K., Sullivan, M.M., and Marin-Padilla, M.: Size and number of umbilical vessels: a study of multiple pregnancy in man and the armadillo. Obstet. Gynecol. 24:819–834, 1964.

Bergman, P., Lundin, P., and Malmström, T.: Mucoid degeneration of Wharton's jelly: an umbilical cord anomaly threatening foetal life. Acta Obstet. Gynecol. Scand. 40:372–378, 1961.

Bergström, H.: Intrauterin fosterdöd genom förblödning. Nord. Med. 4:592–593, 1963.

Bhargava, I., and Raja, P.T.K.: Arteriovenous crossings on the chorial surface of the human placenta in abnormal pregnancy and development. Experientia 25:831–832, 1969.

Bhargava, I., Chakravarty, A., and Raja, P.T.K.: Anatomy of foetal blood vessels on the chorial surface of the human placenta. IV. With absence of one umbilical artery. Acta Anat. (Basel) 80:620–635, 1971.

Bilek, K., Roth, K., and Piskazeck, K.: Insertio-velamentosa-Blutung vor dem Blasensprung. Zentralbl. Gynäkol. 84: 1536–1541, 1962.

Blackburn, W., Cooley, N.R., and Manci, E.A.: Correlations between umbilical cord structure-composition and normal and abnormal fetal development. In, Proceedings of the Greenwood Genetics Conference. Vol. 7. R.A. Saul, ed., pp. 180–181. Jacobs Press, Clinton, SC, 1988.

Blanc, W.A., and Allan, G.W.: Intrafunicular ulceration of persistent omphalomesenteric duct with intra-amniotic hemorrhage and fetal death. Am. J. Obstet. Gynecol. 82: 1392–1396, 1961.

Bobitt, J.R.: Abnormal antepartum fetal heart rate tracings, failure to intervene, and fetal death: review of five cases reveals potential pitfalls of antepartum monitoring programs. Am. J. Obstet. Gynecol. 133:415–421, 1979.

Bodelsson, G., Sjöberg, N.-O., and Stjernquist, M.: Contractile effect of endothelin in the human uterine artery and autoradiographic localization of its binding sites. Am. J. Obstet. Gynecol. 167:745–750, 1992.

Bourne, G.L.: The Human Amnion and Chorion. Lloyd-Luke, London, 1962.

Boyd, J.D., and Hamilton, W.J.: The Human Placenta. Heffer & Sons, Cambridge, 1970.

Brady, A.G.: Knotted umbilical cord as a cause of death in a Cercopithecus aethiops fetus. Lab. Anim. Sci. 33:375–376, 1983.

Brant, H.A., and Lewis, B.V.: Prolapse of the umbilical cord. Lancet 2:1443–1445, 1966.

Brar, H.S., Medearis, A.L., DeVore, G.R., and Platt, L.D.: Maternal and fetal blood flow velocity waveforms in patients with preterm labor: effect of tocolytics. Obstet. Gynecol. 72:209–214, 1988.

Bret, A.J., and Bardiaux, M.: Hématome du cordon. Rev. Fr. Gynecol. Obstet. 55:240–249, 1956.

Broome, D.L., Kellogg, B., Weiss, B.A., and Wilson, M.G.: Needle puncture of the fetus during amniocentesis. Lancet 2:604, 1975.

Broome, D.L., Wilson, M.G., Weiss, B., and Kellogg, B.: Needle puncture of the fetus: a complication of second-trimester amniocentesis. Am. J. Obstet. Gynecol. 126:247–252, 1976.

Browne, F.J.: On the abnormalities of the umbilical cord which may cause antenatal death. J. Obstet. Gynaecol. Br. Emp. 32:17–48, 1925.

Busacca, M., Dejana, E., Balconi, G., Olivieri, S., Pietra, A., Vergara-Dauden, M., and de Gaetano, G.: Reduced prostacyclin production by cultured endothelial cells from umbilical arteries of babies born to women who smoke. Lancet 2:609–610, 1982.

Cai, W.Q., Bodin, P., Loesch, A., Sexton, A., and Burnstock, G.: Localization of vasoactive substances in the endothelial cells of human umbilical vessels [abstract]. Histochem. J. 14:600, 1992.

Cai, W.Q., Bodin, P., Sexton, A., Loesch, A., and Burnstock, G.: Localization of neuropeptide Y and atrial natriuretic peptide in the endothelial cells of human umbilical blood vessels. Cell Tissue Res. 272:175–181, 1993a.

Cai, W.Q., Terenghi, G., Bodin, P., Burnstock, G., and Polak, J.M.: In situ hybridization of atrial natriuretic peptide mRNA in the endothelial cells of human umbilical vessels. Histochemistry 100:277–283, 1993b.

Camilleri, A.P.: Umbilical cord. B.M.J. 2:757, 1964.

Cardosos, L.E.M., Erlich, R.B., Rudge, M.C., Peracoli, J.C., and Mourao, P.A.S.: A comparative analysis of glycosaminoglycans from human umbilical arteries in normal subjects and in pathological conditions affecting pregnancy. Lab. Invest. 67:588–595, 1992.

Carp, H.J.A., Mashiach, S., and Serr, D.M.: Vasa previa: a major complication and its management. Obstet. Gynecol. 53:273–275, 1979.

Chantler, C., Baum, J.D., and Scopes, J.W.: Giant umbilical cord associated with a patent urachus and fused umbilical arteries. J. Obstet. Gynaecol. Br. Commonw. 76:273–274, 1969.

Chasnoff, I.J., and Fletcher, M.A.: True knot of the umbilical cord. Am. J. Obstet. Gynecol. 127:425–427, 1977.

Chaurasia, B.D., and Agarwal, B.M.: Helical structure of the umbilical cord. Acta Anat. (Basel) 103:226–230, 1979.

Clapp, J.F., Peress, N.S., Wesley, M., and Mann, L.I.: Brain damage after intermittent partial cord occlusion in the chronically instrumented fetal lamb. Am. J. Obstet. Gynecol. 159:504–509, 1988.

Clare, N.M., Hayashi, R., and Khodr, G.: Intrauterine death from umbilical cord hematoma. Arch. Pathol. Lab. Med. 103:46–47, 1979.

Clarke, J.A.: An x-ray microscopic study of the vasa vasorum of the human umbilical arteries. Z. Zellforsch. 66:293–299, 1965.

Colgan, T.J., and Luk, S.C.: Umbilical-cord torsion, thrombosis, and intrauterine death of a twin. Arch. Pathol. Lab. Med. 106:101, 1982.

Collins, J.H.: Two cases of multiple umbilical cord abnormalities resulting in stillbirth: prenatal observation with ultrasonography and fetal heart rates. Am. J. Obstet. Gynecol. 168:125–128, 1993.

Collins, J.C., Muller, R.J., and Collins, C.L.: Prenatal observation of umbilical cord abnormalities: a triple knot and torsion of the umbilical cord. Am. J. Obstet. Gynecol. 169:102–104, 1993.

Cook, F.G., Taylor, R., and Gillan, J.E.: Placental venous thrombosis—a clinically significant finding in intrauterine death. Lab. Invest. 56:1P, 1987.

Cordero, D.R., Helfgott, A.W., Landy, H.J., Reik, R.F., Medina, C., and O'Sullivan, M.J.: A non-hemorrhagic manifestation of vasa previa: a clinicopathologic case report. Obstet. Gynecol. 82:698–700, 1993.

Corkill, T.F.: The infant's vulnerable life-line. Aust. N.Z. J. Obstet. Gynaecol. 1:154–160, 1961.

Corridan, M., Kendall, E.D., and Begg, J.D.: Cord entanglement causing premature separation and amniotic fluid embolism: case report. Br. J. Obstet. Gynaecol. 87:935–940, 1980.

Coulter, J.B.S., Scott, J.M., and Jordan, M.M.: Oedema of the umbilical cord and respiratory distress in the newborn. Br. J. Obstet. Gynaecol. 82:453–459, 1975.

Crawford, J.M.: A study of human placental growth with observations on the placenta in erythroblastosis foetalis. J. Obstet. Gynaecol. Br. Emp. 66:885–896, 1959.

Crawford, J.S.: Cord round the neck: incidence and sequelae. Acta Paediatr. (Stockh.) 51:594–603, 1962.

Crawford, J.S.: Cord around the neck: further analysis of incidence. Acta Paediatr. (Stockh.) 53:553–557, 1964.

Crichton, J.L.: Tensile strength of the umbilical cord. Am. J. Obstet. Gynecol. 115:77–80, 1973.

Critchlow, C.W., Leet, T.L., Benedetti, T.J., and Daling, J.R.: Risk factors and infant outcomes associated with umbilical cord prolapse: a population-based case-control study among births in Washington state. Am. J. Obstet. Gynecol. 170:613–618, 1994.

Cullen, T.S.: Embryology, Anatomy, and Disease of the Umbilicus Together with Diseases of the Urachus. Saunders, Philadelphia, 1916.

Dadak, C., Kefalides, A., Sinzinger, H., and Weber, G.: Reduced umbilical artery prostacyclin formation in complicated pregnancies. Am. J. Obstet. Gynecol. 144:792–795, 1982.

Davignon, J., Lorenz, R.R., and Shepherd, J.T.: Response of human umbilical artery to changes in transmural pressure. Am. J. Physiol. 209:51–59, 1965.

De Sa, D.J.: Rupture of fetal vessels on placental surface. Arch. Dis. Child. 46:495–501, 1971.

De Sa, D.J.: Diseases of the umbilical cord. In, Pathology of the Placenta. E.V.D.K. Perrin, ed. Churchill Livingstone, New York, 1984.

De Sa, M.F., and Meirelles, R.S.: Vasodilating effect of estrogen on the human umbilical artery. Gynecol. Invest. 8:307–313, 1977.

DeVore, G.R., Mayden, K., Tortora, M., Berkowitz, R.L., and Hobbins, J.C.: Dilation of the umbilical vein in rhesus hemolytic anemia: a predictor of severe disease. Am. J. Obstet. Gynecol. 141:464–466, 1981.

Didolkar, S.M., Hal, J., Phelan, J., Gutberlett, R., and Hill, J.L.: The prenatal diagnosis and management of a hepato-omphalocele. Am. J. Obstet. Gynecol. 141:221–222, 1981.

Dildy, G.A., and Clark, S.L.: Umbilical cord prolapse. Contemp. Obstet. Gynecol. 38:23–31, 1993.

Dillon, W.P., and O'Leary, L.A.: Detection of fetal cord compromise secondary to umbilical cord hematoma with the nonstress test. Am. J. Obstet. Gynecol. 141:102–1103, 1981.

Dippel, A.L.: Hematomas of the umbilical cord. Surg. Gynecol. Obstet. 70:51–57, 1940.

Dippel, A.L.: Maligned umbilical cord entanglements. Am. J. Obstet. Gynecol. 88:1012–1018, 1964.

Di Terlizzi, G., and Rossi, G.F.: Studio clinico-statistico sulle anomalie del funiculo. Ann. Obstet. Ginecol. 77:459–474, 1955 [see Fox, 1978].

Dolff, M.: Die sogenannten Rekanalisationen der Stammzottengefäße bei Endarteritis obliterans der Plazentagefäße. Arch. Gynecol. 226:325–332, 1978.

Dombrowski, M.P., Budev, H., Wolfe, H.M., Sokol, R.J., and Perrin, E.: Fetal hemorrhage from umbilical cord hemangioma. Obstet. Gynecol. 70:439–442, 1987.

Doshi, N., and Klionsky, B.: Pathology of disseminated intravascular coagulation in the newborn. Lab. Invest. 40:303, 1979.

Dreyfus, M., Magny, J.F., Bridey, F., Schwarz, H.P., Planché, C., Dehan, M., and Tchernia, G.: Treatment of homozygous protein C deficiency and neonatal purpura fulminans with a purified protein C concentrate. N. Engl. J. Med. 325:1565–1568, 1991.

Dunn, P.M., Fraser, I.D., and Raper, A.B.: Influence of early cord ligation on the transplacental passage of foetal cells. J. Obstet. Gynaecol. Br. Commonw. 73:757–760, 1966.

Dyer, D.C.: Comparison of the constricting actions produced by serotonin and prostaglandins on isolated sheep umbilical arteries and veins. Gynecol. Invest. 1:204–209, 1970.

Earn, A.A.: The effect of congenital abnormalities of the umbilical cord and placenta on the newborn and mother: a survey of 5676 consecutive deliveries. J. Obstet. Gynaecol. Br. Emp. 58:456–459, 1951.

Eastman, N.J.: Editorial comments. Surg. Gynecol. Obstet. 22:16, 1967.

Eastman, N.J., and Hellman, L.M., eds.: Williams Obstetrics. 12th Ed. Appleton, New York, 1961.

Eddleman, K.A., Lockwood, C.J., Berkowitz, G.S., Lapinski, R.H., and Berkowitz, R.L.: Clinical significance and sonographic diagnosis of velamentous umbilical cord insertion. Am. J. Perinatol. 9:123–126, 1992.

Editorial: Closure of umbilical blood-vessels. Lancet 2:381, 1966.

Edmonds, H.W.: The spiral twist of the normal umbilical cord in twins and in singletons. Am. J. Obstet. Gynecol. 67:102–120, 1954.

Eggens, J.H., and Bruins, H.W.: An unusual case of fetal distress. Am. J. Obstet. Gynecol. 148:219–220, 1984.

Ellison, J.P.: The nerves of the umbilical cord in man and the rat. Am. J. Anat. 132:53–60, 1971.

Ente, G., Penzer, P.H., and Kenigsberg, K.: Giant umbilical cord associated with patent urachus. Am. J. Dis. Child. 120:82–83, 1970.

Feinstein, S.J., Lodeiro, J.G., Vintzileos, A.M., Weinbaum, P.J., Campbell, W.A., and Nochimson, D.J.: Intrapartum ultrasound diagnosis of nuchal cord as a decisive factor in management. Am. J. Obstet. Gynecol. 153:308–309, 1985.

Ferrazzi, E., Brambati, B., Lanzani, A., Oldrini, A., Stripparo, L., Guerneri, A., and Makowski, E.L.: The yolk sac in early pregnancy failure. Am. J. Obstet. Gynecol. 158:137–142, 1988.

Fisk, N.M., Maclachlan, N., Ellis, C., Tannirandorn, Y., Tonge, H.M., and Rodeck, C.H.: Absent end-diastolic flow in first trimester umbilical artery. Lancet 2:1256–1257, 1988.

Fletcher, S.: Chirality in the umbilical cord. Brit. J. Obstet. Gynaecol. 100:234–236, 1993.

Foldes, J.J.: Spontaneous intrauterine rupture of the umbilical cord: report of a case. Obstet. Gynecol. 9:608–609, 1957.

Fortune, D.W., and Östör, A.G.: Umbilical artery aneurysm. Am. J. Obstet. Gynecol. 131:339–340, 1978.

Fortune, D.W., and Östör, A.G.: Angiomyxomas of the umbilical cord. Obstet. Gynecol. 55:375–378, 1980.

Fox, H.: Thrombosis of foetal arteries in the human placenta. J. Obstet. Gynaecol. Br. Commonw. 73:961–965, 1966.

Fox, H.: Abnormalities of the foetal stem arteries in the human placenta. J. Obstet. Gynaecol. Br. Commonw. 74:734–738, 1967.

Fox, H.: Pathology of the Placenta. Saunders, London, 1978.

Fox, H., and Jacobson, H.N.: Innervation of the human umbilical cord and umbilical vessels. Am. J. Obstet. Gynecol. 103:384–389, 1969.

Fox, H., and Khong, T.Y.: Lack of innervation of human umbilical cord: an immunohistochemical and histochemical study. Placenta 11:59–62, 1990.

Fribourg, S.: Cord length and complications. Obstet. Gynecol. 58:533, 1981.

Froehlich, L.A., and Fujikura, T.: Significance of a single umbilical artery: report from the collaborative study of cerebral palsy. Am. J. Obstet. Gynecol. 94:274–279, 1966.

Fujikura, T., and Benson, R.C.: Placentitis and fibrous occlusion of fetal vessels in the placenta of stillborn infants. Am. J. Obstet. Gynecol. 89:225–229, 1964.

Fujikura, T., and Carleton, J.H.: Unilateral thickening of fetal arteries on the placenta resembling arteriosclerosis. Am. J. Obstet. Gynecol. 100:843–845, 1968.

Fujikura, T., and Hosoda, Y.: Unilateral thickening of placental fetal veins. Placenta 11:241–245, 1990.

Fujinaga, M., Chinn, A., and Shepard, T.H.: Umbilical cord growth in human and rat fetuses: evidence against the "stretch hypothesis." Teratology 41:333–339, 1990.

Gad, C.: A case of haemorrhage in labour from a placental vessel causing foetal death. Acta Obstet. Gynecol. Scand. 47:342–344, 1968.

Galle, P.C., and Meis, P.J.: Complications of amniocentesis: a review. J. Reprod. Med. 27:149–155, 1982.

Gardiner, J.P.: The umbilical cord: normal length; length in cord complications; etiology and frequency of coiling. Surg. Gynecol. Obstet. 34:252–256, 1922.

Gardner, D.G., Hedges, B.K., Lapointe, M.C., and Deschapper, C.F.: Expression of the atrial natriuretic peptide gene in human fetal heart. J. Clin. Endocrinol. Metab. 69:729–737, 1989.

Gardner, R.F.R., and Trussell, R.R.: Ruptured hematoma of the umbilical cord. Obstet. Gynecol. 24:791–793, 1964.

Gassner, C.B., and Paul, R.H.: Laceration of umbilical cord vessels secondary to amniocentesis. Obstet. Gynecol. 48:627–630, 1976.

Gebrane-Younes, J., Minh, H.N., and Orcel, L.: Ultrastructure of human umbilical vessels: a possible role in amniotic fluid formation? Placenta 7:173–185, 1986.

Genest, D.R.: Estimating the time of death in stillborn fetuses. II. Histologic evaluation of the placenta; a study of 71 stillborns. Obstet. Gynecol. 80:585–592, 1992.

Gerlach, H.: Kongenitales Nabelarterienaneurysma. Z. Allg. Pathol. 111:420–423, 1968.

Ghosh, K.G., Ghosh, S.N., and Gupta, A.B.: Tensile properties of human umbilical cord. Indian J. Med. Res. 79:538–541, 1984.

Giacoia, G.P.: Body stalk anomaly: congenital absence of the umbilical cord. Obstet. Gynecol. 80:527–529, 1992.

Giacomello, F.: Ultrasound determination of nuchal cord in breech presentation. Am. J. Obstet. Gynecol. 159:531–532, 1988.

Gianopoulos, J., Carver, T., Tomich, P.G., Karlman, R., and Gadwood, K.: Diagnosis of vasa previa with ultrasonography. Obstet. Gynecol. 69:488–491, 1987.

Gilbert, E.: The short cord syndrome. Pediatr. Pathol. 5:96, 1986.

Gill, P., Jarjoura, D., and VanHook, J.: Wharton's jelly in the umbilical cord: a study of its quantitative variation and clinical correlates [abstract 124]. Am. J. Obstet. Gynecol. 168:334, 1993.

Glanfield, P.A., and Watson, R.: Intrauterine death due to umbilical cord torsion. Arch. Pathol. Lab. Med. 110:357–358, 1986.

Goerttler, K.: Die Bedeutung der funktionellen Struktur der Gefäßwand. I. Untersuchungen an der Nabelschnurarterie des Menschen. Gegenbaurs Morphol. Jahrb. 91:368–393, 1951.

Golden, A.S.: Umbilical cord-placental separation: a complication of IUD failure. J. Reprod. Med. 11:79–80, 1973.

Gonzalez-Crussi, F., and Roth, L.M.: The human yolk sac and yolk sac carcinoma. Hum. Pathol. 7:675–691, 1976.

Goodlin, R.C.: Fetal dysmaturity, "lean cord," and fetal distress. Am. J. Obstet. Gynecol. 156:1357, 1987.

Goodlin, R.C., and Clewell, W.H.: Sudden fetal death following amniocentesis. Am. J. Obstet. Gynecol. 118:285–288, 1974.

Grange, K., Arya, S., Opitz, J., Laxova, R., Herrmann, J., and Grieco, A.: Rilievi clinico-statistici sulla inserzione velamentosa ed a racchetta del cordone ombellicale. Monit. Obstet. Ginecol. Endocrinol. Metab. 8:89–102, 1936 [see Fox, 1978].

Graumann, W.: Polysaccharide. Ergebnisse der Polysaccharidhistochemie: Mensch und Säugetier. In, Handbuch der Histochemie. Vol. II/2. W. Graumann and K. Neumann, eds. Fischer, Stuttgart, 1964.

Grieco, A.: Rilievi clinico-statistici sulla inserzione velamentosa ed a racchetta del cordone ombellicale. Monit. Ostet. Ginecol. Endocrin. Metabol. 8:89–102, 1936.

Grosser, O.: Frühentwicklung, Eihautbildung und Placentation des Menschen und der Säugetiere. Bergmann, Munich, 1927.

Gruber, F.H.: Gas in the umbilical vessels as a sign of fetal death. Radiology 89:881–882, 1967.

Gruenwald, P.: The amount of fetal blood remaining in the placenta at birth. Proc. Soc. Exp. Biol. Med. 130:326–329, 1969.

Gu, J., Pinheiro, J.M.B., Yu, C.Z., D'Andrea, M., Muralidharan, S., and Malik, A.: Detection of endothelinlike immunoreactivity in epithelium and fibroblasts of the human umbilical cord. Tissue Cell 23:437–444, 1991.

Guidetti, A.A., Divon, M.Y., Cavaleri, R.L., Langer, O., and Merkatz, I.R.: Fetal umbilical artery flow velocimetry in postdate pregnancies. Am. J. Obstet. Gynecol. 157:1521–1523, 1987.

Hall, S.P.: The thin cord syndrome: a review with a report of two cases. Obstet. Gynecol. 18:507–509, 1961.

Harold, J.G., Siegel, R.J., Fitzgerald, G.A., Satoh, P., and Fishbein, M.C.: Differential prostaglandin production by human umbilical vasculature. Arch. Pathol. Lab. Med. 112:43–46, 1988.

Harris, L.E., and Wenzl, J.E.: Heterotopic pancreatic tissue and intestinal mucosa in the umbilical cord. N. Engl. J. Med. 268:721–722, 1963.

Hartman, K.R., Rawlings, J.S., and Feingold, M.: Protein C deficiency. Am. J. Dis. Child. 144:1353–1354, 1990.

Hathout, H.: The vascular pattern and mode of insertion of the umbilical cord in abortion material. J. Obstet. Gynaecol. Br. Commonw. 71:963–964, 1964.

Heckmann, U., Cornelius, H.V., and Freudenberg, V.: Das Teratom der Nabelschnur: ein kasuistischer Beitrag zu den echten Tumoren der Nabelschnur. Geburtshilfe Frauenheilkd. 32:605–607, 1972.

Heifetz, S.A.: Single umbilical artery: a statistical analysis of 237 autopsy cases and review of the literature. Perspect. Pediatr. Pathol. 8:345–378, 1984.

Heifetz, S.A.: Thrombosis of the umbilical cord: analysis of 52 cases and literature review. Pediatr. Pathol. 8:37–54, 1988.

Heifetz, S.A., and Rueda-Pedraza, M.E.: Hemangiomas of the umbilical cord. Pediatr. Pathol. 1:385–398, 1883a.

Heifetz, S.A., and Rueda-Pedraza, M.E.: Omphalomesenteric duct cysts of the umbilical cord. Pediatr. Pathol. 1:325–335, 1983b.

Hempel, E.: Die ultrastrukturelle Differenzierung des menschlichen Amnionepithels unter besonderer Berücksichtigung des Nabelstrangs. Anat. Anz. 132:356–370, 1972.

Hemsen, A., Gillis, C., Larsson, O., Haegerstrand, A., and Lundberg, J.M.: Characterization, localization and actions of endothelins in umbilical vessels and placenta. Acta Physiol. Scand. 143:395–404, 1991.

Herberz, O.: Über die Insertio furcata funiculi umbilicalis. Acta Obstet. Gynecol. Scand. 18:336–351, 1938.

Herrmann, U.J., and Sidiropoulos, D.: Single umbilical artery: prenatal findings. Prenat. Diagn. 8:275–280, 1988.

Hersh, J., and Buchino, J.J.: Umbilical cord torsion/constriction sequence. In, Proceedings of the Greenwood Genetics Conference. Vol. 7. R.A. Saul, ed., pp. 181–182, Jacobs Press, Clinton, SC, 1988.

Hertig, A.T.: The placenta: some new knowledge about an old organ. Obstet. Gynecol. 20:859–866, 1962.

Hertig, A.T.: Human Trophoblast. Charles C Thomas, Springfield, IL, 1968.

Hey, A., and Röckelein, G.: Die sogenannten Endothelvakuolen der Plazentagefäße—Physiologie oder Krankheit. Pathologe 10:66–67, 1989.

Hitschold, T., Weiss, E., Beck, T., Hüntefering, H., and Berle, P.: Low target birth weight or growth retardation? Umbilical Doppler flow velocity waveforms and histometric analysis of fetoplacental vascular tree. Am. J. Obstet. Gynecol. 168:1260–1264, 1993.

Hoag, R.W.: Fetomaternal hemorrhage associated with umbilical vein thrombosis. Am. J. Obstet. Gynecol. 154:1271–1274, 1986.

Hobel, C.J., Emmanouilides, G.C., Townsend, D.E., and Yashiro, K.: Ligation of one umbilical artery in the fetal lamb: experimental production of fetal malnutrition. Obstet. Gynecol. 36:582–588, 1970.

Hoboken, W.: Anatomia Secundinae. Ribbium, Ultrajecti, 1669.

Hong, C.B., Donahue, J.M., Giles, R.C., Petrites-Murphy, M.B., Poonacha, K.B., Roberts, A.W., Smith, B.J., Tramontin, R.R., Tuttle, P.A., and Swerczek, T.W.: Equine abortion and stillbirth in central Kentucky during 1988 and 1989 foaling seasons. J. Vet. Diagn. Invest. 5:560–566, 1993.

Horwitz, S.T., Finn, W.F., and Mastrota, V.F.: A study of umbilical cord encirclement. Am. J. Obstet. Gynecol. 89:970–974, 1964.

Howorka, E., and Kapczynski, W.: Unusual thickness of the fetal end of the umbilical cord. J. Obstet. Gynaecol. Br. Commonw. 78:283, 1971.

Hoyes, A.D.: Ultrastructure of the epithelium of the human umbilical cord. J. Anat. 105:149–162, 1969.

Hoyme, H.E., Jones, K.L., Allen, M.I.V., Saunders, B.S., and Benirschke, K.: Vascular pathogenesis of transverse limb reduction defects. J. Pediatr. 101:839–843, 1982.

Hyrtl, J.: Die Blutgefäße der menschlichen Nachgeburt in normalen und abnormen Verhältnissen. Braumüller, Wien, 1870.

Inglis, C.G., Kingdom, J.C.P., and Nelson, D.M.: Atrial natriuretic hormone: a paracrine or endocrine role within the human placenta? J. Clin. Endocrinol. Metab. 76:1014–1018, 1993.

Irani, P.K.: Haematoma of the umbilical cord. B.M.J. 2:1436–1437, 1964.

Ivemark, B.I., Lagergren, C., and Ljungqvist, A.: Generalized arterial calcification associated with hydramnios in two stillborn infants. Acta Paediatr. Suppl. (Stockh.) 135:103–110, 1962.

James, J.D., and Nickerson, C.W.: Laceration of umbilical artery and abruptio placentae secondary to amniocentesis. Obstet. Gynecol. 48:44s–45s, 1976.

Janosco, E.O., Lona, J.Z., and Belin, R.P.: Congenital anomalies of the umbilicus. Am. Surg. 43:177–185, 1977.

Jauniaux, E., De Munter, C., Vanesse, M., Wilkin, P., and Hustin, J.: Embryonic remnants of the umbilical cord: morphologic and clinical aspects. Hum. Pathol. 20:458–462, 1989a.

Jauniaux, E., Donner, C., Simon, P., Vanesse, M., Hustin, J., and Rodesch, F.: Pathological aspects of the umbilical cord after percutaneous umbilical blood sampling. Obstet. Gynecol. 73:215–218, 1989b.

Javert, C.T., and Barton, B.: Congenital and acquired lesions of the umbilical cord and spontaneous abortion. Am. J. Obstet. Gynecol. 63:1065–1077, 1952.

Jimenez, E., Unger, M., Vogel, M., Lobeck, H., Wagner, G., Schwiermann, J., Schäfer, A., and Grosch-Wörner, I.: Morphologische Untersuchungen an Plazenten HIV-positiver Mütter. Pathologe 9:228–234, 1988.

Jogee, M., Myatt, L., and Elder, M.G.: Decreased prostacyclin production by placental cells in culture from pregnancies complicated by fetal growth retardation. Br. J. Obstet. Gynaecol. 90:247–250, 1983.

Jones, C.J.P., Jauniaux, E., and Campbell, S.: Development and degeneration of the secondary human yolk sac. Placenta 14:A32, 1993.

Jones, K.P., Wheater, A.W., and Musgrave, W.: Simple test for bleeding from vasa previa. Lancet 2:1430–1431, 1987.

Jones, T.B., Sorokin, Y., Bhatia, R., Zador, I.E., and Bottoms, S.F.: Single umbilical artery: accurate diagnosis? Am. J. Obstet. Gynecol. 169:538–540, 1993.

Kan, P.S., and Eastman, N.J.: Coiling of the umbilical cord around the foetal neck. J. Obstet. Gynaecol. Br. Emp. 64:227–228, 1957.

Kaplan, C., August, D., and Mizrachi, H.: Single umbilical artery and cord accidents. [abstract 17]. Mod. Pathol. 3(1):4P, 1990.

Karbowski, B., Bauch, H.J., and Schneider, H.P.G.: Functional differentiation of umbilical vein endothelial cells following pregnancy complicated by smoking or diabetes mellitus. Placenta 12:405, 1991.

Katz, V., Blanchard, G., Dingman, C., Bowes, W.A., and Cefalo, R.C.: Atenolol and short umbilical cords. Am. J. Obstet. Gynecol. 156:1271–1272, 1987.

Katz, Z., Shosham, Z., Lancet, M., Blickstein, I., Mogilner, B.M., and Zalel, Y.: Management of labor with umbilical cord prolapse: a 5-year study. Obstet. Gynecol. 72:278–280, 1988.

Kelber, R.: Gespaltene "solitäre" Nabelschnurarterie. Arch. Gynecol. 220:319–323, 1976.

Kernbach, M.: Das neuroektoblastische System der Plazenta des Menschen. Anat. Anz. 113:259–269, 1963.

Kernbach, M.: Existe-t-il du tissu nerveux dans le placenta? Rev. Fr. Gynecol. 64:357–361, 1969.

Kessler, A.: Blutungen aus den Nabelschnurgefässen in der Schwangerschaft. Gynaecologia 150:353–365, 1960.

Khong, T.Y., and Dilly, S.A.: Calcification of umbilical artery: two distinct lesions. J. Clin. Pathol. 42:931–934, 1989.

King, D.L.: Placental migration demonstrated by ultrasonography: a hypothesis of dynamic placentation. Radiology 109:167–170, 1973.

King, E.L.: Intrauterine death of the fetus due to abnormalities of the umbilical cord: report of three cases. Am. J. Obstet. Gynecol. 12:812–816, 1926.

King, S.: Patent omphalomesenteric duct. Arch. Surg. 96:545–548, 1968.

Kishore, N., and Sarkar, S.C.: The arterial patterns of placenta: a postpartum radiological study. J. Obstet. Gynaecol. India 17:9–13, 1967.

Kjeldsen, J., and Pedersen, J.: Relation of residual placental blood-volume to onset of respiration and the respiratory-distress syndrome in infants of diabetic and non-diabetic mothers. Lancet 1:180–184, 1967.

Klebe, J.G., and Ingomar, C.J.: Placental transfusion in infants of diabetic mothers elucidated by placental residual blood volume. Acta Paediatr. (Stockh.) 63:59–64, 1974. The influence of the method of delivery and the clamping technique on the red cell volume in infants of diabetic and non-diabetic mothers. Acta Paediatr. (Stockh.) 63:65–69, 1974.

Kouyoumdjian, A.: Velamentous insertion of the umbilical cord. Obstet. Gynecol. 56:737–742, 1980.

Kreibich, D.: Über eine grosse Urachuscyste bei einer 80 jährigen Frau. Zentralbl. Gynäkol. 69:523–528, 1947.

Kreyberg, L.: A teratoma-like swelling in the umbilical cord possibly of acardiac nature. J. Pathol. Bacteriol. 75:109–112, 1958.

Kristiansen, F.V., and Nielsen, V.T.: Intra-uterine fetal death and thrombosis of the umbilical vessels. Acta Obstet. Gynecol. Scand. 64:331–334, 1985.

Krone, H.-A.: Die Bedeutung der Nidationsstörungen für die Pathologie der Embryonalentwicklung. Bibl. Microbiol. Fasc. 1:111–116, 1960 [Wiener Colloqium: Pränatale Infektionen, 1959].

Krone, H.-A.: Die Bedeutung der Plazenta für die Entstehung von Mißbildungen. Wien. Med. Wochenschr. 117:393–397, 1967.

Krone, H.A., Jopp, H., and Schellerer, W.: Die Bedeutung anamnestischer Befunde für die verschiedenen Formen des Nabelschnuransatzes. Z. Geburtshilfe Gynäkol. 163:205–213, 1965.

Labarrere, C., Sebastiani, M., Siminovich, M., Torassa, E., and Althabe, O.: Absence of Wharton's jelly around the umbilical arteries: an unusual cause of perinatal mortality. Placenta 6:555–559, 1985.

Lachenmayer, L.: Adrenergic innervation of the umbilical vessels: light- and fluorescence microscopic studies. Z. Zellforsch. 120:120–136, 1971.

Lacro, R.V., Jones, K.L., and Benirschke, K.: The umbilical cord twist: origin, direction, and relevance. Am. J. Obstet. Gynecol. 157:833–838, 1987.

Lang, I., Hartmann, M., Blaschitz, A., Dohr, G., Skofitsch, G., and Desoye, G.: Immunohistochemical evidence for the heterogeneity of maternal and fetal vascular endothelial cells in human full-term placenta. Cell Tissue Res. 274:211–218, 1993.

Lange, I.R., Manning, F.A., Morrison, I., Chamberlain, P.F., and Harman, C.R.: Cord prolapse: is antenatal diagnosis possible. Am. J. Obstet. Gynecol. 151:1083–1085, 1985.

Las Heras, J., and Haust, D.: Ultrastructure of fetal stem arteries of human placenta in normal pregnancy. Virchows Arch. 393:133–144, 1981.

Lauweryns, J.M., deBruyn, M., Peuskens, J., and Bourgeois, N.: Absence of intrinsic innervation of the human placenta. Experientia 25:432, 1969.

LeDonne, A.T., and McGowan, L.: Effect of an oxytocic on umbilical cord venous pressure. Obstet. Gynecol. 30:103–107, 1967.

Lee, M.C.L., and Aterman, K.: An intestinal polyp of the umbilical cord. Am. J. Dis. Child. 116:320–323, 1968.

Lee, S.T., and Hon, E.H.: Fetal hemodynamic response to umbilical cord compression. Obstet. Gynecol. 22:553–562, 1963.

Leff, M.: Hemorrhage from a ruptured varicosity in the placenta causing the death of the fetus. Am. J. Obstet. Gynecol. 22:117–118, 1931.

Lehman, R.E.: Umbilical cord prolapse following external cephalic version with tocolysis. Am. J. Obstet. Gynecol. 146:963–964, 1983.

Leinzinger, E.: Varixthrombose der Nabelschnur. Z. Geburtshilfe Gynäkol. 171:82–87, 1969.

Leinzinger, E.: Totaler Nabelschnurabriss intra partum bei Hydramnion. Zentralbl. Gynäkol. 94:1233–1238, 1972.

Lemtis, H.: Über eine seltene Nabelschnurmißbildung. Geburtshilfe Frauenheilkd. 26:986–993, 1966.

Lemtis, H.: Über Aneurysmen im fetalen Gefäßapparat der menschlichen Plazenta. Arch. Gynecol. 206:330–347, 1968.

Lenke, R.R., Ashwood, E.R., Cyr, D.R., Gravett, M., Smith, J.R., and Stenchever, M.A.: Genetic amniocentesis: significance of intraamniotic bleeding and placental location. Obstet. Gynecol. 65:798–801, 1985.

Leu, A.J., and Leu, H.J.: Spezielle Probleme bei der histologischen Altersbestimmung von Thromben und Emboli. Pathologe 10:87–92, 1989.

Leung, A.K.C., and Robson, W.L.M.: Single umbilical artery: a report of 159 cases. Am. J. Dis. Child. 143:108–111, 1989.

Levy, H., Meier, P.R., and Makowski, E.L.: Umbilical cord prolapse. Obstet. Gynecol. 64:499–502, 1984.

Loquet, P., Broughton-Pipkin, F., Symonds, E.M., and Rubin, P.C.: Blood velocity waveforms and placental vascular formation. Lancet 2:1252–1253, 1988.

Ludwig, K: Ein weiterer Beitrag zum Bau der Gorilla-Placenta. Acta Anat. (Basel) 46:304–310, 1961.

Macara, L.M., Kingdom, J.C.P., and Kaufmann, P.: Control of the fetoplacental circulation. Fetal Maternal Med. Rev. 5:167–179, 1993.

Maclean, M.R., Templeton, A.G.B., and McGrath, J.C.: The influence of endothelin-1 on human foeto-placental blood vessels: a comparison with 5-hydroxytryptamine. Br. J. Pharmacol. 106:937–941, 1992.

Mäkilä, U.M., Jouppila, P., Kirkinen, P., Viinikka, L., and Ylikorkala, O.: Relation between umbilical prostacyclin production and blood-flow in the fetus. Lancet 1:728–729, 1983.

Mallard, E.C., Gunn, A.J., Williams, C.E., Johnston, B.M., and Gluckman, P.D.: Transient umbilical cord occlusion causes hippocampal damage in fetal sheep. Am. J. Obstet. Gynecol. 167:1423–1430, 1992.

Malpas, P.: Length of the umbilical cord at term. B.M.J. 1:673–674, 1964.

Malpas, P., and Symonds, E.M.: Observations on the structure of the human umbilical cord. Surg. Obstet. Gynecol. 123:746–750, 1966.

Manci, E.A., Ulmer, D.R., Nye, D.M., Shah, A., and Mvumbi, L.: Variations in normal umbilical cord length following birth [abstract 33]. Mod. Pathol. 6:p6p, 1993.

Marchetti, A.A.: A consideration of certain types of benign tumors of the placenta. Surg. Gynecol. Obstet. 68:733–743, 1939.

Marciniak, E., Wilson, H.D., and Marlar, R.A.: Neonatal purpura fulminans: a genetic disorder related to the absence of protein C in blood. Blood 65:15–20, 1985.

Marco-Johnson, M.J., Marlar, R.A., Jacobson, L.J., Hays, T., and Warady, B.A.: Severe protein C deficiency in newborn infants. J. Pediatr. 113:359–363, 1988.

Matheus, M., and Sala, M.A.: The importance of placental examination in newborns with single umbilical artery. Z. Geburtshilfe Perinatol. 184:231–232, 1980.

McCoshen, J.A., Tulloch, H.V., and Johnson, K.A.: Umbilical cord is the major source of prostaglandin E_2 in the gestational sac during term labor. Am. J. Obstet. Gynecol. 160:873–978, 1989.

McCowan, L.M., Mullen, B.M., and Ritchie, K.: Umbilical artery flow velocity waveforms and the placental vascular bed. Am. J. Obstet. Gynecol. 157:900–902, 1987.

McCurdy, C., Anderson, C., Borjon, N., Brzechffa, P., Miller, H., McNamara, M., Newman, A., and Seeds, J.: Antenatal sonographic diagnosis of nuchal cord [abstract 329]. Am. J. Obstet. Gynecol. 170:366, 1994.

McKay, D.G., Roby, C.C., Hertig, A.T., and Richardson, M.V.: Studies of the function of early human trophoblast. II. Preliminary observations on certain chemical constituents of chorionic and early amniotic fluid. Am. J. Obstet. Gynecol. 69:735–741, 1955.

McLennan, J.E.: Implications of the eccentricity of the human umbilical cord. Am. J. Obstet. Gynecol. 101:1124–1130, 1968.

McLennan, H., Price, E., Urbanska, M., Craig, N., and Fraser, M.: Umbilical cord knots and encirclements. Aust. N.Z. J. Obstet. Gynaecol. 28:116–119, 1988.

Merttens, J.: Beiträge zur normalen und pathologischen Anatomie der menschlichen Placenta. Z. Geburtshilfe Gynäkol. 30:1–97, 1894.

Messer, R.H., Gomez, A.R., and Yambao, T.J.: Antepartum testing for vasa previa: current standard of care. Am. J. Obstet. Gynecol. 156:1459–1462, 1987.

Meyenburg, M.: Gibt es Veränderungen des Plazentasitzes im Bereich kaudaler Uterusabschnitte während der Schwangerschaft? Eine echographische Verlaufsstudie. Geburtshilfe Frauenheilkd. 36:715–721, 1976.

Meyer, A.W.: On the structure of the human umbilical vesicle. Am. J. Anat. 3:155–166, 1904.

Meyer, W.J., Blumenthal, L., Cadkin, A., Gauthier, D.W., and Rotmensch, S.: Vasa previa: prenatal diagnosis with transvaginal color Doppler flow imaging. Am. J. Obstet. Gynecol. 169:1627–1629, 1993.

Miller, M.E., Higginbottom, M., and Smith, D.A.: Short umbilical cord: its origin and relevance. Pediatrics 67:618–621, 1981.

Mills, J.L., Harley, E.E., and Moessinger, A.C.: Standards for measuring umbilical cord length. Placenta 4:423–426, 1983.

Mishriki, Y.Y., Vanyshelbaum, Y., Epstein, H., and Blanc, W.: Hemangioma of the umbilical cord. Pediatr. Pathol. 7:43–49, 1987.

Mitchell, A.P.B., Anderson, G.S., and Russell, J.K.: Perinatal death from foetal exsanguination. B.M.J. 1:611–614, 1957.

Mochizuki, M., Maruo, T., Masuko, K., and Ohtsu, T.: Effects of smoking on fetoplacental-maternal system during pregnancy. Am. J. Obstet. Gynecol. 149:413–420, 1984.

Moessinger, A.C., Blanc, W.A., Marone, P.A., and Polsen, D.C.: Umbilical cord length as an index of fetal activity: experimental study and clinical implications. Pediatr. Res. 16:109–112, 1982.

Moessinger, A.C., Mills, J.L., Harley, E.E., Ramakrishnan, R., Berendes, H.W., and Blanc, W.A.: Umbilical cord length in Down's syndrome. Am. J. Dis. Child. 140:1276–1277, 1986.

Moise, K.J., Carpenter, R.J., Huhta, J.C., and Deter, R.L.: Umbilical cord hematoma secondary to in utero intravascular transfusion for Rh isoimmunization. Fetal Ther. 2:65–70, 1987.

Moncrieff, D., Parker-Williams, J., and Chamberlain, G.: Placental drainage and fetomaternal transfusion. Lancet 2:453, 1986.

Monie, I.W.: Velamentous insertion of cord in early pregnancy. Am. J. Obstet. Gynecol. 93:276–281, 1965.

Monie, I.W., and Khemmani, M.: Absent and abnormal umbilical arteries. Teratology 7:135–142, 1973.

Moore, R.D.: Mast cells of the human umbilical cord. Am. J. Pathol. 32:1179–1183, 1956.

Murdoch, D.E.: Umbilical-cord doubling. Obstet. Gynecol. 27:555–557, 1966.

Myatt, L., Brockman, D.E., Eis, A.L.W., and Pollock, J.S.: Immunohistochemical localization of nitric oxide synthase in the human placenta. Placenta 14:487–495, 1993.

Naaktgeboren, C., and van Wagtendonk, A.M.: Wahre Knoten in der Nabelschnur nebst Bemerkungen über Plazentophagie bei Menschenaffen. Z. Säugetierk. 31:376–382, 1966.

Nadkarni, B.B.: Innervation of the human umbilical artery: an electron-microscope study. Am. J. Obstet. Gynecol. 107:303–312, 1970.

Naeye, R.L.: Umbilical cord length: clinical significance. J. Pediatr. 107:278–281, 1985.

Naeye, R.L., and Tafari, N.: Noninfectious disorders of the placenta, fetal membranes and umbilical cord. In, Risk Factors in Pregnancy and Disease of the Fetus and Newborn. Williams & Wilkins, Baltimore, pp. 145–172, 1983.

Nanaev, A.K., Domogatsky, S.P., and Milovanov, A.P.: Immunohistochemical study of the extracellular matrix and intermediate filaments in the human umbilical cord. Placenta 13:A48, 1992.

Newton, M., and Moody, A.R.: Fetal and maternal blood in the human placenta. Obstet. Gynecol. 18:305–308, 1961.

Nieder, J., and Link, M.: Ein Beitrag zur Pathologie der Nabelschnurgeschwülste. Z. Gynäkol. 92:420–428, 1970.

Nielsen, T.P., Nelson, R.M., Lee-Green, B., Lowe, P.N., and Reese, L.A.: Patent urachus complicating pregnancy: a review and report of a case. Am. J. Obstet. Gynecol. 143:61–68, 1982.

Nikolov, S.D., and Schiebler, T.H.: Über das fetale Gefäßsystem der reifen menschlichen Placenta. Z. Zellforsch. 139:333–350, 1973.

Nöldeke, H.: Geburtskomplikationen bei Insertio velamentosa. Zentralbl. Gynäkol. 58:351–356, 1934.

Novack, A.H., Mueller, B., and Ochs, H.: Umbilical cord separation in the newborn. Am. J. Dis. Child. 142:220–223, 1988.

Obolensky, W.: Durch Blasensprung bedingte Blutung aus dem Fötalkreislauf, ihre Erkennung und Verhütung. Gynaecologia 164:279–282, 1967.

Omar, H.A., Figueroa, R., Omar, R.A., and Wolin, M.S.: Properties of an endogenous arachidonic acid-elicited relaxing mechanism in human placental vessels. Am. J. Obstet. Gynecol. 167:1064–1070, 1992.

Ornoy, A., Crone, K., and Altshuler, G.: Pathological features of the placenta in fetal death. Arch. Pathol. Lab. Med. 100:367–371, 1976.

Otto, A.W.: Lehrbuch der pathologischen Anatomie des Menschen und der Thiere. Ruecker, Berlin, 1830.

Ottow, B.: Interpositio velamentosa funiculi umbilicalis, eine bisher übersehene Nabelstranganomalie, ihre Entstehung und klinische Bedeutung. Arch. Gynecol. 116:176–199, 1922.

Ottow, B.: Über die Insertio furcata der Nabelschnur. Arch. Gynecol. 118:378–382, 1923.

Oudesluys-Murphy, A.M., Eilers, G.A.M., and deGroot, C.J.: The time of separation of the umbilical cord. Eur. J. Pediatr. 146:387–389, 1987.

Painter, D., and Russell, P.: Four-vessel umbilical cord associated with multiple congenital anomalies. Obstet. Gynecol. 50:505–507, 1977.

Panigel, M.: Réactions vaso-motrices de l'arbre vasculaire foetal au cours de la perfusion de cotylédons placentaires isolés maintenus en survie. C. R. Acad. Sci. (Paris) 255: 3238–3240, 1962.

Panizza, V.H., Alvarez, H., and Benedetti, W.L.: The in vitro contractility of the human placental chorial vessels. J. Reprod. Med. 26:478–482, 1981.

Papaloucas, A., Avgoustiniatos, J., and Paisios, P.: Innervation of the umbilical cord in full term foetuses. IRCS Med. Sci. Anat. Hum. Biol. 3:117–118, 1975.

Parry, E.W.: Some electron microscope observation on the 'mesenchymal structures of full-term umbilical cord. J. Anat. 107:505–518, 1970.

Parry, E.W., and Abramovich, D.R.: Some observations on the surface layer of full-term human umbilical cord epithelium. J. Obstet. Gynaecol. Br. Commonw. 77:878–884, 1970.

Parry, E.W., and Abramovich, D.R.: The ultrastructure of human umbilical vessel endothelium from early pregnancy to full term. J. Anat. 111:29–42, 1972.

Patel, D., Dawson, M., Kalyanam, P., Lungus, E., Weiss, H., Flaherty, E., and Nora, E.G.: Umbilical cord circumference at birth. Am. J. Dis. Child. 143:638–639, 1989.

Pearson, A.A., and Sauter, R.W.: The innervation of the umbilical vein in human embryos and fetuses. Am. J. Anat. 125:345–352, 1969.

Pearson, A.A., and Sauter, R.W.: Nerve contributions to the pelvic plexus and the umbilical cord. Am. J. Anat. 128: 485–498, 1970.

Pent, D.: Vasa previa. Am. J. Obstet. Gynecol. 134:151–155, 1979.

Perrin, E.V.D., and Bel, J.K.-V.: Degeneration and calcification of the umbilical cord. Obstet. Gynecol. 26:371–376, 1965.

Petrikovsky, B.M., Nochimson, D.J., Campbell, W.A., and Vintzileos, A.M.: Fetal jejunoileal atresia with persistent omphalomesenteric duct. Am. J. Obstet. Gynecol. 158: 173–175, 1988.

Phelan, J.P., Ahn, M.O., Korst, L., and Martin, G.I.: Nucleated red blood cells: a marker for fetal asphyxia [abstract 49]. Am. J. Obstet. Gynecol. 170:286, 1994.

Philip, A.G.S.: Further observations on placental transfusion. Obstet. Gynecol. 42:334–343, 1973.

Philip, A.G., Yee, A.B., Rosy, M., Surti, N., Tsamtsouris, A., and Ingall, D.: Placental transfusion as an intrauterine phenomenon in deliveries complicated by foetal distress. B.M.J. 1:11–13, 1969.

Pinto, A., Sorrentino, R., Sorrentino, P., Guerritore, T., Miranda, L., Biondi, A., and Martinelli, P.: Endothelial-derived relaxing factor released by endothelial cells of human umbilical vessels and its impairment in pregnancy-induced hypertension. Am. J. Obstet. Gynecol. 164:507–513, 1991.

Potter, E.L.: Pathology of the Fetus and Infant. Year Book, Chicago, 1961.

Priman, J.: A note on the anastomosis of the umbilical arteries. Anat. Rec. 134:1–5, 1959.

Quek, S.P., and Tan, K.L.: Vasa previa. Aust. N.Z. J. Obstet. Gynaecol. 12:206–209, 1972.

Quinlan, D.K.: Coarctation in cord of twenty-one-week-old fetus, with atresia, fibrosis, secondary torsion. S. Afr. J. Obstet. Gynaecol. 3:1–2, 1965.

Qureshi, F., and Jacques, S.M.: Marked segmental thinning of the umbilical cord vessels. Arch. Pathol. Lab. Med. 118:826–830, 1994.

Radcliffe, P.A., Sindelair, P.J., and Zeit, P.R.: Vasa previa with marginal placenta previa of an accessory lobe: report of a case. Obstet. Gynecol. 16:472–475, 1961.

Rath, W., Osterhage, G., Kuhn, W., Gröne, H.J., and Fuchs, E.: Visualization of ¹²⁵I-endothelin-1 binding sites in human placenta and umbilical vessels. Gynecol. Obstet. Invest. 35:209–213, 1993.

Ratten, G.J.: Spontaneous haematoma of the umbilical cord. Aust. N.Z. J. Obstet. Gynaecol. 9:125–126, 1969.

Rayburn, W.F., Beynen, A., and Brinkman, D.L.: Umbilical cord length and intrapartum complications. Obstet. Gynecol. 57:450–452, 1981.

Reece, E.A., Pinter, E., Green, J., Mahoney, M.J., Naftolin, F., and Hobbins, J.C.: Significance of isolated yolk sac visualised by ultrasonography. Lancet 1:269, 1987.

Reeves, T.B.: A double umbilicus. Anat. Rec. 10:15–18, 1916.

Reiss, H.E.: Umbilical cord. B.M.J. 2:511, 1964.

Resta, R.G., Luthy, D.A., and Mahony, B.S.: Umbilical cord hemangioma associated with extremely high alpha-fetoprotein levels. Obstet. Gynecol. 72:488–491, 1988.

Rey, E.: Effects of methyldopa on umbilical and placental artery flow velocity waveforms. Obstet. Gynecol. 80:783–787, 1992.

Reynolds, S.R.M.: The proportion of Wharton's jelly in the umbilical cord in relation to distention of the umbilical arteries and vein, with observations on the folds of Hoboken. Anat. Rec. 113:365–377, 1952.

Rhen, K., and Kinnunen, O.: Ante-partum rupture of the umbilical cord. Acta Obstet. Gynecol. Scand. 41:86–89, 1962.

Rissmann, D.: Aneurysma der Nabelschnurarterie. Zentralbl. Gynäkol. 55:550–551, 1931.

Rizos, N., Doran, T.A., Miskin, M., Benzie, R.J., and Ford, J.A.: Natural history of placenta previa ascertained by diagnostic ultrasound. Am. J. Obstet. Gynecol. 133:287–291, 1979.

Robaut, C., Mondon, F., Bandet, J., Ferre, F., and Cavero, I.: Regional distribution and pharmacological characterization of [¹²⁵I]endothelin-1 binding sites in human fetal placental vessels. Placenta 12:55–67, 1991.

Robertson, R.D., Rubinstein, L.M., Wolfson, W.L., Lebherz, T.B., Blanchard, J.B., and Crandall, B.F.: Constriction of the umbilical cord as a cause of fetal demise following midtrimester amniocentesis. J. Reprod. Med. 26:325–327, 1981.

Robinson, L.K., Jones, K.L., and Benirschke, K.: The nature of structural defects associated with velamentous and marginal insertion of the umbilical cord. Am. J. Obstet. Gynecol. 146:191–193, 1983.

Röckelein, G., and Hey, A.: Ultrastrukturelle Untersuchungen der Vakuolenbildung in arteriellen Choriongefäßen der reifen menschlichen Plazenta. Z. Geburtshilfe Perinat. 189:65–68, 1985.

Röckelein, G., and Scharl, A.: Scanning electron microscopic investigations of the human umbilical artery intima: a new conception on postnatal arterial closure mechanism. Virchows Arch. [A] 413:555–561, 1988.

Röckelein, G., Kobras, G., and Becker, V.: Physiological and pathological morphology of the umbilical and placental circulation. Pathol. Res. Pract. 186:187–196, 1990.

Rolschau, J.: The relationship between some disorders of the umbilical cord and intrauterine growth retardation. Acta Obstet. Gynecol. Scand. Suppl. 72:15–21, 1978.

Romero, R., Chervenak, F.A., Coustan, D., Berkowitz, R.L., and Hobbins, J.C.: Antenatal sonographic diagnosis of umbilical cord laceration. Am. J. Obstet. Gynecol. 143:719–720, 1982.

Rucker, M.P., and Tureman, G.R.: Vasa previa. Va. Med. Monthly 72:202–207, 1945.

Rust, W.: Seltsame Veränderungen an den Nabelschnurgefässen. Arch. Gynecol. 165:58–62, 1937.

Ruvinski, E.D., Wiley, T.L., Morrison, J.C., and Blake, P.G.: In utero diagnosis of umbilical cord hematoma by ultrasonography. Am. J. Obstet. Gynecol. 140:833–834, 1981.

Salas, S.P., Power, R.F., Singleton, A., Wharton, J., Polak, J.M., and Brown, J.: Heterogeneous binding sites for α-atrial natriuretic peptide in human umbilical cord and placenta. Am. J. Physiol. 261:R633–R638, 1991.

Sander, C.H.: Hemorrhagic endovasculitis and hemorrhagic villitis of the placenta. Arch. Pathol. Lab. Med. 104:371–373, 1980.

Scheffel, T., and Langanke, D.: Die Nabelschnurkomplikationen an der Universitäts-Frauenklinik von 1955 bis 1967. Zentralbl. Gynäkol. 92:429–434, 1970.

Schellong, G., and Pfeiffer, R.A.: Persistierender Ductus omphalo-mesentericus als Ursache ungewöhnlicher Komplikationen bei der Austauschtransfusion. Arch. Kinderheilkd. 175:204–209, 1967.

Scheuner, G.: Über die Verankerung der Nabelschnur an der Plazenta. Morphol. Jahrb. 106:73–89, 1964.

Scheuner, G.: Über die mikroskopische Struktur der Insertio velamentosa. Zentralbl. Gynäkol. 87:38–49, 1965.

Schiebler, T.H., and Kaufmann, P.: Reife Plazenta. In, Die Plazenta des Menschen. V. Becker, T.H. Schiebler, and F. Kubli, eds. Thieme, Stuttgart, 1981.

Schiff, I., Driscoll, S.G., and Naftolin, F.: Calcification of the umbilical cord. Am. J. Obstet. Gynecol. 126:1046–1048, 1976.

Schordania, J.: Der architektonische Aufbau der Gefässe der menschlichen Nachgeburt und ihre Beziehungen zur Entwicklung der Frucht. Arch. Gynecol. 135:568–598, 1929a.

Schordania, J.: Über das Gefäßsystem der Nabelschnur. Z. Ges. Anat. 89:696–726, 1929b.

Schreier, R., and Brown, S.: Hematoma of the umbilical cord: report of a case. Obstet. Gynecol. 20:798–800, 1962.

Schreiner, C.A., and Hoornbeek, F.K.: Developmental aspects of sirenomelia in the mouse. J. Morphol. 141:345–358, 1973.

Schwalbe, E.: Allgemeine Mißbildungslehre (Teratologie). Gustav Fischer, Jena, 1906.

Scott, J.M., and Jordan, J.M.: Placental insufficiency and the small-for-dates baby. Am. J. Obstet. Gynecol. 113:823–832, 1972.

Scott, J.M., and Wilkinson, R.: Further studies on the umbilical cord and its water content. J. Clin. Pathol. 31:944–948, 1978.

Scott, J.S.: Placenta extrachorialis (placenta marginata and placenta circumvallata). J. Obstet. Gynaecol. Br. Emp. 67:907–918, 1960.

Seeds, J.W., Chescheir, N.C., Bowes, W.A., and Owl-Smith, F.A.: Fetal death as a complication of intrauterine intravascular transfusion. Obstet. Gynecol. 74:461–463, 1989.

Seifert, D.B., Ferguson, J.E., Behrens, C.M., Zemel, S., Stevenson, D.K., and Ross, J.C.: Nonimmune hydrops fetalis in association with hemangioma of the umbilical cord. Obstet. Gynecol. 66:283–286, 1985.

Seligsohn, U., Berger, A., Abend, M., Rubin, L., Attias, D., Zivelin, A., and Rapaport, S.I.: Homozygous protein C deficiency manifested by massive venous thrombosis in the newborn. N. Engl. J. Med. 310:559–362, 1984.

Shanklin, D.R.: The influence of placental lesions on the newborn infant. Pediatr. Clin. North Am. 17:25–42, 1970.

Shaw, A., and Pierog, S.: "Ectopic" liver in the umbilicus: an unusual focus of infection in a newborn infant. Pediatrics 44:448–450, 1969.

Shen-Schwarz, S., Macpherson, T., and Mueller-Heubach, E.: Hemorrhagic endovasculitis of the placenta: incidence and clinical features in an unselected population. Pediatr. Pathol. 5:112, 1986.

Shen-Schwarz, S., Macpherson, T.A., and Mueller-Heubach, E.: The clinical significance of hemorrhagic endovasculitis of the placenta. Am. J. Obstet. Gynecol. 159:48–51, 1988.

Shepherd, J.T.: Bayliss response in the umbilical artery. Fed. Proc. 27:1408–1409, 1968.

Shepherd, A.J., Richardson, C.J., and Brown, J.P.: Nuchal cords as a cause of neonatal anemia. Am. J. Dis. Child. 139:71–73, 1985.

Sibulkin, M.: A note on the bathtub vortex and the earth's rotation. Am. Sci. 71:352–353, 1983.

Siddall, R.S.: Spontaneous rupture of the umbilical cord. Am. J. Obstet. Gynecol. 10:836–840, 1925.

Siddiqi, T.A., Bendon, R., Schultz, D.M., and Miodovnik, M.: Umbilical artery aneurysm: prenatal diagnosis and management. Obstet. Gynecol. 80:530–533, 1992.

Silva, P. de, Stoskopf, C.G., Keegan, K.A., and Murata, Y.: Use of fetal scalp hematocrit in the diagnosis of severe hemorrhage from vasa previa. Am. J. Obstet. Gynecol. 153:307–308, 1985.

Silver, R.K., Dooley, S.L., Tamura, R.K., and Depp, R.: Umbilical cord size and amniotic fluid volume in prolonged pregnancy. Am. J. Obstet. Gynecol. 157:716–720, 1987a.

Silver, M.M., Yeger, H., and Lines, L.D.: Hemorrhagic endovasculitis-like lesion in placental organ culture. Lab. Invest. 56:6P, 1987b.

Silver, M.M., Yeger, H., and Lines, L.D.: Hemorrhagic endovasculitis-like lesion induced in placental organ culture. Hum. Pathol. 19:251–256, 1988.

Sinha, A.A.: Ultrastructure of human amnion and amniotic plaques of normal pregnancy. Z. Zellforsch. 122:1–14, 1971.

Sinnathuray, T.A.: The nuchal cord incidence and significance. J. Obstet. Gynaecol. Br. Commonw. 73:226–231, 1966.

Slijper, E.J.: Die Geburt der Säugetiere. In, Handbuch der Zoologie, Vol. 8. W. Kükenthal, ed., pp. 1–108. de Gruyter, Berlin, 1960.

Smart, P.J.G.: Some observations on the vascular morphology of the foetal side of the human placenta. J. Obstet. Gynaecol. Br. Commonw. 69:929–933, 1962.

Smith, D., and Majmudar, B.: Teratoma of the umbilical cord. Hum. Pathol. 16:190–193, 1985.

Soernes, T., and Bakke, T.: The length of the human umbilical cord in vertex and breech presentations. Am. J. Obstet. Gynecol. 154:1086–1087, 1986.

Spatz, W.B.: Nabelschnur-Längen bei Insektivoren und Primaten. Z. Säugetierk. 33:226–239, 1968.

Spellacy, W.N., Gravem, H., and Fisch, R.O.: The umbilical cord complications of true knots, nuchal coils, and cords around the body. Am. J. Obstet. Gynecol. 94:1136–1142, 1966.

Spiteri, M., Anh, N.H., and Panigel, M.: Ultrastructure du muscle lisse des artères du cordon ombilical humain. Pathol. Biol. (Paris) 14:348–357, 1966.

Spivack, M.: On the anatomy of the so-called "valves" of umbilical vessels, with especial reference to the valvulae Hobokenii. Anat. Rec. 66:127–148, 1936.

Spivack, M.: On the presence or absence of nerves in the umbilical blood vessels of man and guinea pig. Anat. Rec. 85:85–109, 1943.

Stevens, N.G., and Sander, C.H.: Placental hemorrhagic endovasculitis: risk factors and impact on pregnancy outcome. Lab. Invest. 50:57A, 1984.

Stevenson, R.E., Jones, K.L., Phelan, M.C., Jones, M.C., Barr, M., Clericuzio, C., Harley, R.A., and Benirschke, K.: Vascular steal: the pathogenetic mechanism producing sirenomelia and associated defects of the viscera and soft tissues. Pediatrics 78:451–457, 1986.

Strassmann, P.: Placenta praevia. Arch. Gynecol. 67:112–275, 1902.

Strong, T.H., Elliott, J.P., and Radin, T.R.: Non-coiled umbilical blood vessels: A new marker for the fetus at risk. Obstet. Gynecol. 81:409–411, 1993.

Strong, T.H., Jarles, D.L., Vega, J.S., and Feldman, D.B.: The umbilical coiling index. Am. J. Obstet. Gynecol. 170:29–32, 1994.

Swanberg, H., and Wiqvist, N.: Rupture of the umbilical cord during pregnancy. Acta Obstet. Gynecol. Scand. 30:323–337, 1951.

Szécsi, K.: Beiträge zur spontanen Zerreißung der zu kurzen Nabelschnur. Zentralbl. Gynäkol. 77:1024–1028, 1955.

Takagi, T., Toda, T., Leszczynski, D., and Kummerow, F.: Ultrastructure of aging human umbilical artery and vein. Acta Anat. (Basel) 119:73–79, 1984.

Takechi, K., Kuwabara, Y., and Mizuno, M.: Ultrastructural and immunohistochemical studies of Wharton's jelly umbilical cord cells. Placenta 14:235–245, 1993.

Ten Berge, B.S.: Nervenelemente in Plazenta und Nabelschnur. Gynaecologia 156:49–53, 1963.

Tharakan, T., Baxi, L.V., and Diuguid, D.: Protein S deficiency in pregnancy: a case report. Am. J. Obstet. Gynecol. 168:141–142, 1993.

Theuring, F.: Fibröse Obliterationen an Deckplatten- und Stammzottengefäßen der Placenta nach intrauterinem Fruchttod. Arch. Gynecol. 206:237–251, 1968.

Thomas, J.: Untersuchungsergebnisse über die Aplasie einer Nabelarterie unter besonderer Berücksichtigung der

Zwillingsschwangerschaft. Geburtshilfe Frauenheilkd. 21: 984–992, 1961.

Thomas, J.: Die Entwicklung von Fetus und Placenta bei Nabelgefäßanomalien. Arch. Gynecol. 198:216–223, 1963.

Torpin, R.: Classification of human pregnancy based on depth of intrauterine implantation of ovum. Am. J. Obstet. Gynecol. 66:791–800, 1953.

Torrey, W.E.: Vasa previa. Am. J. Obstet. Gynecol. 63:146–152, 1952.

Tortora, M., Chervenak, F.A., Mayden, K., and Hobbins, J.C.: Antenatal sonographic diagnosis of single umbilical artery. Obstet. Gynecol. 63:693–696, 1984.

Trudinger, B.J., and Cook, C.M.: Different umbilical artery flow velocity waveforms in one patient. Obstet. Gynecol. 71:1019–1021, 1988.

Trudinger, B.J., Stevens, D., Connelly, A., Hales, J.R.S., Alexander, G., Bradley, L., Fawcett, A., and Thompson, R.S.: Umbilical artery flow velocity waveforms and placental resistance: the effects of embolization of the umbilical circulation. Am. J. Obstet. Gynecol. 157:1443–1448, 1987.

Tuggle, A.Q., and Cook, W.A.: Laceration of a placental vein: an injury possibly inflicted by the fetus. Am. J. Obstet. Gynecol. 131:220–221, 1978.

Ukeshima, A., Hayashi, Y., and Fujimoto, T.: Surface morphology of the human yolk sac: endoderm and mesothelium. Arch. Histol. Jpn. 49:483–494, 1986.

Uyanwah-Akpom, P.O., and Fox, H.: The clinical significance of marginal or velamentous insertion of the cord. Br. J. Obstet. Gynaecol. 84:941–943, 1977.

Vandriede, D.M., and Kammeraad, L.A.: Vasa previa: case report, review and presentation of a new diagnostic method. J. Reprod. Med. 26:577–580, 1981.

Vanhaesebrouck, P., Vanneste, K., de Praeter, C., and van Trappen, Y.: Tight nuchal cord and neonatal hypovolemic shock. Arch. Dis. Child. 62:1276–1277, 1987.

Vardi, P.: Placental transfusion: an attempt at physiological delivery. Lancet 2:12–13, 1965.

Virgilio, L.A., and Spangler, D.B.: Fetal death secondary to constriction and torsion of the umbilical cord. Arch. Pathol. Lab. Med. 102:32–33, 1978.

Von Hayek, H.: Der funktionelle Bau der Nabelarterien und des Ductus Botalli. Z. Anat. Entwicklungsgesch. 105:15–24, 1936.

Vu, T., Baldwin, V.J., Perrin, E.V.D.K., and Shanklin, D.R.: Major umbilical vessel rupture in utero. Pediatr. Pathol. 2:494, 1984.

Waidl, E.: Zur Genese und Klinik der Insertio velamentosa. Zentralbl. Gynäkol. 82:1902–1906, 1960.

Walker, C.W., and Pye, B.G.: The length of the umbilical cord; a statistical report. B.M.J. 1:546–548, 1960.

Walsh, S.Z.: Maternal effects of early and late clamping of the umbilical cord. Lancet 1:996–997, 1968.

Walz, W.: Über das Ödem der Nabelschnur. Zentralbl. Gynäkol. 69:144–148, 1947.

Weber, J.: Constriction of the umbilical cord as a cause of foetal death. Acta Obstet. Gynecol. Scand. 42:259–268, 1963.

Wentworth, P.: Some anomalies of the foetal vessels of the human placenta. J. Anat. 99:273–282, 1965.

White, R.P.: Pharmacodynamic study of maturation and closure of human umbilical arteries. Am. J. Obstet. Gynecol. 160:229–237, 1989.

Widholm, O., and Nieminen, U.: Prolapse of umbilical cord. Acta Obstet. Gynecol. 42:21–29, 1963.

Wigger, H.J., Kiu, T.W., Moessinger, A.C., Marboe, C.C., and Blanc, W.A.: Effect of cigarette smoking on the ultrastructure of the placenta. Lab. Invest. 50:14P, 1984.

Williams, J.H., and Benirschke, K.: Chorionic vessel thrombosis: a possible etiology of neonatal purpura. J. Reprod. Med. 20:285–288, 1978.

Williams, J., Katzman, G.H., and Kripke, S.S.: Neck compression by nuchal cord. Am. J. Obstet. Gynecol. 140:345–346, 1981.

Winter, R.: Die Rolle regressiver Veränderungen der Plazenta bei der sogenannten Plazentamigration. Geburtshilfe Frauenheilkd. 38:1093–1098, 1978.

Winters, R.H.: Unique vascular relationship in human umbilical cord. Nature 226:656, 1970.

Wolf, P.L., Jones, K.L., Longway, S.R., Benirschke, K., and Bloor, C.: Prenatal death from acute myocardial infarction and cardiac tamponade due to embolus from the placenta. Am. Heart J. 109:603–605, 1985.

Wolfman, W.L., Purohit, D.M., and Self, S.E.: Umbilical vein thrombosis at 32 weeks' gestation with delivery of a living infant. Am. J. Obstet. Gynecol. 146:468–470, 1983.

Woods, D.L., and Malan, A.F.: The site of umbilical cord insertion and birth weight. Br. J. Obstet. Gynaecol. 85: 332–333, 1978.

Yamada, K., and Shimizu, S.: Concanavalin A–peroxidase–diaminobenzidine (con A-PO-DAB)-alcian blue (AB): a reliable method for dual staining of complex carbohydrates. Histochemistry 47:159–169, 1976.

Yang, H.Y., Shum, A.Y.C., Ng, H.T., and Chen, C.F.: Effect of ethanol on human umbilical artery and vein in vitro. Gynecol. Obstet. Invest. 21:131–135, 1986.

Yao, A.C., and Lind, J.: Placental transfusion: review. Am. J. Dis. Child. 127:128–141, 1974.

Yao, A.C., and Lind, J.: Placental Transfusion. A Clinical and Physiological Study. Charles C Thomas, Springfield, IL, 1982.

Yao, A.C., Hirvensalo, M., and Lind, J.: Placental transfusion-rate and uterine clamping. Lancet 1:380–383, 1968.

Yao, A.C., Moinian, M., and Lind, J.: Distribution of blood between infant and placenta after birth. Lancet 2:871–873, 1969.

Yao, A.C., Lind, J., and Lu, T.: Closure of the human umbilical artery: a physiological demonstration of Burton's theory. Eur. J. Obstet. Gynecol. Reprod. Biol. 7:365–368, 1977.

Yavner, D.L., and Redline, R.W.: Angiomyxoma of the umbilical cord with massive cystic degeneration of Wharton's jelly. Arch. Pathol. Lab. Med. 113:935–937, 1989.

Young, A.: The primate umbilical cord with special reference to the transverse communicating artery. J. Hum. Evol. 1:345–359, 1972.

Young, G.B.: The peripatetic placenta. Radiology 128:183–188, 1978.

14
Placental Shape Aberrations

In recent years it has become practical to record and follow the location of the placenta during the course of gestation by sonography. This methodology has shown that a "dynamic placentation" occurs. That is, the original location of the implanting blastocyst may be modified during the course of its development to a term placenta. These concepts are examined in this chapter, and the various types of abnormal placental developments are discussed. The chapter also considers the morphology of placenta accreta and that of ectopic implantation.

The factors that determine the site of nidation of the human blastocyst are not fully understood. The human blastocyst implants normally in the upper portion of the uterus; nevertheless, abnormal implantation is frequent and may lead to pregnancy complications, such as placenta previa. It has been suggested, for instance, that the site of placental implantation influences the frequency of fetal malpresentation. Wingate and Pauls (1968) studied this subject using chromium 51 as tracer in placental localization in 85 patients. They found no correlation between either fundal or lower uterine implantation and fetal malpresentations. Previous authors, on the other hand, had suggested that an abnormal location of the blastocyst in the endometrium may lead to abnormal forms of the mature placenta. An early proponent of such thoughts was Schatz (1886), who envisaged normal, broad, and superficial implantation. Later these ideas were particularly strongly championed by Torpin (1969b), who related the depth of implantation and its location in the uterus to the development of circumvallate placentation. Location of the implantation may be important and could be better correlated now with sonography. We have seen two circumvallate placenta in cornual implantations. Others have suggested that the placental location is instrumental in triggering the normal impulse for the initiation of labor and that it is correlated with the length of gestation.

SITE OF PLACENTAL ATTACHMENT

There are several means by which investigators have approached localization of the implantation and the ultimate placental site. Hertig and Rock (1973) summarized their findings from the successful search of 34 early human ova; they obtained the following results.

Tubal location	1
Free in uterus	7
Implanted, normal	17
Implanted, abnormal	9

The normal embryos were more often on the posterior wall than were the implantations of abnormal blastocysts.

When the placental site is determined by postpartum palpation, as was done by Booth et al. (1962) in 200 patients, the following distribution emerged.

Anterior	53%
Posterior	39%
Lateral	8%

When these data are expressed with respect to the height of placental location, the following distributions were found.

Fundal position	2%
Fundal and upper segment	42%
Upper segment	47%
Upper and lower segments	9%

A fundal attachment was found in 44% of primigravidae and 20% of multigravidae; preeclampsia was twice as common in fundal placentas, which may merely reflect the fact that this condition is commoner with a first pregnancy. There was no relation to the length of pregnancy and labor. Scipiades and Burg (1930), in an extensive study on placentation, cited Orsini (1928), who found an anterior placenta in 26.6%, a posterior implantation in 41.6%, a fundal site in 2.2%, a lower uterus site in 23.0%, and at other sites in 3.5%. Later methods have used the distance of the membrane rupture site to the edge of the placenta as an indicator of placental localization (Little, 1962; Little & Friedman, 1964). This method, of course, needs to take into consideration that the placenta must be carefully extracted and not disturbed after delivery. Among the 10,101 placentas correlated during the evaluation by Little and Friedman (1964), the mean rupture site was between 5 and 9 cm (39.3%). In 11% it was 0 cm (possible marginal placenta previa), and in only 0.3% was it more than 19 cm. These authors were unable to confirm the relation of high

378

uterine position and preeclampsia but did not make a distinction with the parity of their patients. They found a twofold higher frequency of vaginal bleeding with low-lying placentas, but otherwise no influence on the length of labor, type of delivery, or neonatal outcome was identified. Torpin (1958) used his method of distending the membranous sac in a bucket of water after birth and determined, in 147 cases, that when the placenta had implanted in the "crease made by the reflection of the anterior and posterior uterine walls, the resulting placenta is almost invariably bilobate."

Indium isotope scanning and sonography were employed by Harris (1975) in 401 patients for placental localization in an effort to ascertain whether localization over the putative uterine "pacemaker" (Larks et al., 1959) influences the length of pregnancy. It was found in the right upper quadrant in about the same frequency as in the left (85/79), although the former had statistically slightly significantly shorter pregnancies. This finding disagrees with the theory that location in the right upper quadrant lengthens pregnancy.

More incisive results come from studies using sonographic localization of the placenta (Gottesfeld et al., 1966), which is now almost routinely ascertained during the course of pregnancy. These studies stimulated interest, and King (1973) was the first to show that a placenta previa of early pregnancy changes to one that does not require surgery for placenta previa at term, and that this change takes place in most cases. He termed this phenomenon dynamic placentation. In none of his 14 cases of marginal placenta previa, observed near midgestation, was there a true placenta previa at term, although several had a near cervical implantation. He reasoned that this change in position comes about largely by uterine growth and its changing shape as gestation advances. Nearly the same conclusions were arrived at independently by Meyenburg (1976) and have since been confirmed by many other investigators (e.g., Winters, 1978). Young (1978), who studied the same features with arteriography, located the placenta twice as often in the upper uterine segment as a placenta previa. He also noted the disappearance of most placentas previa with term approaching. He suggested that those placentas that do not move may represent accretas, but there was no histological support for this concept. In a large study of ultrasono-graphic findings prior to amniocentesis between 16 and 18 weeks, Rizos et al. (1979) found the following locations.

Site	Previas (%)	All Placentas (%)
Anterior	69	37
Posterior	10	24
Anterior and Posterior	21	5
Fundal	0	34

Their incidence of placenta previa at midterm was 5.3%, and it converted to a nonprevia in 90.4% by term. Their overall term previa incidence was 0.58%, similar to that of other studies.

A similar, large study of placental localization by sonography was reported by Fried (1978). When he followed the location over the three trimesters, he observed the following.

Site	10–20 Weeks(%)	21–31 Weeks(%)	32–40 Weeks(%)
Anterior	25	41	44
Posterior	37	28	26
Anterior-fundal	9	6	8
Posterior-fundal	17	18	15
Fundal	12	7	7

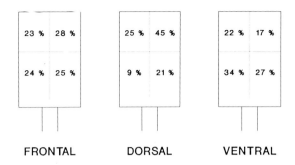

23 %	28 %	25 %	45 %

FRONTAL   DORSAL   VENTRAL

FIGURE 267. Distribution of placental locations in quadrants when viewed from the side (frontal) and with respect to anterior and posterior portions of the uterus. (From Nordlander et al., 1977, with permission.)

In other words, little change occurred in the overall location of placentas. Parenthetically, he found many more cephalic presentations with anterior than posterior placentas.

Gallagher et al. (1987) performed sonography during the second trimester of pregnancy in 1,239 women and found a central placenta previa in 3 patients and marginal or partial previa in 48 (5%). At term, only four (0.3%) of the patients had a placenta previa: the three patients with the central previa previously identified and one with marginal previa found during the second trimester. The authors chose therefore to name this condition "potential previa" when it is so identified during midgestation in order to clearly distinguish this sonographic condition from the true placenta previa at term. Studies have shown that transvaginal ultrasonography is informative with respect to the presence of placenta previa when third trimester hemorrhage necessitates diagnosis (Lim et al., 1989). Of considerable interest is the study by Guy et al. (1990) on patients with antepartum bleeding. These authors showed by transvaginal sonography of many patients with persistent previas that the intervillous blood flow is predominantly lacunar. These patients also had a greater requirement for blood replacement subsequent to delivery. Oppenheimer et al. (1994) documented the "migration" by transvaginal sonography during the third trimester. When more migration occurred, cesarean section was much less often needed.

An incisive study of localization by indium scintigraphy and cobalt cervical marker comes from Nordlander et al. (1977; see also Nelp & Larson, 1967; Gustafson et al., 1974). Their rather clear-cut data are redrawn in Figure 267; they showed an anterior placenta in 98 instances and a posterior placenta in 80. An anterior placenta had a significantly greater chance of being low-lying, and the distance of the placental edge from the uterine internal cervical os increased with the age of the gestation. Attempts at making the exact diagnosis of placenta previa during early gestation have ramifications for therapy. Thus Arias (1988) reported that the use of cervical cerclage in the treatment of vaginal bleeding due to placenta previa has merits as a temporary measure.

Volumetric Growth

Sonography has also remedied the absence of data about growth of the human placenta. In 1967 Boyd and Hamilton lamented that few studies on the in situ placenta had been published; they presented their findings of 151 such specimens beyond the third month of gestation and found striking variations in the thickness of the placentas; they also reviewed the published data from many countries on placental growth. Their findings refuted the then prevalent thought of Grosser (1927) that placental expansion ceases after the 4th month of gestation. In their study, it was evident that continuous growth of the placental diameter could be measured up to 17.2 cm, with a surface area of 23,245 mm² at term. Conversely, Bleker et al. (1977), who measured the placental volume from 23 weeks on and expressed it from sonographic determinations of cross sections, found that growth in volume ceased well before term, peaking at 250 days and then even decreasing. Hoogland et al. (1980), from their sonographic study of placental size at 150 days' menstrual age, suggested that this methodology is reliable only when the placenta occupies an anterior position. It is interesting to note that a small placenta foreshadowed low birth weight even at that early age. Reliable data on placental volume were also obtained sonographically by Wolf et al. (1979), who compared their measured volume with that of the delivered placenta in a waterbath.

Abnormal Shapes ("Errors in Outline")

The term "error in outline" (Shanklin, 1958) is a descriptive, appropriate designation for a variety of placental forms. The placenta is rarely truly circular. More often it is oval, and not infrequently it has an irregular, often triangular shape that is presumably determined by its site of location, areas of atrophy, and perhaps the manner of its original implantation. The most striking

abnormality is the placenta bilobata, two lobes being separated by a segment of membranes (Figure 268). It stands to reason that these membranous vessels occasionally thrombose, or that they present clinically as vasa previa with bleeding. The second lobe is not always as large as the main lobe; it varies, becoming occasionally a much smaller lobe, which is then called a succenturiate (accessory) lobe. Of course, when the placental halves are connected by a broad or even a narrow band, one may classify the misshapen organ differently, according to the whim of the observer. Firm rules do not exist. It must also be acknowledged that vasa previa may not bleed but may still cause fetal problems because of compression of the vessels (Cordero et al., 1993).

Succenturiate lobes may occur singly or multiply, have a tendency to infarct, and present as placenta previa (Roth, 1957) (Figure 269); they may also be retained in utero after delivery. A wide spectrum of abnormalities exists here and the incidence differs with the series published. Thus Fujikura et al. (1970) found a "bipartite" (duplex) placenta in 4.2% of 8,505 specimens collected in the Collaborative Perinatal Study. They found both multiparity and sterility overrepresented in these women, as well as prenatal bleeding, placenta previa (Figure 270), and retained placentas. They also commented on the fact that the cord usually inserts between the two lobes, as in Figure 270. Torpin and Barfield (1968), who clearly had their greatest interest in this condition, found that in one-third of bilobed placentas the cord inserts on the larger lobe, and in two-thirds it has a velamentous insertion. Occasionally, though, it takes its position on the smaller lobe (Figure 271). Torpin and Hart (1941) found twice the incidence (8.6%) in their extensive historical review

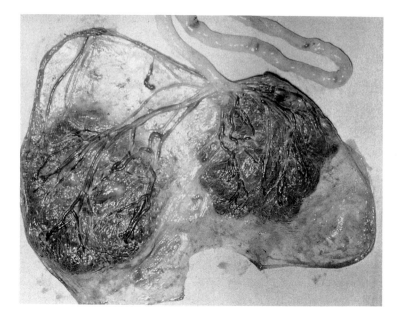

FIGURE 268. Bilobed placenta (duplex; bipartite). One disk was attached anteriorly, and the other was on the posterior wall of the uterus. Membranous vessels course from the characteristically velamentous insertion of the umbilical cord.

FIGURE 269. Succenturiate lobes in an immature placenta. Some of these lobes are infarcted (pallor) and would atrophy in time.

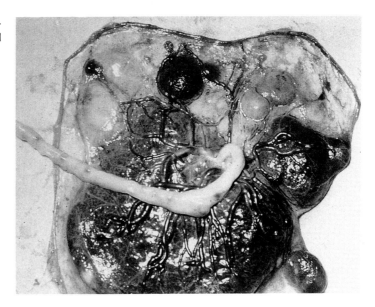

and reported on 355 cases. Usually, the placental lobes of bilobed organs had an anterior and a posterior location, and the larger lobe was usually marginate. The collar-shaped placenta reported by Keeler and Cope (1963) is but a variation of the theme. Likewise, the "pendulous placental polyp" described by Thomas (1962), although unusual, probably merely represents an exceptional succenturiate lobe.

In our experience, succenturiate lobes occur in 5% to 6% of routinely examined placentas. One-third of them are associated with some type of infarction of placental tissue, and occasional atrophy occurs between the extra

lobe and the main placenta. This situation contrasts with the 13% overall incidence of infarcts without succenturiate lobes. Succenturiate lobes have been recognized by ultrasonography (Hata et al., 1988).

Other unusual shapes occur. Thus Bergman (1961) reported on a placenta whose surface looked as though it was a loosely tied sac (a circumvallate placenta) and found that it was caused by a bicornuate uterus. Figure 272 shows a placenta fenestrata, one in which a central portion is atrophied sufficiently to appear like the membranes. There was no cotyledon missing, and the cause (?myoma, possible site of cornual tubal orifice)

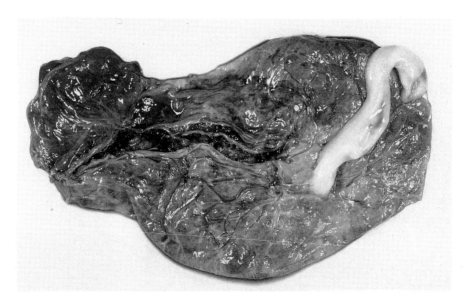

FIGURE 270. Succenturiate lobe (attached to the main placenta by a broad bridge) necessitated cesarean section because it was positioned as a placenta previa. It is one of a number of such specimens. The accessory lobe is remarkably hemorrhagic.

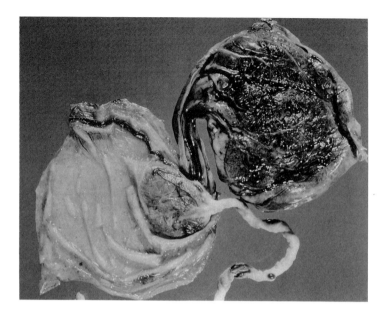

could not be ascertained. A similar condition must have prevailed in Greig's case (1950) of a central placenta previa with bulging membranes and hemorrhage.

The mechanism by which succenturiate lobes and duplex placentas develop is unclear. It is relevant, however, that this placentation occurs nearly regularly in many catarrhine monkeys and has best been studied in the rhesus monkey. Torpin (1969a) found 75% of rhesus monkey placentas to be bidiscoid, whereas the other 25% had a single lobe; and he observed that the connecting vessels always course laterally, never otherwise.

He made the important notation that atrophic villi are found in the membranes, implying that the blastocyst must have originally implanted interstitially and not, as had been assumed, only superficially so as to reach both uterine surfaces. Because baboons are close relatives—indeed may mate and hybridize with rhesus monkeys—but have a single-disk placenta, their placental evolution was of interest to Chez et al. (1972). These authors found single disks in 22% of the 121 rhesus monkey placentas studied. They suggested that implantation is partially under genetic influence because some males

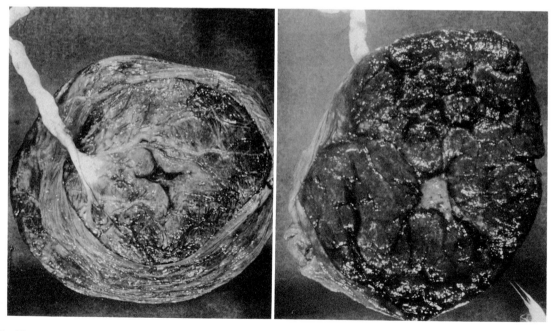

FIGURE 272. Placenta fenestrata. The central area of the placenta has a distinct defect, with only chorionic membranes being present. No explanation was evident. (Courtesy Dr. L.F. Moreno, Caracas, Venezuela.)

were much more prone to father the single placentas. A clear-cut mode of genetic transmission was absent, but they searched for membranous villi, as did we (Benirschke & Miller, 1982), and found none. They concluded that these monkeys (but also baboons) have a more superficial implantation, supporting Heuser and Streeter's finding (1941) that the primary disk implants on day 9 and the secondary disk on day 14, but on the opposite side of the uterus. This differs clearly from human placentation; and to date, then, a decisive answer as to the origin of placentas with accessory lobes is outstanding. It is interesting, however, that at least one-half of the placentas with succenturiate lobes have areas of atrophy or frank infarction. This finding much supports the notion of a secondary conversion from more normal placentation. As with other anomalies, we await studies of the births of offspring from such abnormal placentas in order to ascertain possible genetic causes.

The condition "capped placenta" has been described by Defoort and Thiery (1988). This abnormal shape is characterized by having a cup or bell shape and curvatures in two axes. These investigators studied the uncommon (0.8%) feature of bleeding during the second trimester. Previously, bleeding at that time had been considered to be most frequently a feature of a placenta previa-like implantation. Defoort and Thiery did not find it to be so. Circumvallate placentation, succenturiate lobes, low-lying placentas, and retroamnionic bleeding were found instead. In addition, 27% (17) of their 63 cases were due to "capped placentas"—placentas with implantation on lateral, anterior, and posterior walls of the uterus. The lower portion of the placenta did not reach the uterine isthmus.

Placenta Previa

The term placenta previa refers to the location of the placenta over the internal os. The placenta is thus being "previous" to the delivering part of the baby. Low implantation is the cause, and the condition is of great medical concern. Placenta previa is the principal cause of third trimester bleeding, and it often necessitates an emergency cesarean section. Both mother and fetus may bleed in a life-threatening manner. The incidence has variably been given as between 0.3% and 1.0% (even 3.0%) since the first publication of a large database by Strassmann (1902). Abnormal cord insertion and circumvallation are frequently present as well. Nielsen and colleagues (1989) found an incidence of 0.33% among 26,644 patients of placenta previa that necessitated abdominal delivery. The risk was 0.25% in "unscarred" uteri, compared to 1.22% in patients with previous cesarean section(s). These authors concluded that previous section predisposes to placenta previa and

antenatal hemorrhage. A large national statistical review by Iyasu et al. (1993) described the overall incidence of placenta previa to be 4.8 per 1,000 deliveries with a fatality of 0.03% of the cases; it was higher in black than white women. In addition, these authors ascertained a higher risk for abruptio, fetal malpresentation, postpartum hemorrhage, and of course cesarean section.

Placenta previa has been the topic of a large body of literature. Many authors are concerned with optimal clinical management (Kellogg, 1943; Schmitz et al., 1954; Scott, 1964; Brenner et al., 1978; many others). Some investigators concern themselves mostly with the origin of the blood in the vaginal hemorrhage (Bartholomew et al., 1953; Hartemann et al., 1962; McShane et al., 1985). Yet others address fetal prematurity, early diagnosis, and its causes and relation to cervical pregnancy and placenta accreta.

It has become customary to subdivide placenta previa into several categories, such as "central" (total) and "partial" (lateral or marginal) placenta previa. Strassmann (1902) criticized rigid subdivisions and questioned their terminology. Despite this criticism, everyone understands the terms central previa and marginal previa. The former generally poses the greater threat and requires early diagnosis. Schmitz et al. (1954) classified their 112 cases (0.6%) into 31% total, 27% partial, and 42% low-lying previas. (The latter are somewhat dubiously included in this group.)

Tatum and Mulé (1965) evolved a complex "overlay" method of grading the previas (depending on cervical canal coverage if the cervix were allowed to completely efface). They found that their classification did not correlate well with effective clinical management. The term low-lying previa therefore is not a well defined entity.

Brenner et al. (1978) surveyed 31,070 pregnancies (185 previas) and found an 0.6% overall frequency, with 0.12% of total previas. They confirmed the long-suspected correlation with multiparity (also older women), previous abortion, multiple births, and male infant. Surprisingly, prolapsed cord was also three times more common. Fetal and placental weights were not affected when corrected for fetal age. There was a significant association with fetal mortality, fetal anomalies, and low Apgar scores. Gabert (1971) also found normal fetal weights. Jopp and Krone (1966) reported significant fetal weight depression and increases in placental weight, which they attributed to compensatory placental hyperplasia. Higginbottom et al. (1975) also found lower than expected fetal weights and associated dysmaturity.

It is easy to understand that the maternal hemorrhage may originate from the placental margin or the disrupted intervillous space. There is, however, also significant neonatal anemia associated with the birth from a placenta previa, and it is the case more so when the maternal bleeding has been excessive (Wickster, 1952; McShane et al., 1985). This anemia is clearly due to the well recognized, but rarely recorded, fetal bleeding that is due to disrupted placental villous vessels during labor (Bromberg et al., 1957; Hartemann et al., 1962; Bar-David et al., 1984). However, it may be difficult to detect the defects by placental examination (Wiener, 1948). Some authors find that fetomaternal bleeding also occurs (Zilliacus, 1964; Huntington, 1968). The neonatal anemia can result, of course, from the disruption that occurs when the placenta is cut during cesarean section, aspects that are well discussed by Schellong (1969).

The early diagnosis of placenta previa was once accomplished by arteriography (Borell et al., 1963) but is now readily made sonographically. Evidence for the frequent finding of previa placentation during early pregnancy and the subsequent "conversion" of such placentas previa to low-lying, nonprevias is reviewed in the section above. Wexler and Gottesfeld (1977, 1979) went so far as to consider this previa position as a "normal" variant of placentation, and Ballas et al. (1979) stated that it frequently causes midtrimester vaginal bleeding. From their evaluation of the location of the placenta, these authors prognosticated the ultimate outcome by the extent of previa placental tissue. Many other investigators (e.g., Comeau et al., 1983) subsequently addressed this topic with an aim to improve fetal outcome in this common condition. Bartholomew et al. (1953) suggested a novel mechanism of bleeding in central placenta previa. They observed that in the central villous portion of the tissue that overlies the internal os there were numerous old clots, apparently from former bleeding episodes. They held these clots to be evidence of placental villous disruption and assumed that it is not the detachment of placenta from the

decidua that causes the bleeding. Moreover, at the edge of the placenta, disruption of the "marginal sinus" may take place in marginal placenta previa and thus lead to bleeding when the endocervix dilates during late gestation.

The pathology of placenta previa is easy to understand. The membranes have no free margin in the vaginally delivered placenta, and the edge of the placenta is frequently disrupted and hemorrhagic. Because there are often old clots at this site, varying from being laminated and brown, friable loose blood to partly decomposed material that is sometimes green from hemosiderin (Figures 273, 274), the fetal vessels of the chorionic surface, when at the edge, may be disrupted.

According to Strassmann (1902), one often encounters some degree of circumvallation or margination. It is rarely reported in other series and is also not our experience. Strassmann also correlated the insertion of the umbilical cord with previas and found that the cord may insert anywhere but is more often near the site of the cervical os. That problem is certainly not the case in the placenta shown in Figure 273, and examples of the eccentric placental growth that caused Strassmann to be such an ardent champion of the trophotropic expansion theory of placental tissue (expanding toward the better endometrial grounds above) are not often clearly seen.

Low-lying portions of placenta are occasionally either atrophied or infarcted. It is most often the case when the initially marginal previa has failed to develop, has undergone atrophy, and has thus become a "marginal" previa or better, a low-lying placenta. An intact uterus with an immature fetus from a placenta previa complication is seen in Figure 275. The cervical canal and the forelying placental tissue betray the bleeding that had occurred. That the bleeding can be due to a succenturiate placental lobe has been described several times

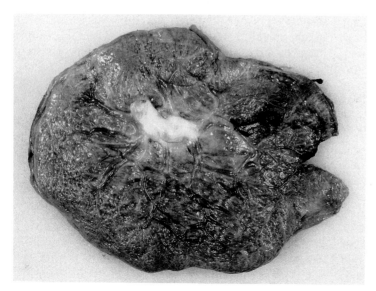

FIGURE 273. Placenta previa from a cesarean section. Note the disruption and discoloration of the right, previa pole of the placenta. The cord is centrally inserted in a disperse vasculature arrangement.

FIGURE 274. Maternal surface of the placenta in Figure 273. The old marginal clot is brown and friable, and the edge of the placenta is disrupted; the membranes are torn.

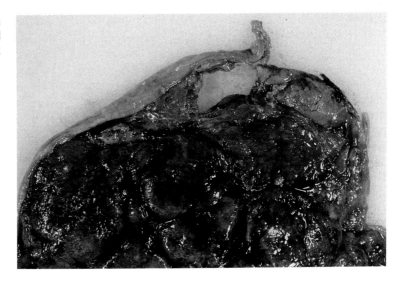

(Radcliffe et al., 1961; van Huysen, 1961), and the condition has been observed in a variety of animals as well. These reports even include cases where placenta previa caused fetal exsanguination (Kingsley & Martin, 1979).

The cause of placenta previa is perhaps the most widely debated aspect of this anomaly. Obstetricians of the last century suggested much the same pathophysiology that we know today. It is aptly summarized in the long article by Strassmann (1902). Multiparity,

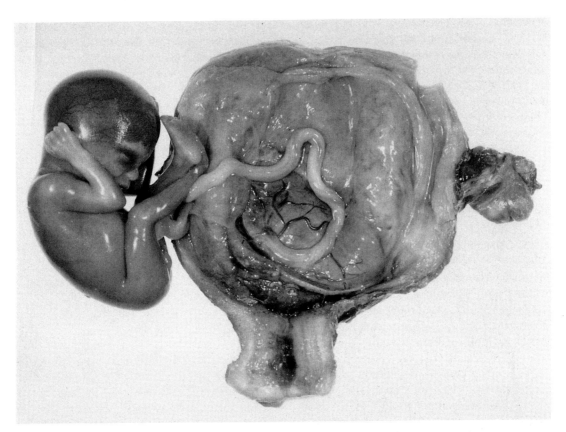

FIGURE 275. Placenta previa accreta. Hysterectomy was done at approximately 14 weeks (fetus is 10 cm crown-rump length). Note the endocervical blood and congested sickle-shaped previa (arrows).

advanced maternal age, previous abortions, and rapid succession of pregnancies are the principal factors. Studies have been contradictory as to whether induced abortions were (Barrett et al., 1981) or were not (Grimes & Techman, 1984) precursors of placenta previa. Grimes and Techman reviewed the early literature that reported no such correlation; they also found no risk from preceding curettage. Thus there is still dispute as to the main reasons for this condition. Strassmann believed that the placenta implanted low because of unsuitability of the fundal endometrium. He reasoned that in rapidly successive pregnancies the endometrium had not reconstituted sufficiently to become a site of implantation. His discussion included the putative *Haftfleck* (point of attachment) of Schatz that was disturbed by a previous pregnancy or abortion. Similar notions were reiterated by Nieminen and Klinge (1963), who discuss Iffy's 1962 theory of abnormal endocrine support. Although occasionally disputed, the dependence of placenta previa on maternal age and parity has been solidly supported by the findings of Penrose (1939) and Kalmus (1947). Rarely is a placenta previa found in association with incompetent cervix, but such may be difficult to diagnose as an independent condition when the previa has already led to hemorrhage (Ringrose, 1976). An extensive analysis of correlative factors has emerged from the oft-mentioned Collaborative Perinatal Study and was published by Naeye (1978). This author found no increase in fetal anomalies, and there was no association with maternal age in placenta previa. There was relatively high perinatal mortality (11%), and increased fetal hematopoiesis (? anemia, stress) and growth retardation were found. Moreover, contrary to many earlier reports, the placentas and fetal organs were lighter. The placental villi were interpreted to show hyperplasia. Nielsen et al. (1989) found a greater incidence after cesarean section in a large cohort.

There can be no doubt, however, that placenta previa is often associated with placenta accreta. With placenta accreta, the placenta fails to dislodge from the uterus after delivery of the newborn. When such a uterus is studied histologically, it is found that the villous tissue had not been attached to decidua, but that it has grown onto the myometrium without intervening decidua. There is good evidence that placenta accreta is due to the failure of normal decidua to form, usually because the endometrium is deficient and cannot transform. Kistner et al. (1952) stated that the absence of the "spongious layer" of the decidua is the important feature. Thus the trophoblast does not stop invading when it should, and it penetrates more broadly into muscle than is normal. Placenta accreta is also a regular finding in abdominal and tubal pregnancies, where there is also no normal endometrium to transform into decidua. A

similar situation arises in the lower uterine segment and endocervix. Despite the thick nature of the endocervical mucosa, it does not follow the normal hormonal signals for decidualization, and when implantation occurs here a placenta accreta forms. Although placenta previa accreta and cervical pregnancy are rare (only about 150 cases having been reported), many of these reports (reviews by Kistner et al., 1952; Friesen, 1961) attest to the importance of this condition, which may endanger the mother's life because of afibrinogenemia, in addition to the hemorrhage (Rosa et al., 1956; Koren et al., 1961). Some authors have noted the frequency of prior cesarean section and curettage as being important (Rubenstone & Lash, 1963; Clark et al., 1985). Clark et al. believed that placenta previa and its variants are not rare and cited a steady rise in case reports.

It is then surprising to find the study from Khong and Robertson (1987) that purports to negate the previous theories on the pathogenesis of placenta accreta and placenta previa accreta. Their novel view, which requires more discussion, is based on study of the placental bed in placenta accreta (inappropriately referred to as "creta"). Here they found a deficiency of the usual placental bed giant cells, a preponderance of uninuclear trophoblast, and a difference in the maternal vasculature in the areas of adherence. Moreover, they (as did other investigators) found that accretas may be focal, that there may be normal decidua next to areas of adherence, and that the decidua parietalis of such cases is also normal. From these findings they deduced that "there is a defective interaction between maternal tissues, particularly decidua, and migratory trophoblast in early stages of placentation resulting in undue adherence of the placenta or penetration into the uterus coupled with the development of an abnormal uteroplacental circulation." In other words, they believed that absent decidua is not the primary event, as is our belief and the opinion held by most previous students of the matter. Their concept is contrary to all other findings made in studies of this disease. For example, similar findings of accreta placentation are regularly made with ectopic pregnancy, both the tubal and abdominal varieties. Although occasional decidualization of tubal mucosa does occur, it is uncommon; and true decidua in ectopic pregnancy is rare. One must, of course, be able to differentiate decidual cells from X cells, which is not always done with ease.

Placenta accreta is also typical for endocervical implantation and in uteri that were altered focally by curettage or by the scars of cesarean section. Khong and Robertson (1987) dismissed the analogy of deficient decidua in tubal pregnancy by saying that these pregnancies rarely go to term. [Augensen (1983) described an exception and reviewed the literature; see below.] True enough, but the reason for the usual failure of ectopic pregnancies to reach term is that the accretas of tubal pregnancy usually become placentas percreta with bleeding. This point has also been emphasized by Pauerstein et al. (1986), who recommended local resection on that basis. Moreover, many term tubal pregnancies have indeed been observed (e.g., Frachtmann, 1953; Miller, 1987).

In our opinion, the adherent placental bed morphology betrays the ill-understood interactions between trophoblast and normal decidua. After all, why is it that not every pregnancy results in placenta accreta? The trophoblast stops destroying the endometrium or decidua at a given point during placentation and leaves (in humans) a portion of decidua basalis untouched. It is not so in all species, as in the Dasypodidae, where the superficial myometrium is also differently constructed. This failure to destroy all of the decidua basalis may be related to temporal changes in the trophoblast's behavior, carefully timed genetically; or it may be that the decidua plays a specific role in this delimitation of the advancing invasion by trophoblastic cells. It is not to say that some of the advancing trophoblast does not reach deeper into the mouths of vessels and into the myometrium; it certainly does. However, a primary deficiency of decidual transformation or of the depth of endometrium/decidua still best explains the placenta accreta. The findings described by Khong and Robertson (1987) may be explained as *sequelae* of absent decidua, rather than its cause. Parenthetically, we agree with their statement that the presence of adenomyosis as a basis of placenta accreta has been vastly overrated.

Cramer (1987) described a placenta increta that had invaded and partially destroyed the leiomyoma on which it rested. From this finding he deduced that accretas/incretas are due to overly aggressive trophoblast, rather than decidual deficiency. He believed it to be the cause, not only in this case but also of other accretas. He reasoned that the ability of decidua to produce laminin, fibronectin, collagen type IV, and proteoglycans (Wewer et al., 1986) may be defective and suggested that the normal balance of the placental invasiveness and the decidua to resist invasion may be disturbed in accretas. Rice et al. (1989), who studied pregnancies complicated by leiomyomas, found that retroplacental tumors were significantly frequently complicated by abruptio placentae.

Placenta Accreta

Placenta accreta is an important condition clinically. It may be life-threatening (Manyonda & Varma, 1991). As has just been described, with placenta accreta the villous tissue is in direct contact with the myometrium, and the placental villi are anchored to muscle fibers rather than to intervening decidual cells. The deficiency of decidua prevents normal separation of the placenta after delivery. Normally, the placenta separates from the uterine musculature in a plane just peripheral to Nitabuch's fibrin layer. It is accomplished by the shearing action of contracting myometrium against the stationary, noncontracting placenta and occurs in irregular planes of friable decidual cells. Thus either the entire placenta is retained, or when the focus of adherence is small only a portion of placenta is retained. These adherent areas tend to bleed; fibrin and clot continue to accumulate around such retained placental tissue, and in time a "placental polyp" develops that may necessitate operative removal. Lester et al. (1956) found placental fragments to be an unimportant feature of immediate postpartum hemorrhage (4.5%). When hemorrhage occurred in a later stage of the puerperium, however, placental polyp was the cause in 44.4% of affected mothers.

Placenta accreta cannot easily be diagnosed from the delivered placenta, but it has been shown that it is often (in 45%) associated with elevated maternal serum α-fetoprotein levels (Zelop et al., 1992; Kupferminc et al., 1993). The placenta may be disrupted during the delivery because of the accretion, and there may thus be missing cotyledons. Occasionally, one can palpate these retained cotyledons by manual exploration in the postpartum uterus. When histological sections of such a placenta are made, however, the deficiency of endometrium that underlies placenta accreta is not evident. For such a diagnosis one must examine the entire uterus or curettings that include the myometrium. Even then it may be difficult to orient the lesion, and a firm diagnosis may be difficult to render. It is much easier done when whole specimens are available, which of course is the less acceptable outcome for the patient. Nevertheless, hysterectomy is a frequent sequela when large areas of placenta accreta exist. If the site of attachment is fixed before trimming the tissues for histology, the lesion is easily diagnosed microscopically (Figure 276). Pathologists must be aware of the difficulties of distinguishing the populations of cells that make up the placental floor, especially when they do not examine many placentas. For this differential diagnosis the pathologist must distinguish between the basal decidual cells and the unicellular trophoblast (mostly X cells), which are abundant at the site of placenta previa implantation. There is usually an abundance of basal fibrin, and the maternal vessels show the focally deficient "physiologic change" described by Khong and Robertson (1987). It may be of parenthetical interest here to mention that successful treatment with methotrexate has been undertaken in cervical accretas (Oyer et al., 1988; Palti et al., 1989; Bakri et al., 1993). Also, microembolization through the internal iliac artery (Kivikoski et al., 1988)

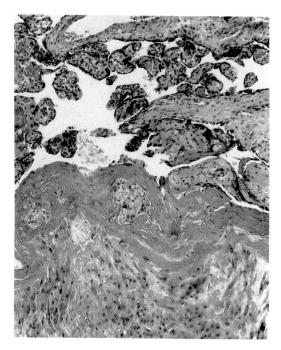

FIGURE 276. Placenta accreta at term. Villi are attached to myometrium, and the cellular layer at the bottom is composed of only cellular trophoblast (X cells). There is still a large amount of Nitabuch's fibrin layer. H&E. ×125.

predisposing factors. The fact that 57 maternal deaths occurred in these women (9.5%) with 9.6% fetal deaths attests to the gravity of the condition.

The frequent antecedent of cesarean section was also stressed by Breen et al. (1977), who reviewed the literature and found an overall incidence of 1 in 7,000 pregnancies. This figure is only a rough estimate, however; the higher frequency reported from Thailand (1:540) by Sumawong et al. (1966) was speculated to relate possibly to their higher incidence of proliferative trophoblastic disease. This argument is unjustified, we believe, as there is no evidence that accretas are the result of an overly aggressive trophoblast. Conversely, all correlations point to a defective uterus. Another comprehensive study of placenta accreta comes from Millar's pen (1959). He reviewed not only the morphology of this condition but its etiology. The decidua was always absent at the attachment site, and it was frequently deficient elsewhere in the uterus. Fox (1972) pointed out correctly that there is usually a deficiency of placental septum formation with placenta accreta. When septa are present in a placenta accreta, they are comprised of uterine muscle. He considered that there may be an endocrine deficiency that fails to support

has been used to treat these abnormal implantation sites.

Various antecedents to placenta accreta have been described, such as "constitutional endometrial defect," scars, diverticula, cornual implantation, leiomyoma (Figure 277), and previous curettage (Sumawong et al., 1966). The classical paper on placenta accreta is by Irving and Hertig (1937). They studied 18 cases of this condition, and reviewed 80 cases from the literature. They reported an incidence of 1 in 1,956 deliveries. Deficiency of endometrium, as they were once incurred during endometrial cautery (e.g., steam), is no longer a problem, but endometrial defects caused by curettage and by cesarean section have become prevalent. A familial occurrence was once described in Eskimos, but it has not been confirmed (Schaefer, 1960). Patients "successfully" treated for Asherman syndrome (intrauterine adhesions) often develop accretas and other complications (Friedman et al., 1986).

Fox (1972) presented a comprehensive review of this relatively frequent condition and chose to combine all stages of accretion, including increta and percreta. He reiterated that it is a condition of elderly multigravidas, many of whom have uterine malformations (septa) or other complications listed earlier. Of the 622 reported cases covered by his 25-year review, 213 were associated with placenta previa (34%) and 7 were placentas membranaceas (see below); in only 43 cases were there no

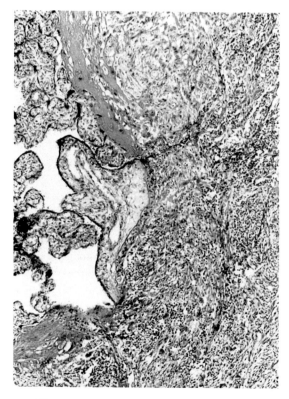

FIGURE 277. Placenta accreta over a leiomyoma. The leiomyoma (right) was delivered with the placenta at term (see also Cramer, 1987). H&E. ×100. (Courtesy Dr. Ralph Richart, New York, New York.)

normal endometrial growth. Fox also reported some early cases in which decidua was already lacking. One very young placenta accreta was also found accidentally at hysterectomy by Begneaud et al. (1965). The histological features were identical to those of other accretas.

It has been suggested that the clinical picture associated with placenta previa has been changing (Read et al., 1980); certainly, associated fetal mortality figures have improved. Weckstein et al. (1987) reported a case of placenta percreta and stated their belief that this condition is increasing in frequency because of increased cesarean section rates.

Placenta Increta and Percreta

Many authors, Fox (1972) for instance, do not distinguish accretas from incretas and percretas, and Luke et al. (1966) criticized terms that have become fairly accepted in the medical nomenclature, when they recalled 427 cases from the literature of accretas, incretas, and percretas. In contrast to placenta accreta, with incretas the myometrium is invaded by the placental villous tissue, whereas with percretas the villi penetrate the entire wall and the uterus ruptures. The latter may then become an acutely life-threatening condition. In general, the causes of such "invasive" placentas are similar to those of the "placenta accreta vera." These conditions are nearly always present when tubal ectopic pregnancies rupture. Placenta percreta has also been reported to follow tubal reconstructive surgery at the uterine fundus (Stromme, 1963), with septate uteri (Ries & Middleton, 1972), complicating therapy for "missed abortion" (Harden et al., 1990), and of course through former cesarean section sites (Berchuck & Sokol, 1983). The invading placenta may be intramural in position (Cava & Russell, 1978; Fait et al., 1987), perhaps its rarest site. Although adenomyosis is an attractive and often proposed cause of such rare cases, it has rarely been found. McGowan (1965) proposed previous instrumental injury as a possibility because he saw two cases that were interpreted to have resulted from curettage. Ayers et al. (1971) have even reported the presence of fetal tissues within placenta increta sites of women who had previously suffered abortion. Dessouky (1980) found viable abdominal villi in the omentum after an instrumental abortion; the patient recovered after resection.

The most demonstrative pictures of placenta accreta to percreta were produced by Morison (1978). Among a population of 645,000 deliveries from his institution, he found 67 uteri thus affected. Of them, 31 were accretas (14 focal, 17 partial), 3 were incretas, and 3 were percretas; 17 were placentas previa accreta, 11 were placenta previa increta, and 2 were placenta previa percreta. In most of these cases, there was massive hemorrhage. Maternal death (twice only in his series) is a possible outcome. The fetus also often dies, but Gribble and Fitzsimmons (1985) described fetal survival (890 g) with such a complication.

Placenta accreta (vera) is usually detected after delivery when the placenta fails to separate or is incompletely delivered. Incretas and percretas more frequently manifest during earlier gestation because of hemorrhage or uterine rupture. They have even been diagnosed by ultrasonography (Cox et al., 1988; Finberg & Williams, 1992; Hoffman-Tretin et al., 1992; Shapiro et al., 1992). Cox et al. diagnosed the event at 16 weeks, closed the disrupted uterus, and allowed the pregnancy to continue another 8 weeks. The infant was then delivered by cesarean section. After a stormy course over 2 months, the malformed neonate died. Five other conservatively managed cases were reviewed by Cox et al. as well. Other instances of young percretas have been described at 19 weeks' gestation (DeWane & McCubbin, 1981) and 22 weeks' gestation (Bateman, 1967). The etiology of percreta, however, was not always clearly documented. On the other hand, Hassim et al. (1968) treated a mother with uterine rupture that occurred at 26 weeks; the patient expired. Another case involved rupture through a cesarean section scar at 37 weeks' gestation. Percreta with hemorrhage was documented by Hornstein et al. (1984) as occurring during elective termination of a 16-week pregnancy. The mother was 40 years of age and had leiomyomas but no other known risk factor. Rupture of the uterus is sometimes associated with the presence of an intrauterine device (Axelsson & Winblad, 1976), and it has occurred with pregnancy in bicornuate uteri (Zabrieskie, 1962). Zabrieskie reviewed the outcome of pregnancy in 92 patients with malformed uteri; he found that retained placentas occurred in 15% of patients, and that rupture occurred in four. Placenta percreta that invades the bladder and causes hematuria or massive hemorrhage has also been described, and it is being seen more frequently with sonography or magnetic resonance imaging (MRI) (Taefi et al., 1970; Silber et al., 1973; Thorp et al., 1992). Nagy (1989) described a primigravida with placenta percreta at 23 weeks' gestation. The placenta had implanted at the fundus and it had spontaneously penetrated. He believed that percretas in primigravidae, at this stage of gestation, to be exceptionally rare events.

Two cases of percreta are shown in Figures 278 and 279. The first was a patient whose erythroblastotic placenta would not separate after delivery. Hemorrhage necessitated hysterectomy. The mother's obstetrical history included five previous cesarean sections. The bulging placenta can readily be seen in Figure 278 at the arrows. In this case, only the peritoneum separated the villous tissue from the cul-de-sac. The specimen was much disrupted during the traumatic event. The "invasive" nature of the placenta into the lower uterine segment is seen in Figure 279, it being actually a placenta increta. The placenta in Figure 280, on the other hand, comes from what was thought to be an abdominal pregnancy near term with a surviving infant. Most of the placenta had an abdominal position and was attached to a defect in the uterus. The placenta had more or less herniated through a uterine defect. It was covered with old blood and hemosiderin. There was no basal decidua, and there were virtually no free membranes. This case then represented nearly a placenta membranacea with the final implantation on the peritoneum (Figure 281); there was significant salpingitis present also. In another, nearly fatal case of placenta previa, the pregnancy had followed curettage and therapy for postabortal endometritis. Because such cases usually require hysterectomy, it is not common that one can evaluate possible future reproductive events. We had the opportunity to examine material from a first trimester percreta that nearly led to fatal hemorrhage. The tissue was excised, and the patient had a successful second pregnancy. During her third pregnancy, however, another percreta developed at 14 weeks, necessitating hysterectomy. Despite careful search, we were unable to identify

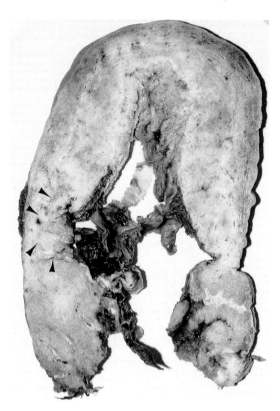

FIGURE 279. Same specimen as Figure 278 after fixation and sagittal sectioning. Placental outline is indicated by arrows where it is invasive. The blood overlying this area is visible. Also seen are the scars from preceding cesarean sections in the anterior wall (right).

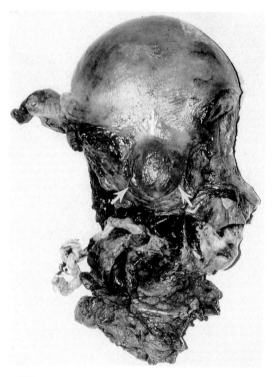

FIGURE 278. Placenta increta-near-percreta. The patient bled during delivery, and the placenta would not separate, so a hysterectomy was done. At the posterior aspect of the lower uterine segment, one can see the nodular protrusion (arrows) of peritoneum-covered placenta.

adenomyosis or other predisposing factors (Mulligan, personal communication, 1962).

Placenta Membranacea

Placenta membranacea is an unusual abnormality of placental form. Some authors have estimated its occurrence to be 1 in 3,300 pregnancies, but this approximation is a gross overestimate. Although the entity was described as early as 1807, only a handful of references can be found on placenta membranacea. Many cases are hidden in the literature on placenta accreta. Thus of the 622 cases of placenta accreta gathered by Fox (1972) for his report, seven were placentas membranacea. Although it is true that some membranaceas are also accretas, it is not the case for all. The placenta membranacea (diffusa) is an organ in which all, or nearly all, of the circumference of the fetal sac is covered by villous tissue. The placental mass is generally thin (1–2 cm), and it is often disrupted (Figures 282, 283). It has been suggested that placenta membranacea is a variant of extensive succenturiate lobe formation, but I do not

FIGURE 280. Placenta percreta from the maternal side with much old blood covering the protruding tissue. (Courtesy Dr. J. Carey, San Diego, California.)

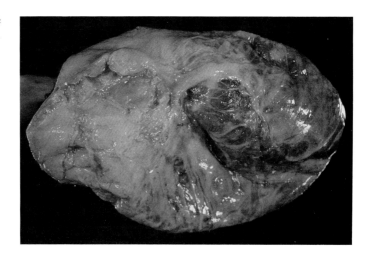

believe it to be the case. There is never a separation or even a hint of segregation of tissue from a main placental disk; and the tissue is uniformly thin. This type of placental anomaly has been likened to the placenta found in Suidae, Equidae, and Cetacea. However, it is not an appropriate comparison because these orders of mammals do not have an invasive placenta. Only a

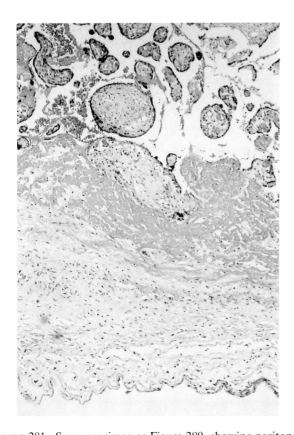

FIGURE 281. Same specimen as Figure 280, showing peritoneal implantation. The villi are anchored to the connective tissue of the peritoneum (below) by a broad band of fibrin. H&E. ×60.

superficial macroscopic similarity to the animals' placentas exists, and it is thus not appropriate to speak of "atavism."

Placenta membranacea frequently manifests clinically as early bleeding and placenta previa. Affected pregnancies often terminate in premature delivery but not invariably. They also may incur difficulties with placental separation after delivery. The literature on placenta membranacea has been reviewed by Finn (1954) and by Janovski and Granowitz (1961); more recent cases have been reported by Mathews (1974), Las Heras et al. (1982), and Hurley and Beischer (1987). The etiology of placenta membranacea is not understood. It is easy to state that those villi destined to become the chorion laeve do not atrophy normally and that there is endometrial hypoplasia on "constitutional" or other grounds; but, in general, no author has presented support for these hypotheses. The fact that the anomaly often presents with midtrimester bleeding and is thus often diagnosed with placenta accreta may merely reflect the fact that placenta membranacea also overlies the internal os and thereby has a chance of becoming a placenta previa accreta. Occasional cases, such as the one depicted in the previous edition of this book, may have other areas of accretion. Most reported patients delivered their placentas without evidence of accreta. There has not been any associated fetal growth retardation.

One of the cases, described by Finn (1954), is of particular interest. Finn was the obstetrician for this "infant" 27 years after her birth. This now-adult woman delivered a macerated, stillborn fetus at 5 months after several weeks of bleeding. This placenta, just like that associated with her own birth, was a typical placenta membranacea (Finn, personal communication, 1976). Thus either genetic influences determined this abnormal placenta, or it was the result of an abnormal uterine environment that was under genetic control. It seems

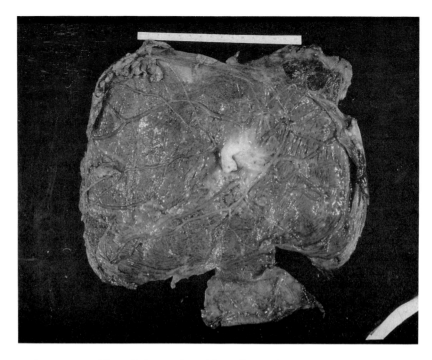

FIGURE 282. Placenta membranacea at 35 weeks' gestation. Virtually no free membranes are seen, and the placenta is thin. Patient had recurrent bleeding necessitating hysterotomy.

highly improbable that such a rare anomaly would occur twice within this one pedigree by accident.

PLACENTA IN ECTOPIC PREGNANCY

The placenta of ectopic pregnancies is relevant here because ectopic pregnancies are also placentas accreta and percreta. Additionally, the problem of removing the placenta accreta associated with an abdominal fetus poses interesting issues.

Virtually all tubal pregnancies are at least placentas accreta. When they rupture, they do so because the placenta almost always has become a placenta percreta. Overdistension of the tube is not the primary cause of tubal rupture in ectopic pregnancy, which is somewhat in contrast to what has been reported by Philippe et al. (1970). In a review of 112 tubal pregnancies, these authors observed that ectopic implantation is often superficial and that it leads to bleeding at the site of attachment. They did not specifically discuss the rupture. Numerous case reports of viable term fetuses from tubal pregnancies testify to tubal expansibility.

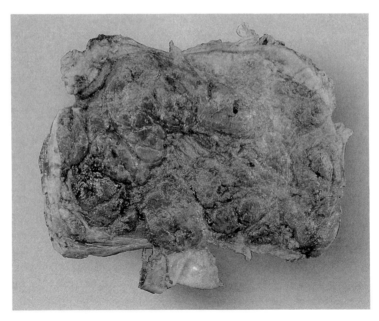

FIGURE 283. Maternal surface of the placenta in Figure 282, showing old clot but the absence of accreta in this placenta membranacea.

McElin and Randall (1951) established criteria for this entity and collected 45 cases from the literature. The placenta they reported was clearly an accreta and was difficult to separate at operation. The associated fetal mortality reported in the literature was 75% and the maternal mortality 10%. Frachtman (1953) reviewed this topic extensively. He found at least 75 reported cases, to which he added his own. His case had a thin placenta. Large infarcts were found in O'Connell's case (1952). Sunde (1965) emphasized the need to attempt complete removal of the placenta. Augensen (1983) found the placenta to possess a short cord (22 cm) and observed extensive decidualization of the sac's wall as well as many placental infarcts. One wonders if the "decidualization" was truly endometrium or if it could have been X cells. Short cords are expected because of the inability of the fetus to move. Thus Willemen et al. (1965) recorded 31 cm for the cord's length, and a case described by Chokroverty et al. (1986) had a 38 cm long cord with a macerated fetus. Many areas of placental degeneration were found as well.

The report by Gustafson et al. (1953) included a color picture of a placenta with velamentous cord insertion. It described a decidual reaction, but it actually depicted a typical placenta accreta with many X cells. We believe that, as is not uncommon, these cells were mistakenly interpreted to be decidua. This consideration is an important one that was once specifically studied by Moritz and Douglass (1928), who claimed that they regularly found decidua in tubal pregnancies at the villous attachment site "if the chorionic villi are intact." This finding is contrary to our experience. True decidual transformation is rare in the tubal mucosa except at term, and all tubal pregnancies in our patients have been accretas. The connection to the tubal musculature is afforded by X cells, or the "placental site cells." They often have a superficial resemblance to decidual cells but are of trophoblastic origin. It was for this reason that they were referred to as X cells in the first place—because of the difficulty of differentiating them from maternal tissue elements.

It is also surprising to find striking contradictions in a study of 90 placentas (young abortions) of tubal pregnancies by Laufer et al. (1962). In their introduction, these authors wrote that decidua was lacking in the tube, but in their summary they stated that, aside from the hydropic degeneration and placental infarcts that are expected, decidua was found in all cases. Not only are tubal ectopic pregnancies accretas, when they rupture (as is commonly the case) they do so because the placenta becomes a placenta percreta with blood issuing from the intervillous space into the peritoneal cavity.

Reports of intraligamentary pregnancy (Vierhout & Wallenburg, 1985) merge with the next topic, abdominal pregnancy. The patient Vierhout and Wallenburg described was presumed to have developed interstitial placentation from rupture of a tubal implantation; the patient suffered severe toxemia, and the placenta was left behind and resorbed spontaneously. Interstitial implantation also occurred in the case described by Schmitt and Dittrich (1973), probably secondary to an abdominal pregnancy. As in so many other abdominal pregnancies, there was no amniotic fluid, and the child had deformations. The placenta had succenturiate lobes, many infarcts, and intervillous thrombi. It was small and had unusually thick membranes. Similar cases of "interstitial" tubal pregnancy, related to previous tubal surgery, were recorded by Kalchman and Meltzer (1966) and Woolam et al. (1967); these authors reviewed the literature and provided good illustrations.

PLACENTA IN ABDOMINAL PREGNANCY

Implantation in the abdominal cavity, particularly when associated with term fetuses, has long been a topic of heated discussion. It may be associated with tubal disease and contraceptive devices,

as in the case described by Tisdall et al. (1970). Early diagnosis is a matter of concern, as it is difficult (Atrash et al., 1987). Ultrasonography and MRI studies have been advocated (Spanta et al., 1987). This complication of pregnancy is estimated to occur once in 3,000 to 8,000 births, according to the review of Martin et al. (1988). It also is associated with high fetal (83%) and some maternal mortality, according to these authors. They described nine cases of early and six cases of advanced abdominal pregnancy and provided an excellent review of current management.

Abdominal pregnancy also causes concern because of the unanswered question of how to deliver the placenta (Hreshchyshyn et al., 1961), as it does not deliver spontaneously because it is a placenta accreta. There is extraordinary local vascular development in response to implantation. When that tissue is dislodged, exsanguinating hemorrhage may occur. These authors analyzed 101 such cases and found that attempted placental removal was the commonest practice; they also advocated it when it is surgically feasible. They found a high morbidity when the placenta was retained; for example, Caruso et al. (1963) reported a patient who had subsequent bowel perforation.

St. Clair et al. (1969) intentionally left the placenta in the abdomen and perfused the umbilical vessels with methotrexate. They undertook this measure because methotrexate is highly toxic to trophoblast. The placenta involuted rapidly, and the gonadotropin titers fell. They believed that this therapy may have improved the involution, which otherwise may take as long as 50 days. Rahman et al. (1982) have also reported use of this agent, but they were less enthusiastic about its benefit. These authors reported that 10 cases occurred among 102,000 deliveries. Somewhat similar figures were obtained in other large series dealing with ectopic pregnancy (Hallatt & Grove, 1985). Many abdominal pregnancies are secondary to tubal abortion; Hallatt and Grove depicted the typical accreta on uterine muscle and described the distribution of the major implantation sites.

The placenta in abdominal pregnancy is rarely described in detail. It has been mentioned that the placental floor lacks decidua, that a large vascular supply supports the intervillous space, and that the placenta may develop on many maternal organs. Holzer and Pickel (1976) found such a case to have a large succenturiate lobe and a velamentous cord insertion. A remarkable vascular attachment to the mother was described by Norén and Lindblom (1986), where a normal, term infant had a thickened placental sac over which many islands of placenta were distributed. The only connection to the mother was a 2 cm wide and 3 cm long vascular pedicle that connected the placenta to the uterine fundus. It was easily ligated. The placenta membranacea had many intervillous thrombi and infarcts. Fetal growth retardation (Shott et al., 1973), anomalies and deformations (Paintin, 1970; Guha-Ray & Hamblin, 1977), and occasionally pulmonary hypoplasia (Cartwright et al., 1986) are often described. Several reports of abdominal pregnancy have appeared in which the condition occurred after hysterectomy (Kornblatt, 1968; Niebyl, 1974; Nehra & Loginsky, 1984). The latter authors collected 30 such cases from the literature.

The fate of the retained placenta is also rarely described in detail. When complications such as perforations and adhesions necessitate reoperation, the placental tissue is usually not described. Only sonographic studies of the atrophy are available (Belfar et al., 1986). An interesting report comes from Spinnato et al. (1987), who saw a cyst develop 3 weeks after the term delivery of a normal infant from an abdominal pregnancy. The umbilical cord was tied near its base, and the chorion laeve was not removed, nor was it closed. Despite the absence of a fetus, the membranes reaccumulated a large amount of fluid. When the mass was finally excised, the fluid was brown and thick. It contained much necrotic debris and the remains of a macerating umbilical cord with its ligature, which were clearly depicted. Regrettably, no histology is available.

Ovarian pregnancies usually abort. The definition of ovarian pregnancy generally follows the strict criteria set in the past. These criteria are often attributed to Spiegelberg (1878), but they were actually delineated by Cohnstein the year before. A term pregnancy has rarely been reported in the ovary, although Williams et al. (1982) described such a case. As expected, the umbilical cord was short (22 cm) but the placenta unusually large (1,500 g). When sections are made of the implantation site of ovarian pregnancies, the placental villi often insert on the cells of the corpus luteum. The cellular component of the placental floor is the X cell, frequently mistakenly identified (Yu et al., 1984). The English literature of ovarian pregnancy was reviewed by Boronow et al. (1965), who found 62 cases in 13 years. In other words, it is not an uncommon entity. They noted that the usual antecedents of ectopic pregnancy (pelvic and tubal inflammation, sterility, and endometriosis) are not important in this disease. The site of implantation often contains much hemorrhage and only some trophoblastic giant cells. True placental tissue is frequently absent, except for some degenerating villi.

Circumvallate Placenta (Extrachorial and Circummarginate Placentas)

Some writers have regarded the circumvallate placenta as clinically important; others have stated that it is a clinically meaningless deviation from normal. In circumvallate placentas, the membranes of the chorion laeve do not insert at the edge of the placenta but at some inward distance from the margin, toward the umbilical cord. At the margin, one usually finds variable amounts of fibrin and recent and old blood. At times, a striking number of such deposits are present. In typical circumvallate placentas, there is a truly complete circumferential ring that severely restricts the total surface of the chorion frondosum. At the periphery, "naked" placental tissue protrudes, which is the reason for the designation placenta extrachorialis. This condition should not be confused with an extramembranous fetus, a placental anomaly that occurs after early rupture of the membranes, with the fetus lying in the endometrial cavity and outside the membranous sac. This situation is not the case with ordinary circumvallate placentas, although, as is seen with the extramembranous pregnancy, there is also a striking circumvallation present. When no typical plication of the membranes occurs at the margin, and when the edge of the protruding placenta is covered only by some fibrin, we speak of a circummarginate placenta.

These two forms blend into each other, and partial circumvallation is common. The incidences of these common conditions are listed in Table 19, which was compiled from several large prospectively and retrospectively collected series. Circumvallate placentas are rarely found during the first trimester, although Meyer (1909) and Torpin (1966) depicted uteri at 3.5 months with intact circumvallate placentas. Most authors agree

TABLE 19. Reported frequency of circumvallate and circummarginate placentas.

Author	No. of studies	Frequency (%)	
		Circumvallate	Circummarginate
Scott (1960)	3,161	18.3 (extrachorial)	
Ziel (1963)	40,143	0.62	
Wilson & Paalman (1967)	10,927	1.0	
Wentworth (1968)	895	6.5	25.5
Benson & Fujikura (1969)	39,514	3.6	3.3
Whites		2.0	3.4
Blacks			
Fox & Sen (1972)	3,000	2.4	22.0
Benirschke	13,537	5.25	

that circumvallation is often complicated by prenatal bleeding and premature delivery.

Two characteristic circumvallate placentas with different amounts of extrachorial tissue are illustrated in Figures 284 and 285, and Figure 286 shows a typical circummarginate placenta. Variations between these degrees are frequent. Gross examination of such placentas often shows yellow-brown discolored marginal fibrin, testifying to its origin from hematomas. In cases where this anomaly is the cause of midtrimester hemorrhage and premature delivery, one may find a substantial amount of blood at the margin. It may undermine the margin of the placenta and thus initiate a clinical picture of abruptio placentae. Although much of this blood comes from the maternal vessels, the bleeding may be significant enough to elevate the chorion laeve from the site of its insertion and then disrupt the fetal vessels (Figure 287). Thus the hematoma and vaginal bleeding are frequently of mixed maternal and fetal origin. In some cases, it is the mechanism of neonatal anemia (Mitchell et al., 1957). Scott (1960) superbly investigated the structure of the margins of extrachorial pregnancies and found evidence that the chorion, once upon a time, must have been more marginally inserted. When he injected placental vessels with radiopaque dye and placed a wire around the insertion sites of the membranes, he found pictures such as that shown in Figure 288. Here one can see that the fetal surface vessels pursue a horizontal course way past the wire circumference before they dip vertically into the placental tissue. This picture indicates that the vessels must have been running in chorion initially, before this membrane was dislodged by the hematoma; this point is dramatically illustrated in Figure 287. The bleeding was so acute in this case that many fetal vessels were severed. This old blood accumulated at the margin, hemolyzed, and changed into fibrin-like deposits that cover up the old horizontal vessels. It is also the

FIGURE 284. Typical circumvallate placenta at approximately 35 weeks' gestation. Note the small surface area of the remaining chorion frondosum and the large white fibrin ring at the periphery.

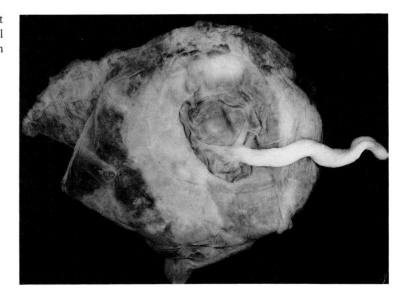

cause of the discoloration. Hemosiderin is often found in the more extensive cases. This fibrin causes the plica to form that is so characteristic of circumvallate placentas (Figures 289, 290). The amnion may follow the chorion into this plica, or most commonly, it flatly covers the plica without infolding.

Because circumvallation occurs so frequently, this anomaly has been investigated many times to explain its formal genesis. As a result, numerous theories have been proposed. Several opposing ideas have been presented without, it is fair to say, firm resolution that would be acceptable to all. Schatz (1886) reviewed older writings with which he strongly disagreed. He contended that circumvallate placentas arise because the embryonic mass implants too superficially. That concept was supported by Hertig and Gore (1969). The

opposite view has been defended by Torpin (1953, 1955, 1965, 1966). He confessed a life-long preoccupation with understanding the etiology of these abnormal placental forms. Torpin believed that the evidence points to excessively deep implantation of the blastocyst into a "fungating," hyperplastic decidua. He concurred with Gottschalk's (1891) opinion. That viewpoint, expressed many years earlier, was a dissenting voice against Schatz's superficial ("polypoid") placentation theory. Nevertheless, this superficial implantation theory has become the predominant thought in our texts, perhaps because of the eminence of Schatz (1886) and Meyer (1909). Likewise, the pronouncements of Williams (1927) carried much weight in the United States. Williams had done a study of circumvallate placentas and then opined that "all had been said"

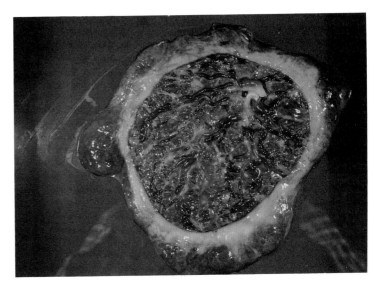

FIGURE 285. There is a lesser degree of circumvallation in this placenta than in the one shown in Figure 284.

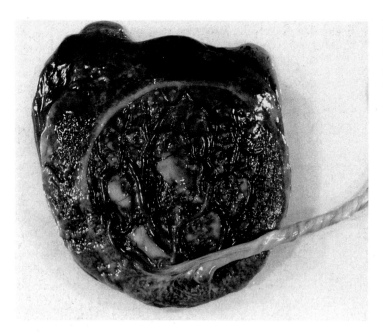

FIGURE 286. Sickle-shaped circummarginate placenta, with free villous tissue protruding beyond the membrane insertion. This point, combined with the near-marginal insertion of the cord at the opposite end, is considered to reflect trophotropism.

about the theories of its genesis. He further suggested that we discard the term marginata (circummarginate). His opinions included claims that true circumvallation occurs in fewer than 2% of deliveries, and he supported the notion of superficial implantation.

A challenging consideration of pathogenesis is that originally enunciated by Liepmann (1906). He saw several early circumvallate placentas, one of which

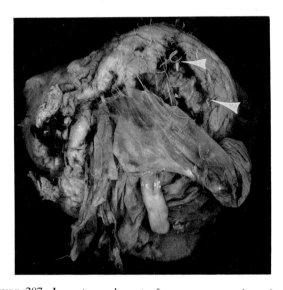

FIGURE 287. Immature placenta from an exsanguinated premature infant. Massive old and recent blood clot was circumferentially present; it has been partially removed, showing the stretched and occasionally interrupted fetal vessels (arrowheads) through which the fetus bled. The membranes were brown from deposits of hematoidin and hemosiderin, and from hemolyzed blood.

clearly related to premature loss of amnionic fluid. Exactly the same mechanism takes place in all extramembranous pregnancies, which are some of the most classical examples of circumvallate placentation (see Chapter 12). Liepmann proposed that the marginal infolding derives from *Stauchung* (impaction, collision, jamming), the failure of the sac to be held open. Later students have either confirmed Torpin's view (Wentworth, 1968), or they were noncommittal (Scott, 1960).

All theories seem to suggest that there is only one way for circumvallates to originate, whereas in fact there may be different types and origins. Reduced amnionic fluid pressure distending the sac in extramembranous pregnancy clearly speaks as an etiological moment in that case. When significant hemorrhage occurs circumferentially, as can happen with midtrimester abortion, it may be the primary cause of circumvallation. When a midtrimester placenta previa changes to a marginal insertion at the lower segment and the fundal portion expands, it may be the origin of the sickle-shaped, so-called placenta marginata. This term, placenta marginata (or circummarginate placenta), is a poor one, and most authors consider these placentas to be part of the spectrum of circumvallation. The term should be abandoned. When the apposing membranous sacs of twins exert differential pressures on one another, the meeting point is often discordant with the placental bed. That is, the membranes often do not meet exactly over the place where the respective placental areas terminate. They are frequently pushed away from this "equator," and "bare" placental tissue exists; at least it is covered by the membranes of the other twin. It, too, is a form of extrachorial placenta. If, as has been sug-

FIGURE 288. Radiograph of placenta "extra-chorialis" (circumvallate) whose fetal vessels were injected with barium sulfate. The circular wire marks the edge of the chorionic plate. Note the many chorionic vessels pursuing a straight course past the edge of the membranes' insertion. (Reprinted with permission from Scott, J.S., Placenta extra-chorialis: a factor in antepartum haemorrhage. J. Obstet. Gynaecol. Brit. Emp. 67:904–918, Blackwell Scientific Publications, Osney Mead, Oxford, UK, 1960.)

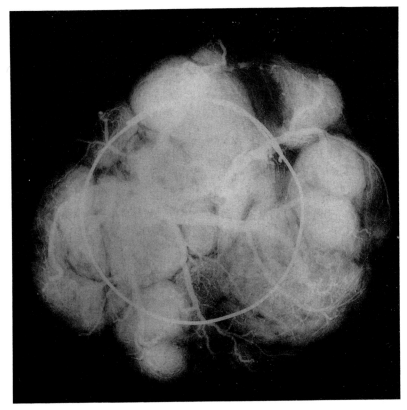

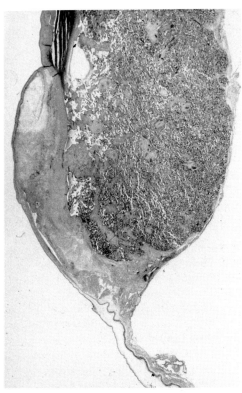

FIGURE 289. Margin of circumvallate placenta. The gray, homogeneous material under the plica represents fibrin and degenerating clot. Note that the amnion is not infolding with the chorion in this example, as is otherwise so often the case. H&E. ×4.

gested, a polypoid, superficial implantation were the cause of circumvallation, one might find fewer atrophied villi in the chorion laeve. This possibility had already been entertained by Torpin (1969b), and we have looked for such a possible deficiency in rolled membranes of normal and circumvallate placentas as well. We found that there was a high degree of variation in the villi so discovered, but circumvallate placentas often had such villi. Harbert et al. (1970) described three circumvallate placentas in rhesus monkeys that had only a single disk (instead of their normal two-disk placenta). Harbert et al. evaluated the respective interrelations of these anomalies and concluded that if they were indeed related it would mean that the cause must have been aberrant trophoblastic behavior before the 17th day of pregnancy. Johnson et al. (1978) reported two similar cases in stumptailed macaques. Suzuki (1971), however, found two circumvallates in two-disk rhesus placentas. This finding negates the hypothesis of Harbert and colleagues (1970). Because of the relative frequency of single-disk placentas in macaques (25%), the concurrences of the two conditions may be merely happenstance.

As stated earlier, "true" circumvallate placentas are correlated with prenatal bleeding, premature termination of pregnancy, multiparity, abruptio, and early fluid loss (Ziel, 1963; Naftolin et al., 1973), and occasionally they are familial (Deacon et al., 1974). For a consideration of clinical significance, it must be cautioned that

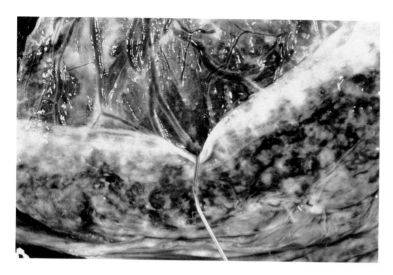

FIGURE 290. Plica of the circumvallate margin with a wire holding up the overhanging margin of the membrane insertion. Note the simultaneous infolding of the amnion.

the term "circumvallate" is not used uniformly by all pathologists and obstetricians, which is perhaps one reason for the marked differences in the reported incidence (1–7%) and for the confusion with the so-called placentas marginata. Our data include only cases such as are shown in Figures 284, 285, and 287 but not Figure 286. Lademacher et al. (1981), who favored a genetic etiology of this anomaly, identified significantly higher frequencies of perinatal death (11% versus 3%), premature deliveries (37% versus 13%), congenital anomalies (15% versus 4%), and single umbilical artery with circumvallate placentation. It was true also for circummarginate placentation, where the figures were 3%, 25%, and 4%, respectively. In a study of 3,000 consecutive deliveries, Fox and Sen (1972) again suggested that circummarginate placentas have no clinical importance but that circumvallate placentas associate significantly frequently with threatened abortion, premature labor, and fetal growth retardation. To this list some authors (Morgan, 1955) have added that circumvallation is associated with a higher maternal morbidity rate due to postpartum hemorrhage and a more frequent need for manual removal of the placenta. Repeated occurrence of circumvallate placentas in successive pregnancies has been reported occasionally (Wilson & Paalman, 1967).

Benson and Fujikura (1969) concluded, after an exhaustive analysis of the 39,514 pregnancies in the Collaborative Perinatal Study, that "despite some well-documented obstetric-pediatric complications, extrachorial placenta is an uncommon, rarely serious clinical problem." They further believed that "our finding of minimal correlation between these morphologic variations and clinical abnormalities is due to the prospective nature of the study." We doubt that everyone would agree with this statement. Rolschau (1978), for instance, found this placentation to be correlated with

single umbilical artery, growth retardation, and an increased incidence of prematurity. Other authors found similar results from large studies of prospectively collected placentas.

References

Arias, F.: Cervical cerclage for temporary treatment of patients with placenta previa. Obstet. Gynecol. 71:545–548, 1988.

Atrash, H.K., Friede, A., and Hogue, C.J.R.: Abdominal pregnancy in the United States: frequency and maternal mortality. Obstet. Gynecol. 69:333–337, 1987.

Augensen, K.: Unruptured tubal pregnancy at term with survival of mother and child. Obstet. Gynecol. 61:259–261, 1983.

Axelsson, H., and Winblad, B.: Dislocated IUD and intrauterine ectopic pregnancy with uterine rupture. Obstet. Gynecol. 47:365–366, 1976.

Ayers, L.R., Drosman, S., and Saltzstein, S.L.: Iatrogenic paracervical implantation of fetal tissue during therapeutic abortion: a case report. Obstet. Gynecol. 37:755–760, 1971.

Bakri, Y.N., Rifai, A., and Legarth, J.: Placenta previa-percreta: magnetic resonance imaging findings and methotrexate therapy after hysterectomy. Am. J. Obstet. Gynecol. 169:213–214, 1993.

Ballas, S., Gitstein, S., Jaffa, A.J., and Peyser, M.R.: Midtrimester placenta previa: normal or pathologic finding. Obstet. Gynecol. 54:12–14, 1979.

Bar-David, J., Piura, B., Leiberman, J.R., and Kaplan, H.: Discrimination between fetal and maternal blood. Am. J. Obstet. Gynecol. 148:352, 1984.

Barrett, J.H., Boehm, F.H., and Killam, A.P.: Induced abortion: a risk factor for placenta previa. Am. J. Obstet. Gynecol. 141:769–772, 1981.

Bartholomew, R.A., Colvin, E.D., Grimes, W.H., Fish, S.S., and Lester, W.M.: Hemorrhage in placenta previa: a new concept of its mechanism. Obstet. Gynecol. 1:41–45, 1953.

Bateman, D.E.R.: Spontaneous rupture of uterus at 22 weeks' pregnancy. B.M.J. 2:844, 1967.

Begneaud, W., Dougherty, C.M., and Mickal, A.: Placenta accreta in early gestation; report of 2 cases. Am. J. Obstet. Gynecol. 92:267–268, 1965.

Belfar, H.L., Kurtz, A.B., and Wagner, R.J.: Long-term follow-up after removal of an abdominal pregnancy. J. Ultrasound Med. 5:521–523, 1986.

Benirschke, K., and Miller, C.J.: Anatomical and functional differences in the placenta of primates. Biol. Reprod. 26: 29–53, 1982.

Benson, R.C., and Fujikura, T.: Circumvallate and circummarginate placenta: unimportant clinical entities. Obstet. Gynecol. 34:799–804, 1969.

Berchuck, A., and Sokol, R.J.: Previous cesarean section, placenta increta, and uterine rupture in second-trimester abortion. Am. J. Obstet. Gynecol. 145:766–767, 1983.

Bergman, P.: Accidental discovery of uterus bicornis on examination of placenta. Obstet. Gynecol. 17:649, 1961.

Bleker, O.P., Kloosterman, G.J., Breur, W., and Mieras, D.J.: The volumetric growth of the human placenta: a longitudinal ultrasonic study. Am. J. Obstet. Gynecol. 127:657–661, 1977.

Booth, R.T., Wood, C., Beard, R.W., Gibson, J.R.M., and Pinkerton, J.H.M.: Significance of site of placental attachment in uterus. B.M.J. 1:1732–1734, 1962.

Borell, U., Fernström, I., and Ohlson, L.: Diagnostic value of arteriography in cases of placenta previa. Am. J. Obstet. Gynecol. 86:535–547, 1963.

Boronow, R.C., McElin, T.W., West, R.H., and Buckingham, J.C.: Ovarian pregnancy: report of four cases and a thirteen-year survey of the English literature. Am. J. Obstet. Gynecol. 91:1095–1106, 1965.

Boyd, J.D., and Hamilton, W.J.: Development and structure of the human placenta from the end of the 3rd month of gestation. J. Obstet. Gynaecol. 74:161–226, 1967.

Breen, J.L., Neubecker, R., Gregori, C.A., and Franklin, J.E.: Placenta accreta, increta, and percreta: a survey of 40 cases. Obstet. Gynecol. 49:43–47, 1977.

Brenner, W.E., Edelman, D.A., and Hendricks, C.H.: Characteristics of patients with placenta previa and results of "expectant management." Am. J. Obstet. Gynecol. 132:180–191, 1978.

Bromberg, Y.M., Salzberger, M., and Abrahamov, A.: Foetal blood in genital haemorrhage due to placenta praevia and abruptio placentae. Lancet 1:767, 1957.

Cartwright, P.S., Brown, J.E., Davis, R.J., Thieme, G.A., and Boehm, F.H.: Advanced abdominal pregnancy associated with fetal pulmonary hypoplasia: report of a case. Am. J. Obstet. Gynecol. 155:396–397, 1986.

Caruso, L.J., Liegner, B., and Tamis, A.B.: Advanced abdominal pregnancy: report of a case. Obstet. Gynecol. 22:795–797, 1963.

Cava, E.F., and Russell, W.M.: Intramural pregnancy with uterine rupture: a case report. Am. J. Obstet. Gynecol. 131:214–216, 1978.

Chez, R.A., Schlesselman, J.J., Salazar, H., and Fox, R.: Single placentas in the rhesus monkey. J. Med. Primatol. 1:230–240, 1972.

Chokroverty, M., Caballes, R.L., and Gear, P.E.: An unruptured tubal pregnancy at term. Arch. Pathol. Lab. Med. 110:250–251, 1986.

Clark, S.L., Koonings, P.P., and Phelan, J.P.: Placenta previa/accreta and prior cesarean section. Obstet. Gynecol. 66:89–92, 1985.

Comeau, J., Shaw, L., Marcell, C.C., and Lavery, J.P.: Early placenta previa and delivery outcome. Obstet. Gynecol. 61:577–580, 1983.

Cordero, D.R., Helfgott, A.W., Landy, H.J., Reik, R.F., Medina, C., and O'Sullivan, M.J.: A non-hemorrhagic manifestation of vasa previa: a clnicopathologic case report. Obstet. Gynecol. 82:698–700, 1993.

Cox, S.M., Carpenter, R.J., and Cotton, D.B.: Placenta percreta: ultrasound diagnosis and conservative surgical management. Obstet. Gynecol. 71:454–456, 1988.

Cramer, S.F.: Letter to the editor: case report. Pediatr. Pathol. 7:473–475, 1987.

Deacon, J.S.R., Gilbert, E.F., Visekul, C., Herrmann, J., and Opitz, J.M.: Polyhydramnios and neonatal hemorrhage in three sisters: a circumvallate placenta syndrome. Birth Defects 10:41–49, 1974.

Defoort, S.S., and Thiery, W.M.: Capping placenta: a new etiologic factor in midtrimester bleeding. Z. Geburtshilfe Perinatol. 192:33–35, 1988.

Dessouky, D.A.: Ectopic trophoblast as a complication of first-trimester induced abortion. Am. J. Obstet. Gynecol. 136:407–408, 1980.

DeWane, J.C., and McCubbin, J.H.: Spontaneous rupture of an unscarred uterus at 19 weeks' gestation. Am. J. Obstet. Gynecol. 141:222–223, 1981.

Fait, G., Goyert, G., Sundareson, A., and Pickens, A.: Intramural pregnancy with fetal survival: case history and discussion of etiologic factors. Obstet. Gynecol. 70:472–474, 1987.

Finberg, H.J., and Williams, J.W.: Placenta accreta: prospective sonographic diagnosis in patients with placenta previa and prior cesarean section. J. Ultrasound Med. 11:333–343, 1992.

Finn, J.L.: Placenta membranacea. Obstet. Gynecol. 3:438–440, 1954.

Fox, H.: Placenta accreta, 1945–1969. Obstet. Gynecol. Surv. 27:475–490, 1972.

Fox, H., and Sen, D.K.: Placenta extrachorialis: a clinico-pathologic study. J. Obstet. Gynaecol. Br. Commonw. 79: 32–35, 1972.

Frachtman, K.G.: Unruptured tubal term pregnancy. Am. J. Surg. 86:161–168, 1953.

Fried, A.M.: Distribution of the bulk of the normal placenta: review and classification of 800 cases by ultrasonography. Am. J. Obstet. Gynecol. 132:675–680, 1978.

Friedman, A., deFazio, J., and deCherney, A.: Severe obstetric complications after aggressive treatment of Asherman syndrome. Obstet. Gynecol. 67:864–867, 1986.

Friesen, R.F.: Placenta previa accreta. Can. Med. Assoc. J. 84:1247–1253, 1961.

Fujikura, T., Benson, R.C., and Driscoll, S.G.: The bipartite placenta and its clinical features. Am. J. Obstet. Gynecol. 107:1013–1017, 1970.

Gabert, H.A.: Placenta previa and fetal growth. Obstet. Gynecol. 38:403–406, 1971.

Gallagher, P., Fagan, C.J., Bedi, D.G., Winsett, M.Z., and Reyes, R.N.: Potential placenta previa: definition, frequency, and significance. Am. J. Roentgenol. 149:1013–1015, 1987.

Gottesfeld, K.R., Thompson, H.E., Holmes, J.H., and Taylor, E.D.: Ultrasonic placentography—a new method for placental localization. Am. J. Obstet. Gynecol. 96:538–547, 1966.

Gottschalk, S.: Weitere Studien über die Entwicklung der menschlichen Placenta. Arch. Gynecol. 40:169–244, 1891.

Greig, C.: Central placenta previa with bulging bag of membranes. J. Obstet. Gynaecol. Br. Emp. 57:251–252, 1950.

Gribble, R.K., and Fitzsimmons, J.M.: Placenta previa percreta with fetal survival. Am. J. Obstet. Gynecol. 153:314–316, 1985.

Grieco, A.: Rilievi clinico-statistici sulla inserzione velamentosa ed a racchetta del cordone ombellicale. Monit. Ostet.-Ginecol. Endocrin. Metabol. 8:89–102, 1936.

Grimes, A.A., and Techman, T.: Legal abortion and placenta previa. Am. J. Obstet. Gynecol. 149:501–504, 1984.

Grosser, O.: Frühentwicklung, Eihautbildung und Placentation des Menschen und der Säugetiere. Bergmann, Munich, 1927.

Guha-Ray, D.K., and Hamblin, M.H.: Arthrogryposis multiplex congenita in an abdominal pregnancy. J. Reprod. Med. 18:109–112, 1977.

Gustafson, G.W., Bowman, H.E., and Stout, F.E.: Extrauterine pregnancy at term. Obstet. Gynecol. 2:17–21, 1953.

Gustafson, H., Nordlander, S., Westin, B., and Asard, P.-E.: Placenta praevia and abruptio placentae. Acta Obstet. Gynecol. Scand. 53:235–241, 1974.

Guy, G.P., Peisner, D.P., and Timor-Tritsch, I.E.: Ultrasonographic evaluation of uteroplacental blood flow patterns of abnormally located and adherent placentas. Am. J. Obstet. Gynecol. 163:723–727, 1990.

Hallatt, J.G., and Grove, J.A.: Abdominal pregnancy: a study of twenty-one consecutive cases. Am. J. Obstet. Gynecol. 152:444–449, 1985.

Harbert, G.M., Martin, C.B., and Ramsey, E.M.: Extrachorial (circumvallate) placentas in rhesus monkeys. Am. J. Obstet. Gynecol. 108:98–104, 1970.

Harden, M.A., Walters, M.D., and Valente, P.T.: Postabortal hemorrhage due to placenta increta: a case report. Obstet. Gynecol. 75:523–526, 1990.

Harris, V.G.: Relation between placental site and length of gestation. Br. J. Obstet. Gynaecol. 82:581–584, 1975.

Hartemann, J., Dellestable, P., and Pierce, A.: L'anémie des enfants de placenta praevia. Bull. Fed. Soc. Gynecol. Fr. 14:422–424, 1962.

Hassim, A.M., Lucas, C., and Elkabbani, S.A.M.: Spontaneous uterine rupture caused by placenta percreta. B.M.J. 2:97–98, 1968.

Hata, K., Hata, T., Aoki, S., Takamori, H., Takamiya, O., and Kitao, M.: Succenturiate placenta diagnosed by ultrasound. Gynecol. Obstet. Invest. 25:273–276, 1988.

Hertig, A.T., and Gore, H.: Die Implantation, die Frühentwicklung des befruchteten Eies und ihre Störungen. In, Gynäkologie und Geburtshilfe. Vol. I. O. Käser, V.

Friedberg, K.G. Ober, K. Thomsen, and J. Zander, eds., pp. 565–584. Georg Thieme, Stuttgart, 1969.

Hertig, A.T., and Rock, J.: Searching for early fertilized human ova. Gynecol. Invest. 4:121–139, 1973.

Heuser, C.H., and Streeter, G.L.: Development of the macaque embryo. Contrib. Embryol. Carnegie Inst. 29:15–55, 1941.

Higginbottom, J., Slater, J., and Porter, G.: The low-lying placenta and dysmaturity. Lancet 1:859, 1975.

Hoffman-Tretin, J.C., Koenigsberg, M., Rabin, A., and Anyaegbunam, A.: Placenta accreta: additional sonographic observations. J. Ultrasound Med. 11:29–34, 1992.

Holzer, E., and Pickel, H.: Ausgetragene ektopische Schwangerschaft mit lebendem Kind. Zentralbl. Gynäkol. 98:52–55, 1976.

Hoogland, H.J., deHaan, J., and Martin, C.B.: Placental size during early pregnancy and fetal outcome: A preliminary report of a sequential ultrasonographic study. Am. J. Obstet. Gynecol. 138:441–443, 1980.

Hornstein, M.D., Niloff, J.M., Snyder, P.F., and Frigoletto, F.D.: Placenta percreta associated with a second-trimester pregnancy termination. Am. J. Obstet. Gynecol. 150:1002–1003, 1984.

Hreshchyshyn, M.M., Bogen, B., and Loughran, C.H.: What is the actual present-day management of the placenta in late abdominal pregnancy? Am. J. Obstet. Gynecol. 81:302–317, 1961.

Huntington, K.M.: Foetal cells in antepartum haemorrhage. Lancet 2:682, 1968.

Hurley, V.A., and Beischer, N.A.: Placenta membranacea: case reports. Br. J. Obstet. Gynaecol. 94:798–802, 1987.

Iffy, L.: Contribution to the etiology of placenta previa. Am. J. Obstet. Gynecol. 83:969–975, 1962.

Irving, F.C., and Hertig, A.T.: A study of placenta accreta. Surg. Gynecol. Obstet. 64:178–200, 1937.

Iyasu, S., Saftlas, A.K., Rowley, D.L., Koonin, L.M., Lawson, H.W., and Atrash, H.K.: The epidemiology of placenta previa in the United States, 1979 through 1987. Am. J. Obstet. Gynecol. 168:1424–1429, 1993.

Janovski, N.A., and Granowitz, E.T.: Placenta membranacea: report of a case. Obstet. Gynecol. 18:206–212, 1961.

Johnson, W.D., Hughes, H.C., and Stenger, V.G.: Placenta extrachorialis in the stumptailed macaque (Macaca arctoides). Lab. Anim. Sci. 28:81–84, 1978.

Jopp, H., and Krone, H.: Das Verhältnis zwischen Kindesgewicht und Plazentagewicht bei Placenta praevia. Geburtshilfe Frauenheilkd. 26:403–408, 1966.

Kalchman, G.G., and Meltzer, R.M.: Interstitial pregnancy following homolateral salpingectomy. Am. J. Obstet. Gynecol. 96:1139–1143, 1966.

Kalmus, H.: The incidence of placenta praevia and antepartum haemorrhage according to maternal age and parity. Ann. Eugen. 13:283–290, 1947.

Keeler, F.J., and Cope, P.H.: Placenta of unusual shape. Obstet. Gynecol. 22:679, 1963.

Kellogg, F.S.: Eight years of placenta previa at the Boston Lying-in Hospital. Med. Rec. Ann. Houston 37:502–507, 1943.

Khong, T.Y., and Robertson, W.B.: Placenta creta and placenta praevia creta. Placenta 8:399–409, 1987.

King, D.L.: Placental migration demonstrated by ultrasonography. Radiology 109:167–170, 1973.

Kingsley, S.R., and Martin, R.D.: A case of placenta praevia in an orang-utan. Vet. Rec. 104:56–57, 1979.

Kistner, R.W., Hertig, A.T., and Reid, D.E.: Simultaneously occurring placenta previa and placenta accreta. Surg. Gynecol. Obstet. 94:141–151, 1952.

Kivikoski, A.I., Martin, C., Weyman, P., Picus, D., and Giudice, L.: Angiographic arterial embolization to control hemorrhage in abdominal pregnancy: A case report. Obstet. Gynecol. 71:456–457, 1988.

Koren, Z., Zuckerman, H., and Brzezinski, A.: Placenta previa accreta with afibrinogenemia: report of 3 cases. Obstet. Gynecol. 18:138–145, 1961.

Kornblatt, M.B.: Abdominal pregnancy following a total hysterectomy: report of a case. Obstet. Gynecol. 32:488–489, 1968.

Kupferminc, M.J., Tamura, R.K., Wigton, T.R., Glassenberg, R., and Socol, M.L.: Placenta accreta is associated with elevated maternal serum alpha-fetoprotein. Obstet. Gynecol. 82:266–269, 1993.

Lademacher, D.S., Vermeulen, R.C.W., Harten, J.J.v.d., and Arts, N.F.: Circumvallate placenta and congenital anomalies. Lancet 1:732, 1981.

Larks, S.D., Dasgupta, K., Assali, N.S., and Morton, D.G.: The human electrohysterogram: electrical evidence for the existence of pacemaker function in the parturient uterus. J. Obstet. Gynaecol. Br. Emp. 66:229–238, 1959.

Las Heras, J.L., Harding, P.G., and Haust, M.D.: Recurrent bleeding associated with placenta membranacea partialis: report of a case. Am. J. Obstet. Gynecol. 144:480–482, 1982.

Laufer, A., Sadovsky, A., and Sadovsky, E.: Histologic appearance of the placenta in ectopic pregnancy. Obstet. Gynecol. 20:350–353, 1962.

Lester, W.M., Bartholomew, R.A., Colvin, E.D., Grimes, W.H., Fish, J.S., and Galloway, W.H.: Role of retained placental fragments in immediate and delayed postpartum hemorrhage. Am. J. Obstet. Gynecol. 72:1214–1226, 1956.

Liepmann, W.: Beitrag der Placenta circumvallata. Arch. Gynecol. 80:439–454, 1906.

Lim, B.H., Tan, C.E., Smith, A.P.M., and Smith, N.C.: Transvaginal ultrasonography for diagnosis of placenta praevia. Lancet 1:444, 1989.

Little, W.A.: Toxaemia and placental attachment. B.M.J. 2:387, 1962.

Little, W.A., and Friedman, E.A.: Significance of the placental position: A report from the collaborative study of cerebral palsy. Obstet. Gynecol. 23:804–809, 1964.

Luke, R.K., Sharpe, J.W., and Greene, R.R.: Placenta accreta: the adherence or invasive placenta. Am. J. Obstet. Gynecol. 95:660–668, 1966.

Manyonda, I.T., and Varma, T.R.: Massive obstetric hemorrhage due to placenta previa/accreta with prior cesarean section. Int. J. Gynecol. Obstet. 34,183–186, 1991.

Martin, J.N., Sessums, J.K., Martin, R.W., Pryor, J.A., and Morrison, J.C.: Abdominal pregnancy: current concepts of management. Obstet. Gynecol. 71:549–557, 1988.

Mathews, J.: Placenta membranacea. Aust. N.Z. J. Obstet. Gynaecol. 14:45–47, 1974.

McElin, T.W., and Randall, L.M.: Intratubal term pregnancy without rupture: review of the literature and presentation of diagnostic criteria. Am. J. Obstet. Gynecol. 61:130–137, 1951.

McGowan, L.: Intramural pregnancy. J.A.M.A. 192:637–639, 1965.

McShane, P.M., Heyl, P.S., and Epstein, M.F.: Maternal and perinatal morbidity resulting from placenta previa. Obstet. Gynecol. 65:176–182, 1985.

Meyenburg, M.: Gibt es Veränderungen des Plazentasitzes im Bereich kaudaler Uterusabschnitte während der Schwangerschaft? Eine echographische Verlaufsstudie. Geburtshilfe Frauenheilkd. 36:715–721, 1976.

Meyer, R.: Zur Anatomie und Entstehung der Placenta marginata s. partim extrachorialis. Arch. Gynecol. 89:542–573, 1909.

Millar, W.G.: A clinical and pathological study of placenta accreta. J. Obstet. Gynaecol. Br. Emp. 66:353–364, 1959.

Miller, E.D.: A 2,000 gm tubal pregnancy. Am. J. Obstet. Gynecol. 156:1152–1153, 1987.

Mitchell, A.P.B., Anderson, G.S., and Russell, J.K.: Perinatal death from foetal exsanguination. B.M.J. 1:611–614, 1957.

Morgan, J.: Circumvallate placenta. J. Obstet. Gynaecol. Br. Emp. 62:899–900, 1955.

Morison, J.E.: Placenta accreta: A clinicopathologic review of 67 cases. Obstet. Gynecol. Annu. 7:107–123, 1978.

Moritz, A.R., and Douglass, M.: A study of uterine and tubal decidual reaction in tubal pregnancy: based on the histological examination of the tubes and endometria of fifty-three cases of ectopic gestation. Surg. Gynecol. Obstet. 47:785–790, 1928.

Naeye, R.L.: Placenta previa: predisposing factors and effects on the fetus and surviving infants. Obstet. Gynecol. 52:521–525, 1978.

Naftolin, F., Khudr, G., Benirschke, K., and Hutchinson, D.L.: The syndrome of chronic abruptio placentae, hydrorrhea, and circumvallate placenta. Am. J. Obstet. Gynecol. 116:347–350, 1973.

Nagy, P.S.: Placenta percreta induced uterine rupture and resulted in intraabdominal abortion. Am. J. Obstet. Gynecol. 161:1185–1186, 1989.

Nehra, P.C., and Loginsky, S.J.: Pregnancy after vaginal hysterectomy. Obstet. Gynecol. 64:735–737, 1984.

Nelp, W.B., and Larson, S.M.: Diagnosis of placenta praevia by photoscanning with albumin labeled with technetium Tc 99m. J.A.M.A. 200:158–162, 1967.

Niebyl, J.R.: Pregnancy following total hysterectomy. Am. J. Obstet. Gynecol. 119:512–515, 1974.

Nielsen, T.F., Hagberg, H., and Ljungblad, U.: Placenta previa and antepartum hemorrhage after previous cesarean section. Gynecol. Obstet. Invest. 27:88–90, 1989.

Nieminen, U., and Klinge, E.: Placenta praevia and low implantation of the placenta. Acta Obstet. Gynecol. Scand. 42:339–357, 1963

Nordlander, S., Sundberg, B., Westin, B., and Asard, P.-E.: Scintigraphic studies of uterine and placental growth and placental migration during pregnancy. Acta Obstet. Gynecol. Scand. 56:483–486, 1977.

Norén, H., and Lindblom, B.: A unique case of abdominal pregnancy: what are the minimal requirements for placental contact with the maternal vascular bed? Am. J. Obstet. Gynecol. 155:394–396, 1986.

O'Connell, C.P.: Full-term tubal pregnancy. Am. J. Obstet. Gynecol. 63:1305–1311, 1952.

Oppenheimer, L.W., Mackenzie, F., Girard, J., Dabrowski, A., and Yossef, E.: Migration rate of low lying placenta in the third trimester—can it predict outcome? [abstract 309]. Am. J. Obstet. Gynecol. 170:361, 1994.

Orsini, A.: La sede della placenta nella specie umana. Riv. Ital. Ginecol. 8:19–63, 1928.

Oyer, R., Tarakjian, D., Lev-Toaff, A., Friedman, A., and Chatwani, A.: Treatment of cervical pregnancy with methotrexate. Obstet. Gynecol. 71:469–471, 1988.

Paintin, D.B.: Abdominal pregnancy carried to term following the treatment of pelvic tuberculosis. Proc. R. Soc. Med. 63:54–55, 1970.

Palti, Z., Rosenn, B., Goshen, R., Ben-Chitrit, A., and Yagel, S.: Successful treatment of a viable cervical pregnancy with methotrexate. Am. J. Obstet. Gynecol. 161:1147–1148, 1989.

Pauerstein, C.J., Croxatto, H.B., Eddy, C.A., Ramzy, I., and Walters, M.D.: Anatomy and pathology of tubal pregnancy. Obstet. Gynecol. 67:301–308, 1986.

Penrose, L.S.: Maternal age, order of birth and developmental abnormalities. J. Ment. Sci. 85:1141–1150, 1939.

Philippe, E., Ritter, J., Lefakis, P., Laedlein-Greilsammer, D., Itten, S., and Foussereau, S.: Grossesse tubaire, ovulation tardive et anomalie de nidation. Gynecol. Obstet. (Paris) 69:617–628, 1970.

Radcliffe, P.A., Sindelair, P.J., and Zeit, P.R.: Vasa previa with marginal placenta previa of an accessory lobe: report of a case. Obstet. Gynecol. 16:472–475, 1961.

Rahman, M.S., Al-Suleiman, S.A., Rahman, J., and Al-Sibai, M.H.: Advanced abdominal pregnancy: observations in 10 cases. Obstet. Gynecol. 59:366–372, 1982.

Read, J.A., Cotton, D.B., and Miller, F.C.: Placenta accreta: changing clinical aspects and outcome. Obstet. Gynecol. 56:31–33, 1980.

Rice, J.P., Kay, H.H., and Mahony, B.S.: The clinical significance of uterine leiomyomas in pregnancy. Am. J. Obstet. Gynecol. 160:1212–1216, 1989.

Ries, K.J., and Middleton, E.B.: Rupture of septate uterus due to placenta percreta. Obstet. Gynecol. 39:705–712, 1972.

Ringrose, C.A.: Placenta previa in association with an incompetent cervix. Am. J. Obstet. Gynecol. 124:659, 1976.

Rizos, N., Doran, T.A., Miskin, M., Benzie, R.J., and Ford, J.A.: Natural history of placenta previa ascertained by diagnostic ultrasound. Am. J. Obstet. Gynecol. 133:287–291, 1979.

Rolschau, J.: Circumvallate placenta and intrauterine growth retardation. Acta Obstet. Gynecol. Scand. Suppl. 72:11–14, 1978.

Rosa, P., Ghilain, A., and Dumont, A.: Placenta praevia accreta et afibrinogénémie secondaire. Bull. Soc. R. Belge Gynecol. Obstet. 26:588–594, 1956.

Roth, L.G.: Central placenta previa due to a succenturiate lobe. Am. J. Obstet. Gynecol. 74:447–449, 1957.

Rubenstone, A.I., and Lash, S.R.: Placenta previa accreta. Am. J. Obstet. Gynecol. 87:198–202, 1963.

Schaefer, O.: Familial occurrence of abnormal placentation and fetal malformations, observed in Baffin Island Eskimos. Can. Med. Assoc. J. 83:437–438, 1960.

Schatz, F.: Die Gefässverbindungen der Placentarkreisläufe eineiiger Zwillinge, ihre Entwicklung und ihre Folgen. Arch. Gynecol. 27:1–72, 1886.

Schellong, G.: Anämie und Schock beim Neugeborenen durch fetalen Blutverlust. Monatsschr. Kinderheilkd. 117:578–579, 1969.

Schmitt, R., and Dittrich, A.: Ausgetragene Extrauteringravidität bei lebendem Kind. Zentralbl. Gynakol. 95:28–31, 1973.

Schmitz, H.E., O'Dea, N.J., and Isaacs, J.H.: Placenta previa: A survey at the Lewis Memorial Maternity Hospital. Obstet. Gynecol. 3:3–10, 1954.

Scipiades, E., and Burg, E.: Über die Morphologie der menschlichen Placenta mit besonderer Rücksicht auf unsere eigenen Studien. Arch. Gynecol. 141:577–619, 1930.

Scott, J.S.: Placenta extra-chorialis (placenta marginata and circumvallata): a factor in antepartum haemorrhage. J. Obstet. Gynaecol. Br. Emp. 67:904–918, 1960.

Scott, J.: Ante-partum haemorrhage-2. B.M.J. 1:1231–1234, 1964.

Shanklin, D.R.: The human placenta: a clinicopathologic study. Obstet. Gynecol. 11:129–138, 1958.

Shapiro, J.L., Sherer, D.M., Hurley, J.T., Metlay, L.A., and Amstey, M.S.: Postpartum ultrasonographic findings associated with placenta accreta . Am. J. Obstet. Gynecol. 167:601–601, 1992.

Shott, R.J., Cook, L.N., and Andrews, B.F.: Intra-abdominal pregnancy: an unusual cause of fetal growth retardation. Am. J. Dis. Child. 126:361–362, 1973.

Silber, S.J., Breakey, B., Campbell, D., Williams, H., and Fellman, S.: Placenta percreta invading bladder. J. Urol. 109:615–618, 1973.

Spanta, R., Roffman, L.E., Grissom, T.J., Newland, J.R., and McManus, B.M.: Abdominal pregnancy: magnetic resonance identification with ultrasonographic follow-up of placental involution. Am. J. Obstet. Gynecol. 157:887–889, 1987.

Spiegelberg, O.: Zur Casuistik der Ovarialschwangerschaft. Arch. Gynecol. 13:73–79, 1878.

Spinnato, J.A., Aksel, S., and Mendenhall, H.W.: Postpartum polyhydramnios: a unique complication of advanced pregnancy. Obstet. Gynecol. 70:490–492,1987.

St. Clair, J.T., Wheeler, D.A., and Fish, S.A.: Methotrexate in abdominal pregnancy. J.A.M.A. 208:529–531, 1969.

Strassmann, P.: Placenta praevia. Arch. Gynecol. 67:112–275, 1902.

Stromme, W.B.: Placenta increta: report of a case with unusual etiology. Obstet. Gynecol. 21:133–135, 1963.

Sumawong, V., Nondasuta, A., Thanapath, S., and Budthimedhee, V.: Placenta accreta: a review of the literature and a summary of 10 cases. Obstet. Gynecol. 27:511–516, 1966.

Sunde, A.: Advanced extrauterine pregnancy. Acta Obstet. Gynecol. Scand. 44:159–162, 1965.

Suzuki, K.: Concomitant occurrence of circumvallate placenta with single disc and bidiscoid placentas. Am. J. Obstet. Gynecol. 110:1147–1148, 1971.

Taefi, P., Kaiser, T.F., Sheffer, J.B., Courey, N.G., and Hodson, J.M.: Placenta percreta with bladder invasion and massive hemorrhage: report of a case. Obstet. Gynecol. 36:686–687, 1970.

Tatum, H.J., and Mulé, J.G.: Placenta previa: a functional classification and a report on 408 cases. Am. J. Obstet. Gynecol. 93:767–774, 1965.

Thomas, J.: Der gestielte Plazentarkotyledo—eine Bauanomalie der Nachgeburt. Zentralbl. Gynäkol. 84:684–690, 1962.

Thorp, J.M., Councell, B., Sandridge, D.A., and Wiest, H.H.: Antepartum diagnosis of placenta previa percreta by magnetic resonance imaging. Obstet. Gynecol. 80:506–508, 1992.

Tisdall, L., Nichols, R.A., and Sicuranza, B.J.: Abdominal pregnancy associated with an intrauterine contraceptive device . Am. J. Obstet. Gynecol. 106:937–939, 1970.

Torpin, R.: Classification of human pregnancy based on depth of intrauterine implantation of the ovum. Am. J. Obstet. Gynecol. 66:791–800, 1953.

Torpin, R.: Placenta circumvallata and placenta marginata. Obstet. Gynecol. 6:277–284, 1955.

Torpin, R.: Human placental anomalies: etiology, evolution and historical background. Mo. Med. 55:353–357, 1958.

Torpin, R.: An explanation of placental marginal infarct rings: a significant summary of a life-long evaluation of a concept of placental formation. J. Med. Assoc. Ga. 54:274–276, 1965.

Torpin, R.: Evolution of a placenta circumvallata. Obstet. Gynecol. 27:98–101, 1966.

Torpin, R.: Placentation in the rhesus monkey (Macaca mulatta). Obstet. Gynecol. 34:410–413, 1969a.

Torpin, R.: The Human Placenta. Its Shape, Form, Origin and Development. Charles C Thomas, Springfield, IL, 1969b.

Torpin, R., and Barfield, W.E.: Placenta duplex. J. Med. Assoc. Ga. 57:78–80, 1968.

Torpin, R., and Hart, B.F.: Placenta bilobata. Am. J. Obstet. Gynecol. 42:38–49, 1941.

Van Huysen, W.T.: Placenta previa of a succenturiate lobe. N. Engl. J. Med. 265:284–286, 1961.

Vierhout, M.E., and Wallenburg, H.C.S.: Intraligamentary pregnancy resulting in a live infant. Am. J. Obstet. Gynecol. 152:878–879, 1985.

Weckstein, L.N., Masserman, J.S.H., and Garite, T.J.: Placenta accreta: a problem of increasing clinical significance. Obstet. Gynecol. 69:480–482, 1987.

Wentworth, P.: Circumvallate and circummarginate placentas. Am. J. Obstet. Gynecol. 102:44–47, 1968.

Wewer, U.W., Faber, M., Liotta, L.A., and Albrechtsen, R.: Immunochemical and ultrastructural assessment of the nature of the pericellular basement membrane of human decidual cells. Lab. Invest. 53:624–633, 1986.

Wexler, P., and Gottesfeld, K.R.: Second trimester placenta previa: an apparently normal placentation. Obstet. Gynecol. 50:706–709, 1977.

Wexler, P., and Gottesfeld, K.R.: Early diagnosis of placenta previa. Obstet. Gynecol. 54:231–234, 1979.

Wickster, G.Z.: Posthemorrhagic shock in the newborn. Am. J. Obstet. Gynecol. 63:524–537, 1952.

Wiener, A.S.: Diagnosis and treatment of anemia of the newborn caused by occult placental hemorrhage. Am. J. Obstet. Gynecol. 56:717–722, 1948.

Willemen, D.F.W., Bol, J.J., Unnik, A.J.M., and Breda, A.T.: Een voldragen tubaire Zwangerschap. Nederl. Tijdschr. Geneesk. 109:2339–2341, 1965.

Williams, J.W.: Placenta circumvallata. Am. J. Obstet. Gynecol. 13:1–16, 1927.

Williams, P.C., Malvar, T.C., and Kraft, J.R.: Term ovarian pregnancy with delivery of a live female infant. Am. J. Obstet. Gynecol. 142:589–591, 1982.

Wilson, D., and Paalman, R.J.: Clinical significance of circumvallate placenta. Obstet. Gynecol. 29:774–778, 1967.

Wingate, M.B., and Pauls, F.: Effect of the placental site on fetal presentation at term. Can. Med. Assoc. J. 99:531–532, 1968.

Winters, R.: Die Rolle regressiver Veränderungen der Plazenta bei der sogenannten Plazentamigration. Geburthilfe Frauenheilkd. 38:1093–1098, 1978.

Wolf, H., Oosting, H., and Treffers, P.E.: Placental volume measurements by ultrasonography: evaluation of the method. Am. J. Obstet. Gynecol. 156:1191–1194, 1979.

Woolam, G.I., Pratt, J.H., and Wilson, R.B.: Uterine rupture following tubal implantation: report of 2 cases. Obstet. Gynecol. 29:415–419, 1967.

Young, G.B.: The peripatetic placenta. Radiology 128:183–188, 1978.

Yu, T.J., Iwasaki, I., Teratani, T., Tanaka, T., and Aoki, M.: Primary ovarian pregnancy in a cystic teratoma. Obstet. Gynecol. 64:52s–54s, 1984.

Zabrieskie, J.R.: Pregnancy and the malformed uterus. West. J. Surg. Obstet. Gynecol. 70:293–296, 1962.

Zelop, C., Nadel, A., Frigoletto, F.D., Pauker, S., MacMillan, M., and Benacerraf, B.R.: Placenta accreta/percreta/increta: A cause of elevated maternal serum alpha-fetoprotein. Obstet. Gynecol. 80:693–694, 1992.

Ziel, H.A.: Circumvallate placenta, a cause of antepartum bleeding, premature delivery, and perinatal mortality. Obstet. Gynecol. 22:798–802, 1963.

Zilliacus, H.: The detection of foetal blood in haemorrhage of late pregnancy. Gynaecologia 157:103–109, 1964.

15
Histopathological Approach to Villous Alterations

Microscopic Evaluation

Evaluation of the placental villous tissue during routine evaluation of the placenta is important in order to gain an overall understanding of the normalcy of the placenta and to ascertain possible disorders. If the villous structure is abnormal, it helps to direct one's attention to certain pregnancy disturbances that may require further study.

In addition, one needs to consider the influence of the method of fixation on the villous structure. Different fixatives produce different histological appearances with which one must be familiar. Moreover, the rapidity of fixation is important if such features as edema are to be evaluated properly. All these findings are crucial for a proper microscopic evaluation of villous tissue, which is peculiarly subject to artifacts.

The placental examination can then lead to significant insight as to the pathogenesis of many disorders. Salafia et al. (1992) found, for instance, an excellent correlation of various features with intrauterine growth retardation (IUGR). Importantly, the associated or causative villous pathology were chronic villitis, infarcts, so-called hemorrhagic endovasculitis, and thromboses. In their quantitative study of placentas from undefined growth-retarded newborns and appropriate controls, Wong and Latour (1966) found only minor changes that would not allow characterization by ordinary microscopy. It was possible to show only that the placentas of growth-retarded neonates have a reduced villous surface area when quantitative measurements of villi and trophoblast were made. Since then, however, a much better understanding of IUGR has been gained, and one cannot help but believe that the cases these authors studied had a mixed etiology. Likewise, one must then presume that the placental changes might differ markedly.

Such scrutiny presupposes a considerable familiarity with the normal structure of the placenta and that sufficient tissue samples have been collected for this study.

For instance, it must be appreciated that the center of a placental lobule differs in its villous appearance from that of the lobular periphery. In the central areas and under the chorion the villi are more widely separated, and they may have an appearance different from that of the villi at the periphery of a lobule. This organization of the "placentone," as the German histologists have named this area (Schuhmann, 1981) is particularly well shown in Figure 24 of Becker and Röckelein (1989). Misinterpretation of that feature alone may lead to an assessment of so-called dysmaturity of villi. Altshuler and Herman (1989) characterized villous dysmaturity thus: "Third trimester placentas that have large villi with numerous stromal cells, a lack of syncytiotrophoblast, and syncytiotrophoblastic knots . . . examples are chorangiosis, diabetes, and immunohemolytic anemia." It must be said, however, that there is no unifying hypothesis to define, let alone explain, "dysmaturity." We prefer not to use this term at all because it is not specific enough. Rather, we employ the term villous maldevelopment to mean similar abnormalities in structure when no specific cause is apparent. What is meant is that the villous architecture is admixed; there are perhaps mature villi mixed with edematous or hypercellular immature villi, scarred avascular villi with chorangiosis (Figures 291, 294, 296), and so on. Dysmaturity is not a precise diagnosis, and it would be better to describe the abnormality specifically rather than to use the ill-defined term dysmaturity.

Assessment of Villous Maturation

Other considerations concerning errors in villous development have been summarized by Vogel (1992). He suggested that these maturational disturbances occur as often as in 25% of otherwise normal placentas, albeit in only confined, small areas of the placentone. Most did not have a known fetal impact, although their frequency was much increased in problem pregnancies. Because

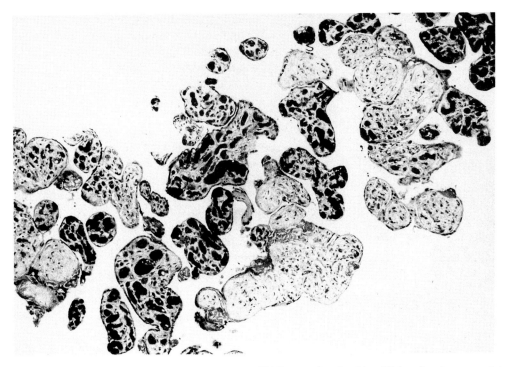

FIGURE 291. Chorangiosis (grade 2, according to Altshuler, 1984) associated with villitis of unknown origin. H&E. ×90. (Courtesy Dr. G. Altshuler, Oklahoma City.)

there exists no uniform, agreed-upon terminology, Vogel (1992) produced a table (see below) that may be helpful.

The term "placental dysfunction" was perhaps first used by Clifford (1954), when he described the features of *postmature gestations*. He suggested that postmature delivery occurred then as often as in 5% of gestations, and he indicated that the perinatal mortality increased after term significantly. He was emphatic that much of this mortality reflected intrauterine fetal demise and suggested that it resulted from the supposed decrease of placental function. Clifford addressed fetal function but had little to say about placental findings. The meconium discharge, deficient water transfer, and meconium aspiration seem to have been the principal aspects of postmaturity he considered, although oxygen deficiency was

Becker (1981)	Schweikhart (1985)	Kloos & Vogel (1974)	Vogel (1984)
Normal maturation	Synchronous maturation	Mature, age-corresponding	Mature gestation, age-appropriate
Delayed maturation		Discontinuous vascularization	Dissociated villous maturation, mostly mature
Retarded maturation	Terminal villi deficiency	Concordant retarded villi	Dissociated villous maturation, mostly immature
Arrested maturation	Persisting immaturity	Persisting embryonal structure	Arrest of villous maturation
Premature maturation	Asynchronous postterm maturity	Premature maturation	Villous premature maturation
Chorioangiosis		Chorangiomatosis	Chorangiosis, type I
Pseudochorioangiosis		Angiomatosis	Chorangiosis, type II
Chorioangiomatosis		Chorangiosis	

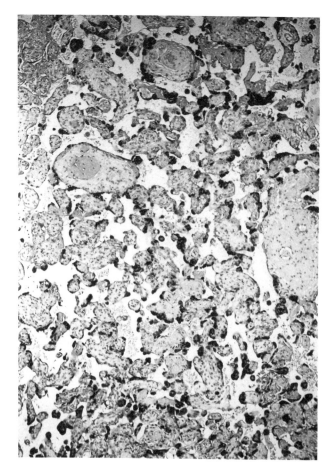

FIGURE 292. "Tenney-Parker changes" at 25 weeks' gestation. This placenta is from a preeclamptic pregnancy and shows features of accelerated maturation. Large numbers of syncytial knots (Tenney-Parker) are present everywhere. H&E. ×64.

inferred. From the pathologist's point of view there are no truly characteristic histological findings that allow one to make the diagnosis of postmaturity in placental examination.

The term accelerated maturation (Figure 292) has often been used, but it is not synonymous with postmaturity. Another term, maturitas praecox placentae, was used by Becker (1960) to indicate that some villous features indicated more development than expected for the gestational age. Naeye (1992) made the point that this concept of accelerated maturation has often led to confusion and that it is difficult to define precisely. Statistically speaking, the truly postmature placenta is more calcified, but because not all postmature placentas have an excess of calcification it is a difficult parameter to judge. They are also more frequently meconium stained, and they more often have chorioamnionitis (Naeye, 1992), although not all are so altered. The villi may appear to be slightly more cellular but they are not

characteristically so changed, and immature intermediate villi are usually absent (see Chapter 4). For these reasons we summarize much of the villous maturation at the end of this chapter.

Abnormal-appearing villi occur frequently in *prematurely delivered placentas* of abnormal pregnancies, especially in those of preeclamptic women. They primarily manifest as an increase of syncytial knots, smaller villi, and perhaps an increase in the cross sections of capillary lumens. Despite the subtle and irregular changes, however, there are no uniform changes that characterize premature villous tissue precisely. Schweikhart et al. (1986) were impressed with the proliferation of terminal villi in premature placentas, likening their architecture to bonsai trees; they found hypermature placentas as frequently as in 43% of placentas delivered between 29 and 32 weeks.

Placental Insufficiency

The term placental insufficiency is a difficult one to define precisely. One might expect that placental weight bears on this question, and placental weight has often been used to suggest that the placental function is "adequate" or "insufficient." Ratios to fetal weight have then been used to correlate placental function. Sinclair (1948) found the placental weight to increase linearly as gestation progresses; he was unable to account for the great microscopic variability among placentas. He indicated also that birth weights were lower when a marginal insertion of the umbilical cord was present, a feature that is often neglected in published studies as the cord insertion is usually not recorded.

Garrow and Hawes (1971) examined the proposition of placental weight increases in some detail. They showed that after 42 weeks there was no accumulation of structural proteins in the placenta but that the increasing weight resulted from pooling of fetal blood, a variable that also needs to be carefully controlled for meaningful analysis. After much effort at quantitative analysis they concluded that studies such as the ones reported are "a laborious task, and the yield of additional information is relatively small." Mayhew and colleagues (1993) assessed placental growth from 12 weeks to term and demonstrated linear growth by "hyperplasia" rather than by ultimate hypertrophy. Generally, the weight ratio given for such comparisons is that of fetus/placenta. Normally this ratio lies between 7.0 and 7.5, but alterations of the ratio are so frequent one cannot deduce placental dysfunction from an altered ratio. It is now possible to ascertain sonographically the placental volume (thickness and circumference) and relate it to fetal growth. Perhaps more appropriate correlations will be made in the future with this modality. That these parameters are useful was impressively shown by early results of studies by Jauniaux et al. (1994).

A consideration of the entity placental insufficiency fits well into the context of this discussion. As can be imagined, we prefer not to use this term. It implies a specific *placental* disease when in fact the malady is usually due to one of a variety of factors. They include an abnormal fetal genome, chronic infection, and a large number of maternal diseases; they may also relate to the site of the placenta in the uterus. A good case in point to illuminate the semantic complexity is the discussion by Fejgin et al. (1993). These authors suggested that the low gonadotropin secretion of triploid placentas was due to placental insufficiency. A much more cogent and persuasive argument was supplied by Goshen and Hochberg (1994). They explained the secretory levels as being due to the genetic contribution in the two types of partial hydatidiform moles (PHMs), and in complete hydatidiform moles (CHMs). Thus two *maternal* genomes (in triploidy) leads to low human chorionic gonadotropin (hCG) values; two *paternal* genomes (in some cases of PHM and usually in CHM) leads to excessive secretion of this hormone because of the genetic expression of specific genes.

For somewhat different reasons, others have also spoken against the use of this all-inclusive term (Gille, 1985; Kuss, 1987), as was quoted in some detail by Vogel (1992). Conversely, Becker and Röckelein (1989) made cogent pleas to retain the term placental insufficiency. They then produced a complex tabular account of the possible causes of placental insufficiency and stated that an insufficient placenta is one in which there is a critical reduction of placental exchange membrane. This entity then encompasses all those features discussed under their special headings: preeclamptic changes, chorangiosis, tumors, avascular villi, excessive fibrin deposits, and so on. We prefer to specify and name the lesions rather than to embrace them all in the imprecise terminology of placental insufficiency.

For routine examination of the histological picture, it is important to study various areas in the placenta, as they do not all have the same appearance. For example, the peripheral edge of the placenta often has some increased fibrinoid deposition as a normal feature, and some degree of infarction may be present that is not representative of the remainder of the organ. The villi underneath the chorionic plate are also more widely spaced than those of the floor, and this anatomical difference often leads to focal coagulation that is not necessarily pathological. At the margin of the placenta, infarction and excessive fibrin deposits are common and should be considered normal events, if that is the only location of these changes.

Examination of Fetal Stem Vessels

When assessing the adequacy of villous tissue for fetal growth, it is our practice to proceed in an orderly fashion with the examination so all aspects are inspected and evaluated. We begin with the assessment of the umbilical cord and its vessels. Here it is of interest to know if the vasculature is congested, there is a sufficient amount of blood within the vessels, and, importantly, there are nucleated red blood cells (NRBCs) within the fetal blood. The presence of NRBCs is abnormal and connotes anemia or previous hypoxia of some duration. When NRBCs are found, we make it a practice to check the newborn blood smear to enumerate these cells (see Chapter 9). At this time we also examine the vessels of the umbilical cord for thrombi, inflammation, and possible meconium damage.

The vascular system is next studied in the surface of the placenta. Here the presence or absence of thrombi is carefully assessed. These frequent, important aspects of prenatal pathology are most commonly found in the veins. These surface veins are difficult to differentiate from arteries by histological study alone. Veins lie below the arteries, but it is best to identify them macroscopically. When thrombi are old, they transform ultimately into "cushions" (see Chapter 13) (De Sa, 1973), or organized thickenings of the vascular wall. It must be emphasized that some of these "cushions" are readily misinterpreted as they may represent bifurcations of vessels. The thrombi may be occlusive, and they may also calcify; this change is prominently found in cytomegalovirus (CMV) infections and also when the thrombi are old. Calcification occurs also in the walls of vessels when thrombi have been long-standing. Altshuler (1993) has stated that he finds cushions "associated with clinically diagnosed neonatal asphyxia."

More often than obliterative thrombosis one finds only mural fibrin deposits. These deposits usually betray long-standing diseases and correlate primarily with stasis from cord problems such as knots, entangling, or prolapse. Occasionally, mural thrombosis of surface veins results solely from marked twisting of the umbilical cord.

The main stem villous vessels are next inspected. It is in these vessels that, hemorrhagic endovasculitis (HEV) is most commonly seen (Sander, 1980). HEV is primarily associated with stillbirths. They represent in our opinion a postmortem or postthrombotic phenomenon; the lesion is discussed in greater detail on p. 364 and in Chapter 20.

Examination of the Fetal Capillary Bed

The number of capillaries in the terminal villi is next evaluated. They may be markedly congested when the cord has been clamped soon after delivery of the

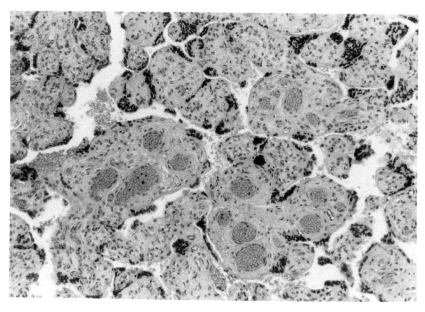

FIGURE 293. Marked congestion of villous capillaries and veins in a 30-week placenta from a preeclamptic pregnancy. There is also associated increased knotting. H&E. ×100.

neonate and also when maternal diabetes has complicated the pregnancy. Congestion as shown in Figure 293, however, must not be confused with the more ominous condition known as chorangiosis (Altshuler, 1984). The designation chorangiosis makes reference to a numerical increase of capillaries within the peripheral placental villi. Although chorangiosis can be an impressive feature, it does not relate to neoplastic changes, such as angiomas, as has been suggested. This condition is presently underrated as an indicator of chronic prenatal hypoxia. When studying the placentas of infants admitted to the neonatal intensive care unit of his hospital, Altshuler found that 5.5% had chorangiosis in their placentas. He provided criteria for the evaluation that have not yet been challenged.

What is important about chorangiosis is its relative rarity and that it is strongly correlated with perinatal mortality and a wide variety of pregnancy and placental disorders. It is definitely a pathological feature. The appearance is characteristic, and it is obvious that weeks must be required for the degree of capillary proliferation to take place that produces chorangiosis. It is perhaps for these reasons that the lesion had been termed chorangiomatosis in the past (see Chapter 24).

Chorangiosis occurs also in women who have pregnancies at high altitudes (Reshetnikova et al., 1993). That the proliferation of villous capillaries is an adaptation to chronic oxygen deficiency is further supported by the experimental results in guinea pigs described by Scheffen et al. (1990) (p. 143). They demonstrated an increase of capillaries when guinea pigs were chronically

(45 days) deprived of normal oxygen tension in their environment. This point is relevant also to the long history of placental studies at high altitude, where the smaller size of infants and placentas found has much interested investigators. Jackson and her coworkers (1987) have studied the placentas of women at high altitude in Bolivia and compared them with those at sea level. The total villous length was smaller at high altitude, whereas capillary cross sections were increased. Thus an altered capillary/villus ratio emerged as being characteristic. Kaufmann et al. (1993) had earlier shown that cytotrophoblast proliferates in the presence of hypoxia. Now they have placed it into the context of possible cytokine-regulated phenomena, perhaps regulated by villous stromal (?Hofbauer) cells. Subsequent to the villous cytotrophoblast proliferation, the syncytium increases; teleologically, perhaps it occurs in order to increase oxygen delivery to the fetus. This increase is followed by capillary endothelial proliferation, although, admittedly, mitoses were rarely found. Fibrosis is another sequela, processes that are similar to those seen with preeclampsia (see Chapter 19).

The terminal villi may lack all capillaries, markedly reducing the available exchange area, and its quantity must be estimated. Such avascular villi are commonest following chronic villitis, as with CMV infection. Next most commonly, avascular villi result from main stem and surface vessel thrombosis (Figure 294) (Altshuler & Herman, 1989). In similar degenerative events, McDermott et al. (1993) have shown that a chronic reduction of fetal blood flow precedes villous infarction.

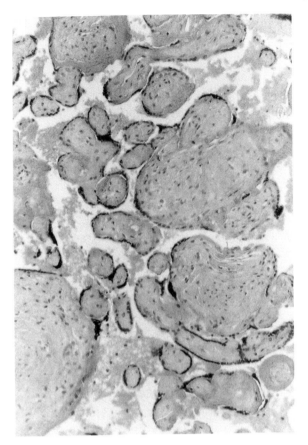

FIGURE 294. Marked fibrosis and "avascularity" of a villous district due to obliteration of a large surface vessel. Note the extremely thin trophoblastic cover of villi and pyknotic nuclei. H&E. ×160.

They suggested that siderosis of villous basement membranes, seen so prominently in cases of arterial thrombosis, was a good marker for this reduced flow. Calcifications of villous basement membranes, having a similar appearance, are discussed below. An increase in the number of villous cytotrophoblast has been observed with conditions that are related to hypoxia, for instance, anemia, preeclampsia and related disorders, and pregnancy at high altitude (see p. 78f and p. 142 for more details).

Villous Architecture and Fibrinoid

Having studied the vasculature, we prefer next to evaluate the low-power appearance of the villous architecture. It is at this time that structural abnormalities are identified that have an only focal distribution. Focal edema (Naeye et al., 1983; Shen-Schwarz et al., 1989; Naeye, 1992; Altshuler, 1993) is easiest to identify at this time, and its abundance can then be estimated. Naeye et al. (1983) had described villous edema to occur especially in placentas affected by chorioamnionitis but

believed it to correlate best with fetal hypoxia. The extent of edema also correlated with low Apgar scores and other features leading to perinatal mortality. Naeye (1992) specifically suggested that severe villous edema may interfere with oxygen delivery to the fetus by compression of capillaries within villi. Edema would also allow one to recognize possibly increased numbers of Hofbauer cells, especially in association with Rh incompatibility, chronic infections, and maternal diabetes. Focal areas of chronic villitis, especially those at the placental floor, are identified; and structurally abnormal villi are seen.

During this survey with low power inspection of the villous tissue, the maturity of villi is adjudicated, perhaps representing the most difficult task during placental examination for the novice. It must be admitted that it is often impossible to accomplish this task accurately, mostly because of preparative problems. Thus the diagnosis of postmature villi cannot easily be made correctly from villous examination alone. Maternal factors, fixation, and storage strongly affect the histological villous appearance and must be weighed. The influence of maternal conditions is perhaps best seen with preeclampsia when the reduced intervillous blood flow leads to Tenney-Parker changes (Tenney & Parker, 1940). These changes are exemplified by a diffuse increase in syncytial knotting and a decreased size of terminal villi due to lack of interstitial fluid.

An examination of the villous tissue under low power also allows one to identify irregular maturation of villi, foci of fibrosis, and the quantity of fibrin deposited. A diffuse increase of fibrin is sometimes interpreted as reflecting chronic intervillous perfusional problems (Altshuler, 1993). Alternatively, excessive fibrinoid deposition is a striking feature of the so-called maternal floor infarction syndrome (see p. 245ff). With this condition, not only is the decidual floor heavily infiltrated by "fibrinoid," this material often disseminates throughout the villous tissue and is associated with proliferation of extravillous trophoblast. The villous tissue in such cases is stiff during macroscopic study, is diffusely penetrated with gray fibrin masses (*Gitterinfarkt*), and may show many microcysts in the increased extravillous trophoblast deposits. Microscopically, the fibrin encases villi that are being strangled, consequently lack vessels, and ultimately die. It strongly correlates with IUGR and intrauterine fetal demise. Naturally, true infarcts are also noted during this survey, and their age is estimated as well (see Chapter 19).

Intervillous Space, Infarcts

Finally, the intervillous space is evaluated. Does it contain thrombi, especially underneath the chorionic plate? Are they fresh or old, and are they the possible sites of fetal bleeding? Are there tumor metastases or other abnormal features that need study with higher magnification? Are the maternal cells perhaps sickled? Subchorionic thrombi are common, as was discussed extensively in Chapter 11 (p. 242). Sonographers have often referred to the subchorionic space as being "lucent" and have speculated that sonographic lucencies are meaningful abnormalities of placentation. In most, the sonographically identified subchorionic lucencies disappear with delivery. Nevertheless, large laminated thromboses may occur in this location and can interfere with fetal development. Growth retardation, vascular compromise, and lateral expansion of these thrombi with abruptio have been described and were discussed in some detail earlier (see p. 242ff). What is not clear from the current literature is the etiology of large "thrombohematomas," as these abnormalities have been referred to. Some authors consider them to be related to abruptio placentae, whereas others have likened them to Breus' mole. We consider it possible that they are accidental expansions of the normal subchorionic thrombi that make up the fibrinous plaques of term placental surface and that arise most likely by eddying and rheological aberrations in the intervillous circulation. None of these lesions is related to the angioma, even though sonographically they may have similar appearances.

True placental infarcts result from occlusion of the maternal vascular supply. They have different qualities sonographically and are also clearly different from thromboses. They involve actual placental tissue, whereas the thromboses push the villous structures aside. There may be some infarction of villi adjacent to the thromboses, but it is not a major feature. Infarcts are generally the result of disturbances of intervillous circulation, usually secondary to obstruction of maternal arteries in the placental floor. They also accompany most abruptios. With a true infarct the trophoblast dies first, and subsequently the stroma, vessels, and all other components of the villi undergo necrosis. Initially, there is still some nuclear dusting from karyorrhexis, but eventually that disappears too. Early infarcts still possess some fetal red blood cells with hemoglobin, and they are therefore red; later the hemoglobin lyses and the infarcts turn white or yellowish. Eventually, infarcts atrophy remarkably and may focally calcify. In the adjacent villous tissue there is frequently some degree of Tenney-Parker change because of the circulatory disturbance and the ensuing local hypoxia. Virtually all infarcts have the same appearance, and it is uncommon that their microscopic evaluation makes a useful contribution to the understanding of the placental pathology. Therefore we have recommended that few of them be examined microscopically and, rather, that more non-infarcted tissue be sampled in placentas affected by infarcts. One can reliably identify infarcts macroscopi-

cally and then make a judgment as to their volumetric contribution to the whole organ.

Abruptio Placentae

More problematic is the evaluation of abruptio placentae. When it is fresh, no histopathology may be visible. The retroplacental hematoma may have the same appearance as that of the blood that normally appears after placental detachment. Older abruptios tend to compress the villous tissue, and they are then more easily identified microscopically. The blood cells are degenerating, there is laminated fibrin, pigmented macrophages may be present after a few days, and the decidua basalis is degenerated and often replaced by the hematoma. Indeed, this destruction of the decidua basalis usually makes it impossible to identify the maternal blood vessels and the atherosis or thrombosis within them that were responsible for the abruptio.

It is noteworthy that small areas of abruptio placentae are much more common than is usually stated (Benirschke & Gille, 1977). The reason is that most retroplacental hemorrhages do not produce the usually cited clinical symptomatology of sudden abdominal pain and bleeding. Their contribution to fetal well-being may also be much less significant than is that of the large retroplacental hemorrhage with detachment of a major portion of placental tissue. Because most abruptios are considered to be the result of trauma or maternal vascular disease, an assessment of the decidual spiral arterioles is desirable. In the locale of the abruption, however, it is usually impossible. The vessels here are often destroyed by the process, or they have remained behind during delivery of the placenta. One must therefore look in adjacent portions of decidua and especially in the decidua capsularis. Atherosis and thrombosis are often well displayed in these vessels. It must be cautioned that their absence is not meaningful. These lesions are often irregularly distributed; and to determine their status with certainty requires blunt curettage after delivery of the placenta. That procedure is not a favorite part of obstetrical care, and it is thus not often undertaken. It is therefore frequently impossible to rule out vascular changes as the cause of abruptions, and their etiology remains obscure.

Major Histopathological Findings

This brief survey lists the major histopathological observations that should be made during placental microscopy.

Syncytiotrophoblast

The syncytiotrophoblastic cover of the villous trees usually shows considerable variations in thickness, distribution of nuclei, and structure of nuclei. Extremely thin anuclear areas (epithelial plates) and accumulations of nuclei (syncytial knots) are arranged in a mosaic-like pattern. *Homogeneous trophoblastic thickness* and numerous Langhans' cells (villous cytotrophoblast) are found in immature placentas (Figure 46), with persisting villous immaturity, with erythroblastosis (Figure 102), and in most placentas from diabetic mothers (Figure 340).

Homogeneous trophoblastic thickness combined with loss of villous cytotrophoblast is a typical feature of "terminal villi deficiency," which is discussed in detail in Chapter 10 (Figures 103, 295). Extremely thin syncytiotrophoblast with evenly distributed pyknotic nuclei locally forming large knots (Figures 262, 294, 295) are additional important features. When they are combined with the absence of villous cytotrophoblast, it usually points to deficient fetal perfusion of the villi (e.g., fetal death, thrombosis of stem vessels). This malperfusion leads to an increased intravillous oxygen partial pressure and failure of villous cytotrophoblast to proliferate and to regenerate the syncytium (see p. 142).

Knotting of the Syncytiotrophoblast

Increased numbers of syncytial knots, sprouts, and bridges are called syncytial knotting, or Tenney-Parker changes. As discussed in Chapter 10 (p. 176f), these features have to be interpreted with care because they are influenced by the thickness of the section. Küstermann (1981), Burton (1986a,b), and Cantle et al. (1987) showed that most of these nuclear accumulations are flat sections of irregularly shaped villous surfaces. An *increased incidence of knotting* thus points to abnormal villous shapes (increased branching and bulging of villi) (see Chapter 10), and they can usually be found under hypoxic conditions. Typical clinical examples include hypertensive disorders (Alvarez et al., 1969) (Figure

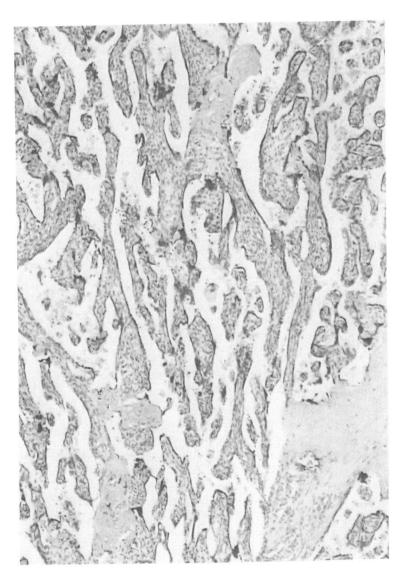

FIGURE 295. "Terminal villi deficiency" near term. Note the slender, straight sections of mature intermediate villi arranged in parallel and the absence of terminal villi with sinusoidally dilated capillaries. This feature is common in postmature placentas combined with IUGR. H&E. ×30.

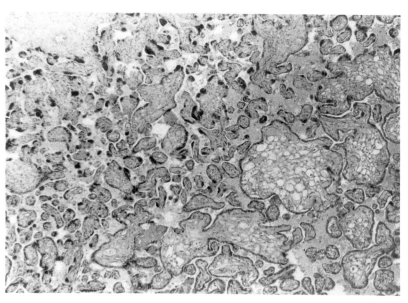

FIGURE 296. Immature placenta at 30 weeks from a patient with preeclampsia. Note the accelerated maturity (left) with numerous syncytial knots (Tenney-Parker change) associated with small terminal villi and large immature intermediate villi at right. The latter are not edematous in nature but, rather, display a reticular stroma. H&E. ×64.

296), maternal anemia (Piotrowicz et al., 1969), and pregnancy at high altitude (Jackson et al., 1987). Some cases of prolonged pregnancy (Figure 106) (Essbach & Röse, 1966; Emmrich & Mälzer, 1968) and many cases of preterm delivery (maturitas precox placentae) (Becker, 1981; Schweikhart et al., 1986) show similar features. When groups of small terminal villi with increased knotting alternate with groups of severely immature villi (Figure 296), preeclampsia is a prominent possibility (see Chapter 19).

The syncytial knots just discussed are usually concentrated in groups of terminal villi. Similar trophoblastic features around the surfaces of immature villous types (Figure 101) represent, in most cases, *villous sprouting*. Abnormal degrees of this phenomenon can be seen in moles and in several of the chromosomal aberrations (Figure 471) (Chapters 21, 22).

Langhans' Cells

The villous cytotrophoblast is difficult to identify in routine paraffin sections. Despite the fact that Langhans' cells are present at about 20% of the villous surfaces at term, one usually finds only one clearly identifiable Langhans' cell per cross section of any peripheral villus. *Lower frequencies of Langhans' cells* (fewer than one in two villous cross sections) are found in terminal villi deficiency (Schweikhart & Kaufmann, 1987) (see p. 173), in cases of IUGR that are combined with absent end-diastolic umbilical flow (Macara et al., 1994) (see p. 175), and in fetally malperfused villi (fetal death, thrombosis of stem vessels) (see p. 360ff).

In contrast, *increased numbers of Langhans' cells* (more than two per peripheral villous cross section) are usual findings in immature placentas; they also exist in the presence of "persisting immaturity" (Becker & Röckelein, 1989) (see p. 171ff), erythroblastosis (Wentworth, 1967; Pilz et al., 1980) (see Chapter 16), and maternal diabetes mellitus (Werner & Schneiderhan, 1972) (see Chapter 19). It is said that their number increases with the severity and duration of preeclampsia (Fox, 1978).

Vasculosyncytial Membranes

Vasculosyncytial membranes are the result of sinusoidal dilatation of the terminal villous capillaries, which bulge against the trophoblastic surfaces and attenuate them to thin lamellae (Figures 29, 33). The incidence is closely related to fetal villous vascularization. Immature placentas, cases of "persisting immaturity," and "terminal villi deficiency" (Figures 80, 295) (see pp. 171–174) show reduced villous capillarization and, consequently, a *paucity of vasculosyncytial membranes*.

On the other hand, increased capillarization of terminal villi is found at high altitude (Jackson et al., 1987; Reshetnikova et al., 1993) and with some other hypoxic disorders (preeclampsia, maternal heart failure, maternal anemia) (Alvarez et al., 1970, 1972; Beischer et al., 1970) (see p. 142ff). It results in an *increase of the vasculosyncytial membranes*; it can come about, of course, only when these conditions have existed for some time. In IUGR with absent end-diastolic umbilical blood flow, similar features are observed. Here, normal or possibly even increased capillarization are combined with reduced diameters of terminal villi (Macara et al., 1994). Finally, fetal villous congestion (Figure 291) can increase vasculosyncytial membranes.

Trophoblastic Basement Membrane

In routine paraffin sections of normal villi, the trophoblastic basement membrane is usually seen only when special stains are applied (aldehyde-fuchsin, periodic acid-Schiff, immunohistochemistry for collagen IV or laminin). *Marked thickening of the basement membrane* that becomes clearly visible has been described with various pathological conditions, such as preeclampsia and essential hypertension (Fox, 1968c), maternal diabetes (Liebhart, 1971, 1974), and IUGR with absent end-diastolic umbilical blood flow (Macara et al., 1994). The reason for these basement membrane changes presumably is that constituents of the basal lamina are secretory products of the villous trophoblast; the increased thickness indicates altered trophoblastic activity (e.g. increased secretion or decreased turnover of basal lamina molecules).

Perivillous Fibrinoid

Most perivillous fibrinoid is a blood clotting product (p. 94ff). It is found in defects of the villous trophoblastic cover (see p. 204) and here may act as a substitute for damaged trophoblast. The deposition of perivillous fibrinoid is a regular phenomenon, occurring in every placenta; and the amount increases with advancing pregnancy. This increase is particularly true for the stem villi, whose trophoblastic surface is largely replaced by fibrinoid at term (Figures 92, 93). One normally finds some increase of fibrin encasing larger groups of villi below the chorionic plate (subchorionic laminated fibrin, bosselation) and in the marginal zone.

Macroscopically visible deposits that embed larger parts of villous trees are abnormal. They are referred to as Gitterinfarkts (Becker & Röckelein, 1989), and increased amount of fibrinoid at the base of the placenta belong to the entity known as "maternal floor infarction," an important placental disease (see p. 245ff). By obstructing large parts of the maternofetal exchange surface they may endanger fetal growth and survival. Otherwise, disseminated perivillous fibrinoid deposition has no pathological significance (Fox, 1967).

Intravillous Fibrinoid

Intravillous fibrinoid has also been referred to as villous fibrinoid necrosis. It must not be confused with the perivillous fibrinoid just discussed. It is a fibrinoid patch that replaces villous stroma and vasculature underneath

a more or less intact trophoblastic cover (Figure 19F). It occurs occasionally in normal mature placentas, but its incidence is increased in placentas from diabetic mothers and in cases of erythroblastosis fetalis (Fox, 1968b). Its genesis has been discussed in context with immune attacks (Burstein et al., 1973).

Villous Calcification

Villous calcifications are relatively uncommon and different from the minute calcium deposits in fibrinoid that occur with advancing gestation. The latter is found mostly in the floor and septa and was discussed in Chapter 11. Villous calcification may occur when villi have been destroyed by processes of the past, such as thrombosis, CMV infection, infarction, and others (Figure 297). Calcifications of villous tissues are also observed in some retained placental fragments or when the placenta of a fetus papyraceus is retained to term. Quantitatively they may play no important role in placental pathology.

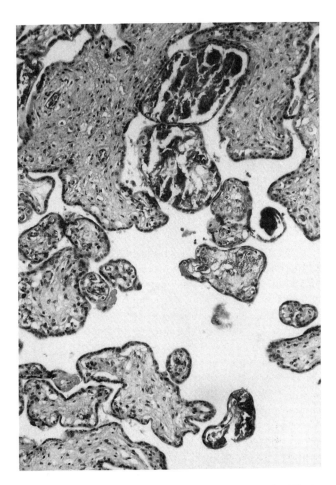

FIGURE 297. Immature placenta with degenerated villi that contain conspicuous areas of calcification (black, irregular, and fragmented intravillous foci). H&E. ×160.

An entirely different type of calcification is the finely granular deposition of purple-staining precipitate in basement membranes of abortuses. It is currently not certain that it represents calcium salts, as other salts have similar staining characteristics. This fine stippling is perhaps the result of deficient transport of materials transported through the trophoblast but not consumed after fetal death with its cessation of capillary flow. It has no known etiological role.

Stem Vessels

It was suggested that the number of arteries in peripheral stem villi is decreased in association with umbilical Doppler high resistance (Giles et al., 1985). Since then, the topic of fetal villous arteries has attracted much attention. Studies by other investigators have not corroborated this finding (Jackson et al., personal communication; Macara & Leiser, personal communication).

The most conspicuous pathological changes of fetal stem vessels comprise *thromboses*. They are common features and affect mostly superficial veins. Laminated mural thrombi are our most common finding. They result primarily from obstruction of venous return to the fetus (cord knots, spirals, prolapse), velamentous insertion, and accompany long-standing chorioamnionitis and CMV infection. The main stem vessels and further distal vascular structures may atrophy or disappear completely. Thrombosis may thus lead to complete atrophy of portions of the villous tissue (Figure 262).

Thrombosis of large arteries is less common, and usually it remains unclear what the etiology might have been. Protein C and S deficiencies have been entertained as possible causes but have never been proved. They are extremely serious for fetal development and survival.

Obliterative endarteritis (Figure 280) and especially hemorrhagic endovasculitis (HEV) (Figure 264), are prominent aspects of this area. HEV is found nearly exclusively in stillborn infants and most often results from postmortem dissolution of the large blood vessels and those of stem villi. Identical changes accompany local obliterations (velamentous vessels); there is no convincing evidence that they represent an infection (see p. 360ff).

Other vascular phenomena, such as fibromuscular sclerosis, also occur in stem vessels, primarily arteries. They have been extensively discussed by Fox (1978) and other placentologists. We see them as secondary features of vascular phenomena and usually find them in the "localized" form. It is uncommon to identify such lesions in widespread distribution. They are then related to Doppler flow anomalies and growth retardation (Fok et al., 1990), but a precise etiology has not been iden-

tified. Occlusions of this type are found after infarcts and primarily with long-standing thrombosis. Indeed, when they occur in infarcts we find it unlikely that they are "proliferative" in nature; it is more probable that they come about by the condensation of dying tissues. These obliterations are usual findings in placentas associated with fetal demise. We believe them to be secondary features because other diseases nearly always explain the fetal death.

The extensive discussion of endarteritis obliterans by Fox (1978) includes a photograph of a vessel depicting *endothelial edema*. It represents an artifact and has no relation to endarter*itis*. Similar discussions occurred in considerations of human immunodeficiency virus (HIV)-related vascular alterations (see p. 324). Indeed, the entity has been widely discussed as occurring with diabetes, preeclampsia, erythroblastosis, and other conditions. Rapid fixation and the use of Bouin's solution usually prevents "endarteritis" from being recognizable. It must also be said that the peripheral districts of so-called endarteritis are usually not disturbed, negating its importance as a primary disease of the placenta.

Nucleated Red Blood Cells

The fetal blood vessels may contain nucleated red blood cells (NRBCs). It is a normal finding in gestations of less than 3 months' duration (Figure 18C). These elements are abnormal during the last trimester, however, especially when they are identified by routine histology. They then betray the fetal response to erythropoietin, a hormone that is now frequently measured in neonates. When NRBCs are present one must enumerate them in neonatal blood smears as they rapidly decline after birth. They signify fetal anemia, infection, erythroblastosis, transplacental hemorrhage, or, importantly, prenatal hypoxia. Because it takes time for the secretion of these cells from precursor stores (liver, marrow) through the intervention of erythropoietin and perhaps other signals, the presence of NRBCs suggests that fetal tissue "hypoxia" of whatever type has occurred many hours, perhaps days, before birth. The topic is dealt with more extensively in Chapter 9 (p. 162f).

Villous Capillarization

The vasculature of villi is difficult to adjudicate, as the capillaries tend to collapse after delivery. The degree of collapse depends on the mode of delivery, the mode of cord clamping, the time elapsed between cessation of umbilical circulation and fixation, and the composition of the fixative (see Tables 9–11). Moreover, when the tissue is fixed in inadequate volumes of fixative the tissue becomes compressed. Thus asymmetrical compression or distortion of the placenta during fixation may cause considerable shifts of intravascular volume with complete collapse in one part of the fetal vascular bed and apparent overdistension in another. Therefore conclusions concerning villous capillarization must always take these potential errors into consideration.

Reduced capillarization of the terminal villous tree is a typical sign of terminal villi deficiency (Figure 100), providing it is seen in an otherwise mature placenta. This feature is always combined with a uniformly thin trophoblastic cover of the villi that has stromal fibrosis and unusually straight and parallel sections of peripheral villous branches (Figure 295) (see Chapter 10).

Complete atrophy of capillaries can be found peripheral to obstructive lesions in the stem vessels (see Chapter 13). Small groups of avascular villi are seen in every placenta (Figure 294), but a higher incidence is often combined with IUGR or intrauterine fetal death.

Hypercapillarization may show different features, some of which have already been considered. Cases of *hypoxic hypercapillarization* are usually characterized by numerous but small capillary cross sections, a feature often referred to as chorangiosis (Figures 98, 105, 291) (see Chapter 24) (Bacon et al. 1984; Jackson et al., 1985, 1988). Three-dimensional reconstruction revealed richly branched capillary nets (Scheffen et al., 1990).

One sometimes finds cases in which fewer but enormously dilated capillary cross sections occupy the villi (Figure 104). They have long, unbranched capillary loops (Figure 99) and usually exist among premature deliveries (Schweikhart et al., 1986). Salvatore (1968) has named this condition *hypermaturity*, and Becker (1981) described it as maturitas praecox. We observed the most impressive cases of this kind association with severe IUGR with absent umbilical end-diastolic blood flow (Macara et al., 1994) (p. 175; Figure 298).

These features are difficult to differentiate from *villous congestion* (Figure 293), also resulting in overdistended peripheral vessels. The loss of plasma between the erythrocytes, extravasations, and signs of hemolysis may be helpful for the diagnosis. Congestion may be the result of cord complications (see p. 350ff) and of thrombosis of major villous stem veins. Finally, we have often observed congestion in cases of premature rupture of the membranes, perhaps because of loss of amnionic fluid thus altering venous umbilical blood flow.

Stromal Architecture and Stromal Fibrosis

Fibrosis of stem villi is a good indicator of placental maturity (Figures 83–93). Fibrosis starts on about the 15th week p.m., begins around the stem vessels, and should be complete a few weeks before term (Table 13). When reticular, unfibrosed connective tissue persists under the trophoblastic membrane, as in Figures 86 and 87, it signifies immaturity.

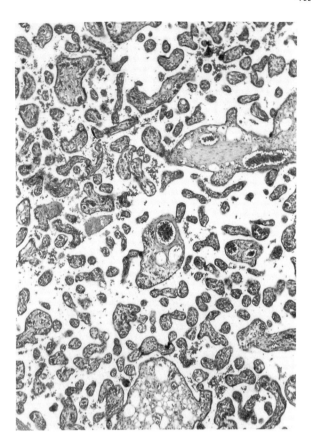

FIGURE 298. Placenta at 29 weeks' gestation associated with severe fetal growth retardation (neonatal death), showing marked accelerated maturation of the villous branches. As is typical for many cases of accelerated maturation, stem villi remain in their normal immature condition. Their appearance must not be confused with edema. H&E. ×64.

Extensive stromal fibrosis is abnormal especially when it is not restricted to the stem villi (i.e., those with media-endowed vessels). It can be found in the condition known as terminal villi deficiency (Figure 295) (Kaufmann et al., 1987), in IUGR combined with absent umbilical end-diastolic blood flow (Macara et al., 1994), in avascular villi following stem vessel obstruction (Figure 294) (Veen et al., 1982), in CMV infection, and in a few other conditions. It has been speculated that increased intravillous oxygen partial pressure stimulates collagen synthesis when it occurs in the maternally well oxygenated but fetally malperfused placenta (Fox, 1968c; for review see Kaufmann et al., 1993). In contrast, intraplacental hypoxia has been inferred to be responsible for reduced villous fibrosis (Fox, 1978), for example, unfibrosed, immature villi in preeclampsia (Figure 296).

Hofbauer Cells (Macrophages)

Hofbauer cells can easily be seen within the stromal channels of the immature intermediate villi (Figures 67,

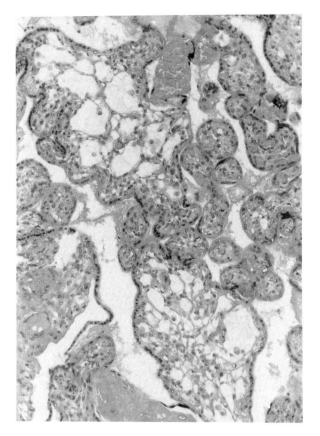

FIGURE 299. Placenta at 26 weeks' gestation from a patient with congenital epidermolysis bullosa. The villous architecture, appropriate for this gestational age, is composed of immature intermediate villi with reticular stroma surrounded by small mesenchymal villi. H&E. ×160.

72). When one uses immunohistochemical markers it becomes evident that they are present in all villous types throughout all stages of pregnancy, although they may be difficult to see. Therefore the impression of

increased numbers of Hofbauer cells is usually the result of increased numbers of immature intermediate villi. It thus points to an immature placenta or persisting immaturity in a term organ (p. 171ff). Other associations are unknown.

An apparent deficiency of macrophages is observed in moles and some chromosomal aberrations, especially in their large, pale villi that have the appearance of immature intermediate villi. In these cases, the pale stroma is loose and hydropic and does not belong to the reticular type—that with stromal channels and containing macrophages (Figures 451, 485, 497) (see Chapters 21, 22).

Inflammatory Changes

Villi may participate in infectious diseases by infiltration of mononuclear and polymorphonuclear leukocytes (polys). Polys are rarely within villi; they are commonest in the amnionic sac infection syndrome, chorioamnionitis. When polys are present within villi, it signifies an acute infectious bacterial disease. *Acute villitis* is a prominent feature of listeriosis, a disease disseminated by maternal septicemia. Other maternal bacterial infections, such as staphylococcal sepsis and other bacterial septicemias, are uncommon. They all produce abscesses in the placenta with dissolution of villous tissue.

Much the commonest placental infection recognized is that with *CMV*. The picture this virus produces is variable. When one finds plasma cells concentrated in a few villi, especially when they are accompanied by hemosiderin-laden macrophages and villous sclerosis, CMV infection is likely. One may then have to search for the typical inclusion bodies, a sometimes difficult task, or stain with immunoprobes or identify the virus with a polymerase chain reaction technique. The typical "owl-eye cells" are found in endothelium, trophoblast,

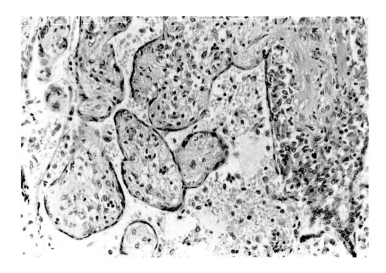

FIGURE 300. Placenta from a patient with VUE at 36 weeks' gestation. A stillborn infant resulted from this pregnancy. There is marked infiltration of chronic inflammatory cells and simultaneous destruction of villous integrity (right). H&E. ×250.

and unidentified stromal cells (Figure 419). Other chronic villitides are due to toxoplasma and syphilis; they are rarely due to rubella and other viruses (see Chapter 20).

Much the most problematic is the entity known as *villitis of unknown etiology* (VUE), which is also discussed at length in Chapter 20. With this villitis chronic inflammatory cells predominate but plasma cells and polys are generally absent. The villi may, however, disintegrate, as Figure 300 shows. VUE is frequent and has no known etiology. It may recur during subsequent gestations; and when extensive it may cause fetal death. No microorganisms have been discovered as its cause, and suggestions of the possible infiltration with maternal immunocytes are still inconclusive. They may signal immune recognition of the fetal antigen, but that is far from certain.

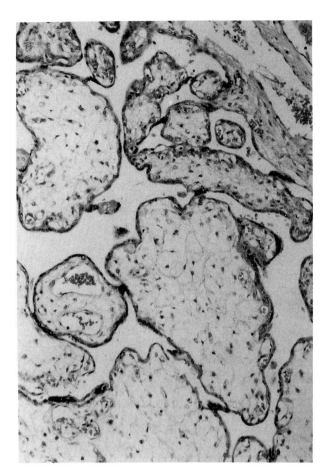

FIGURE 302. Villi of hydropic fetus with Finnish nephrosis. Most villi are severely hydropic, but they are not different from villi in placentas from other hydrops cases. Compare with Figure 301. H&E. ×160.

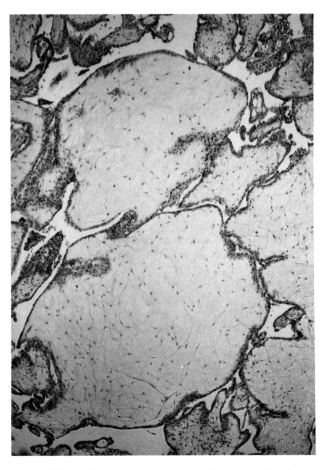

FIGURE 301. Villi in a partial hydatidiform mole due to triploidy. There is marked villous distension with edematous fluid. At first glance, this appearance is similar to that of immature intermediate villi (Figures 299, 303), but the macrophages of normal intermediate villi are lacking here. H&E. ×64.

Villous Edema or Immaturity

Many authors call every large, pale-staining villus an edematous villus following the description by Naeye et al. (1983). It is our experience that most of these villi are in fact normal immature intermediate villi (Figure 299) (Pilz et al., 1980; Kaufmann et al., 1987). They may cause diagnostic problems, as their reticular stromal core has only a weak affinity for conventional stains because they lack collagen. The resulting histological picture is that of a seemingly edematous villus that had accumulated much interstitial fluid.

True *edematous villi* indeed exist, however, as well. They are particularly impressive in hydatidiform moles and hydatid degeneration of abortion specimens (Figure 301), but some are found occasionally in conjunction with infections such as syphilis, toxoplasmosis, CMV infection, and a variety of cases of

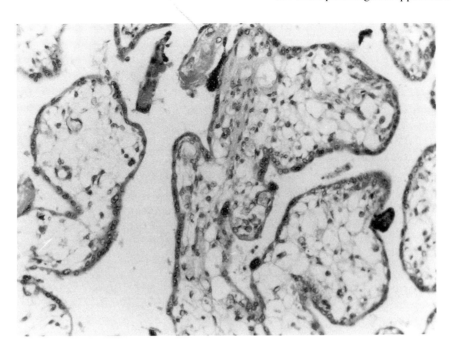

FIGURE 303. Immature placenta from a pregnancy with hydrops fetalis due to fetal endocardial fibroelastosis. The placenta shows a combination of normal immaturity with edema. The villi exhibit partly normal immature reticular stroma with an abundance of macrophages (Hofbauer cells, dark cells in reticular spaces), which is normal for immature intermediate villi. In other villi the reticular pattern is partially destroyed by various degrees of edema. H&E. ×256.

hydrops (Figure 302). Placentas from erythroblastosis and other causes of hydrops may show a combination of the two features, as most villi display a retarded maturation and many are additionally edematous (Figure 303).

Small numbers of *immature intermediate villi* are found in the centers of the villous trees in nearly every mature placenta. These are the still proliferating villi and may represent a kind of growth reserve. When they occur in disseminated fashion, or even when there is only a prevalence of this villous type, it indicates immaturity, synchronous or asynchronous. It may be found in many cases of prolonged pregnancy (Fox, 1968d; Kemnitz & Theuring, 1974; Mikolajczak et al., 1987).

References

Altshuler, G.: Chorangiosis: an important placental sign of neonatal morbidity and mortality. Arch. Pathol. Lab. Med. 108:71–74, 1984.

Altshuler, G.: Some placental considerations related to neurodevelopmental and other disorders. J. Child Neurol. 8:78–94, 1993.

Altshuler, G., and Herman, A.A.: The medicolegal imperative: placental pathology and epidemiology. In, Fetal and Neonatal Brain Injury: Mechanisms, Management and the Risk of Malpractice. D.K. Stevenson and P. Sunshine, eds., pp. 250–263. B.C. Decker, Toronto, 1989.

Alvarez, H., Morel, R.L., Benedetti, W.L., and Scavarelli, M.: Trophoblast hyperplasia and maternal arterial pressure at term. Am. J. Obstet. Gynecol. 105:1015–1021, 1969.

Alvarez, H., Benedetti, W.L., Morel, R.L., and Scavarelli, M.: Trophoblast development gradient and its relationship to placental hemodynamics. Am. J. Obstet. Gynecol. 106:416–420, 1970.

Alvarez, H., Medrano, C.V., Sala, M.A., and Benedetti, W.L.: Trophoblast development gradient and its relationship to placental hemodynamics. II. Study of fetal cotyledons from the toxemic placenta. Am. J. Obstet. Gynecol. 114:873–878, 1972.

Bacon, B.J., Gilbert, R.D., Kaufmann, P., Smith, A.D., Trevino, F.T., and Longo, L.D.: Placental anatomy and diffusing capacity in guinea pigs following long-term maternal hypoxia. Placenta 5:475–487, 1984.

Becker, V.: Über maturitas praecox placentae. Verh. Dtsch. Ges. Pathol. 44:256–260, 1960.

Becker, V.: Pathologie der Ausreifung der Plazenta. In, Die Plazenta des Menschen. V. Becker, T.H. Schiebler, and F. Kubli, eds., pp. 266–281. Thieme, Stuttgart, 1981.

Becker, V., and Röckelein, G.: Pathologie der weiblichen Genitalorgane I. Pathologie der Plazenta und des Abortes. Springer-Verlag, Heidelberg, 1989.

Beischer, N.A., Sivasamboo, R., Vohra, S., Silpisornkosal, S., and Reid, S.: Placental hypertrophy in severe pregnancy anaemia. J. Obstet. Gynaecol. Br. Commonw. 77:398–409, 1970.

Benirschke, K., and Gille, J.: Placental pathology and asphyxia. In, Intrauterine Asphyxia and the Developing Fetal Brain. L. Gluck, ed. Year Book, Chicago, 1977.

Burstein, R., Frankel, S., Soule, S.D., and Blumenthal, H.T.: Aging of the placenta: autoimmune theory of senescence. Am. J. Obstet. Gynecol. 116:271–276, 1973.

Burton, G.J.: Intervillous connections in the mature human placenta: instances of syncytial fusion or section artifacts? J. Anat. 145:13–23, 1986a.

Burton, G.J.: Scanning electron microscopy of intervillous connections in the mature human placenta. J. Anat. 147: 245–254, 1986b.

Cantle, S.J., Kaufmann, P., Luckhardt, M., and Schweikhart, G.: Interpretation of syncytial sprouts and bridges in the human placenta. Placenta 8:221–234, 1987.

Clifford, S.H.: Postmaturity—with placental dysfunction. Am. J. Obstet. Gynecol. 44:1–13, 1954.

De Sa, D.J.: Intimal cushions in foetal placental veins. J. Pathol. 110:347–352, 1973.

Emmrich, P., and Mälzer, G.: Zur Morphologie der Plazenta bei Übertragung. Pathol. Microbiol. 32:285–302, 1968.

Essbach, H., and Röse, I.: Plazenta und Eihäute. Fischer, Jena, 1966.

Fejgin, M.D., Amiel, A., Goldberger, S., Barnes, I., Zer, T., and Kohn, G.: Placental insufficiency as a possible cause of low maternal serum human gonadotropin and low maternal serum unconjugated estriol levels in triploidy. Am. J. Obstet. Gynecol. 167:766–767, 1993.

Fok, R.Y., Pavlova, Z., Benirschke, K., Paul, R.H., and Platt, L.D.: The correlation of arterial lesions with umbilical artery Doppler velocimetry in the placentas of small-for-dates pregnancies. Obstet. Gynecol. 75:578–583, 1990.

Fox, H.: Perivillous fibrin deposition in the human placenta. Am. J. Obstet. Gynecol. 98:245–251, 1967.

Fox, H.: Basement membrane changes in the villi of the human placenta. J. Obstet. Gynaecol. Br. Commonw. 75: 302–306, 1968a.

Fox, H.: Fibrinoid necrosis of placental villi. J. Obstet. Gynaecol. Br. Commonw. 75:448–452, 1968b.

Fox, H.: Fibrosis of placental villi. J. Pathol. Bacteriol. 95: 573–579, 1968c.

Fox, H.: Villous immaturity in the term placenta. Obstet. Gynecol. 31:9–12, 1968d.

Fox, H.: Pathology of the Placenta. Saunders, London, 1978.

Garrow, J.S., and Hawes, S.F.: The relationship of the size and composition of the human placenta to its functional capacity. J. Obstet. Gynaecol. Br. Commonw. 78:22–28, 1971.

Giles, W.B., Trudinger, B.J., and Baird, P.J.: Fetal umbilical artery flow velocity waveforms and placental resistance: pathological correlation. Br. J. Obstet. Gynaecol. 92: 31–38, 1985.

Gille, J.: Kritische Gedanken zur "Plazentainsuffizienz." Med. Klin. 80:148–152, 1985.

Goshen, R., and Hochberg, A.A.: The genomic basis of the β-subunit of human chorionic gonadotropin diversity in triploidy. Am. J. Obstet. Gynecol. 170:700–701, 1994.

Jackson, M.R., Joy, C.F., Mayhew, T.M., and Haas, J.D.: Stereological studies on the true thickness of the villous membrane in human term placentae: a study of placentae from high altitude pregnancies. Placenta 6:249–258, 1985.

Jackson, M.R., Mayhew, T.M., and Haas, J.D.: Morphometric studies on villi in human term placentae and the effects of altitude, ethnic grouping and sex of newborn. Placenta 8:487–495, 1987.

Jackson, M.R., Mayhew, T.M., and Haas, J.D.: On the factors which contribute to thinning of the villous membrane in human placentae at high altitude. II. An increase in the degree of peripheralization of fetal capillaries. Placenta 9: 9–18, 1988.

Jauniaux, E., Ramsay, B., and Campbell, S.: Ultrasonographic investigation of placental morphologic characteristics and size during the second trimester of pregnancy. Am. J. Obstet. Gynecol. 170:130–137, 1994.

Kaufmann, P., Luckhardt, M., Schweikhart, G., and Cantle, S.J.: Cross-sectional features and three-dimensional structure of human placental villi. Placenta 8:235–247, 1987.

Kaufmann, P., Kohnen, G., and Kosanke, G.: Wechselwirkungen zwischen Plazentamorphologie und fetaler Sauerstoffversorgung. Versuch einer zellbiologischen Interpretation pathohistologischer und experimenteller Befunde. Gynäkologe 26:16–23, 1993.

Kemnitz, P., and Theuring, F.: Makroskopische, licht und elektronenmikroskopische Plazentabefunde bei Uebertragung. Zentralbl. Allg. Pathol. 118:43–54, 1974.

Kloos, K., and Vogel, M.: Pathologie der Perinatalperiode. Thieme, Stuttgart, 1974.

Kuss, E.: Was ist "Das Plazentainsuffizienzsyndrome"? Geburtshilfe Frauenheilkd. 47:664–670, 1987.

Küstermann, W.: Über "Proliferationsknoten" und "Syncytialknoten" der menschlichen Placenta. Anat. Anz. 150: 144–157, 1981.

Liebhart, M.: The electron microscopic pattern of placental villi in diabetes of the mother. Acta Med. Pol. 12:133–137, 1971.

Liebhart, M.: Ultrastructure of the stromal connective tissue of normal placenta and of placenta in diabetes mellitus of mother. Pathol. Eur. 9:177–184, 1974.

Macara, L., Kingdom, J.C.P., Hair, J., More, I.A.R., Lyall, F., Kohnen, G., Greer, I.A., and Kaufmann, P.: Ultrastructure of placental terminal villi from pregnancies complicated by intrauterine growth retardation. (1994, submitted).

Mayhew, T.M., Wadrop, E., and Simpson, R.A.: Growth of villous sub-compartments in human placenta from 12 weeks to term. Placenta 14:A49, 1993.

McDermott, M., O'Malley, F., and Gillan, J.E.: Chronic reduction of fetal blood flow precedes placental infarction. Mod. Pathol. [abstract 34]. 6:6P, 1993.

Mikolajczak, J., Ruhrberg, A., Fetzer, M., Kaufmann, P., and Goecke, C.: Irreguläre Zottenreifung bei Frühgeburtlichkeit und Übertragung, und ihre Darstellbarkeit im Ultraschall. Gynäkol. Rundsch. 27:145–146, 1987.

Naeye, R.L.: Disorders of the Placenta, Fetus, and Neonate. Diagnosis and Clinical Significance. Mosby Year Book, St. Louis, 1992.

Naeye, R.L., Maisels, J., Lorenz, R.P., and Botti, J.J.: The clinical significance of placental villous edema. Pediatrics 71:588–594, 1983.

Pilz, I., Schweikhart, G., and Kaufmann, P.: Zur Abgrenzung normaler, artefizieller und pathologischer Strukturen in reifen menschlichen Plazentazotten. III. Morphometrische

Untersuchungen bei Rh-Inkompatibilität. Arch. Gynecol. Obstet. 229:137–154, 1980.

Piotrowicz, B., Niebroj, T.K., and Sieron, G.: The morphology and histochemistry of the full term placenta in anaemic patients. Folia Histochem. Cytochem. 7:436–444, 1969.

Reshetnikova, O.S., Burton, G.J., and Milovanov, A.P.: Hypoxia at altitude and villous vascularisation in the mature human placenta [abstract]. Placenta 14:A62, 1993.

Salafia, C.M., Vintzileos, A.M., Silberman, L., Bantham, K.F., and Vogel, C.A.: Placental pathology of idiopathic intrauterine growth retardation at term. Am. J. Perinatol. 9:179–184, 1992.

Salvatore, C.A.: The placenta in acute toxemia: a comparative study. Am. J. Obstet. Gynecol. 102:347–353, 1968.

Sander, C.H.: Hemorrhagic endovasculitis and hemorrhagic villitis of the placenta. Arch. Pathol. Lab. Med. 104: 371–373, 1980.

Scheffen, I., Kaufmann, P., Philippens, L., Leiser, R., Geisen, C., and Mottaghy, K.: Alterations of the fetal capillary bed in the guinea pig placenta following long-term hypoxia. Adv. Exp. Med. Biol. 277:779–790, 1990.

Schuhmann, R.: Plazenton: Begriff, Entstehung, funktionelle Anatomie. In, Die Plazenta des Menschen. V. Becker, T.H. Schiebler, and F. Kubli, eds., pp. 192–207. Thieme, Stuttgart, 1981.

Schweikhart, G.: Morphologie des Zottenbaumes der menschlichen Plazenta—Orthologische und pathologische Entwicklung und ihre klinische Relevanz. Thesis, Medical Faculty, University of Mainz, 1985.

Schweikhart, G., and Kaufmann, P.: Endzottenmangel und klinische Relevanz. Gynäkol. Rundsch. 27(suppl. 2): 147–148, 1987.

Schweikhart, G., Kaufmann, P., and Beck, T.: Morphology of placental villi after premature delivery and its clinical relevance. Arch. Gynecol. 239:101–114, 1986.

Shen-Schwarz, S., Ruchelli, E., and Brown, D.: Villous oedema of the placenta: a clinicopathological study. Placenta 10:297–307, 1989.

Sinclair, J.G.: Significance of placental and birthweight ratios. Anat. Rec. 102:245–258, 1948.

Tenney, B., and Parker, F.: The placenta in toxemia of pregnancy. Am. J. Obstet. Gynecol. 39:1000–1005, 1940.

Veen, F., Walker, S., and Fox, H.: Endarteritis obliterans of the fetal stem arteries of the human placenta: an electron microscopic study. Placenta 3:181–190, 1982.

Vogel, M.: Pathologie der Schwangerschaft, der Plazenta und des Neugeborenen. In, Pathologie. Vol. 3. W. Remmele, ed. Springer-Verlag, Heidelberg, 1984.

Vogel, M.: Atlas der Morphologischen Plazentadiagnostik. Springer-Verlag, Heidelberg, 1992.

Wentworth, P.: The placenta in cases of hemolytic disease of the newborn. Am. J. Obstet. Gynecol. 98:283–289, 1967.

Werner, C., and Schneiderhan, W.: Plazentamorphologie und Plazentafunktion in Abhaengigkeit von der diabetischen Stoffwechselfuehrung. Geburtshilfe Frauenheilkd. 32:959–966, 1972.

Wong, T.-C., and Latour, J.P.A.: Microscopic measurement of the placental components in an attempt to assess the malnourished newborn infant. Am. J. Obstet. Gynecol. 94: 942–950, 1966.

16
Erythroblastosis Fetalis and Hydrops Fetalis

ERYTHROBLASTOSIS FETALIS

Erythroblastosis fetalis, or hemolytic disease of the newborn, is a condition caused by specific antibodies of the mother directed against red blood cell antigens of the fetus. They are largely Rh-(D) antigens, but rare cases of sensitization against other antigens (e.g., Kell), and ABO incompatibility with fetal hemolytic disease have been described. Leventhal and Wolf (1956) have presented Kell isoimmunization as a cause of fatal erythroblastosis (EF). This form was also found in the well illustrated case of Ivemark et al. (1959). Anti-K antibodies usually arise as a result of transfusion, and the fetal disease is usually mild. Of 194 pregnancies complicated by this antibody constellation, only 16 affected babies were identified, of which 3 were severely affected by hemolytic disease (Leggat et al., 1991). The difficulty in this situation is the identification of the pregnancies at risk, an aspect discussed in some detail in an Editorial (1991). Anti-K hemolytic disease does not differ pathologically from the erythroblastosis caused by anti-D. Relatively few cases of typical, severe EF have been described as being due to ABO incompatibility. These cases are summarized by Freda and Carter (1962), and a fatal case is delineated in the paper by Miller and Petrie (1963); but usually the hemolytic disease of ABO incompatibility is mild. The pathological findings of infant and placenta are the same as those in EF due to Rh incompatibility; in the case described by Miller and Petrie, the placenta weighed 900 g and had typical features of erythroblastosis. Other types of hemolysis occur that produce similar pathological features of infant and placenta. Thus hemolysis in fetal blood may rarely result because of glucose-6-phosphate dehydrogenase (G-6-PD) deficiency, virus infection, or for other uncommon reasons. These causes of fetal hemolysis must be differentiated from the classical erythroblastosis.

As RhoGam prophylaxis (Mittendorf & Williams, 1991) has become more widespread, the typical disease has become relatively uncommon. Pathologists and clinicians are now challenged to unravel the causes and therapy of nonimmunologic hydrops fetalis (see below) and of other causes of prenatal anemia, such as transplacental bleeding (see below and Chapter 17). From a pathologist's view, these conditions are often indistinguishable, and additional tests are needed to identify the many specific disease entities that comprise this complex fetal condition.

The cause of typical erythroblastosis is the transplacental transfer of maternal antibodies that cause hemolysis in the fetus. As a consequence, the fetus attempts to repair this loss of red blood cells by overproduction and premature dissemination of immature red cell precursors (nucleated red blood cells, or NRBCs). The hematopoietic tissue becomes increasingly activated in the fetus, and the peripheral blood thus contains an increased number of NRBCs and erythroblasts, elegantly demonstrated by Nicolaides et al. (1988a,b). These authors performed reticulocyte counts in 127 pregnancies with isoimmunization, from 17 to 36 weeks, and suggested that it may be the extensive hepatic red blood cell production that causes the hydrops by obstructing sinusoidal blood flow. In our opinion, it is not the most likely mechanism to cause hydrops to develop. We believe that fetal cardiac failure is the main cause of hydrops and of the placental changes. The high-output congestive heart failure results from anemia and is the presumed cause of cardiomegaly in EF (Naeye, 1967). The issue is not completely resolved, however, as there is no strict correlation between the severity of anemia and cardiac hypertrophy (Carter et al., 1990). Because of the frequently extensive hemolysis, large iron stores may occur in the liver and spleen while the fetus becomes progressively anemic. When the hematocrit falls below 15%, edema, ascites, and eventually anasarca develop, the condition known as hydrops fetalis (Saltzman et al., 1989). Normative values for hemoglobin and NRBC and reticulocyte counts, ascertained by cordocentesis, are to be found in the contribution by Nicolaides et al. (1989). They discovered that hemoglobin and red blood cell counts increased linearly from 17 to 40 weeks' gestation. Importantly, the "erythroblast count decreased exponentially from a mean of 83/100 leukocytes at 17 weeks to 4/100 leukocytes at 40 weeks." Similar values obtained by other investigators were reviewed by Weiner et al. (1992), who also measured protein levels, enzymes, pH, gases, and venous pressure. Thilaganathan and collaborators (1992) found that erythropoietin levels were significantly increased only in the presence of severe fetal anemia. Moya and his colleagues (1993) found that erythropoietin levels were elevated in erythroblastosis also, but before 24 weeks' gestation this response was much smaller.

Fetal hydrops due to hemolysis may be quickly and completely reversed when the anemic fetus is transfused intravascularly before birth, thus restoring oxygenation (Socol et al., 1987; Grannum et al., 1988). The latter authors documented the impressive changes in protein and hemoglobin levels that occur. Nicolaides et al. (1988a,b), who provided the normative values for fetal hemoglobin levels from 17 to 40 weeks' gestation (11–15 g/dl), found that hydropic fetuses had hemoglobin values of 7 to 10 g/dl. A study investigating the possible mechanism of fetal death occurring in such pregnancies during transfusion showed that acute increases in hematocrit were associated with substantial mortality (Radunovic et al., 1992), and Nicolini et al. (1989) implicated increases in venous pressure during transfusion. The bilirubin, liberated by hemolysis, is effectively exchanged transplacentally, and the neonate rarely has much jaundice, which is a later, usually neonatal, development in erythroblastosis.

Other fetal changes are worth mentioning. Hepatosplenomegaly is prominent; usually the infants have some hypoproteinemia. They also often suffer severe thrombocytopenia (Harman et al., 1988) and display increased beta cell activity in their islets of Langerhans. The islet cell hyperplasia, which is combined with a greater islet insulin content (Driscoll & Steinke, 1967), was explained to result from insulin binding by the circulating hemoglobin (Steinke et al., 1967). The occasional presence of large maternal ovarian lutein cysts with hydrops fetalis is more difficult to explain. These cysts are clearly associated with an usually enlarged placenta, as was shown by Burger (1947), Christie (1961), Rabinowitz et al. (1961), and Hatjis (1985). Ovarian lutein cysts are also found in nonimmune hydrops, and they occasionally accompany fetal triploidy. These varied observations have led to the suggestion that, similar to women with hydatidiform moles, the fetal ovarian cysts result from elevated titers of human chorionic gonadotropin (hCG), produced because of the enlargement of the placenta. Christie (1961) and Hatjis (1985) have determined that the maternal serum levels of hCG are significantly above normal in the presence of fetal hydrops. Initially, this elevation of hCG titers was thought to result from the persistent presence of the Langhans layer of trophoblast or from its exaggerated appearance. Now that the origin of hCG has clearly been determined to be the syncytium, the abundance of hCG with fetal hydrops must be assumed to result from placental enlargement alone. In this connection, it is relevant to point out that human placental lactogen (hPL) and placental protein 5 (PP5) are also elevated in fetal hydrops (Lee et al., 1984). The elevation of hPL and hCG levels may relate to a larger placental mass, as suggested by Lee et al. (1984), but the increased PP5 levels are not so readily understood.

Placental Pathology in Erythroblastosis

The striking features of the placenta in erythroblastosis fetalis are its pallor, uniform enlargement, and villous "immaturity" (Figure 304). Because of the edema and enlargement, placentas of erythroblastosis are also friable. The changes were delineated early by Hellman and Hertig (1937) prior to knowledge of the nature of the disease. They enumerated syncytial degeneration, persistence of Langhans' layer, prominence of Hofbauer cells, the presence of erythropoietic cells in the vascular spaces, and stromal edema of villi. Since then, many studies have been conducted, all with essentially the same results. It is now apparent that the placental alterations are largely secondary to the fetal anemia and cardiac failure. Wentworth (1967) studied the placentas with the Gough large-section technique and affirmed that "the more severely the baby was affected, the larger the placenta was in relation to the baby." In the severe cases, the placentas were extremely pale and more friable than normal. Additional diagnostic histological features in the placenta were a marked decrease in the number of fetal vessels and an increase in the number of NRBCs in these vessels. Langhans' layer persisted in all cases but in itself it was not considered to be a specific change. Wentworth believed that the changes resulted from a direct effect of antibodies on the placenta. Montemagno et al. (1966) suggested from immunofluorescent antibody studies that the syncytium possesses the Rh antigen, and that antibodies localized to these antigens damage the syncytium and produce the pathological change seen in the placenta of EF. On occasion, one finds small amounts of hemosiderin deposited in chorionic macrophages, betraying the long-standing hemolysis. It is not a prominent finding, however. Rarely, one observes some icteric staining of placental surface vessels and umbilical cord. We now know that these nonspecific changes are essentially similar in placentas of unrelated types of hydrops fetalis (e.g., α-thalassemia). We believe that it is impossible, without history or specific immunological tests, to make the specific diagnosis of EF from a placental examination alone, an opinion similar to that expressed by Bouissou et al. (1969). The latter authors suggested, however, that the crowding of hematopoietic elements in the

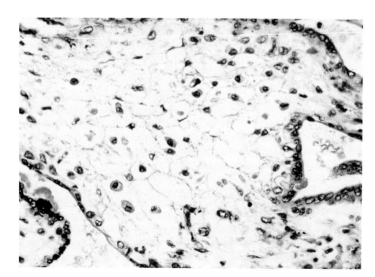

FIGURE 304. Villus in a stillborn with typical erythroblastosis fetalis. Note the edema, abundance of Hofbauer cells, and persistent cytotrophoblast. The fetal vessels are obliterated because of fetal demise. H&E. ×250.

hepatic parenchyma caused the fetal edema, which is contrary to our views.

Wentworth (1967) provided an excellent photograph of the anemic and normal placental portions of a set of dizygotic (DZ) twins in which only one twin was affected. Becker and Bleyl (1961) performed fluorescence microscopy on such placentas and believed that it demonstrated the increased permeability of the erythroblastotic placentas. The authors demonstrated a "condensation of . . . the interfibrillary substance of the connective tissue" of villi and believed it to be due to an increase in interfibrillary substance. This reaction, we believe, is largely the result of edema and of the accumulation of Hofbauer cells. It has occasionally been suggested that extramedullary hematopoiesis also takes place within the villous stroma. We believe that this suggestion is not the case. To be sure, the abundance of erythroblasts in some cases so much crowds the fetal capillaries that a villous production site is simulated. There is normally a large number of bone marrow-like elements in the fetal capillaries in EF; Alenghat and Esterly (1983) even found some of these cells to contain mitoses in abortion specimens. Burstein and Blumenthal (1962) found that the abundance of syncytial knots was about the same as in normal controls but that the villi were much expanded; by their method, this expansion resulted in a decreased villous count. They also emphasized the occurrence of fetal capillary proliferative lesions. There was no mention as to whether any of the placentas came from stillborn births. Apparently similar pathological findings were presented in a Russian paper

that was not accessible to us (Iakovtsova, 1964). Busch and Vogel (1972) provided a complete review of the historical aspects of the placental changes theretofore described and added their own observations of 58 cases. They found that these changes related to the severity of the hemolytic disease (i.e., the degree of anemia) and emphasized the occurrence of "maturational changes of villi." Finally, they found that about one-third of their cases had intervillous thrombi. This lesion is indeed common in the placentas of erythroblastosis fetalis, and it is not easily explained. One may postulate that intervillous thrombi are the sequelae of an increased hydrostatic pressure within the fetal capillaries and resultant bleeding. This hypothesis would be supported by finding many NRBCs within the thrombi (Figure 305). Intervillous thrombi are, however, also frequent in hydatidiform moles that have no fetal vasculature. We believe that the mechanism of the formation of intervillous thromboses in both conditions is similar. The villous edema so alters the intervillous blood flow as to cause local eddying and stasis, with thrombosis the end result. Nevertheless, because NRBCs are often found in the thrombi, fetal bleeding must occur at times. It may result from local villous hypoxic injury, as it has been repeatedly demonstrated that distension of fetal vessels and necrosis at the surface of the villi take place. This subject is further discussed in Chapter 17 in the consideration of fetal hemorrhage. Busch and Vogel (1972) contended that the placental enlargement was the result of real growth. The investigations by Vidyasagar and Haworth (1973), however, negated this

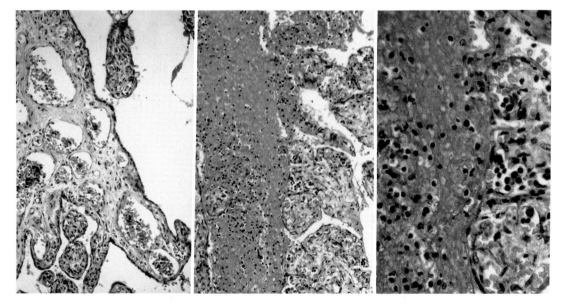

FIGURE 305. Immature placenta from a live infant with edema. Note the marked villous vascular distension and numerous erythroblasts in the fetal circulation (left). Inter- villous thrombi with nucleated red blood cells are seen in the same placenta (middle, right). H&E. left ×60; middle ×40; right ×160.

explanation. They found no differences when they compared the weights of non-EF placentas with those from nonhydropic cases of EF. Their decidual surfaces and DNA, water, and protein contents were similar.

An electron microscopic study of the placentas from erythroblastotic infants was undertaken by Jones and Fox (1978). These investigators found characteristic syncytial necrosis, cytotrophoblastic hyperplasia, thickening of basement membranes of villi and vessels, and immature endothelial cells. They did not identify a distinct pathogenesis of these alterations but ruled out immunologically mediated changes. Rather, they believed that the syncytial degeneration was the result of villous enlargement with consequent decrease of the intervillous space. The most detailed study of villous alterations in EF comes from the investigations by Pilz et al. (1980). They insisted that in order to obtain reproducible results it is necessary for protocols to provide specific fixation and other data. They obtained their material from in situ aspiration biopsies of eight cases of EF and compared them with 20 normal organs. Their morphometry showed an enlargement of "intermediate villi" that depended on the severity of the disease. They also observed an increase in cytotrophoblast; the terminal villi were not altered, and there was an increase in Hofbauer cells. These investigators

believed that the increased number and size of Hofbauer cells probably relate to the increased antigen–antibody reaction that must take place in the stroma of villi. They were unable to find the alterations in capillary lumens that were suggested to exist by other authors. There was no chorangiosis. They further emphasized that the changes they observed may represent a true maturational disturbance of the villi. In this regard, it is noteworthy that calcifications of the placenta are uncommon in EF.

Modern management of the isoimmunized gravida requires supervision of fetal progress. It includes sonography for the detection of edema, evaluation of amnionic bilirubin concentration, and the ascertainment of umbilical vein diameter. When these parameters were correlated, Reece et al. (1988) showed that umbilical venous dimension does not parallel the other, time-honored methods of prenatal evaluation. Prenatal intraabdominal transfusion, for the therapy of affected fetuses (e.g., Queenan & Douglas, 1965), is gradually being displaced by intravascular transfusion. This technique is usually done near the site of cord insertion on the placental surface (Rodeck et al., 1984); it allows sampling of fetal blood and estimation of total blood volume (Macgregor et al., 1988). The survival of transfused blood in the fetus is approximately similar with

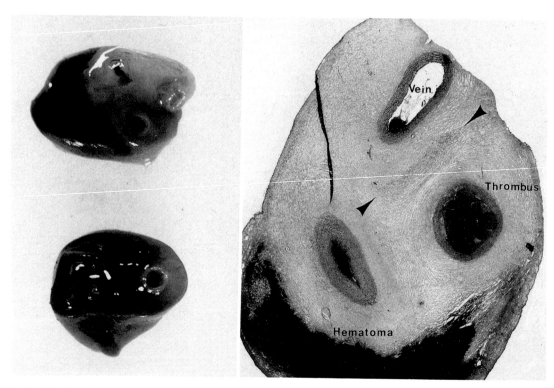

FIGURE 306. Umbilical cord with thrombosis of one artery at 3 weeks after cordocentesis. A new attempt caused infusion of blood into the cord substance. A line of leukocytic exudate

(arrows), coming from the umbilical vein, has formed between the vein and the occluded artery, whose wall is dead. H&E. ×3.

the two techniques (Pattison & Roberts, 1989). With the introduction of cordocentesis, newly observed pathological features in the placenta have been noted. Berkowitz et al. (1986), presented their results of 18 such transfusions, weighed the advantages and disadvantages of cordocentesis, and drew attention to the problems that ensue from the need for repeated puncture. The complications mainly involved injury to the umbilical cord; they witnessed stillbirth as a result. Pielet et al. (1988) also drew attention to the possible dangers accruing from cordocentesis. They found two stillbirths without recognizable cord injury; in another neonate with postnatal developmental delay, however, one umbilical artery was clotted after transfusion had been performed into the umbilical vein. A similar case is shown in Figure 306. This patient had unsuccessful cord blood sampling at 28 weeks' gestation. At 29.5 weeks successful transfusion of 45 ml blood was accomplished into the vein. At 32 weeks another transfusion was attempted; it ended with infusion of blood into the cord, and emergency cesarean section was necessary. The child survived. The cord had a superficial hematoma that extended onto the placental surface. The entire cord was stained with hemolyzed blood; hemosiderin was found in the chorionic macrophages. One umbilical artery was necrotic and had old obliterative thrombosis. Interestingly, there was a line of polymorphonuclear leukocytic exudation extending between the vein and the occluded artery, in the absence of chorioamnionitis. We concluded that the degenerating vessel caused the (sterile) inflammation. This occlusion had presumably occurred 3 weeks earlier. Figure 307 shows the result of needle puncture of the fetal surface in a relevant case. During amniocentesis, the posteriorly located placenta was accidentally injured, and an "upwelling" of blood was seen sonographically. Two weeks later, a stillborn fetus was delivered. The placental surface showed the site of needle injury to a surface vessel. We have also seen a stillborn fetus whose third transfusion was given into the cord. During that procedure, bradycardia developed after the needle was inserted. The procedure was stopped, and abdominal blood was given instead, but the fetus succumbed. There was a tense, placental portion of the cord with hematoma, and fresh occlusive thrombi were found within superficial arterial ramifications. Moreover, within this thrombotic material, typical squames were found (Figure 308), presumably introduced by the needle from the amnionic cavity. Our interpretation was that after needle insertion a cord hematoma and vascular spasm ensued, followed by arterial thrombosis. Seeds and his colleagues (1989) asserted that the demonstration of "echogenic venous turbulence" was an important feature of successful intravascular transfusion. When they found it absent in a fetus that developed bradycardia, a hematoma of

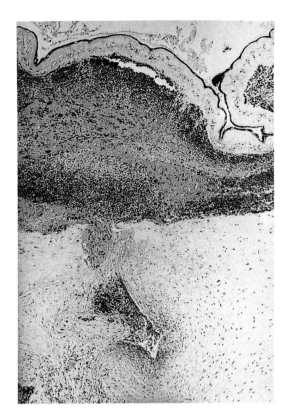

FIGURE 307. Midgestation placental surface 2 weeks after amniocentesis. The needle injured the chorionic vessel below. Note the fresh hematoma with hemosiderin and the attempted repair of the vascular wall. H&E. ×16.

the cord was found to have developed. James (1970) measured villous size in EF placentas after intrauterine (abdominal) transfusions had been given and correlated the findings with hemoglobin levels. Normal values were found when the hemoglobin was above 11 g/dl, but the mean villous volume was increased in more severely affected infants. Houston and Brown (1966) reported a case of fetal gas bacillus infection after fetal transfusion; the edematous placenta was colonized by large numbers of gram-positive bacterial rods, and there was chorioamnionitis. When it is necessary to traverse the placenta in order to gain access to the fetus, the placenta may be injured and may bleed, which may enhance maternal immunization. These aspects were described by Friesen et al. (1967), who identified puncture marks in the placenta in such cases. These investigators found significant bleeding into the mother in 7.5% of cases when transgression of an anterior placenta was necessary in order to gain access to the amnionic sac.

Twins may be discordant (Figures 309, 310) or concordant for EF. When discordant, the severity of the disease often differs markedly (Beischer et al., 1969). In one such case with marked discrepancy, a difference in ABO compatibility was held to be responsible. The

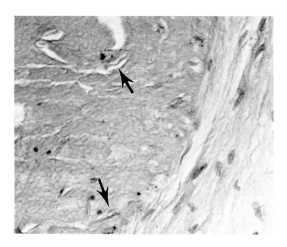

FIGURE 308. Arterial thrombus at the placental surface in a hydropic stillborn, days after cordocentesis for transfusion. Note the typical squames (arrows), presumably introduced by the needle during transfusion. H&E. ×256.

authors postulated that undetermined factors may be operative in producing discordance. A similarly discordant set of DZ twins with EF was detailed by Wiener et al. (1962). Manning et al. (1985) reported on the prenatal transfusions in a number of such twins. It is remarkable that maternal Rh isoimmunization may occur after fetal demise. Stedman et al. (1988) described three cases. They assumed that transplacental bleeding had occurred early during this unsuccessful pregnancy

and was thus causally related to the fetal demise by the production of antibodies. This situation most likely was true in their first patient who had torsion of the umbilical cord; the others had negative placental findings. This observation brings into question the mechanism of primary immunization against Rh antigens, usually held to occur most frequently at the time of delivery or immediately thereafter. It is the rationale for postpartum RhoGam prophylaxis, which has been highly effective in preventing isoimmunization. Injury to the placenta, such as occurs during manual removal of the placenta and during cesarean section, enhances fetal blood transfer. Queenan and Nakamoto (1964) found that spontaneous placental delivery and previous drainage of cord blood minimize the probability of isoimmunization. Although it is possible that occasional fetal bleeding during early pregnancy may lead to immunization of primigravidas, the commonest time of sensitization is at delivery (Scott et al., 1977).

Maternal bleeding into a female fetus presumably accounts only for few immunizations in their future gestations, when an Rh-negative infant is delivered to an Rh-positive mother (Taylor, 1967). Such mother-to-fetus transfer of blood, however, was said to occur in as many as 43% of samples analyzed by Luca et al. (1978). This subject is further discussed at the end of Chapter 17.

The amount of immunogen needed for isoimmunization has been debated. Attempts to elucidate it with experimental findings have been made in Rh-negative

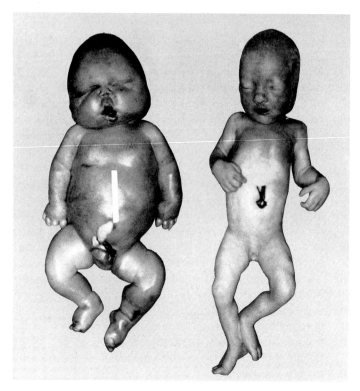

FIGURE 309. Immature, fraternal twins: one with erythroblastosis, the other normal. The placenta of the erythroblastotic twin (Figure 310) is markedly enlarged and unusually pale.

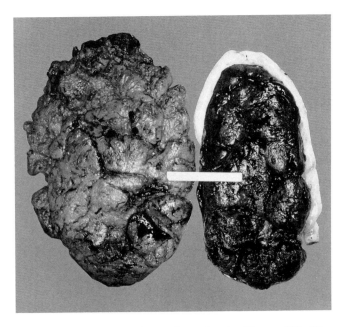

FIGURE 310. Placentas from the twins in Figure 309. The enlarged, edematous placenta of the DiDi twins, one with erythroblastosis (left), shows the pallor and bulky cotyledons.

volunteers. Zipursky and Israels (1967) suggested that repeated injections of as little as 0.1 ml ABO compatible Rh-positive blood suffice to immunize Rh-negative individuals. (That amount is presumably frequently attained in normal pregnancies.) Mollison (1968) opined that the minimum amount needed for immunization is 0.25 ml of fetal blood.

These deliberations are particularly important when one considers whether a hydatidiform mole, spontaneous abortion, or ectopic pregnancy can immunize an Rh-negative woman. Price (1968) reported a case of hydatidiform mole followed by a normal pregnancy in which antibodies were detected at about 6 months; the neonate succumbed from EF. It was assumed that the mole had immunized the primigravida. It seems unlikely to us that a bloodless structure is capable of Rh immunization unless the original tissue was a partial mole with triploidy. These moles often contain fetal vessels with blood. It has also been debated about when, in patients with "abortion," it becomes necessary to provide RhoGam to patients. Freda et al. (1970) came to the conclusion that it was indicated only after the second month of pregnancy. Regrettably, their data do not specify whether the abortions they studied were terminations of pregnancy or true spontaneous abortions. Most of the latter cases have no circulating fetal blood, as they are due to chromosomal errors that led to embryonic death. They should not deliver sufficient antigen for sensitization; there is no doubt, however, that embryonic erythrocytes are capable of

immunization. Examples are the cases of therapeutic terminations of early pregnancy studied by Matthews et al. (1969), Jorgensen (1969), Murray and Barron (1971), and Eklund (1981). To be sure, the risk of sensitization is small, and it depends on the use and type of instrumentation used for the termination of pregnancy, such as suction versus dilatation and curettage. It also depends on fetal age. Ectopic pregnancies present a significantly higher risk for isoimmunization than that which occurs with spontaneous abortion (Grimes et al., 1981), presumably because of their less frequent cytogenetic abnormalities and fewer embryonic deaths. Whether chorionic villous sampling (CVS) presents a risk is yet to be determined. When Warren et al. (1985) studied α-fetoprotein (AFP) levels and Kleihauer stains following CVS, they found AFP levels to rise. They believed that the Kleihauer technique was not sufficiently sensitive to detect possible fetal bleeding. To our knowledge, the risk incurred for isoimmunization due to CVS has not been sufficiently investigated. It is generally thought that Rh-positive fetal red blood cells represent the only immunogen to Rh-negative women, but trophoblastic cells may contain Rh antigen and produce sensitization. Direct immunofluorescence studies with fluorescent anti-Rh D antibodies have shown that fluorescence may localize to the syncytium (Jarkowski et al., 1964). Goto et al. (1980) extended these studies. They impressively demonstrated, with appropriate controls, that the amount of trophoblastic Rh antigen decreases with advancing gestation, in contrast to the increasing prevalence on fetal red blood cells. They also showed that it localizes on trophoblastic surfaces, and that it is present in hydatidiform mole. Whether it can be the cause of sensitization remains elusive.

There is no answer to the obvious question as to why it is that not all Rh-negative women with Rh-positive conceptuses become immunized. Trophoblast is invasive and embolizes to the maternal lung in all pregnancies; perhaps it does not gain access to the antigen-processing machinery of lymph nodes. Complete absence of AB antigens from trophoblast was demonstrated by studies of Szulman (1972), who did, however, readily identify the antigen in fetal epithelium and in placental capillaries, including in a chorangioma.

Nonimmune Hydrops

In many cases of hydrops fetalis, the etiology is different from that of EF discussed above. Santolaya et al. (1992) found that of the 76 fetuses with hydrops (among 12,572 ultrasound examinations) only 10 were due to immunological causes, and 66 had nonimmune hydrops fetalis. They were unable to assign a cause in 17 cases.

Some of the other hydropic fetuses result from fetal anemia and heart failure, trisomies, and other abnormalities. Many other hydropic fetuses, however, are idiopathic, a euphemism for our lack of knowledge of their precise etiology. It must also be cautioned that ascites alone is insufficient for the diagnosis of hydrops, in which case generalized edema and fluid in cavities exists. This fluid accumulation in the pleural spaces often leads to pulmonary hypoplasia, which condition is not the cause of the hydrops, however (Green et al., 1990). The placental pathology is similar to that of EF, but substantial differences are also identified in individual cases. Novak et al. (1991) have described "hemorrhagic endovasculitis" of the placental vessels, an entity that is more fully discussed elsewhere. They depicted obliterated main stem vessels amidst rather nonhydropic villi, which is usually regarded as a postmortem phenomenon; 8 of their 14 cases were stillborn, and most were complicated by hydramnios. In some unexplained cases of fetal hydrops the pathologist may be able to exclude specific causes. Often pathologists are confronted with a stillborn, frequently a macerated, hydropic fetus and are asked to provide an idea as to the mechanism that led to the fetal hydrops. In the following pages we review many of the currently known entities of nonimmunological hydrops and then discuss idiopathic hydrops fetalis. Larger series dealing with causes of hydrops fetalis are the following: Macafee et al. (1970), Moerman et al. (1982), Hutchison et al. (1982), Nakamura et al. (1987), and Machin (1989). Watson and Campbell (1986) provided a detailed management protocol for such pregnancies. A large review of 600 cases is provided by Jauniaux et al. (1990), who ascertained that more than 35% of cases could be ascribed to a genetically transmitted disease. Chromosomal disorders ranked first with 15.7%, α-thalassemia was second (10.3%), with a wide variety of anomalies following. Jauniaux et al. suggested that chromosomal analysis was needed in such cases. Mallmann and colleagues (1991) suggested that perhaps 49 of their 324 cases of nonimmune hydrops represent an expression of immunological rejection.

α-Thalassemia

Normal adult hemoglobin molecules contain two unlike pairs of polypeptide (globin) chains: α-chains and β-chains. During embryonic and fetal life, special forms of hemoglobin are prevalent at different and carefully scheduled times. Abnormal construction of the globin chains that make up fetal hemoglobin results in altered hemoglobins that may be deficient in oxygen-carrying capacity. This situations, in turn, can lead to abnormal red blood cell shapes, such as occurs in sickle cell disease. In the thalassemias (α- and β-thalassemias), anemia results from a decreased production of normal hemoglobin. These disorders are classified according to the chain that is depressed. Examples include α-, β-, δ-, and γ-thalassemia (Nathan, 1973).

α-Thalassemia is a lethal inherited abnormality of hemoglobin structure that often causes hydrops fetalis. It was the first type of nonimmunologic hydrops for which an innovative explanation was identified. This complication of pregnancy has occupied much more attention in the United States in recent years because of the immigration of Indochinese with this genetic background. It is also a model in which prenatal marrow transplantation and gene therapy are being considered. Thus, diagnosis is important, as the homozygous condition is lethal and the recurrence rate is at least 1:4. Detailed screening methods (cresyl blue staining, erythrocyte indices, and iron study) have been described for the couples at risk for this disease (Skogerboe et al., 1992). The pathology seen in the newborn is essentially identical to that of Rh disease. Lie-Injo and her colleagues (1959, 1962, 1968) reported the association of hydrops fetalis and Bart's (Bartholomew) hemoglobin in Indonesian families. Since then, this disease has been recognized in Filipinos (Pearson et al., 1965; Nakayama et al., 1986), Thais (Pootrakul et al., 1967; Thumasathit et al., 1968), Chinese (Kan et al., 1967), Germans (Rönisch & Kleihauer, 1967), and Canadian Orientals (with hemoglobin H disease: Ing et al., 1968; Gray et al., 1972). It probably occurs in other races. The α-thal₁ gene has been identified in Kurdish Jews (Horowitz et al., 1966) and in Ashkenazi Jews, but it has not been associated with hydrops (Goldschmidt et al., 1968). The same is true of American Blacks. The frequency of this deletion of α-chain genes is greatest in Indonesians and Chinese (Zeng & Huang, 1985). Hydrops is caused by the homozygous presence of the gene for Bart's hemoglobin. The four α-chains are herein replaced by four τ-chains. The γ-chains are often heterogeneous (Vedvick et al., 1979), and different chain composition causes different severities of the disease. In hemoglobin-Bart's disease, or α-thalassemia, the defective hemoglobin is unable to release its oxygen effectively, causing tissue hypoxia, fetal cardiac failure, and hydrops (Orkin & Nathan, 1976). It is essentially lethal at birth or shortly thereafter. The fetal red blood cells in this disorder are frequently misshapen; they may, for instance, be sickled. Cardiac hypertrophy is often striking, as is the extensive and widespread extramedullary hematopoiesis. The substitution of various types of hemoglobin chain during development and the location of their production in the fetus are complex and have been lucidly portrayed by Nalbandian et al. (1971). Orkin and Michelson (1980) showed, by DNA sequence analysis, that the 5'-portion of the α-globin structural gene was deleted in a case of α-thalassemia.

The switching of hemoglobins during embryonic development is regulated in a complex manner; it has been studied by Peschle et al. (1985) and by Wood and his colleagues (1985). Different states of DNA methylation have been identified, but the mechanism that initiates this switch remains unknown. Many other types of neonatal hemoglobinopathies are known, for instance hemoglobin H disease, in which four β-chains constitute the molecule. This particular hemoglobinopathy is prevalent in Orientals. It causes neonatal anemia, but hydrops has not been described (Milner et al., 1971). The same is true of sickle cell anemia and sickle cell β-thalassemia. Both are associated with poor reproductive outcome but do not feature hydrops as a complication (Laros & Kalstone, 1971). A detailed review of many of these considerations was provided by Jonxis (1965), who described details on the switching from embryonic to fetal hemoglobins and from fetal to adult hemoglobins; he also listed the then known abnormal hemoglobins.

Louderback and Shanbrom (1967) indicated that hemoglobin electrophoresis is perhaps the simplest and most widely available tool for the differential diagnosis of the various types of cord blood hemoglobin. Sexauer et al. (1976) described a simple, rapid electrophoretic method for the analysis of cord bloods. They found that 11% of their 7,500 cord blood samples from black newborns contained an abnormal hemoglobin. The methods for genetic diagnosis have now been considerably simplified (Lebo et al., 1990), and they have been successfully applied to prenatal diagnosis as well. Kan et al. (1976) accomplished it by molecular hybridization. Rubin and Kan (1985) presented a rapid, decisive method based on slot-blot analysis. Williamson et al. (1981) and Chang and Kan (1981) showed that with CVS it is possible to accurately diagnose sickle cell disease in the fetus, and many cases of thalassemia can be diagnosed by direct globin gene analysis. Appropriate samples of blood must be saved for such studies at autopsy when the etiology of hydrops is uncertain. The aforementioned methods also facilitate the diagnosis of heterozygotes, which was previously so difficult to accomplish (Terheggen & Kleihauer, 1968). Unusual causes of hemolytic disease of the newborn, such as the γ-β-thalassemia reported by Kan et al. (1972), are also thus delineated.

The placenta in the presence of thalassemia differs little from that of pregnancies with classical erythroblastosis, and histology alone cannot provide the differential diagnosis: The placenta is, however, usually even more enlarged than in erythroblastosis; it is pale, friable, and edematous. The cytotrophoblast is prominent; and in the much enlarged fetal circulation large numbers of red blood cell precursors are found (Figures 311, 312). Hemosiderin is occasionally seen within chorionic macrophages but it may also be bilirubin pigment from bilirubinuria and liver damage. The placental enlargement has often been massive. The

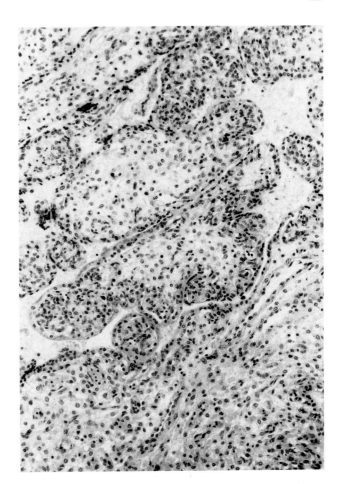

FIGURE 311. Placenta from a pregancy in a woman with α-thalassemia. There were severe edema, "immature" villi, and large numbers of nucleated red blood cells and erythroblasts in the circulation. The placenta weighed 1,005 g, had hemosiderin staining of the chorion, and was disrupted, friable and pale. The fetus was growth-retarded and hydropic, and it succumbed. H&E. ×100.

placenta shown in Figure 312 weighed 1,900 g. Lie-Injo et al. (1968) described weights up to 3,500 g (!), most of which, of course, is water. They observed a set of fraternal twins, wherein one of the placentas was normal and the other abnormal, which conclusively established that the pathological changes in the placenta have a fetal cause. Pregnancy-induced hypertension (preeclampsia) is a frequent corollary of this condition, presumably because of the massive placental enlargement.

It is of related interest to be aware of the complex relations that exist between placental weight (and edema) and fetal and maternal anemia. These aspects have been studied by Beischer and his colleagues (1968). These investigators found that the placental weight of mothers with various types of anemia was in an approximately normal range, whereas the placental weight in cases of EF was much increased, even when compared

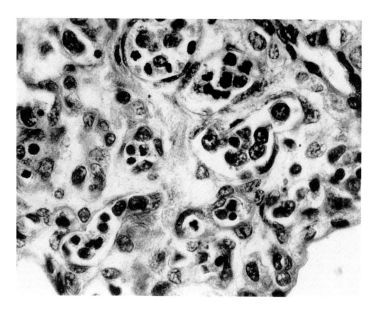

FIGURE 312. Placenta from a case of maternal α-thalassemia and fetal hydrops. This placenta weighed 1,900 g and had macroscopic features similar to those seen in the placenta shown in Figure 311. Note the large number of marrow-like elements in the fetal capillaries. H&E. ×640.

with the enhanced placental weight found usually in the pregnancies of diabetic mothers. Other aspects of clinical management are important. Guy and colleagues (1985) studied five pregnant Oriental women sonographically and found that sonographic surveillance for hydrops was an invaluable tool in clinical management (see also Saltzman et al., 1989, for criteria). These investigators emphasized that the pregnancies were frequently complicated by preeclampsia and by retained placenta, which necessitated manual removal. Miller et al. (1987) reported theca-lutein cysts in a Vietnamese mother who had hydramnios and a hydropic 1,290 g infant who died immediately after birth. The placenta weighed 1,600 g. The ovarian cysts are attributed to elevated hCG levels from an enlarged placenta. The mother's β-chain hCG levels were 1.12 million mIU/ml. The gonadotropin levels fell rapidly to 83.8 mIU/ml within 15 days, and her ovarian masses disappeared. This case is not unlike the cases of ovarian cysts that sometimes accompany EF. Mouse models of this disorder have been described. Their potential usefulness for the elucidation of yet unknown aspects of this disease were discussed by Whitney and Popp (1984). With the increasing population of Vietnamese and other Orientals in the United States α-thalassemia is being seen more frequently and must be routinely considered in the differential diagnosis of hydrops (Suh, 1994).

Fetal Hemorrhage

Hydrops fetalis has repeatedly been the result of massive and chronic fetomaternal hemorrhage, and it is for that reason that it has been our practice to examine maternal blood for fetal cells (Kleihauer technique; see Chapter 17) in all cases of unexplained stillbirths. As in EF, when the hemoglobin levels fall below a certain point (about 7 g/dl, or a hematocrit of approximately 15% or less), cardiac failure may cause hydrops. When fetal exsanguination is rapid, it does not as quickly produce hydrops and more likely results in fetal death. Ensuing heart failure and transudation is required for hydrops to occur. This aspect was discussed in the case presented by Herman et al. (1987), where the fetal hematocrit was 15% and the hemoglobin 3 g/dl at term. In this case, the mother had a 2.8% Kleihauer test result (approximately 150 ml fetal blood), and no placental abnormalities were found. Bowman et al. (1984) considered it to be an exceptional cause of fetal hydrops. They reviewed the few cases from the literature and described a neonate in whom large, chronic, bidirectional blood exchange must have occurred. The placenta showed major fetal vessels to have ruptured, which were believed to explained this phenomenon, and there were also many placental infarcts. The placenta was not markedly enlarged (560 g). No untoward accidents had occurred until 31 weeks, when the mother experienced a rapidly increasing abdominal girth. The authors considered that the hydrops resulted from fetal hypervolemic heart failure. Cardwell (1988) described a hydropic 2,750 g liveborn infant who had been treated by prenatal transfusion at 21 weeks' gestation. The Kleihauer test had been 0.4%, which corresponded to a 50% loss of fetal blood. The finding of NRBCs in the fetal circulation is herein also an important pathological finding (Fox, 1967). Villaespesa and colleagues (1990), who investigated 59 cases of nonimmune hydrops, believed that right-sided cardiovascular failure should be investigated, as 50% of their cases were due to this mechanism. Their point was borne out by direct measurement of venous pressures in hydropic fetuses (Johnson et al., 1992).

We have now seen many hydropic neonates with verified fetomaternal hemorrhage. One had the hemorrhage after an amniocentesis performed to ascertain fetal maturity (0.3% Kleihauer; hematocrit 19% three days later). Another fetus exsanguinated for no known reason (shown in Chapter 17). A third newborn had an 18% hematocrit at birth and could not be revived. Many NRBCs were found in villous vessels. All three placentas were pale and edematous but were not as overtly hydropic as in thalassemia. Zwi and Becroft (1986) reported a patient with ulcerative colitis who was on prednisone and sulfasalazine therapy; the fetus developed hydrops fetalis at 24 weeks' gestation, after 4 weeks of vaginal bleeding. No fetal red blood cells were identified in this blood, but a marginal separation of a 460 g edematous placenta had occurred. The macerated fetus weighed 1,070 g. It had a dilated and enlarged heart, and there was complete absence of hematopoiesis in the liver and bone marrow. The latter finding led the authors to suggest that aplastic anemia was the cause of the fetal hydrops and placentomegaly. The cause of the anemia was not determined, but it is noteworthy that the mother's sulfasalazine therapy had been discontinued during early pregnancy.

Fetal Tumors

Congenital neuroblastoma has repeatedly been shown to cause fetal death. Birner (1961) described such a fetus and found an unusually enlarged placenta (1,240 g). The 3,925 g fetus was slightly edematous and macerated, but the placenta did not contain neuroblastoma cells. The villi were enlarged and edematous and had an increased number of Hofbauer cells. Additionally, Langhans' cells had persisted to term. Strauss and Driscoll (1964) were the first authors to draw attention to the involvement of the placenta with neuroblastoma metastases. Their first fetus was edematous and resembled an erythroblastotic infant. The placenta was markedly enlarged and friable, and it resembled that of erythroblastosis fetalis. Cords of neuroblastoma cells were found in fetal capillaries. Their second reported infant was born at term accompanied by a 1,030 g placenta. Typical neuroblastoma cells and erythroblasts crowded the fetal capillaries (Figure 313). The fetal heart was enlarged. The first mother had theca lutein cysts, similar to those mentioned earlier in the chapter. Other cases of fetal hydrops with congenital neuroblastoma and placentomegaly have since been described (Anders et al., 1973; Moss & Kaplan, 1978; Perkins et al., 1980; Slikke & Balk, 1980; Smith et al., 1981; Newton et al., 1985). A possible immune hypothesis for the development of the hydrops was entertained by Strauss and Driscoll (1964), but most authors have discounted this possibility. Hydrops and placentomegaly were present in Birner's case (1961), but there was no placental neoplasm. This finding suggested that it was not the plugging of fetal capillaries with tumor cells that caused the placentomegaly and could not be the etiology of hydrops. The case described by Newton et al. (1985) may have relevance to the considerations of pathogenesis. It was associated with maternal hypertension, presumed to be produced by the production of catecholamines from the fetal neuroblastoma. Perhaps similar changes of blood pressure occur in the fetus and contribute to fetal heart failure. Perkins et al. (1980) found, in a case of congenital neuroblastoma, that the villous tissue too was infiltrated by neuroblastoma cells, and that these cells contained cytoplasmic granules that electron microcopically were typical of neuroblastoma cells. We have seen placental hydrops with a severely hydropic and macerated fetus in whose placental vessels there were many malignant small cells. A positive diagnosis of the neoplasm was impossible (Figure 314). No tumor mass existed in the fetus.

Sacrococcygeal teratomas also produce placentomegaly and fetal edema. They are frequently accompanied by hydramnios and elevated hCG levels (Barentsen, 1975). In the first two such cases described,

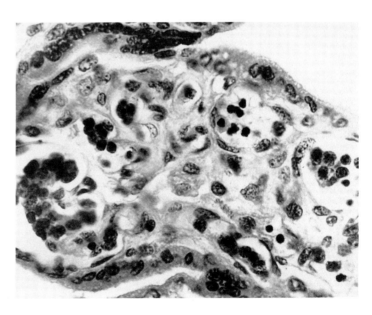

FIGURE 313. Villus from a case of congenital neuroblastoma. The enlarged villus has numerous neuroblastoma cells in the fetal vessels, some of which show some rosetting. H&E. ×400.

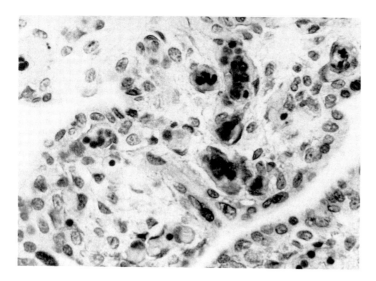

FIGURE 314. Villi of a macerated, hydropic fetus. Note the edema and numerous hyperchromatic cells intravascularly. Neuroblastoma was suspected but could not be proved. H&E. ×350.

the placental edema and large number of NRBCs in the villous capillaries were identical to those seen in placental erythroblastosis (Kohga et al., 1980). When we wrote this paper, we considered that high-output cardiac failure produced the hydrops. This diagnosis was confirmed by the study of Langer et al. (1989). These authors observed such a tumor at 21 weeks' gestation with hydrops and placental edema. After they attempted to remove the tumor they observed a diminution of hydrops and reduction in placental thickness. Other cases of sacrococcygeal teratoma, hydramnios, hydrops, and placentomegaly (occasionally associated with preeclampsia) are reviewed in this publication and those of Perlin et al. (1981), Feige et al.

(1982), Pringle et al. (1987), Holzgreve et al. (1987), Kuhlmann et al. (1987), and Bock et al. (1990), in which additional cases are also described.

Fetal placental *leukemia* is rare. Macroscopically, it resembles erythroblastosis fetalis and causes placentomegaly. Figure 315 illustrates a 1,000 g placenta in presumed fetal leukemia that came with a severely macerated fetus who was not autopsied. We have seen only one other similar case, which involved a fetus with trisomy 21.

Various *angiomas* have repeatedly caused hydrops fetalis and placentomegaly. For instance, Imakita et al. (1988) described a patient with severe hydramnios at 31 weeks' gestation; there were sonographic features of

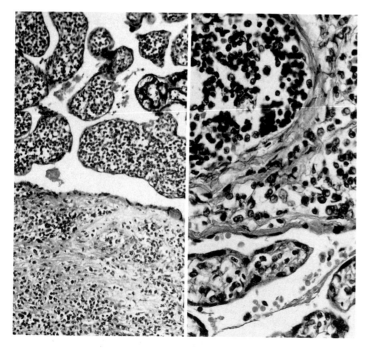

FIGURE 315. Placenta from a macerated stillborn with presumed leukemia. The villous capillaries are packed with leukemic cells, and some stromal infiltration is seen. H&E. left ×60; right ×160. (Courtesy Dr. E.V. Perrin).

FIGURE 316. Edematous villi (left) in a 27-week-old fetus with hydrops due to cystic adenomatoid malformation of the lung (right). H&E. left ×150; right ×100.

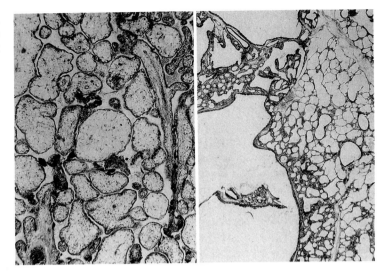

hydrops fetalis and a large chorangioma. The patient delivered 2 days after an amniocentesis. The infant died at 2 days of age. The neonate's hemoglobin content was 15 g/dl; there was hypoproteinemia but no evidence of isoimmunization. The fetal heart was markedly hypertrophied and dilated, and the 840 g placenta had a 5.5 × 4.5 × 3.0 cm chorangioma. The authors conjectured that the location of the angioma may have been such as to have obstructed the venous return from the placenta. They also reviewed many previously reported cases of this association of chorangioma with hydrops. No doubt high-output cardiac failure of the fetus was responsible for the hydramnios and the placentomegaly. An interesting case of fetal hydrops, resulting from a complex hemangioma of the umbilical cord, was presented by Seifer et al. (1985). It occurred in one of dichorionic female twins who weighed 2,100 g at birth but who lost her edema over the course of the first month of life. The birth weight of the co-twin was 1,670 g. High output failure was thought to have been caused by an angioma in the umbilical cord that measured 9 cm in diameter and 18 cm in length. This enlargement was mainly due to edema, however. The placenta was otherwise normal. Hepatic angiomas of the fetus are occasionally so large as to cause fetal heart failure (Gonen et al., 1989; Skopec & Lakatua, 1989) and may be associated with significant neonatal thrombocytopenia. In cases of prenatally recognized nonimmune hydrops fetalis, sonographic study may identify such tumors as a cause of hydrops. Dr. A. James McAdams has shown us a 7-month-old child with a presumed hepatic "hamartoma" in whom the hydropic placenta had weighed 1,320 g.

Cystic adenomatoid malformation of the lung, although not a true neoplasm, is another well recognized cause of fetal hydrops and placental edema. Figure 316 shows the markedly hydropic placenta of the case published by Gottschalk and Abramson (1957). In this case, autopsy findings indicated that the mediastinum had shifted and had thus caused a chronic impediment to venous return from the placenta. The fetal heart was one-half the expected size; the placenta was edematous and weighed 1,105 g at 27 weeks' gestation. The authors cited additional similar cases. We saw a similar case in one twin sonographically, with shift of the mediastinum; and Bromley et al. (1992) reported such a set of twins as well. An infant with anasarca, whose placenta was not described, underwent successful removal of a similar large tumor (Aslam et al., 1970). Clark et al. (1987) even operated successfully on a hydropic child with cystic adenomatoid malformation after having placed an intrathoracic shunt prenatally. Ascites and subcutaneous edema disappeared, and the child delivered normally 17 weeks later. The tumor was removed on the first day of life. These authors and Kohler and Rymer (1973) cited additional cases of hydrops with adenomatoid malformations of the fetal lung. Occasional other tumors are associated with or cause fetal hydrops. Gray (1989) reported fetal hydrops with a *mesoblastic nephroma*. It was associated with hydramnios, but the placenta was not described.

Congenital Anomalies and Hydrops Fetalis

Aside from the adenomatoid malformation of the lung, numerous other congenital anomalies have been causally or otherwise related to the development of fetal hydrops. Benacerraf and Frigoletto (1986) diagnosed the presence of a diaphragmatic hernia and then drained a large right hydrothorax: the fetus survived and was born without further complications. The placenta was not described. The Klippel-Trenaunay syndrome (angioosteohypertrophy) has occurred with hydrops fetalis (Mor et al., 1988). The placenta weighed 760 g and was bulky and friable. The newborn had giant port-wine nevi and high-output cardiac failure. Seward and Zusman (1978) reported the case of a hydropic newborn who had fetal anemia, perhaps due to a small bowel volvulus. Brinson and Goldsmith (1988) reported a child with intrauterine intussusception and intestinal perforation; hypoproteinemia was therein presumed to have caused the hydrops. Pulmonary sequestration has often caused nonimmune hydrops (Weiner et al., 1986), presumably also because of obstructed venous return to the heart. The placenta in this case was normal. Several cases of hydrops associated with Noonan syndrome have been described (Bawle & Black, 1986; Oudesluys-Murphy, 1987); the associated placentas were not mentioned. Koffler et al. (1978) described two cases of chylothorax that were associated with hydramnios, in the absence of hydrops; the placenta was not mentioned. Both infants survived. A similar case comes from Sacks et al. (1983), who stated that the placenta was not enlarged. Chylothorax and lymphangiectasis are occasionally the causes of hydrops. Abnormal development of lymphatics may be responsible for generalized edema (Windebank et al., 1987). The latter authors identified abnormal connections of lymphatics and vessels in an hydropic infant. They were also associated with cystic hygroma, a feature that may be at the basis of the edema in 45,X fetuses (Turner syndrome). Alternatively, coarctation of the aorta may be causative (Lacro et al., 1988). The placenta in Turner syndrome, however, is not hydropic. If anything, it is smaller, and occasionally has the features of a Breus' mole (subchorionic tuberous hematoma). We have observed a set of monozygotic (MZ) twins with abnormal chromosomes. One was 46,XX and normal; the other was 45,X and had massive edema, ascites, and cervical hygroma. A similar set of discordant MZ twins (46,XY and 45,X) with hydrops in the latter twin was reported by Gonsoulin et al. (1990). Many reports on chromosomal trisomies suggest that these anomalies are an occasional cause of hydrops. Landrum et al. (1986) found that 17 cases of hydrops with trisomy 21, six with trisomy 18, and two with trisomy 13 had been reported. They added their own cases: three with trisomy 21 and one with trisomy 13. Hendricks et al. (1993) also found two cases of hydrops with trisomy 21 and an associated but transitory myeloproliferative disorder and anemia. It is of interest to note here that in a case of chromosome 18p- syndrome the fetal hydrops was probably due to a complete heart block, resulting from calcifications in the atrioventricular node (Bridge et al., 1989). Schwanitz and colleagues (1988) have reported hydrops fetalis in a child with duplications of the long arms of chromosomes 15 and 17, offspring of a parent with balanced 15/17 translocation. They suggested that a chromosomal analysis should be undertaken in every case of non-

immune hydrops in which the cause has remained obscure. The cause of hydrops in these infants is unknown (see also Watson & Campbell, 1986), and the placenta is rarely discussed. Gropp (1984) found similar conditions of edema in the experimentally induced mouse trisomy. He evaluated the various reported suggestions that seek to explain the fetal hydrops. The Neu-Laxova syndrome is another cause of hydrops; it is accompanied by multiple anomalies, hydramnios, and occasional placental edema (Broderick et al., 1988). It has also been reported that congenital myotonic dystrophy may lead to hydrops and pleural effusions, but the status of the placenta was not described (Curry et al., 1988). Tuberous sclerosis has also been implicated in the genesis of hydrops fetalis. Östör and Fortune (1978) described such a case but did not mention the placenta. The hydrops was presumably secondary to the cardiac rhabdomyoma present.

Congenital Heart Disease

Numerous cases of congenital heart disease have been described to have hydrops fetalis. Best known among them perhaps are Ebstein's anomaly of the tricuspid valve (Moller et al., 1966), endocardial fibroelastosis (Ben Ami et al., 1986), premature closure of the foramen ovale (Rodin & Nichols, 1975; Olson et al., 1987), and some forms of hypoplastic left heart (Leake et al., 1973). Many other anomalies have been listed, too numerous for this discussion. Some were noted by Kleinman et al. (1982), who did not have any cases of "idiopathic" hydrops. They reported 10 cardiovascular anomalies, and 3 with supraventricular tachycardia. These authors emphasized the importance of fetal echocardiography. McFadden and Taylor (1989), in a review of a large series of congenital heart disease and nonimmune hydrops, expressed the view that the two conditions were not causally related. They were especially emphatic to point out that premature closure of the foramen ovale was not a cause of hydrops fetalis. Groves and Baskett (1984) reviewed 26 cases of nonimmune hydrops fetalis. They found 11 cases with anomalies and 5 with primary heart malformation. There were also four cases of the twin transfusion syndrome. In a set of twins whose placenta did not show anastomoses, Mogilner et al. (1982) attributed the hydrops to prolonged maternal indomethacin therapy and ductal closure. There is even a report of a massively edematous rhesus monkey fetus with hydrops fetalis due to a complex anomaly of the heart (Cukierski et al., 1986). The placenta was circumvallate and monodiscoid, and it had numerous infarcts and features of placenta previa. The fetus was no longer edematous at autopsy, long after fetal death, but its thickened, edematous features had been identified sonographically. Rare cases of hydrops with generalized arterial calcification (Williams syndrome) have occurred (Jones et al., 1972; Carles et al., 1992). Pulmonary hemorrhage (blood clot) was believed to be the cause in the last case. In one such fetus, prenatal blood sampling allowed the diagnosis of fetal hypercalcemia (Westgren et al., 1988). Its placenta was markedly edematous. In other cases, calcifications extended along the cord and placental vessels. In a case with massive calcifications of the placental villous cores that we saw, fetal fructokinase deficiency was diagnosed. It is unknown as to whether it was the cause of hydrops.

Cardiac Arrhythmias

A variety of arrhythmias has been documented to cause anasarca and placentomegaly. Some of them, when recognized by sonography or other means, have been treated successfully before birth. Fetal heart block and other rhythm disturbances have occasionally been attributed to specific antibodies, such as occur with lupus, Sjögren syndrome, and other autoimmune diseases. Vetter and Rashkind (1983) have summarized this phenomenon. Specific morphological alterations in the atrioventricular node or localized deposits of antibodies and other globulins have occasionally been thus identified. Veille et al. (1985) described such a child in a mother with Sjögren syndrome, wherein antinuclear antibodies against the Ro (SSA) and La (SSB) antigens were detected during pregnancy. Despite fetal heart block, a normal child was born; and the placenta was apparently normal. Taylor et al. (1986) showed that these antibodies cross the placental barrier. In fatal cases these authors found the antibodies localized in all portions of the fetal hearts. Scheib and Waxman (1989) described recurrent congenital heart block without hydrops. Supraventricular tachycardia has often caused hydrops and placental enlargement. This point is particularly important for pathologists to appreciate because in such stillborns no specific pathological findings explain the placentomegaly and hydrops. Clinical observations are necessary for the diagnosis. One of the first reported cases of severe hydrops, hydramnios, and placentomegaly (1,025 g) was described by Silber and Durnim (1969). The reduced cardiac output was believed to result in the fetal edema. Lingman et al. (1986) reviewed 113 cases of fetal cardiac arrhythmia. Ninety-four cases had supraventricular arrhythmias, consisting mostly of extrasystoles. None had heart failure. Five cases had heart block; of these fetuses, three died from congestive heart failure. Fourteen cases had ventricular arrhythmias. In 2% there were associated congenital anomalies; 13.5% had fetal distress with 0.7% mortality; and four fetuses required in utero therapy for congestive heart failure. In 72% of cases the arrhythmias

disappeared spontaneously during the perinatal period. Vintzileos et al. (1985) found that atrial flutter complicated a case of familial vitamin D-resistant rickets, in which edema and placentomegaly were observed prenatally. The fetus was resistant to therapy. The authors reviewed the previously described cases of prenatally recognized atrial flutter. Fetal hydrops was rare among them, whereas cardiomegaly and hepatomegaly were common.

Since the initial report by Klein et al. (1979) of attempted cardioversion with propanolol, numerous hydropic fetuses with atrioventricular tachycardia have been successfully treated before birth. The treatment was primarily with digitalis (Hallack et al., 1991) but also with quinidine (Guntheroth et al., 1985), verapamil, and other agents (reviewed by Wiggins et al., 1986; DeLia & Emery, 1986). An important consideration is that with severely hydropic fetuses placental drug transport may be insufficient for effective digitalization (Younis & Granat, 1987). Direct fetal injections have also been given (Weiner & Thompson, 1988). In some of the many reported cases, disappearance of hydrops and placental enlargement has been witnessed sonographically, indicating that the placental edema results from fetal heart failure. Hydrops and its subsequent resolution have also been induced experimentally in fetal sheep by atrial pacing (Stevens et al., 1982; Nimrod et al., 1987).

Placental edema and enlargement have been reported following periods of acute fetal tachypnea (Manning et al., 1981). Such rapid respirations are probably the result of the edema rather than its cause.

Nephrotic Syndrome

Congenital nephrosis is another well recognized cause of fetal hydrops with placentomegaly. It is an autosomal recessive condition characterized by anasarca, hypoproteinemia, and albuminuria. Despite the commonly used designation as "Finnish type" of nephrosis, the first case was probably described from Switzerland in 1942 (Giles et al., 1957). The familial nature, a frequent Finnish background of families, and electron microscopic findings have been summarized by Hoyer et al. (1967, 1973) and Seppälä et al. (1976). The latter authors found that more than one-half of the more than 200 cases reported came from Finnish ancestry. They also reported that amnionic fluid α-fetoprotein levels are elevated in this condition, and that fetal death may occur. Whereas the placenta in their case was described to be grossly and microscopically normal, that of a Chinese patient reported by Hung et al. (1977) was enlarged (700 g) and edematous. Milunsky et al. (1977) also saw a normal placenta with an aborted specimen at 14 weeks' gestation. Kaplan et al. (1985), who reported

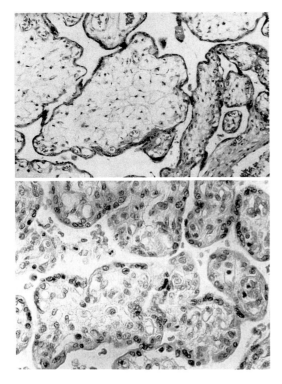

FIGURE 317. Villi of a hydropic fetus with Finnish nephrosis. All villi are severely hydropic but are not different from hydropic placentas with other types of hydrops. The cyto-trophoblast (Langhans' layer) is unusually prominent. H&E. Top ×160; bottom ×400.

several cases and performed electron microscopy of the glomeruli, found only mild placental edema. Presumably, the placentomegaly that has been observed occasionally is dependent on the degree of hypoproteinemia in the fetus. There are no characteristic features in the placental pathology (Figure 317). An electron micrograph of the placental barrier in a case with recurrent congenital nephrosis is shown in Figure 318 after a therapeutic abortion at 19 weeks. No gross or microscopic abnormalities were present in the fetus or placenta. The kidneys showed the typical abnormality of the glomeruli.

Parvovirus Anemia

Pattison et al. (1981) recognized that human parvovirus B19 may cause severe anemia and a hypoplastic crisis in patients with sickle cell anemia. A succinct review of the diseases caused by this virus may be found in the editorial by Anderson and Török (1989). Infection with this highly contagious virus is now known to be an important cause of second trimester abortion and hydrops fetalis. Infections by many types of parvoviruses have been reviewed by Anderson and Pattison (1984). In children, infection with parvovirus B19 causes the so-called fifth disease, or erythema infectiosum (Pillay et

al., 1992). The affliction is commonly referred to as "slapped cheeks" (or face) syndrome because of the appearance of infected children, a disease that is usually self-limited; 40% to 60% of adults have antibodies (IgG) from a previous infection. Asymptomatic women may transmit the virus to their fetuses, and anemia and hydrops may thus result (Brown et al., 1984). These authors cited other infectious causes of hydrops as well (e.g., Chagas' disease, cytomegalovirus infection), which are discussed in Chapter 20. Similarly, listeriosis has been an occasional cause of nonimmune hydrops (Gembruch et al., 1987).

Parvovirus infection does not always cause maternal symptoms, nor does maternal infection always lead to fetal hydrops. It can usually be diagnosed, however, by the typical groundglass inclusion bodies of NRBCs it produces. These bodies are composed of crystals of small (20 nm) virus particles. The inclusion bodies may also be seen in stillborn hydropic fetuses, as they are resistant to autolysis; and often, but not always, they can be identified in their placentas, as was pointed out in the review by Rogers (1992) (Figure 319). Additionally, one often observes hemosiderin in chorionic macrophages. We have seen a macerated fetus with this condition, with typical placental pathology and intestines that had ruptured before birth. Bond et al. (1986) reported a woman with this infection at 15 weeks' gestation. She had a skin rash, and 12 weeks later she delivered a hydropic fetus. DNA hybridization studies and electron microscopy showed many parvovirus particles in the placenta. Some were coated with antibody. Knisely et al. (1988) have also shown that the virions are readily identified in erythroid precursor cells by electron microscopy, even when only formalin-fixed tissues were available. The virus has a preferential attraction to hematopoietic (erythroid) precursor cells (Srivastara & Lu, 1988) but inclusion bodies have been observed in other tissues (e.g., hepatocytes, myocardium, endothelium) (Knisely, 1990).

The characteristic feature of this infection, then, is the presence of lightly staining, eosinophilic intranuclear inclusion bodies in circulating normoblasts (identification from fetal cord samples by Nerlich et al., 1991) and in their precursors in fetal organs (Anand et al., 1987). Cordocentesis was employed by Peters and Nicolaides (1990) for the identification of the virus by DNA hybridization. Immunoglobulins were negative, and the hydrops due to fetal parvovirus infection resolved following prenatal transfusions. Kovacs et al. (1992), working with fetal blood samples and amnionic fluid, developed a sensitive, rapid polymerase chain reaction (PCR) test for the detection of the antigen. The inclusion bodies contain the B19 antigen, whose serological detection is now also widely available (Gray, 1987). In general, elevated IgG titers in maternal blood denote

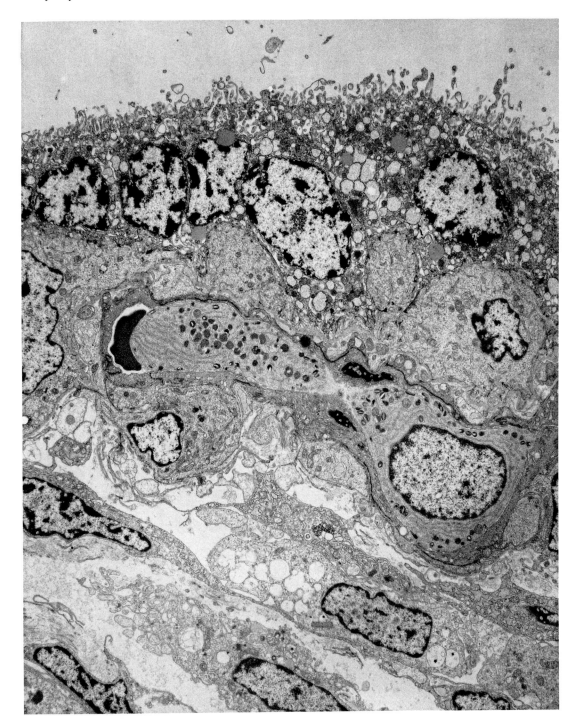

FIGURE 318. Electron micrograph of the villous surface in a case of fetal hydrops due to the nephrotic syndrome. The villous surface (above), microvilli, basement membranes, and fetal capillaries are all normal. ×4,800. (Courtesy Dr. G. Altshuler, Oklahoma City).

former infection, whereas an elevated IgM titer diagnoses recent or active disease. Diagnostic criteria on histological material from marrow were well described and beautifully depicted by Krause et al. (1992). The diagnosis is feasible even in autolyzed specimens because

of the resistance of the virus particles. Generally, the fetal tissues show little or no inflammatory reaction. Elsacker-Niele and collaborators (1989) reported an exception. They found two aborted fetuses in one tissues other than the erythroid cells were involved, and

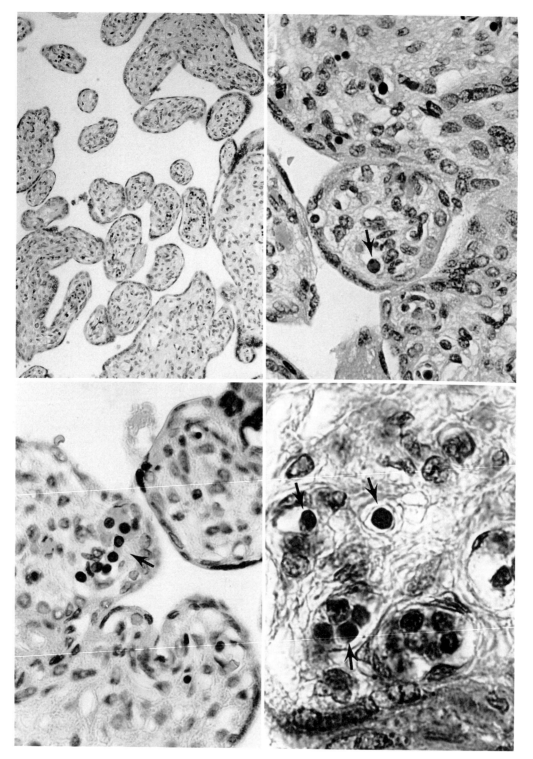

FIGURE 319. Hydrops caused by fetal human parvovirus B19 infection. The villi are edematous, fetal capillaries are filled with normoblasts, and many normoblastic nuclei have smudged amphophilic, intranuclear inclusion bodies (arrows). H&E. Top left ×160; top right ×240; bottom left ×400; bottom right ×640.

in a terminated pregnancy they discovered extensive ocular malformations and inflammation of all fetal and placental tissue. One wonders if these could have been another infection superimposed on parvovirus disease.

Although this virus was believed to lack teratogenicity, Weiland et al. (1987) also found an infected fetus with myocarditis and ocular anomalies. Other cases with identification of the virus were described by Briner et al. (1987) and Franciosi and Tattersall (1987), who used paraffin-embedded tissue for DNA hybridization. Carrington et al. (1987) and Bernstein and Capeless (1989) found elevated maternal serum α-fetoprotein-levels in this condition. Rogers et al. (1993) and Mark et al. (1993) reviewed their 32 cases of hydrops fetalis and found 16% to have been due to this infection. Sections of liver were most productive, whereas only two of five placentas had diagnostic inclusions. In their analysis the inclusion bodies were so characteristic that PCR with DNA hybridization was unnecessary.

The reason for the severe anemia of fetuses was explored by Gray et al. (1987) and Kinney et al. (1988) in prospective studies of cord blood during an outbreak of the infection. This investigation of the frequency of stillbirths during an outbreak showed that the risk of stillbirth or abortion is not high. Similar prospective studies were reported by Hall et al. (1990) in England and Rodis et al. (1990) in the United States. They indicated a rather low risk of fetal hydrops development. Although intrauterine transfusion therapy has been shown to be beneficial (Soothill, 1990; Sahakian et al., 1991), recovery from this infection has also been witnessed without therapy. Humphrey et al. (1991) observed one such case with recovery from hydrops after a 26-week infection, and Pryde et al. (1992) observed two cases that resolved spontaneously. A similar case with ascites and spontaneous resolution was described early by Morey and colleagues (1991), and two others observed by Sheikh et al. (1992) had normal postnatal development. Maeda et al. (1988) depicted the intense hepatic iron deposits in these hydropic infants, perhaps related to the hemolysis. Schwarz et al. (1988), who observed 42 pregnancies with parvovirus infection, found that the infection was inapparent in one-third of the gravidas. In about one-fourth there were fetal complications; the authors thought that the ascites, rather than the anemia, led to fetal death. Burton and Caul (1988) emphasized that the placenta represents "a most fruitful source of nucleated red cells containing parvovirus inclusions and is worthy of study in all cases of hydrops fetalis caused by infection with human parvovirus B19." Macroscopically, the placenta is not different from that in other cases of hydrops fetalis. It is pale, friable, enlarged, and edematous. A complete review of the topic is available from Anand et al. (1987). Rodis et al. (1988), in a study of pregnant women during an outbreak in Connecticut, drew attention to the potential dangers of this disease for pregnant teachers because of their contact with infected children. Further annotations are to be found by Stocker and Singer (1988). Anderson et al. (1988) reported a hydrops due to this infection, and Porter et al. (1988) showed by immunohistochemistry that fetal myocardial nuclei are also infected. Metzman and

colleagues (1989) showed that this infection may cause severe liver disease. They reported a neonatal death with growth retardation and severe hepatic destruction in an infected infant whose mother suffered a rash during the 21st week of pregnancy. It has now also been reported that villous destruction may be the result of parvovirus infection. Samra et al. (1989), who reviewed the world literature of this fetal infection, observed that there is "a high risk to the fetus once the virus crosses the placenta." Their 20 weeks' gestation hydropic stillborn was accompanied by a placenta that showed villous necrosis and calcification.

Hydrops of Unknown Etiology

As more and more causes of fetal edema and hydrops have become known, hydrops of unknown etiology, a baffling entity, is disappearing rapidly. The recognition of syphilis as one such occasional cause (Barton et al., 1992) is representative of the many unusual etiologies one must consider. We believe that the term idiopathic hydrops fetalis should be used with restraint. It merely betrays that we have not yet discovered its etiology and must probe further to assign a specific cause. Drogendijk (1963), who considered this topic in some detail, was of the opinion that hydrops of unknown etiology probably results from some placental malfunction. He illustrated trophoblastic mitoses and other microscopic alterations of villi, but it is our conviction that these conditions are secondary to the fetal condition and that placental edema follows fetal decompensation. Mostoufi-Zadeh et al. (1985) have compiled a thoughtful review of the topic and bring together much of the literature of this "challenge to the perinatal pathologist." Another review and presentation of 11 cases comes from Evron et al. (1985). Some of the rarer entities identified to cause fetal hydrops are discussed by Gloster et al. (1984), including the Beckwith-Wiedeman syndrome with omphalocele and unusual tumors. Ginsburg and Groll (1973) and Rice et al. (1984) found that fetal Gaucher's disease was a cause, and Davis (1982) presented a long list for the differential diagnosis. It included fetal G-6-PD deficiency (in males) with hemolysis resulting from maternal ingestion of fava beans and ascorbic acid (Mentzer & Collier, 1975) or sulfonamides (Perkins, 1971), myocarditis, renal vein thrombosis, achondroplasia, and other conditions. We have seen a case of myocarditis causing hydrops in an 18 weeks' gestation pregnancy. The mother had a "bad cold" during early pregnancy. In the fetus, myocarditis and thyroiditis were present with many plasma cells. The placenta was edematous but otherwise normal. Coxsackie B5 virus infection was believed to be responsible (Benirschke et al., 1986). Ravindranath et al. (1987) identified glucose-phosphate-isomerase deficiency as a cause of hydrops fetalis. Appelman et al. (1988) found I-cell disease (mucolipidosis type II), pterygium syndrome, and α-thalassemia as causes of hydrops and suggested that elevated optical density levels (Δ OD_{450}) may be associated with hydrops fetalis of nonimmune etiology. Other essays on hydrops of nonimmune etiology have been provided by Verger et al. (1963), Giacoia (1980), and Maidman et al. (1980). The latter authors encountered 5 cases in 12,830 deliveries (1:2,566) and suggested management principles. A case of hydrops with unknown etiology was successfully managed by abdominal albumen injection (Shimokawa et al., 1988). Several perplexing instances of recurrent hydrops of unknown etiology have been published by Silverstein and Kanbour (1981). We have seen such a case wherein there were large thrombi in the umbilical cord vessels whose ultimate etiology remained elusive. Cumming (1979) reported two recurrent cases. We autopsied three immature infants with hydrops in whose livers (only) there was massive and unexplained iron deposition. The anemic fetuses had numerous prenatally acquired encephaloclastic lesions, although in one the hematocrit was 23%. This condition may be similar to the perinatal hemochromatosis described by Silver et al. (1989) and Hardy et al. (1990) in several sibships. Although some of their cases had neonatat edema and ascites, hydrops was not described. The placentas of four of their cases was described as being hydropic, with numerous NRBCs in vessels. The iron and copper contents were not increased in them. Schwartz et al. (1981) had two of their four cases in a sibship; they suggested that hypoproteinemia is an important aspect, and that it is perhaps the reason for successful therapy with albumen. Turski et al. (1978) also found markedly decreased serum albumin in a case of unexplained hydrops with hepatosplenomegaly and a 1,900 g edematous placenta. Although it may have been speculated that fetal deficiency of α-fetoprotein could be a cause of fetal hydrops, it has not been found to be so in two cases with such deficiency described by Greenberg et al. (1992). Seeds et al. (1984) attempted, unsuccessfully, to prevent pulmonary hypoplasia in a hydropic fetus with single umbilical artery. They placed a shunt from the peritoneum to the amnionic sac at 29 weeks' gestation. The measured amniotic fluid pressure ranged from 17 to 26 cm H_2O. The investigators determined various constituents in the ascitic fluid as well. Other genetic metabolic diseases have been associated with hydrops but it is not always certain that the disorder was also the true cause of the hydrops. Meizner et al. (1990) found it in Niemann-Pick disease, Uno et al. (1973) reported hydrops in Wolman's disease, and Gillan et al. (1984) found it in another lysosomal storage disorder; glucuronidase deficiency has been the apparent cause in

cases described by Nelson et al. (1982) and Irani and colleagues (1983).

References

Alenghat, E., and Esterly, J.R.: Intravascular hematopoiesis in chorionic villi. Amer. J. Clin. Pathol. 79:225–227, 1983.

Anand, A., Gray, E.S., Brown, T., Clewley, J.P., and Cohen, B.J.: Human parvovirus infection in pregnancy and hydrops fetalis. N. Engl. J. Med. 316:183–186, 1987.

Anders, D., Kindermann, G., and Pfeifer, U.: Metastasizing fetal neuroblastoma with involvement of the placenta simulating fetal erythroblastosis. J. Pediatr. 82:50–53, 1973.

Anderson, M.J., and Pattison, J.R.: The human parvoviruses: brief review. Arch. Virol. 82:137–148, 1984.

Anderson, L.J., and Török, T.J.: Human parvovirus B19. N. Engl. J. Med. 321:536–538, 1989.

Anderson, M.J., Khousam, M.N., Maxwell, D.J., Gould, S.J., Happerfield, L.C., and Smith, W.J.: Human parvovirus B19 and hydrops fetalis. Lancet 1:535, 1988.

Appelman, Z., Blumberg, B.D., Golabi, M., and Golbus, M.S.: Nonimmune hydrops fetalis may be associated with an elevated delta OD_{450} in the amniotic fluid. Obstet. Gynecol. 71:1005–1008, 1988.

Aslam, P.A., Korones, S.B., Richardson, R.L., and Pate, J.W.: Congenital cystic adenomatoid malformation with anasarca. J.A.M.A. 212:622–624, 1970.

Barentsen, R.: Sacrococcygeal teratoom en hydramnion. Nederl. Tidschr. Geneesk. 119:1168–1169, 1975.

Barton, J.R., Thorpe, E.M., Shaver, D.C., Hager, W.D., and Sibai, B.M.: Nonimmune hydrops fetalis associated with maternal infection with syphilis. Am. J. Obstet. Gynecol. 167:56–58, 1992.

Bawle, E.V., and Black, V.: Nonimmune hydrops fetalis in Noonan's syndrome: Am. J. Dis. Child. 140:758–760, 1986.

Becker, V., and Bleyl, U.: Placentarzotte bei Schwangerschaftstoxikose und fetaler Erythroblastose im fluorescenzmikroskopischen Bilde. Virchows Arch. [Pathol. Anat.] 334:516–527, 1961.

Beischer, N.A., Holsman, M., and Kitchen, W.H.: Relation of various forms of anemia to placental weight. Am. J. Obstet. Gynecol. 101:801–809, 1968.

Beischer, N.A., Pepperell, R.J., and Barrie, J.U.: Twin pregnancy and erythroblastosis. Obstet. Gynecol. 34:22–29, 1969.

Benacerraf, B.R., and Frigoletto, F.D.: In utero treatment of a fetus with diaphragmatic hernia complicated by hydrops. Am. J. Obstet. Gynecol. 155:817–818, 1986.

Ben-Ami, M., Shalev, E., Romano, S., and Zuckerman, H.: Midtrimester diagnosis of endocardial fibroelastosis and atrial septal defect: a case report. Am. J. Obstet. Gynecol. 155:662–663, 1986.

Benirschke, K., Swartz, W.H., Leopold, G., and Sahn, D.: Hydrops due to myocarditis in a fetus. Am. J. Cardiovasc. Pathol. 1:131–133, 1986.

Berkowitz, R.L., Chitkara, U., Goldberg, J.D., Wilkins, I., Chervenak, F.A., and Lynch, L.: Intrauterine intravascular transfusions for severe red blood cell isoimmunization:

ultrasound-guided percutaneous approach. Am. J. Obstet. Gynecol. 155:574–581, 1986.

Bernstein, I.M., and Capeless, E.L.: Elevated maternal serum alpha-fetoprotein and hydrops fetalis in association with fetal parvovirus B-19 infection. Obstet. Gynecol. 74: 456–457, 1989.

Birner, W.F.: Neuroblastoma as a cause of antenatal death. Am. J. Obstet. Gynecol. 82:1388–1391, 1961.

Bock, B., Riess, R., Wünsch, P.H., and Feige, A.: Pränatale Diagnostik eines Steißbeinteratoms mit Hydrops fetalis und Plazentahypertrophie—Konsequenzen für den weiteren Schwangerschaftsverlauf. Geburtshilfe Frauenheilkd. 50: 647–649, 1990.

Bond, P.R., Caul, E.O., Usher, J., Cohen, B.J., Clewley, J.P., and Field, A.M.: Intrauterine infection with human parvovirus. Lancet I:448–449, 1986.

Bouissou, H., Kanoun, T., Bierme, S., and Bierme, R.: Foie et placenta au cours de la maladie hémolytique par iso-immunisation Rh (étude histologique et déductions). Pathol. Biol. (Paris) 17:109–120, 1969.

Bowman, J.M., Lewis, M., and de Sa, D.J.: Hydrops fetalis caused by massive maternofetal transplacental hemorrhage. J. Pediatr. 104:769–772, 1984.

Bridge, J.A., McManus, B.M., Remmenga, J., and Cuppage, F.P.: Complete heart block in the 18p- syndrome: congenital calcification of the atrioventricular node. Arch. Pathol. Lab. Med. 113:539–541, 1989.

Briner, J., Hassam, S., Girsberger, M., and Tratschin, J.D.: Demonstration of parvovirus infection in human fetuses and infants by in situ hybridization. Pediatr. Pathol. 7:479–480, 1987.

Brinson, R.A., and Goldsmith, J.P.: Nonimmune hydrops fetalis associated with intrauterine intussusception. J. Perinatol. 8:225–227, 1988.

Broderick, K., Oyer, R., and Chatwani, A.: Neu-Laxova syndrome: a case report. Am. J. Obstet. Gynecol. 158:574–575, 1988.

Bromley, B., Frigoletto, F.D., Estroff, J.A., and Benacerraf, B.R.: The natural history of oligohydramnios/polyhydramnios sequence in monochorionic diamniotic twins. Ultrasound Obstet. Gynecol. 2:317–320, 1992.

Brown, T., Anand, A., Ritschie, L.D., Clewley, J.P., and Reid, T.M.S.: Intrauterine parvovirus infection associated with hydrops fetalis. Lancet 2:1033–1034, 1984.

Burger, K.: Mit Hydrops foetus et placentae einhergehende Luteinzysten. Zentralbl. Gynäkol. 69:533–536, 1947.

Burstein, R.H., and Blumenthal, H.T.: Vascular lesions of the placenta of possible immunogenic origin in erythroblastosis fetalis. Am. J. Obstet. Gynecol. 83:1062–1068, 1962.

Burton, P.A., and Caul, E.O.: Fetal cell tropism of human parvovirus B19. Lancet 1:767, 1988.

Busch, W., and Vogel, M.: Die Plazenta beim "morbus haemolyticus neonatorum." Z. Geburtshilfe Perinatol. 176:17–28, 1972.

Cardwell, M.S.: Successful treatment of hydrops fetalis caused by fetomaternal hemorrhage: a case report. Am. J. Obstet. Gynecol. 158:131–132, 1988.

Carles, D., Serville, F., Dubecq, J.-P., Alberti, E.M., Horowitz, J., and Weichwold, W.: Idiopathic arterial calci-fication in a stillborn complicated by pleural hemorrhage and hydrops fetalis. Arch. Pathol. Lab. Med. 116:293–295, 1992.

Carrington, D., Gilmore, D.H., Whittle, M.J., Aitken, D., Gibson, A.A.M., Patrick, W.J.A., Brown, T., Caul, E.O., Field, A.M., Clewley, J.P., and Cohen, B.J.: Maternal serum α-fetoprotein—a marker of fetal aplastic crisis during intrauterine human parvovirus infection. Lancet 1:433–435, 1987.

Carter, B.S., DiGiacomo, J.E., Balderston, S.M., Wiggins, J.W., and Merenstein, G.B.: Disproportionate septal hypertrophy associated with erythroblastosis. Am. J. Dis. Child. 144:1225–1228, 1990.

Chang, J.C., and Kan, Y.W.: Antenatal diagnosis of sickle cell anaemia by direct analysis of the sickle mutation. Lancet 2:1127–1129, 1981.

Christie, R.W.: Lutein cysts of ovaries associated with erythroblastotic hydrops fetalis. Assay of gonadotropin in serum of Rh-sensitized women in later stages of pregnancy. Am. J. Clin. Pathol. 36:518–523, 1961.

Clark, S.L., Vitale, D.J., Minton, S.D., Stoddard, R.A., and Sabey, P.L.: Successful fetal therapy for cystic adenomatoid malformation associated with second-trimester hydrops. Am. J. Obstet. Gynecol. 157:294–295, 1987.

Cukierski, M.A., Tarantal, A.F., and Hendrickx, A.G.: A case of nonimmune hydrops fetalis with a rare cardiac anomaly in a rhesus monkey. J. Med. Primatol. 15:227–234, 1986.

Cumming, D.C.: Recurrent nonimmune hydrops fetalis. Obstet. Gynecol. 54:124–126, 1979.

Curry, C.J.R., Chopra, D., and Finer, N.N.: Hydrops and pleural effusions in congenital myotonic dystrophy. J. Pediatr. 113:555–557, 1988.

Davis, C.L.: Diagnosis and management of nonimmune hydrops fetalis. J. Reprod. Med. 27:594–600, 1982.

DeLia, J.E., and Emery, M.G.: Digoxin therapy in the fetus. Am. J. Dis. Child. 140:974–975, 1986.

Driscoll, S.G., and Steinke, J.: Pancreatic insulin content in severe erythroblastosis fetalis. Pediatrics 39:449–450, 1967.

Drogendijk, A.C.: The pathogenesis of foetal hydrops. Gynaecologia 156:129–139, 1963.

Editorial: Dangers of anti-Kell in pregnancy. Lancet 337: 1319–1320, 1991.

Eklund, J.: Embryonic rhesus-positive red cells stimulating a secondary response after early abortion. Lancet 2:748, 1981.

Elsacker-Niele, A.M.W., Salimans, M.M.M., Weiland, H.T., Vermey-Keers, C., Anderson, M.J., and Versteeg, J.: Fetal pathology in human parvovirus B19 infection. Br. J. Obstet. Gynaecol. 96:768–775, 1989.

Evron, S., Yagel, S., Samueloff, A., Margaliot, E., Burstein, P., and Sadovsky, E.: Nonimmunologic hydrops fetalis: a review of 11 cases. J. Perinat. Med. 13:147–151, 1985.

Feige, A., Gille, J., Maillot, K.v., and Mulz, D.: Pränatale Diagnostik eines Steißbeinteratoms mit Hypertrophie der Plazenta. Geburtshilfe Frauenheilkd. 42:20–24, 1982.

Fox, H.: The incidence and significance of nucleated erythro-cytes in the foetal vessels of the mature human placenta. J. Obstet. Gynaecol. Br. Commonw. 74:40–43, 1967.

Franciosi, R., and Tattersall, P.: Human parvovirus (B19) causing hydrops fetalis. Pediatr. Pathol. 7:485–486, 1987.

Freda, V.J., and Carter, B.-A.: Placental permeability in the human for anti-A and anti-B isoantibodies. Am. J. Obstet. Gynecol. 84:1351–1367, 1962.

Freda, V.J., Gorman, J.G., Galen, R.S., and Treacy, N.: The threat of Rh immunisation from abortion. Lancet 1: 147–148, 1970.

Friesen, R.F., Bowman, J.M., Barnes, P.H., Grewar, D., Mcinnis, C., and Bowman, W.D.: Intrauterine transfusions for erythroblastosis. Am. J. Obstet. Gynecol. 97:343–339, 1967.

Gembruch, U., Niesen, M., Hansmann, M., and Knöpple, G.: Listeriosis: a cause of non-immune hydrops fetalis. Prenat. Diagn. 7:277–282, 1987.

Giacoia, G.P.: Hydrops fetalis (fetal edema): a survey. Clin. Pediatr. 19:334–339, 1980.

Giles, H.M., Ough, R.C.B., Darmady, E.M., Stranack, F., and Woolf, L.I.: The nephrotic syndrome in early infancy: a report of three cases. Arch. Dis. Child. 32:167–180, 1957.

Gillan, J.E., Lowden, J.A., Gaskin, K., and Cutz, E.: Congenital ascites as a presenting sign of lysosomal storage disease. J. Pediatr. 104:225–231, 1984.

Ginsburg, S.J., and Groll, M.: Hydrops fetalis due to infantile Gaucher's disease. J. Pediatr. 82:1046–1048, 1973.

Gloster, E.S., Jimenez, J.F., Godoy, G., Burrows, P., Hill, D., Mollitt, D.L., and Grunow, W.A.: Nonimmune hydrops fetalis: the Arkansas Children's Hospital experience for 1982–1983. Lab. Invest. 50:3P, 1984.

Goldschmidt, E., Cohen, T., Isacsohn, M., and Freier, S.: Incidence of hemoglobin Bart's in a sample of newborn from Israel. Acta Genet. (Basel) 18:361–368, 1968.

Gonen, R., Fong, K., and Chiasson, D.A.: Prenatal sonographic diagnosis of hepatic hemangioendothelioma with secondary nonimmune hydrops fetalis. Obstet. Gynecol. 73:485–487, 1989.

Gonsoulin, W., Copeland, K.L., Carpenter, R.J., Hughes, M.R., and Elder, F.B.: Fetal blood sampling demonstrating chimerism in monozygotic twins discordant for sex and tissue karyotype (46,XY and 45,X). Prenat. Diagn. 10: 25–28, 1990.

Goto, S., Nishi, H., and Tomoda, Y.: Blood group Rh-D factor in human trophoblast determined by immunofluorescent method. Am. J. Obstet. Gynecol. 137:707–712, 1980.

Gottschalk, W., and Abramson, D.: Placental edema and fetal hydrops: a case of congenital cystic and adenomatoid malformation of the lung. Obstet. Gynecol. 10:626–631, 1957.

Grannum, P.A.T., Copel, J.A., Moya, F.R., Scioscia, A.L., Robert, J.A., Winn, H.N., Coster, B.C., Burdine, C.B., and Hobbins, J.C.: The reversal of hydrops fetalis by intravascular intrauterine transfusion in severe isoimmune fetal anemia. Am. J. Obstet. Gynecol. 158:914–919, 1988.

Gray, E.S.: Human parvovirus infection. J. Pathol. 153:310–311, 1987.

Gray, E.S.: Mesoblastic nephroma and non-immunological hydrops fetalis [letter to the editor]. Pediatr. Pathol. 9:607–609, 1989.

Gray, E.S., Davidson, R.J.L., and Anand, A.: Human parvovirus and fetal anaemia. Lancet 1:1144, 1987.

Gray, G.R., Towell, M.E., Wright, V.J., and Hardwick, D.F.: Thalassemic hydrops fetalis in two Chinese-Canadian families. Can. Med. Assoc. J. 107:1186–1190, 1972.

Green, D.W., Donovan, E.F., and Wood, B.P.: Radiological cases of the month. Am. J. Dis. Child. 144:93–94, 1990.

Greenberg, F., Faucett, A., Rose, E., Bancalari, L., Kardon, N.B., Mizejewski, G., Haddon, J.E., and Alpert, E.: Congenital deficiency of α-fetoprotein. Am. J. Obstet. Gynecol. 167:509–511, 1992.

Grimes, D.A., Geary, F.H., and Hatcher, R.A.: Rh immuno-globulin utilization after ectopic pregnancy. Am. J. Obstet. Gynecol. 140:246–249, 1981.

Gropp, A.: Fetal hydrops in chromosome disorders as principle of damage in developmental pathology: clinical observations in man and experimental studies in the mouse. In, One Medicine. O.A. Ryder and M.L. Byrd, eds., pp. 84–95, Chapter 8. Springer-Verlag, New York, 1984.

Groves, G.R., and Baskett, T.F.: Nonimmune hydrops fetalis: antenatal diagnosis and management. Am. J. Obstet. Gynecol. 148:563–569, 1984.

Guntheroth, W.G., Cyr, D.R., Mack, L.A., Benedetti, T., Lenke, R.R., and Petty, C.N.: Hydrops from reciprocating atrioventricular tachycardia in a 27-week fetus requiring quinidine for conversion. Obstet. Gynecol. 66:29S–33S, 1985.

Guy, G., Coady, D.J., Jansen, V., Snyder, J., and Zinberg, S.: α-Thalassemia hydrops fetalis: clinical and ultrasonographic considerations. Am. J. Obstet. Gynecol. 153:500–504, 1985.

Hall, S.M., Cohen, B.J., Mortimer, P.P., Caul, E.O., Cradock-Watson, J., Anderson, M.J., Pattison, J.R., Shirley, J.A., and Peto, T.E.A.: Prospective study of human parvovirus (B19) infection in pregnancy. B.M.J. 300:1166–1170, 1990.

Hallak, M., Neerhof, M.G., Perry, R., Nazir, M., and Hulka, J.C.: Fetal supraventricular tachycardia and hydrops fetalis: combined intensive, direct, and transplacental therapy. Obstet. Gynecol. 78:523–525, 1991.

Hardy, L., Hansen, J.L., Kushner, J.P., and Knisely, A.S.: Neonatal hemochromatosis: genetic analysis of transferrin-receptor, H-apoferritin, and L-apoferritin loci and of the human leukocyte antigen class I region. Am. J. Pathol. 137:149–153, 1990.

Harman, C.R., Bowman, J.M., Menticoglou, S.M., Pollock, J.M., and Manning, F.A: Profound fetal thrombocytopenia in rhesus disease: serious hazard at intravascular transfusion. Lancet 2:741–742, 1988.

Hatjis, C.G.: Nonimmunologic fetal hydrops associated with hyperreactio luteinalis. Obstet. Gynecol. 65:11S–13S, 1985.

Hellman, L.M., and Hertig, A.T.: Pathological changes in the placenta associated with erythroblastosis of the fetus. Am. J. Pathol. 14:111–120, 1937.

Hendricks, S.K., Sorensen, T.K., and Baker, E.R.: Trisomy 21, fetal hydrops, and anemia: prenatal diagnosis of transient myeloproliferative disorder? Obstet. Gynecol. 82: 703–705, 1993.

Herman, A., Bukovsky, Y., Benson, L., Weinraub, Z., and Caspi, E.: Intrapartum use of fetal scalp hematocrit in the diagnosis of profound fetal anemia caused by fetomaternal hemorrhage. Am. J. Obstet. Gynecol. 157:1182–1183, 1987.

Holzgreve, W., Miny, P., Anderson, R., and Golbus, M.S.: Experience with 8 cases of prenatally diagnosed sacrococcygeal teratomas. Fetal Ther. 2:88–94, 1987.

Horowitz, A., Cohen, T., Goldschmidt, E., and Levene, C.: Thalassemia among Kurdish Jews in Israel. Br. J. Haematol. 12:555–568, 1966.

Houston, C.S., and Brown, A.B.: An unusual complication of intrauterine transfusion. Can. Med. Assoc. J. 94:1274–1277, 1966.

Hoyer, J.R., Michael, A.F., Good, R.A., and Vernier, R.L.: The nephrotic syndrome of infancy: clinical, morphologic, and immunologic studies of four infants. Pediatrics 40:233–246, 1967.

Hoyer, J.R., Mauer, S.M., Kjellstrand, C.M., Buselmeier, T.J., Simmons, R.L., Michael, A.F., Najarian, J.S., and Vernier, R.L.: Successful renal transplantation in 3 children with congenital nephrotic syndrome. Lancet 1:1410–1413, 1973.

Humphrey, W., Magoon, M., and O'Shaughnessy, R.: Severe nonimmune hydrops secondary to parvovirus B-19 infection: spontaneous reversal in utero and survival of a term infant. Obstet. Gynecol. 78:900–902, 1991.

Hung, P.-L., Huang, C.-C., and Huang, T.,-S.: Nephrotic syndrome in a Chinese infant. Am. J. Dis. Child. 131:557–559, 1977.

Hutchison, A.A., Drew, J.H., Yu, V.Y.H., Williams, M.L., Fortune, D.W., and Beischer, N.A.: Nonimmunologic hydrops fetalis: a review of 61 cases. Obstet. Gynecol. 59:347–352, 1982.

Iakovtsova, A.G.: Morphologic changes in the placenta in isoantigenic incompatibility of maternal and fetal blood. Pediatr. Akhush. Ginekol. 1:53–55, 1964.

Imakita, M., Yutani, C., Ishibashi-Ueda, H., Murakami, M., and Chiba, Y.: A case of hydrops fetalis due to placental chorangioma. Acta Pathol. Jpn. 38:941–945, 1988.

Ing, R.Y.K., Crookston, J.H., Dworatzek, J.A., and Burnie, K.L.: Alpha thalassemia: five cases of hemoglobin H disease in Oriental-Canadian families. Can. Med. Assoc. J. 99:49–56, 1968.

Irani, D., Kim, H.S., El-Hibri, H., Dutton, R.V., Beaudet, A., and Armstrong, D.: Postmortem observations on β-glucuronidase deficiency presenting as hydrops fetalis. Ann. Neurol. 14:486–490, 1983.

Ivemark, B.I., Högman, C., Rudert, P.O., and Andersen, B.: Kell-iso-immunization as the cause of fatal erythroblastosis fetalis. Acta Pathol. Microbiol. Scand. 45:193–202, 1959.

James, G.B.: Histology of the placenta after repeated intrauterine transfusions. Proc. R. Soc. Med. 63:54, 1970.

Jarkowski, T.L., Rosenblatt, M., Wolf, P., and Pearson, B.: Tissue-fixed antigens of the Rh blood group system in placentae and fetuses; with particular reference to hemolytic disease of the newborn. Lab. Invest. 13:937, 1964.

Jauniaux, E., Maldergem L.v., Munter, C. de, Moscoso, G., and Gillerot, Y.: Nonimmune hydrops fetalis associated with genetic abnormalities. Obstet. Gynecol. 75:568–572, 1990.

Johnson, P., Sharland, G., Allan, L.D., Tynan, M.J., and Maxwell, D.J.: Umbilical venous pressure in nonimmune hydrops fetalis: correlation with cardiac size. Am. J. Obstet. Gynecol. 167:1309–1313, 1992.

Jones, C.J.P., and Fox, H.: An ultrastructural study of the placenta in materno-fetal rhesus incompatibility. Virchows Arch. Pathol. Anat. Histol. 379:229–241, 1978.

Jones, D.E.D., Pritchard, K.I., Gioannini, C.A., Moore, D.T., and Bradford, W.D.: Hydrops fetalis associated with idiopathic arterial calcification. Obstet. Gynecol. 39:435–440, 1972.

Jonxis, J.H.P.: The development of hemoglobin. Pediatr. Clin. North Am. 12:535–550, 1965.

Jorgensen, J.: Rhesus-antibody development after abortion. Lancet 2:1253–1254, 1969.

Kan, Y.W., Allen, A., and Lowenstein, L.: Hydrops fetalis with alpha thalassemia. N. Engl. J. Med. 276:18–23, 1967.

Kan, Y.W., Forget, B.G., and Nathan, D.G.: Gamma-beta thalassemia: a cause of hemolytic disease of the newborn. N. Engl. J. Med. 286:129–134, 1972.

Kan, Y.W., Golbus, M.S., and Dozy, A.M.: Prenatal diagnosis of α-thalassemia: clinical application of molecular hybridization. N. Engl. J. Med. 295:1165–1167, 1976.

Kaplan, C., Lane, B., Miller, F., Baker, D., and Trunca, C.: Renal pathology of prenatally diagnosed nephrosis. Pediatr. Pathol. 3:271–281, 1985.

Kinney, J.S., Anderson, L.J., Farrar, J., Strikas, R.A., Kumar, M.L., Kliegman, R.M., Sever, J.L., Hurwitz, E.S., and Sikes, R.K.: Risk of adverse outcomes of pregnancy after human parvovirus B19 infection. J. Infect. Dis. 157:663–667, 1988.

Klein, A.M., Holzman, I.R., and Austin, E.M.: Fetal tachycardia before the development of hydrops-attempted cardioversion: a case report. Am. J. Obstet. Gynecol. 134:347–348, 1979.

Kleinman, C.S., Donnerstein, R.L., Devore, G.R., Jaffe, C.C., Lynch, D.C., Berkowitz, R.L., Talner, N.S., and Hobbins, J.C.: Fetal echocardiography for evaluation of in utero congestive heart failure: a technique for study of nonimmune hydrops. N. Engl. J. Med. 306:568–575, 1982.

Knisely, A.S.: Parvovirus B19 infection in the fetus. Lancet 336:443, 1990.

Knisely, A.S., O'Shea, P., McMillan, P., Singer, D.B., and Magid, M.S.: Electron microscopic identification of parvovirus virions in erythroid-line cells in fatal hydrops fetalis. Pediatr. Pathol. 8:163–170, 1988.

Kohga, S., Nambu, T., Tanaka, K., Benirschke, K., Feldman, B.H., and Kishikawa, T.: Hypertrophy of the placenta and sacrococcygeal teratoma: report of two cases. Virchows Arch. A Pathol. Anat. Histol. 386:223–229, 1980.

Kohler, H.G., and Rymer, B.: Congenital cystic malformation of the lung and its relation to hydramnios. J. Obstet. Gynaecol. Br. Commonw. 80:130–134, 1973.

Koffler, H., Papile, L.-A., and Burstein, R.: Congenital chylothorax: two cases associated with maternal polyhydramnios. Am. J. Dis. Child. 132:638, 1978.

Kovacs, B.W., Carlson, D.E., Shahbahrami, M.S., and Platt, L.D.: Prenatal diagnosis of human parvovirus B19 in nonimmune hydrops fetalis by polymerase chain reaction. Am. J. Obstet. Gynecol. 167:461–466, 1992.

Krause, J.R., Penchansky, L., and Knisely, A.S.: Morphological diagnosis of parvovirus B19 infection. Arch. Pathol. Lab. Med. 116:178–180, 1992.

Kuhlmann, R.S., Warsof, S.L., Levy, D.L., Flake, A.J., and Harrison, M.R.: Fetal therapy 2:95–100, 1987.

Lacro, R.V., Jones, K.L., and Benirschke, K.: Coarctation of the aorta in Turner syndrome: a pathologic study of fetuses with nuchal hygromas, hydrops fetalis, and female genitalia. Pediatrics 81:445–451, 1988.

Landrum, B.G., Johnson, D.E., Ferrara, B., Boros, S.J., and Thompson, T.R.: Hydrops fetalis and chromosomal trisomies. Am. J. Obstet. Gynecol. 154:1114–1115, 1986.

Langer, J.C., Harrison, M.R., Schmidt, K.G., Silverman, N.H., Anderson, R.L., Goldberg, J.D., Filly, R.A., Crombleholme, T.M., Longaker, M.T., and Golbus, M.S.: Fetal hydrops and death from sacrococcygeal teratoma: rationale for fetal surgery. Am. J. Obstet. Gynecol. 160:1145–1150, 1989.

Laros, R.K., and Kalstone, C.E.: Sickle cell β-thalassemia and pregnancy. Obstet. Gynecol. 37:67–71, 1971.

Leake, R.D., Strimling, B., and Emmanouilidis, G.C.: Intrauterine cardiac failure with hydrops fetalis: case report in a twin with the hypoplastic left heart syndrome and review of the literature. Clin. Pediatr. 12:649–651, 1973.

Lebo, R.V., Saiki, R.K., Swanson, K., Montano, M.A., Erlich, H.A., and Golbus, M.S.: Prenatal diagnosis of α-thalassemia by polymerase chain reaction and dual restriction enzyme analysis. Hum. Genet. 85:293–299, 1990.

Lee, J.-N., Huang, S.-C., Ouyang, P.-C., and Chard, T.: Circulating placental proteins in pregnancies complicated by Rh isoimmunization. Obstet. Gynecol. 64:131–132, 1984.

Leggat, H.M., Gibson, J.M., Barron, S.L., and Reid, M.M.: Anti-Kell in pregnancy. Br. J. Obstet. Gynaecol. 98:162–165, 1991.

Leventhal, M.L., and Wolf, A.M.: Erythroblastosis (hydrops) fetalis from Kell sensitization. Am. J. Obstet. Gynecol. 71:452–454, 1956.

Lie-Injo, L.E.: Haemoglobin of new-born infants in Indonesia. Nature 183:1125–1126, 1959.

Lie-Injo, L.E.: Alpha-chain thalassemia and hydrops fetalis in Malaysia; report of 5 cases. Blood 20:581–590, 1962.

Lie-Injo, L.E., Lopez, C.G., and Dutt, A.K.: Pathological findings in hydrops foetalis due to alpha-thalassemia: a review of 32 cases. Trans. R. Soc. Trop. Med. Hyg. 62:874–879, 1968.

Lingman, G., Lundström, N.R., Marsal, K., and Ohrlander, S.: Fetal cardiac arrhythmia—clinical outcome in 113 cases. Acta Obstet. Gynecol. Scand. 65:263–267, 1986.

Louderback, A.L., and Shanbrom, E.: Hemoglobin electrophoresis. J.A.M.A. 202:718–719, 1967.

Luca, E.C. de, Casadei, A.M., Pascone, R., Tardi, C., and Pacioni, C.: Maternofetal transfusion during delivery and sensitization of newborn against the rhesus D-antigen. Vox Sang. 34:241–243, 1978.

Macafee, C.A.J., Fortune, D.W., and Beischer, N.A.: Non-immunological hydrops fetalis. J. Obstet. Gynaecol. Br. Commonw. 77:226–237, 1970.

Macgregor, S.N., Socol, M.L., Pielet, B.W., Sholl, J.T., and Minogue, J.P.: Prediction of fetoplacental blood volume in isoimmunized pregnancy. Am. J. Obstet. Gynecol. 159:1493–1497, 1988.

Machin, G.A.: Hydrops revisited: literature review of 1,414 cases published in the 1980s. Am. J. Med. Genet. 34:366–390, 1989.

Maeda, H., Shimokawa, H., Saton, S., Nakano, H., and Nunoue, T.: Nonimmunologic hydrops fetalis resulting from intrauterine human parvovirus B-19 infection: report of two cases. Obstet. Gynecol. 72:482–485, 1988.

Maidman, J.E., Yeager, C., Anderson, V., Makabali, G., O'Grady, J.P., Arce, J., and Tishler, D.M.: Prenatal diagnosis and management of nonimmunologic hydrops fetalis. Obstet. Gynecol. 56:571–576, 1980.

Mallmann, P., Gembruch, U., Mallmann, R., and Hansmann, M.: Investigations into a possible immunological origin of idiopathic non-immune hydrops fetalis and initial results of prophylactic immune treatment of subsequent pregnancies. Acta Obstet. Gynecol. Scand. 70:35–40, 1991.

Manning, F.A., Heaman, M., Boyce, D., and Carter, L.J.: Intrauterine fetal tachypnea. Obstet. Gynecol. 58:398–400, 1981.

Manning, F.A., Bowman, J.M., Lange, I.R., and Chamberlain, P.F.: Intrauterine transfusion in an Rh-immunized twin pregnancy: a case report of successful outcome and a review of the literature. Obstet. Gynecol. 65:2S–6S, 1985.

Mark, Y., Rogers, B.B., and Oyer, C.E.: Diagnosis and incidence of fetal parvovirus infection in an autopsy series. II. DNA amplification. Pediatr. Pathol. 13:381–386, 1993.

Matthews, C.D., Matthews, A.E.B., and Gilbey, B.E.: Antibody development in rhesus-negative patients following abortion. Lancet 2:318–319, 1969.

McFadden, D.E., and Taylor, G.P.: Cardiac abnormalities and nonimmune hydrops fetalis: a coincidental, not causal, relationship. Pediatr. Pathol. 9:11–17, 1989.

Meizner, I., Levy, A., Carmi, R., and Robinsin, C.: Niemann-Pick disease associated with nonimmune hydrops fetalis. Am. J. Obstet. Gynecol. 163:128–129, 1990.

Mentzer, W.C., and Collier, E.: Hydrops fetalis associated with erythrocyte G-6-PD deficiency and maternal ingestion of fava beans and ascorbic acid. J. Pediatr. 86:565–567, 1975.

Metzman, R., Anand, A., DeGiulio, P.A., and Knisely, A.S.: Hepatic disease associated with intrauterine parvovirus B19 infection in a newborn premature infant. J. Pediatr. Gastroenterol. Nutr. 9:119–114, 1989.

Miller, D.F., and Petrie, S.J.: Fatal erythroblastosis fetalis secondary to ABO incompatibility. Obstet. Gynecol. 22:773–777, 1963.

Miller, P.D., Smith, B.C., and Marinoff, D.N.: Theca-lutein ovarian cysts associated with homozygous α-thalassemia. Am. J. Obstet. Gynecol. 157:912–914, 1987.

Milner, P.F., Clegg, J.B., and Weatherall, D.J.: Haemoglobin-H disease due to a unique haemoglobin variant with an elongated α-chain. Lancet 1:729–732, 1971.

Milunsky, A., Alpert, E., Frigoletto, F.D., Driscoll, S.G., McCluskey, R.T., and Colvin, R.B.: Prenatal diagnosis of the congenital nephrotic syndrome. Pediatrics 59:770–773, 1977.

Mittendorf, R., and Williams, M.A.: RH$_0$(D) immunoglobulin (RhoGAM): how it came into being. Obstet. Gynecol. 77:301–303, 1991.

Moerman, P., Fryns, J.P., Goddeeris, P., and Lauweryns, J.M.: Nonimmunologic hydrops fetalis: a study of ten cases. Arch. Pathol. Lab. Med. 106:635–640, 1982.

Mogilner, B.M., Ashkenazy, M., Borenstein, R., and Lancet, M.: Hydrops fetalis caused by maternal indomethacin treatment. Acta Obstet. Gynecol. Scand. 61:183–185, 1982.

Moller, J.H., Lynch, R.P., and Edwards, J.E.: Fetal cardiac failure resulting from congenital anomalies of the heart. J. Pediatr. 68:699–703, 1966.

Mollison, P.L.: Suppression of Rh-immunization by passively administered anti-Rh. Br. J. Haematol. 14:1–4, 1968.

Montemagno, U., Stefano, M. di, and Cardone, A.: Aspetti istoimmunologici della placenta nella incompatibilita Rh. In, Simpos. Sui Problemi Ostetrico-Pediatrici della Sofferenza Fetale. pp. 649–655. Offic. Grafiche Stianti-Sanscasciano, Siena, Italy, 1966.

Mor, Z., Schreyer, P., Wainraub, Z., Hayman, E., and Caspi, E.: Nonimmune hydrops fetalis associated with angioosteohypertrophy (Klippel-Trenaunay) syndrome. Am. J. Obstet. Gynecol. 159:1185–1186, 1988.

Morey, A.L., Nicolini, U., Welch, C.R., Economides, D., Chamberlain, P.F., and Cohen, B.J.: Parvovirus B19 infection and transient fetal hydrops. Lancet 337:496, 1991.

Moss, T.J., and Kaplan, L.: Association of hydrops fetalis with congenital neuroblastoma. Am. J. Obstet. Gynecol. 132:905–906, 1978.

Mostoufi-Zadeh, M., Weiss, L.M., and Driscoll, S.G.: Nonimmune hydrops fetalis: a challenge in perinatal pathology. Hum. Pathol. 16:785–789, 1985.

Moya, F.R., Grannum, P.A.T., Widness, J.A., Clemons, G.K., Copel, J.A., and Hobbins, J.C.: Erythropoietin in human fetuses with immune hemolytic anemia and hydrops fetalis. Obstet. Gynecol. 82:353–358, 1993.

Murray, S., and Barron, S.L.: Rhesus isoimmunization after abortion. B.M.J. 3:87–89, 1971.

Naeye, R.L.: New observations in erythroblastosis fetalis. J.A.M.A. 200:105–110, 1967.

Nakamura, Y., Komatsu, Y., Yano, H., Kitazono, S., Hosokawa, Y., Fukuda, S., Kawano, S., Nagasue, N., Matsunaga, T., Aiko, Y., Hashimoto, T., and Morimatsu, M.: Nonimmunologic hydrops fetalis: a clinicopathological study of 50 autopsy cases. Pediatr. Pathol. 7:19–30, 1987.

Nakayama, R., Yamada, D., Steinmiller, V., Hsia, E., and Hale, R.W.: Hydrops fetalis secondary to Bart hemoglobinopathy. Obstet. Gynecol. 67:176–180, 1986.

Nalbandian, R.M., Henry, R.L., Camp, F.R., Wolf, P.L., and Evans, T.N.: Embryonic, fetal, and neonatal hemoglobin synthesis: relationship to abortion and thalassemia. Obstet. Gynecol. Surv. 26:185–191, 1971.

Nathan, D.G.: Thalassemia: a progress report on applied molecular biology. N. Engl. J. Med. 288:1122–1123, 1973.

Nelson, A., Peterson, L.A., Frampton, B., and Sly, W.S.: Mucopolysaccharidosis VII (β-glucuronidase deficiency) presenting as nonimmune hydrops fetalis. J. Pediatr. 101:574–576, 1982.

Nerlich, A., Schwarz, T.F., Roggendorf, M., Roggendorf, H., Ostermeyer, E., Schramm, T., and Gloning, K.-P.: Parvovirus B19-infected erythroblasts in fetal cord blood. Lancet 337:310, 1991.

Newton, E.R., Louis, F., Dalton, M.E., and Feigold, M.: Fetal neuroblastoma and catecholamine-induced maternal hypertension. Obstet. Gynecol. 65:49S–52S, 1985.

Nicolaides, K.H., Soothill, P.W., Clewell, W.H., Rodeck, C.H., Mibashan, R.S., and Campbell, S.: Fetal haemoglobin measurement of red cell isoimmunization. Lancet 1:1073–1075, 1988a.

Nicolaides, K.H., Thilaganathan, B., Rodeck, C.H., and Mibashan, R.S.: Erythroblastosis and reticulocytosis in anemic fetuses. Am. J. Obstet. Gynecol. 159:1063–1065, 1988b.

Nicolaides, K.H., Thilaganathan, B., and Mibashan, R.S.: Cordocentesis in the investigation of fetal erythropoiesis. Am. J. Obstet. Gynecol. 161:1197–1200, 1989.

Nicolini, U., Talbert, D.G., Fisk, N.M., and Rodeck, C.H.: Pathophysiology of pressure changes during intrauterine transfusion. Am. J. Obstet. Gynecol. 160:1139–1145, 1989.

Nimrod, C., Davies, D., Harder, J., Iwanicki, S., Kondo, C., Takahashi, Y., Maloney, J., Persaud, D., and Nicholson, S.: Ultrasound evaluation of tachycardia-induced hydrops in the fetal lamb. Am. J. Obstet. Gynecol. 157:655–659, 1987.

Novak, P.M., Sander, M., Yang, S.S., and Oeyen, P.V.v.: Report of fourteen cases of nonimmune hydrops fetalis in association with hemorrhagic endovasculitis of the placenta. Am. J. Obstet. Gynecol. 165:945–950, 1991.

Olson, R.W., Nishibatake, M., Arya, S., and Gilbert, E.F.: Nonimmunologic hydrops fetalis due to intrauterine closure of fetal foramen ovale. Birth Defects 23:433–442, 1987.

Orkin, S.H., and Michelson, A.: Partial deletion of the α-globin structural gene in human α-thalassemia. Nature 286:538–540, 1980.

Orkin, S.H., and Nathan, D.G.: Current concepts in genetics. N. Engl. J. Med. 295:710–714, 1976.

Östör, A.G., and Fortune, D.W.: Tuberous sclerosis initially seen as hydrops fetalis: report of a case and review of the literature. Arch. Pathol. Lab. Med. 102:34–39, 1978.

Oudesluys-Murphy, A.M.: Nonimmune hydrops fetalis in Noonan's syndrome. Am. J. Dis. Child. 141:478–479, 1987.

Pattison, J.R., Jones, S.E., Hodgson, J., Davis, L.R., White, J.M., Stroud, C.E., and Murtoza, L.: Parvovirus infections and hypoplastic crisis in sickle-cell anaemia. Lancet 1:664–665, 1981.

Pattison, N., and Roberts, A.: The management of severe erythroblastosis fetalis by fetal transfusion: survival of transfused adult erythrocytes in the fetus. Obstet. Gynecol. 74:901–904, 1989.

Pearson, H.A., Shanklin, D.R., and Brodine, C.R.: Alpha-thalassemia as cause of nonimmunological hydrops. Am. J. Dis. Child. 109:168–172, 1965.

Perkins, R.P.: Hydrops fetalis and stillbirth in a male glucose-6-phosphate dehydrogenase-deficient fetus possibly due to maternal ingestion of sulfisoxazole. Am. J. Obstet. Gynecol. 111:379–381, 1971.

Perkins, D.G., Kopp, C.M., and Haust, M.D.: Placental infiltration in congenital neuroblastoma: a case study with ultrastructure. Histopathology 4:383–389, 1980.

Perlin, B.M., Pomerance, J.J., and Schifrin, B.S.: Nonimmunologic hydrops fetalis. Obstet. Gynecol. 57:584–588, 1981.

Peschle, C., Mavilio, F., Care, A., Migliaccio, G., Migliaccio, A.R., Salvo, G., Samoggia, P., Petti, S., Guerriero, R., Marinucci, M., Lazzaro, D., Russo, G., and Mastroberardino, G.: Haemoglobin switching in human embryos: asynchrony of θ → α and epsilon → gamma-globin switches in primitive and definitive erythropoietic lineage. Nature 313:235–238, 1985.

Peters, M.T., and Nicolaides, K.H.: Cordocentesis for the diagnosis and treatment of human fetal parvovirus infection. Obstet. Gynecol. 75:501–504, 1990.

Pielet, B.W., Socol, M.L., Macgregor, S.N., Ney, J.A., and Dooley, S.L.: Cordocentesis: an appraisal of risks. Am. J. Obstet. Gynecol. 159:1497–1500, 1988.

Pillay, D., Patou, G., Hurt, S., Kibbler, C.C., and Griffiths, P.D.: Parvovirus B19 outbreak in a children's ward. Lancet 339:107–109, 1992.

Pilz, I., Schweikhart, G., and Kaufmann, P.: Zur Abgrenzung normaler, artefizieller und pathologischer Strukturen in reifen menschlichen Plazentarzotten. III. Morphometrische Untersuchungen bei Rhesus-Inkompabilität. Arch. Gynecol. 229:137–154, 1980.

Pootrakul, S., Wasi, P., and Na-Nakorn, S.: Haemoglobin Bart's hydrops foetalis in Thailand. Ann. Hum. Genet. 30:293–311, 1967.

Porter, H.J., Quantrill, A.M., and Flehming K.A.: B19 parvovirus infection of myocardial cells. Lancet 1:535–536, 1988.

Price, J.R.: Rh sensitization by hydatidiform mole. N. Engl. J. Med. 278:1021, 1968.

Pringle, K.C., Weiner, C.P., Soper, R.T., and Kealey, P.: Sacrococcygeal teratoma. Fetal Ther. 2:80–87, 1987.

Pryde, P.G., Nugent, C.E., Pridjian, G., Barr, M., and Faix, R.G.: Spontaneous resolution of nonimmune hydrops fetalis secondary to human parvovirus B19 infection. Obstet. Gynecol. 79:859–861, 1992.

Queenan, J.T., and Douglas, G.R.: Intrauterine transfusion: a preliminary report. Obstet. Gynecol. 25:308–321, 1965.

Queenan, J.T., and Nakamoto, M.: Postpartum immunization: the hypothetical hazard of manual removal of the placenta; report of a study. Obstet. Gynecol. 23:392–395, 1964.

Rabinowitz, P., Harris, E.J., and Friedman, I.S.: Thecalutein cysts of the ovaries: a case of erythroblastosis with abruptio placentae and acute renal failure. J.A.M.A. 177:509–510, 1961.

Radunovic, N., Lockwood, C.J., Alvarez, M., Plecas, D., Chitkara, U., and Berkovitz, R.L.: The severely anemic and hydropic isoimmune fetus: changes in fetal hematocrit associated with intrauterine death. Obstet. Gynecol. 79:390–393, 1992.

Ravindranath, Y., Paglia, D.E., Warrier, I., Valentine, W., Nakatani, M., and Brockway, R.A.: Glucose phosphate isomerase deficiency as a cause of hydrops fetalis. N. Engl. J. Med. 316:258–261, 1987.

Reece, E.A., Gabrielli, S., Abdalla, M., O'Connor, T.Z., and Hobbins, J.C.: Reassessment of the utility of fetal umbilical vein diameter in the management of isoimmunization. Am. J. Obstet. Gynecol. 159:937–938, 1988.

Rice, G.E., Mostoufi-Zadeh, M., Kolodny, E.H., and Driscoll, S.G.: Hydrops fetalis in Gaucher's disease. Teratology 29:53A–54A, 1984.

Rodeck, C.H., Nicolaides, K.H., Warsof, S.L., Fysh, W.J., Gamsu, H.R., and Kemp, J.R.: The management of severe rhesus isoimmunization by fetoscopic intravascular transfusions. Am. J. Obstet. Gynecol. 150:769–774, 1984.

Rodin, A.E., and Nichols, M.M.: Congestive heart failure in the fetus and during the first day of life. Texas Med. 72:44–48, 1975.

Rodis, J.F., Hovick, T.J., Quinn, D.L., Rosengren, S.S., and Tattersall, P.: Human parvovirus infection in pregnancy. Obstet. Gynecol. 72:733–738, 1988.

Rodis, J.F., Quinn, D.L., Gary, G.W., Anderson, L.J., Rosengren, S., Cartter, M.L., Campbell, W.A., and Vintzileos, A.M.: Management and outcomes of pregnancies complicated by human B19 parvovirus infection: a prospective study. Am. J. Obstet. Gynecol. 163:1168–1171, 1990.

Rogers, B.B.: Histopathologic variability of finding erythroid inclusions with intranuclear parvovirus B19 infection. Pediatr. Pathol. 12:883–889, 1992.

Rogers, B.B., Mark, Y., and Oyer, C.E.: Diagnosis and incidence of fetal parvovirus infection in an autopsy series. I. Histology. Pediatr. Pathol. 13:371–379, 1993.

Rönisch, P., and Kleihauer, E.: Alpha-Thalassämie mit HbH und Bart's in einer deutschen Familie. Klin. Wochenschr. 45:1193–1200, 1967.

Rubin, E.M., and Kan, Y.W.: A simple sensitive prenatal test for hydrops fetalis caused by α-thalassemia. Lancet 1:75–77, 1985.

Sacks, L.M., Polin, J.I., and Breckenridge, J.: Congenital chylothorax presenting as hydrops fetalis: a case report. J. Reprod. Med. 28:341–344, 1983.

Sahakian, V., Weiner, C.P., Naides, S.J., Williamson, R.A., and Scharosch, L.L.: Intrauterine transfusion treatment of nonimmune hydrops fetalis secondary to human parvovirus B19 infection. Am. J. Obstet. Gynecol. 164:1090–1091, 1991.

Saltzman, D.H., Frigoletto, F.D., Harlow, B.L., Barss, V.A., and Benacerraf, B.R.: Sonographic evaluation of hydrops fetalis. Obstet. Gynecol. 74:106–111, 1989.

Samra, J.S., Obhrai, M.S., and Constantine, G.: Parvovirus infection in pregnancy. Obstet. Gynecol. 73:832–834, 1989.

Santolaya, J., Alley, D., Jaffe, R., and Warsof, S.L.: Antenatal classification of hydrops fetalis. Obstet. Gynecol. 79:256–259, 1992.

Scheib, J.S., and Waxman, J.: Congenital heart block in successive pregnancies: a case report and evaluation of risk with therapeutic consideration. Obstet. Gynecol. 64:30S–33S, 1984.

Seeds, J.W., Bowes, W.A., and Chescheir, N.C.: Echogenic venous turbulence is a critical feature of successful intravascular transfusion. Obstet. Gynecol. 73:488–490, 1989.

Schwanitz, G., Zerris, K., Niesen, M., Haverkamp, F., and Schmid, G.: Hydrops fetalis as an indication for prenatal chromosome analysis with the example of the diagnosis of a duplication 15q11 and 17q25 due to familial translocation 15/17. Ann. Genet. 31:186–189, 1988.

Schwartz, S.M., Visekul, C., Laxova, R., McPherson, E., and Gilbert, E.F.: Idiopathic hydrops fetalis report of 4 patients including 2 affected sibs. Am. J. Med. Genet. 8:59–66, 1981.

Schwarz, T.F., Roggendorf, M., Hottenträger, Deinhardt, B., Enders, G., Gloning, K.P., Schramm, T., and Hansmann, M.: Human parvovirus B19 infection in pregnancy. Lancet 2:566–567, 1988.

Scott, J.R., Beer, A.E., Guy, L.R., Liesch, M., and Elbert, G.: Pathogenesis of Rh immunization in primigravidas: fetomaternal versus maternofetal bleeding. Obstet. Gynecol. 49:9–14, 1977.

Seeds, J.W., Herbert, W.N.P., Bowles, W.A., and Cefalo, R.C.: Recurrent idiopathic fetal hydrops: results of prenatal therapy. Obstet. Gynecol. 64:30S–33S, 1984.

Seeds, J.W., Bowes, W.A., and Chescheir, N.C.: Echogenic venous turbulence is a critical feature of successful intravascular transfusion. Obstet. Gynecol. 73:488–490, 1989.

Seifer, D.B., Ferguson, J.E., Behrens, C.M., Zemel, S., Stevenson, D.K., and Ross, J.: Nonimmune hydrops fetalis in association with hemangioma of the umbilical cord. Obstet. Gynecol. 66:283–286, 1985.

Seppälä, M., Aula, P., Rapola, J., Karjalainen, O., Huttunen, N.-P., and Ruoslahti, E.: Congenital nephrotic syndrome: prenatal diagnosis and genetic counselling by estimation of amniotic-fluid and maternal serum alpha-fetoprotein. Lancet 1:123–125, 1976.

Seward, J.F., and Zusman, J.: Hydrops fetalis associated with small-bowel volvulus. Lancet 2:52–53, 1978.

Sexauer, C.L., Graham, H.L., Starling, K.A., and Fernbach, D.J.: A test for abnormal hemoglobins in umbilical cord blood. Am. J. Dis. Child. 130:805–806, 1976.

Sheikh, A.U., Ernest, J.M., and O'Shea, M.: Long-term outcome in fetal hydrops from parvovirus B19 infection. Am. J. Obstet. Gynecol. 167:337–341, 1992.

Shimokawa, H., Hara, K., Fukuda, A., and Nakano, H.: Idiopathic hydrops fetalis successfully treated in utero. Obstet. Gynecol. 71:984–986, 1988.

Silber, D.L., and Durnim, R.E.: Intrauterine atrial tachycardia: associated with massive edema in a newborn. Am. J. Dis. Child. 117:722–726, 1969.

Silver, M.M., Beverley, D.W., Valberg, L.S., Cutz, E., Phillips, M.J., and Shaheed, W.A.: Perinatal hemochromatosis: clinical, morphologic, and quantitative iron studies. Am. J. Pathol. 128:538–554, 1989.

Silverstein, A.J., and Kanbour, A.I.: Repetitive idiopathic fetal hydrops. Obstet. Gynecol. 57:18S–21S, 1981.

Skogerboe, K.J., West, S.F., Smith, C., Terashita, S.T., LeCrone, C.N., Detter, J.C., and Tait, J.F.: Screening for α-thalassemia: correlation of hemoglobin H inclusion bodies with DNA-determined genotype. Arch. Pathol. Lab. Med. 116:1012–1018, 1992.

Skopec, L.L., and Lakatua, D.J.: Non-immune fetal hydrops with hepatic hemangioendothelioma and Kasabach-Merritt syndrome: a case report. Pediatr. Pathol. 9:87–93, 1989.

Slikke, J.W. v.d., and Balk, A.G.: Hydramnios with hydrops fetalis and disseminated fetal neuroblastoma. Obstet. Gynecol. 55:250–253, 1980.

Smith, C.R., Chan, H.S.L., and DeSa, D.J.: Placental involvement in congenital neuroblastoma. J. Clin. Pathol. 34:785–789, 1981.

Socol, M.L., Macgregor, S.N., Pielet, B.W., Tamura, R.K., and Sabbagha, R.E.: Percutaneous umbilical transfusion in severe rhesus isoimmunization: resolution of fetal hydrops. Am. J. Obstet. Gynecol. 157:1369–1375, 1987.

Soothill, P.: Intrauterine blood transfusion for non-immune hydrops fetalis due to parvovirus B19 infection. Lancet 336: 121–122, 1990.

Srivastara, A., and Lu, L.: Replication of B19 parvovirus in highly enriched haematopoietic progenitor cells from normal human bone marrow. J. Virol. 62:3059–3063, 1988.

Stedman, C.M., Quinlan, R.W., Huddleston, J.F., Cruz, A.C., and Kellner, K.R.: Rh sensitization after third-trimester fetal death. Obstet. Gynecol. 71:461–463, 1988.

Steinke, J., Gries, F.A., and Driscoll, S.G.: In vitro studies of insulin inactivation with reference to erythroblastosis fetalis. Blood 30:359–363, 1967.

Stevens, D.C., Hilliard, J.K., Schreiner, R.L., Hurwitz, R.A., Murrell, R., Mirkin, L.D., Bonderman, P.W., and Nolen, P.A.: Supraventricular tachycardia with edema, ascites, and hydrops in fetal sheep. Am. J. Obstet. Gynecol. 142:316–322, 1982.

Stocker, J.T., and Singer, D.B.: Human parvovirus B19 infection, hydrops fetalis, and possibly myocarditis: annotated bibliography. Pediatr. Pathol. 8:356–358, 1988.

Strauss, L., and Driscoll, S.G.: Congenital neuroblastoma involving the placenta: reports of two cases. Pediatrics 34: 23–31, 1964.

Suh, Y.K.: Alpha thalassemia—differential diagnosis. J. Perinatol. (in press, 1994).

Szulman, A.E.: The A, B and H blood-group antigens in human placenta. N. Engl. J. Med. 286:1028–1031, 1972.

Taylor, J.F.: Sensitization of Rh-negative daughters by their Rh-positive mothers. N. Engl. J. Med. 276:547–551, 1967.

Taylor, P.V., Scott, J.S., Gerbis, L.M., Esscher, E., and Scott, O.: Maternal antibodies against fetal cardiac antigens in congenital complete heart block. N. Engl. J. Med. 315: 667–672, 1986.

Terheggen, H.G., and Kleihauer, E.: Die α-Thalassämie: eine kasuistische Mitteilung. Z. Kinderheilkd. 103:182–191, 1968.

Thilaganathan, B., Salvesen, D.R., Abbas, A., Ireland, R.M., and Nicolaides, K.H.: Fetal plasma erythropoietin concentration in red blood cell-isoimmunized pregnancies. Am. J. Obstet. Gynecol. 167:1292–1297, 1992.

Thumasathit, B., Nondasuta, A., Silpisornkosol, S., Lousuebsakul, B., Unchalipongse, P., and Mangkornkanok, M.: Hydrops fetalis associated with Bart's hemoglobin in northern Thailand. J. Pediatr. 73:132–138, 1968.

Turski, D.M., Shahidi, N., Visekul, C., and Gilbert, E.: Nonimmunologic hydrops fetalis. Am. J. Obstet. Gynecol. 131:586–587, 1978.

Uno, Y., Taniguchi, A., and Tanaka, E.: Histochemical studies in Wolman's disease—report of an autopsy case accompanied with a large amount of milky ascites. Acta Pathol. Jpn. 23:779–790, 1973.

Vedvick, T.S., Wheeler, S.A., and Koenig, H.M.: Heterogeneity of fetal hemoglobin in severe α-thalassemia. Biol. Neonate 36:181–184, 1979.

Veille, J.C., Sunderland, C., and Bennett, R.M.: Complete heart block in a fetus associated with maternal Sjögren's syndrome. Am. J. Obstet. Gynecol. 151:660–661, 1985.

Verger, P., Martin, C., Dubecq, J.-P., Kermarec, Y., and Lomazzi, R.: Étude pathologique et therapeutique de l'anasarque foeto-placentaire. Arch. Fr. Pediatr. 20:417–436, 1963.

Vetter, V.L., and Rashkind, W.J.: Congenital complete heart block and connective-tissue disease. N. Engl. J. Med. 309:236–238, 1983.

Vidyasagar, D., and Haworth, J.C.: Placental dimensions, cell size, and cell number in erythroblastosis fetalis. Am. J. Obstet. Gynecol. 115:267–270, 1973.

Villaespesa, A.R., Mier, M.P.S., Ferrer, P.L., Baleriola, I.A., and Gonzalez, J.I.R.: Nonimmunologic hydrops fetalis: an etiopathogenetic approach through the postmortem study of 59 patients. Am. J. Med. Genet. 35:274–279, 1990.

Vintzileos, A.M., Campbell, W.A., Soberman, S.M., and Nochimson, D.J.: Fetal atrial flutter and X-linked dominant vitamin D-resistant rickets. Obstet. Gynecol. 65:39S–44S, 1985.

Warren, R.C., Butler, J., Morsman, J.M., Mckenzie, C., and Rodeck, C.H.: Does chorionic villus sampling cause fetomaternal hemorrhage? Lancet 1:691, 1985.

Watson, J., and Campbell, S.: Antenatal evaluation and management in nonimmune hydrops fetalis. Obstet. Gynecol. 67:589–593, 1986.

Weiland, H.T., Vermey-Keers, C., Salimans, M.M.M., Fleuren, G.J., Verwey, R.A., and Anderson, M.J.: Parvovirus B19 associated with fetal abnormality. Lancet 1:682–683, 1987.

Weiner, C., Varner, M., Pringle, K., Hein, H., Williamson, R., and Smith, W.L.: Antenatal diagnosis and palliative treatment of nonimmune hydrops fetalis secondary to extralobar sequestration. Obstet. Gynecol. 68:275–280, 1986.

Weiner, C.P, and Thompson, I.B.: Direct treatment of fetal supraventricular tachycardia after failed transplacental therapy. Am. J. Obstet. Gynecol. 158:570–573, 1988.

Weiner, C.P., Sipes, S.L., and Wenstrom, K.: The effect of fetal age upon normal fetal laboratory values and venous pressure. Obstet. Gynecol. 79:713–718, 1992.

Wentworth, P.: The placenta in cases of hemolytic disease. Am. J. Obstet. Gynecol. 98:283–289, 1967.

Westgren, M., Eastman, W.N., Ghandourah, S., and Woodhouse, N.: Intrauterine hypercalcaemia and non-immune hydrops fetalis—relationship to the Williams syndrome. Prenat. Diagn. 8:333–337, 1988.

Whitney, J.B., and Popp, R.A.: Thalassemia: alpha-thalassemia in laboratory mice. Am. J. Pathol. 116:523–525, 1984.

Wiener, A.S., Wexler, I.B., and Schutta, E.J.: A pair of male fraternal twins with contrasting manifestations of Rh hemolytic disease. Acta Genet. Med. Gemell. 11:17–28, 1962.

Wiggins, J.W., Bowes, W., Clewell, W., Manco-Johnson, M., Manchester, D., Johnson, R., Appareti, K., and Wolfe, R.R.: Echocardiographic diagnosis and intravenous digoxin management of fetal tachyarrhythmias and congestive heart failure. Am. J. Dis. Child. 140:202–204, 1986.

Williamson, R., Eskdale, J., Coleman, D.V., Niazi, M., Loeffler, F.E., and Modell, B.M.: Direct gene analysis of chorionic villi: a possible technique for first-trimester antenatal diagnosis of haemoglobinopathies. Lancet 2:1125–1127, 1981.

Windebank, K.P., Bridges, N.A., Ostman-Smith, I., and Stevens, J.E.: Hydrops fetalis due to abnormal lymphatics. Arch. Dis. Child. 62:198–200, 1987.

Wood, W.G., Bunch, C., Kelley, S., Gunn, Y., and Breckon, G.: Control of haemoglobin switching by a developmental clock? Nature 313:320–323, 1985.

Younis, J.S., and Granat, M.: Insufficient transplacental digoxin transfer in severe hydrops fetalis. Am. J. Obstet. Gynecol. 157:1268–1269, 1987.

Zeng, Y.-T., and Huang, S.-Z.: α-Globin gene organisation and prenatal diagnosis of α-thalassemia in Chinese. Lancet 1:304–307, 1985.

Zipursky, A., and Israels, L.G.: The pathogenesis and prevention of Rh immunization. Can. Med. Assoc. J. 97:1245–1257, 1967.

Zwi, L.J., and Becroft, D.M.O.: Intrauterine aplastic anemia and fetal hydrops: a case report. Pediatr. Pathol. 5:199–205, 1986.

17
Transplacental Hemorrhage, Cell Transfer, Trauma

Transplacental Blood and Cell Transfer

A century ago, considerable controversy raged as to whether the fetal and maternal circulations were united or separate. In an interesting essay, Baer (1828) discussed this dispute in great detail; and in order to settle the issue once and for all he performed experiments on dogs. These studies showed conclusively that the two vascular beds are separate from one another. The early history of this topic is covered in excellent detail in the historical review of De Witt (1959).

Although transfer of maternal cells to the fetus is a rare event, the fetus often bleeds into the maternal circulation, despite the anatomical separation of the two circulations. The reason for this fetal bleeding is often obscure. It is an important aspect of placentation, however, whose pathogenesis must be further explored. Pathologists who examine placentas must make the appropriate observations at placental examination, as is herein explained. They must also be familiar with the methodology that enables a positive diagnosis of fetal blood loss, and they may then be in the position to add new knowledge about the mechanism of transplacental fetal bleeding from the detailed study of relevant cases.

Trauma

Fetal bleeding across the placenta occurs for many reasons. One reason that has been well substantiated is trauma to the placenta; in fact, *transplacental fetal bleeding* and *abruptio placentae* are the two major complications of severe trauma during pregnancy. It has been alleged that: "Blunt abdominal trauma during pregnancy occurs in 0.62 per 1,000 deliveries, with 26% of such cases involving assault" (Rodgers et al., 1992). These authors presented such a case in which a conviction for negligent homicide was obtained: A 60 ml (46%) fetomaternal hemorrhage had occurred after the patient had been kicked in the abdomen. A complete overview of blunt trauma during pregnancy can be found in the review by Pearlman et al. (1990b). The same group of authors also undertook a prospective study of 85 women with trauma during pregnancy (Pearlman et al., 1990a). They found significantly more fetomaternal hemorrhages than in controls, especially when the placenta was located anterior in the uterus. Abruptio occurred also frequently and could not be predicted by the severity of the trauma. On the other hand, among 233 hospitalizations for blunt trauma to the pregnant abdomen, Dahmus and Sibai (1993) found preterm delivery in 1%, fetal distress in 1.7%, and abruptio in 2.6%. In their experience, Kleihauer tests were not predictive of outcome. Williams et al. (1990) found that preterm labor was the principal sequela of trauma during pregnancy. They studied 84 relevant cases and observed abruptio and rupture of the uterus but no cases of delayed abruptio. Premature labor occurred in 28% of their cases, but there were no fetal injuries.

On the other hand, it has been substantiated that the fetus may sustain injuries, such as skull fracture. The placenta itself may also actually rupture from various insults. Buchsbaum (1968, 1979) and Crosby (1974) have competently reviewed the numerous descriptions from the literature. Buchsbaum pointed out that abruptio is only rarely caused by trauma (0.49–1.30%). Much more commonly it is the result of maternal vascular disease, appearing as a complication of preeclampsia. These studies must be consulted for a comprehensive overview of the topic; they are not restricted to physical trauma but include topics such as hypovolemia and sports injuries. Crosby emphatically stated that abruptio due to accidents, if it occurs, leads invariably to fetal death within 48 hours. Moreover, it is his opinion that a causal relation between trauma and fetal injury is often difficult to establish. Goodwin and Breen (1990) studied 205 patients with noncatastrophic trauma during pregnancy and found complications in 18 (8.8%).

Premature labor was seen in ten, abruptio in five, fetal injury in one, and fetal death in two. Although fetal hemorrhage occurred significantly more commonly than in a control population, they opined that when no obstetrical complications are evident the quantitation of transplacental bleeding is unnecessary.

Amniocentesis is a frequently discussed topic when considering placental trauma. Transplacental hemorrhage not infrequently occurs after amniocentesis. It happens not only when amniocentesis is done for genetic diagnosis during the second trimester (Blajchman et al., 1974; Goodlin & Clewell, 1974; Young et al., 1977; Lele et al., 1982) but also near term, when it is done to determine fetal maturity or to evaluate Rh disease (Zipursky et al., 1963a,b). With improved localization of the placenta by sonography, this hazard has diminished. Nevertheless, it remains an important complication that may lead to fetal exsanguination, stillbirth, and maternal immunization against fetal Rh antigens (Bowman & Pollock, 1985). Herrmann and Sidiropoulos (1986) found a 1.5% incidence of transplacental bleeding when amniocentesis was done during the second trimester (See below).

Examination of the placenta in such cases may be rewarding, as was shown in Figure 237. In that patient, repeated amniocentesis for the assessment of fetal maturity in a diabetic patient had led to several disruptions of the fetal surface vessels; it eventually necessitated cesarean section because of fetal bleeding. Bleeding of the fetus may take place into the amnionic cavity or transplacentally into the mother. For its avoidance, the value of placental localization prior to amniocentesis has been well established. Pauls and Boutros (1970) localized the placenta with chromium 51-tagged red blood cells. They found that bleeding of the fetus occurred much more frequently when the placenta had not been localized (11% versus 0%). More recently, ultrasonographic localization has achieved the same results but is more easily accomplished (Gottesfeld et al., 1966; Mennuti et al., 1983). Herrmann and Sidiropoulos (1986) evaluated their results in 209 Rh-negative women who came to amniocentesis during the second trimester. Significant hemorrhages occurred in three patients (i.e., Kleihauer-positive findings of more than 2 per 100 cells in the maternal circulation). There was no correlation with anterior placentas and bloody amnionic fluid. It is their opinion that the rarity of this occurrence, the ability to predict sensitization accurately with Kleihauer stains, and the use of prophylactic RhoGham therapy have made amniocentesis a safe procedure.

A positive Kleihauer-Betke test (Kleihauer et al., 1957) quickly establishes the presence of fetal blood in the maternal circulation. Assessment of α-fetoprotein levels, also reflecting fetal blood transfer, as done by

Mennuti et al. (1983) is perhaps preferable. Lele et al. (1982) found this test to be more sensitive than the Kleihauer technique. For example, when maternal and fetal major blood group incompatibilities exist, the fetal red blood cells may quickly lyse in the mother's circulation, which causes misleading results in Kleihauer tests. Placental injury following amniocentesis has also been described by Goodlin and Clewell (1974). They found two defects in a large placental surface vein from which the fetus had exsanguinated into the amnionic cavity. Figure 320 shows the placenta of a stillborn fetus at 30 weeks. This fetus was transfused 4 days before delivery as therapy for Rh disease. Three large defects (holes) were found on the fetal surface. Exsanguination had thus occurred. The placenta had a posterior uterine location; and hemosiderin macrophages were located near the sites of injury. Retromembranous hematomas have also been identified following amniocentesis, a complication discussed in Chapter 12.

Fetal bleeding into the mother often occurs during *therapeutic abortion*, even during early pregnancy (Voigt & Britt, 1969; Walsh & Lewis, 1970; Lakoff et al., 1971; Leong et al., 1979). Because there is complete disruption of the placenta, the bleeding is not surprising. Curettage for abortion of Rh-negative women is thus now routinely followed by prophylactic RhoGam therapy. Warren et al. (1985) found, in a study of 161 chorionic villous sampling (CVS) procedures, that fetomaternal hemorrhage occurred as often as in 49%. They found all Kleihauer test evaluations to be negative and therefore judged this procedure to be too insensitive. Positive results were obtained by measuring α-fetoprotein levels in maternal blood before and after the curettage. Los et al. (1993) observed the first case of fetal demise following transabdominal CVS, occurring

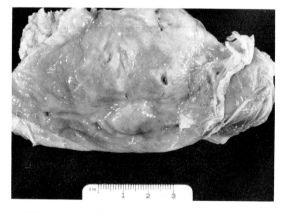

FIGURE 320. Fetal surface of a placenta from a 30-week gestation with three holes through which exsanguination occurred. The fetus had been transfused 4 days earlier. There are many hemosiderin-laden macrophages in the chorion and amnion that obscure the vascular architecture.

1 week after the procedure; and Pozniak et al. (1988) observed rapid retromembranous bleeding during CVS from "venous lakes," although it was apparently composed of maternal blood. Litwak et al. (1970) reported that 32% of patients with spontaneous abortion had fetal bleeding. More surprising is that 11% of women with threatened abortion before 20 weeks' gestation had a positive Kleihauer test, in contrast to 4% of the controls (Stein et al., 1992).

Fernandez-Rocha and Oullette (1976) depicted the placenta in a fetal hemorrhage produced by insertion of a *pressure catheter*. In an effort to secure fetal monitoring, the catheter was introduced with a stiff guide. The amnionic cavity contained much blood, and the fetal surface had disrupted vessels and contained a hematoma.

That the placenta bleeds into the mother during labor and delivery, of course, has long been recognized (Lloyd et al., 1980), and it is the reason for prophylactic, passive immunization. In 14.5% of the patients reported by Lloyd et al., fetal cells were recognized in postpartum maternal blood; in 1% of deliveries a larger hemorrhage was diagnosed. Manual removal of the placenta was even more disruptive.

Doolittle (1963) studied placentas after delivery to identify the nature of the fetal vascular disruptions. He first cannulated the umbilical veins during labor and then measured pressures of 30 to 60 mm/Hg, which increased to 90 to 115 mm/Hg just prior to extrusion of the placenta. The cannulated placentas were then insufflated with air under water, and the pressures exerted were recorded. In 23% of these placentas, air leaks were identified, usually near the chorionic surface. Pressures of up to 300 mm/Hg did not burst the villous circulation within intact vessels. Doolittle opined that traction on the cord was a probable mechanism of the frequent placental disruption that leads to fetal bleeding. He suggested that most such bleeding would be prevented by opening the cord clamp before extrusion of the placenta. This measure, in his experience, allowed an average of 70 ml of fetal blood to escape.

Cesarean section, of course, may also allow fetal bleeding to occur from the placenta. This fact was recognized as early as 1888 according to Smith and Benjamin (1968). Feldman and her collaborators (1990) found that some fetal hemorrhage occurred in 18% of patients undergoing cesarean section, with 2.5% losing more than 30 ml of blood. They discussed at some length the possible mechanism of this bleeding and could exclude that blood loss occurred during manual separation of the placenta. Alternatively, Pilkington et al. (1966) had identified fetal bleeding *before* cesarean section, so the possibility remains that the clinical reasons for the section are in part responsible for the hemorrhage. The important aspect of this study is to recognize that a

single dose of RhoGam may not suffice for immunoprophylaxis after cesarean section.

Pollack (1968) first found that external fetal version, done for breech presentation, may injure the placenta with fetal bleeding into the mother. This report described a pregnancy at 35 weeks' gestation in which the patient experienced hemoglobinuria 4 hours after version. The placenta showed "a small area of separation." This cause of fetal bleeding is an infrequent but serious event. To prevent the risk of exsanguination, external fetal rotation is now commonly followed by fetal monitoring and Kleihauer studies. Gjode et al. (1980) found that during the first attempt of version, which they investigated in 50 women, 28% had fetal hemorrhage of 0.1 to 1.5 ml. In Rh-negative women, therefore, prophylaxis is needed. A fatal case of transplacental bleeding after fetal version was described by Luyet et al. (1976). In a case of "spontaneous" massive fetomaternal hemorrhage with a meconium-stained but otherwise normal placenta, the fetus developed extensive infarctions of various organs (Naeye et al., 1964).

Buchsbaum and Staples (1985) reported two self-inflicted *gunshot injuries* that caused fetal death, and they reviewed many other similar cases. The placenta was not described in this report, but in Buchsbaum's extensive summary of 1968 several placental injuries from gunshot wounds were cited. Awwad et al. (1994) reviewed 14 cases of penetrating wounds of the pregnant uterus. Two women died, and one-half of the fetuses were stillborn. Fetal fractures were witnessed, and abruptio placentae and placental tears were also seen.

Automobile accidents are now the commonest cause of traumatic transplacental hemorrhage. Skull fractures, fetal death, and vaginal bleeding were reviewed and a case was reported by Theurer and Kaiser (1963), but the placenta of that case was not discussed. Abruptio placentae and uterine disruption led to fetal death in a case reported by Eaton and Danzinger (1967). Exsanguination into the amnionic sac from a complete radial tear of the placenta occurred in the case of Peyser and Toaff (1969). We have documented another case of blunt trauma received in an automobile accident during the 34th week of a normal pregnancy (Benirschke & Gille, 1977). Fetal heart tones were absent 3 hours after the accident. The uterus and spleen were lacerated, and the placenta had a 50% retroplacental hematoma with early infarction 2 days after the accident. Figure 321 shows a relevant case. This term pregnancy eventuated in the precipitous birth of a stillborn infant with cardiac arrest and intraventricular hemorrhage. A 7-cm fresh retroplacental hematoma was found that had compressed a large portion of the placenta, causing it to be acutely infarcted. The mother had worn a seatbelt.

Crosby and Costiloe (1971) found that pregnant women who are involved in car accidents have a high

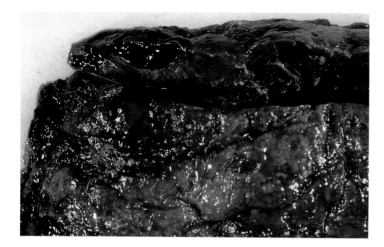

FIGURE 321. Retroplacental hematoma after an automobile accident at term. The infant was stillborn with intraventricular hemorrhage. The placental area of abruptio is depressed, and there is early infarction. See text.

fetal loss. Separation of the placenta was found to be the most common cause of fetal death when the mother lived. Fetal death was commonest in car accidents as a result of maternal demise. The question of the efficacy of wearing seatbelts to avoid possible uterine injury was also answered in this study of Crosby and Costiloe (1971). They concluded that, despite occasional fetal loss from abruptio, seat belts should be worn by pregnant mothers. Crosby (1968) had earlier found that abortion occurred in 20% of patients pregnant 20 weeks or less when they were in automobile accidents. In unselected cases of car accidents, fetal loss was 25%, but 50% of these losses were due to maternal death. In an apparently trivial car accident near term suffered by a patient described by Cumming and Wren (1978), multiple fetal surface placental hemorrhages were identified, and fetal skull fracture led to fetal death. Larroche (1986) has provided evidence of a relation between car accidents and prenatal encephaloclastic lesions. A 75% placental abruptio, with a surviving immature infant, occurred in a pregnancy in which a delayed retroplacental hemorrhage had developed. The patient had not worn a seat belt and suffered a steering wheel injury to the abdomen (Lavin & Miodovnik, 1981). Delayed abruptio was also reported by Higgins and Garite (1984). It occurred 5 days after an automobile accident, and there was old, clotted blood behind the placenta. Kettel et al. (1988) reported varying amounts of abruption in three patients who were in car accidents. Crosby (1974) had opined that abruptio following trauma usually leads to fetal demise within 48 hours or not at all.

Murray (1964) described a patient with fetal death who delivered 6 hours after a car accident and where the mother suffered severe fibrinogenopenia, presumably due to consumption coagulopathy. Because defibrination with disseminated intravascular coagulation is often a sequela of eclampsia, and hypotheses relating the two have been formed, it is relevant to emphasize

that this patient had no evidence of preeclampsia. She was a gravida 14 without hypertension. Chibber et al. (1984) have documented that inapparent placental injury during a car accident may lead to transplacental bleeding with rhesus immunization. The placenta of their case was not described. In a woman who delivered a 2,100 g infant, a transplacental hemorrhage of 42% estimated blood volume occurred after a car accident; despite this bleeding, Bickers and Wennberg (1983) judged the placenta to be normal grossly and microscopically. Stafford et al. (1988) described eight cases of fetal death following automobile accidents; they found four abruptios, three placentas with severe infarction, and miscellaneous lacerations. Umbilical thrombosis was present in one fetus. Cardwell and Snyder (1989), in reply, drew attention to the perhaps more important aspect of transplacental hemorrhage in such cases. A patient with whom we are familiar had a car accident with immediate cessation of fetal movements. The patient received a blow to the right abdomen, whereupon she noted the fetus to have shifted to the left. She was admitted to hospital 1.5 hours later, where fetal monitoring recorded a sudden drop of heart rate. An emergency cesarean section was performed 6 hours after the accident. The 7.5 months' gestation fetus was stillborn, and a small laceration of uterus and placental contusions were noted. No abruptio was found, and there was no blood in the amnionic sac. Portions of the placenta were dark (Figure 322). The mother had been wearing a lap and cross-chest seatbelt. This fetus clearly exsanguinated into the mother, as the Kleihauer stain yielded 2.05% of fetal red blood cells in the maternal circulation, representing 60 to 75 ml of fetal blood; his hematocrit was 36%.

The nature of placental injury that may lead to transplacental bleeding in car accidents is depicted in Figure 323. This patient had an automobile accident at 33 weeks' gestation; she was admitted and was found to

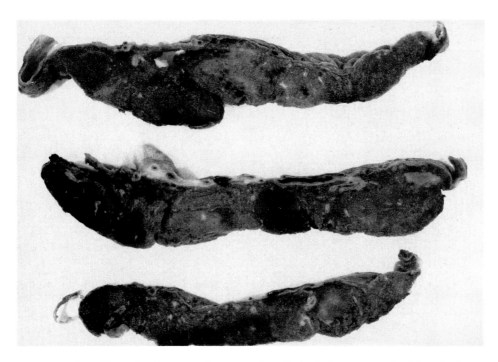

FIGURE 322. Appearance of a 37-week placenta after an automobile accident 6 hours earlier, with fetal death due to exsanguination. Note the dark, areas of the villous tissue that had intravillous hemorrhages. Bleeding into the decidua basalis had also occurred, although there was no abruptio. Fetal hematocrit was 36%. (Courtesy Dr. D.J. Carlson, Exeter, New Hampshire.)

have normal fetal heart tones. She was then discharged, but precipitous labor ensued and she delivered 14 hours after the accident. The infant's depressed Apgar scores (5/5), subsequent stormy course, and intraventricular hemorrhage presumably stemmed from the acute anemia (hemoglobin 8 g/dl, hematocrit 24%). Some nucleated red blood cells in the fetal circulation indicated the fetal response to anemia. There was a large bruise of villous tissue with focal massive intravillous hemorrhage. In addition, an intervillous hematoma and small laceration of the placenta were found. If Kleihauer studies had been done shortly after the accident they would have forewarned the treating physician of the fetal blood loss.

Fetal hemorrhage occurred in 28% of patients who experienced *other types of abdominal trauma* (e.g., falling). Rose et al. (1985) reviewed this subject in one of the few reports with case controls. The extent of bleeding (average volume 16 ml) was not related to the nature of the trauma or to the gestational age. Fort and Harlin (1970) produced similar figures and discussed the poor fetal prognosis of such trauma. When reading these various reports, one is impressed by the frequency with which relatively minor trauma can cause fetal transplacental hemorrhage. Of course, "spontaneous" hemorrhage also occurs. We have always believed that such spontaneous hemorrhages can result from trauma to the placenta inflicted by the fetus (e.g., by kicking). This

assumption was strengthened when Eden (1987) reported two cases of maternal vaginal bleeding during pregnancy, associated with severe pain caused by fetal movements. Upon sonographic study, it became apparent that the fetus was "punching" the area of the placenta from which (marginal) bleeding occurred. Rare cases of umbilical cord hemorrhage and laceration, following trauma, have been summarized by Buchsbaum (1968). The management of trauma during pregnancy has been detailed by Higgins (1988).

Quintero et al. (1993) have searched for fetal trauma by embryoscopy. They found hemorrhagic lesions of the fetus, especially of the skull, in 30% of cases during CVS. Thrombi were not seen. Shulman and colleagues (1990) believed it was the amount of villous tissue sampled, rather than the method employed, that correlated with the extent of fetomaternal bleeding during CVS. Unfortunately, in most cases the cause of spontaneous transplacental hemorrhage remains obscure. Punching or turning by the fetus may injure the placenta, much as the placenta is occasionally injured with external version of a fetus in breech presentation. We have seen a stillbirth in a near term pregnancy that was complicated by sudden maternal hemoglobinuria. A Kleihauer-Betke stain was done, and 15 ml of fetal blood was detected in the maternal circulation. The baby died shortly thereafter. It was blood group A+, the mother being O Rh-negative. The placenta was pale and had

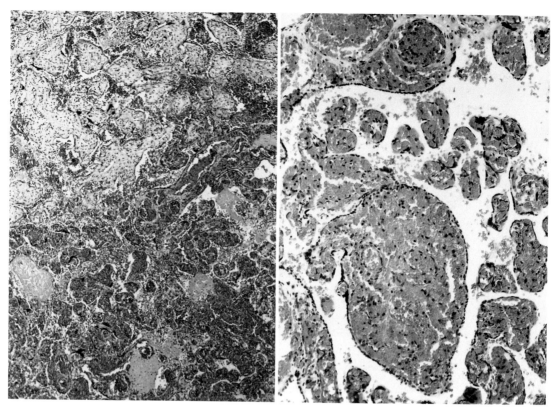

FIGURE 323. Massive, focal villous hemorrhage ("bruise") in an immature placenta 14 hours after an automobile accident. The mother had been discharged, but fetal hemorrhage into the mother led to severe, disabling anemia. H&E. left ×40; right ×160.

several intervillous thromboses but no other lesions to account for the transplacental hemorrhage.

Other causes of transplacental hemorrhage include placental disease, such as chorangioma, choriocarcinoma, placenta previa, and abruptio placentae. Perhaps other conditions exist that have yet to be identified. Huff (1988) found that "fetal" (placental) bleeding occurred more often after cesarean section when the placenta had not been "drained" of fetal blood from the cord.

Placenta in Hemorrhage

One should suspect transplacental bleeding when the villous tissue of the placenta is unusually pale. This observation presupposes that the examiner is familiar with the "normal" color of the placental tissue at the different stages of gestation. Immature placentas are paler than are those at term. The presence of intervillous thrombi may be another clue signaling that bleeding through the placenta has occurred; they may even signify the point of origin of hemorrhage and should be noted for that reason. The temporal aspects of the development of fetal anemia due to transplacental hemorrhage are usually not known. One might think that given

hematocrit and hemoglobin values for the newborn would provide detailed information as to the precise time the hemorrhage took place. It is unfortunately not true, as specific studies to ascertain the decrease of hematocrit have not been made. It would be desirable to collect information in cases where the timing is well known (from trauma) and the amount estimated (from Kleihauer stains) in order to estimate just how long it takes to reduce the hematocrit to a given level. This information would aid in assessing doubtful cases, some of which end in litigation. When placental or neonatal anemia are apparent, the maternal blood must be studied promptly for the possible presence of fetal red blood cells and perhaps for α-fetoprotein levels as well.

Another concern is how rapid is the response of red blood cell replacement when blood is lost. It is known that *nucleated red blood cells* (NRBCs) appear in the circulation of anemic fetuses, best exemplified by erythroblastosis fetalis. The same happens when acute blood loss occurs and when fetuses are hypoxic. This feature plays an important role in current medicolegal decisions. What we need to know is how rapid is the response of the appearance of NRBCs to the loss of red blood cells and hypoxia, and if this response is quantitatively reflected in the number of NRBCs in the circulation. Considerable confusion exists as to the number of NRBCs in the neonatal circulation. It is our opinion that NRBCs should not be observed in the term placenta during the histological evaluation. When NRBCs are present in the fetal blood, and it is obviously important that they be diagnosed correctly, it is a distinctly abnormal finding. The pathologist should then try to find the reason for their presence. Geissler and Japha (1901) stated emphatically that "contrary to the dogma" NRBCs are not found in young children. Ryerson and Sanes (1934) undertook an incisive study of NRBCs in placentas. They attempted to ascertain the parameters that would allow the age of gestation to be determined histologically. All NRBCs had disappeared by the end of the third month of pregnancy; and if more than 1% NRBCs are found, it indicated immaturity to them. Fox (1967) also published on this phenomenon and related NRBCs to hypoxia or asphyxia. We concur with the interpretation of a relation to fetal tissue hypoxia; indeed, it is our practice to take note of the presence of NRBCs when examining placentas. Green and Mimouni (1990) provided criteria and suggested that "a value greater than 1×10^9/L. should be considered a potential index of intrauterine hypoxia." Normally, there were no NRBCs in term neonates, and the 95th percentile had 1.7 in absolute counts. Diabetic mothers' babies had increased numbers, as did infants with hypoxia and growth-retarded neonates. Shurin (1987) concluded that there are about 200 to 600 NRBCs/mm^3 and 10,000 to 30,000 WBCN/mm^3; she also stated that the normal infant has 4% to 5% of NRBCs in cord blood samples, which is a higher figure than is our experience. Shurin reflected that this number indicates the erythroid hyperplasia due to high levels of erythropoietin production. In general, it is our belief that because of the complex sequence of signals that initiate erythropoiesis and release of NRBCs many hours pass from a hypoxic (anemic) stimulus to the appearance of NRBCs in the circulation. Thus the identification of NRBCs suggests a significant fetal problem many hours prior to birth. Quantitative and temporal sequences must be obtained in future studies, and two relevant cases that provide some guide are discussed in Chapter 27. Shields et al. (1993), in the laboratory of R.A. Brace, have reviewed what is known of this aspect of red blood cell restoration after hemorrhage in sheep. Despite an initial rise in erythropoietin level, a significant hemorrhage (40%) is not followed by a significant increase in reticulocyte count, nor are the former blood volume and hematocrit restored before birth. Thus the ovine model may not be an adequate one to settle this important topic.

Jauniaux et al. (1990) have made an important clinicopathological correlation in a case of significant fetomaternal hemorrhage. They observed sonographically a 3×3 cm heterogeneic, hypoechoic placental lesion when, at 18 weeks' gestation, a pregnant patient was found to have elevated maternal serum α-fetoprotein levels. The Kleihauer test was positive. At 22 weeks there was only peripheral turbulent flow around the lesion, which at about 30 weeks' gestation was found to represent a laminated white lesion of fibrin. It represented the presumed area of intervillous thrombosis whence the fetal hemorrhage occurred.

It should also be mentioned that intervillous thromboses are not necessarily due to fetomaternal hemorrhages. When the blood systems are compatible, agglutination may not take place. Conversely, intervillous hematomas may occur for entirely different reasons also. They may result when the intervillous perfusion is significantly altered, as for instance because of the presence of placental edema (erythroblastosis, Chapter 16; hydatidiform moles, Chapter 22), and for local, structural reasons. This type of intervillous thrombosis is considered in greater detail in Chapter 11.

TECHNIQUE FOR IDENTIFICATION OF FETAL RED BLOOD CELLS

Fetal red blood cells in the maternal blood are best identified with the Kleihauer-Betke technique (Kleihauer et al., 1957). Since that seminal contribution, the original method has undergone many refinements. Moreover, there are currently several commercial kits available for detecting fetal cells in the maternal circulation (e.g., Boehringer Mannheim; Simmler, St. Louis; Fetaldex of Ortho Diagnostics, Raritan, NJ). Some of these techniques were mentioned by Virgilio and Simon (1977), who evaluated several methods. Simon et al. (1978) used two techniques to evaluate the risk of fetal bleeding in 200 Rh-negative women. Six women experienced significant fetal hemorrhages that necessitated RhoGam administration. The Fetaldex and Kleihauer techniques compared favorably in the assessment.

The Kleihauer-Betke technique depends on the fact that fetal hemoglobin, in an acidic milieu of pH 3, is less soluble than maternal (adult) hemoglobin. For its execution, air-dried blood films are first fixed in 80% alcohol for 5 minutes and then eluted in several possible buffers for 7 to 10 minutes. Usually, the buffer is freshly made from 0.2 M Na_2PO_4 and 0.1 M citric acid. The slides are rinsed twice with water, stained for 10 minutes in hematoxylin solution, rinsed, and covered with a 1% eosin solution (or a similar dye) for 10 minutes. They are then rinsed in water and air-dried. Palliez et al. (1970) successfully used 1% safranin and a 1:20 dilution of Ziehl fuchsin. Fetal red blood cells maintain their color; but because the maternal hemoglobin is eluted, the maternal cells appear as mere shadows (Figure 324). The quantity of fetal blood loss is estimated from counts of these respective cell populations. Mollison (1972) suggested a formula that simplifies the estimation of fetal blood loss: If it is assumed that the maternal red cell volume is 1,800 ml:

$$\text{Fetal hemorrhage (ml)} = \frac{2,400}{\text{maternal cells (light)/fetal cells (dark)}}$$

In this careful survey of stains, executed under standard conditions by various laboratories, Mollison emphasized that any enumeration of the fetal (stained) cells alone underestimates the fetal blood loss, as only 90% of fetal cells stain positively; the

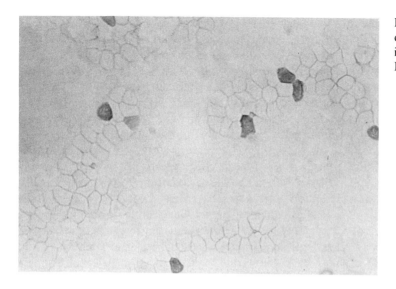

FIGURE 324. Kleihauer stain of maternal blood. The darkly stained cells are fetal erythrocytes. Fetal cells in this blood film numbered approximately 5%. Eosin, Kleihauer. ×1,000.

remainder possess hemoglobin A. He recommended a standardized approach to the estimation of fetal blood loss, as otherwise large errors would invalidate results. The method of enumeration used by Kleihauer, for instance, would underestimate the amount of fetal blood lost. Mollison suggested that five fields be counted under low power and compared with an appropriate reference slide. If more than 10 darkly stained cells are found in a field, a quantitative analysis was recommended. Grobbelaar (1968) also quantitated the red blood cell contamination of maternal blood and recommended that $50 \, \text{mm}^2$ of blood film be scanned and that reports note the precise methodology of enumeration, lest the results not be interpretable.

For the purposes of rapidly identifying mothers in need of RhoGam immunoprophylaxis, Nance and her colleagues (1989) presented a flow cytometry methodology that is effective in identifying quickly and accurately the contamination with D+ cells in maternal blood.

Zipursky et al. (1959) found that 21% of postpartum patients had fetal cells in the circulation, but other authors have found that a much greater percentage of postpartum women have fetal red blood cell contamination (McLarey & Fish, 1966; Sullivan & Jennings, 1966). Fraser and Raper (1962) made the important observation that ABO-incompatible cells disappear much more rapidly than do compatible cells. Their observation was affirmed later by the findings of Palliez et al. (1970). Indeed, Zilliacus (1963) found occasional agglutinated and partially disintegrated fetal cells in maternal blood in women who had experienced transplacental hemorrhage from the fetus. An important study of fetal blood transfer to the mother comes from Owen et al. (1989). These investigators undertook a prospective analysis of Kleihauer stains before and after normal delivery in 66 patients. They found that "three patients (4.6%) had a massive feto-maternal hemorrhage. None of the post-delivery stains showed evidence of a significant feto-maternal hemorrhage unless results of the antepartum stain had also been positive. We conclude that the delivery process itself does not stimulate a massive feto-maternal hemorrhage in cases of fetal death." Massive hemorrhage in three women presented as decreased fetal movements, nonreactive fetal heart rates, and positive Kleihauer tests (Kosasa et al., 1993). This situation led the authors to recommend immediate delivery for such pregnancies. The cause of the hemorrhage remained unknown.

Some authors have doubted that the Kleihauer test truly evaluates fetal cells in the maternal circulation. This aspect was studied and the techniques verified by the large investigation undertaken by Freese and Titel (1963). They made some modification of the Kleihauer technique and reviewed improvements of methods from other authors that they collected from the literature. As with other investigators, these authors found a high incidence of fetal blood contamination in postpartum maternal circulating blood, and they established a quantitative relation of this contamination to the ABO status of mother and infant. When the mother was blood group O and the fetus A, B, or AB, the fetal cells disappeared more rapidly from the maternal blood. Other authors who have demonstrated frequent, but small, "leaks" of fetal blood; they have also made modifications of the technique (Léwi et al., 1961; Brown & Cowles, 1963; Keenan & Pearse, 1963; Fielding, 1968). Virgilio and Simon (1977) provided a quantitative assessment of the number of red blood cells and compared commercial kits with the original method. Two reports specifically evaluated the methods that enumerate small numbers of contaminating fetal red blood cells. Thus Schneider and Ludwig (1963) showed that they were able to quantitate fetal blood volumes of between $50 \, \text{mm}^3$ and $50 \, \text{ml}$ in the maternal circulation with the Kleihauer technique. Jones (1969) described a simple "machine" that obtains comparably thin blood films for the better quantitation of fetal blood loss. Stonehill and LaFerla (1986) emphasized that in 25% of pregnancies from 10 to 28 weeks' gestation the maternal blood contains increasing amounts of fetal hemoglobin, a finding originally emphasized as a possible cause of erroneous Kleihauer tests by Pembrey et al. (1973). During that gestational period, maternal cells with fetal hemoglobin should not be confused with fetal cells. Woodrow and Finn (1966) also studied the staining reaction of red blood cells in pregnant and nonpregnant women. They concluded that, because of occasional staining of cells in nonpregnant women, only findings of more than 2 cells per 50 low-power fields are of significance. They found no increased transplacental bleeding during the third trimester and suggested that most cases of Rh isoimmunization take place during labor. Finally, Leiberman et al. (1989) also noted that 25% of pregnant women produce hemoglobin F. Other interfering factors are the prevalence of β-thalassemia minor, which occurs in 1.4% of American Blacks, and the fact that 1.7% of white Americans may have increased numbers of hemoglobin F-containing red blood cells. These findings make it mandatory that elevated Kleihauer results be carefully evaluated. Leiberman et al. also suggested the use of the more sensitive measurement of α-fetoprotein for an evaluation of cases with

FIGURE 325. Section of an intervillous thrombus stained with antifetal hemoglobin peroxidase methodology. Fetal hemoglobin-containing erythrocytes (dark cells) are particularly evident in the fetal capillaries (right). Numerous fetal red blood cells are present in the fresh intervillous thrombus (left). Peroxidase. ×250. (Courtesy Dr. C. Kaplan, New York.)

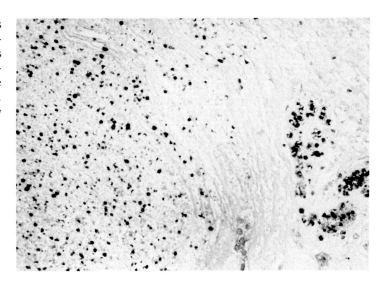

presumed transplacental bleeding. The possible confusion here, in cases of fetal anomalies that may be another cause of elevated α-fetoprotein levels, is obvious.

That errors in assessment of transplacental bleeding occur was shown in a case described by LaFerla et al. (1981), and these errors are the reason the authors recommended that the Kleihauer test be supported with findings from other tests. These other techniques, however, have fully validated the concept of transplacental bleeding. It is true for the test developed by Ness (1982), an enzyme-linked antiglobulin reaction, which can also be useful for evaluating the potential recipients of Rh-immune globulin. Tomoda (1964) demonstrated that fluorescent antibodies against fetal hemoglobin can be employed to enumerate the fetal cells in the maternal circulation. Streiff et al. (1964) used a variety of techniques to demonstrate fetal cells in the maternal system; Zilliacus et al. (1975) found that fluorescent Y chromosome stains often showed fetal (male) lymphocytes in pregnant mothers' blood; and Lee and Vazquez (1962) showed that fluorescent antibodies against the A and B blood groups stained appropriately marked fetal cells in maternal blood with blood group O. Thus the warning issued by Stonehill and La Ferla (1986) may have been too cautious. It is imperative, of course, that the quantity of fetal cells be assessed accurately for the judgment of quantities of antiglobulin administration in rhesus-negative mothers (Eich & Tripoldi, 1974).

The life-span of fetal cells in the maternal circulation has been studied by Kleihauer and Brandt (1964). They determined that fetal cells can be maintained for a long time in the maternal circulation. Although the life-span of fetal cells in the maternal circulation is somewhat shorter than that of normal cells, the cause of neonatal anemia due to transplacental bleeding may be ascertained as long as 4 to 6 weeks after delivery by Kleihauer tests alone. The survival of fetal red blood cells is naturally strongly correlated with the constellation of fetal and maternal red blood cell compatibilities. Fetal red blood cells can also be identified in amnionic fluid and vaginal blood with the aforementioned techniques (e.g., in cases of presumed placenta previa).

Occasional failure to identify fetal red blood cells by the Kleihauer technique in cases that strongly suggest their presence has led to the development of alternate methods. Thus failing to identify fetal cells in blood-stained amnionic fluid in a patient with

elevated α-fetoprotein levels led Ahmed and Brown (1986) to perform hemoglobin electrophoresis; they thereby identified predominantly fetal hemoglobin. Chamberlain et al. (1982) compared the results from Kleihauer stains with α-fetoprotein levels. They found that the latter method gave more accurate results. In this connection, the Apt test is occasionally mentioned without there generally being a clear understanding of its usefulness. The Apt-Downey test was primarily designed to differentiate between fetal and maternal blood in the stomachs of newborns; it has also been used to examine vaginal blood. Apt and Downey (1955) first described the method to allow rapid determination of the origin of blood in stools of neonates (melena). The method is generally less satisfactory than the others mentioned for distinguishing fetal red blood cells from maternal cells. The procedure depends on alkali denaturation of hemoglobin. Crissinger et al. (1987) described it as follows: "Specimen is mixed with tap water (1 part of hemorrhagic fluid to 5 parts water), centrifuged, and 1 ml of 0.25 M sodium hydroxide is added to 5 ml of the supernatant. Brown-yellow color indicates adult hemoglobin, and pink indicates fetal hemoglobin."

Another method for identifying fetal red blood cells was employed by Kaplan et al. (1982). These investigators were interested in ascertaining whether placental intervillous thrombi (IVT) contain fetal or maternal erythrocytes. Potter (1948) had earlier assumed these thrombi to be made up of mainly maternal cells. She based her deduction on macroagglutination findings with differing ABO blood groups of mother and fetus. Cells that were presumably NRBCs were interpreted as lymphocytes. Javert and Reiss (1952) had shown that the so-called red infarcts of an earlier nomenclature were intervillous coagulation events. Because they found NRBCs in 48.7% of these thrombi, they discouraged the use of the term intervillous thrombus. Kaplan et al. (1982) used Sternberger's technique of peroxidase labeling to study histological sections with intervillous coagulation. They found that more than 85% of intervillous thrombi contained irregularly distributed fetal erythrocytes (Figure 325). Often they were present in large numbers, and the authors deduced from these findings that intervillous thrombi may be one entry point for fetal cells into the maternal circulation. Devi et al. (1968) had previously established that a good correlation exists between the presence of fetal red blood cells in the maternal circulation and the number of intervillous thrombi.

Significant Transplacental Hemorrhage

The diagnosis of anemia in the newborn due to occult hemorrhage was first seriously considered by Wiener (1948). He had observed three newborns with low hemoglobin values, two of them being 6.5 g and 8.7 g. One patient had been delivered by cesarean section because of a placenta previa; the other was born normally. The third patient was an unusual case of erythroblastosis, a disease that was under intensive study at that time and whose cause was then being defined. There was much interest in this new phenomenon of a putative transplacental passage of fetal blood to the mother. Wiener remarked that "the main objection to this concept is the difficulty of demonstrating such postulated placental defects in pathologic specimens." He referred to the known hemorrhages due to vasa previa but found no good explanation for his observations of neonatal anemia. This "interesting and recent hypothesis" was discussed by Wickster (1952). He reviewed some cases of abruptio and placenta previa. He also presented the case of an unexplained fetal blood loss—enough to cause shock in the neonate but recent enough not to have caused isoimmunization of the mother. Only after Chown's papers were published in 1954 and 1955 was there wider interest in the topic of prenatal bleeding. Chown (1954) reported two cases of neonatal anemia. I examined the placentas and found intervillous thrombi and noted many NRBCs in the fetal circulation. A transfusion reaction had occurred in one mother; the other suffered "pain at 8.5 months' gestation."

It is now widely recognized that significant fetomaternal hemorrhages may cause fetal anemia, even exsanguination, hydrops fetalis, maternal isoimmunization, and fetal cardiac rhythm irregularities, and that fetal death may result from it (Saber, 1977; Shahar et al., 1981; Laube & Schauberger, 1982; Fay, 1983; Almeida & Bowman, 1994). Indeed, there is a report of a patient who had at least three consecutive pregnancies complicated by this event, without explanation for the occurrence of their significant transplacental hemorrhage (Catalano & Capeless, 1990). The neonate often displays significant morbidity; and severe anemia and shock are common during the neonatal period (Moya et al., 1987; Li & Bromham, 1988) (see also below). It has also been reported that cerebral palsy has resulted from prenatal hemorrhage (Fay, 1983), presumably due to acute hypotension; and neonatal death is frequent (e.g., Griffin, 1969). The documentation of fetal microcephaly following such an event is especially important. Del Valle and colleagues (1992) documented a fascinating event of this nature. The patient sustained a motor vehicle accident at 27 weeks with fetal distress ensuing. Kleihauer tests were negative, but amniocentesis yielded bloody fluid and cordocentesis a hematocrit of 17%. The fetus was transfused and a mature fetus delivered at 37 weeks. Its Apgar scores were 8/9 and the hematocrit 50%. There was a 25% infarction of the placenta that the authors believed to have been caused by a rupture of a fetal vessel at the time of the accident. It may well also have been the cause of hemorrhage and central nervous system insult. The frequency and magnitude of transplacental hemorrhage were well evaluated in a large study by Almeida and Bowman (1994). They stated in their comprehensive study that "there appear to be two important factors in clinical outcome: the amount of and rate of bleeding."

To make the precise diagnosis of fetal hemorrhage prenatally may be difficult in the clinical arena. Cardwell (1987) has reviewed this aspect and also provided management suggestions (Leiberman et al., 1989). Similarly, Mor-Yosef and his colleagues (1984) considered the sinusoidal rhythm of fetal heart tracings as being the result of massive transplacental hemorrhage near term. The anemic neonate had a marked reticulocytosis and elevated globin synthesis; the cause may have been an exceedingly tightly entangled cord. Ellis and Kohler (1976) found marked thymic atrophy in these neonates at autopsy. The thymic atrophy certainly is not specific for hemorrhage but is found in a wide variety of infants who have experienced prenatal "stress." It should be considered a result of ACTH-cortisol stimulation, as is also the maturation found in the fetal adrenal cortex. Following an initial review of the topic by Fynaut (1960), Renaer et al. (1976) gathered many of the reported cases of significant prenatal hemorrhage into a large review article. There were 11 cases of massive transplacental transfusion. The reviewers concluded that the incidence of transfer of blood increases with gestational age, and that it occurs as commonly as in 1 of 300 pregnancies. The phenomenon accounts for fetal death in approximately 1:2,000 deliveries. Renaer et al. (1976) also observed one maternal transfusion reaction and described a wide range of hematocrit and hemoglobin values for the newborns. Etiological factors included cesarean section, external fetal version, amniocentesis, placement of a Drew-Smythe catheter, trauma, and tumultuous labor (see also Finn et al., 1963; Zipursky et al., 1963a,b). A catalogue of other associated or causative conditions, including those in a large number of European references, may be found in Rosta's (1978) review.

Separate from the aforementioned literature, many other cases have been described in individual case reports. Gunson (1957) provided six such observations. Borum et al. (1957) reported two cases, one of which had a normal placenta; in the other, a cord was wrapped twice around the neck. Perhaps the venous congestion from this obstruction caused the transplacental bleeding.

Mannherz (1960) observed a neonatal red blood cell count of 2.05 million and 7.3% Kleihauer-positive cells in the maternal circulation. He estimated that, over time, the fetus must have lost 250 ml of blood. The placental surface was brownish and the villous tissue pale. Grimes and Wright (1961) reported an anemic, distressed newborn from an uncomplicated pregnancy. They drew attention to a case in which the mother suffered hemolysis, fibrinogenopenia, and acute renal tubular necrosis. In that case, there was an ABO incompatibility between mother and fetus. Donaldson (1962) found a recently stillborn, postmature baby who had died owing to transplacental hemorrhage and whose placenta had a large retroplacental hematoma. In that case, the retroplacental bleeding occurred in the absence of toxemia. Rudolph et al. (1962) reported a fetal death in which an intervillous thrombus in the placenta was accompanied by hemosiderin deposits. Paros (1962) described an anemic term infant in whom he estimated that 400 ml of fetal blood had been lost into the maternal circulation over a period of time. Most recently, Willis and Foreman (1988) observed massive, chronic fetal bleeding with fetal cardiac irregularities and later, persistent late decelerations. The Kleihauer-Betke stains showed 14.5% fetal cells in the maternal circulation, an estimated 700 ml of fetal blood; the fetus had a hematocrit of 17% and hemoglobin of 5.1 g/dl, was meconium-stained, but had a normal neonatal course. It must have bled over a prolonged period. These authors reviewed several other cases not listed here and found an essentially normal placenta in their case. No untoward events had been noted during the 38-week pregnancy. Rouse and Weiner (1990) saw the development of fetal hydrops and attempted treatment with serial transfusions. The placenta they found was large, but it had no characteristic lesions to explain the fetal hemorrhage. Another case of fetomaternal hemorrhage treated with repeated transfusion was reported by Fischer et al. (1990). There also had been a sinusoidal pattern of heart tracings, and the fetus' movements improved immediately after transfusions. The placenta had a subchorionic hematoma 2 cm from the cord insertion, perhaps due to needle insertion. Thrombi were found in stem vessels of the placenta.

Cohen et al. (1964) stated that the placenta rarely accomplishes a perfect separation of the maternal and fetal bloodstreams and estimated that 1% of pregnancies are complicated by significant fetal bleeding. Despite these repetitious reports in the literature, Keller et al. (1980) still considered this entity to be a frequently overlooked cause of perinatal morbidity and mortality. They reported on five cases with two deaths, and one of the infants had cerebral infarcts at birth. Schellong (1969), who discussed the causes and therapy of neonatal anemia, thought that transfusion of the neonate is indicated only when the observed neonatal hemoglobin value falls below 8% to 10% of normal. Shiller (1957) observed shock in an anemic neonate whose placenta had a retroplacental blood clot. He drew attention to the presence of many NRBCs in the fetal circulation, a maternal vein, and the intervillous space. Because of the known risk factors for transplacental bleeding (e.g., cesarean section, trauma.), Ness et al. (1987) prospectively studied a cohort of D-negative women for fetal hemorrhage and isoimmunization. The investigators were unable to predict reliably the occurrence of such hemorrhage, nor were they able to use historical events from the patient to form a basis for the administration of prophylactic antibodies (RhoGam). Fliegner et al. (1987) also thought that occult fetomaternal hemorrhage was an important cause of fetal mortality and morbidity that should be investigated in otherwise unexplained stillbirths.

Fetal Consequences of Massive Hemorrhage Across the Placenta

Severe fetal anemia is a prominent sequela of transplacental hemorrhage. Sections of the placenta from such a case are shown in Figure 326. The villous tissue is unusually thick and pale; and one large, fresh intervillous hematoma is seen within the middle section. The villous capillary bed of this placenta was markedly distended and had the appearance of chorangiosis. This pregnancy was the first of a patient whose 2,040 g infant had Apgar scores of 8/8, a neonatal hemoglobin level of 4.5 g/dl, and a hematocrit of 14%. An excessive number of NRBCs were present in the fetal blood. The maternal and fetal blood groups were compatible. The child was edematous and had cardiomegaly but improved markedly after prompt transfusions were given. By Kleihauer stains, there were 3% to 5% of fetal cells in the maternal circulation. No history of trauma or other untoward event had occurred during the pregnancy that could have been held responsible for the massive fetal bleeding. Many similar cases have been reported in the literature (e.g., Debelle et al., 1977), and every perinatal pathologist has seen such cases (reviewed by Smith & Benjamin, 1968; See also Freese, 1965; McGowan, 1968; Pai et al., 1975). For example, Carper and O'Donnell (1967) described a neonate with shock attributable to protracted fetal anemia; there were 4.5% positive cells in Kleihauer stains of maternal blood. The mother and fetus were blood group compatible, and the infant survived after transfusion. The placenta was not overtly unusual, but the mother had sustained two falls during pregnancy that may have been the cause of trauma to the placenta. Naeye et al. (1964) observed a neonate with prenatal exsanguination

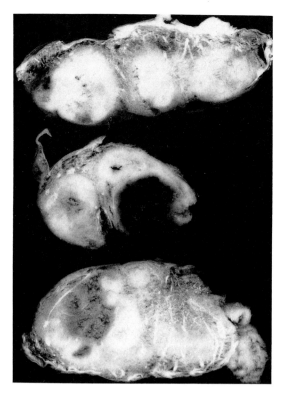

FIGURE 326. Three slices of formalin-fixed placenta of neonate with edema and severe anemia (hemoglobin 4.5 g/dl; hematocrit 14%) due to transplacental hemorrhage. Note the thickness of the placenta, the severe pallor, and, in the central section, the large intervillous hematoma.

manifested by a hematocrit of 15%, hemoglobin of 7.4 g/dl, and 48 NRBCs per 100 white blood cells. Despite therapy, the infant died. Autopsy findings included widespread infarctive necroses in many organs. The placenta was meconium stained but was not otherwise described. It is important to emphasize in this connection that it may be difficult for the pathologist to identify fetal anemia in a stillborn at autopsy. Thus in every stillborn coming to autopsy the possibility of fetal transplacental hemorrhage should be considered and must be properly excluded if such cases are not to be missed. This is the point of the contribution by Laube and Schauberger (1982). They found that 3.4% of all fetal deaths and 0.04% of all births among 9,223 deliveries were due to this cause. Walter et al. (1965) found a severely anemic 3,100 g newborn, rapidly and successfully treated with transfusion, whose placenta weighed 1,920 g. It had no specific lesions other than distension of all villous vessels. Because transplacental bleeding may result in necrosis of a variety of fetal organs, including the brain, its documentation is of particular importance at a time when medicolegal claims abound. Reference to such cases has been made in an earlier portion of this chapter. It must here be remembered

also that fetal blood is often transferred across the placenta at the time of delivery, which is the basis for RhoGam prophylaxis after delivery. Owen et al. (1989), conscious of the possible misinterpretation of fetal hemorrhage (as evidenced by Kleihauer stains) as the cause of prenatal death, compared predelivery versus postdelivery Kleihauer stain results. Their findings indicated that puerperal collection of blood for Kleihauer stains is satisfactory. Their contribution and others suggested that 10% to 15% of otherwise unexplained fetal deaths and perhaps 4% of all fetal deaths were the result of massive transplacental hemorrhage.

Prenatal blood loss has been associated with the clinical identification of specific prenatal disturbances. Clark and Miller (1984) observed a sinusoidal fetal heart rate pattern during labor that they associated with the occurrence of a fetal to maternal hemorrhage. The mother had spontaneous rupture of membranes; and because of the fetal heart rate patterns a cesarean section was performed. The neonate had a hematocrit of 16%, and Kleihauer stains showed 7.6% fetal cells in the maternal circulation. Because of the large quantity of fetal blood in the mother (265 ml), a chronic hemorrhage was suspected. In a pregnancy where fetal tachycardia, atrial dilatation, and atrial fibrillation were present, Bacevice et al. (1985) observed 45 to 60 ml of fetal red blood cells in the maternal circulation before birth. It led to digitalization, cesarean section, and the delivery of an infant with a 37% hematocrit. Unfortunately, the placenta was not described. There had been no risk factors associated with the fetal hemorrhage.

In the cases of fetal bleeding that complicates *cordocentesis* (Feinkind et al., 1990; Ghidini et al., 1993), local hemorrhage or abruptio can be identified, although it is not the case for most spontaneous transplacental hemorrhages. Most of the pathological changes found in these placentas are a result of the fetal anemia rather than being its cause. The pallor, edema, chorangiosis, and placentomegaly result from prolonged fetal cardiac failure. Many of the placentas cannot be shown to have overt abnormalities that could be the cause of the fetal bleeding. This was, for instance, the case in the well studied infant described by Léwi et al. (1965). This infant had a neonatal hematocrit of only 17% and a hemoglobin concentration of 4.8 g/dl. Likewise, Desbuquois et al. (1962) observed a normal placenta associated with fetal anemia in a 3,400 g neonate; they cited similar cases from the literature. We have observed an exsanguinated, term stillborn infant in whose subamnionic space a large amount of fresh blood separated the amnion (4 cm) from the chorion. At cesarean section, 500 ml of blood was removed, and the placenta was 50% abrupted. No risk factors were identified. To be sure, many of the placentas of cases with fetal exsanguination possess intervillous thrombi. They have often been thought of as the possible sites of fetal bleeding, as suspected in the earliest cases described by Chown (1955), the case of Debelle et al. (1977), and the case illustrated in Figure 326. Devi et al. (1968) studied the placentas of 120 normal deliveries, 264 complicated deliveries, 98 pregnancies of Rh-negative women without antibodies, and 35 Rh-negative patients with antibodies. Their findings indicated that the so-called Kline's hemorrhages (see below) positively correlated with the presence of fetal cells in the maternal circulation. The more frequently such lesions were present, the greater was the size of the transplacental hemorrhage. The authors presented their findings in several tables; and their results impressively support the notion that Kline's lesions, intervillous thrombi, operative delivery, infarcts, and abruptio placentae statistically correlate with fetal bleeding.

Kline had described in 1948 that specific microscopic lesions in the placenta correlate with bleeding of the fetus. In the placentas of 15 erythroblastotic fetuses he found "numerous breaks," with NRBCs in the adjacent intervillous space. He deduced that these "breaks" occurred in the peripheral capillaries or even in larger blood vessels. After agglutination of red blood cells and deposition of fibrin, the overlying trophoblastic epithelium appeared to degenerate, serving as a nidus for clots to form. We believe that this alleged causality of the capillary occlusion is incorrect. In many fetal vascular occlusions, there is no trophoblastic degeneration; nor can breaks in blood vessels and villous surfaces be identified. It is also noteworthy that, despite the presence of a 2.7 cm spherical "cyst" with NRBCs in one of Chown's cases (1955), no trophoblastic damage was found on the villous surfaces. The integrity of the villous surface trophoblast is dependent solely on the intervillous circulation. It is not dependent on the fetal circulation. Occlusions of fetal capillaries do not cause trophoblastic necrosis; they cause the villus to atrophy and occasionally to become edematous, eventually making it fibrotic.

Nevertheless, the term Kline hemorrhage has become associated with the putative lesions that are believed to initiate transplacental hemorrhage. When defects in the trophoblast occur, fibrinoid deposits across the defects; the trophoblast disruptions increase in frequency with advancing gestation normally, as does the fibrin (see Chapter 11). The fibrin deposits may calcify and eventually become part of the diffuse microcalcification of term placentas. Breaks of villi also occur frequently throughout gestation. Presumably, they are "healed" by this maternal fibrin deposition.

We believe that, in vivo, the fetal blood flow and its pressure maintain the placental villi in an "erected" position. They are thus more susceptible to injury from fetal kicking than if they are empty, or "deflated." We can readily envisage that small breaks can then occur spontaneously and when the villi are injured by the fetus. To us, this more readily explains the frequency of fetal bleeding in otherwise normal placentas. Wentworth (1964) has advocated the use of flat, large (Gough) sections of the delivered and formalin-fixed placenta for the observation of Kline hemorrhages. The cases he studied were correlated with Kleihauer stains of maternal blood, and the Kline hemorrhages could be evaluated by gross inspection. A positive correlation between the number of Kline lesions and the finding of positive Kleihauer stains was observed by Wentworth. Some of the illustrated "lesions" indicate that the author considered the normal villous lakes to be Kline lesions. These are the sites of primary injection of the maternal jets, the "holes" one observes in most delivered placentas. Wentworth (1964) found no correlation with infarcts, calcification, or other placental lesions.

Large intervillous thrombi may occur during labor (Figure 327). They are then fresh clots and without structure. There may be older, laminated clots with a similar appearance (Figures 328–330). When these clots contain fetal cells, their older age may be revealed by the presence of macrophages that have engulfed fetal

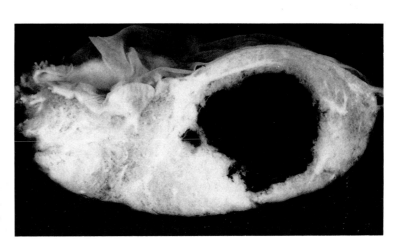

FIGURE 327. Fresh intervillous thrombus in the center of villous tissue is presumed to have occurred during the delivery. Note the extreme pallor of this placenta from an erythroblastotic infant.

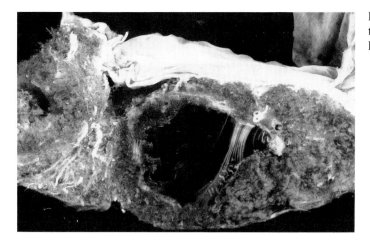

FIGURE 328. Intervillous thrombus in the center of a term placenta. It is somewhat older than the thrombus in Figure 327. Note the laminated fibrin at right.

red blood cells (Figure 331). We are here referring to intervillous thrombi that occur in the centers of the villous mass and that do not relate to lesions in the floor of the placenta, as those shown in Figures 328 and 329. The latter intervillous thrombi are associated with maternal vascular lesions, often occur in preeclampsia, and are frequently laminated and pale. They differ from infarcts, which are granular in macroscopic appearance and invariably involve villi. Typical intervillous thrombi merely displace adjacent villi. Of course, if intervillous thrombi become large or if they are of longer duration, the compressed adjacent villous tissue also becomes infarcted. Other intervillous thrombi occur underneath the fetal surface. Those subchorionic fibrin masses increase with gestation and result from eddying of the intervillous blood as it is reflected underneath the chorion. In some placentas they protrude into the amnionic cavity and may become Breus' moles. These features are discussed in Chapter 11. Finally, more

remarkable subchorionic fibrin deposits occur with some maternal cardiac diseases (see Chapter 19). In addition, subchorionic fibrin deposits are regularly present in the immature placentas delivered after intraamnionic saline and urea instillation for therapeutic abortion. It is of parenthetical interest to note that intervillous thrombi and placental infarcts never undergo the repair process known to pathologists as "organization." That is to say, unlike other organs, the placenta never manifests the fibrous tissue ingrowth and neovascularization that occurs in other organs whose infarcts organize and become scars. Even the larger thrombi of surface vessels and in the umbilical cord do not "organize" frequently.

In occasional cases of fatal fetomaternal bleeding, the placenta has exhibited specific lesions that may explain

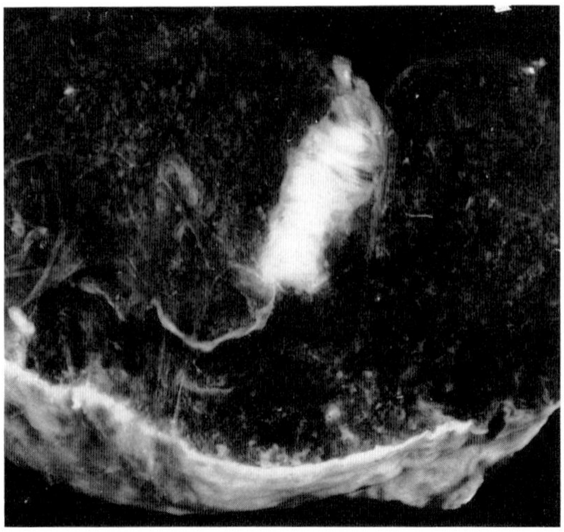

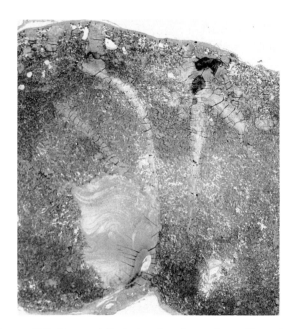

FIGURE 329. Layered fibrin residue of an old intervillous thrombus originating from cotyledonary septum.

FIGURE 330. Layered fibrin in a basal-type intervillous thrombus, associated with decidual necrosis and thrombosis of a decidual vein. There is no adjacent infarction yet. H&E. ×6.

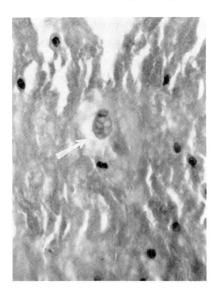

FIGURE 331. Old intervillous thrombus. Note the maternal erythrocytophagocytic macrophage (arrow). H&E ×400.

the hemorrhage. Santamaria et al. (1987) found a "choriocarcinoma in situ" in the pale placenta of an otherwise normal stillborn. The trophoblast was clearly invasive and had presumably caused some fetal vascular discontinuity. More importantly, perhaps, the lesion was not identifiable by macroscopic examination as a tumor. Small "infarcts" were seen and sampled, but grossly they were not deemed to be exceptional. The discovery of this (and other) placental choriocarcinomas in situ was fortuitous. Perhaps other "unexplained" transplacental hemorrhages would have yielded similar lesions had the placenta been examined in more detail.

A small chorioangioma of the placenta was found in another fetus with transplacental hemorrhage (Figure 332). There was no tumorous destruction of villi in this case, but the adjacent vessels were severely distended. They may have bled. Stiller and Skafish (1986) also reported on transplacental hemorrhage in association with a chorioangioma of the placenta, fetal distress, and maternal hemolysis. Brown (1963) found that large placentas and excessively calcified organs have an increased association with transplacental hemorrhage. Pollack and Montague (1968), on the other hand, stated that postmature placentas did not allow fetal hemorrhage to occur more frequently. The occurrence of fetal hemoglobin (>5%) in retroplacental hematomas was demonstrated in 29 of 93 cases by Oehlert et al. (1960).

Other Fetal Blood Elements Passing Through the Placenta

Although transplacental red blood cell passage has the most serious consequences (anemia, immunization), transplacental white blood cell transfer is also of interest. For instance, do tumor cells readily pass the placental villi? As was reviewed in Chapter 19, maternal leukemia cells do not usually pass the placental "barrier." Of the solid neoplasms, only occasional melanoma cells are known to have traversed the placenta to the fetus with certainty. It is thus surprising to learn that some studies have suggested that lymphocyte traffic may occur across the placenta, and that it is alleged to take place in both directions. This topic has been reviewed in some detail by Schröder (1975), who concluded that the question of fetal leukocytes in the ma-

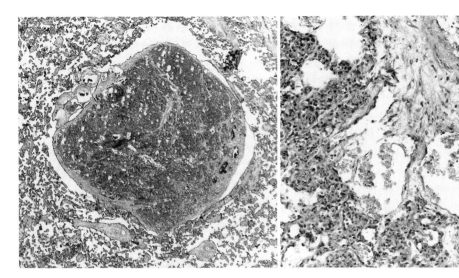

FIGURE 332. Small chorangioma in a mature placenta (maternal sickle cell disease) has caused transplacental hemorrhage (hematocrit 22%; 120 ml blood loss). The markedly distended fetal vessels, seen at right with extreme thinning of their walls, may be the sites of hemorrhage. H&E. Left ×12.5; right ×50.

ternal circulation was still controversial, at least at that time. In part, the results of such studies are difficult to interpret because the mitotic inhibition of maternal leukocytes, when admixed with fetal lymphocytes, prevents ready identification of fetal cells (Olding et al., 1974). The conclusion of Schröder, however, was that fetal lymphocytes frequently pass to the mother, and that they probably do so in most normal pregnancies. They may be found up to years postpartum in the maternal blood or bone marrow, but they do not respond to the usual mitogens (Schröder et al., 1977).

Selypes and Lorencz (1988) have developed a methodology with which to identify fetal lymphocytes in the maternal circulation. They used this technique to identify fetal sex and diagnosis of possibly aberrant fetal karyotypes. Other techniques are now being used to identify fetal cells in the maternal blood. Adinolfi et al. (1989) and Lo et al. (1989) have used the polymerase chain reaction (PCR) for DNA amplification and the identification of Y chromosome-bearing cells in maternal venous blood. No contamination with fetal cells was found in six samples from pregnancies of 24 to 36 weeks' gestation by the first investigators. Deported syncytiotrophoblast was apparently trapped in the maternal lung. Their deportation, of course, had long been known (Schmorl, 1893, 1905; Raafat et al., 1975). In the investigation by Lo et al. (1989) Y sequences were found in the cells of all 12 women with male conceptuses but in none of the seven cases with female fetuses. The possibility of contamination in this study was criticized by Holzgreve et al. (1990). Isolation of fetal DNA from maternal blood, contaminated by fetal NRBCs has been amply documented also by Bianchi et al. (1990). In later studies she suggested that these cells traverse the placenta at different times (Bianchi et al., 1991). The reliability of Lo's technique was further questioned by the study of Suzumori et al. (1992). On the other hand, a carefully designed and cautiously executed study of peripheral blood for Y-specific ZFY sequences showed conclusively that nucleated fetal cells nearly regularly contaminate maternal blood (Kao et al., 1992). In a prospective study, Hamada et al. (1993) found by fluorescence in situ hybridization (FISH) in 50 male conceptuses that NRBCs were regularly found in the maternal circulation after 15 weeks. During the first trimester their incidence was 1:100,000 nucleated cells, whereas it was 1:10,000 at term. Elias and colleagues (1992) have even made the diagnosis of trisomy 21 and trisomy 18 by the FISH method by demonstrating three fluorescent markers in nucleated cells. Cell sorting of nucleated cells and other techniques are now in use to enrich the fetal cells contaminating the maternal blood (Gänshirt-Ahlert et al., 1992a,b). Surprisingly, Bertero et al. (1988) have found some maternal (definitely *not*

fetal) antigens on the surface of these circulating cells. They deduced from this finding that the prenatal diagnosis of β-thalassemia they attempted was not feasible. The topic of prenatal diagnosis from maternal blood contaminated by fetal cells is under intense study. Many approaches were evaluated at a conference held in September 1993. It seems likely that the nearly regular, if small, contamination of NRBCs in the maternal circulation even during early pregnancy is suitable for this purpose. Concentration methods exist, clinical trials are under way, and verification of the cells under study as being cells from the current fetus are assured. Less optimal (because somewhat invasive) are the methods to obtain cells from washings of the endocervical canal.

MOTHER TO FETUS TRANSFER OF CELLS

Although occasional cases of such cellular exchange have been well documented, much less good evidence has been adduced that maternal cells frequently pass to the fetus in significant numbers. Schröder (1975), in the same review mentioned above, noted the observation of Kadowaki et al. (1965) of the prenatally incurred lymphocytic chimerism in a neonate with presumed immunological incompetence. This child later developed graft-versus-host disease as a result of his lymphocyte chimerism. Similar chimerism, induced by prenatal maternal lymphocyte transfer in a child with thymic alymphoplasia, reported by Githens et al. (1969), had no ill effect. Oehme et al. (1966) were able to show maternal leukocyte transfer to the rabbit fetus, with striking accumulation of these cells in the fetal lung. A few other reports of 46,XX cells in the circulation of male fetuses have been forthcoming (El-Alfi & Hathout, 1969; Moszkowski et al., 1971). Such passage is clearly exceptional, and graft-versus-host rejection of the immunologically compromised fetus, as in Kadowaki's case, must be exceedingly uncommon. Moreover, when lymphocyte co-cultivation of maternal and fetal cells is experimentally studied, the maternal cell response is markedly reduced (Kawagoe et al., 1971; Olding et al., 1974). This problem may also have been the cause of Olding's (1972) failure to identify 46,XX cells in the cord blood of male infants.

Interestingly, there have been occasional reports of fetal plethora that were apparently due to mother-to-fetus blood transfer. Wong and Cann (1972) described a fatal transfusion reaction with fetal renal tubular necrosis in such a putative case of maternal-fetal transfusion. The child was born at 43 weeks' gestation after a normal pregnancy, and the placenta was not infarcted; nor was it abrupted. The neonatal hemoglobin concentration was 16.8% g/dl, there was hemoglobinuria, and the fetal blood did not clot. Immunological studies of the fetal red blood cells suggested that maternal cells were circulating at birth. Chronic maternofetal transfusion was found in a case of hydrops fetalis described by Bowman et al. (1984). The mother had received fetal cells transplacentally (5.4% Kleihauer-positive cells). The hydropic infant was plethoric, with a hemoglobin of 20.5 g/dl and a 63% hematocrit. The placenta accompanying this fetus had extensive areas of infarction and intervillous thrombi; and microscopically there were torn fetal vessels. The authors concluded that such cases must be rare, and they were able to refer to only one previously described case of fetal plethora, that of Michael and Mauer (1961). They suggested that this bidirectional exchange was possible due to the disrupted large fetal placental vessels, an otherwise uncommon phenomenon. Michael and Mauer (1961) found three newborns of normal pregnancies with hematocrits of 73%, 79%, and 80% respectively, and hemoglobin values of 21.2, 21.8, and 24.6 g/dl. In two of these cases the fetal and maternal blood groups differed, and differential agglutination allowed proof of maternal red blood cell transfer to the fetus. The placentas were not described, and the mechanism of transplacental transfer was only speculated upon. There are, however, numerous studies that affirm the nearly regular transfer of *some* maternal red blood cells to the fetus, albeit in smaller numbers than those needed to induce fetal plethora. They are not accompanied by abnormal placentas; and they have also been found to occur in mice (Holliday & Barnes, 1973). They obviously embody the importance of possible fetal Rh-isoimmunization when the fetus is Rh-negative and the mother Rh-positive (Jennings & Clauss, 1978). Messer et al. (1966) found that parenteral administration of carbazochrome to the mother decreased the transfer. Red blood cell transfer from mother to fetus was affirmed by Smith et al. (1961) and Zarou et al. (1964) using chromium 51-labeled red blood cells. Macris et al. (1958) and Fujikura and Klionsky (1975) identified such transfer, with the marker being sickled erythrocytes. Many other studies have been summarized by additional investigators (Megapanos et al., 1966; Eimer & Weiland, 1969) and leave no doubt that this phenomenon is relatively frequent and perhaps occasionally important. Mayer et al. (1965) demonstrated, in an impressive electron micrograph, the apparent passage of a red blood cell through a fetal villous capillary.

References

Adinolfi, M., Camporeses, C., and Carr, T.: Gene amplification to detect fetal nucleated cells in pregnant women. Lancet 2:328–329, 1989.

Ahmed, J., and Brown, C.: Failure of the Kleihauer test to detect red blood cells in amniotic fluid. Lancet 1:1393, 1986.

Almeida, V. de, and Bowman, J.M.: Massive fetomaternal hemorrhage: Manitoba experience. Obstet. Gynecol. 83: 323–328, 1994.

Apt, L., and Downey, W.S.: "Melena" neonatorum: the swallowed blood syndrome; a simple test for the differentiation of adult and fetal hemoglobin in bloody stools. J. Pediatr. 47:6–12, 1955.

Awwad, J.T., Azar, G.B., Seoud, M.A., Mroueh, A.M., and Karam, K.S.: High-velocity penetrating wounds of the gravid uterus: review of 16 years of civil war. Obstet. Gynecol. 83:259–264, 1994.

Bacevice, A.E., Dierker, L.J., and Wolfson, R.N.: Intrauterine atrial fibrillation associated with fetomaternal hemorrhage. Am. J. Obstet. Gynecol. 153:81–82, 1985.

Baer, K.E.v.: Untersuchungen ueber die Gefaessverbindungen zwischen Mutter und Frucht in den Saeugethieren. L. Voss, Leipzig, 1828.

Benirschke, K., and Gille, J.: Placental pathology andasphyxia. In, Intrauterine Asphyxia and the Developing Fetal Brain. L. Gluck, ed., pp. 117–136. Year Book, Chicago, 1977.

Bertero, M.T., Camaschella, C., Serra, A., Bergui, L., and Caligaris-Cappio, F.: Circulating trophoblast cells in pregnancy have maternal genetic markers. Prenat. Diagn. 8:585–590, 1988.

Bianchi, D.W., Flint, A.F., Pizzimenti, M.F., Knoll, J.H.M., and Latt, S.A.: Isolation of fetal DNA from nucleated

erythrocytes in maternal blood. Proc. Natl. Acad. Sci. U.S.A. 87:3279–3283, 1990.

Bianchi, D.W., Stewart, J.E., Garber, M.F., Lucotte, G., and Flint, A.F.: Possible effect of gestational age on the detection of fetal nucleated erythrocytes in maternal blood. Prenat. Diagn. 11:523–528, 1991.

Bickers, R.G., and Wennberg, R.P.: Fetomaternal transfusion following trauma. Obstet. Gynecol. 61:258–259, 1983.

Blajchman, M.A., Maudsley, R.F., Uchida, I., and Zipursky, A.: Diagnostic amniocentesis and fetal-maternal bleeding. Lancet 1:993, 1974.

Borum, A., Loyd, H.O., and Talbot, T.R.: Possible fetal hemorrhage into maternal circulation: report of two cases. J.A.M.A. 164:1087–1088, 1957.

Bowman, J.M., and Pollock, J.M.: Transplacental fetal hemorrhage after amniocentesis. Obstet. Gynecol. 66: 749–754, 1985.

Bowman, J.M., Lewis, M., and de Sa, D.J.: Hydrops fetalis caused by massive maternofetal transplacental hemorrhage. J. Pediatr. 104:769–772, 1984.

Brown, E.S.: Foetal erythrocytes in the maternal circulation. B.M.J. 1:1000–1001, 1963.

Brown, W.E., and Cowles, G.T.: Fetal cells in maternal blood. South. Med. J. 56:782–783, 1963.

Buchsbaum, H.J.: Accidental injury complicating pregnancy. Am. J. Obstet. Gynecol. 102:752–769, 1968.

Buchsbaum, H.J.: Trauma in Pregnancy. Saunders, Philadelphia, 1979.

Buchsbaum, H.J., and Staples, P.P.: Self-inflicted gunshot wound to the pregnant uterus: report of two cases. Obstet. Gynecol. 65:32S–65S, 1985.

Cardwell, M.S.: Fetomaternal hemorrhage: when to suspect, how to manage. Postgrad. Med. 82:127–130, 1987.

Cardwell, M.S., and Snyder, S.W.: Feto-maternal hemorrhage—possible cause of fetal distress. Am. J. Obstet. Gynecol. 161:1744, 1989.

Carper, J.M., and O'Donnell, W.M.: Severe neonatal anemia due to massive transplacental hemorrhage. Am. J. Clin. Pathol. 47:444–447, 1967.

Catalano, P.M., and Capeless, E.L.: Fetomaternal bleeding as a cause of recurrent fetal morbidity and mortality. Obstet. Gynecol. 76:972–73, 1990.

Chamberlain, E.M., Scott, J.R., Wu, J.T., Rote, N.S., and Egger, M.J.: A comparison of acid elution techniques and alpha-fetoprotein levels for the detection of fetomaternal bleeding. Am. J. Obstet. Gynecol. 143:912–917, 1982.

Chibber, G., Zacher, M., Cohen, A.W., and Kline, A.J.: Rh immunization following abdominal trauma: a case report. Am. J. Obstet. Gynecol. 149:692, 1984.

Chown, B.: Anaemia from fetal bleeding of the fetus into the mother's circulation. Lancet 1:1213–1215, 1954.

Chown, B.: The fetus can bled: three clinicopathological pictures. Am. J. Obstet. Gynecol. 70:1298–1308, 1955.

Clark, S.L., and Miller, F.C.: Sinusoidal fetal heart rate pattern associated with massive fetomaternal transfusion. Am. J. Obstet. Gynecol. 149:97–99, 1984.

Cohen, F., Zuelzer, W.W., Gustafson, D.C., and Evans, M.M.: Transplacental bleeding from the fetus. Blood 23: 621–646, 1964.

Crissinger, K.D., Ryckman, F.C., and Balisteri, W.F.: Necrotizing enterocolitis and gastrointestinal hemorrhage. In, Neonatal-Perinatal Medicine. Diseases of the Fetus and Infant. A.A. Fanaroff, and R.J. Martin, eds., pp. 928–932. Mosby, St. Louis, 1987.

Crosby, W.M.: Pathology of obstetric injuries in pregnant automobile-accident victims. In, Accident Pathology. Proceedings of an International Conference. K.M. Brinkhous, ed., pp. 204–207. U.S. Government Printing Office, Washington, D.C., 1968.

Crosby, W.M.: Trauma during pregnancy: maternal and fetal injury. Obstet. Gynecol. Surv. 29:683–699, 1974.

Crosby, W.M., and Costiloe, J.P.: Safety of lap-belt restraint for pregnant victims of automobile collisions. N. Engl. J. Med. 284:632–636, 1971.

Cumming, D.C., and Wren, F.D.: Fetal skull fracture from an apparently trivial motor vehicle accident. Am. J. Obstet. Gynecol. 132:342–343, 1978.

Dahmus, M.A., and Sibai, B.M.: Blunt abdominal trauma: are there any predictive factors for abruptio placentae or maternal-fetal distress? Am. J. Obstet. Gynecol. 169: 1054–1059, 1993.

Debelle, G.D., Gillam, G.L., and Tauro, G.P.: A case of hydrops foetalis due to foeto-maternal haemorrhage. Austr. Paediatr. J. 13:131–133, 1977.

Del Valle, G.O., Joffe, G.M., Izquierdo, L.A., Smith, J.F., Kasnic, T., Gilson, G.J., Chatterjee, M.S., and Curet, L.B.: Acute posttraumatic fetal anemia treated with fetal intravascular transfusion. Am. J. Obstet. Gynecol. 166: 127–129, 1992.

Desbuquois, G., Boulard, P., and Grenier, B.: Hemorrhage foetale dans la circulation maternelle. Arch. Fr. Pediatr. 19:1341–1346, 1962.

Devi, B., Jennison, R.F., and Langley, F.A.: Significance of placental pathology in transplacental hemorrhage. J. Clin. Pathol. 21:322–331, 1968.

De Witt, F.: An historical study on theories of the placenta to 1900. J. Hist. Med. Allied Sci. 14:360–374, 1959.

Donaldson, I.: Intrauterine haemorrhage as a cause of foetal death. Lancet 1:1351, 1962.

Doolittle, J.E.: Placental vascular integrity related to third-stage management. Obstet. Gynecol. 22:468–472, 1963.

Eaton, C.J., and Danzinger, R.F.: Traumatic disruption of pregnancy: report of a case and its legal implications. Obstet. Gynecol. 30:16–22, 1967.

Eden, J.A.: Fetal-induced trauma as a cause of antepartum hemorrhage. Am. J. Obstet. Gynecol. 157:830–831, 1987.

Eich, F.G., and Tripoldi, D.: Screening and quantitating fetal-maternal hemorrhages. Am. J. Clin. Pathol. 61:192–198, 1974.

Eimer, H., and Weiland, A.: Untersuchungen über die Placentapassage mütterlicher Erythrocyten. Arch. Gynecol. 208:113–122, 1969.

El-Alfi, O., and Hathout, H.: Maternofetal transfusion: Immunologic and cytogenetic evidence. Am. J. Obstet. Gynecol. 103:599–600, 1969.

Elias, S., Price, J., Dockter, M., Wachtel, S., Tharapel, A., Simpson, J.L., and Klinger, K.W.: First trimester prenatal diagnosis of trisomy 21 in fetal cells from maternal blood. Lancet 340:1033, 1992.

Ellis, J., and Kohler, H.G.: Small infant thymus in cases of fatal feto-maternal transfusion. B.M.J. 1:694, 1976.

Fay, R.A.: Feto-maternal haemorrhage as a cause of fetal morbidity and mortality. Br. J. Obstet. Gynaecol. 90:443–446, 1983.

Feinkind, L., Nanda, D., Delke, I., and Minkoff, H.: Abruptio placentae after percutaneous umbilical cord sampling: a case report. Am. J. Obstet. Gynecol. 162:1203–1204, 1990.

Feldman, N., Skoll, A., and Sibai, B.: The incidence of significant fetomaternal hemorrhage in patients undergoing cesarean section. Obstet. Gynecol. 163:855–858, 1990.

Fernandez-Rocha, L., and Oullette, R.: Fetal bleeding: an unusual complication of fetal monitoring. Am. J. Obstet. Gynecol. 125:1153–1154, 1976.

Fielding, J.: Detecting foetal cells. Lancet 1:202, 1968.

Finn, R., Harper, D.T., Stallings, S.A., and Krevans, J.R.: Transplacental hemorrhage. Transfusion 3:114–124, 1963.

Fischer R.L., Kuhlman, K., Grover, J., Montgomery, O., and Wapner, R.J.: Chronic, massive fetomaternal hemorrhage treated with repeated fetal intravascular transfusions. Am. J. Obstet. Gynecol. 162:203–204, 1990.

Fliegner, J.R.H., Fortune, D.W., and Barrie, J.U.: Occult fetomaternal hemorrhage as a cause of fetal mortality and morbidity. Aust. N.Z.J. Obstet. Gynecol. 27:158–161, 1987.

Fort, A.T., and Harlin, R.S.: Pregnancy outcome after noncatastrophic maternal trauma during pregnancy. Obstet. Gynecol. 35:912–915, 1970.

Fox, H.: The incidence and significance of nucleated erythrocytes in the foetal vessels of the mature human placenta. J. Obstet. Gynaecol. Br. Commonw. 74:40–43, 1967.

Fraser, I.D., and Raper, A.B.: Observation of compatible and incompatible foetal red cells in the maternal circulation. B.M.J. 2:303–304, 1962.

Freese, U.E.: Massive fetal hemorrhage into the maternal circulation. Obstet. Gynecol. 26:848–851, 1965.

Freese, U.E., and Titel, J.H.: Demonstration of fetal erythrocytes in maternal circulation. Obstet. Gynecol. 22: 527–532, 1963.

Fujikura, T., and Klionsky, B.: Transplacental passage of maternal erythrocytes with sickling. J. Pediatr. 87:781–783, 1975.

Fynaut, J.: Anémie par hémorragie transplacentaire. Bull. Soc. R. Belge Gynecol. Obstet. 30:198–206, 1960.

Gänshirt-Ahlert, D., Basak, N., Aidynli, K., and Holzgreve, W.: Fetal DNA in uterine vein blood. Obstet. Gynecol. 80:601–603, 1992a.

Gänshirt-Ahlert, D., Burschyk, M., Garritsen, H.S.P., Helmer, L., Miny, P., Horst, J., Schneider, H.P.G., and Holzgreve, W.: Magnetic cell sorting and the transferrin receptor as potential means of prenatal diagnosis from maternal blood. Am. J. Obstet. Gynecol. 166:1350–1355, 1992b.

Geissler, D., and Japha, A.: Beitrag zu den Anämieen junger Kinder. Jahrb. Kinderheilkd. 56:627–647, 1901.

Ghidini, A., Sepulveda, W., Lockwood, C.J., and Romero, R.: Complications of fetal blood sampling. Am. J. Obstet. Gynecol. 168:1339–1344, 1993.

Githens, J.H., Muschenheim, F., Fulginiti, V.A., Robinson, A., and Kay, H.E.M.: Thymic alymphoplasia with XX/XY lymphoid chimerism secondary to probable maternal-fetal transfusion. J. Pediatr. 75:87–94, 1969.

Gjode, P., Rasmussen, T.B., and Jorgensen, J.: Fetomaternal bleeding during attempts at external version. Br. J. Obstet. Gynaecol. 87:571–573, 1980.

Goodlin, R.C., and Clewell, W.H.: Sudden fetal death following diagnostic amniocentesis. Am. J. Obstet. Gynecol. 118:285–288, 1974.

Goodwin, T.M., and Breen, M.T.: Pregnancy outcome and fetomaternal hemorrhage after noncatastrophic trauma. Am. J. Obstet. Gynecol. 162:665–671, 1990.

Gottesfeld, K.R., Thompson, H.E., Holmes, J.H., and Taylor, E.D: Ultrasonic placentography—a new method for placental localization. Am. J. Obstet. Gynecol. 96:538–547, 1966.

Green, D.W., and Mimouni, F.: Nucleated erythrocytes in healthy infants and in infants of diabetic mothers. J. Pediatr. 116:129–131, 1990.

Griffin, W.T.: Occult fetal-maternal transfusion. Am. J. Obstet. Gynecol. 105:993, 1969.

Grimes, H.G., and Wright, F.S.: Fetomaternal transfusion: a case report. Am. J. Obstet. Gynecol. 82:1371–1374, 1961.

Grobbelaar, B.G.: Transplacental haemorrhage in Rh-haemolytic disease. B.M.J. 1:300, 1968.

Gunson, H.H.: Neonatal anemia due to fetal hemorrhage into the maternal circulation. Pediatrics 20:3–6, 1957.

Hamada, H., Arinami, T., Kubo, T., Hamaguchi, H., and Iwasaki, H.: Fetal nucleated cells in maternal peripheral blood: frequency and relationship to gestational age. Hum. Genet. 91:427–432, 1993.

Herrmann, U., and Sidiropoulos, D.: Amniocentese bei rhesusnegativen Frauen: Häufigkeit und Konsequenzen fetomaternaler Transfusionen. Arch. Gynecol. 239:241–243, 1986.

Higgins, S.D.: Trauma in pregnancy. J. Perinatol. 8:288–292, 1988.

Higgins, S.D., and Garite, T.J.: Late abruptio placenta in trauma patients: implications for monitoring. Obstet. Gynecol. 63:10S–12S, 1984.

Holliday, J., and Barnes, R.D.: The normal transplacental passage of maternal red cells in mice. Cell Tissue Kinet. 6:455–459, 1973.

Holzgreve, W., Gänshirt-Ahlert, D., Burschyk, M., Horst, J., Miny, P., Gal, A., and Pohlschmidt, M.: Detection of fetal DNA in maternal blood by PCR. Lancet 335:1220–1221, 1990.

Huff, D.L.: Fetal-maternal hemorrhage and management of the third stage of labor at cesarean section—a prospective study. Okla. Obstet. Gynecol. J. Club 4:92, 1988.

Jauniaux, E., Gibb, D., Moscoso, G., and Campbell, S.: Ultrasonographic diagnosis of a large placental intervillous thrombosis associated with elevated maternal serum α-fetoprotein level. Am. J. Obstet. Gynecol. 163:1558–1560, 1990.

Javert, C.T., and Reiss, C.: The origin and significance of macroscopic intervillous coagulation hematomas (red infarcts) of the human placenta. Surg. Gynecol. Obstet. 94:257–269, 1952.

Jennings, E.R., and Clauss, B.: Maternal-fetal hemorrhage: its incidence and sensitizing effects. Am. J. Obstet. Gynecol. 131:725–727, 1978.

Jones, P.: Assessment of size of small volume foeto-maternal bleeds: a new method of quantification of the Kleihauer technique. B.M.J. 1:85–88, 1969.

Kadowaki, J., Thompson, R.I., Zuelzer, W.W., Wooley, P.V., Brough, A.J., and Gruber, D.: XX/XY lymphoid chimaerism in congenital immunological deficiency syndrome with thymic aplasia. Lancet 2:1152–1156, 1965.

Kao, S.-M., Tang, G.-C., Hsieh, T.-T., Young, K.-C., Wang, H.-C., and Pao, C.C.: Analysis of peripheral blood of pregnant women for the presence of fetal Y chromosome-specific ZFY gene deoxyribonucleic acid sequences. Am. J. Obstet. Gynecol. 166:1013–1019, 1992.

Kaplan, C., Blanc, W.A., and Elias, J.: Identification of erythrocytes in intervillous thrombi: a study using immuno-peroxidase identification of hemoglobins. Hum. Pathol. 13:554–556, 1982.

Kawagoe, K., Koresawa, M., Ohama, K., and Kadotani, T.: A preliminary study of immunological tolerance in human newborn baby based on mixed leucocyte cultures. Jpn. J. Genet. 46:191–194, 1971.

Keenan, H., and Pearse, W.H.: Transplacental transmission of fetal erythrocytes. Am. J. Obstet. Gynecol. 86:1096–1098, 1963.

Keller, J.L., Baker, D.A., and Clemmons, J.J.: Massive fetal-maternal hemorrhage: an overlooked cause of perinatal morbidity and mortality. Lab. Invest. 42:32, 1980.

Kettel, L.M., Branch, D.W., and Scott, J.R.: Occult placental abruption after maternal trauma. Obstet. Gynecol. 71:449–453, 1988.

Kleihauer, E., and Brandt, G.: Zur Lebensdauer fetaler Erythrocyten im mütterlichen Kreislauf nach feto-maternaler Transfusion. Klin. Wochenschr. 42:458–459, 1964.

Kleihauer, E., Braun, H., and Betke, K.: Demonstration von fetalem Hämoglobin in den Erythrocyten eines Blutausstriches. Klin. Wochenschr. 35:637–638, 1957.

Kline, B.S.: Microscopic observations of the placental barrier in transplacental erythrocytotoxic anemia (erythroblastosis fetalis) and in normal pregnancy. Am. J. Obstet. Gynecol. 56:226–237, 1948.

Kosasa, T.S., Ebesugawa, I., Nakayama, R.T., and Hale, R.W.: Massive fetomaternal hemorrhage preceded by decreased fetal movement and a nonreactive fetal heart rate pattern. Obstet. Gynecol. 82:711–714, 1993.

LaFerla, J.J., Butch, S.H., and Cooley, J.R.: Utilization of specific mixed agglutination in a case of apparent feto-maternal hemorrhage. Am. J. Obstet. Gynecol. 141:581–582, 1981.

Lakoff, K.M., Klein, J., Bolognese, R.J., and Corson, S.L.: Transplacental hemorrhage during voluntary interruption of pregnancy. J. Reprod. Med. 6:260–261, 1971.

Larroche, J.-C.: Fetal encephalopathies of circulatory origin. Biol. Neonate 50:61–74, 1986.

Laube, D.W., and Schauberger, C.W.: Fetomaternal bleeding as a cause for "unexplained" fetal death. Obstet. Gynecol. 60:649–651, 1982.

Lavin, J.P., and Miodovnik, M.: Delayed abruption after maternal trauma as a result of an automobile accident. J. Reprod. Med. 26:621–624, 1981.

Lee, R.E., and Vazquez, J.J.: Immunocytochemical evidence for transplacental passage of erythrocytes. Lab. Invest. 11:580–584, 1962.

Leiberman, J.R., Mazor, M., and Cohen, A.: Detection of fetal blood. Am. J. Obstet. Gynecol. 161:257–258, 1989.

Lele, A.S., Carmody, P.J., Hurd, M.E., and O'Leary, J.A.: Fetomaternal bleeding following diagnostic amniocentesis. Obstet. Gynecol. 60:60–64, 1982.

Leong, M., Duby, S., and Kinch, R.A.H.: Fetal-maternal transfusion following early abortion. Obstet. Gynecol. 54: 424–426, 1979.

Léwi, S., Clarke, T.K., Guéritat, Walker, P., and Mayer, M.: Less érythrocytes foetaux dans la circulation maternelle. Bull. Gynecol. Obstet. 13:535–545, 1961.

Léwi, S., Barrier, J., Ducas, P., and Clarke, T.K.: Nouvelle observation de transfusion foeto = maternelle. Bull. Fed. Soc. Gynecol. Obstet. 17:130–136, 1965.

Li, T.C., and Bromham, D.R.: Fetomaternal macrotransfusion in the Yorkshire region. 2. Perinatal outcome. Br. J. Obstet. Gynaecol. 95:1152–1158, 1988.

Litwak, O., Taswell, H.F., Banner, E.A., and Keith, L.: Fetal erythrocytes in maternal circulation after spontaneous abortion. J.A.M.A. 214:531–534, 1970.

Lloyd, L.K., Miya, F., Hebertson, R.M., Kochenour, N.K., and Scott, J.R.: Intrapartum fetomaternal bleeding in Rh-negative women. Obstet. Gynecol. 56:285–288, 1980.

Lo, Y.-M.D., Patel, P., Wainscoat, J.S., Sampietro, M., Gillmer, M.D.G., and Fleming, K.A.: Prenatal sex determination by DNA amplification from maternal peripheral blood. Lancet 2:1363–1365, 1989.

Los, F.J., Jahoda, M.G.J., Wladimiroff, J.W., and Brezinka, C.: Fetal exsanguination by chorionic villus sampling. Lancet 342:1559, 1993.

Luyet, F., Schmid, J., Maroni, E., and Duc, G.: Massive feto-maternal transfusion during external version with fatal outcome. Arch. Gynecol. 221:273–275, 1976.

Mannherz, K.H.: Feto-maternale Blutung als Ursache von Neugeborenenanämie. Zentralbl. Gynäkol. 82:1252–1257, 1960.

Macris, N.T., Hellman, L.M., and Watson, R.J.: Transmission of transfused sickle-trait cells from mother to fetus. Am. J. Obstet. Gynecol. 76:1214–1218, 1958.

Mayer, M.M., Anh, J.N.H., and Panigel, M.M.: Observation au microscope électronique du passage d'hématies a travers la paroi des capillaires foetaux dans le placenta humain. C. R. Acad. Sci. Paris 260:4605–4606, 1965.

McGowan, G.W.: Massive transplacental hemorrhage with neonatal death. J.A.M.A. 203:599–601, 1968.

McLarey, D.C., and Fish, S.A.: Fetal erythrocytes in the maternal circulation. Am. J. Obstet. Gynecol. 95:824–830, 1966.

Megapanos, E.N., Rettos, A.S., Sfontouris, I.G., and Statholoulos, A.I.: La perméabilité du placenta aux érythrocytes maternels au terme grossesse. Gynecol. Obstet. (Paris) 65:233–240, 1966.

Mennuti, M.T., DiGaetano, A., McDonnell, A., Cohen, A.W., and Liston, R.M.: Fetal-maternal bleeding asso-ciated with genetic amniocentesis: real-time versus static ultrasound. Obstet. Gynecol. 62:26–30, 1983.

Messer, R.H., Pearse, W.H., and Keenan, H.: Effect of carbazochrome salicylate on transplacental transmission of fetal erythrocytes. Obstet. Gynecol. 27:83–88, 1966.

Michael, A.F., and Mauer, A.M.: Maternal-fetal transfusion as a cause of plethora in the neonatal period. Pediatrics 28:458–461, 1961.

Mollison, P.L.: Quantitation of transplacental haemorrhage. B.M.J. 3:31–34, 1972 (correction p. 115).

Mor-Yosef, S., Granat, M., Cividalli, G., and Peleg, O.: Acute feto-maternal transfusion—diagnostic considerations. Aust. N.Z. J. Obstet. Gynaecol. 24:219–222, 1984.

Moszkowski, E.F., Eby, B., Shocket, C., and Givila, V.: Cytogenetic evidence for materno-fetal transfusion of polymorphonuclears. J. Reprod. Med. 6:49–51, 1971.

Moya, F.R., Perez, A., and Reece, E.A.: Severe fetomaternal hemorrhage: a report of four cases. J. Reprod. Med. 32: 243–246, 1987.

Murray, D.J.: Severe abruptio placentae initiated by trauma and assciated with hypofibrinogenemia. Can. Med. Assoc. J. 91:1316–1317, 1964.

Naeye, R.L., Lambert, K.C., and Durfee, H.A.: Widespread infarcts following fetomaternal hemorrhage: report of case. Obstet. Gynecol. 23:115–117, 1964.

Nance, S.J., Nelson, J.M., Arndt, P.A., Lam, H.-T.C., and Garratty, G.: Quantitation of fetal-maternal hemorrhage by flow cytometry: a simple and accurate method. Am. J. Clin. Pathol. 91:288–292, 1989.

Ness, P.M.: The assessment of fetal-maternal hemorrhage by an enzyme-linked antiglobulin test for Rh-immune globulin recipients. Am. J. Obstet. Gynecol. 143:788–792, 1982.

Ness, P.M., Baldwin, M.L., and Niebyl, J.R.: Clinical high-risk designation does not predict excess fetal-maternal hemorrhage. Am. J. Obstet. Gynecol. 156:154–158, 1987.

Oehlert, G., Mohrmann, J.E., and Michel, C.F.: Untersuchungen zur Plazentapassage fetaler Blutelemente. Zentralbl. Gynäkol. 82:1544–1551, 1960.

Oehme, J., Hundeshagen, H., and Eschenbach, C.: Über die Passage markierter Leukocyten vom Muttertiere zum Feten—zugleich ein Beitrag zur Runt-Disease. Klin. Wochenschr. 44:430–433, 1966.

Olding, L.: The possibility of materno-foetal transfer of lymphocytes in man. Acta Paediatr. Scand. 61:73–75, 1972.

Olding, L., Benirschke, K., and Oldstone, M.B.A.: Inhibition of mitosis of lymphocytes from human adults by lymphocytes from human newborns. Clin. Immunol. Immunopathol. 3:79–89, 1974.

Owen, J., Stedman, C.M., and Tucker, T.L.: Comparison of predelivery versus postdelivery Kleihauer-Betke stains in cases of fetal death. Am. J. Obstet. Gynecol. 161:663–666, 1989.

Pai, M.K.R., Bedritis, I., and Zipursky, A.: Massive transplacental hemorrhage: clinical manifestations in the newborn. Can. Med. Assoc. J. 112:585–589, 1975.

Palliez, R., Delecour, M., Monnier, K.-C., Hutin, A., and Abdelatif, M.: Passage transplacentaire des hématies foetales durant la grossesse et dans le post-partum. Rev. Fr. Gynecol. 65:579–584, 1970.

Paros, N.L.: Case of foetal anaemia due to transplacental bleeding seen in general practice. B.M.J. 1:839–840, 1962.

Pauls, F., and Boutros, P.: The value of placental localization prior to amniocentesis. Obstet. Gynecol. 35:175–177, 1970.

Pearlman, M.D., Tintinalli, J.E., and Lorenz, R.P.: A prospective controlled study of outcome after trauma during pregnancy. Am. J. Obstet. Gynecol. 162:1502–1510, 1990a.

Pearlman, M.D., Tintinalli, J.E., and Lorenz, R.P.: Blunt trauma during pregnancy. N. Engl. J. Med. 323:1609–1613, 1990b.

Pembrey, M.E., Weatherhall, D.J., and Clegg, J.B.: Maternal synthesis of haemoglobin F in pregnancy. Lancet 1:1350–1355, 1973.

Peyser, M.R., and Toaff, R.: Traumatic rupture of the placenta: a rare cause of fetal death. Obstet. Gynecol. 34:561–563, 1969.

Pilkington, R., Knoz, E.G., Russell, J.K., and Walker, W.: Foetal-maternal transfusion and rhesus sensitisation. J. Obstet. Gynaecol. Br. Commonw. 73:909–916, 1966.

Pollock, A.: Transplacental haemorrhage after external cephalic version. Lancet 1:612, 1968.

Pollack, M., and Montague, A.C.W.: Transplacental hemorrhage in postterm pregnancies. Am. J. Obstet. Gynecol. 102:383–387, 1968.

Potter, E.L.: Intervillous thrombi in the placenta and their possible relation to erythroblastosis fetalis. Am. J. Obstet. Gynecol. 56:959–961, 1948.

Pozniak, M.A., Cullenward, M.J., Zickuhr, D., and Curet, L.B.: Venous lake bleeding: a complication of chorionic villus sampling. J. Ultrasound Med. 7:297–299, 1988.

Quintero, R.A., Romero, R., Mahoney, M.J., Abuhamad, A., Vecchio, M., Holden, J., and Hobbins, J.C.: Embryoscopic demonstration of hemorrhagic lesions on the human embryo after placental trauma. Am. J. Obstet. Gynecol. 168:756–759, 1993.

Raafat, M., Brayton, J.B., Apgar, V., and Borgaonkar, D.S.: A new approach to prenatal diagnosis using trophoblastic cells in maternal blood. Birth Defects 11:295–302, 1975.

Renaer, M., Putte, I.V. de, and Vermylen, C.: Massive feto-maternal hemorrhage as cause of perinatal mortality and morbidity. Eur. J. Obstet. Gynecol. Reprod. Biol. 6:125–140, 1976.

Rodgers, B.D., Marusak, J.J., and Rodgers, D.E.: Criminal prosecution for prenatal injury. Obstet. Gynecol. 80:522–523, 1992.

Rose, P.G., Strohm, P.L., and Zuspan, F.P.: Fetomaternal hemorrhage following trauma. Am. J. Obstet. Gynecol. 153:844–847, 1985.

Rosta, J.: Feto-maternal hemorrhage during pregnancy and delivery. In, Perinatal Medicine, Part II. E. Kerpel-Fronius, P.V. Véghelyi, and J. Rosta, eds. Akademiai Kiado, Budapest, 1978.

Rouse, D., and Weiner, C.: Ongoing fetomaternal hemorrhage treated by serial fetal intravascular transfusions. Obstet. Gynecol. 76:974–975, 1990.

Rudolph, A.J., Abrahamov, A.A., and deVenecia, J.F.: Another case of fetomaternal transfusion. J. Philippine Med. Assoc. 38:134–137, 1962.

Ryerson, C.S., and Sanes, S.: The age of pregnancy. Histologic diagnosis from percentage of erythroblasts in chorionic capillaries. Arch. Pathol. 17:548–651, 1934.

Saber, R.S.: Stillbirth due to extensive feto-maternal transfusion. N.Y. State J. Med. 77:2249–2250, 1977.

Santamaria, M., Benirschke, K., Carpenter, P.M., Baldwin, V.J., and Pritchard, J.A.: Transplacental hemorrhage associated with placental neoplasms. Pediatr. Pathol. 7:601–615, 1987.

Schellong, G.: Anämie und Schock beim Neugeborenen durch fetalen Blutverlust. Monatsschr. Kinderheilkd. 117:578–579, 1969.

Schmorl, G.: Pathologisch-Anatomische Untersuchungen über Puerperale Eklampsie. F.C.W. Vogel, Leipzig, 1893.

Schmorl, G.: Über das Schicksal embolisch verschleppter Plazentarzellen. Verh. Dtsch. Pathol. Ges. 8:39–46, 1905.

Schneider, J., and Ludwig, G.A.: Eine neue Zählmethode zur quantitativen Erfassung kleinster Mengen fetaler, in den mütterlichen Kreislauf eingeschwemmter Erythrocyten. Klin. Wochenschr. 41:563–565, 1963.

Schröder, J.: Review article: transplacental passage of blood cells. J. Med. Genet. 12:230–242, 1975.

Schröder, J., Schröder, E., and Cann, H.M.: Fetal cells in the maternal blood: lack of response of fetal cells in maternal blood to mitogens and mixed leukocyte culture. Hum. Genet. 38:91–97, 1977.

Selypes, A., and Lorencz, R.: A noninvasive method for determination of the sex and karyotype of the fetus from the maternal blood. Hum. Genet. 79:357–359, 1988.

Shahar, E., Birenbaum, E., Inbar, D., and Brish, M.: Hypovolemic shock at birth due to extensive fetomaternal hemorrhage. Isr. J. Med. Sci. 17:441–444, 1981.

Shields, L.E., Widness, J.A., and Brace, R.A.: Restoration of fetal red blood cells and plasma proteins after a moderately severe hemorrhage in the ovine fetus. Am. J. Obstet. Gynecol. 169:1472–1478, 1993.

Shiller, J.G.: Shock in the newborn caused by transplacental hemorrhage from fetus to mother. Pediatrics 20:7–11, 1957.

Shulman, L.P., Meyers, C.M., Simpson, J.L., Andersen, R.N., Tolley, E.A., and Elias, S.: Fetomaternal transfusion depends on amount of chorionic villi aspirated but not on method of chorionic villus sampling. Am. J. Obstet. Gynecol. 162:1185–1188, 1990.

Shurin, S.B.: The blood and the hematopoietic system. In, Neonatal-Perinatal Medicine. A.A. Fanaroff & R.J. Martin, eds. pp. 826–827. Mosby, St. Louis, 1987.

Simon, N.V., Virgilio, L.A., Beaverson, M.L., and Deveney, L.B.: Detection of large fetal-maternal transfusions. Obstet. Gynecol. 52:249–252, 1978.

Smith, J.J., and Benjamin, F.: Post-hemorrhagic anemia and shock in the newborn at birth. Obstet. Gynecol. Surv. 23:511–521, 1968.

Smith, K., Duhring, J.L., Greene, J.W., Rochlin, D.B., and Blakemore, W.S.: Transfer of maternal erythrocytes across the human placenta. Obstet. Gynecol. 18:673–676, 1961.

Stafford, P.A., Biddinger, P.W., and Zumwalt, R.E.: Lethal intrauterine fetal trauma. Am. J. Obstet. Gynecol. 159:485–489, 1988.

Stein, G.A.v., Munsick, R.A., Stiver, K., and Ryder, K.: Fetomaternal hemorrhage in threatened abortion. Obstet. Gynecol. 79:383–386, 1992.

Stiller, A.G., and Skafish, P.R.: Placental chorangioma: a rare cause of fetomaternal transfusion with maternal hemolysis and fetal distress. Obstet. Gynecol. 67:296–298, 1986.

Stonehill, L.L., and LaFerla, J.J.: Assessment of fetomaternal hemorrhage with Kleihauer-Betke test. Am. J. Obstet. Gynecol. 155:1146, 1986.

Streiff, F., Peters, A., and Vincent, D.: La perméabilité placentaire aux hématies. Pathol. Biol. 12:963–972, 1964.

Sullivan, J.F., and Jennings, E.R.: Transplacental fetal-maternal hemorrhage. Am. J. Pathol. 46:36–42, 1966.

Suzumori, K., Adachi, R., Okada, S., Narukawa, T., Yagami, Y., and Sonta, S.: Fetal cells in the maternal circulation: detection of Y-sequence by gene amplification. Obstet. Gynecol. 80:150–154, 1992.

Theurer, D.E., and Kaiser, I.H.: Traumatic fetal death without uterine injury: report of a case. Obstet. Gynecol. 21:477–480, 1963.

Tomoda, Y.: Demonstration of foetal erythrocyte by immunofluorescent staining. Nature 202:910–911, 1964.

Virgilio, L.A., and Simon, N.V.: Measurement of fetal cells in the maternal circulation. Obstet. Gynecol. 50:364–366, 1977.

Voigt, J.C., and Britt, R.P.: Feto-maternal haemorrhage in therapeutic abortion. B.M.J. 2:395–396, 1969.

Walsh, J.J., and Lewis, B.V.: Transplacental haemorrhage due to termination of pregnancy. J. Obstet. Gynaecol. Br. Commonw. 77:133–136, 1970.

Walter, P., Lewi, S., Loewe-Lyon, S., and Clarke, T.K.: Transfusion foeto-maternelle avec hypertrophie du placenta. Gynecol. Obstet. (Paris) 64:103–110, 1965.

Warren, R.C., Butler, J., Morsman, J.M., McKenzie, C., and Rodeck, C.H.: Does chorionic villus sampling cause fetomaternal haemorrhage? Lancet 1:691, 1985.

Wentworth, P.: A placental lesion to account for foetal haemorrhage into the maternal circulation. J. Obstet. Gynaecol. Br. Commonw. 71:379–387, 1964.

Wickster, G.Z.: Posthemorrhagic shock in the newborn. Am. J. Obstet. Gynecol. 63:524–537, 1952.

Wiener, A.S.: Diagnosis and treatment of anemia of the newborn caused by occult placental hemorrhage. Am. J. Obstet. Gynecol. 56:717–722, 1948.

Williams, J.K., McCalin, L., Rosemurgy, A.S., and Colorado, N.M.: Evaluation of blunt abdominal trauma in the third trimester of pregnancy: maternal and fetal considerations. Obstet. Gynecol. 75:33–37, 1990.

Willis, C., and Foreman, C.S.: Chronic massive fetomaternal hemorrhage: a case report. Obstet. Gynecol. 71:459–461, 1988.

Wong, T.T.T., and Cann, M.C.K.: Transfusion reaction following ABO-incompatible maternofetal transfusion. J. Pediatr. 80:479–483, 1972.

Woodrow, J.C., and Finn, R.: Transplacental haemorrhage. Br. J. Haematol. 12:297–309, 1966.

Young, P.E., Matson, M.R., and Jones, O.W.: Fetal exsanguination and other vascular injuries from midtrimester amniocentesis. Am. J. Obstet. Gynecol. 129:21–24, 1977.

Zarou, D.M., Lichtman, H.C., and Hellman, L.M.: The transmission of chromium-51 tagged maternal erythrocytes from mother to fetus. Am. J. Obstet. Gynecol. 88:565–571, 1964.

Zilliacus, H.: Agglutinated incompatible fetal erythrocytes in the maternal circulation. Am. J. Obstet. Gynecol. 86:1093–1095, 1963.

Zilliacus, R., Chapelle, A. de la, Schröder, J., Tilikainen, A., Kohne, E., and Kleihauer, E.: Transplacental passage of foetal blood cells. Scand. J. Haematol. 15:333–338, 1975.

Zipursky, A., Hull, A., White, F.D., and Israel, L.G.: Foetal erythrocytes in the maternal circulation. Lancet 1:451–452, 1959.

Zipursky, A., Pollock, J., Chown, B., and Israels, L.G.: Transplacental foetal haemorrhage after placental injury during delivery or amniocentesis. Lancet 2:493–494, 1963a.

Zipursky, A., Pollock, J., Neelands, P., Chown, B., and Israels, L.G.: The transplacental passage of foetal red blood-cells and the pathogenesis of Rh immunisation during pregnancy. Lancet 2:489–493, 1963b.

18
Fetal Storage Disorders

Many of the so-called errors in metabolism, the storage diseases, produce inclusions or vacuoles in the tissues of affected individuals. The placenta is often similarly involved, and chorionic villous biopsy (CVS) is now often employed to make the diagnosis prenatally, as for instance when diagnosing lipofuscinosis (Rapola et al., 1990). Electron microscopy and special enzyme studies may be necessary for the precise diagnosis of the defect involved. Thus appropriate fixation is needed and must be anticipated at the time of CVS, as many of the inclusions are highly water- and lipid-solvent-soluble. An excellent ultrastructural study of 11 cases has been reported by Jones et al. (1990) that details procedures and findings. It also depicts the findings in admirable detail and provides additional literature.

Gaucher's disease, as mentioned in Chapter 18, may cause fetal hydrops. It is a heterogeneous disease whose genetics and clinical manifestations were well described by Sidransky and Ginns (1993). In the case described by Ginsburg and Groll (1973), polyhydramnios complicated the second pregnancy of a patient in the second trimester. At 34 weeks she delivered a macerated, hydropic fetus. The large, edematous placenta had the macroscopic features of erythroblastosis fetalis. The mother's third pregnancy also resulted in neonatal demise due to Gaucher's disease. The fetal findings were characteristic of type II Gaucher's disease in the hydropic, 21-week fetus described by Rice et al. (1984). The placenta was not described.

Mucolipidosis type II, or *I cell disease*, is a rare and fatal disorder whose genetic transmission is autosomal recessive. Gellis and Feingold (1977) delineated the principal features of affected children. Hanai et al. (1971) emphasized the abundance of periodic acid-Schiff (PAS)-positive lysosomal inclusions in the cells of affected children. In 1974 Granström et al. and Rapola et al. separately reported that affected newborns may have coarse features similar to those of Hurler syndrome and demonstrated inclusions in leukocytes. Aula

et al. (1975) made the first prenatal diagnosis of this disease from an increase of amnionic fluid hydrolases. Later they used fibroblasts of the aborted fetus to confirm the diagnosis. The investigators emphasized that paraffin sections do not allow visualization of the inclusions, which are obvious, however, in epoxy-embedded material. The inclusions of this disorder are preferentially located in kidney and mesenchymal cells. Terashima et al. (1975) presented an extensive differential diagnosis of these inclusions in their description of three cases. Placental involvement with inclusion-bearing cells was demonstrated in a case report of Powell et al. (1976). The syncytium and Hofbauer cells were primarily affected; the vacuoles of formerly mucolipid-containing lysosomes were readily apparent in paraffin sections of the placenta (Figure 333), but the features were much enhanced by processing the tissues in epoxy resin. The authors of this paper emphasized that only fetal cells contained the vacuoles. Affected tissue included the X cells of cell columns. There were no inclusions in decidual cells, and the authors used this characteristic to further identify X cells as being of fetal origin. The placenta was grossly pale and somewhat enlarged; the fetus was not hydropic. The same report contains three additional and similar storage diseases that affected the placenta, but the precise nature of their storage disorders could not be identified. Abe et al. (1976) and Nagashima et al. (1977) have described other morphological studies. Several investigators have further elaborated on placental aspects of mucolipidosis type II. Thus Rapola and Aula (1977) beautifully demonstrated the ultrastructural changes of the syncytium and suggested that the diagnosis could easily be made from this material alone (Figure 334). Diagnosis would now be possible with CVS alone, without having to resort to enzyme study. Gehler et al. (1976) have reported biochemical studies of I cell disease. The differential diagnosis of mucolipidosis types I and III was discussed in a study by Herd et al. (1978). Hug

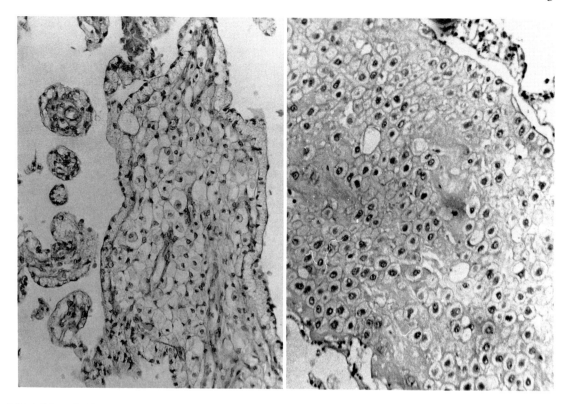

FIGURE 333. Villus (left) and X cell column of placenta affected by mucolipidosis II (I cell disease). Note the abundance of vacuoles in the syncytium and Hofbauer cells; similar inclusions are present in the cytoplasm of X cells. H&E. ×240.

et al. (1984) have shown that maternal serum hexosaminidase levels are increased in pregnancies affected by I cell disease, which allows diagnosis without uterine invasion. We strongly disagree with the interpretation of Cozzutto (1983), however, who reported on a macerated stillborn whose placenta also had extensive vacuolar changes. The placenta was structurally typical of I cell disease. Cozzutto found vacuolated "stromal decidual cells," but he did not depict them. He interpreted the changes as "convincingly demonstrating"

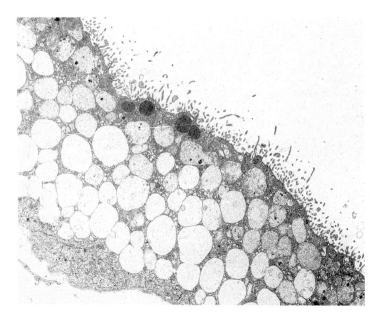

FIGURE 334. Electron micrograph of syncytium in a case of I cell disease. Note the extensive fine vacuolation, the storage sites of washed-out glycolipids in the syncytial cytoplasm. ×6,700. (Courtesy Dr. J. Rapola, Helsinki, Finland.)

that the foam cells are a transformation secondary to edema or fetal death. In our experience, such vacuolation never results from fetal death or edema. The abundance of foam cells, the disposition of trophoblastic vacuoles, and irregular calcifications observed by him (and us as well) are indicative of an unidentified fetal storage disorder. Because the cellular glycolipids are highly water-soluble, the empty appearance of the vacuoles is the usual finding in many fetal storage disorders.

Hurler syndrome (mucopolysaccharidosis I) showed "striking vacuolation of stromal cells," including Hofbauer cells (Jones et al., 1990).

Other storage diseases affect fetal and placental tissue. By amniocentesis at 14 weeks, Lowden et al. (1973) identified the absence of β-galactosidase. That absence is diagnostic of type 1 GM1 *gangliosidosis*. The pregnancy was terminated; typical inclusions (zebra bodies) were ultrastructurally identified in the fetal ganglion cells. Although other fetal cells were unremarkable in paraffin sections, vacuoles were seen in epon-embedded material. The placenta showed numerous "empty vacuoles" in the syncytial cytoplasm. They were visible even in paraffin sections. Presumably, they contain the water-soluble storage product and galactose-rich mucopolysaccharide. Other case descriptions of the disease do not include descriptions of the placenta (Giugliani et al., 1985).

Absence of α-galactosidase A results in Fabry's disease, a disorder of glycosphingolipid metabolism. The tissues accumulate ceramide trihexose. A pregnancy in a patient with this disease was described by Popli et al. (1990) after she had received a renal allograft. The placenta of the term fetus was normal, but the decidual cells contained argyrophilic granules that, electron micrographically had an appearance similar to that of zebra bodies. The fetal portions of the placenta were normal. O'Brien (1982) has reviewed many lysosomal disorders and their enzymatic deficiencies and provided details of the enzymatic defect.

In the studies by Jones et al. (1990), *Tay Sachs' disease* (GM2 gangliosidosis type I) was found to produce vacuolation of syncytiotrophoblast, with occasional myelin bodies in villous stromal cells. In *Sandhoff's disease* (type II) "the most striking feature . . . was the occurrence of parallel membranous arrays in occasional lysosomes within stromal cells." Myelin bodies were found in trophoblast and endothelium.

Mucolipidosis IV (Morquio syndrome type B) is due to the deficiency of β-galactosidase and also referred to as GM1-gangliosidosis. This disease has been diagnosed from cultured amnionic fluid cells by Kohn et al. (1977). The amnion cells contained multiple single-membrane bounded inclusions. Mesodermal elements, however, were negative. Although it may appear superficially

that this disease is similar to I-cell disease, in this condition the amnion, not the syncytium and Hofbauer cells, has the vacuolation. The placenta of a case we saw was much enlarged (950 g) and much paler and softer than normal. Its amnionic epithelium, trophoblast, Hofbauer cells, and circulating lymphocytes showed striking vacuolation, similar to those of I cell disease. Calcified thrombi were found in large surface vessels. The 4,050 g neonate had massive ascites but no organomegaly.

Morquio's disease (mucopolysaccharidosis type IVA) has also been diagnosed from enzyme analysis of CVS (Applegarth et al., 1987). Within the family reported by these authors, nonimmune hydrops fetalis had occurred during previous pregnancies. The authors drew attention to earlier reports of hydrops with Gaucher's, Wolman's, and Salla's diseases, sialidosis, and mucopolysaccharidosis type VII. In their family, they had an hydropic fetus with a bulky placenta. Vacuolar villous edema and prominent Hofbauer cells were found, but there was no histological evidence of storage products in the trophoblast.

Maroteaux et al. (1978) and See et al. (1978) have described the general features of *sialidosis* ("nephrosialidosis"; mucolipidosis type I). They depicted the inclusions in the neuraminidase-deficient cells but did not describe the placenta. In other case reports (Aylsworth et al., 1980; Stevenson et al., 1983) the inclusions of tissues and cultured cells are all well depicted, but these authors did not describe the associated placentas either. Laver et al. (1983) found typical storage vacuoles in Hofbauer cells and the villous syncytium. Amniocyte morphology in this disease has been reported to be normal by electron microscopic study (Stevenson et al., 1983). In a similar disorder, hydrops fetalis resulted in two pregnancies from a combined deficiency of neuraminidase and β-galactosidase (Kleijer et al., 1979). The placenta of these fetuses was not described. Gillan et al. (1984), who discussed congenital ascites in various storage disorders (sialidosis, Salla's disease, gangliosidosis, Gaucher's disease), depicted a placental villus with vacuolated syncytial cytoplasm of a fetus with Salla's disease.

Niemann-Pick disease (type C) does not result in visible storage products of the placenta. When tissue is obtained from CVS and cultured under special conditions, however, the tissue-cultured cells of affected fetuses have been shown to accumulate laminated inclusions of nonesterified cholesterol (myelin bodies), which can then be stained with filipin for unesterified cholesterol, and the diagnosis may thus be secured (Vanier et al., 1989; Jones et al., 1990). Nonimmune hydrops with hydramnios commencing at 19 weeks' gestation has been described by Meizner et al. (1990) in Niemann-Pick disease. Fetal death occurred at 36 weeks, and the inclusions were identified electron microscopically in the enlarged spleen. The placenta was not described.

Desai et al. (1985) found lysosomal lipid deposits in *cholesterol ester storage disease* in which the fetal adrenal glands had foci of necrosis, and many other tissues possessed a vacuolated cytoplasm.

Bendon and Hug (1985) reported placental abnormalities in five cases of *Pompe's disease (glycogen storage disease type II; α-1,4-glucosidase deficiency)*. During routine examination of the placenta, the only unusual finding was the cytoplasmic vacuolation of amnionic connective tissue cells. Electron microscopy, however, showed typical membrane-bound, glycogen-filled inclusions in capillary endothelial cells and the villous stroma. They were present even in midtrimester abortuses. Hug et al. (1991) described the diagnosis from CVS at 10 weeks. The previous pregnancy had resulted in an affected child. Electron microscopic examination 5 days after biopsy identified the typical glycogen-packed membrane-enclosed inclusions in many fetal cells, including fibrocytes, that appear as vacuoles during histological study. These authors insisted that the demonstration of vacuoles alone is insufficient for the diagnosis. Jones and her collaborators (1990) reported similar findings of lysosomal glycogen accumulation. They were seen in cytotrophoblast, endothelium, fibrocytes, and pericytes. We have seen the placenta of a neonate with *glycogen storage disease type IV (amylopectinase deficiency)*. It had vacuoles in the amnionic epithelium, but no specific lesions were identified. There were none of those cells that had been identified in Pompe's disease. The pregnancy was complicated by hydramnios. The newborn had Lafora bodies in heart, liver, and muscle, had pleural transudate, was dysmorphic, and suffered fatal pulmonary hypoplasia. The placenta was enlarged. A second pregnancy was similarly involved. Similarly, in *sialic acid storage disease*, Jones et al. (1990) noted that the Hofbauer cells, endothelium, and syncytium were packed with clear, membrane-bound vacuoles (Jauniaux et al., 1987).

It is apparent from these descriptions that many congenital enzyme deficiencies can be diagnosed from amnionic fluid cultures or CVS samples, and that they may be accompanied by placental manifestations. The location and type of inclusion cannot always be anticipated. Thus the inclusions of lipofuscinosis were mainly in the fetal capillary endothelium, although they had earlier been suggested to be in syncytiotrophoblast (Rapola et al., 1990). The villous specimens should therefore be processed for optimal ultrastructural studies. CVS has become of great value in selected cases, especially prenatal counseling. In this area of research, some published animal models closely parallel the human disease. Their use may be of value, particularly for study of the placenta (Baker et al., 1976).

References

Abe, K., Matsuda, I., Arashima, S., Mitsuyama, T., Oka, Y., and Ishikawa, M.: Ultrastructural studies in fetal I-cell disease. Pediatr. Res. 10:669–676, 1976.

Applegarth, D.A., Toone, J.R., Wilson, R.D., Long, S.L., and Baldwin, V.J.: Morquio disease presenting as hydrops fetalis and enzyme analysis of chorionic villus tissue in a subsequent pregnancy. Pediatr. Pathol. 7:593–599, 1987.

Aula, P., Rapola, J., Autio. S., Raivio, K., and Karjalainen, O.: Prenatal diagnosis and fetal pathology of I-cell disease (mucolipidosis type II). J. Pediatr. 87:221–226, 1975.

Aylsworth, A.S., Thomas, G.H., Hood, J.L., Malouf, N., and Libert, J.: A severe infantile sialidosis: clinical, biochemical, and microscopic features. J. Pediatr. 96:662–668, 1980.

Baker, H.J., Mole, J.A., Lindsey, J.R., and Creel, R.M.: Animal models of human ganglioside storage diseases. Fed. Proc. 35:1193–1201, 1976.

Bendon, R.W., and Hug, G.: Morphologic characteristics of the placenta in glycogen storage disease type II (β-1,4-glucosidase deficiency). Am. J. Obstet. Gynecol. 152:1021–1026, 1985.

Cozzutto, C.: Case report. Foamy degeneration of placenta. Virchows Arch. [Pathol. Anat.] 401:363–368, 1983.

Desai, P.K., Astrin, K.H., Gordon, R.E., Thung, S., Strauss, L., and Desnick, R.J.: Cholesterol ester storage disease: prenatal diagnosis and fetal pathology. Lab. Invest. 52:4P, 1985.

Gehler, J., Cantz, M., Stoeckenius, M., and Spranger, J.: Prenatal diagnosis of mucolipidosis II (I-cell disease). Eur. J. Pediatr. 122:201–206, 1976.

Gellis, S.S., and Feingold, M.: Picture of the month. I-cell disease (mucolipidosis II). Am. J. Dis. Child. 131: 1137–1138, 1977.

Gillan, J.E., Lowden, J.A., Gaskin, K., and Cutz, E.: Congenital ascites as a presenting sign of lysosomal storage disease. J. Pediatr. 104:225–231, 1984.

Ginsburg, S.J., and Groll, M.: Hydrops fetalis due to infantile Gaucher's disease. J. Pediatr. 82:1046–1048, 1973.

Giugliani, R., Dutra, J.C., Pereira, M.L.S., Rotta, N., Drachler, M.d.L., Ohlweiler, L., Neto, J.M.d.P., Pinheiro, C.E., and Breda, D.J.: GM1 gangliosidosis: clinical and laboratory findings in eight families. Hum. Genet. 70: 347–354, 1985.

Granström, M.-L., Aula, P., and ja Rapola, J.: Kliinis-patologinen kokousselostus XY: kudosviljelyn avulla selvitetty aineenvaihduntasairaus. Duodecim 90:421–430, 1974.

Hanai, J., Leroy, J., and O'Brien, J.S.: Ultrastructure of cultured fibroblasts in I-cell disease. Am. J. Dis. Child. 122:34–38, 1971.

Herd, J.K., Dvorak, A.D., Wiltse, H.E., Eisen, J.D., Kress, B.C., and Miller, A.L.: Mucolipidosis type II: multiple elevated serum and urine enzyme activities. Am. J. Dis. Child. 132:1181–1186, 1978.

References   475

Hug, G., Bove, K.E., Soukup, S., Ryan, M., Bendon, R.,
Babcock, D., Warren, N.S., and Dignan, P.S.J.: Increased
serum hexosaminidase in a woman pregnant with a fetus
affected by mucolipidosis II (I-cell disease). N. Engl. J.
Med. 311:988–989, 1984.

Hug, G., Chuck, G., Chen, Y.-T., Kay, H.H., and Bossen,
E.H.: Chorionic villus ultrastructure in type II glycogen
storage disease (Pompe's disease). N. Engl. J. Med. 324:
342–343, 1991.

Jauniaux, E., Vamos, E., Libert, J., Elkhazen, N., Wilkin,
P., and Hustin, J.: Placental electron microscopy and histochemistry in a case of sialic acid storage disorder. Placenta
8:433–442, 1987.

Jones, C.J.P., Lendon, M., Chawner, L.E., and Jauniaux, E.:
Ultrastructure of the human placenta in metabolic storage
disease. Placenta 11:395–411, 1990.

Kleijer, W.J., Hoogeveen, A., Verheijen, F.W., Niermeijer,
M.F., Galjaard, H., O'Brien, J.S., and Warner, J.G.:
Prenatal diagnosis of sialidosis with combined neuraminidase and β-galactosidase deficiency. Clin. Genet.
16:60–61, 1979.

Kohn, G., Livni, N., Ornoy, A., Sekeles, E., Beyth, Y.,
Legum, C., Bach, G., and Cohen, M.M.: Prenatal diagnosis of mucolipidosis IV by electron microscopy. J. Pediatr.
90:62–66, 1977.

Laver, J., Fried, K., Beer, S.l., lancu, T.C., Heyman, E.,
Bach, G., and Zeiger, M.: Infantile lethal neuraminidase
deficiency (sialidosis). Clin. Genet. 23:97–101, 1983.

Lowden, J.A., Cutz, E., Conen, P.E., Rudd, N., and Doran,
T.A.: Prenatal diagnosis of GM1-gangliosidosis. N. Engl. J.
Med. 288:225–228, 1973.

Maroteaux, P., Humbel, R., Strecker, G., Michalski, J.-C.,
and Mande, R.: Un nouveau type de sialidose avec atteinte
renale: la nephrosialidose. Arch. Fr. Pediatr. 35:819–829,
1978.

Meizner, I., Levy, A., Carmi, R., and Robinsin, C.: Niemann-
Pick disease associated with nonimmune hydrops fetalis.
Am. J. Obstet. Gynecol. 163:128–129, 1990.

Nagashima, K., Sakakibara, K., Endo, H., Konishi, Y.,
Nakamura, N., Suzuki, Y., and Abe, T.: I-cell disease

(mucolipidosis II): pathological and biochemical studies of
an autopsy case. Acta Pathol. Jpn. 27:251–264, 1977.

O'Brien, J.F.: The lysosomal storage diseases. Mayo Clin.
Proc. 57:192–197, 1982.

Popli, S., Leehey, D.J., Molnar, Z.V., Nawab, Z.M., and
Ing, T.S.: Demonstration of Fabry's disease deposits in
placenta. Am. J. Obstet. Gynecol. 162:464–465, 1990.

Powell, H.C., Benirschke, K., Favara, B.E., and Pflueger,
O.H.: Foamy changes of placental cells in fetal storage
disorders. Virchows Arch. A Pathol. Anat. Histol. 369:
191–196, 1976.

Rapola, J., and Aula, P.: Morphology of the placenta in fetal
I-cell disease. Clin. Genet. 11:107–113, 1977.

Rapola, J., Autio, S., Aula, P., and Nanto, V.: Lymphocytic
inclusions in I-cell disease. J. Pediatr. 85:88–90, 1974.

Rapola, J., Salonen, R., Ämmälä, P., and Santavuori, P.:
Prenatal diagnosis of the infantile type of neuronal ceroid
lipofuscinosis by electron microscopic investigation of
human chorionic villi. Prenat. Diagn. 10:553–559, 1990.

Rice, G.E., Mostoufi-Zadeh, M., and Driscoll, S.G.: Hydrops
fetalis in Gaucher's disease. Teratology 29:53A–54A,
1984.

See, G.L., Stanescu, R., and Lyon, G.: Un nouveau type de
sialidose avec atteinte renale: la nephrosialidose. Arch. Fr.
Pediatr. 35:830–844, 1978.

Sidransky, E., and Ginns, E.I.: Clinical heterogeneity among
patients with Gaucher's disease. J.A.M.A. 269:1154–1157,
1993.

Stevenson, R.E., Lubinsky, M., Taylor, H.A., Wenger,
D.A., Schroer, R.J., and Olmstead, P.M.: Sialic acid
storage disease with sialuria: clinical and biochemical
features in the severe infantile type. Pediatrics 72:441–449,
1983.

Terashima, Y., Tsuda, K., Isomura, S., Sugiura, Y., and
Nogami, H.: I-cell disease: report of three cases. Am. J.
Dis. Child. 129:1083–1090, 1975.

Vanier, M.T., Rousson, R.M., Mandon, G., Choiset, A.,
Lake, B.D., and Pentchev, P.G.: Diagnosis of Niemann-
Pick disease type C on chorionic villus biopsy. Lancet
1:1014–1015, 1989.

19
Maternal Diseases Complicating Pregnancy: Diabetes, Tumors, Preeclampsia, Lupus Anticoagulant

Numerous diseases may complicate pregnancy. The most important of those that affect placental development and function are herein reviewed. Our own experience with some of these entities is added. With some of these complications of pregnancy, the placental findings may simply be confirmatory of the disease. With others, placental pathology may be the first indication of an abnormality. Despite many reports of diseases that complicate pregnancy, associated placentas are often not examined, or they are not reported in the descriptions. It is unfortunate because those placentas could aid in diagnosis and knowledge of the pathogenesis of these conditions. Moreover, a better understanding of the placenta could allow us better insight into the mechanisms of the effects that certain conditions have on the fetus. Burrow and Ferris (1988) have written a comprehensive text on medical complications of pregnancy but have also almost totally excluded placental considerations. Because of their particular importance, some entities (e.g., Rh isoimmunization disease and hydrops, pyelonephritis, and infections in general are presented in other chapters).

Maternal Diseases

Scleroderma has been reported on many occasions in pregnancy, although the usually late onset of this disease makes it an uncommon association. Slate and Graham (1968) observed six patients with generalized scleroderma and followed their nine pregnancies. When reviewing all pregnancies of their scleroderma patients, irrespective of the time of onset of the disease before or during pregnancy, stillbirths, abortions, and premature births were found to be common. Pregnancies occurring after the onset of scleroderma ended in 2 premature births, 2 stillborns, and 12 abortions. When they reviewed the literature, these authors also found five maternal deaths among 72 women. These investigators

thought that preeclampsia was not an unduly common complication of scleroderma. In the discussion following their paper, additional cases were presented. None, however, was accompanied by a placental description.

Spellacy (1964), who reported a case with premature labor, found that the placenta had small infarcts; and he gathered 11 additional cases from the literature. Abruptio placentae was described in a case by Hayes et al. (1962). Maternal (decidual) vascular changes have not been described with scleroderma, which is remarkable because scleroderma is occasionally complicated by lupus erythematosus, and abruptios have been reported to occur with scleroderma. In the two patients whom we saw extensive fibrin deposits gave the appearance of maternal floor infarction. One such placenta is shown in Figure 335. This 34-year-old gravida 4, para 1, aborta 2, had a precipitous labor at 38 weeks' gestation. Her obstetricians suspected abruptio placentae. The pregnancy terminated with a growth-retarded stillbirth. The placenta was also unusually small (310 g) and had numerous infarcts and X cell proliferations. Many nucleated red blood cells (NRBCs) were present in the fetal circulation, and the marked X cell proliferation was accompanied by many cysts. A similarly cystic placenta associated with scleroderma was seen by us previously, but that pregnancy was associated with a normal child. Neither placenta had decidual vascular lesions. Gunther and Harer (1964) observed three pregnancies in a patient with scleroderma. Each was complicated by placenta previa.

Dermatomyositis during pregnancy was reported by Barnes and Link (1983). The patient became ill at age 15, had a therapeutic abortion at age 22, and developed significant subcutaneous calcinosis while being treated. The successful pregnancy occurred at age 24, three months after cessation of methotrexate medication. Vaginal spotting took place at 3 months, but she remained normotensive and had no proteinuria. A

476

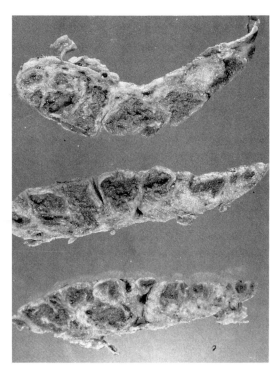

FIGURE 335. Placenta of a patient with scleroderma at 38 weeks' gestation. Numerous infarcts, *Gitterinfarcts*, maternal floor infarction, and X cell proliferation were seen. The placenta and stillborn fetus were growth-retarded. (Courtesy Dr. Bonnie Bobzien.)

cesarean section was performed at 42 weeks with a healthy infant delivered. The placenta had "subamnionic necrosis and hemorrhage involving 30% of the fetal surface." There also was an infarct, but no decidual arteriolopathy was present. The authors referred to a few other case reports, with similar findings of infarcts in the placenta the only pathological lesions. We saw the placenta of such a patient who had a spontaneous demise of a growth-retarded fetus at 38 weeks. The placenta had the typical appearance of massive *Gitterinfarcts* (see Chapter 11).

Ehlers-Danlos syndrome is not a homogeneous disease entity. Many types have been differentiated and a foundation concerned with this disease collects data, including those of pregnancy. One or another form occurs occasionally during pregnancy. Atalla and Page (1988) estimated Ehlers-Danlos disease to occur once in 150,000 pregnancies, of which 35% were of type II. Barabas (1966) found that 14 of his 18 patients delivered prematurely because of premature rupture of the membranes. He suggested that the membranes were exceptionally fragile, but there are no actual measurements of the strength of membranes and no pathological data. Normal members of the families did not suffer from this putative lack of membrane strength. In the pedigrees reported by Barabas, the premature membrane ruptures

were nearly always restricted to affected fetuses. Atalla and Page (1988) reported a case of Ehlers-Danlos syndrome type III with pregnancy and reviewed the sparse literature. Their patient never developed abdominal striae; but because of increasing pains during pregnancy, she had a cesarean section at 35 weeks' gestation. Her membranes were then ruptured artificially. Thus with the possible exception of true increased fragility of the fetal membranes in affected offspring, the placenta has not been reported to be abnormal.

Rheumatoid arthritis has rarely been observed during pregnancy, according to the report of Duhring (1970). He described the successful outcome of pregnancy in a para 3 patient who had suffered the disease for 17 years. The fetus was markedly growth-retarded, and the placenta was small, infarcted, and calcified. The umbilical cord was grossly virtually devoid of Wharton's jelly, but a histological study was not reported.

Nine cases of *periarteritis nodosa* had been reported before Nagey et al. (1983) described another case. Their patient was a 28-year-old woman who had experienced many complications of the disease for 5 years. This mother had had one previous abortion, and this pregnancy was therapeutically terminated at 16 weeks. The placenta appeared to be normal by light and electron microscopic examination. Decidual vessels, however, were not present in the specimen. Previous reports had commented on the high risk for maternal survival but did not include descriptions of the placenta. Owen and Hauth (1989) reported another case, but they did not include a description of the placenta.

A report of maternal *Takayasu's arteritis* complicating pregnancy indicates that normal gestation may yield a normal infant. Winn et al. (1988) observed a woman who had this disease diagnosed 3 years earlier and who had significant arterial disease as a consequence. She was delivered of a healthy infant at 33 weeks. The placenta was not described.

A patient with progressive, severe *myositis ossificans* posed serious problems in pregnancy management but delivered a healthy neonate. The pregnancy was complicated by premature rupture of membranes and infection with group B β-hemolytic streptococci. The placenta was not described (Thornton et al., 1987).

Patients in *acute renal failure* not only may survive pregnancy and have normal infants when appropriately managed, but their placentas are found to be normal (Soyannwo et al., 1966). It is, of course, the case only when the renal failure is independent of pregnancy-induced hypertension and its decidual vascular disease. Renal injury may occur after a *spider bite* (Martinez, 1967) and *snake bites* (James, 1985). The latter author suggested that the venom may cross the placenta and kill the fetus. Renal failure and abruptio placentae have also been produced by the bite of *Bothrops jararaca*, a species of snake (Zugaib et al., 1985). This accident occurred during the 32nd week of gestation and, despite antiserum administration within 6 hours the fetus died in utero from a 75% abruption. *Mushroom poisons* (amatoxins) have been described to cause maternal intoxication, but they do not cross the placenta. A fetus appeared to progress normally after such intoxication, and there was no detectable amnionic fluid toxin; the placenta was not described (Belliardo et al., 1983).

Pregnant women with *chronic renal failure*, on the other hand, have a high perinatal mortality rate (Hou, 1985). Many placental lesions are then found. Most notable among them is retarded growth of the placenta, presumably secondary to maternal decidual vascular disease and hypertension.

Patients with successful *renal transplantation* have a 30% incidence of preeclampsia during pregnancy and suffer occasional rejection of the transplant (Penn et al., 1980; Davison, 1987). It is interesting that toxemia of pregnancy develops frequently in these patients, who usually are medicated with steroids and immunosuppressive agents. Intercurrent infection is a serious hazard, but cyclosporin immunosuppression apparently does not interfere with placentation. The placenta, however, is rarely described (Burrows et al., 1988). Beller et al. (1976) made efforts to differentiate the clinical identification of *malignant nephrosclerosis* from preeclampsia but did not provide information on the placentas in the two patients they described.

Although *acute fatty liver of pregnancy* has a dismal outcome (the survival rate has improved to 18–23%), placental abnormalities remain undescribed (Kaplan, 1985). Hemolysis, coagulation, and other disturbances occur clinically, and toxemia may result with its complications; but the primary disease does not apparently affect the placenta. When maternal bilirubin is high, gross examination of the placenta can identify the pigmentation, particularly in the perivascular connective tissue of the fetal surface. Microscopically, however, no abnormalities are detected, and visible pigment-laden macrophages are rare.

Cholestasis of pregnancy has been associated with a high rate of stillbirth and other perinatal complications. Fisk and Storey (1988) reviewed 83 such cases and found meconium staining in 45%, preterm labor in 44%, and fetal distress in 22%. In their opinion, the low mortality achieved (3 of 83) was due to intensive monitoring of the end stages of pregnancy and the result of judicious intervention. Other than the frequent meconium staining of the placenta, there were no abnormal placental findings.

Patients with *hyperemesis gravidarum* who were treated with total parenteral alimentation were studied by Levine and Esser (1988). Their fetuses all matured to at least 38 weeks' gestation and were not growth-retarded. Examination of the placentas showed no lipid deposits or other abnormalities.

A direct effect of *alcohol ingestion* on the placenta is disputed, although fetal growth retardation and other consequences of the fetal alcohol syndrome are well delineated in the offspring of patients with alcohol abuse during pregnancy (Jones et al., 1973). Several studies have shown that the placenta is smaller than that of controls. Kaminski et al. (1978) found the placentas to weigh 591 g when 45 to 67 ml of alcohol was consumed daily and 581 g when more than 67 ml was consumed daily. Control placental weights were 611 g with less than 44 ml daily alcohol consumption. That the placenta transports alcohol readily has been shown on numerous occasions (Ditts, 1970), with fatal fetal intoxication having been reported (Jung et al., 1980). The influence of alcoholism on the length of umbilical cords (shortening in experimental systems) was mentioned in Chapter 13. Baldwin et al. (1982) reviewed placentas of pregnancies with alcohol abuse and found an increased incidence of chorioamnionitis, chronic villitis, meconium staining, chorioangiomas, and especially persistence of embryological remnants in the umbilical cords. The significance of these lesions is unknown. The inflammatory complications indicate that the social circumstances of the population differed from those of the controls. Other investigators (Sokol et al., 1980) observed no abnormalities in placentas of alcoholics. Marbury et al. (1983), on the other hand, found a significant increase in the incidence of abruptio placentae and a correlation with the amount of alcohol consumed. Blakley (1983), who reviewed the topic extensively, referred to evidence that alcohol consumption leads to fetal hypoxia and compensatory placental enlargement.

The use of *cocaine* (benzoylmethylecgonine) and "*crack*" (the free base smokable form of cocaine) during pregnancy has increased appreciably. A survey conducted in Florida indicated that some 15% of pregnant women tested positive for urinary metabolites of controlled substances (Chasnoff et al., 1990), but in a community study of South Carolina it was 1% (Weathers et al., 1993). Consuming cocaine during pregnancy has been linked to abruptio placentae (Acker et al., 1983; Chasnoff et al., 1985; Dombrowski et al., 1991; Hoskins et al., 1991). In vitro enzyme studies by Roe et al. (1990) showed that placental microsomal fractions biotransform cocaine to inactive compounds. Fetal growth retardation, transient hypertension, severe placental vasoconstriction (Lederman et al., 1978), and other deleterious outcomes of pregnancy have been reported (Cregler & Mark, 1986). Mercado et al. (1989) observed a patient with repeated abruptios, abortions, and continued cocaine use who ultimately had a postpartum cerebral hemorrhage, presumably due to hypertension.

In the placentas of 20 crack users Page et al. (1989) found abruptio placentae in 12 (ten with large clots, one with retroplacental depression, six with recent and old clots). Eight had normal placentas, and ten of the abrupted placentas had liveborn babies; two had placenta previa, and five had chorioamnionitis. Much of the effect of cocaine, at least during pregnancy, seems to be mediated through its known hypertensive and vasoconstrictive activity (Woods et al., 1987). Specific effects on placental structure have not been reported, nor have they been present in our experience; moreover, the frequency of abruptio placentae is, in our experience, not as excessive as given in the many reports. The reported series of abruptio placentae that are a complication of cocaine exposure (occasionally remote exposure) do not provide data on the pathological examination of the placentas. Thus it cannot be ascertained whether the alleged abruptios are recent or old, or if they are related to chorioamnionitis, as this problem is more frequent in these patients. Chorioamnionitis, as discussed in Chapter 20, often causes marked deciduitis with bleeding and clots from that site that mimics abruptio, but it is a different mechanism. We are therefore still skeptical that cocaine exposure produces abruptio placentae often (Gilbert et al., 1990). Moreover, the vasculature that *might* be affected by the putative constriction of cocaine, the spiral arterioles, should be inviolate because of its structural change from trophoblast infiltration. There is, however, no question of the increased frequency of fetal growth retardation. Little et al. (1989), who studied outcome in 53 cocaine abusers, found a significant increase only of prematurity and preeclampsia. There was also a slight increase of congenital heart disease; but in contrast to other studies they reviewed and that showed more abruptios, this problem was not found in their population. The authors suggested that it may be due to the fact that placentas are not routinely examined or are examined only when stillbirths occur. It must be admitted also, and was commented on by these investigators, that cocaine abuse is often combined with alcohol and other drug abuse and with maternal cigarette smoking; this has also been pointed out by Donvito (1988) and Frank et al. (1988). Moreover, the social makeup of the population may predispose to intrauterine infection. The vasoconstriction caused by these agents may be transmitted to the fetus, in whom cerebral infarction has occasionally been observed (Chasnoff et al., 1986). In a study of 75 pregnant women with cocaine use, the patterns of preterm delivery, growth retardation, and abruptio was affirmed, but the cause of abruptio was questioned (Chasnoff et al., 1989). When women stopped using cocaine after the first trimester, there was no reduction in the incidence of abruptio placentae. Fulroth et al.

(1989) reported a significantly higher incidence (34%) of meconium staining when compared with that (10%) of a control population. The cardiovascular effect of cocaine injection has been studied in pregnant sheep by Moore et al. (1986). They found a rise of maternal arterial pressure (32–37%), combined with a 36% to 42% reduction of uterine blood flow, lasting 15 minutes after injection, at levels comparable to those seen with human usage. Fetal arterial pressure also rose to 12.6%. Chávez et al. (1989) reported that offspring of cocaine abusers suffer an increased risk of urinary tract anomalies, but it has not been our experience.

Effects on pregnancy somewhat similar to those seen with cocaine usage have been made with maternal *heroin* abuse. Nacye et al. (1973) studied this complication of pregnancy in detail and found that 60% of these mothers had intrauterine infection (chorioamnionitis) as the principal finding. Also, there was frequent meconium staining of the fetus and placenta, and growth retardation.

Lysergic acid diethylamide (LSD) administration during pregnancy is associated with an increased abortion rate (McGlothlin et al., 1970), but the placenta has not been described to be abnormal. The abortions and fetal damage have been inferred to be secondary to chromosome breakage (Warren et al., 1970). Later studies negated this effect. An extensive investigation of drug-related injury on the placenta was undertaken by Freese (1978). He found that no consistent changes take place, and that any effect is one of direct action on the fetus, rather than on the placenta. Blanc et al. (1971) described a case of amnionic bands with amputations of digits in an LSD user. This finding prompted their review of six malformed infants born to LSD users and led them to caution that a causal relation may exist between LSD and amnionic bands.

Smoking during pregnancy has been the topic of numerous studies, and many have yielded contradictory results. It is often considered to be the cause of an increased frequency of abortions (Kline et al., 1977), low birth weight, and some morphological placental changes. A study of 7,651 patients from California indicated that smokers' placentas had more calcifications and more subchorionic fibrin deposits (Christianson, 1979). This investigator found the placental weight not to be decreased, as did so many other students. He likened the result to placentas of higher altitude and made reference to the self-selection of smokers and the difficulties inherent in ascertaining true alterations that might be due only to smoking. An early review of the topic (Editorial, 1968) suggested that the adverse effects may be mediated through reduced blood flow to placenta and fetus. When umbilical and uterine blood flow velocities were studied, the effect on fetal growth appeared to result from a highly significant rise in fetal placental vascular resistance (Morrow et al., 1988). Other causes (hypoxia and cation changes) have also been held responsible. The data relating to reduction of birth weight, often considered as being controversial, were reviewed by Murphy et al. (1977) and Alberman et al. (1977). Asmussen (1979) found fetal weight to be reduced by 325 g and the placenta by 123 g, similar to the later findings of Wen et al. (1990). Studies of the endothelium obtained from umbilical arteries and vein showed widening of the basement membrane; in heavy smokers this change is said to have been visible even by light microscopy. Additionally, there was deposition of other materials, edema, reduction of smooth endoplasmic reticulum of muscle cells, and loss of intercellular junctions between endothelial cells. Heavy smokers had marked dilatation of the rough endoplasmic reticulum. The microvillous surface of the syncytial cells was reduced, and there was a reduction in cytotrophoblastic elements. The villi had decreased vascularization and increased collagen content. The author inferred that similar changes may take place in the vessels of the fetus. Wingerd et al. (1976) reported that the placental/fetal ratio was increased in smokers, presumably due to the reduced fetal weight. On the other hand, Teasdale and Ghislaine (1989), who undertook a careful quantitative morphometric study with appropriate controls, found only minor changes in the placenta. There was a "tendency for the placentas . . . to contain proportionally more nonparenchymal and less parenchymal tissue." The authors concluded that the effect of smoking was more related to ischemic or toxic effects of several compounds in tobacco smoke than to significant alterations in the functional structure of the placenta. This opinion was also voiced in an editorial (Anonymous, 1989b), whose author pleaded that "it is dishonest to say there is serious evidence that her fetus is at risk if she does not give up smoking." Jauniaux and Burton (1992), on the other hand, found that smokers developed increased mean thicknesses of the villous membrane and trophoblast. They believed that these changes may account for the biological disturbances during gestation.

Naeye (1978) has reported an increased frequency of single umbilical artery (SUA) and abnormal cord insertions in the anomalous fetuses of smokers. Kuhnert et al. (1987b) showed that placental cadmium and zinc levels were increased in smokers, with a 9% reduction in zinc levels of fetal red blood cells (and a decrease in fetal weight) (Kuhnert et al., 1987a). A significant reduction of umbilical arterial prostacyclin production was reported in the umbilical cords of smoking mothers by Dadak et al. (1981). They likened this effect to a similar finding in women with preeclampsia and speculated that this potent vasodilator may be involved in growth retardation of the fetus. The immunohistological study of Sanyal et al. (1993) indicated that smokers' placentas have an increased hydrocarbon hydroxylase activity within the trophoblast, presumably stimulated by the toxins in the smoke. Rubin et al. (1986) and some other authors have reported that significant passive smoking has a similar deleterious effect on fetal development. The difficulties of such correlation were examined by Chen et al. (1989), who conducted a study in Chinese women. They did not find that passive smoking posed a risk to the fetus.

A variety of ultrastructural observations were made on the umbilical blood vessels in smoking women's pregnancies. Thus Asmussen (1978) found the intima and media of the vein to be edematous, and the elastic membranes were partially destroyed. Fewer changes were identified in the umbilical arteries (Asmussen, 1982b); but in heavy smokers, scanning electron microscopy delineated more general changes (Bylock et al., 1979). Intercellular "holes" were seen in the intima that were interpreted to result from cellular injury, and Asmussen (1982a) found glycogen and lipid accumulation in the muscular wall cells. He also reported an increase of mitochondria in the endothelial cells of arteries of smoking mothers (Asmussen, 1984). In the villous basement membranes of such pregnancies, this author observed thickening and an increase in villous stromal collagen (Asmussen, 1980). Pinette et al. (1989) reported that the placentas of smoking mothers had increased maturation, as graded by sonographic scanning methodology.

Additionally, there have been numerous investigations concerning the putative relation of abruptio placentae to smoking; most have suggested that a relation exists, most recently the large prospective study of Raymond and Mills (1993). It is troublesome, however, that few of these studies have actually examined the placentas, that an increased frequency of premature rupture of membranes is found, and that it is thus possible that chorioamnionitis may be the mechanism of possible "abruptio." The most recent study of smoking and abruptio is that by Voigt et al. (1990). This population-based case-control study endeavored to ascertain if smoking, abruptio, and small-for-gestational-age (SGA) status were correlated, using data from birth certificates. Importantly, the placentas were not examined. An increased frequency of abruptio was found with smoking and an increase of SGA infants, but the latter was not correlated with smoking. These authors suggested that 38% of abruptios was "attributable to maternal smoking." Perhaps the first authors to suggest an increase of "accidental hemorrhage" (abruptio) with smoking were Andrews and McGarry (1972), whose paper is replete with a variety of tabular information. Goujard et al. (1975) opined that abruptios were perhaps due to "serious spasm, the release of which, by surge of blood, would cause arterial rupture." Their point is difficult to follow as the rate of stillbirth in smokers was much increased (250%) in their study population, but that of abruptios was lower than in controls. In a later study (Goujard et al., 1978) the authors provide additional evidence for a relation to stillbirths and make an further correlation with alcohol intake. As is true for most studies, however, the placentas were not studied for inflammation, and the cause of true abruptio is difficult to evaluate. Underwood and colleagues found no increase in abruptio placentae among smokers, while Meyer and Tonascia (1977) found a dose-related increase in abruptio, placenta previa, and premature rupture of membranes. Most of the abruptios occurred before 32 weeks' gestation, which leads us to consider that inflammation, rather than true retroplacental bleeding, may be the significant problem. The increase in placental ratio in smokers, studied by Wingerd et al. (1976), was found to be the result of lower fetal weight, rather than larger placentas. Naeye et al. (1977) reviewed the data from the Collaborative Study regarding the influence of smoking on placental/fetal development. They found an increase in abruptios and infarcts and lighter placentas in smokers. All in all, there appears to be a larger body of evidence to suggest that smoking has some deleterious effect on placenta and fetal development.

Few other *drugs* have shown well recorded effects on placental structure, the notable exception being methotrexate (Li et al., 1956; Goldstein & Berkowitz, 1987) with its severe trophoblast toxicity. Severe fetal growth retardation occurred with a patient who attempted to cause abortion by taking much aminopterin; the placenta was not described (Shaw & Rees, 1980). Alkylating agents have been used successfully for the therapy of malignancies during pregnancy, and usually they have been attended with no ill effect. Lacher and Geller (1966) reported a successful gestation in a pregnant patient with Hodgkin's disease who was given therapeutic doses of cyclophosphamide and vinblastine. The placenta was not specifically mentioned. The size of the infant (3,060 g) and its development, however, suggested that the placenta must have been normal. Hennessey and Rottino (1963) concluded from personal observations on 35 patients with Hodgkin's disease complicating pregnancy that there was no need to interrupt the pregnancy. They did not describe the associated placentas. Knörr et al. (1969) found no abnormalities of placental structure after therapy with alkylating agents during pregnancy, and Nordlund et al. (1968), also found that pregnancy progresses without fetal toxicity. Nicholson (1968) reviewed the cytotoxic agents used during pregnancy. In the villi of a therapeutic abortion of an epileptic patient medicated with diphenylhydantoin, large clusters of lymphocytes were

found in the fetal capillaries; it is unknown if this finding resulted from the lymphoproliferative effect of the drug (Greco et al., 1973), as the specimen did not contain an embryo.

Irradiation during pregnancy is usually avoided, of course, because of the deleterious effects it has on the fetus. In two gestations complicated by squamous cell carcinoma of the cervix, Driscoll et al. (1963) reported the effects of therapeutic irradiation on two fetuses, 16 and 22 weeks' gestational age. In the first, hydronephrosis was present, and the decidua showed foci of necrosis and inflammation, as well as necrosis of the amnion and chorion laeve. In the older fetus, scattered degenerative changes were observed, but the placenta was normal. Likewise, when rat placentas were irradiated with the fetus shielded, the exposure had no effect on fetal growth. Relative "radioresistance" of the gestationally older placenta was inferred from these experiments (see also Brent, 1960).

Whether treatment with the β-adrenergic blocking agent *propranolol* has an effect on placental development is uncertain. Fiddler (1974) described the pregnancy of a patient who had been taking 30 mg of propranolol three times daily for 3 years for treatment of obstructive hypertrophic cardiomyopathy. The patient delivered a severely growth-retarded infant accompanied by a 200-g placenta. He quoted other authors who found no ill effect from this medication and yet others who witnessed spontaneous abortions. Reduction of maternal cardiac output is speculated to have caused this fetal growth retardation, but the disease itself may also have been causative.

Maternal heart disease has been the topic of many studies, and because of its complexity the outcome of fetal growth and placental development is variable. Only one of five patients with aortic stenosis were reported to have fetal growth retardation (Easterling et al., 1988). McFaul et al. (1988) found no increased fetal mortality, growth retardation, or congenital anomalies among 519 pregnancies of 405 women treated for heart disease during pregnancy. Feraboli (1951) described placental infarcts and intervillous thromboses in six patients with "cardiopathy" and opined that the lesions are not specific but resulted from "slowing of the general circulation." He suggested that the fetal vessels were sclerosed, and that placental villous fibrosis occurred. We have seen several placentas of patients with severe rheumatic cardiac disease, especially with mitral stenosis, in whose placentas there were large subchorionic intervillous thromboses. In some of them adjacent infarcts were present. Nunez (1963) studied 15 placentas of women with "cardiac disease" properly classified according to New York Heart Association standards. He performed a quantitative assessment of villous structures and found the villous surface to be reduced, with simultaneous reduction of the fetal/ maternal placental weight ratio. Because the villous capillary bed was expanded, Nunez inferred that there was an expanded fetal blood volume. Kerber et al. (1968) found a normal placenta and normal-sized fetus with choanal atresia in a patient who was being treated with warfarin and heparin for a prosthetic mitral valve.

Pregnancy complicated by *hypercholesterolemia* resulted in an entirely normal placenta, despite fetal growth retardation (Barss et al., 1985). Cholesterol deposits were sought but not found. In a patient with *hypobetalipoproteinemia* also a normal placenta was found (Parker et al., 1986). Numerous lipid-laden macrophages were present in the intervillous space of a patient with extreme *hyperlipemia* that complicated pregnancy (Nielsen et al., 1973). The foam cells measured up to 35 µm in diameter and were concentrated at the maternal floor of the placenta. No foam cells were found within the placental villi. The infant delivered normally, had a birth weight of 3,650 g, and was normal. The placenta also had a normal gross appearance. The placenta of a patient with "well controlled" *phenylketonuria*, provided by Dr. B.H Landing, was entirely normal. In a case of *Gordon syndrome* (short stature, defective dentition, hyperkalemic hyperchloremic acidosis, and chronic hypertension), Kirshon et al. (1987) reported normal fetal development and, it is assumed, a normal placenta. We have seen a patient with *Smith-Lemli-Opitz syndrome* whose pregnancy ended prematurely (courtesy Dr. S. Sadowinski, Los Angeles). The placenta showed slight edema but had no other findings of note. As is regrettably so often the case, the placental findings were not documented in a case of *cystic fibrosis* reported by Rosenow and Lee (1968). The infant developed normally, as did two term infants born to a patient with *Wilson's disease*, but the placenta was not reported (Dreifuss & McKinney, 1966). Oga et al. (1993) reported on the birth of a child who had hepatomegaly from this maternal disease and continued to suffer abnormal liver function tests. The "maternal side of the placenta" had an increased copper content. Their illustration suggests that the copper is contained in the cytoplasm of the decidua basalis.

With *pruritus gravidarum*, the associated cholestasis is frequently accompanied by premature birth and fetal death; the placenta is commonly meconium-stained (Sasseville et al., 1981). The same authors discussed many other dermatoses seen during pregnancy and reported that *impetigo herpetiformis* is associated with frequent stillbirths and "placental insufficiency." With *papular dermatitis* of pregnancy, it has been suggested that the lesions are due to a hypersensitivity reaction to an abnormal placenta. High human chorionic gonadotropin (hCG) levels are believed to reflect this abnormality, but the evidence does not appear to be firm. *Pruritus* during pregnancy (of undefined etiology) was thought to be the cause of "hyperplacentosis" (placentas of more than 600 g) with increased hCG levels (Goodlin et al., 1985). This association, however, also seems ill-defined, and specific placental lesions were not reported.

Several contributions have elucidated the pathology of *sarcoidosis* during pregnancy. Altchek et al. (1955) found uterine involvement by sarcoidosis granulomas and established that despite active, widespread sarcoidosis normal pregnancy may ensue. Dines and Banner (1967) and other authors they quoted found that the pulmonary complication of sarcoidosis may improve during pregnancy. From his review of 54 pregnancies, O'Leary (1968) was unable to agree. Kelemen and Mándi (1969) were the first authors to report typical sarcoid granulomas in the term placenta of a normal infant. Small, grossly visible granulomas were seen in the floor of that placenta.

Normal fetal development occurred in a patient with maternal *cystinosis* that had much earlier been complicated by nephropathy and renal allografts at age 8. The maternal cells in the decidua capsularis had numerous vacuolated, cystine-containing cells. The placenta was normal (Reiss et al., 1988). Cystinuria, on the other hand, has occasionally been associated with mild fetal growth retardation. *Fetal cystinosis* may be diagnosed from placental specimens. Smith et al. (1989) found that homozygous cystinosis patients' placentas had significantly elevated cystine content, as did fetal leukocytes; heterozygotes could not be clearly distinguished from normals.

Maternal *Gaucher's disease* complicating pregnancy has been associated with hemorrhagic complications that resulted from thrombocytopenia. Houlton and Jackson (1978) described it to be due to extensive infiltration with foamy macrophages throughout the marrow spaces. In another case (Addleman & Gold, 1963) with good outcome, the placenta appeared grossly normal (W. Addleman, personal communication, 1963). Watov and de Sandre (1964) reported another four pregnancies, two of which resulted in placenta previa. The authors did not report the placental histology. These reports referred to other cases in the literature, but a definitive study of the placenta with maternal Gaucher's disease has not come to our attention.

Pheochromocytoma complicating pregnancy has serious implications for the fetus and mother. A review made in our department (S.A. Russo, personal communication, 1986) encountered 120 case reports with 45% fetal deaths, 12% abortions, and 25% maternal mortality. Thrombosis of the umbilical cord was found in one case (Fox et al., 1969) and abruptio placentae in four cases (Pestelek & Kapor, 1963). Most of the deaths could not be adequately explained. The disease is often mistaken for toxemia of pregnancy because of the hypertension and frequent albuminuria (Cannon, 1958). Cannon described several abortions that occurred in a patient with pheochromocytoma. Combs et al. (1989) found that there was marked fall (40%) in cardiac output during paroxysmal attacks due to pheochromocytoma and suggested that it may compromise the fetus.

Hematological Disorders

Sickle cell anemia occurs, with few exceptions, in Blacks. It is characterized by the presence of sickle-shaped red blood cells, which result from crystallization into "tactoids" of the abnormal hemoglobin S, particularly under conditions of reduced oxygen tension. Formalin fixation allows microscopic identification of sickle cells in histological sections (Figure 336). Fujikura and Froehlich (1968) suggested that the hypoxia of postpartum placental separation induces sickling in the intervillous space. They examined 2,117 placentas of black women and found sickling in 9.4%. They remarked that formalin fixation was superior for preservation; Bouin's solution causes too much red blood cell lysis, and Zenker's solution causes a reversal of the sickling phenomenon. No associated pathological findings were reported in their large study.

The heterozygous condition (trait) of S hemoglobinopathy occurs with a frequency of 9% in the United States black population and is as high as 45% in central Africa. In infants with sickle cell thalassemia (hemoglobin SC disease), infarcts of the placenta have been reported (Bentsi-Enchill & Konotey-Ahulu, 1969).

Patients with the homozygous disease have many serious problems. Urinary tract infection (45%), pre-eclampsia (25%), and puerperal sepsis (20%) are the main complications. In heterozygotes these complications occur significantly less frequently and are less severe (Winston & Mastroianni, 1953). Whalley et al. (1963) found no difference in the outcome of pregnancy in heterozygotes when compared to controls. Platt (1971) found increased perinatal mortality, and Brown et al. (1972) observed lower birth weights. Blister cells (erythrocytes with vacuoles) were found in a patient with sickle cell disease who died after giving birth to a growth-retarded child (Krayalcin et al., 1972). Prophylactic transfusion reduces the frequency of painful crises but does not secure a beneficial pregnancy outcome (Koshy et al., 1988), presumably because the significant placental lesions have already been produced prior to this therapy.

The placentas of patients with SS disease may have Tenney-Parker changes, infarcts, increased fibrin, abruptios, and villous edema (Anderson et al., 1960; Shanklin, 1976; Koshy et al., 1988). These placentas are relatively small, and the associated fetuses have growth retardation. Fox (1978) did not encounter those lesions; he reported that most of the changes are histological alterations of the intervillous red blood cells. A single pregnancy with SE disease has been reported, but the placenta was not described (Ramahi et al., 1988). The 2,310 g neonate had hydrocephalus. T. Fujikura (personal communication, 1976) found that sickle cells occasionally traverse the placenta to the fetal side. He indicated that in about one-half of the placentas examined sickle cells were found in aspirated cord blood; in addition, he identified occasional deported villi (Figure 337) in this blood. Doubtless, it is a traumatic

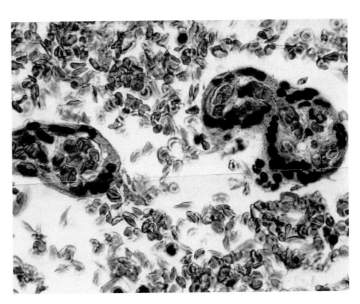

FIGURE 336. Sickle-shaped red blood cells in the intervillous space of a patient with SS disease at term. The fetal capillaries, of course, contain normal red blood cells, containing mostly fetal hemoglobin. H&E. ×640.

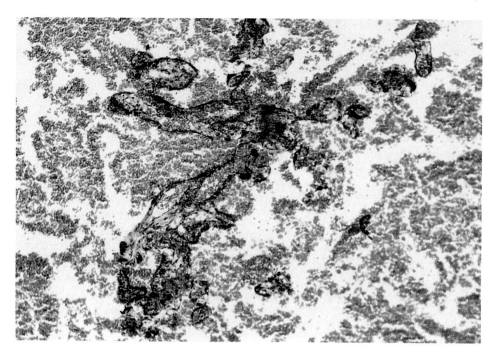

FIGURE 337. Mature villi and sickle cells in aspirated blood from the umbilical cord. It is probably an artifact that occurred during delivery of the placenta. H&E. ×150. (Courtesy Dr. T. Fujikura.)

feature of delivery of the placenta and has no bearing on fetal life.

Mordel et al. (1989) reviewed the literature of pregnancy complicated by maternal β-thalassemia. Their patient was transfusion-dependent but delivered a normal term infant. They referred to other patients who suffered fetal growth retardation and abortion. The placenta was not described.

Idiopathic thrombocytopenia (ITP) is a rare complication of pregnancy. It carries with it the risk of postpartum hemorrhage and, less commonly, neonatal hemorrhagic complications (Jones et al., 1961). The latter may be a hazard when obtaining fetal scalp samples for the purpose of fetal pH determination. More recently, however, cordocentesis has been practiced successfully in maternal thrombocytopenic states to assess the fetal platelet count (Kaplan et al., 1990). On rare occasion, the placenta has had intervillous thrombi, but most commonly the disease is not associated with placental lesions (Kaibara et al., 1985). In other cases, infarcts and decidual vascular lesions have been reported in the placenta (Scott, 1966; Mercer et al., 1988). It is not clear, however, whether they were caused by the ITP or were perhaps the result of preeclampsia and steroid therapy (Schenker & Polishuk, 1968).

Thrombotic thrombocytopenic purpura (TTP) during pregnancy has been described by Wurzel (1979). The pregnancy ended with a macerated fetus. The placenta showed many hyaline thrombi in the decidual arterioles

that presumably caused the fetal death. TTP is a serious disease and carries a high mortality rate. Fewer than 70 cases have been described, according to Ambrose et al. (1985). Often the disease is mistaken for severe preeclampsia; perhaps some aspects of their clinical presentations are shared because of the similarity of their occlusive vascular lesions. In a case of maternal TTP, we have seen fibrin deposits in decidual vessels, resembling atherosis. An apparently normal placenta with an infant having no thrombocytopenia was described in the first report of *Evans syndrome* during pregnancy (Silverstein et al., 1966).

Neonatal thrombocytopenia has many causes, including the transfer of maternal *HLA antibodies* (Sharon & Amar, 1981; Sørensen et al., 1982; Morales & Stroup, 1985), maternal *thiazide* administration (Rodriguez et al., 1964), and alloimmunization (Deaver et al., 1986). The latter condition has special dangers of fetal intracranial hemorrhage and is now being treated with prenatal platelet transfusions (Daffos et al., 1988; Mueller-Eckhardt et al., 1988). Despite these advances, the placenta remains usually unstudied or it was found to be normal.

Messer (1987) and Handin (1981) have reviewed bleeding disorders during pregnancy. *Leukoagglutinins* cause neonatal neutropenia but have no known effect on the placenta (Payne, 1964). A pregnancy complicated by *von Willebrand's disease* was reported by Leone et al. (1975), but the placenta was not reported; the infant was normal. A patient with *factor VII deficiency* was successfully treated by Fadel and Krauss (1989), whose main concern was possible abruptio. A retrospective study of pregnancy outcome of 32 patients with *hemorrhagic hereditary telangiectasia* showed a slightly higher frequency of abortions. The placentas were not reported (Goodman et al., 1967). *Protein C deficiency* during pregnancy was studied by Vogel et al. (1989). No complications occurred. In a pedigree that contained 15 pregnancies no excess fetal loss but an increased incidence of thrombosis were observed (Trauscht-VanHorn et al., 1992). A somewhat different outcome in fetal protein C deficiency is discussed in Chapter 13, under thromboses of the fetal circulation. Milo et al. (1989) reported on a patient with acute intermittent *porphyria* during pregnancy believed to be secondary to the antiemetic drug metoclopramide. When the drug was discontinued, the symptoms disappeared and a normal infant was delivered. We saw a case of alleged porphyria developing during pregnancy that after examination of the placenta was shown to be due to acute cytomegalovirus infection.

Folate deficiency has been incriminated in many complications of pregnancy, including abortion, abruptio placentae, and other diseases (Streiff & Little, 1967; Hibbard & Hibbard, 1968). In two large studies of women with folic acid deficiency severe enough to cause megaloblastic anemia in the mother, no measurable effect on fetal well-being or placentation were observed (Kitay, 1968; Pritchard et al., 1970).

Beischer et al. (1970) evaluated the effect of *anemia* on pregnancy and the placenta. They prospectively studied of a large number of placentas obtained from different localities. The investigators found that severe maternal anemia caused highly significant placental hypertrophy. In their interpretation, the "anemia causes inadequate oxygenation of the fetoplacental unit, which in turn, in a proportion of patients, evokes a physiological response which results in compensatory placental hypertrophy." Some placentas weighed in excess of 700 g. We have seen, however, placentas of severely anemic patients with hemoglobin values of 4 g/dl that were small and had pronounced Tenney-Parker changes (i.e., increased knotting of syncytium).

The finding of placental hypertrophy with anemia has raised the question as to what changes may be observed in placentas of chronic oxygen deficiency at *high altitude.* Metcalfe et al. (1966) have summarized the adaptation of the pregnant organism to the rarified atmosphere; placental changes were not then identified with certainty. Alzamora (1958), on the other hand, has reported that the placenta at high altitude is considerably larger than normal. This point is of particular interest in relation to the important studies carried out by Tominaga and Page (1966). These investigators experimentally studied placental effects of oxygen depriva-tion. They exposed explanted human placental tissue to low and high oxygen tension in vitro and found that low oxygen exposure led to increased syncytial knotting (the Tenney-Parker change of preeclampsia). Contrary to the findings of later investigators (Ong & Burton, 1991), they found a reversibility of this phenomenon. This trophoblastic change was believed to cause thinning of the exchange membrane and thus considered to enhance oxygen transfer to the fetus. Quantitative studies on the effect of high altitude on the placenta were carried out by Jackson et al. (1987, 1988) and their results are different. They also reviewed the relevant literature and found that infants at high altitude were smaller but that the placental weight was not enlarged (at 3,600 m in Bolivia). There was, however, a histological (measured and quantitated) alteration in the disposition of villous capillaries. Mean villous length was reduced at high altitude, villous capillaries were thinner, and cross sections of capillaries were more numerous. This effect (presumably due to chronic hypoxia) led to an altered capillary/villous ratio at high altitude in these Bolivian samples. The capillaries were also more closely applied to the trophoblastic surface than is the case at sea level. This finding was particularly evident in the histometric study of Reshetnikova et al. (1993). These investigators found a significantly larger capillary volume in placentas of high altitude; the findings were at times similar to chorangioma, presumably representing chorangiosis (see Chapter 24). Kaufmann et al. (1993) reviewed this topic in some detail and suggested that a first effect of hypoxia is an effect on cytotrophoblast with its proliferation, to be followed by syncytiogenesis (knots). They suggested that various cytokines of yet undetermined nature and sequence affect the connective tissue of the villi (perhaps Hofbauer cells) to mediate these effects.

In a case of *fetal Letterer-Siwe's disease* described by Ahnquist and Holyoke (1960), the placenta was entirely normal. The stillborn fetus had widespread involvement of reticuloendothelial cell proliferation with numerous giant cells. The mother had been vaccinated against poliomyelitis and influenza during pregnancy, but the authors considered a causal relation unlikely.

Endocrine Disorders

Thyroid diseases have no direct known impact on placental structure and function. Many thyroid disorders enhance the probability of preeclampsia. Placental infarcts and abruptio are thus found more commonly than normal. Scott (1966) stated that hyperthyroidism is not infrequent during pregnancy and mentioned that hydramnios occasionally complicates such pregnancies. Davis et al. (1989) found an incidence of hyperthyroidism of 1 per 2,000 deliveries. Vulsma et al. (1989)

suggested that substantial amounts of maternal thyroxine may be transferred to the fetus; however, Bachrach and Burrows (1989) provided evidence that the amounts transferred, in fact, may be much smaller than was suggested. Infants of hyperthyroid patients may be growth-retarded or hyperthyroid (Elsas et al., 1967; Cove & Johnson, 1985). They also more frequently have prenatal distress, meconium staining, and fetal demise (Page et al., 1988). Page et al. encountered chronic villitis in one of their perinatal deaths, but it probably bears no relation to the maternal hyperthyroidism. Diabetes is also more frequent in hyperthyroid patients during pregnancy (Bruner et al., 1988). All aspects of the physiology of thyroid metabolism and thyroid diseases are well reviewed in the ACOG Bulletin (1993).

Untreated hypothyroidism renders most patients anovulatory. It is therefore not often encountered as a complication of pregnancy. Davis et al. (1988) reviewed 14 pregnancies in overtly hypothyroid patients. Anemia (31%), toxemia (44%), abruptio (19%), and postpartum hemorrhage (19%) were found. Fetal death occurred in 12% and growth retardation in 31%. The frequent abortions, congenital anomalies, and maternal infertility associated with hypothyroid states were discussed in some detail by Hoet et al. (1960).

Cushing's disease rarely complicates pregnancy. Grimes et al. (1973) adequately reviewed the literature of 26 reported pregnancies that resulted in only 11 term births. There were four abortions and four stillbirths; premature deliveries made up the remainder. The placentas of these pregnancies were not reported. Likewise, Aron et al. (1990), in an extensive review of complications of this disease, failed to indicate if placental pathological features are seen. These authors and Buescher et al. (1992) suggested that the ACTH-like material from the placenta and its corticotropin-releasing hormone-like compound may exacerbate the clinical state of Cushing's disease during pregnancy. Occasionally, Cushing's disease has its onset during pregnancy and disappears after its termination. Wieland et al. (1971) reported such a case and referred to others in the literature. Upon termination of pregnancy during the 14th week, their patient improved remarkably. Normal placental tissue was obtained.

Diabetes During Pregnancy

Abnormalities of glucose metabolism, such as gestational and overt diabetes, are certainly among the commonest medical complications of pregnancy. These conditions cause increased fetal wastage such as abortion, prematurity, macrosomia, and congenital anomalies (Cheung et al., 1990; White & Beischer, 1990). The placenta of women with diabetes is often severely

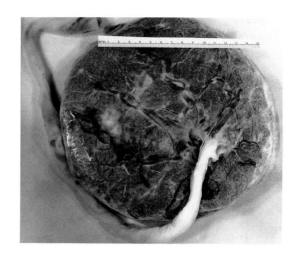

Figure 338. Plethoric, thick, somewhat edematous placenta from a patient with treated class A diabetes.

abnormal. The results of placental investigations, however, must be considered with caution. There have been dramatic changes in the management of maternal diabetes and in surveillance for gestational diabetes over the years. Thus the results of early placental studies are not necessarily expected currently. Also, because of the high fetal mortality during the last 2 weeks of pregnancy, most pregnant diabetic patients are now delivered before term, which perhaps helps explain why most diabetic mothers' placentas are not calcified in current observations. Older publications state that diabetic mothers' placentas showed increasing amounts of calcium deposits. We have the impression, however, that the usual calcifications in the floor of the placenta and in the septa are decreased in diabetics' placentas. A comprehensive review of diabetic pregnancies, fetal outcome, anomalies, and placental changes is to be found in the exhaustive review by Haust (1981). It is thoroughly referenced and illustrated, and it contains a large section on placental changes in the presence of maternal diabetes. In particular, there is a detailed consideration of the ultrastructural pathology of the associated placenta.

The placenta of most poorly controlled diabetics is enlarged, thick, and plethoric (Figure 338), which are manifestations of fetal hypervolemia and maternal hyperglycemia. The hypervolemia is also reflected in the considerably higher residual blood volume of the delivered placenta (Kjeldsen & Pedersen, 1967; Klebe & Ingomar, 1974a,b). When diabetes is well controlled during pregnancy, the placental weight does not deviate from normal (Clarson et al., 1989). The villous structure of the placenta in maternal diabetes is focally "dysmature" or relatively immature. An increased frequency of cytotrophoblastic mitoses may be ob-

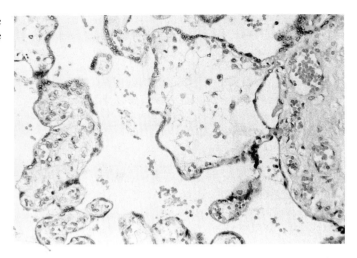

FIGURE 339. Focal immaturity and villous edema of the placenta in a class A diabetic mother. Note the large Hofbauer cells in the edematous villus. H&E. ×160.

served. These placentas are also often edematous, and their appearance has occasionally been likened to that of placentas from erythroblastotic pregnancies (Maqueo et al., 1965), although they lack the anemia, of course. Maqueo et al. also observed a high frequency of preeclampsia in this population, which is not our observation. There is also frequently some degree of chorangiosis in the placentas of diabetics (Figures 339, 340). In the offspring, there is a slight increase in the frequency of single umbilical artery (SUA; 3–5% in diabetic progeny compared to ±1% average incidence) (Driscoll, 1965). This increase is particularly seen in gestations complicated by acidosis (Emmrich et al., 1974). When the pregnancy is complicated by nephropathy (class F diabetes), fetal growth retardation and placental infarcts may be found with increased frequency. Infarcts are otherwise uncommon in diabetic mothers' placentas. It is our opinion that none of these changes are *specific* for maternal diabetes and that they reflect primarily the altered glucose availability and

fetal adjustments to the intermittent excessive glucose load. Perhaps most characteristic of diabetes is the greater probability of fetal and placental vascular thrombosis. This problem is occasionally reflected in fetal renal vein thrombosis, and it may also be the cause of thromboses in the fetal-placental surface and mainstem vessels. From their detailed study of growth and maturation of villi in controlled diabetics, Mayhew and collaborators (1994) suggested that the villous tissue shows many adaptations in diabetes. The placentas had weights similar to those of the controls, presumably because of excellent maternal diabetic control. They found increased fetal capillary length and distension and shorter maternofetal diffusion distances.

The umbilical cord is usually more "edematous"; more accurately, it contains more Wharton's jelly. No specific placental anomalies are associated with the one highly characteristic fetal anomaly of maternal diabetes: sacral agenesis (the so-called caudal regression syndrome). Salafia and Silberman (1989) made the point

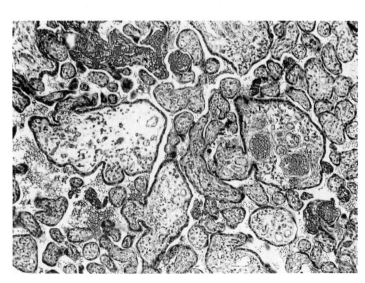

FIGURE 340. Placenta of a diabetic mother. Note the marked plethora and chorangiosis. H&E. ×160.

that funisitis is common in diabetic pregnancies and that it is correlated with irregular fetal heart rate patterns. The placentas they studied were also heavier.

There is no longer doubt that the placenta possesses specific insulin-binding receptors (Haour & Bertrand, 1974), and that these receptors are reduced in number in placentas of SGA babies (Potau et al., 1981). Despite earlier assertions that transplacental insulin traffic occurs (Gitlin et al., 1965), it is now clear that insulin does not normally pass the placenta in quantities sufficient to have a metabolic effect (Adam et al., 1969; Wolf et al., 1969; Kalhan et al., 1975). There is, however, antibody-bound insulin transferred in significant quantities, and it correlates with fetal macrosomia (Menon et al., 1990). This transfer suggested to the authors that immunogenic insulin should not be used during pregnancy. Another interpretation of the data was provided by Kimmerle and Chantelau (1991). Glucose passes the placenta readily, and the fetus responds to hyperglycemia with hyperplasia of the islets of Langerhans (Driscoll, 1965) and increased insulin secretion (Jørgensen et al., 1966; Thomas et al., 1967). The hyperplastic islets contain an increased amount of insulin (Steinke & Driscoll, 1965). Periodic hyperglycemia was thought to be the cause of fetal polyuria and hydramnios. That this assertion is probably an oversimplification has been demonstrated by the ultrasonographic study of fetal urination in the presence of diabetes-induced hydramnios (Wladimiroff et al., 1975).

Robb and Hytten (1976) have rigorously studied placental glycogen content throughout gestation. They found that glycogen concentrations normally decreased toward term, when it was around 1.5 mg/g of blood-free placental tissue. There were no significant changes when diabetic mothers' placentas were compared with those of normal pregnancies or those from toxemic gestations (see also Fischer & Horky, 1966). Thus the larger size of the placenta is not attributable to glycogen storage. Most of the large fetal size is due to obesity. A valuable test to ascertain maternal hyperglycemia during pregnancy is the concentration of glycohemoglobin in maternal blood. It adequately reflects the degree of maternal control, and higher concentrations significantly correlate with abortions in diabetics (Miodovnik et al., 1985). When strict control is exercised, pregnant diabetics are no more liable to lose a pregnancy than normal women, and they have normal amounts of glycosylated hemoglobin in their circulation (Mills et al., 1988). In pregnancies complicated by maternal diabetes, there is also much enhanced secretion of hCG by the placenta, as reflected in blood and amnionic fluid levels. Elkind-Hirsch and colleagues (1989) have found that the placenta of diabetics contains more gonadotropin-releasing hormone than normal placentas. The hCG concentration, on the other

hand, was not elevated. Greco et al. (1989) asserted from their immunocytochemical studies of proteins in diabetic placentas that β-hCG staining was increased, whereas other proteins (PLAP, SP1, and hPL) were decreased. It must be cautioned that the evaluation of these staining reactions is subjective (visual) only.

Thomsen and Lieschke (1958) were among the earliest investigators to study the placental structure in maternal diabetes. They found increased weight, plethora, calcifications, and "villous regenerations." The latter manifests as "immaturity" of the villi, more abundant and obvious cytotrophoblastic investment of villi, and villous edema. These nonspecific changes were found randomly distributed throughout the placenta. Burstein et al. (1963) claimed that major fetal vessels of the placenta have insulin bound to their walls. These authors studied diabetic placentas using insulin antibodies and fluorescence microscopy. They observed that placentas from diabetics had increased knotting of the syncytium. Aladjem (1967a) examined villi with phase microscopy and found no specific changes in diabetes, although many minor placental alterations were described. Vogel (1967), on the other hand, believed that the changes he found were so characteristic he coined the term plakopathia diabetica. This condition consists of persistent embryonic villi, discordant maturation of villous structure, disorders of villous ramification, and chorangiosis. Decreases in collagen content and mucopolysaccharides in diabetic mothers' placentas were found by Liebhardt (1968). We also believe that collagen content is much decreased. Winick and Noble (1967) observed that an increase in the number of normal-sized cells caused increased placental size. In the study of 48 placentas from diabetic mothers, Fox (1969) observed some abnormalities of villous maturation as well as "obliterative endarteritis of fetal stem arteries," thickening of trophoblast membrane, and an increase in villous fibrinoid necrosis. He speculated that these changes may result from "an immunologic reaction." Thickening of stem arterial walls was shown by Samaan et al. (1974), who correlated it with the degree of the diabetic metabolic disturbance. Jácomo et al. (1976) described similar vascular changes and attempted to quantitate them. In our experience quantitation is a difficult endeavor, and to evaluate villous vessels without establishing some rigid criteria for measurement produces problematical results. Thus we do not believe that they are "real" changes, and certainly none is specific for maternal diabetes. If they were real, they could be related only to fetal hypervolemia, perhaps to a high fetal blood pressure.

Differences of opinion and interpretation, reflected in a voluminous literature on the placenta of diabetic pregnancies, have been reviewed by Teasdale (1981, 1983, 1984). This author studied, with carefully controlled quantitative tools, the histomorphometry of placentas of diabetics from classes A, B, and C, classified according to White (1978). Teasdale's principal findings were that the placental exchange membrane (fetal vascular and villous surfaces) increases with maternal diabetes, but that few other significant changes (other than enlargement) could be detected.

Somewhat similar findings of an increased surface membrane for exchange were observed with planimetry by Böjrk and Persson (1984). These investigators paid particular attention to taking samples from similar areas of the placenta, as the villous structure in the center of a cotyledon differs from that at its periphery. This normally orderly organization of the cotyledonary structure was found to be somewhat disrupted in diabetic mothers' placentas. Driscoll (1965) found that the weight increase of placentas from class F diabetics was smaller than that from nondiabetics. This difference of class A to C placentas from class F placentas is mostly subject to the influence of maternal renal disease. Driscoll also observed that the decidua is often unusually thick; and of course with preeclampsia and hypertension the decidual vessels show characteristic arteriolar angiopathy (see also Horký, 1968). Parenthetically, it may be mentioned that the placentas of experimentally induced diabetes in rats share the enlarged size with the human counterpart (Pitkin et al., 1971). In addition, Padmanabhan et al. (1988) found cystic degeneration in the labyrinthine area. They interpreted it to result from glycogen depletion and coalescence of cellular degenerations. Both investigators observed preservation of normal architecture when insulin therapy was instituted. The cystic degenerations occurred even in the placentas of spontaneously diabetic BB-Wistar rats (Brownscheidele & Davis, 1981).

A number of electron microscopic studies have been undertaken to gain a better understanding of the morphological alterations of diabetic mothers' placentas. Okudaira et al. (1966) found no specific changes in these placentas. Minor, irregular degenerative changes were recorded, such as mitochondrial and endoplasmic reticulum degeneration in the syncytial cells. Some thickening of the basement membranes was observed, but it was not uniform. Widmaier (1970) added the finding of persistence of a nearly complete Langhans' cytotrophoblastic layer. Jones and Fox (1976) were more emphatic about ultrastructural changes in placentas of diabetics. Although they investigated mainly gestational diabetes, these investigators described patchy syncytial necrosis, dilated rough endoplasmic reticulum, cytotrophoblastic hyperplasia, focal thickening of basement membranes, and narrowing of small vessels. Others had reported dilatation of capillaries to be a prominent finding. Jones and Fox (1976) suggested

that the changes they observed may occur only patchily, and that they were similar to those of overt diabetes. Laurini et al. (1984) reported that, despite strict control of diabetes during pregnancy, ultrastructural changes in the placenta continue to persist: "blebs," thickened basement membranes, endothelial proliferation, and increased collagen content. Their deduction was that the commonest pathological feature is "dysmaturity," defined as "relative immaturity" of the placenta. Kaufmann and Stark (1977) reported that characteristic placental alterations occur with maternal diabetes. During cesarean section, they obtained biopsy specimens from the placenta for electron microscopy. In these tissues they observed the following characteristic features: 75 Å thick intratrophoblastic filaments, an abundance of smooth endoplasmic reticulum, and collapsed mitochondria in relatively edematous cells. Thus there is good evidence that the placenta, in a somewhat variable fashion, undergoes some minor morphological alterations in response to maternal diabetes. The significance of these findings remains uncertain, especially vis-à-vis their relation to the altered physiological states experienced by mothers and infants affected by this condition.

Congenital, hereditary *fructose intolerance* during pregnancy was studied by Marks et al. (1989), who also discussed the difficult management of such patients. Two children succumbed neonatally, and the most recent pregnancy was associated with a livebirth and a calcified placenta.

Maternal Neoplasms

Many maternal neoplasms have complicated pregnancy and some have caused placental disease. Pulitzer et al. (1985) have even reported that, on rare occasion, implantation takes place on endometrial adenocarcinoma; there was no associated placental development, however. Implantation over leiomyomas caused abruptio placentae in 57% of cases observed by Rice et al. (1989). We have seen placenta accreta in such locations. Carcinoma of the breast and cervix, gastrointestinal neoplasms, and melanoma have occurred during pregnancy, in that order of frequency (Donegan, 1983). Delerive et al. (1989) reported the metastasis of a pulmonary oat cell carcinoma to the placenta. In their review they found that 39% of the 38 cases of placental metastases reported were of melanoma. The tumor of their case lay free in the intervillous space and had not invaded the villi; the neonate was free of disease. Macroscopically, the placenta was entirely normal. In our experience, metastasis to the fetus is rare. Although metastases of several cancers and lymphomas have been found in the placenta, and in leukemias the intervillous space may be filled with leukemic cells, few neoplasms

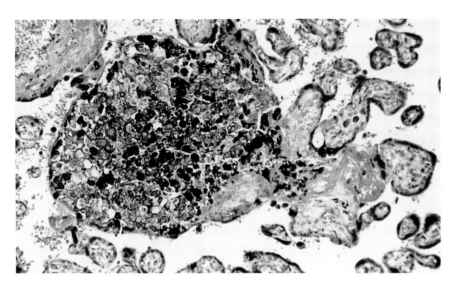

FIGURE 341. Term placenta with malignant melanoma metastasis. Pigmented tumor cells invade the villous tissue, and many pigmented Hofbauer cells are present. H&E. ×160. (Courtesy Drs. W.L. Freedman and F.J. McMahon.)

have traversed the placental barrier and seeded to the fetus.

The most important of these neoplasms is *malignant melanoma*. A melanoma metastasis was described and well illustrated by Holland (1949); and Reynolds (1955) described a placental metastasis of a malignant melanoma. The placenta appeared grossly normal but contained many microscopic amelanotic nodules. The infant remained normal for at least 10 months. George et al. (1960) reviewed 115 cases of melanoma that complicated pregnancy. They found two cases with placental metastases; all of the infants remained normal. The difficulty cells have traversing the placenta was studied experimentally. Working with experimental melanoma cell lines, Retik et al. (1962) were able to induce widespread maternal metastases, but the placenta and fetuses remained free of tumor. Cavell (1963) identified melanoma metastases in an infant of 2 months. Apparently, the infant had acquired the metastases transplacentally from the mother, but they disappeared spontaneously. The placenta was described as having been scarred and infarcted, but it did not undergo microscopic study. Aronson (1963) observed a muscular swelling that contained melanin pigment in an infant whose mother died from melanoma 4 days after parturition. Those lesions also disappeared spontaneously. Another case of transplacental metastatic melanoma was described by Brodsky et al. (1965). In umbilical cord blood, cells were identified that were consistent with melanoma, and many placental intervillous spaces were filled with melanoma cells. The maternal surface of the placenta appeared brown, with "rare foci of black pigmentation." Both mother and infant died with widespread metastases.

Heite and Kaden (1972) collected 27 cases of metastatic placental cancer, three of which were placental melanoma metastases, of which two metastasized to the fetus. A case of metastatic amelanotic melanoma in the placenta, the ninth reported melanoma of the placenta, was published by Sokol et al. (1976). These authors found that 28 cases of metastatic cancer in the placenta had been reported, five of which had involved the fetus. Their patient had undergone a cesarean section at 31 weeks. She died with widespread tumor 8 days postpartum. The neonate, who died from respiratory disease, had no tumor. Multiple firm nodules, 0.5 cm in diameter, were found in the villous tissue. They were comprised of cells that contained melanin and were similar to the maternal tumor cells. The placental villi were focally invaded by the neoplasm.

The placental melanoma metastasis shown in Figure 341 was in a patient described by Freedman and McMahon (1960). Despite villous infiltration with melanophages and some tumor cells, no fetal metastases were found, nor did the infant have melanuria. Widespread placental metastases from a maternal melanoma were found by Stephenson et al. (1971). The infant developed hepatomegaly, but metastatic tumor was never found. Melanoma metastases in the placenta were identified immunohistochemically with the S100 protein probe by Machin (1987). The infant was growth-retarded but had no evidence of tumor. A maternal melanoma was first diagnosed by placental metastases in the case described by Anderson et al. (1989). The tumor was metastatic to intervillous space and present in villi; the infant remained normal, but the mother died 6 months after delivery. The authors suggested in their review of 16 cases that a more unfavorable prog-

FIGURE 342. Widely disseminated fetal giant cell nevus cells in placental villi. H&E. ×250. (Courtesy Dr. G. Monif.)

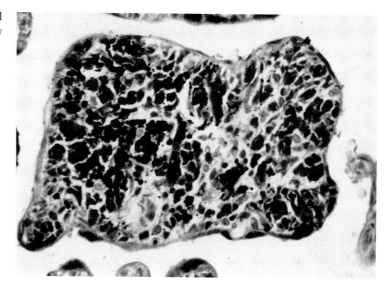

nosis exists when maternal age is under 30, the tumor is present in the lower extremity, and the neoplastic disease commenced during the 3 years before the affected pregnancy. They asserted that the extent of villous involvement had no influence on prognosis.

Fetal giant pigmented nevi were described by Holaday and Castrow (1968) and later by Demian et al. (1974) and Campbell et al. (1987). In the placenta of the first case, multiple foci of pigmented nevus cells were present in the villi. The neoplasm was considered to be benign despite these deposits. In the second case of extensive *fetal* giant nevus, the placenta was grossly unremarkable but was extensively involved microscopically (Figure 342). Because of this large amount of placental tumor, the authors suggested that the cells had arrived there by early neural crest cell migration. The last case may actually have been a malignant melanoma. At autopsy, metastases were found in the fetus. Its skin lesion, a large nevus, was detected sonographically. By light microscopy, the enlarged but grossly normal placenta was densely infiltrated with neoplastic cells. In contrast to the finding of maternal melanoma, these cells were confined to the villi. They did not invade the intervillous space, nor were they metastatic to the mother.

Metastatic *breast carcinoma* is depicted in Figure 343. It was confined to the intervillous space. Similar cases have been described by Cross et al. (1951) and Rewell and Whitehouse (1966). Many adenocarcinomas of the breast have been reported as having metastasized to the placenta, according to the reviews of Freedman and McMahon (1960), Potter and Schoeneman (1970), McGowan (1964), and Lemtis and Hörmann (1969). The latter authors drew attention to the absence of

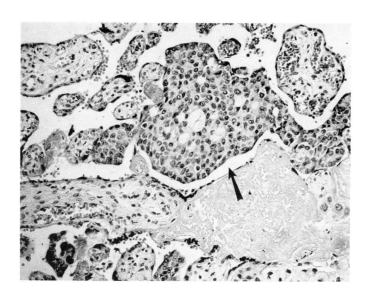

FIGURE 343. Adenocarcinoma of the breast metastatic to the intervillous space (arrow). Note the absence of vascularization in the nests of tumor cells. H&E. ×160.

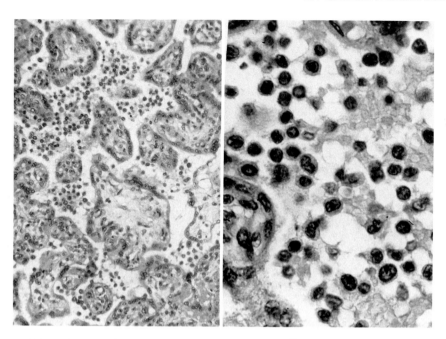

FIGURE 344. Placenta at 36 weeks' gestation from a patient who died from acute myelogenous leukemia the day after cesarean section. The white blood cell count at delivery was 147,200/mm^3. The child was well at 10 years. Note the large number of leukemic cells in the intervillous space but not within the villi. H&E. Left ×160; right ×640.

vascularization of these intervillous tumor colonies. For that reason, they suggested that these deposits be called pseudometastases. The following other *solid tumors* have been found in the placenta.

1. Pancreas (Smythe et al., 1976)
2. Lung (Jones, 1969; Read & Platzer, 1981)
3. Ovary (Horner, 1960)
4. Rectum (Rothman et al., 1973)
5. Skin: squamous cell carcinoma (Orr et al., 1982)
6. Medulloblastoma (Pollack et al., 1993)

Several of these reviewers referred to single additional cases of rare other tumors that were present in the placenta but that did not metastasize to the fetus. With the exception of melanoma, no documented case of transplacental seeding by a malignant maternal neoplasm has been identified. Hörmann and Lemtis (1965a,b) gathered a number of cases of metastatic tumors. They opined that the placenta has "remarkable defense mechanisms" against passing neoplasms from the mother to the fetus. In the rare cases where *multiple myeloma* has complicated pregnancy, the placentas were not described. The associated fetuses and infants developed normally, despite maternal chemotherapy with urethane (Kosova & Schwartz, 1966; Rosner et al., 1968). When Hodgkin's disease was treated during pregnancy, the infants also developed normally. Of the 35 cases reviewed by Hennessy and Rottino (1963), the placenta was not studied, except in the case of non-

Hodgkin lymphoma described by Tsujimura et al. (1993). The placenta showed numerous yellow, partially necrotic lesions, and the tumor had massively invaded the intervillous space; the premature infant succumbed. It is unknown if the placental substance was invaded or if the fetus became affected by the tumor. On occasion though, it has been described that the fetus has acquired the disease transplacentally (Priesel & Winkelbauer, 1926). A pregnancy complicated by a diffuse cavernous *hemangioma of the uterus* was described by Lotgering et al. (1989). They delivered the patient at 35 weeks and found the placenta to separate only with difficulty and with much loss of blood. Possible hemorrhage from placental invasion of the angioma is a possibility in this condition.

Many reports have dealt with the question of transplacental transfer of cells in the presence of maternal *leukemia*. At times the intervillous space is filled with leukemic cells (Figure 344), and yet no malignant cells can be identified in the fetal vessels of the placenta. Usually, these cells are not present in blood aspirated from the umbilical cord. Extreme idiopathic maternal leukocytosis occasionally occurs during pregnancy only to disappear after parturition. The intervillous spaces may then be crowded with maternal leukocytes, giving the appearance of leukemia. Care must thus be taken to differentiate this phenomenon from maternal leukemia. Bierman et al. (1956) found 50 reported cases of maternal leukemia during pregnancy. Not a single infant had been affected with the disease. In their case of

acute lymphocytic leukemia, the maternal white blood cell count at birth was 154,000 mm^3, but that of the neonate was only 3,300 mm^3. The placenta had severe leukemic cell infiltration that was confined to the inter-villous space. Ask-Upmark (1964) followed six children born to leukemic mothers for 9 to 41 years. Leukemia developed in none. Rigby and his colleagues (1964) quinacrine-labeled the buffy coat cells of a mother with acute myelogenous leukemia and reinjected them before birth. They then examined the fetal blood 7 hours after injection, when the infant had delivered. Occasional fluorescing forms were seen. Such findings, however, are not convincing evidence of transplacental transfer of leukemic cells. Diamandopoulos and Hertig (1963) studied the placenta of a leukemic patient and the offspring of 48 pregnancies. They did not find any transfer of cells. These authors estimated that about 400 patients with leukemia complicating pregnancy had been reported. Only a few cases of transplacental trans-mission seemed possible, but they were not well sup-ported. One such case is that of a mother who was diagnosed as having lymphocytic leukemia postpartum. Her child developed leukemia at age 9 months (Cramblett et al., 1958). The placenta and neonatal studies were not described. Thus there can be only speculation as to transplacental transfer of leukemic cells in that particular case. Other larger reviews of the literature also have shown no fetal acquisition of the disease, despite the presence of large numbers of leukemia cells in the intervillous space and despite the fact that a variety of maternal leukemia types were studied (Ask-Upmark, 1961; Lee et al., 1962; Johnson, 1972; Nummi et al., 1973). In another case, despite massive intervillous invasion by myeloid leukemia cells, the villi of a partial hydatidiform mole were not invaded (Honor & Brown, 1990).

Primary fetal leukemia has been reported only rarely; the Cabott case no. 37-1976 of myelogenous leukemia in a neonate is a good example (Scully et al., 1976). Finally, intrauterine growth retardation and a mecon-ium-stained placenta were found in a patient with adult T cell leukemia/lymphoma by Ohba et al. (1988).

Hypertensive Disorders

Preeclampsia

This common disease of pregnancy is now most fre-quently referred to as pregnancy-induced hypertension (PIH). The terms are interchangeable. One reason to be as specific as possible about the terminology is that the disease process may produce symptoms similar to those of circulating lupus anticoagulant, discussed below. Moreover, to our veterinary colleagues, toxemia denotes a different disorder, usually a condition of ruminants. In fact, classical PIH is uncommon in animals. It has there been diagnosed primarily in primates, especially in Patas monkeys (Gille et al., 1977; Palmer et al., 1979), but its effects are seen in other primate species, such as the gorilla, chimpanzee, and langur. Chesley (1985), a master of this disease, is adamant that strict criteria should be used in the defini-tion of this condition. He asserted that many patients with mild *preeclampsia* later suffer eclampsia. He also emphasized that all of the abnormal clinical findings in the pregnancy-induced disease disappear after gesta-tion, and that there are no sequelae to be expected in renal or vascular involvement in the future lives of the patient. His conclusions contrast with those of Epstein (1964) who found that women with a history of PIH had a significantly higher risk of developing "late hypertension."

Two recent classifications of preeclampsia and hyper-tensive disorders of pregnancy have been offered: a relatively simple definition, primarily based on blood pressure changes and put forth by Redman and Jef-feries (1988), and the more complex systematics published by Davey and MacGillivray (1988). Both proposals are aimed at providing a better delineation of the various hypertensive diseases, so that the effect of treatment can be more meaningfully assessed. These classifications may simplify diverse designations of the past and make some order of chaos, but that they are unlikely to be generally useful has been the topic of an Editorial (Anonymous, 1989a) and correspondence by Davey and MacGillivray (1989), Roberts (1989), and Lilford (1989).

Pregnancy-induced hypertension presents clinically as hypertension, edema, and proteinuria. Typically, after the uterus has been emptied of fetus and placenta, the disease ceases. Indeed, Hunter et al. (1961) found that immediate postpartum curettage of the placental bed causes maternal blood pressures to return to normal much more quickly than when curettage was not done. Inasmuch as PIH occurs in the absence of a fetus (as with hydatidiform moles), it is clearly dependent on the presence of placental tissue. The ultimate pathogenesis of PIH, however, has not yet been fully defined. Eas-terling and Benedetti (1989) have suggested that the disease is the result of a "hyperdynamic condition in which the characteristic hypertension and proteinuria are mediated by renal hyperperfusion." Numerous other possible etiological factors exist and were analyzed by authors.

Animal Models

Because of the frequency of toxemia, and to better understand its pathogenesis, several animal models have been used with the intent to simulate the human disease. It has been a difficult under-taking, and many of these models have primarily addressed the mechanism of abruptio placentae. Haynes (1963) induced abruptio placentae in the rabbit by temporary occlusion of the inferior vena cava. Fibrinoid degeneration and aneurysmal dilatation were produced in the decidual vessels, simulating human toxemic pathology. An interesting discussion of the paper further elu-cidated this relation. Abitbol et al. (1976b) have used the rabbit in a more extensive model study. They constricted the lower aorta, causing hypertension, proteinuria, and fetal growth retardation. They also demonstrated changes in liver and kidney similar to those of human PIH. The placenta contained infarcts and other changes resembling PIH, but these changes were also seen in some animals that did not exhibit toxemic symptoms (Abitbol et al., 1976a). Several years before, Howard and Goodson (1953) pro-duced abruptio placentae in dogs when they ligated the dogs' lower vena cava during pregnancy. Combs et al. (1993) con-stricted the aorta in rhesus monkeys and produced a "syndrome resembling preeclampsia", presumably due to the reduced lower aortic blood pressure. Interestingly, this group of investigators found that in these animals the depth of cytotrophoblastic infiltra-tion into the endomyometrium was markedly enhanced (Zhou et al., 1993). When Hodari (1967) constricted uterine arteries of dogs before their pregnancy occurred, progressive hypertension and proteinuria were produced, which ceased after delivery. Abitbol et al. (1976c) also used strictures (of aortas) before dogs became pregnant; they observed proteinuria, hypertension, and some fluid retention. The placentas of these animals showed diffuse hemor-rhagic infarction; in addition, typical renal lesions were induced. Many investigators have attempted to produce PIH and placental abruption in nonhuman primates. Thus Myers and Fujikura (1968), during the course of studies on the effect of ligation of interco-tyledonary vessels in rhesus monkeys, found that ablation of the "accessory lobe" invariably led to fetal death. They found that ligation of intercotyledonary vessels caused placental villi to con-tinue their growth and to develop increased syncytial knotting, a common feature of PIH. Wallenburg et al. (1973a) identified and ligated one to four uteroplacental arteries in the floor of rhesus monkey placentas. This measure was invariably followed by necrosis and typical infarction. The earliest identifiable lesions occurred 23 hours after ligation. The infarction closely resembled that seen in human placentas of PIH. Cavanagh et al. (1974) have long worked to develop a suitable model in baboons, placing clips about uterine arteries before pregnancy. Primarily renal lesions were thus produced. In later experiments, the investigators were able to produce hypertension and proteinuria that simulated human PIH (Cavanagh et al., 1977). When they subsequently con-stricted aortic blood flow in baboons, fetal and placental growth retardation and a reduction of amnionic fluid were induced; the placental morphology was not described (Cavanagh et al., 1985). Abitbol et al. (1977) also induced PIH in rhesus monkeys. They restricted aortic flow only during the last month of gestation. Resultant lesions included diffuse hemorrhagic infarction of the placenta, as well as renal and hepatic lesions. In general, the primate models more closely simulate the PIH seen in women, certainly the placental infarcts and glomerular lesion were iden-tical. Spiral arterioles in the placental bed, characteristically al-tered in human PIH, however, have usually not been investigated in these experiments. In the sporadic cases of primate toxemia that we have seen, the atherosis lesions were not fully expressed.

Placental Pathology of Preeclampsia

The principal pathological changes of the placenta in PIH are (1) decidual arteriolopathy; (2) infarcts in

central portions of the placenta; (3) abruptio placentae; (4) Tenney-Parker changes; and (5) retarded growth. These pathological features are not all invariably present. Also, one observes occasional cases with severe placental changes in which no maternal symp-toms relative to PIH have been elicited. Fetal and placental growth retardation, Couvelaire uterus, defi-brination, and the nephropathy of glomerular capillary endotheliosis, are frequently encountered manifesta-tions of PIH and are secondary features. Wynn (1977) concluded correctly that "conventional gross and histo-logic examinations of the fetal portion of the placenta have not uncovered a pathognomonic lesion of pre-eclampsia." This statement is particularly pertinent now that the lesions of lupus anticoagulant have been found to be identical to those previously ascribed solely to toxemia. Sletnes et al. (1992) studied preeclamptic women and found that 19% had antiphospholipid anti-bodies, with growth retardation of the offspring a pro-minent feature. A central issue in the understanding of pathological changes in PIH is whether these placental features allow a clean differentiation of PIH from other states of hypertensive disease. Wynn's review is one of the most critical essays to examine this point. Other reviews may be consulted: for example, that by Muller et al. (1971), which is based on their study of 168 cases of PIH. They attempted to correlate villous changes with the severity of PIH. The studies by Schuhmann and Geier (1972) and by Hölzl et al. (1974) also examined the severity of the clinical disease in relation to per-fusional and villous alterations. Another review of the placenta in toxemia was by Soma and his colleagues (1982). They gave the following tabular presentation of placental lesions in 53 cases of severe toxemia.

Lesion	Cases (%)	Controls (%)
Infarcts	54.7	32.8
Intervillous thrombi	20.7	10.0
Circumvallation	26.4	10.0
Abruptio	11.3	0
Decidual necrosis	16.9	9.6
Abnormal cord insertion	12.1	4.1
Meconium staining	18.9	12.8

Decidual Arteriopathy

Hertig (1945) was the first investigator to describe the pathological changes of PIH in the spiral arterioles at the implantation site. Since then, "atherosis" has be-come the hallmark of the disease, and it is generally believed that the other major placental changes are the result of specifically altered placental bed vessels (Figures 345, 346). Zeek and Assali (1950) found "acute

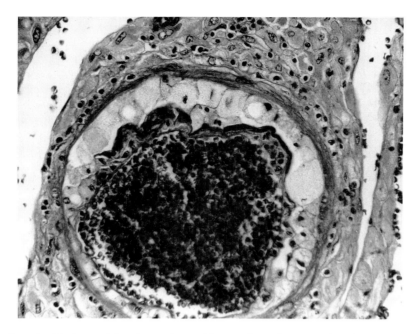

FIGURE 345. Atherosis in a decidual arteriole of a patient with preeclampsia. Note that the vessel wall has been replaced by fibrin, the intima is replaced by cholesterol-laden macrophages, and there is mural thrombosis. H&E. ×250.

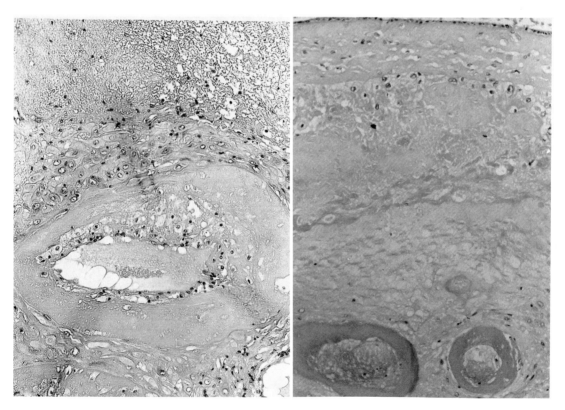

FIGURE 346. Hyalinized vessels with thrombosis and old atherosis in the decidua capsularis; there is also adjacent decidual necrosis. The pregnancy was at 33 weeks, and a 920 g SGA infant was delivered with severe PIH and abruptio. H&E. ×60.

atherosis" in the placental bed of 34 toxemic patients; none was present in 37 other cases, and only 3 of 143 nontoxemic patients had early atherosis. Eighteen nontoxemic hypertensive patients did not have atherosis. They considered the lesion to be an early change of the spiral arterioles; fibrinoid necrosis and lumen obstruction by thrombosis were considered to be later events. Zeek and Assali believed this lesion to be the primary cause of placental infarcts. They also emphasized that the fetal circulation does not maintain the integrity of the placental villous tissue; rather, this integrity is contingent on the intervillous blood flow. This *maternal* blood supply brings oxygen and nutrients. When the *fetal* circulation is obliterated, the villi merely shrink; only much later do they atrophy and degenerate. The typical infarcts, however, have maternal vascular disruption as their cause. Many other investigators have made the same observations, and they summarize the vast literature of this topic. Here the systematic studies of Marais (1962a,b,c,d, 1963a,b) must be mentioned. He was the first investigator to describe the appearance of spiral arteries in some detail using the colposcope. Marais determined the nature of intervillous flow by simultaneously injecting the maternal and fetal circulations of an intact uterus; he reaffirmed the independence of the two circulations. Atherosis, fibrin deposition, and arteriosclerosis were delineated by Marais, who contended that acute thrombosis of placental bed vessels is the principal lesion that ultimately leads to placental ablation. Because he observed obliterative lesions in the absence of hypertension, Marais also concluded that the obliterative changes of these vessels were not caused by the maternal hypertension. Nadji and Sommers (1973) found decidual vascular changes in 14% of induced first trimester abortuses and suggested that they represent precursors of future PIH lesions. Likewise, Lichtig et al. (1984) described atherosis during the first trimester of pregnancy, but its significance remains uncertain. Shanklin and Sibai (1989) have undertaken a systematic electron microscopic study of maternal vessels in women with PIH and controls. They found extensive endothelial injury especially in placental site venules with some fibrin deposition. No relationship to degree of hypertension could be established, and they found no atherosis. They were emphatic to state that the lesions they found were venous endothelial, and not confined to the placental site, let alone the arterioles.

Brosens et al. (1967, 1972) and Robertson et al. (1967) have led a major group of investigators who studied the pathogenesis of the decidual vascular lesions in PIH. They documented the normal response to implantation of placental bed vessels, and the alterations that occur during hypertensive pregnancies. The principal tenet of these investigators is that, under phy-

siological conditions, trophoblast of the placental shell infiltrates the arterial bed of decidua and myometrium and destroys the walls with fibrinoid changes. This infiltration of the 100 or so arterial mouths of the implantation site ultimately renders these vessels incapable of reacting to mediators by constriction, as they normally would have. With preeclampsia, on the other hand, the invasion of the proximal, myometrial branches is impeded. Whether this failure of the "second wave" of invading cells is an intrinsic trophoblastic failure or is mediated by maternal influences is still unknown. With PIH, trophoblast merely penetrates the decidual vessels; it fails to alter the myometrial vasculature's constrictive reactivity to mediators. Under "physiological" conditions, the arteries are changed into "large, tortuous channels by replacement of the normal musculoelastic wall with a mixture of fibrinoid material and fibrous tissue" (Brosens et al., 1967). The interactions of toxemia with or without preexisting hypertension were also detailed and well illustrated by these investigators. The changes and interpretations are complex and hypothetical. They must be read in the original text or in the summary review (Brosens et al., 1972). Similar findings were seen in subsequent investigations by Gerretsen et al. (1981). De Wolf et al. (1975) reported the first electron microscopic studies of the decidual vasculature in PIH. Their findings are important, as they illustrated the imbibition of plasma constituents, the proliferative activity of intimal and muscle cells, and the damage to the vascular endothelium. Fatty infiltration was first observed in the endothelial cells; later, macrophages phagocytose fat from degenerating lipid-laden myogenic foam cells; eventually, medial necrosis occurs. Haust et al. (1977) also found that muscle cells accumulate lipid in the presence of PIH. Their description, however, is not clear. Although they refer to myometrial cells as having accumulated lipid droplets, the electron micrograph suggests this accumulation to occur in the muscular wall of the arterioles at the decidual–myometrial interphase of the placental bed. The difficulties of differentiating smooth muscle cells from lipid-laden macrophages in atherosclerotic lesions has been further investigated by Schaffner et al. (1980). At present we believe it is not certain that the altered elements in atherosis represent typical muscle cells, rather than macrophages. The conclusion that the lipid-laden cells are mostly, if not totally, macrophages was also reached in the immunological studies conducted by Klurfeld (1985) on atheromatous plaques. In further studies of the vascular damage of PIH, Khong et al. (1992) observed that the normal endothelial coat of uteroplacental vessels was disrupted in 8 of 10 patients with PIH. Pijnenborg et al. (1991) observed vascular changes in 47 hypertensive and 17 normal pregnancies. Various states of hypertensive disease, not only PIH,

FIGURE 347. Acute atherosis, fibrinoid degeneration, and early mural thrombosis of a decidual vessel in the presence of PIH. H&E. ×160.

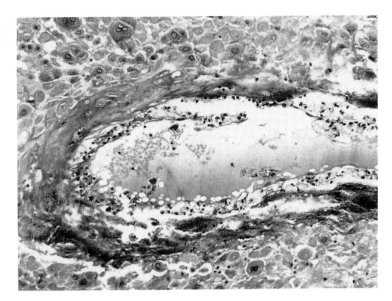

were a cause of atherosis. Zhou et al. (1993) showed in rhesus monkeys with aortic ligatures that the depth of cytotrophoblastic invasion was enhanced, perhaps being mediated by blood pressures.

Because there is so much apparent "fibrinoid" deposition at this site (Figure 347), Kitzmiller and Benirschke (1973) undertook fluorescent labeling studies of placental beds from normal patients and from those with PIH. They found a heavy deposition of γ-globulin and complement C3 in the vascular lesions of PIH (Figure 348). Some fibrin could also be demonstrated, but no Hageman factor or albumin was found here. Two hypertensive patients without preeclampsia and a diabetic primigravida also showed negative staining. In subsequent studies of PIH, Kitzmiller et al. (1981) invalidated the possibility that these deposits were the

result of an immunological "rejection" phenomenon. Only 53% of patients with PIH had such lesions, and some non-PIH patients with hypertension, diabetes or both had indistinguishable vascular changes. Similar investigations, reported by Weir (1981), also showed variable deposits, a predominance of fibrin and C3, but no immunoglobulins. Parenthetically, it may be mentioned here that skin biopsies in patients with PIH have shown deposits of immune complexes (Houwert-de Jong et al., 1982). The review by Wells and Bulmer (1988) should be consulted for additional considerations of the possible immunological delineation of atherosis. Branch et al. (1989) have shown that patients with severe, early-onset toxemia have circulating antibodies to phospholipids. They drew analogies to the lupus anticoagulant syndrome (see below), enhancing the

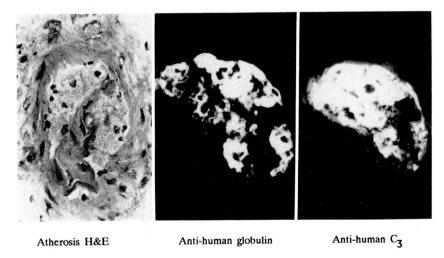

Atherosis H&E   Anti-human globulin   Anti-human C$_3$

FIGURE 348. Atherosis and mural thrombosis in a decidual vessel from a patient with PIH. H&E and immunofluorescence. ×800. (From Kitzmiller & Benirschke, 1973, with permission.)

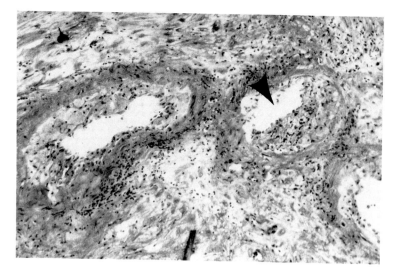

FIGURE 349. Decidual vessels from a patient with PIH, with lymphocyte and macrophage infiltration, atherosis, and an old mural thrombosis (arrow). Globulin and complement were found in these vessels. H&E. ×250.

notion that this common disorder has an immune background.

Although the decidual blood vessels in PIH are often accompanied by a sparse number of lymphoid cells, plasma cells are conspicuously absent (Figure 349). Bardeguez et al. (1991) studied the T lymphocyte population in 62 primigravidas. They found a significant decrease in T-helper cells during the second trimester in women who later developed PIH. This decrease occurred long before clinical symptoms became evident and disappeared 6 to 10 weeks postpartum. Other

immune response studies were cited by these authors. Absence of a significant lymphocyte population from the decidua of PIH patients was the finding in the ultrastructural study of Shanklin and Sibai (1989). On occasion, we have observed a granulomatous reaction at this site (Figure 350). This finding is exceptional; it may be explained on the basis of a possible immune vasculitis and may not be related to PIH. The occasional presence of lymphoid cells at the implantation site and many other features of PIH have repeatedly suggested an immunological basis for this disease. Gusdon et al.

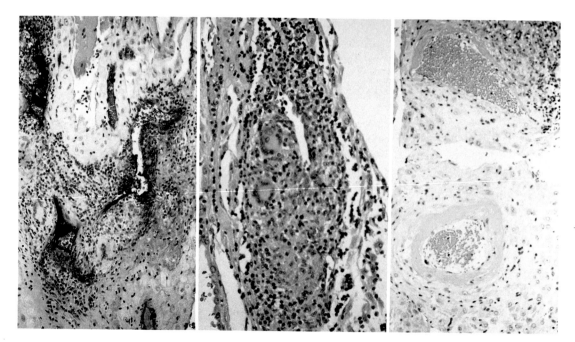

FIGURE 350. Granulomatous reaction around decidual vessels in a 21-year-old patient with eclampsia following severe pre-eclampsia at 31 weeks' gestation. (Left) Antifactor VIII stains show the association with vessels. (Center) Several multi-nucleated giant cells are present. (Right) Typical toxemia changes are present. Left, middle: Anti-VIII. ×160. Right: H&E. 240. (Courtesy Dr. R. V. O'Toole, Columbus, Ohio.)

FIGURE 351. Myometrial vessel of case in Figure 346 showing the thickened artery, presumably exhibiting "spasm," as suggested by Robertson et al. (1986). H&E. ×220.

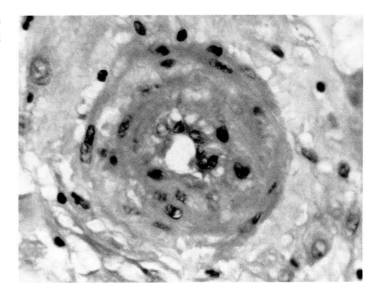

(1977) therefore studied the percentage distribution of T and B cells in normal and toxemic patients. They found no significant differences between the two populations.

Many studies of the vascular lesions in the placenta of patients with PIH have been made of the decidua capsularis that accompanies the membranes (Figure 346), rather than the decidua basalis. The latter is often markedly altered, and at times it is necrotic and is thus less useful for investigation. Placental bed biopsies have now been examined to great advantage. The results from a three-center study extending over 30 years have been published by Robertson et al. (1986). They emphasized that biopsy specimens, usually obtained at cesarean section, should include the myometrium. They gave precise details as to how the specimen should be obtained and processed in order for it to be useful. Even in their experienced hands, decidual bed biopsy specimens were acceptable for interpretation in only 70%. These investigators found the decidua vera to be the most useful tissue for the observation of atherosis; and remarkably they considered the membrane-associated decidua to be decidua vera. This group of investigators paid special attention to the lack of "physiological vascular changes" in the myometrial vessels and to the occurrence of vascular thickening ("spasm") in PIH (Figure 351). Similar changes have been reported in otherwise unexplained fetal growth retardation. When considering all these reports, it must be remembered that the findings made in patients with lupus anticoagulant (see below) may explain some of the still inexplicable results of the past. They have not yet been taken into consideration in these studies as possibly confounding the results.

Khong et al. (1987) attempted a statistical analysis from the study of decidual vessels in 39 patients with PIH. They were unable to relate the lesions to parity, degree of proteinuria, severity and duration of hypertension, or its therapy and found an incidence of 46% atherosis in PIH. This figure is similar to those of other workers cited. Stillbirths, SGA infants, and fetal distress occurred slightly more often in pregnancies whose placentas had atherosis. These results differ from the findings of some other studies, wherein there was a more appreciable increase of pregnancy complications (McFayden et al., 1986). Khong et al. (1987) reaffirmed that hypertension was not the cause of atherosis and suggested that inappropriate immune reactions may be causative. They also found that the presence of atherosis did not affect fetal outcome. The final pathogenesis of this lesion, however, remains unresolved.

Labarrere (1987) also found macrophage and T cell infiltration as well as deposits of immunoglobulins and complement around the spiral arterioles of PIH decidual beds. His observations challenged some of the assertions made by Robertson et al. (1986). These studies mainly indicate that the pathogenesis of atherosis, as well as that of PIH, is still unresolved. Gerretsen et al. (1983) observed, in placental bed biopsies, that the "physiological change" of spiral arteries was present in 95% of normal pregnancies but occurred in only 19% of those complicated by PIH or fetal growth retardation. They observed, nevertheless, that the trophoblastic syncytial giant cell infiltration of the uterine wall in PIH, occurring adjacent to the uterine vessels, was of normal magnitude. The findings of Gerretsen et al. (1983) reaffirmed that pregnancy alterations of the uterine vascular walls are not due to ingrowth of trophoblast from the outside. Rather, this physiological change of vessels is accomplished by upstream growth of cells that originate at the mouths of these vessels. The histochemical studies performed by these investigators confirmed that the cells in the vascular walls are not of the syncytial type but that they represent X cells. We have seen a patient who died from eclampsia and who had typical lesions of atherosis and thrombosis in the central portion of the myometrium under the placental bed. This finding indicates to us that, on occasion, the second wave infiltration of X cells takes place in patients who develop preeclampsia. Moreover, atherosis, infarcts, necrosis, and intrauterine growth retardation (IUGR) can take place long before clinical manifestations allow the diagnosis of preeclampsia.

Infarcts

Placental infarcts are the commonest and most conspicuous lesions observed by the pathologist. They represent necrotic villous tissue. There is no longer any doubt that the tissue has died because of deficient intervillous, maternal circulation. Infarcts are firm, condensed dead villi that often encompass the entire thickness of the placenta (Figure 352). More frequently, however, they involve the base of the placenta. They are particularly common at the placental edge. Here, they signify that the placental edge is "plastic." That is, placental edges often atrophy during late gestation, with the histological picture of infarction ensuing (Figure 353). When infarcts are found in the central portions of the placenta, and particularly when they are randomly thus distributed, PIH or the condition of circulating lupus anticoagulant with anti-cardiolipins are almost invariably present. It is particularly true when infarcts are found during the first and second trimesters, at which time they are otherwise uncommon. The earlier they appear, the more likely the lupus anticoagulant syndrome is to be expected. Placental infarcts differ grossly from intervillous thrombi. They have a granular surface and are much firmer. Intervillous thrombi, in contrast, are either fresh red clots and shiny, or they are laminated and light tan-gray. Their periphery commonly has some infarction of villous tissue.

Placental infarcts are initially dark red. They can be distinguished from living tissue by their firmness and by their lack of a spongy texture (Figure 354). As they age, infarcts lose their fetal hemoglobin and become yellow and then tan-grey. They are never invaded by "organizing" fibrous tissue; during their subsequent evolution they become atrophic. Hemosiderin is often found in early infarcts. The color changes (red and white infarcts) have been especially studied by Bartholomew and his colleagues (1961), who advocated a special method of studying the placenta for the presence of infarcts. They suggested that the entire organ be fixed in formalin and later serially sliced. The value of this method was supported by the studies of Steigrad (1952), who evaluated 716 unselected placentas. He suggested a complex division of infarcts, grading them from types A to H, and attempted a correlation with PIH, especially with its nephropathy. Shanklin (1959), who studied 767 unselected placentas, found no relation of "white or red" infarcts to toxemia, a finding inconsistent with the experience of other authors. He is correct, however, when he emphasized the occurrence of increased trophoblastic knotting (senescence, as he called it) in PIH. Javert and Reiss (1952) studied "red infarcts" (intervillous thrombi); they found them most frequently in conjunction with erythroblastosis, and with toxemia their 49% incidence was substantially increased over the average of 17.6%. These investigators pleaded that the designation "intervillous thrombus" is a misnomer. Because of the frequent (48.7%) contamination with NRBCs, they wished to draw attention to the admixture of maternal and fetal cellular components (further discussed in Chapter 17). Fox (1963) asserted that the term "white infarct" should be

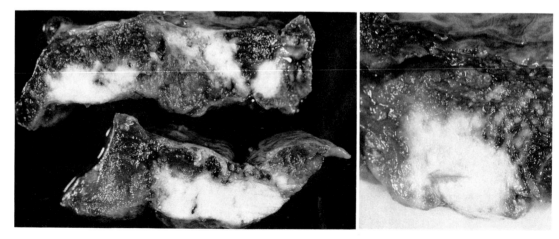

FIGURE 352. Macroscopic aspect of "white" infarcts scattered throughout the placental tissue. There were 40 such infarcts in this patient with PIH. Note that most of the infarcts involve primarily the placental floor.

FIGURE 353. Macroscopic and histological aspects of an old marginal infarct that is not related to preeclampsia. H&E. ×10.

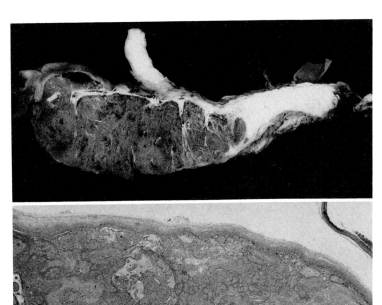

abolished because it is often confused with laminated fibrin/clot accumulation. He found subchorionic fibrin plaques (15%), perivillous fibrin (28%), true infarcts (22%), a central intervillous thrombus (12%), and a basal intervillous thrombus (6%) in a series of 200 normal pregnancies. Huber et al. (1961) also found that intervillous thrombi result from a disturbance of decidual vein perfusion but suggested that they represent different lesions from true infarcts. Bartholomew differed with this view in a discussion of this paper. Marais (1962c) illustrated the lesions with excellent color photographs and succinctly described their pathogenesis. Carter et al. (1963b) presented excellent photomicrographs and affirmed villous dependence on the maternal oxygen supply via the intervillous circulation. In a subsequent contribution (Carter et al., 1963a), the same authors presented a complex classification of infarcts and described a novel entity, the "divergent villous lesion." We believe that there is no need to make such complex distinctions, as they do not aid in prediction or understanding of infarcts, nor do they aid in diagnosis of maternal disease. The "divergent" lesion described is simply an expanding intervillous thrombus

with adjacent villous infarction. Torpin and Swain (1966) interpreted laminated subchorial intervillous thrombi as "infarcts" and thereby confused the nomenclature even more. Stark and Kaufmann (1974) have studied the early changes of placental infarction and examined them with fine structural methods and enzyme analysis. They found that an early process in the genesis of infarcts is the development of "plasma polyp" formation from the syncytium; they beautifully demonstrated this phenomenon by scanning electron microscopy.

Several investigators have attempted to relate the presence of infarcts to preeclampsia. Budliger (1964) reviewed the older literature and made a planimetric and histological study of 95 formalin-fixed placentas. Hemorrhagic and white infarcts were significantly more common, and they were larger in PIH placentas than in controls. Intervillous thrombi were not more common; but, when present, they were larger. Budliger deduced from his findings that a minimum of 190 g placental tissue is needed for fetal survival. Wentworth (1967) examined 679 consecutive placentas with a large section technique after prolonged formalin fixation. Of these placentas, 77 came from patients with mild PIH and 12

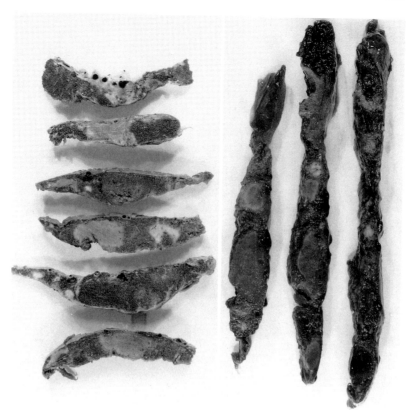

FIGURE 354. Macroscopic aspect of multiple infarcts in a placenta from a patient with severe PIH and a stillborn fetus. Varying ages of infarcts are shown as dark red (fresh), dark gray (intermediate), and white (old). The patient eventually had abruptio placentae.

from those with severe PIH. He found the following: red infarcts 1.3%; old, true infarcts 6.2%. There was a significant increase of infarcts (67.0%) in the severely toxemic patients, whereas the mildly toxemic patients had only a 11.7% incidence of infarction. Some of the villi adjacent to infarcts showed impressive chorangiosis as well (Figures 355, 356) (see Chapter 24). In fact, the massive congestion seen in these early lesions is a necrobiotic change, and it often results in villous hemorrhage before infarction takes place. Wallenburg (1969) also found a significant increase of infarcts with toxemia and noted that the infarcts are commonly

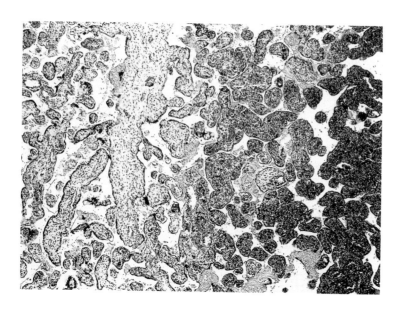

FIGURE 355. Fresh infarct (right) with marked congestion and villous hemorrhages at 27 weeks' gestation in a patient with PIH and abruptio 2 days earlier. H&E. ×60.

FIGURE 356. Same case as in Figure 357, showing an intermediate-aged infarct (left) and an older infarct (right). H&E. ×260.

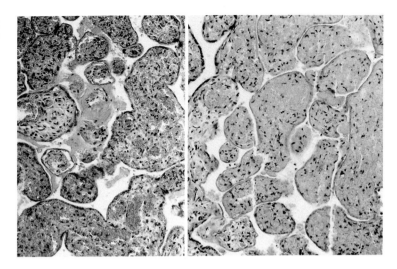

found centrally in the placenta. He also noted a significant correlation with low Apgar scores and low birth weight. In a later contribution, this group of investigators concluded that an infarct represents the death of a fetal cotyledon due to the occlusion of a single decidual blood vessel (Wallenburg et al., 1973b) (Figure 357).

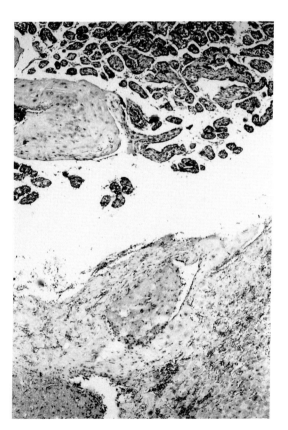

FIGURE 357. This decidual vessel is nearly completely occluded by old thrombus. It is from a patient with PIH and fetal growth retardation. H&E. ×60.

Brosens and Renaer (1972) found in their placental bed biopsy study of the spiral arterioles underlying infarcts that the lesions lacked normal trophoblastic invasion (and thus the physiological reaction of myometrial vessels) and had occlusive thrombosis.

The most ambitious study of the relation of infarcts to perinatal outcome comes from the pen of Naeye (1977). He evaluated 31,494 placentas from the prospective Collaborative Study and endeavored to distinguish infarction from abruptio placentae and to determine their influence on fetal outcome. He deduced that placental infarction caused 2.26 of 1,000 perinatal deaths. "Fatal infarcts were strongly associated with diastolic pressures over 90 mmHg in the gravida," and the situation was augmented when accompanied by proteinuria. Moreover, fatal infarcts were five times commoner with abruptio placentae, and they were also more common in older and overweight gravidas. Naeye believed that infarcts often serve as a nidus for the inception of abruptio. It may also be mentioned here that infarcts and abruptios are not infrequent in patients with sickle cell anemia.

Abruptio Placentae

Abruptio placentae—detachment of the placenta from its decidual seat—has had many names. Holmes (1908) called it ablatio placentae; and it has been referred to as accidental hemorrhage, premature separation of the normally situated placenta, and perhaps other names. Gruenwald et al. (1968) suggested that the term abruptio and premature separation should not be used interchangeably. The former designation he proposed be used only for the cases recognized before birth and premature separation be reserved to the pathologically diagnosed cases. Obviously overlaps occur, which

Gruenwald and colleagues acknowledged, and we consider the two to be identical. It is commonly assumed that this complication of pregnancy represents a sudden, painful event. With total abruptio or when a large retroplacental hematoma suddenly forms, there may indeed be pain due to sudden stretching of the uterine peritoneal covering. More often, abruptio is partial and painless. These cases would be classified as premature separation, according to Gruenwald et al. (1968). Notelvitz et al. (1979) described three cases of painless abruptio placentae characterized by vaginal bleeding and accompanied by backache and a nontender uterus. Because ultrasonographic recognition of the placental separation prevented fetal mortality in their cases, the authors advocated it for diagnostic evaluation. In their large prospective study (primarily relating maternal smoking to abruptio), Raymond and Mills (1993) found that it occurred as often as in 1% of pregnancies past 28 weeks. They also found an association with congenital heart anomalies.

There are many causes of abruptio, such as trauma from accidents or amniocentesis, abnormal uterine structure, separation at the edge in partial placenta previa, and, prominently, preeclampsia. In an occasional placenta one may also recognize the abnormal shape of a bicornuate or otherwise irregular uterus by the configuration of the abrupted placenta (Figure 358). There was an unusual cause, congenital hypofibrinogenemia, with recurrent abruptio placentae in a patient described by Ness et al. (1983). In our experience, when one-half or more of the placenta de-

taches suddenly, the fetus dies. Lemtis (1967) has referred to similar estimates. He made reference to the rare case of fetal survival with as much as 5/6 abruption. Lemtis placed much reliance on the irregular nature of placental perfusion for survival of the fetus. Delivery should be accomplished rapidly in cases of recognized abruptio. If placental detachment takes place over a long period, in stages, and with infarcts ensuing, the fetus may survive but suffers from deficient transplacental oxygen and nutrient supply. It has been shown that trophoblast releases a factor that inhibits platelet aggregation (O'Brien et al., 1987), and it has been postulated that this factor is needed for normal placental blood flow. When it is decreased, abruptio may take place.

The frequency of abruptio placentae in unselected series of pregnancies is estimated to be between 0.17% and 0.96% (Waddington, 1957; Halberstadt et al., 1969). Such figures reflect the obstetrician's ability to make the clinical diagnosis; they are not based on recognition by placental examination. It must be admitted at the outset, however, that the pathologist cannot recognize reliably the presence of an acute abruptio placentae; thus the overall incidence is underestimated by anatomical review. The diagnosis of a recent abruption can only be made clinically. The pathologist relies on alterations in placental structure, and on color changes of the retroplacental blood clot. These changes take time to develop. When we studied 7,038 consecutive placentas past the 20th week of pregnancy, 3.75% of them were found to have features of some degree

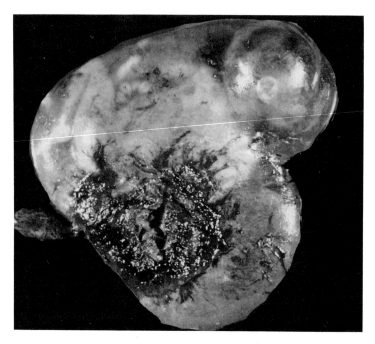

FIGURE 358. Delivery of baby "en caul," with abruptio of a growth-retarded placenta. The bicornuate nature of the uterus is reflected in the abnormally shaped membranes.

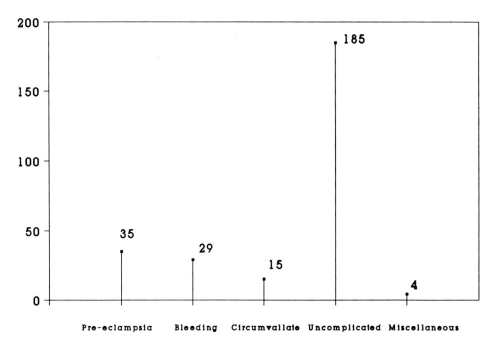

FIGURE 359. Causes of abruptio placentae, pathologically identified.

of abruptio placentae (Benirschke & Gille, 1977). Niswander and Gordon (1972) found evidence of abruption in 2.12% among the prospectively collected cases of the Collaborative Study. They were usually described as retroplacental hematomas. Because not all abruptios bleed externally (the "concealed hemorrhage") or produce the classical signs of a painful, rigid abdomen, the clinical diagnosis is bound to be made less frequently. Our series encountered trauma of various kinds only rarely, whereas preeclampsia and eclampsia were present in 13%; nevertheless, clinically uncomplicated pregnancies predominated (Figure 359). Trauma and, recently, allegedly cocaine abuse are thought to be frequent causes of abruptio. They are covered in other chapters of this book. With regard to trauma, we here relate findings of an important case: The patient had been in a car accident. Her newborn, delivered at 37 weeks, had an Apgar score of 0/1 and a hematocrit of 17%; the infant required transfusion. The maternal Kleihauer test was negative. A fresh, large retroplacental hematoma contained 60% fetal cells. Higgins and Garite (1984) impressively demonstrated that late abruptio is an important sequela of trauma during pregnancy. Abdella et al. (1984) found that abruptio was most commonly associated with eclampsia (23%), chronic hypertension (10%), and preeclampsia (2.3%). Clinical "abruptio" is also mimicked by active peripheral bleeding that ultimately leads to circumvallation, by marginal hemorrhage associated with severe ascending infection, and by the unusual entity marginal sinus thrombosis (Figure 360). The mechanism of marginal

sinus thrombosis was explored and well depicted by Bartholomew (1961). He believed it to be the outstanding cause of first trimester bleeding, but it was

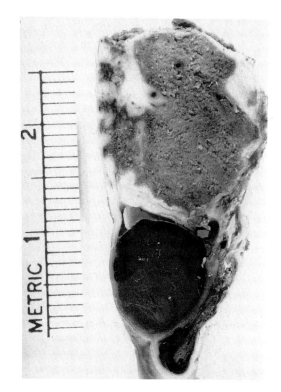

FIGURE 360. Marginal sinus thrombosis, actually a marginal abruption with layered blood clot in an immature placenta.

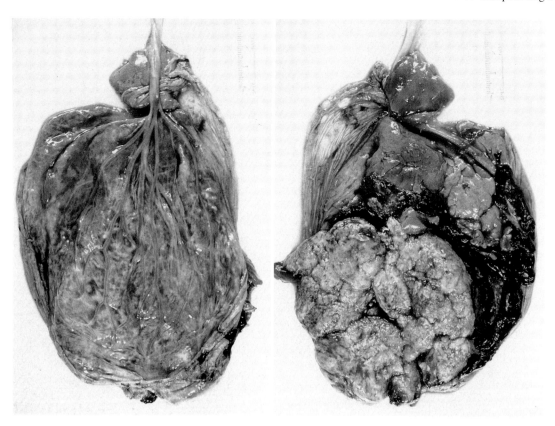

FIGURE 361. Immature placenta with velamentous insertion of the cord and long-standing abruption underneath the cord insertion. The clot is of different ages and has brown, yellow, and red areas. There is associated chorioamnionitis.

also frequent during later pregnancy. With marginal abruptions, Harris et al. (1985) thought that the site of bleeding was venous in nature. In other cases, though, it is undoubtedly related to decidual necrosis and inflammation (Figure 361).

That abruptio is *not* diagnostic of preeclampsia, as earlier contended, has been emphasized by many investigators (Tatum, 1953; Dyer & McCaughey, 1959; Hibbard & Hibbard, 1963). Tatum (1953) discussed the wide spectrum of associated pain and symptoms, whereas Dyer and McCaughey (1959) were more concerned with the appropriate therapy. Hibbard and Hibbard (1963) also denied the overwhelming frequency of toxemia as the etiology of abruptio placentae; they considered folic acid deficiency and grand multiparity to be important etiological factors.

The placenta in classical abruptio placentae has fresh clot attached at the maternal surface. The villous tissue may be compressed; and because of the frequent association with toxemia, infarcts are often found as well. Placental abruptios are most prominent underneath a gradually developing infarct (Figure 362). The clot may be firm if the ablation occurred early. It may be dry and become brown after many hours. Eventually, the clot retracts and has the appearance of fibrinous strands.

Initially, there is a depression with the clot, but it disappears as the overlying placenta infarcts and then atrophies. In old or small abruptions, only minor color changes and infarcts are seen at the maternal aspect of the placenta. When toxemia is the cause of abruptio, the hemorrhage presumably begins with the decidual vascular lesions described above. Thrombosis of the decidual arterioles may lead to decidual necrosis and to subsequent venous hemorrhage (see also Harris et al., 1985). Boe (1951) illustrated the rupture of a spiral arteriole with thrombosis as the cause of a case of abruptio. The patient was not described as being preeclamptic, and several smaller decidual hemorrhages were found. When Hill and Brunton (1968) performed arteriography in pregnant patients, their results suggested that future abruptios could be anticipated because of poor vascular perfusion. It is now agreed that abruptio placentae occurs with increasing frequency in patients with chronic hypertension. Whether the ablation is due to hypertension or to a putative release of vasoactive agents after abruption has been discussed by several investigators. Abdella et al. (1984) spoke out in favor of hypertension as causing the hemorrhage, a point we also espouse. This theory is further supported by the relatively common findings of abruptios

FIGURE 362. Abruptio placentae with a layered retroplacental clot (right) and an adjacent sickle-shaped old
(white) infarct in a patient with preeclampsia.

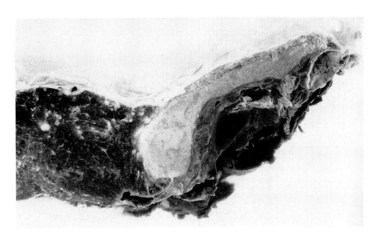

attending pregnancies that are complicated by
pheochromocytomas.

Because abruptio poses a major threat to fetal and
maternal survival, therapeutic regimens have been carefully considered. Sholl (1987) suggested that treatment
should be given according to the gestational age at
which the abruptio occurs. Preterm abruptions, which
often are associated with a poor obstetrical history
and with maternal smoking, may respond to tocolysis;
however, it is a complex clinical problem not easily
discussed fully in this context. Sholl found that his
overall fetal mortality was 17%. He advised the use
of ultrasonography. Cardwell (1987) also made the
diagnosis by ultrasound examination in eight patients
and found significant fetomaternal hemorrhage with the
abruptio. One fetus lost 72 ml into the maternal circulation. Coen et al. (1974) described the remarkable
survival of a 1,630 g premature infant delivered after 75
minutes of complete abruption. They believed that the
attending hypothermia may have aided this infant.
Equally remarkable is the patient described by Lopez-
Zeno et al. (1990). In their case, the fatal injury to the
mother occurred 47 minutes before cesarean delivery,
and the infant was born 22 minutes after maternal
cardiac arrest had occurred. Follow-up at 18 months
revealed no neurological deficit, although focal central nervous system infarction was seen by computed
tomography scan at 5 weeks. Neonatal shock due to
anemia or hypoxia is often a life-threatening problem
for the fetus (Haupt, 1963). Waddington (1957) found
254 abruptios of normally implanted placentas among
26,358 deliveries (1:104). There was one maternal
death and 83.5% fetal survival when aggressive management was used, but only 72.7% fetal survival with passive management. Waddington observed three cases of
Couvelaire uterus and one coagulation defect in this
group of patients. In a prospective study, Naeye et al.
(1977) found an incidence of 3.96 per 1,000 perinatal

deaths due to abruptio. They identified high usage of
cigarettes by the mothers and poor maternal weight
gains during pregnancy. Fetuses often suffered growth
retardation. Important maternal complications are
defibrination (Wisot, 1969) and renal necrosis due to
disseminated intravascular coagulation (DIC) (Sanerkin
& Evans, 1965; Carter, 1967). Impressive deposits of
fibrin may be found in the renal vessels and in other
organs of such patients (Schmorl, 1893; Schneider,
1951). Endotoxin shock is often observed, which has
led to considerations that toxemia of pregnancy results
from a generalized Shwartzman reaction (McKay et al.,
1959). Vassalli et al. (1963) observed deposits of fibrin
and some γ-globulin in the glomeruli of patients with
preeclampsia. The clinical relevance of this finding was
discussed by Dunlop et al. (1978), who found no coagulation problems in patients with essential hypertension.

Kåregård and Gennser (1986) reported an 0.44%
incidence of abruptio in a large Swedish cohort, with
20.2% fetal mortality. Of interest in this study is that a
history of abruptio increased the risk for subsequent
abruptio 10.2-fold. Male conceptuses and twins were
overrepresented among abruptios. In a discussion of
this paper, Grossman and Goldberg (1987) suggested
that the recurrence rate may relate to a high level of
anti-H-Y antibodies, which they found in a patient
with three abruptios. On rare occasions, abruptio with
defibrination occurs long after fetal death (Schneider,
1953). One type of abruptio that has been referred to in
the obstetrical literature is that associated with marked
prematurity and chorioamnionitis (Vintzileos et al.,
1987). We believe that this entity is misdiagnosed as
abruptio because of the presence of a clot accompanying
the placenta. When the placenta is carefully examined,
one finds that the hemorrhage and clot came from
the inflamed decidua capsularis, rather than from a
retroplacental location. Thus the appellation abruptio is
inappropriate.

Fetal Effects of Abruptio Placentae

Early studies suggested that maternal eclampsia may result in vascular damage of their fetuses (König, 1956). This author demonstrated hyalinization and coagulation of small cerebral vessels in such an infant. In a study of 34 cases of placenta previa and 64 cases of abruptio placentae, Robbins et al. (1967) found a high incidence of late cerebral abnormalities of the infants at 1 year of age. Haile (1940) described an infant with eclamptic liver necrosis and referred to the few other reports in the literature of similar injuries. The kidneys were normal, and it is doubtful to us that a coagulation disorder existed in the fetus similar to that observed with maternal DIC. It is not uncommon for neonates, dying from many disorders, to suffer DIC, as was shown by Bleyl and Büsing (1969) and other authors. There are many sporadic reports, however, of thrombocytopenia and other hematological disorders in neonates of mothers with preeclampsia (Mirro & Brown, 1982; Schmidt et al., 1986). Severe defibrination (unmeasurable levels) following abruptio was reported by Edson et al. (1968). The relation of fetal coagulation events in preeclampsia was studied more systematically by Weiner and Keller (1986). They found lowered antithrombin III activity and high fibrinopeptide A concentrations in preeclamptic women; paired samples from fetuses showed normal values. Lau et al. (1964) found abruptio primarily in conjunction with toxemia and reported 68% fetal mortality and 35 maternal deaths among their 100 cases.

Other Placental Changes in Preeclampsia

Aside from the liability of infarcts, abruptio, and the nearly invariable decidual vascular alterations, the placenta of toxemia of pregnancy undergoes some additional and mostly minor structural changes. More often than not, the placenta is smaller and "drier" than expected for that gestational age. When sectioned, the toxemic patient's placenta is much darker than normal organs, reflecting the hemoconcentration of the fetus. Siegel (1962), who unsuccessfully attempted to correlate preeclamptic retinal changes with the degree of toxemia, depicted most of the classical degenerative changes in the placenta. Teasdale (1985) performed histomorphometric studies of the placentas in patients with severe preeclampsia and with moderate fetal growth retardation. He measured a variety of structural features and found only minor quantitative differences from normal controls. Schuhmann and Lehmann (1973) correlated maternal urinary estriol excretion, DHA conversion, and placental morphology with fetal outcome. They found a lack of any such predictability for fetal outcome and suggested that the outcome is primarily dependent on clinical management. Considerably lighter placentas and fetuses were found in hypertensive patients in a study of Cibils (1974). He made teased villous preparations and observed them with a stereomicroscope. There was considerably increased budding of the syncytium in these placentas, similar to the Tenney-Parker change already discussed.

Prominence of syncytial buds has been observed ever since Schmorl (1893) first drew attention to these cells in the pulmonary vessels of patients who died from eclampsia. Earlier, these cells had been interpreted as necrotic, embolized liver cells, but this interpretation was not borne out by Schmorl's detailed studies. Syncytial embolism to the lung is now accepted to be a normal feature of all pregnancies (Bardawil & Toy, 1959; Attwood & Park, 1961). Because these cells have no reproductive potential, they die in situ. In patients with toxemia, and particularly eclampsia, there is enhanced embolization of syncytial cells. Occasional authors have even suggested that excessive pulmonary embolization with syncytial buds may be a cause of maternal death (Marcuse, 1954; Roffman & Simons, 1969). The association of these giant cells in these cases with fibrin thrombi is impressive but does not prove that they have been the cause of DIC in the patients. Jäämeri et al. (1965) found a markedly increased number of circulating syncytial cells in the blood of toxemic patients compared to those seen in normal pregnant women. Iklé (1961, 1964) provided a methodology for the isolation of these cells from the blood and estimated that approximately 100,000 such cells are liberated daily during pregnancy. Wagner (1968) and Wagner et al. (1964) thought that release of these cells was uncommon unless the uterus was "manipulated," and they reported an impressive degree of embolization during curettage for hydatidiform mole. Tedeschi and Tedeschi (1963) showed experimentally that these cells were swiftly disposed of in the lung. Most recently, these cells have been studied with flow cytometry and their DNA content displayed; the suggestion has been made that they might serve as a means for prenatal cytogenetic diagnosis (Covone et al., 1984). Rushton (1984) rightly pointed out, however, that the syncytium has no reproductive potential and is, at present at least, incapable of serving this cytogenetic purpose. It could serve for polymerase chain reaction (PCR) and fluorescence in situ hybridization (FISH), studies, but the cells rarely traverse the lung to become accessible in peripheral blood. Cameron and Park (1965) showed embolized decidua in the lung at necropsy of two pregnant women.

Tenney and Parker (1940) had emphasized that the increased budding of placental syncytium is characteristic of preeclampsia. It is so significant that we now call this finding the Tenney-Parker change. It features

FIGURE 363. Excessive syncytial knotting (budding, sprouting) associated with a 25-week gestation in a pre-eclamptic patient. Almost every tertiary villus has a densely clumped agglomeration of syncytial nuclei and little cytoplasm. H&E. ×160.

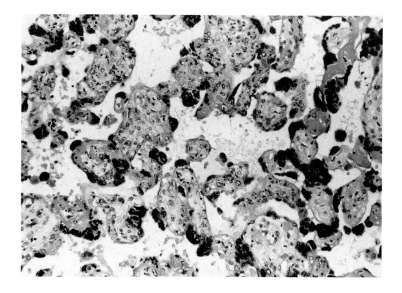

bunching of syncytial cytoplasm and agglomeration of nuclei, which produces characteristic knots at the villous surface (Figure 363). Although some such knots are normally found in preterm and term placentas, their number is much increased in the presence of toxemia. Often this change has incorrectly been referred to as "premature aging" of the villous tissue. The knots may result initially from a loss of villous fluid, and secondary buckling of the covering trophoblast follows. There are also changes of the amount of cytotrophoblast proliferation with subsequent proliferation of syncytium, as discussed earlier. The mechanism of this villous change was studied in vitro by Tominaga and Page (1966). They perfused human placental tissue and observed the response to varying oxygen concentrations of the perfusate. Hypoxia led to vasodilatation of fetal capillaries, and high oxygen-saturation produced fetal capillary vasoconstriction. In long-term organ culture, the reduction of oxygen saturation from 26% to 6% led to the bunching of syncytial nuclei and thinning of the villous trophoblastic covering. This change was found to be reversible when oxygen was increased again. Others have not been able to repeat the reversibility aspect of these experiments (Ong & Burton, 1991). There are light microscopic similarities between the maternal vascular disease of preeclampsia and that of circulating lupus anticoagulant. It must be emphasized that these changes of toxemia are also present in immature placentas in which ordinarily little syncytial budding would be seen. In our experience, when more than 30% of tertiary villi possess syncytial buds, especially in the premature placenta, it is diagnostic of a perfusional compromise. Such features may be associated with abruptio placentae (Figure 364) and can also be seen in the vicinity of fresh infarcts (Figure 365). Alvarez and his colleagues (1967, 1969, 1970) related knotting to an

altered maternal arterial pressure and further supported the notion that it is a diagnostic feature of toxemia; they also quantitated the budding by use of phase contrast microscopy. Aladjem (1967b) made similar observations and suggested that this syncytial change is not caused by cell degeneration. There is also no occlusion of fetal vessels. The sprouting is considered to be an adaptive change to altered maternal blood flow or oxygen content of intervillous blood. Aladjem differentiated between buds and sprouts and called this phenomenon sprouting. Fox (1970) kept villi in organ culture for 10 days; he found markedly increased tritiated thymidine incorporation into cytotrophoblast when the organ culture was hypoxic. This finding suggested to him that the response represents repair of damaged syncytium. A study by Howard et al. (1987) showed that cotyledons, perfused in vitro, responded to hypoxia with acute vasoconstriction rather than the earlier suggested dilatation. This report accords well with findings by Doppler velocimetry, in which maternal and umbilical arterial blood flows were found to be reduced in hypertensive patients who ultimately delivered growth-retarded infants (Giles et al., 1985; Ducey et al., 1987; Hanretti et al., 1988; and critique by Pearce & McParland, 1988). Such clinical studies have led to new insights and a more reliable categorization of risk in hypertensive pregnancies. Rauramo and Forss (1988) have used Doppler velocimetry to show that exercise by women with toxemia and pregnancy diabetes may have a significant deleterious effect on uterine blood flow.

Maternal fibronectin levels are elevated in the presence of preeclampsia, but Anunciado et al. (1987) showed, with fluorescent antibodies, that the villous vascular fibronectin content is decreased. By the use of histochemical techniques, Wielenga and Willighagen

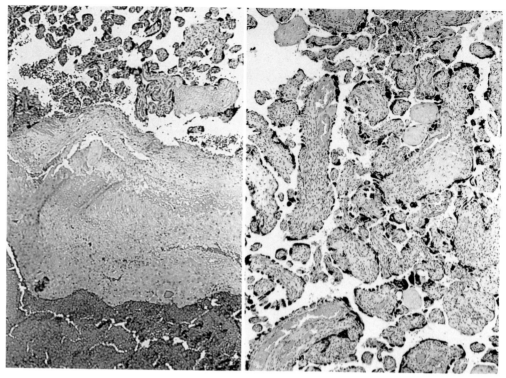

FIGURE 364. Placenta from a 28-week gestation with preeclampsia and abruptio placentae (left). Typical Tenney-Parker change is present in the prematurely "aged" villi. H&E. Left ×16; right ×100.

(1966) demonstrated that toxemic placentas have characteristic losses of enzymes; this change was apparent in areas that required histochemical methods for detection of tissue ischemia. With severe toxemia, the disease process was manifested by increased placental lactate production (Ginsburg & Jeacock, 1967). Furthermore, there are profound microangiopathic alterations of maternal erythrocytes (Cunningham et al., 1985).

Several electron microscopic studies have compared villi of normal placentas with those from preeclamptic patients. No characteristic findings were made in the PIH study reported by Zacks and Blazar (1963).

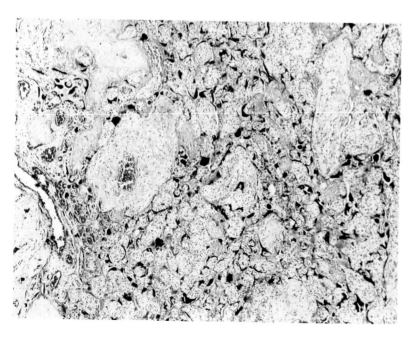

FIGURE 365. Fresh placental infarct, perhaps 1 day old. The intervillous space is obliterated, many villi lack circulation, and preexisting syncytial knotting (Tenney-Parker change) is present. The patient had toxemia of pregnancy. H&E. ×16.

Anderson and McKay (1966) found an increase in cytotrophoblast, thickening of villous basement membranes, and an increase in "bulbous syncytial microvilli." They suggested that only quantitative changes occur but none that characterize the diseased organ. When MacLennan et al. (1972) kept villous tissue in culture for prolonged periods, degenerative changes occurred in the syncytium. The appearances resembled hypoxic alterations seen with preeclampsia. In order to avoid secondary artifacts, Pavelka et al. (1979) obtained biopsy specimens from preeclamptic patients' placentas at cesarean section. They observed a loss of architecture, fibrin deposition, reduction in microvilli, and dilatation of endoplasmic reticulum and of the Golgi apparatus of the syncytium. Their photographs provide superior detail. Similar results were obtained by Jones and Fox (1980), who like most authors came to the conclusion that the lesions are all explicable on the basis of reduced perfusion by maternal blood.

Etiology of Toxemia, PIH, or Preeclampsia

The principal cause of preeclampsia is still unknown. Although it is certain that the disease relates to the presence of placental tissue, the proximate cause is obscure. The fact that the delivery of the placenta (or hydatidiform mole) ends the disease process speaks for this causal relation, however, and many theories have been advanced to explain the mechanism that leads to the symptomatology and pathological features of toxemia. We briefly describe only three of the most recent hypotheses and give references to the general literature. A general review is available by Cunningham and Lindheimer (1992).

1. Lueck et al. (1983) proposed that preeclampsia was the result of an infection by a worm-like "agent." They identified these structures from the peripheral blood of toxemic patients. In a later paper (Aladjem et al., 1983) the authors believed to have shown that they induced a toxemia-like syndrome in dogs by injecting these animals with blood from toxemic patients. These observations caused much subsequent work to be done and provoked intense discussion. Several investigators then found that males have similar structures in the serum (Gau et al., 1983). The structures are now considered to be artifacts of the preparative procedures (Long et al., 1984; Ayala et al., 1986). They do not represent the cause of preeclampsia.

2. The possibility that toxemia of pregnancy represents an immune-mediated disorder has long been an attractive consideration. As was previously discussed in this chapter, immune complexes have been localized in the spiral arterioles of the placental bed and in the renal glomeruli of patients with preeclampsia. Moreover, the lesions of lupus anticoagulant, a condition with identifiable "irregular" antibodies, are indistinguishable from those of toxemia of pregnancy. Hulka and Brinton (1963) suggested that circulating fluorescein-conjugated antibodies localize on trophoblast and signify an immunological conflict. That subsequent pregnancies of patients with toxemia in their first gestation are usually not affected, was overlooked. Sophian (1964) appropriately criticized this simplistic explanation. Much conflicting evidence of the alleged immunopathologic etiology has since been gathered in efforts to clarify this situation. Kitzmiller et al. (1973), Balasch et al. (1981), and Rote and Caudle (1983) found no elevation of complement titers in toxemic pregnancies. Their results

were countered by studies of Vasquez-Escobosa et al. (1982) and Massobrio et al. (1985), who found significant levels of various immunoglobulins and immune complexes in patients with severe toxemia. Alanen et al. (1984), on the other hand, found only a slight increase in circulating immune complexes in patients with severe preeclampsia. Perhaps the tests are not sensitive enough, or they are too dissimilar for the consistent demonstration of an immune reaction. At present, they do not offer much support for the idea that toxemia has an immunological origin.

Two large reviews in 1976 weighed the evidence for and against an immunological disorder. While Scott and Beer (1976) found some relation to a disturbance in the blocking antibodies that normally are believed to protect against placental rejection, their conclusion was that there is no major immunological etiology in toxemia. Scott and Jenkins (1976) elicited evidence for a genetic predisposition; they concluded that the disease probably has a multifactorial etiology. Some support for a genetic predisposition also comes from the findings of Redman et al. (1978); they found that toxemia occurred more often in women who had only one HLA B antigen locus. Perhaps homozygosity at the HLA locus enhances the possibility of developing the disease. Against a simple genetic etiology are the findings of discordance in monozygotic twins and other observations recorded by Thornton and Sampson (1990). Scott and Jenkins (1976) and Willems (1977) postulated a relation to an inadequate production of blocking antibodies in PIH and suggested a possible immunization procedure for the prevention of preeclampsia. Circulating antigen–antibody complexes were sought in toxemic patients by Knox et al. (1978). None was found. McLaughlin et al. (1979), on the other hand, did find circulating complexes in toxemic women and offered suggestions for a resolution of the discrepancies that exist in the literature.

Attention was then directed to study of the cellular components that are often present at the placental–uterine interphase. Scott et al. (1978) reviewed that evidence and found many articles to support the notion that disturbed lymphocyte function exists in association with toxemia. Specifically, it was suggested that patients who exhibit the disease have a high degree of immunological compatibility with their fetus. Hoff and Bixler (1984), from ABO antigen studies of a large cohort, deduced that "the greater the potential for an immune response of the mother to the ABO and HY antigens, the lower is the likelihood of preeclampsia developing in the first pregnancy...." Birkeland and Kristofferson (1979) observed that with toxemia there is a marked hyporesponsiveness of maternal lymphocytes to PHA stimulation. Subsequently, similar findings by Griffin and Wilson (1979) favored the interpretation that this alteration in lymphocyte behavior "may be a consequence rather than the cause of their clinical disease." It should be noted, however, that Musci et al. (1988) found in the serum of preeclamptic patients an increased amount of mitogen. They postulated that this is the result of release from damaged endothelium that occurs in this disease. While Sridama et al. (1983) found a significant decrease in circulating T cells with preeclampsia, there was no good correlation of the severity of the disease with the number of T cells. Moreover, the ratio of helper to suppressor cells was undisturbed. Toder et al. (1983) found the natural killer (NK) cell activity to be increased with toxemia, and that these cells had been preactivated. The question of a change in lymphocyte populations was addressed by Gusdon et al. (1984) using monoclonal antibodies against specific subpopulations of cells. They found that the OKM1 population was normally significantly reduced during the third trimester but not in preeclamptic patients. These cells mediate NK cell activity and antibody-dependent cellular cytotoxicity. Khong (1987) investigated the in situ population of cells that infiltrates the placental attachment site. He was unable to identify any quantitative or qualitative difference between the populations in normal versus preeclamptic patients and suggested that the large population of macrophages may down-regulate a maternal immunological response. Many other contradictory investigations could be cited that serve to emphasize that the simple notion of toxemia, as an immunological disorder, may be erroneous. Kilpatrick (1987) effectively summarized some of these arguments. It should also be noted that recent evidence shows that the "labor-related stress significantly decreases the total number of neonatal T-lymphocytes and the CD4 (helper) T-cell subpopulation in cord blood" (Pittard et al., 1989). Finally, it has been suggested that placental isoferritin, known to be located in the syncytiotrophoblast, acts as an immune mediator during pregnancy. Maymon et al. (1989) found that in preeclamptic women the placental isoferritin concentration in serum was low (7.5 U/ml), compared to that during normal pregnancy (81.6 U/ml) and at term delivery (54.8 U/ml). They suggested it as a useful marker for toxemia.

3. In recent years more attention has been paid to the possibility that preeclampsia may be the result of reduced prostacyclin production or at least that an imbalance of prostaglandin secretion exists. Moreover, as Brosens et al. (1974) pointed out, the response of uterine vessels to vasoactive agents may be significantly different in toxemia, as the "second wave" of trophoblast invasion fails to alter myometrial vessels and so leaves them responsive to constrictive agents. Specifically, lowered prostacyclin production by the placenta and enhanced thromboxane A_2 production have been delineated in numerous detailed studies. Prostacyclin binding and its half-life are reduced during pregnancy. O'Brien et al. (1988) have shown that this decrease is variable, perhaps accounting for some of the conflicting results obtained in the past. There is a significant decrease of prostacyclin in hypertensive pregnancy, which may explain some of the clinical findings in this disease. These aspects have been reviewed. Ylikorkala and Mäkilä (1985) and Mäkilä et al. (1986) discussed their clinical implications.

Demers and Gabbe (1976) found that placentas from preeclamptic women have significantly less prostaglandin E (PGE), and vasoconstrictive PGF is much increased. A marked reduction of prostacyclin production was found in growth-retarded neonates whose mothers had suffered hypertension and preeclampsia (Stuart et al., 1981). Importantly, this reduction was not confined to patients with toxemia. A review of prostaglandins during pregnancy (Anonymous, 1982) brought all findings together and suggested that experimental prostacyclin infusion in preeclampsia may have a beneficial effect. In this review it was suggested that "if normal pregnancy, like normal processes in general, is under the fine control of enzyme systems, abnormal pregnancy, like many other disease states, may reflect the relatively uncontrolled activity of free radicals." Hollister et al. (1988), on the other hand, found that prostacyclin infusion into pregnant sheep did not increase placental vasodilation. Mäkilä et al. (1984) showed that the deficiency of prostacyclin (PGI_2) in preeclampsia is specific for the disease, and that it is not the result of the mode of delivery or anesthesia. Erskine et al. (1985) found evidence to suggest that altered ratios of certain plasma phospholipids may be a useful predictor for the likely development of preeclampsia. In a detailed study of prostacyclin production by placenta, amnion, and chorion, Walsh et al. (1985) showed a marked reduction of the toxemic placenta to produce this enzyme; amnion and chorion did not show this alteration. Jeremy et al. (1986) confirmed this study and offered comments. The deficiency of prostacyclin in toxemia correlates well with its known platelet aggregation effect and hypertension. Prostacyclin has the effect of preventing both of these effects. Walsh (1985) had suggested that preeclampsia represents an imbalance of prostacyclin ($\downarrow$) and thromboxane A_2

($\uparrow$) production. He supported this suggestion with experimental findings. The recognition of these complex interactions has led to successful preventive therapy by Beaufils et al. (1985). Early in pregnancy, they gave antiplatelet medication (150 mg aspirin and 300 mg dipyridamole daily) to mothers who were at high risk for toxemia. They suggested that this treatment prevented toxemia and fetal growth retardation. More extensive studies have borne their theory out, selectively suppressing maternal platelet thromboxane B_2 or (A_2) production (Benigni et al., 1989; Schiff et al., 1989; Uzan et al., 1991). It has also been found that low-dose aspirin inhibits the production of thromboxane from placental surface arteries, whereas the production of prostacyclin is not disturbed (Thorp et al., 1988). Friedman (1988) provided a comprehensive review of all these aspects concerning mediators and their relation to PIH. Rosenfeld (1988) added to this review; he pointed out that during pregnancy angiotension is vasoconstrictive rather than vasodilatory. The primary derangement of these enzymatic changes remains unknown. The interactions of endothelial cell prostanoid release with leukotrienes and complement are probably important (Lundberg et al., 1986; Pober, 1988; Fitzgerald et al., 1990). These topics are being actively investigated in an attempt to unravel the mysteries of this common disease.

4. Other theories concerning the etiology of PIH are too numerous to mention. The idea of excessive salt intake as a cause of toxemia was reviewed by Robinson (1958) and Chalmers (1988) has commented on the subject. The conclusion is that although salt regulation during pregnancy has not been accorded needed attention its causal role for PIH is not secure. Bartholomew et al. (1957) opined that the toxemic aspects of the disease were due to necrosis of placental tissue. This possibility is unlikely because many patients with severe toxemia have few or even no placental infarcts at the time of their first symptoms, and death of one twin's placenta does not induce the disease.

Lupus Erythematosus and Lupus Anticoagulant

Lupus Erythematosus

Systemic lupus erythematosus (SLE) occurs primarily in young women, and it often complicates pregnancy. It has been speculated that this autoimmune disorder is so much more common in women than in men (10:1) because of their sensitization to nuclear antigens to which they are exposed during menstruation (Dameshek, 1958; Grimes et al., 1985; Hulka, 1985). Estrogens exacerbate the disease, because they have a "potent influence on the immune system and therefore an effect on disease processes" (Hayslett & Reece, 1985). These authors reviewed reports of the influence of pregnancy on the course of SLE and found that in 25% to 50% of patients with SLE the disease exacerbates or relapses with pregnancy. In addition, their review indicates that fetal survival is reduced because of an increased number of abortions, maternal renal insufficiency, and placental pregnancy complications. They suggested treatment regimens for women with SLE and pregnancy. It is now believed that pregnancy itself does not constitute a risk to patients with

SLE. Low-dose aspirin therapy is being used but not as yet fully evaluated (Editorial, 1991). Mund et al. (1963) found a 30% abortion rate when SLE began after conception, in contrast to a 14% rate when the disease was already established. A 66% fetal loss among SLE patients was reported by Schenker et al. (1972), who asserted that toxemia and renal disease were the most common complications.

Systemic lupus erythematosus is accompanied by a variety of circulating antibodies, the best known of which is the antinuclear antibody (ANA), which also elicits the LE phenomenon. That the destruction of nuclei and DNA is due to this antibody has been shown by Bennett et al. (1986). These authors identified a "functionally defective receptor for DNA" in most patients with SLE and were able to induce this defect by incubating healthy mononuclear cells with the circulating antibodies of patients with SLE. The defect was manifest by an impaired binding of exogenous DNA to the surfaces of peripheral mononuclear cells. It must be remembered, however, that up to 50% of clinically normal, pregnant women have ANAs at least once during the course of their pregnancy (Rosenberg et al., 1986). Lymphocytotoxic antibodies have been found in about 80% of patients with SLE (Pritchard et al., 1978). Other investigators have reported that these antibodies possess antitrophoblastic activity, which may possibly explain the poor pregnancy outcome that attends the disease (Bresnihan et al., 1977). This idea was particularly attractive because other inflammatory diseases, such as rheumatoid arthritis and scleroderma, are not associated with a high rate of abortion.

The placentas of five patients with SLE were studied by Grennan et al. (1978). They identified fluorescent antibodies against complexes to nuclear antigens on placental villous basement membranes. Grimmer et al. (1988) undertook further studies to define this antitrophoblastic activity. They found IgM antitrophoblast antibodies in a patient with thrombocytopenia and a rash who also exhibited circulating lupus anticoagulant activity, had a twin pregnancy, and had an intrauterine fetal demise. By immunofluorescent antibody techniques, they localized the factor to the placental syncytium and found C3 to be deposited on the basement membranes of villi. The studies were done with the patient's placenta as well as with normal placentas; small vessel deposition of the antibodies was also observed. IgG, IgA, and C3 deposits were not localized to these areas. The twin placenta of this pregnancy was 10% infarcted and had decidual necrosis, but it lacked vascular disease. Perhaps the absence of vascular disease was due to sampling technique, but the authors were cautious about interpreting their findings as having an etiological relation to the fetal demise. This point is particularly pertinent, as deposits of C3 on the villous

basement membranes have been observed in normal placentas (Johnson et al., 1977). The recognition of other circulating antibodies in SLE patients as possible causes of pregnancy mishaps is discussed below. It must be said, however, that despite all the findings of abnormal placentas in SLE, one encounters occasional patients who have neither decidual vascular lesions nor infarcts or fetal growth retardation with this condition. Presumably, these patients are in remission, despite the presence of specific antibodies. SLE patients who have no anticoagulant antibodies have fewer abortions (24.7%) than do those with the antibodies (58.7%) according to the retrospective study of Loizoll et al. (1988).

Some antibodies of patients with SLE are transferred to the fetus, who is often growth-retarded. These antibodies may cause thrombocytopenia, discoid lupus, and a variety of other conditions, including the LE phenomenon. We have seen a term infant weighing 2,000 g born to a mother with discoid lupus whose placenta possessed many infarcts and weighed only 320 g. There was intensive chronic deciduitis in the decidua basalis and decidua vera, with foci of old abruptio placentae. Atherosis was absent, but most decidual vascular walls were infiltrated by chronic inflammatory cells, among which plasma cells predominated. There also was diffuse, moderate chronic villitis. Beck et al. (1966) observed ANAs in neonates of women with SLE with titers approximately the same as those in the mother. Despite this finding, the three neonates they observed remained healthy. LE cells were repeatedly observed in the neonates of mothers with SLE, as reported by Mijer and Olsen (1958) and Gött (1969). These cells disappeared within 7 weeks after delivery, and the infants subsequently developed normally. Jackson (1964) described a third case of a newborn with discoid lupus delivered to a mother with SLE. The neonatal lesions disappeared within 5 months but left small scars. Congenital heart block in such offspring has recently caused concern and is estimated to occur in 1 of 60 SLE pregnancies (Editorial, 1991). Hull et al. (1966) reported a neonatal death; the mother had suffered SLE for 13 years and had been treated with chloroquine throughout pregnancy. The 2,500 g neonate was hydropic at birth, had a complete heart block (45/168 ventricular/atrial contractions), and had skin lesions. At autopsy there was patchy fibrosis of the myocardium. The placenta was bilobed, edematous, and "fibrous-friable." This constellation is now considered to be the "neonatal lupus syndrome." Provost et al. (1987) described two cases and reviewed the literature. In almost all cases, neonatal complications are associated with anti-U_1RNP antibodies, and the mother has anti-La(SS-B)and/or anti-Ro(SS-A) IgG antibodies. For this and other reasons, fetal surveillance has been recommended (Druzin et al., 1987). Another case of heart block was documented by Richards et al. (1990). Their primigravida was not known to have SLE when her fetus developed a complete heart block at 23 weeks' gestation and ascites at 26 weeks. Her ANA titer was then found to be 1:1024. Incipient hydrops led to treatment with betamethasone, which was followed by a reduction of signs of fluid accumulation; the authors attributed the reduction to transplacental steroid antiinflammatory action. The neonate delivered at 37 weeks with retained heart block but did well. Another case of fetal heart block was detailed by Silver et al. (1992a). It caused fetal death, presumably secondary to the extensive placental infarction (>80%) found. Thrombosed vessels with and without atherosis were present in the decidua basalis. In the atrial septum near Koch's triangle, dense fibrosis and calcification were identified and believed to have been responsible for the heart block. The mother possessed anti-Ro and anti-La antibodies. Seip (1960) and Cruveiller et al. (1970), among other investigators, have observed hemolytic anemia, rashes, thrombocytopenia, and leukopenia in neonates of mothers with SLE. Klippel et al. (1974) found inexplicable tubuloreticular cytoplasmic inclusions in the lymphocytes of neonates whose mothers had SLE.

The placentas of patients with SLE may be normal. More often they show changes that are frequently impossible to differentiate from the lesions of preeclampsia. It must be appreciated, however, that preeclampsia is frequently seen in patients with SLE, so it is thus difficult at times to know whether the placental pathology is due to preeclampsia or SLE. The infarctions and retarded placental growth are the result of decidual vascular lesions, which in turn are the cause of the fetal growth retardation found with SLE. Abramowsky and his colleagues (1980) studied ten placentas from patients with SLE and one placenta from a patient with discoid lupus. They found vascular lesions in five placentas. Two placentas exhibited more than 25% infarction, whereas the others showed only discolorations. The outstanding lesion was decidual arteriopathy, with fibrinoid necrosis and infiltration by inflammatory cells. Some vessels appeared aneurysmally dilated and had atherosis. No abruptions were seen grossly, but microscopic study indicated abruption in two cases. Infarction and "premature aging of villi" were the only other pathological findings. In two patients, immunofluorescence study showed massive deposition of IgM and a lesser amount of C3 in the decidual vascular walls. We have had similar experiences with SLE (Benirschke & Driscoll, 1967) and have suggested that the decidual lesions are best observed in retroplacental curettings. Alternatively, the place to find most decidual arterioles with these pathological changes is in the decidua capsularis of the membrane roll. These vessels have lesions similar to those in the maternal floor of the placenta. They are usually less readily found in the decidua basalis that comes with the delivered placenta because not enough of that decidua separates with delivery of the placenta. Moreover, in the floor of the placenta, fibrin and old clot from partial abruptions usually preclude adequate study. Postpartum curettage is required to obtain sufficient material for proper evaluation. Vascular lesions, including atherosis and thrombosis, are clearly the cause of the placental infarcts, the associated abruptions, and the reduced weights of the placenta and the fetus. Between the infarcts of affected placentas, the villous tissue displays Tenney-Parker changes—the increased syncytial knotting best known to accompany preeclampsia and due to reduced maternal perfusion of the intervillous space. This histological state is often referred to as "enhanced aging," but it is simply a reflection of reduced oxygen availability from the decreased intervillous blood flow. Thus there is no need to postulate that specific antitrophoblastic antibodies exert an additional or specific destructive effect. Figure 366 shows the macroscopic appearance of the placenta of a patient with SLE. There are numerous infarcts (55%), which caused fetal death. The placenta was multilobulated because numerous infarcts had caused early atrophy in many areas. The placenta of the case described by Hull et al. (1966) was bilobate, perhaps for the same reasons. Our patient had had a previous spontaneous abortion and a placenta with many decidual vascular lesions. Figures 367 to 370 illustrate vascular lesions of two other patients with SLE. In both cases, fetal death occurred at about 19 weeks' gestation. The macerated fetuses showed no lesions. The placentas were extensively infarcted, had several areas of abruptio, and showed Tenney-Parker changes. Although this change is most commonly seen with preeclampsia, it usually does not appear until the third trimester when pure preeclampsia complicates pregnancy most commonly. There was no clinical evidence of preeclampsia in these patients. Interestingly, with one of these cases mural thrombi were present in vessels of the umbilical cord and in vessels of the placental surface. Branch and Rodgers (1993) found that thrombosis occurred most likely as the result of antibodies to endothelial tissue factor expression.

Because many of these patients have had prednisolone therapy, it may be conjectured that some of the pathological changes can be attributed to this therapy. This question was investigated by Warrell and Taylor (1968). They studied 34 pregnancies of 30 women receiving prednisolone for asthma ($n = 18$), ulcerative colitis ($n = 2$), SLE ($n = 14$), eczema/urticaria ($n = 7$), and arthritis/sarcoidosis ($n = 3$). There were eight fetal deaths and nine fetuses who were at risk of "placental

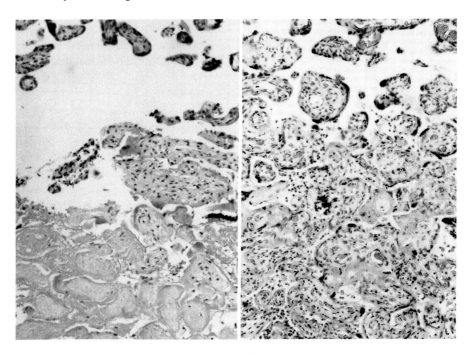

FIGURE 369. Microscopic aspect of villous tissue from the patient with SLE shown in Figure 368. Note the old and recent infarcts and the Tenney Parker change of viable villi. They have the appearance of term villi because of the loss of water and shrinkage. H&E. ×160.

bosis. Lazarchick and Kizer (1989) have given specific details of laboratory procedures necessary for the establishment of this diagnosis. They found that the dilute Russell viper venom test and the tissue thromboplastin inhibition test are sensitive assays. Nevertheless, in several patients the discordance of test results necessitated measurements of specific coagulation factors in order to establish the diagnosis. Apparently wide differences exist in laboratories reporting test results (Peaceman et al., 1992), which must be taken into consideration when prevalence figures and treatment results are evaluated. The antibodies are usually IgG molecules but may be also be IgM. They interfere with the phospholipid-dependent coagulation assays (see also Brandt et al., 1987). Usually considered to be in vitro phenomena (Woodhouse, 1984), their presence is indicative of diverse clinical states, such as thromboses, pregnancy wastage, polyneuritis, and sundry others. A comprehensive review of this complex topic has been provided by Triplett (1989). His paper not only summarizes the basis for the action of various antibodies (see also Reece et al., 1990) but provides a list of reports on pregnancies with and without therapy.

Numerous complications have attended pregnancies with CLAS antibodies, but then there are others in which no pathology is observed. Indeed, the case-control study by Infante-Rivard et al. (1991) indicated that "there is no apparent justification for considering lupus anticoagulants or IgG anticardiolipins to be risk factors for fetal loss among women who present with spontaneous abortion or fetal death and have had no previous spontaneous fetal loss." El-Roeiy and colleagues (1990) ascertained that in normal pregnancies, antiphospholipid antibodies are not observed. Their study also suggested that when these antibodies exist in low titers, they have little or no effect on pregnancy outcome. Aside from fetal wastage, now well recognized in these gestations, a maternal death (following fetal death) has also occurred. It happened in a patient who, at 1 day after the diagnosis of fetal death, suffered disseminated small-vessel thrombosis. Myopericarditis was present in the mother, who had sickle trait and presumably "occult" SLE (Bendon et al., 1987). Farquharson et al. (1985) had reported life-threatening thrombosis that necessitated therapeutic abortion in a pregnant patient. The authors suggested that immunosuppressive therapy may have to be initiated before pregnancy occurs in order to avoid such complications. Not all such patients have clinical symptoms. When abnormal immunological findings with "irregular antibodies" are present in pregnant patients, such as an unexpectedly positive VDRL, further investigation is required. This situation necessitates especially a search for the presence of lupus anticoagulant and anticardiolipins. In the patient just described, many myometrial vessels had lesions at the placental floor; one-third of the placenta had infarcts (30%), and an abruptio placentae was found. The mother also had myocardial

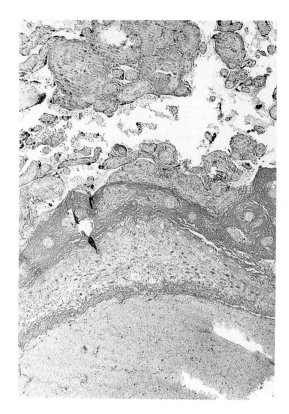

FIGURE 370. Fresh abruptio placentae from a patient with SLE. There is minimal infarction of villous tissue (same case as in Figure 367). The retroplacental clot (below) is elevating the decidua basalis. These changes usually preclude one from observing the vascular lesions in the decidua basalis. H&E. ×60.

and renal lesions. Lockshin et al. (1989) evaluated therapy in 21 patients with high antiphospholipid antibodies and one prior fetal death. They concluded that prednisone does not improve outcome and may in fact worsen it. Branch et al. (1989) showed that an association of antiphospholipid antibodies exists also with severe toxemia of pregnancy, and they suggested that it is one more reason to consider an immune hypothesis for both diseases.

Although there is this well known relation of such irregular antibodies to recurrent fetal wastage, the prevalence of the various types has been disputed and, most importantly, it had not been known if the existence of one or the other types of antibody spells a more sinister prognosis. The study conducted by Lockwood et al. (1989) corrected this deficiency. They ascertained the presence of lupus anticoagulant and anticardiolipin antibodies in a low-risk population and found 2 of 737 patients to have lupus anticoagulant and recurrent abortions. Conversely, 16 of 737 patients had anticardiolipins; 4 of these patients had uncomplicated pregnancies, and 12 had various complications. The authors

concluded that the presence of antiphospholipid antibodies was correlated with unfavorable pregnancy outcome, and that their prevalence is in the range of 0.3%. Two cases of fetal stroke, recognized only later during the neonatal period, were attributed by Silver et al. (1992b) to anticardiolipin antibodies.

Investigations regarding the nature of the CLAS began with the identification of a patient by Nilsson et al. (1975). That mother experienced three pregnancies with intrauterine deaths, and she had circulating lupus anticoagulants. The authors indicated that a relation may exist between this antibody and placental infarction. McVerry et al. (1980) then reported two patients with deficient prostacyclin (PGI_2) production and SLE. Soon after, there was a report of a patient with a history of arterial thromboses, fetal death at 23 weeks, and CLAS (Carreras et al., 1981a). Decreased prostacyclin release could be elicited from that mother's IgG fraction when aortic strips were incubated. The same authors found that 2 of 24 women with repeated abortions, intrauterine fetal growth retardation, and fetal death had lupus anticoagulants (Carreras et al., 1981b). Many reports of essentially similar findings have since followed, as for instance the demonstration by Xu et al. (1990) of the prevalence of low-titer ANA-positive serum in patients with pregnancy losses. There was also a controlled multicenter study by Out et al. (1992) demonstrating conclusively that possession of antiphospholipid antibodies was "a risk factor for adverse pregnancy outcome." Buchanan et al. (1992), who investigated 100 lupus pregnancies with antiphospholipid antibodies, found an 81% pregnancy loss.

Once the causative relation of CLAS to repetitive pregnancy failure had been recognized, various forms of therapy were tried. Lubbe et al. (1963), who treated six patients with CLAS, successfully achieved suppression of the anticoagulant with prednisone therapy. On the other hand, Prentice et al. (1984) managed 15 patients who had three successful pregnancies without immunosuppressive therapy; the results reported by Carp et al. (1989) were much less optimistic. This discrepancy emphasizes the erratic nature of CLAS antibodies in predicting outcome and possibly the differences in laboratory evaluation of this problem. In a later publication, Lubbe and Liggins (1985) reviewed their experience with 49 patients who had 160 unsuccessful pregnancies. They recommended prednisone (40–60 mg/day) and aspirin (75 mg/day) therapy for the management of such pregnancies. Rouget et al. (1982) observed a familial case of anticoagulant in mother and daughter. Branch et al. (1985) reported the frequency of preeclampsia in these patients and recommended steroid and aspirin therapy to improve fetal outcome. The addition of immunoglobulin infusion in the therapy of such patients has been advocated by Wapner et al.

FIGURE 371. Retroplacental hemorrhage with 50% infarction in a 30-week gestation placenta with maternal anticardiolipin antibodies. The 700 g infant survived.

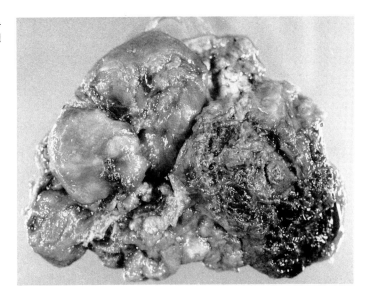

(1989). Unander et al. (1987) studied the sera of 99 patients with habitual abortion and found elevated anticardiolipin antibodies in 42 patients. There was concomitant low C4 activity. Because it is well known that protein C deficiency may lead to thromboses, Cariou et al. (1986) studied the interaction of anticoagulants and protein C. They found inhibition of protein C activation by the antibodies and suggested that it acts against thrombomodulin or its phospholipid moiety. Considerations of the mechanisms of action of the various antibodies in CLAS have been reviewed by Reece et al. (1984) and Lockwood et al. (1986). Two reports have suggested that treatment with high doses of γ-globulin (IgG) not only lowers the levels of antiphospholipid antibodies but also results in improved fetal salvage in severely compromised patients (Carreras et al., 1988; Scott et al., 1988). An interesting "natural experiment" was reported by Stormorken et al. (1988): A patient who had four consecutive miscarriages with the anticoagulant syndrome had a normal, term pregnancy because the mother had spontaneously developed anti-factor II antibody, which had led to hypoprothrombinemia with marked anticoagulation. The authors suggested that one should infer from this case the need for anticoagulation in the usual cases where lupus anticoagulant complicates pregnancy. Randomized trials and prospective studies of the efficacy of various modes of treatment have shown that low-dose aspirin is preferable to prednisone (Cowchock et al., 1992) and that fewer placental infarcts occurred with heparin therapy (Rosove et al., 1990). It has also been suggested that the frequently premature rupture of membranes is related to prednisone medication.

The placenta in patients with CLAS is morphologically indistinguishable from that of patients with severe preeclampsia. With CLAS, the extensive placental infarction and decidual vascular lesions are often found at much younger gestational ages than is the case for preeclampsia. Frequently, the lesions occur before the 20th week of pregnancy. De Wolf et al. (1982) first drew attention to the decidual vascular lesions in this condition. They found multiple microthrombi and typical atherosis in a placenta that had 50% infarction. The authors suggested that because prostacyclin ordinarily is the most important inhibitor of platelet aggregation antibodies to this agent may be held responsible for the thrombosis. Gleicher and Friberg (1985), and Silver (1988) also reported CLAS associated with atherosis and massive placental infarction. The review by Triplett (1989) provides a good chronology of these discoveries. As was mentioned earlier, there is probably no need to incriminate the anti-trophoblastic antibodies detected by Grimmer et al. (1988) in the causality of fetal demise. The degree of infarction and compromise of the intervillous circulation adequately explain resultant stillbirth and growth retardation (Polzin, 1991). Such a placenta is shown in Figure 371. It is the placenta of a severely growth-retarded fetus (30 weeks, 700 g) with placental abruptio and 50% infarction in addition to a velamentous insertion of the umbilical cord. There were many decidual vessels with atherosis, thrombosis, and hyalinization of the thickened walls. The mother had anticardiolipin antibodies but no symptoms of SLE, and the fetus survived. We have also seen atherosis in the decidual vessels of a patient with CLAS, whose pregnancy was considered to have been successfully treated; thus the degree of recognizable vascular lesions in the decidua often does not correspond precisely to the degree of growth retardation of fetus and placenta. Whereas the finding of vascular lesions confirms the diagnosis of CLAS when preeclampsia is absent, it is probably the extent of decidual compromise that de-

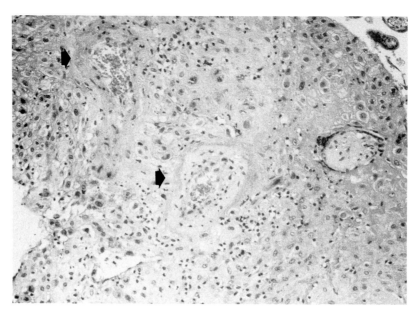

FIGURE 372. Decidua basalis of patient with lupus anticoagulant at 25 weeks' gestation. Decidual arterioles (arrows) show mild mural thrombosis and fibrin deposits, although the placenta was 25% infarcted. H&E. ×160.

termines the fetal and placental growth and pregnancy outcome. However, the degree of vasculopathy is highly variable. It is often difficult to assess quantitatively unless one has adequate placental site curettings available for interpretation. Figure 372 shows mild arteriopathy in the floor of an extensively infarcted placenta. The fetus was stillborn at 25 weeks, but the extent of atherosis poorly correlated with the 25% infarction found in the placenta. Several reviews of the vascular control of placental blood flow are available, especially those by Ylikorkala and Mäkilä (1985) and Mäkilä et al. (1986). These authors suggested that because decidual spiral arterioles are already optimally dilated during pregnancy two agents, prostacyclin and thromboxane A_2, are used to regulate the intervillous blood flow. A disturbance of their finely tuned balance, as accomplished by the antiprostacyclin activity of lupus anticoagulant, may be the principal cause of hypoperfusion of placenta and the subsequent infarction of placental tissue. It is also the best explanation for the efficacy of treatment with aspirin (150 mg/day) and dipyridamole (300 mg/day) in women with preeclampsia or CLAS. Peaceman and Rehnberg (1993) showed that after incubation of the immunoglobulin G fraction of patients with lupus anticoagulant with placental extracts from normal gestations thromboxane was significantly increased.

In addition to decidual vessels with thromboses, vascular occlusions have been observed in the fetus when maternal CLAS was present. Sheridan-Pereira et al. (1988) reported a neonate with aortic thrombosis. We know of a similar case that will soon be re-

ported (Kaplan, personal communication). That fetus had carotid artery obliteration and consequent brain necrosis. As mentioned earlier, Silver et al. (1992b) attributed the cerebral infarction in two infants to transplacentally transmitted antibodies. Trudinger et al. (1988) suggested that the abnormal umbilical artery flow velocity waveforms they identified were the result of "vascular sclerosis evident in the small arteries of the tertiary villi." We have not been able to observe such lesions in the many cases of CLAS we have seen. In our opinion, the degree of infarction and shrinkage of surviving villi associated with the decidual arteriopathy are sufficient to explain the abnormal blood flow.

References

Abdella, T.N., Sibai, B.M., Hays, J.M., and Anderson, G.D.: Relationship of hypertensive disease to abruptio placentae. Obstet. Gynecol. 63:365–370, 1984.

Abitbol, M.M., Driscoll, S.G., and Ober, W.B.: Placental lesions in experimental toxemia in the rabbit. Am. J. Obstet. Gynecol. 125:942–948, 1976a.

Abitbol, M.M., Gallo, G.R., Pirani, C.L., and Ober, W.B.: Production of experimental toxemia in the pregnant rabbit. Am. J. Obstet. Gynecol. 124:460–470, 1976b.

Abitbol, M.M., Pirani, C.L., Ober, W.B., Driscoll, S.G., and Cohen, M.W.: Production of experimental toxemia in the pregnant dog. Obstet. Gynecol. 48:537–548, 1976c.

Abitbol, M.M., Ober, W.B., Gallo, G.R., Driscoll, S.G., and Pirani, C.L.: Experimental toxemia of pregnancy in the monkey, with a preliminary report on renin and aldosterone. Am. J. Pathol. 86:573–590, 1977.

Abramowsky, C.R., Vegas, M.E., Swinehart, G., and Gyves, M.T.: Decidual vasculopathy of the placenta in lupus erythematosus. N. Engl. J. Med. 303:668–672, 1980.

Acker, D., Sachs, B.P., Tracey, K.J., and Wise, W.E.: Abruptio placentae associated with cocaine use. Am. J. Obstet. Gynecol. 146:220–221, 1983.

ACOG: Thyroid disease in pregnancy. ACOG Techn. Bull. 181:1–6, 1993.

Adam, P.A.J., Teramo, K., Raiha, N., Gitlin, D., and Schwartz, R.: Human fetal insulin metabolism early in gestation: response to acute elevation of the fetal glucose concentration and placental transfer of human insulin-I-131. Diabetes 18:409–416, 1969.

Addleman, W., and Gold, S.: Gaucher's disease and pregnancy. Can. Med. Assoc. J. 89:821–823, 1963.

Ahnquist, G., and Holyoke, J.B.: Congenital Letterer-Siwe disease (reticuloendotheliosis) in a term stillborn infant. J. Pediatr. 57:897–904, 1960.

Aladjem, S.: Morphologic aspects of the placenta in gestational diabetes seen by phase-contrast microscopy. Am. J. Obstet. Gynecol. 99:341–349, 1967a.

Aladjem, S.: The syncytial knot: a sign of active syncytial proliferation. Am. J. Obstet. Gynecol. 99:350–358, 1967b.

Aladjem, S., Lueck, J., and Brewer, J.I.: Experimental induction of a toxemia-like syndrome in the pregnant beagle. Am. J. Obstet. Gynecol. 145:27–38, 1983.

Alanen, A., Kekomäki, R., Kero, P., Lindström, P., and Wager, O.: Circulating immune complexes in hypertensive disorders of pregnancy. J. Reprod. Immunol. 6:133–140, 1984.

Alberman, E., Pharoah, P., and Chamberlain, G.: Smoking and the fetus. Lancet 2:36–37, 1977.

Altchek, A., Gaines, J.A., and Siltzbach, L.E.: Sarcoidosis of the uterus. Am. J. Obstet. Gynecol. 70:540–547, 1955.

Alvarez, H.: Prolifration du trophoblaste et sa relation avec l'hypertension artrielle de la toxmie gravidique. Gynecol. Obstet. (Paris) 69:581–588, 1970.

Alvarez, H., Benedetti, W.L., and DeLeons, V.K.: Syncytial proliferation in normal and toxemic pregnancies. Obstet. Gynecol. 29:637–643, 1967.

Alvarez, H., Morel, R.L., Benedetti, W.L., and Scavarelli, M.: Trophoblast hyperplasia and maternal arterial pressure at term. Am. J. Obstet. Gynecol. 105:1015–1021, 1969.

Alzamora, O.: Algunas observaciones sobre las alteraciones de la placenta human en la altura. Rev. Asoc. Med. Prov. Yauli. 3:75, 1958.

Ambrose, A., Welham, R.T., and Cefalo, R.C.: Thrombotic thrombocytic purpura in early pregnancy. Obstet. Gynecol. 66:267–272, 1985.

Anderson, J.F., Kent, S., and Machin, G.A.: Maternal malignant melanoma with placental metastasis: a case report with literature review. Pediatr. Pathol. 9:35–42, 1989.

Anderson, M., Went, L.N., MacIver, J.E., and Dixon, H.G.: Sickle cell disease in pregnancy. Lancet 2:516–521, 1960.

Anderson, W.R., and McKay, D.G.: Electron microscope study of the trophoblast in normal and toxemic placentas. Am. J. Obstet. Gynecol. 95:1134–1148, 1966.

Andrews, J., and McGarry, J.: A community study of smoking in pregnancy. J. Obstet. Gynaecol. Br. Commonw. 79: 1057–1073, 1972.

Anonymous: Pregnancy and the arachidonic-acid cascade. Lancet 1:997–998, 1982.

Anonymous: Classification of hypertensive disorders of pregnancy. Lancet 1:935–936, 1989a.

Anonymous: Smoke screen round the fetus. Lancet 2:1310–1311, 1989b.

Anunciado, A.N., Stubbs, T.M., Pepkowitz, S.H., Lazarchick, J., Miller III, C.M., and Pilia, P.: Altered villus vessel fibronectin in preeclampsia. Am. J. Obstet. Gynecol. 156:898–900, 1987.

Aron, D.C., Schnall, A.M., and Sheeler, L.R.: Cushing's syndrome and pregnancy. Am. J. Obstet. Gynecol. 162: 244–252, 1990.

Aronson, S.: A case of transplacental tumor metastasis. Acta Paediatr. (Stockh.) 52:123–124, 1963.

Asherson, R.A., Khamashta, M.A., Ordi-Ros, J., Derksen, R.H.D.M., Machin, S.J., Barquinero, J., Outt, H.H., Harris, E.N., Vilardell-torres, M., and Hughes, G.R.V.: The "primary" antiphospholipid syndrome: major clinical and serological features. Medicine (Baltimore) 68:366–374, 1989.

Ask-Upmark, E.: Leukemia and pregnancy. Acta Med. Scand. 170:635–658, 1961.

Ask-Upmark, E.: Another follow-up study of children born of mothers with leukemia. Acta Med. Scand. 175:391–394, 1964.

Asmussen, I.: Ultrastructure of human umbilical veins: observations on veins from newborn children of smoking and nonsmoking mothers. Acta Obstet. Gynecol. Scand. 57: 253–255, 1978.

Asmussen, I.: Effects of maternal smoking on the cardiovascular system. Cardiovasc. Med. 4:777–790, 1979.

Asmussen, I.: Ultrastructure of the villi and fetal capillaries in placentas from smoking and nonsmoking mothers. Br. J. Obstet. Gynaecol. 87:239–245, 1980.

Asmussen, I.: Ultrastructure of human umbilical arteries from newborn children of smoking and non-smoking mothers. Acta Pathol. Microbiol. Immunol. Scand. A 90:375–383, 1982a.

Asmussen, I.: Ultrastructure of the umbilical artery from a newborn delivered at term by a mother who smoked 80 cigarettes per day. Acta Pathol. Microbiol. Immunol. Scand. A 90:397–404, 1982b.

Asmussen, I.: Mitochondrial proliferation in endothelium: observations on umbilical arteries from newborn children of smoking mothers. Atherosclerosis 50:203–208, 1984.

Atalla, A., and Page, I.: Ehlers-Danlos syndrome type III in pregnancy. Obstet. Gynecol. 71:508–509, 1988.

Attwood, H.D., and Park, W.W.: Embolism to the lungs by trophoblast. J. Obstet. Gynaecol. Br. Commonw. 68:611–617, 1961.

Averbuch, M., Koifman, B., and Levo, Y.: Lupus anticoagulant, thrombosis and thrombocytopenia in systemic lupus erythematosus. Am. J. Med. 293:2–5, 1987.

Ayala, A.R., De La Fuente, F.R., Loyola, F.D., Gonzalez, E., and Kunhardt, J.: Evidence that a toxemia-related organism (Hydatoxi lualba) is an artifact. Obstet. Gynecol. 67:47–50, 1986.

Bachrach, L.K., and Burrows, G.N.: Maternal-fetal transfer of thyroxine. N. Engl. J. Med. 321:1549, 1989.

Balasch, J., Mirapeix, E., Borche, L., Vives, J., and Gonzalez-Merlo, J.: Further evidence against preeclampsia as an immune complex disease. Obstet. Gynecol. 58:435–437, 1981.

Baldwin, V.J., MacLeod, P.M., and Benirschke, K.: Placental findings in alcohol abuse in pregnancy. Birth Defects 18:89–94, 1982.

Barabas, A.P.: Ehlers-Danlos syndrome: associated with prematurity and premature rupture of foetal membranes; possible increase in incidence. B.M.J. 2:682–684, 1966.

Bardawil, W.A., and Toy, B.L.: The natural history of choriocarcinoma: problems of immunity and spontaneous regression. Ann. N.Y. Acad. Sci. 80:197–261, 1959.

Bardeguez, A.D., McNerney, R., Frieri, M., Verma, U.L., and Tejani, N.: Cellular immunity in preeclampsia: alterations in T-lymphocyte subpopulations during early pregnancy. Obstet. Gynecol. 77:859–862, 1991.

Barnes, A.B., and Link, D.A.: Childhood dermatomyositis and pregnancy. Am. J. Obstet. Gynecol. 146:335–336, 1983.

Barss, V., Phillippe, M., Greene, M.F., and Covell, L.: Pregnancy complicated by homozygous hypercholesterolemia. Obstet. Gynecol. 65:756–757, 1985.

Bartholomew, R.A.: Hemorrhages of late pregnancy. with emphasis on placental circulation and the mechanism of bleeding. Postgrad. Med. 30:397–406, 1961.

Bartholomew, R.A., Colvin, E.D., Grimes, W.H., Fish, J.S., Lester, W.M., and Galloway, W.H.: Facts pertinent to the etiology of eclamptogenic toxemia. Am. J. Obstet. Gynecol. 74:64–84, 1957.

Bartholomew, R.A., Colvin, E.D., Grimes, W.H., Fish, J.S., Lester, W.M., and Galloway, W.H.: Criteria by which toxemia of pregnancy may be diagnosed from unlabeled formalin-fixed placentas. Am. J. Obstet. Gynecol. 82:277–290, 1961.

Beaufils, M., Uzan, S., Donsimoni, R., and Colau, J.C.: Prevention of pre-eclampsia by early antiplatelet therapy. Lancet 1:840–842, 1985.

Beck, J.S., Oakley, C.L., and Rowell, N.R.: Transplacental passage of antinuclear antibody. Arch. Dermatol. 93:656–663, 1966.

Beischer, N.A., Sivasamboo, R., Vohra, S., Silpisornkosal, S., and Reid, S.: Placental hypertrophy in severe pregnancy anaemia. J. Obstet. Gynaecol. Br. Commonw. 77:398–409, 1970.

Beller, F.K., Intorp, H.W., Losse, H., Loew, H., Moenninghoff, W., Schmidt, E.H., and Grundmann, E.: Malignant nephrosclerosis during pregnancy and in the postpartum period (the uremic hemolytic syndrome). Am. J. Obstet. Gynecol. 125:633–639, 1976.

Belliardo, F., Massano, G., and Accomo, S.: Amatoxins do not cross the placental barrier. Lancet 1:1381, 1983.

Bendon, R.W., Wilson, J., Getahun, B., and Bel-Kahn, J.v.d.: A maternal death due to thrombotic disease associated with anticardiolipin antibody. Arch. Pathol. Lab. Med. 111:370–373, 1987.

Benigni, A., Gregorini, G., Frusca, T., Chiabrando, C., Ballerini, S., Valcamonico, A., Orisio, S., Piccinelli, A., Pinciroli, V., Fanelli, R., Gastaldi, A., and Remuzzi, G.: Effect of low-dose aspirin on fetal and maternal generation of thromboxane by platelets in women at risk for pregnancy-induced hypertension. N. Engl. J. Med. 321:357–362, 1989.

Benirschke, K., and Driscoll, S.G.: The Pathology of the Human Placenta. Springer-Verlag, New York, 1967.

Benirschke, K., and Gille, J.: Placental pathology and asphyxia. In, Intrauterine Asphyxia and the Developing Fetal Brain. L. Gluck, ed. Year Book, Chicago, 1977.

Bennett, R.M., Peller, J.S., and Merritt, M.M.: Defective DNA-receptor function in systemic lupus erythematosus and related diseases: evidence for an autoantibody influencing cell physiology. Lancet 1:186–188, 1986.

Bentsi-Enchill, K.K., and Konotey-Ahulu, F.I.D.: Thirteen children from twelve pregnancies in sickle-cell thalassemia. B.M.J. 2:762, 1969.

Bierman, H.R., Aggeler, P.M., Thelander, H., Kelly, K.H., and Cordes, F.L.: Leukemia and pregnancy. J.A.M.A. 161:220–223, 1956.

Birkeland, S.A., and Kristofferson, K.: Pre-eclampsia—a state of mother-fetus immune imbalance. Lancet 2:720–723, 1979.

Björk, O., and Persson, B.: Villous structure in different parts of the cotyledon in placentas of insulin-dependent diabetic women. Acta Obstet. Gynecol. Scand. 63:37–43, 1984.

Blackburn, W.R., Kaplan, H.S., and McKay, D.G.: Morphologic changes in the developing rat placenta following prednisolone administration. Am. J. Obstet. Gynecol. 92:234–246, 1965.

Blakley, P.M.: Experimental teratology of ethanol. In, Issues and Reviews in Teratology. H. Kalter, ed., pp. 237–282. Plenum Press, New York, 1983.

Blanc, W.A., Mattison, D.R., Kane, R., and Chauhan, P.: L.S.D., intrauterine amputations, and amniotic-band syndrome. Lancet 2:158–159, 1971.

Bleyl, U., and Büsing, C.M.: Disseminierte intravasale Gerinnung und perinataler Schock. Verh. Dtsch. Ges. Pathol. 53:495–501, 1969.

Boe, F.: Vascular changes in premature separation of the normally implanted placenta. Acta Obstet. Gynecol. Scand. 38:441–443, 1951.

Bowie, E.J., Thompson, J.H., Pascuzzi, C.A., and Owen, C.A.: Thrombosis in systemic lupus erythematosus despite circulating anticoagulants. J. Lab. Clin. Med. 62:416–430, 1963.

Branch, D.W., Scott, J.R., Kochenour, N.K., and Hershgold, E.: Obstetric complications associated with the lupus anticoagulant. N. Engl. J. Med. 313:1322–1326, 1985.

Branch, D.W., Andres, R., Digre, K.B., Rote, N.S., and Scott, J.R.: The association of antiphospholipid antibodies with severe preeclampsia. Obstet. Gynecol. 73:541–545, 1989.

Branch, D.W., and Rodgers, G.M.: Induction of endothelial cell tissue factor activity by sera from patients with antiphospholipid syndrome: a possible mechanism of thrombosis. Am. J. Obstet. Gynecol. 168:206–210, 1993.

Brandt, J.T., Triplett, D.A., Musgrave, K., and Orr, C.: The sensitivity of different coagulation reagents to the presence of lupus anticoagulants. Arch. Pathol. Lab. Med. 111:120–124, 1987.

Brent, R.L.: The indirect effect of radiation on embryonic development. II. Irradiation of the placenta. Am. J. Dis. Child. 100:103–108, 1960.

Bresnihan, B., Grigor, R.R., Oliver, M., Lewkonia, R.M., Hughes, G.R.V., Lovins, R.E., and Faulk, W.P.: Immunological mechanism for spontaneous abortion in systemic lupus erythematosus. Lancet 2:1205–1207, 1977.

Brodsky, I., Baren, M., Kahn, S.B., Lewis, G., and Tellem, M.: Metastatic malignant melanoma from mother to fetus. Cancer 18:1048–1054, 1965.

Brosens, I., and Renaer, M.: On the pathogenesis of placental infarcts in pre-eclampsia. J. Obstet. Gynaecol. Br. Commonw. 79:794–799, 1972.

Brosens, I., Robertson, W.B., and Dixon, H.G.: The physiological response of the vessels of the placental bed to normal pregnancy. J. Pathol. Bacteriol. 93:569–579, 1967.

Brosens, I.A., Robertson, W.B., and Dixon, H.G.: The role of the spiral arteries in the pathogenesis of preeclampsia. In, Obstetrics and Gynecology Annual: 1972. Vol. 1. R.M. Wynn, ed., pp. 177–191. Appleton-Century-Crofts, East Norwalk, CT, 1972.

Brosens, I., Dixon, H.G., and Robertson, W.B.: Prostaglandins and pre-eclampsia. Lancet 2:412–413, 1974.

Brown, S., Merkow, A., Wiener, M., and Khajezadeh, J.: Low birth weight in babies born to mothers with sickle cell trait. J.A.M.A. 221:1404–1405, 1972.

Brownscheidele, C.M., and Davis, D.L.: Diabetes in pregnancy: a preliminary study of the pancreas, placenta and malformations in the BB Wistar rat. Placenta Suppl. 3:203–216, 1981.

Bruner, J.P., Landon, M.B., and Gabbe, S.: Diabetes and Graves' disease in pregnancy complicated by maternal allergies to antithyroid medication. Obstet. Gynecol. 72:443–445, 1988.

Buchanan, N.M.M., Khamashta, M.A., Morton, K.E., Kerslake, S., Baguley, E., and Hughes, G.R.V.: A study of 100 high risk lupus pregnancies. Am. J. Reprod. Immunol. 28:192–194, 1992.

Budliger, H.: Plazentarveränderungen und ihre Beziehung zur Spättoxikose und perinatalen kindlichen Sterblichkeit. Fortschr. Geburtshilfe Gynäkol. 17:86–110, 1964.

Buescher, M.A., McClamrock, H.D., and Adashi, E.Y.: Cushing syndrome in pregnancy: review. Obstet. Gynecol. 79:130–137, 1992.

Burrow, G.N., and Ferris, T.F.: Medical Complications During Pregnancy. Saunders & Harcourt Brace Jovanovich, Philadelphia, 1988.

Burrows, D.A., O'Neil, T.J., and Sorrells, T.L.: Successful twin pregnancy after renal transplant maintained on cyclosporin A immunosuppression. Obstet. Gynecol. 72:459–461, 1988.

Burstein, R., Berns, A.W., Hirata, Y., and Blumenthal, H.T.: A comparative histo- and immunopathological study of the placenta in diabetes mellitus and in erythroblastosis fetalis. Am. J. Obstet. Gynecol. 86:66–76, 1963.

Bylock, A., Bondjers, G., Jansson, I., and Hansson, H.-A.: Surface ultrastructure of human arteries with special reference to the effects of smoking. Acta Pathol. Microbiol. Scand. A 87:201–209, 1979.

Cameron, H.M., and Park, W.W.: Decidual tissue within the lung. J. Obstet. Gynaecol. Br. Commonw. 72:748–754, 1965.

Campbell, W.A.: Fetal malignant melanoma: ultrasound presentation and review of the literature. Obstet. Gynecol. 70:434–439, 1987.

Cannon, J.F.: Pregnancy and pheochromocytoma. Obstet. Gynecol. 11:43–48, 1958.

Cardwell, M.S.: Ultrasound diagnosis of abruptio placentae with fetomaternal hemorrhage. Am. J. Obstet. Gynecol. 157:358–359, 1987.

Cariou, R., Tobelem, G., Soria, C., and Caen, J.: Inhibition of protein C activation by endothelial cells in the presence of lupus anticoagulant. N. Engl. J. Med. 314:1193–1194, 1986.

Carp, H.J.A., Frenkel, Y., Many, A., Menashe, Y., Mashiach, S., Nebel, L., Toder, V., and Serr, D.M.: Fetal demise associated with lupus anticoagulant: clinical features and results of treatment. Gynecol. Obstet. Invest. 28:178–184, 1989.

Carreras, L.O., Defreyn, G., Machin, S.J., Vermylen, J., Deman, R., Spitz, B., and Assche, A.v.: Arterial thrombosis, intrauterine death and "lupus" anticoagulant: detection of immunoglobulin interfering with prostacyclin formation. Lancet 1:244–246, 1981a.

Carreras, L.O., Vermylen, J., Spitz, B., and Assche, A.v.: "Lupus" anticoagulant and inhibition of prostacyclin formation in patients with repeated abortion, intrauterine growth retardation and intrauterine death. Br. J. Obstet. Gynaecol. 88:890–894, 1981b.

Carreras, L.O., Perez, G.N., Vega, H.R., and Casavilla, F.: Lupus anticoagulant and recurrent fetal loss: successful treatment with gammaglobulin. Lancet 2:393–394, 1988.

Carter, B.: Premature separation of the normally implanted placenta: six deaths due to gross bilateral cortical necrosis of the kidneys. Obstet. Gynecol. 29:30–33, 1967.

Carter, J.E., Vellios, F., and Huber, C.P.: Circulatory factors governing the viability of the human placenta, based on a morphologic study. Am. J. Clin. Pathol. 40:363–373, 1963a.

Carter, J.E., Vellios, F., and Huber, C.P.: Histologic classification and incidence of circulatory lesions of the human placenta, with a review of the literature. Am. J. Clin. Pathol. 40:374–378, 1963b.

Cavanagh, D., Rao, P.S., Tung, K.S.K., and Gastoni L.: Eclamptogenic toxemia: the development of an experimental model in the subhuman primate. Am. J. Obstet. Gynecol. 120:183–196, 1974.

Cavanagh, D., Rao, P.S., Tsai, C.C., and O'Connor, T.C.: Experimental toxemia in the pregnant primate. Am. J. Obstet. Gynecol. 128:75–85, 1977.

Cavanagh, D., Rao, P.S., Knuppel, R.A., Desai, U., and Balis, J.U.: Pregnancy-induced hypertension: development of a model in the pregnant primate (Papio anubis). Am. J. Obstet. Gynecol. 151:987–999, 1985.

Cavell, B.: Transplacental metastasis of malignant melanoma: report of a case. Acta Paediatr. Suppl. 146:37–40, 1963.

Chalmers, I.: Salt, pregnancy, hypertension—and literature searches. Lancet 2:1146, 1988.

Chasnoff, I.J., Burns, W.J., Schnoll, S.H., and Burns, K.A.: Cocaine use in pregnancy. N. Engl. J. Med. 313:666–669, 1985.

Chasnoff, I.J., Bussey, M.E., Savich, R., and Stack, C.M.: Perinatal cerebral infarction and maternal cocaine use. J. Pediatr. 108:210–213, 1986.

Chasnoff, I.J., Griffith, D.R., MacGregor, S., Dirkes, K., and Burns, K.A.: Temporal patterns of cocaine use in pregnancy: perinatal outcome. J.A.M.A. 261:1741–1744, 1989.

Chasnoff, I.J., Landress, H.J., and Barrett, M.E.: The prevalence of illicit-drug or alcohol use during pregnancy and discrepancies in mandatory reporting in Pinellas County, Florida. N. Engl. J. Med. 322:1202–1206, 1990.

Chávez, G.F., Mulinare, J., and Cordero, J.F.: Maternal cocaine use during early pregnancy as a risk factor for congenital urogenital anomalies. J.A.M.A. 262:795–798, 1989.

Chen, Y., Pederson, L.L., and Lefcoe, N.M.: Passive smoking and low birthweight. Lancet 2:54–55, 1989.

Chesley, L.C.: Diagnosis of preeclampsia. Obstet. Gynecol. 65:423–425, 1985.

Cheung, T.H., Leung, A., and Chang, A.: Macrosomic babies. Aust. N.Z. J. Obstet. Gynaecol. 30:319–322, 1990.

Christianson, R.E.: Gross differences observed in the placentas of smokers and nonsmokers. Am. J. Epidemiol. 110:178–187, 1979.

Cibils, L.A.: The placenta and newborn infant in hypertensive conditions. Am. J. Obstet. Gynecol. 118:256–268, 1974.

Clarson, C., Tevaarwerk, G.J.M., Harding, P.G.R., Chance, G.W., and Haust, M.D.: Placental weight in diabetic pregnancies. Placenta 10:275–281, 1989.

Coen, R.W., Papile, L.-A., Figueroa, R., and Henderson, V.M.: Infant survival following protracted fetoplacental separation. Pediatrics 53:760–761, 1974.

Combs, C.A., Easterling, T.R., Schmucker, B.C., and Benedetti, T.J.: Hemodynamic observations during paroxysmal hypertension in a pregnancy with a pheochromocytoma. Obstet. Gynecol. 74:439–441, 1989.

Combs, C.A., Katz, M.A., Kitzmiller, J.L., and Brescia, R.J.: Experimental preeclampsia of the lower aorta: validation with longitudinal blood pressure measurements in conscious rhesus monkeys. Am. J. Obstet. Gynecol. 169:215–223, 1993.

Cove, D.H., and Johnson, P.: Fetal hyperthyroidism: experience of treatment in four siblings. Lancet 1:430–432, 1985.

Covone, A.E., Mutton, D., Johnson, P.M., and Adinolfi, M.: Trophoblast cells in peripheral blood from pregnant women. Lancet 2:841–843, 1984.

Cowchock, F.S., Reece, E.A., Balaban, D., Branch, D.W., and Plouffe, L.: Repeated fetal losses associated with antiphospholipid antibodies: a collaborative randomized trial comparing prednisone with low-dose heparin treatment. Am. J. Obstet. Gynecol. 166:1318–1323, 1992.

Cramblett, H.G., Friedman, J.L., and Najjar, S.: Leukemia in an infant born of a mother with leukemia. N. Engl. J. Med. 259:727–729, 1958.

Cregler, L.L., and Mark, H.: Medical complications of cocaine abuse. N. Engl. J. Med. 315:1495–1500, 1986.

Cross, R.G., O'Connor, M.H., and Holland, P.J.: Placental metastasis of a breast carcinoma. J. Obstet. Gynaecol. Br. Emp. 58:810–811, 1951.

Cruveiller, J., Harpey, J.-P., Vernon, P., Cannat, A., Delattre, A., Hervet, E., Lafourcade, J., and Turpin, R.: Lupus érythémateux systémique: transmission de manifesta-

tions cliniques et de facteurs biologiques de la mère au nouveu-né. Arch. Fr. Pediatr. 27:195–209, 1970.

Cunningham, F.G., and Lindheimer, M.D.: Hypertension in pregnancy. N. Engl. J. Med. 326:927–932, 1992.

Cunningham, F.G., Lowe, T., Guss, S., and Mason, R.: Erythrocyte morphology in women with severe preeclampsia: preliminary observations with scanning electron microscopy. Am. J. Obstet. Gynecol. 153:358–363, 1985.

Dadak, C., Leithner, C., Sinzinger, H., and Silberbauer, K.: Diminished prostacyclin formation in umbilical arteries of babies born to women who smoke. Lancet 1:94, 1981.

Daffos, F., Forester, F., and Kaplan, C.: Prenatal treatment of fetal alloimmune thrombocytopenia. Lancet 2:910, 1988.

Dameshek, W.: Systemic lupus erythematosus: a complex auto-immune disorder? Ann. Intern. Med. 48:707–730, 1958.

Davey, D.A., and MacGillivray, I.: The classification and definition of the hypertensive disorders of pregnancy. Am. J. Obstet. Gynecol. 158:892–898, 1988.

Davey, D.A., and MacGillivray, I.: Classification of hypertensive disorders of pregnancy. Lancet 2:112, 1989.

Davis, L.E., Leveno, K.J., and Cunningham, F.G.: Hypothyroidism complicating pregnancy. Obstet. Gynecol. 72:108–112, 1988.

Davis, L.E., Lucas, M.J., Hankins, G.D.V., Roark, M.L., and Cunningham, F.G.: Thyrotoxicosis complicating pregnancy. Am. J. Obstet. Gynecol. 160:63–70, 1989.

Davison, J.M.: Renal transplantation and pregnancy. Am. J. Kidney Dis. 9:374–380, 1987.

Deaver, J.E., Leppert, P.C., and Zaroulis, C.G.: Neonatal alloimmune thrombocytopenic purpura: a case report. Am. J. Obstet. Gynecol. 154:153–155, 1986.

Delerive, C., Locquet, F., Mallart, A., Janin, A., and Gosselin, B.: Placental metastasis from maternal bronchial oat cell carcinoma. Arch. Pathol. Lab. Med. 113:556–558, 1989.

Demers, L.M., and Gabbe, S.G.: Placental prostaglandin levels in pre-eclampsia. Am. J. Obstet. Gynecol. 126:137–139, 1976.

Demian, S.D.E., Donnelly, W.H., Frias, J.L., and Monif, G.R.G.: Placental lesions in congenital giant pigmented nevi. Am. J. Clin. Pathol. 61:438–442, 1974.

De Wolf, F., Robertson, W.B., and Brosens, I.: The ultrastructure of acute atherosis in hypertensive pregnancy. Am. J. Obstet. Gynecol. 123:164–174, 1975.

De Wolf, F., Carreras, L.O., Moerman, P., Vermylen, J., von Assche, A., and Renaer, M.: Decidual vasculopathy and extensive placental infarction in a patient with repeated thromboembolic accidents, recurrent fetal loss, and lupus anticoagulant. Am. J. Obster. Gynecol. 142:829–834, 1982.

Diamandopoulos, G.T., and Hertig, A.T.: Transmission of leukemia and allied diseases from mother to fetus. Obstet. Gynecol. 21:150–154, 1963.

Dines, D.E., and Banner, E.A.: Sarcoidosis during pregnancy: improvement in pulmonary function. J.A.M.A. 200:726–727, 1967.

Ditts, P.V.: Placental transfer of ethanol. Am. J. Obstet. Gynecol. 112:1195–1198, 1970.

Dombrowski, M.P., Wolfe, H.M., Welch, R.A., and Evans, M.I.: Cocaine abuse is associated with abruptio placentae and decreased birth weight, but not shorter labor. Obstet. Gynecol. 77:139–141, 1991.

Donegan, W.L.: Cancer and pregnancy. CA 33:194–214, 1983.

Donvito, M.T.: Cocaine use during pregnancy: adverse perinatal outcome. Am. J. Obstet. Gynecol. 159:786–787, 1988.

Dreifuss, F.E., and McKinney, W.M.: Wilson's disease (hepatolenticular degeneration) and pregnancy. J.A.M.A. 195:960–962, 1966.

Driscoll, S.G.: The pathology of pregnancy complicated by diabetes mellitus. Med. Clin. North Am. 49:1053–1067, 1965.

Driscoll, S.G., Hicks, S.P., Copenhaver, E.H., and Easterday, C.L.: Acute radiation injury in two human fetuses. Arch. Pathol. 76:113–119, 1963.

Druzin, M.L., Lockshin, M., Edersheim, T.G., Hutson, J.M., Krauss, A.L., and Kogut, E.: Second-trimester fetal monitoring and preterm delivery in pregnancies with systemic lupus erythematosus and/or circulating anticoagulant. Am. J. Obstet. Gynecol. 157:1503–1510, 1987.

Ducey, J., Schulman, H., Farmakides, G., Rochelson, B., Bracero, L., Fleischer, A., Guzman, E., Winter, D., and Penny, B.: A classification of hypertension in pregnancy based on Doppler velocimetry. Am. J. Obstet. Gynecol. 157:680–685, 1987.

Duhring, J.L.: Pregnancy, rheumatoid arthritis, and intrauterine growth retardation. Am. J. Obstet. Gynecol. 108:325–326, 1970.

Dunlop, W., Hill, L.M., Landon, M.J., Oxley, A., and Jones, P.: Clinical relevance of coagulation and renal changes in pre-eclampsia. Lancet 2:346–349, 1978.

Dyer, I., and McCaughey, E.V.: Abruptio placentae: a ten-year survey. Am. J. Obstet. Gynecol. 77:1176–1184, 1959.

Easterling, T.R., and Benedetti, T.J.: Preeclampsia: a hyperdynamic disease model. Am. J. Obstet. Gynecol. 160:1447–1453, 1989.

Easterling, T.R., Chadwick, H.S., Otto, C.M., and Benedetti, T.J.: Aortic stenosis in pregnancy. Obstet. Gynecol. 72:113–118, 1988.

Editorial: Smoking during pregnancy. B.M.J. 2:339–340, 1968.

Editorial: Systemic lupus erythematosus in pregnancy. Lancet 338:87–88, 1991.

Edson, J.R., Blaese, R.M., White, J.G., and Krivit, W.: Defibrination syndrome in an infant born after abruptio placentae. Am. J. Obstet. Gynecol. 72:342–346, 1968.

Elkind-Hirsch, K.E., Raynolds, M.V., and Goldzieher, J.W.: Comparison of immunoreactive gonadotropin-releasing hormone and human chorionic gonadotropin in term placentas from normal women and those with insulin-dependent and gestational diabetes. Am. J. Obstet. Gynecol. 160:71–78, 1989.

El-Roeiy, A., Myers, S.A., and Gleicher, N.: The prevalence of autoantibodies and lupus anticoagulant in healthy pregnant women. Obstet. Gynecol. 75:390–396, 1990.

Elsas, L.J., Whittemore, R., and Burrow, G.N.: Maternal and neonatal Graves' disease. J.A.M.A. 200:250–252, 1967.

Emmrich, P., Amendt, P., and Gödel, E.: Morphologie der Plazenta und neonatale Acidose bei mütterlichem Diabetes mellitus. Pathol. Microbiol. 40:100–114, 1974.

Epstein, F.H.: Late vascular effects of toxemia of pregnancy. N. Engl. J. Med. 271:391–395, 1964.

Erskine, K.J., Iversen, S.A., and Davies, R.: An altered ratio of 18:2(9,11) to 18:2(9,12) linoleic acid in plasma phospholipids as a possible predictor of pre-eclampsia. Lancet 1:554–555, 1985.

Fadel, H.E., and Krauss, J.S.: Factor VII deficiency and pregnancy. Obstet. Gynecol. 73:453–454, 1989.

Farquharson, R.G., Compston, A., and Bloom, A.L.: Lupus anticoagulant: a place for pre-pregnancy treatment? Lancet 2:842–843, 1985.

Feinstein, D.I.: Lupus anticoagulant, thrombosis, and fetal loss. N. Engl. J. Med. 313:1348–1350, 1985.

Feraboli, M.: La placenta nelle cardiopatie. Quad. Clin. Ostet. Ginecol. (Genoa) 6:219–230, 1951.

Fiddler, G.I.: Propranolol and pregnancy. Lancet 2:722–723, 1974.

Fischer, U., and Horký, Z.: Vorläufige Untersuchungen zum Glykogengehalt sowie Sauerstoff- und Glukoseverbrauch der Plazenta in vitro bei Diabetes mellitus. In, Schwangerschaft und Neugeborenes der Zuckerkranken Frau. (IV. Intern. Symp. Diabetesfragen). G. Mohnike, ed., pp. 82–88. VEB Verlag Volk u. Gesundheit, Berlin, 1966.

Fisk, N.M., and Storey, G.N.B.: Fetal outcome in obstetric cholestasis. Br. J. Obstet. Gynaecol. 95:1137–1143, 1988.

Fitzgerald, D.J., Rocki, W., Murray, R., Mayo, G., and Fitzgerald G.A.: Thromboxane A_2 synthesis in pregnancy-induced hypertension. Lancet 335:751–754, 1990.

Fox, H.: White infarcts of the placenta. J. Obstet. Gynaecol. Br. Commonw. 70:980–991, 1963.

Fox, H.: Pathology of the placenta in maternal diabetes mellitus. Obstet. Gynecol. 34:792–798, 1969.

Fox, H.: Effect of hypoxia on trophoblast in organ culture. Am. J. Obstet. Gynecol. 107:1058–1064, 1970.

Fox, H.: Pathology of the Placenta. Saunders, London, 1978.

Fox, L.P., Grandi, J., Johnson, A.H., Watrous, W.G., and Johnson, M.J.: Pheochromocytoma associated with pregnancy. Am. J. Obstet. Gynecol. 104:288–294, 1969.

Frank, D.A., Zuckerman, B.S., Amaro, H., Aboagye, K., Bauchner, H., Cabral, H., Fried, L., Hingson, R., Kayne, H., Levenson, S.M., Parker, S., Reece, H., and Vinci, R.: Cocaine use during pregnancy: prevalence and correlates. Pediatrics 82:888–895, 1988.

Freedman, W.L., and McMahon, F.J.: Placental metastasis: review of the literature and report of a case of metastatic melanoma. Obstet. Gynecol. 16:550–560, 1960.

Freese, U.E.: A placental evaluation of drug addiction in pregnancy. J. Reprod. Med. 20:307–315, 1978.

Friedman, S.A.: Preeclampsia: a review of the role of prostaglandins. Obstet. Gynecol. 71:122–137, 1988.

Fujikura, T., and Froehlich, L.: Diagnosis of sickling by placental examination. Am. J. Obstet. Gynecol. 100:1122–1124, 1968.

Fulroth, R., Phillips, B., and Durand, D.J.: Perinatal outcome of infants exposed to cocaine and/or heroin in utero. Am. J. Dis. Child. 143:905–910, 1989.

Gau, G.S., Bhundia, J., Napier, K., and Ryder, T.A.: The worm that wasn't. Lancet 1:1160–1161, 1983.

George, P.A., Fortner, J.G., and Pack, G.T.: Melanoma with pregnancy: a report of 115 cases. Cancer 13:854–859, 1960.

Gerretsen, G., Huisjes, H.J., and Elema, J.D.: Morphological changes of the spiral arteries in the placental bed in relation to pre-eclampsia and fetal growth retardation. Br. J. Obstet. Gynaecol. 88:876–881, 1981.

Gerretsen, G., Huisjes, H.J., Hardonk, M.J., and Elema, J.D.: Trophoblastic alterations in the placental bed in relation to physiological changes in spiral arteries. Br. J. Obstet. Gynaecol. 90:34–39, 1983.

Gilbert, W.M., Lafferty, C.M., Benirschke, K., and Resnik, R.: Lack of specific placental abnormality associated with cocaine use. Am. J. Obstet. Gynecol. 163:998–999, 1990.

Giles, W.B., Trudinger, B.J., and Baird, P.J.: Fetal umbilical artery blood flow velocity waveforms and placental resistance: pathological correlation. Br. J. Obstet. Gynaecol. 92:31–35, 1985.

Gille, J.H., Moore, D.G., and Sedgwick, C.J.: Placental infarction: a sign of preeclampsia in a Patas monkey (Erythrocebus patas). Lab. Anim. Sci. 27:120–121, 1977.

Ginsberg, J., and Jeacock, M.K.: Placental lactate production in toxemia of pregnancy. Am. J. Obstet. Gynecol. 98:239–244, 1967.

Gitlin, D., Kumate, J., and Morales, C.: Placental insulin transport. Pediatrics 33:65–69, 1965.

Gleicher, N., and Friberg, J.: IgM gammopathy and the lupus anticoagulant syndrome in habitual aborters. J.A.M.A. 253:3278–3281, 1985.

Goldstein, D.P., and Berkowitz, R.S.: Single-agent chemotherapy. In, Gestational Trophoblastic Disease. A.E. Szulman and H.J. Buchsbaum, eds., pp. 135–145. Springer-Verlag, New York, 1987.

Goodlin, R.C., Anderson, J.C., and Skiles, T.L.: Pruritus and hyperplacentosis. Obstet. Gynecol. 66:36S–38S, 1985.

Goodman, R.M., Gresham, G.E., and Roberts, P.L.: Outcome of pregnancy in patients with hereditary hemorrhagic telangiectasia: a retrospective study of 40 patients and 80 matched controls. Fertil. Steril. 18:272–277, 1967.

Gött, E.: Lupus erythematodes disseminatus: Schwangerschaft und Geburt. Dtsch. Med. Wochenschr. 94:274–279, 1969.

Goujard, J., Rumeau, E., and Schwartz, D.: Smoking during pregnancy, stillbirth and abruptio placentae. Biomedicine 23:20–22, 1975.

Goujard, J., Kaminski, M., Rumeau-Rouquette, C., and Schwartz, D.: Maternal smoking, alcohol consumption, and abruptio placenta [letter to the editor]. Am. J. Obstet. Gynecol. 130:738–739, 1978.

Greco, M.A., Klein, S., and Bigelow, B.: Lymphocytosis in the first-trimester placenta of a mother taking diphenylhydantoin. N. Engl. J. Med. 289:867–868, 1973.

Greco, M.A., Kamat, B.R., and Demopoulos, R.I.: Placental protein distribution in maternal diabetes mellitus: an immunocytochemical study. Pediatr. Pathol. 9:679–690, 1989.

Grennan, D.M., McCormick, J.N., Wojtacha, D., Carty, M., and Behan, W.: Immunological studies of the placenta in systemic lupus erythematosus. Ann. Rheum. Dis. 37:129–134, 1978.

Griffin, J.F.T., and Wilson, E.W.: Pre-eclampsia: a state of mother-fetus immune imbalance. Lancet 2:1366–1367, 1979.

Grimes, E.M., Fayez, J.A., and Miller, G.L.: Cushing's syndrome and pregnancy. Obstet. Gynecol. 42:550–559, 1973.

Grimes, D.A., LeBolt, S.A., Grimes, K.R., and Wingo, P.A.: Systemic lupus erythematosus and reproductive function: a case-control study. Am. J. Obstet. Gynecol. 153:179–186, 1985.

Grimmer, D., Landas, S., and Kemp, J.D.: IgM antitrophoblast antibodies in a patient with a pregnancy-associated lupuslike disorder, vasculitis, and recurrent intrauterine fetal demise. Arch. Pathol. Lab. Med. 112:191–193, 1988.

Grossman, R.A., and Goldberg, E.H.: Incidence and recurrence rate of abruptio placentae in Sweden. Obstet. Gynecol. 69:280–281, 1987.

Gruenwald, P., Levin, H., and Yousem, H.: Abruption and premature separation of the placenta. Am. J. Obstet. Gynecol. 102:604–610, 1968.

Gunther, R., and Harer, W.: Systemic scleroderma and pregnancy. Obstet. Gynecol. 23:297–300, 1964.

Gusdon, J.P., Heise, E.R., and Herbst, G.A.: Studies of lymphocyte populations in pre-eclampsia-eclampsia. Am. J. Obstet. Gynecol. 129:255–259, 1977.

Gusdon, J.P., Heise, E.R., Quinn, K.J., and Matthews, L.C.: Lymphocyte subpopulations in normal and preeclampsia pregnancies. Am. J. Reprod. Immunol. 5:28–31, 1984.

Haile, H.: Über Schädigung des Neugeborenen bei Eklampsie. Z. Geburtshilfe Gynäkol. 120:334–352, 1940.

Halberstadt, E., Schneider, D., and Gerber, E.: Über die vorzeitige Lösung der normal inserierten Placenta. Gynaecologia 167:491–502, 1969.

Handin, R.I.: Neonatal immune thrombocytopenia—the doctor's dilemma. N. Engl. J. Med. 305:951–953, 1981.

Hanretti, K.P., Whittle, M.J., and Rubin, P.C.: Doppler uteroplacental waveforms in pregnancy-induced hypertension: a re-appraisal. Lancet 1:850–852, 1988.

Haour, F., and Bertrand, J.: Insulin receptors in the plasma membranes of human placenta. J. Clin. Endocrinol. Metab. 38:334–337, 1974.

Harris, B.A., Gore, H., and Flowers, C.E.: Peripheral placental separation: A possible relationship to premature labor. Obstet. Gynecol. 66:774–778, 1985.

Haupt, H.: Über das Schocksyndrom des Neugeborenen nach vorzeitiger Plazentalösung. Munch. Med. Wochenschr. 105:441–449, 1963.

Haust, M.D.: Maternal diabetes mellitus—effects on the fetus and placenta. In, Perinatal Diseases. R.L. Naeye, J.M. Kissane, and N. Kaufman eds., pp. 201–285. Williams & Wilkins, Baltimore, 1981.

Haust, M.D., Heras, J.L., and Harding, P.G.: Fat-containing uterine smooth muscle cells in "toxemia": possible relevance to atherosclerosis? Science 195:1353–1354, 1977.

Hayes, G.W., Walsh, C.R., and d'Alessandro, E.E.: Scleroderma in pregnancy: report of a case. Obstet. Gynecol. 19:273–274, 1962.

Haynes, D.M.: Experimental abruptio placentae in the rabbit. Am. J. Obstet. Gynecol. 85:626–645, 1963.

Hayslett, J.P., and Reece, E.A.: Systemic lupus erythematosus in pregnancy. Clin. Perinatol. 12:539–549, 1985.

Heite, H.-J., and Kaden, G.: Metastasierung bösartiger Tumoren, insbesondere des malignen Melanomas, in

Plazenta und Kind. Munch. Med. Wochenschr. 114:1909–1913, 1972.

Hennessey, J.P., and Rottino, A.: Hodgkin's disease in pregnancy. Am. J. Obstet. Gynecol. 87:851–853, 1963.

Hertig, A.T.: Vascular pathology in hypertensive albuminuric toxemias of pregnancy. Clinics 4:602–614, 1945.

Hibbard, B.M., and Hibbard, E.D.: Aetiological factors in abruptio placentae. B.M.J. 2:1430–1436, 1963.

Hibbard, B.M., and Hibbard, E.D.: Folate metabolism and reproduction. Br. Med. Bull. 24:10–14, 1968.

Higgins, S.D., and Garite, T.J.: Late abruptio placenta in trauma patients: implications for monitoring. Obstet. Gynecol. 63:10S-12S, 1984.

Hill, J.G., and Brunton, F.J.: Arteriographic assessment of placental vascularity after antepartum haemorrhage. B.M.J. 1:25–26, 1968.

Hodari, A.A.: Chronic uterine ischemia and reversible experimental "toxemia of pregnancy." Am. J. Obstet. Gynecol. 97:597–607, 1967.

Hoet, J.-P., de Meyer, R., and de Meyer-Doyen, L.: Hypothyroïdie et grossesse. Helv. Med. Acta 27:178–195, 1960.

Hoff, C., and Bixler, C.: Maternofetal AB0 antigenic dissimilarity and preeclampsia. Lancet 1:729–730, 1984.

Holaday, W.J., and Castrow, F.F.: Placental metastasis from a fetal giant pigmented nevus. Arch. Dermatol. 98:486–488, 1968.

Holland, E.: A case of transplacental metastasis of malignant melanoma from mother to foetus. J. Obstet. Gynaecol. Br. Emp. 56:529–538, 1949.

Hollister, M.C., Reid, D.L., Phernetton, T.M., Landauer, M., and Rankin, J.H.G.: Dose-response curves of the uterine and placental vascular beds to prostaglandin I_2. Am. J. Obstet. Gynecol. 159:1372–1375, 1988.

Holmes, R.W.: Ablatio placentae. J.A.M.A. 51:1845–1848, 1908.

Hölzl, M., Lüthje, D., and Seck-Ebersbach, K.: Placentaveränderungen bei EPH-Gestose: morphologischer Befund und Schweregrad der Erkrankung. Arch. Gynecol. 217:315–334, 1974.

Honoré, L.H., and Brown, L.B.: Intervillous placental metastasis with maternal myeloid leukemia. Arch. Pathol. Lab. Med. 114:450, 1990.

Horký, Z.: Angiolopathia myometrii bei Diabetes mellitus. Geburtshilfe Frauenheilkd. 28:674–679, 1968.

Hörmann, G., and Lemtis, H.: Abwehrleistungen der "Einheit Fetus und Plazenta" gegenüber hämatogen verschleppten Zellverbänden maligner Blastome der Mutter. Z. Geburtshilfe Gynäkol. 164:129–142, 1965a.

Hörmann, G., and Lemtis, H.: Zur Frage der diaplazentaren Metastasierung maligner Blastome der Mutter. Z. Geburtshilfe Gynäkol. 164:1–8, 1965b.

Horner, E.N.: Placental metastases: case report: maternal death from ovarian cancer. Obstet. Gynecol. 15:566–572, 1960.

Hoskins, I.A., Friedman, D.M., Frieden, F.J., Ordorica, S.A., and Young, B.K.: Relationship between antepartum cocaine abuse, abnormal umbilical artery doppler velocimetry, and placental abruption. Obstet. Gynecol. 78:279–282, 1991.

Hou, S.: Pregnancy in women with chronic renal disease. N. Engl. J. Med. 312:836–839, 1985.

Houlton, M.C.C., and Jackson, M.B.A.: Gaucher's disease and pregnancy. Obstet. Gynecol. 51:619–620, 1978.

Houwert-De Jong, M.H., te Velde, E.R., Nefkens, M.J.J., and Schuurman, H.J.: Immune complexes in skin of patients with pre-eclamptic toxaemia. Lancet 2:387, 1982.

Howard, B.K., and Goodson, J.H.: Experimental placental abruption. Obstet. Gynecol. 2:442–446, 1953.

Howard, R.B., Hosokawa, T., and Maguire, M.H.: Hypoxia-induced fetoplacental vasoconstriction in perfused human placental cotyledons. Am. J. Obstet. Gynecol. 157:1261–1266, 1987.

Huber, C.P., Carter, J.E., and Vellios, F.: Lesions of the circulatory system of the placenta: a study of 234 placentas with special reference to the development of infarcts. Am. J. Obstet. Gynecol. 81:560–573, 1961.

Hulka, J.F.: Discussion of Grimes et al. Am. J. Obstet. Gynecol. 153:185, 1985.

Hulka, J.F., and Brinton, V.: Antibody to trophoblast during early postpartum period in toxemic pregnancies. Am. J. Obstet. Gynecol. 86:130–134, 1963.

Hull, D., Binns, B.A.O., and Joyce, D.: Congenital heart block and widespread fibrosis due to maternal lupus erythematosus. Arch. Dis. Child. 41:688–690, 1966.

Hunter, C.A., Howard, W.F., and McCormick, C.O.: Postpartum curettage effective in reducing hypertension of toxemia. Am. J. Obstet. Gynecol. 81:884–889, 1961.

Iklé, A.: Trophoblastzellen im strömenden Blut. Schweiz. Med. Wochenschr. 91:943, 1961.

Iklé, F.A.: Dissemination von Syncytiotrophoblastzellen im mütterlichen Blut während der Gravidität. Bull. Schweiz. Akad. Med. Wiss. 20:63–72, 1964.

Infante-Rivard, C., David, M., Gauthier, R., and Rivard, G.E.: Lupus anticoagulants, anticardiolipin antibodies, and fetal loss: a case-control study. N. Engl. J. Med. 325:1063–1066, 1991.

Jäämeri, K.E.U., Koivuniemi, A.P., and Carpén, E.O.: Occurrence of trophoblasts in the blood of toxaemic patients. Gynaecologia 160:315–320, 1965.

Jackson, R.: Discoid lupus in a newborn infant of a mother with lupus erythematosus. Pediatrics 33:425–430, 1964.

Jackson, M.R., Mayhew, T.M., and Haas, J.D.: Morphometric studies on villi in human term placentae and the effects of altitude, ethnic grouping and sex of newborn. Placenta 8:487–495, 1987.

Jackson, M.R., Mayhew, T.M., and Haas, J.D.: Effects of high altitude on the vascularization of terminal villi in human placentae. In, Trophoblast Research, Vol. 3. P. Kaufmann and R.K. Miller, eds., pp. 351–360, Plenum, New York, 1988.

Jácomo, K.H., Benedetti, W.L., Sala, M.A., and Alvarez, H.: Pathology of the trophoblast and fetal vessels of the placenta in maternal diabetes mellitus. Acta Diabetol. Lat. 13:216–235, 1976.

James, R.F.: Snake bite in pregnancy. Lancet 2:731, 1985.

Jauniaux, E., and Burton, G.J.: The effect of smoking in pregnancy on early placental morphology. Obstet. Gynecol. 79:645–648, 1992.

Javert, C.T., and Reiss, C.: The origin and significance of macroscopic intervillous coagulation hematomas (red infarcts) of the human placenta. Surg. Gynecol. Obstet. 94: 257–269, 1952.

Jeremy, J.Y., Barradas, M.A., Mikhailidis, D.P., and Dandona, P.: Placental prostaglandin production in normal and toxemic pregnancies (letter). Amer. J. Obstet. Gynecol. 154:212–214, 1986.

Johnson, F.D.: Pregnancy and concurrent chronic myelogenous leukemia. Am. J. Obstet. Gynecol. 112:640–644, 1972.

Johnson, P.M., Natvig, J.B., Ystehede, U.A., and Faulk, W.P.: Immunological studies on human placentae: the distribution and character of immunoglobulins in chorionic villi. Clin. Exp. Immunol. 30:145–153, 1977.

Jones, C.J.P., and Fox, H.: Placental changes in gestational diabetes: an ultrastructural study. Obstet. Gynecol. 48:274–280, 1976.

Jones, C.J.P., and Fox, H.: An ultrastructural and ultrahistochemical study of the human placenta in maternal preeclampsia. Placenta 1:61–76, 1980.

Jones, E.M.: Placental metastases from bronchial carcinoma. B.M.J. 1:491–492, 1969.

Jones, K.L., Smith, D.W., Ulleland, C.N., and Streissguth, A.P.: Pattern of malformation in offspring of chronic alcoholic women. Lancet 1:1267–1271, 1973.

Jones, T.G., Goldsmith, K.L.G., and Anderson, I.M.: Maternal and neonatal platelet antibodies in a case of congenital thrombocytopenia. Lancet 2:1008–1009, 1961.

Jørgensen, K.R., Deckert, T., Pedersen, L.M., and Pedersen, J.: Insulin, insulin antibody and glucose in plasma of newborn infants of diabetic women. Acta Endocrinol. (Copenh.) 52:154–167, 1966.

Jung, A.L., Roan, Y., and Temple, A.R.: Neonatal death associated with transplacental ethanol intoxication. Am. J. Dis. Child. 134:419–420, 1980.

Kaibara, M., Kobayashi, T., and Matsumoto, S.: Idiopathic thrombocythemia and pregnancy: report of a case. Obstet. Gynecol. 65:18S–19S, 1985.

Kalhan, S.C., Schwartz, R., and Adam, P.A.J.: Placental barrier to human insulin-I^{125} in insulin-dependent diabetic mothers. J. Clin. Endocrinol. Metab. 40:139–142, 1975.

Kaminski, M., Rumeau-Rouquette, C., and Schwartz, D.: Effects of alcohol on the fetus. N. Engl. J. Med. 298:55–56, 1978.

Kaplan, M.M.: Acute fatty liver of pregnancy. N. Engl. J. Med. 313:367–370, 1985.

Kaplan, C., Daffos, F., Forestier, F., Tertian, G., Catherine, N., Pons, J.C., and Tchernia, G.: Fetal platelet counts in thrombocytopenic pregnancy. Lancet 336:979–982, 1990.

Kåregård, M., and Gennser, G.: Incidence and recurrence rate of abruptio placentae in Sweden. Obstet. Gynecol. 67:523–528, 1986.

Kaufmann, P., and Stark, J.: Ultrastruktur der Plazenta bei Diabetes, EPH-Gestose und Rh-Inkompatibilität. In, Neue Erkenntnisse über die Orthologie und Pathologie der Plazenta. J.J. Födisch, ed., pp. 53–62. Ferdinand Enke Verlag, Stuttgart, 1977.

Kaufmann, P., Kohnen, G., and Kosanke, G.: Wechselwirkungen zwischen Plazentamorphologie und fetaler Sauerstoffversorgung: Versuch einer zellbiologischen Inter-

pretation pathohistologischer und experimenteller Befunde. Gynäkologe 26:16–23, 1993.

Kelemen, J.T., and Mándi, L.: Sarcoidose in der Placenta. Zentralbl. Allg. Pathol. 112:18–21, 1969.

Kerber, I.J., Warr, O.S., and Richardson, C.: Pregnancy in a patient with a prosthetic mitral valve: associated with a fetal anomaly attributed to Warfarin sodium. J.A.M.A. 203: 223–225, 1968.

Khong, T.Y.: Immunohistologic study of the leukocytic infiltrate in maternal uterine tissues in normal and preeclamptic pregnancies at term. Am. J. Reprod. Immunol. 15:1–8, 1987.

Khong, T.Y., Pearce, J.M., and Robertson, W.B.: Acute atherosis in preeclampsia: maternal determinants and fetal outcome in the presence of the lesion. Am. J. Obstet. Gynecol. 157:360–363, 1987.

Khong, T.Y., Sawyer, I.H., and Heryet, A.: An immunohistologic study of endothelialization of uteroplacental vessels in human pregnancy: evidence that endothelium is focally disrupted by trophoblast in preeclampsia. Am. J. Obstet. Gynecol. 167:751–756, 1992.

Kilpatrick, D.C.: Immune mechanisms and pre-eclampsia. Lancet 2:1460–1461, 1987.

Kimmerle, R., and Chantelau, E.A.: Transplacental passage of insulin. N. Engl. J. Med. 324:198–199, 1991.

Kirshon, B., Edwards, J., and Cotton, D.B.: Gordon's syndrome in pregnancy. Am. J. Obstet. Gynecol. 156:1110–1111, 1987.

Kitay, D.Z.: Folic acid in pregnancy. J.A.M.A. 204:79, 1968.

Kitzmiller, J.L., and Benirschke, K.: Immunofluorescent study of placental bed vessels in pre-eclampsia of pregnancy. Am. J. Obstet. Gynecol. 115:248–251, 1973.

Kitzmiller, J.L., Stoneburner, L., Yelenovsky, P.F., and Lucas, W.E.: Serum complement in normal pregnancy and pre-eclampsia. Am. J. Obstet. Gynecol. 117:312–315, 1973.

Kitzmiller, J.L., Watt, N., and Driscoll, S.G.: Decidual arteriopathy in hypertension and diabetes in pregnancy: immunofluorescent studies. Am. J. Obstet. Gynecol. 141: 773–778, 1981.

Kjeldsen, J., and Pedersen, J.: Relation of residual placental blood-volume to onset of respiratory-distress syndrome in infants of diabetic and non-diabetic mothers. Lancet 1:180–184, 1967.

Klebe, J.G., and Ingomar, C.J.: Placental transfusion in infants of diabetic mothers elucidated by placental residual blood volume. Acta Paediatr. Scand. 63:59–64, 1974a.

Klebe, J.G., and Ingomar, C.J.: The influence of the method of delivery and the clamping technique on the red cell volume in infants of diabetic and non-diabetic mothers. Acta Paediatr. Scand. 63:65–69, 1974b.

Kline, J., Stein, Z.A., Susser, M., and Warburton, D.: Smoking: a risk factor for spontaneous abortion. N. Engl. J. Med. 297:793–796, 1977.

Klippel, J.H., Grimley, P.M., and Decker, J.L.: Lymphocyte inclusions in newborns of mothers with systemic lupus erythematosus. N. Engl. J. Med. 290:96–97, 1974.

Klurfeld, D.M.: Identification of foam cells in human atherosclerotic lesions as macrophages using monoclonal antibodies. Arch. Pathol. 109:445–449, 1985.

Knörr, K., Knörr-Gärtner, H., and Uebele-Kallhardt, B.: Zur Frage der Wirkung alkylierender Substanzen auf die

Entwicklung der Frucht. Geburtshilfe Frauenheilkd. 29: 601–611, 1969.

Knox, G.E., Stagno, S., Volanakis, J.E., and Huddelston, J.F.: A search for antigen-antibody complexes in preeclampsia: further evidence against immunologic pathogenesis. Am. J. Obstet. Gynecol. 132:87–89, 1978.

König, P.A.: Über Eklampsietod und Gefäß wandschaden bei Mutter und Kind. Z. Geburtshilfe Gynäkol. 146:292–307, 1956.

Koshy, M., Burd, L., Wallace, D., Moawad, A., and Baron, J.: Prophylactic red-cell transfusions in pregnant patients with sickle cell disease: a randomized cooperative study. N. Engl. J. Med. 319:1447–1451, 1988.

Kosova, L.A., and Schwartz, S.O.: Multiple myeloma and normal pregnancy: report of a case. Blood 28:102–111, 1966.

Krayalcin, G., Imran, M., and Rosner, F.: "Blister cells": association with pregnancy, sickle cell disease, and pulmonary infarction. J.A.M.A. 219:1727–1729, 1972.

Kuhnert, B.R., Kuhnert, P.M., Debanne, S., and Williams, T.G.: The relationship between cadmium, zinc, and birth weight in pregnant women who smoke. Am. J. Obstet. Gynecol. 157:1247–1251, 1987a.

Kuhnert, P.M., Kuhnert, B.R., Erhard, P., Brashear, W.T., Groh-Wargo, S.L., and Webster, S.: The effect of smoking on placental and fetal zinc status. Am. J. Obstet. Gynecol. 157:1241–1246, 1987b.

Labarrere, C.A.: Placental bed biopsy technique and vascular changes. Am. J. Obstet. Gynecol. 157:1320–1322, 1987.

Lacher, M.J., and Geller, W.: Cyclophosphamide and vinblastine sulfate in Hodgkin's disease during pregnancy. J.A.M.A. 195:486–488, 1966.

Lau, H., Sackreuther, W., Bach, H.G., Grabberr, W., and Hundertmack, R.: Über die vorzeitige Lösung der normal sitzenden Placenta: klinische Beobachtungen an 100 Fällen. Gynaecologia 157:143–160, 1964.

Laurini, R.N., Visser, G.H.A., and Ballegoodie, E. van: Morphological fetoplacental abnormalities despite well-controlled diabetic pregnancy. Lancet 1:800, 1984.

Lazarchick, J., and Kizer, J.: The laboratory diagnosis of lupus anticoagulants. Arch. Pathol. Lab. Med. 113:177–180, 1989.

Lederman, R.P., Lederman, E., Work, B.A., and McCann, D.S.: The relationship of maternal anxiety, plasma catecholamines, and plasma cortisol to progress in labor. Am. J. Obstet. Gynecol. 132:495–500, 1978.

Lee, R.A., Johnson, C.E., and Hanlon, D.G.: Leukemia during pregnancy. Am. J. Obstet. Gynecol. 84:455–458, 1962.

Lemtis, H.: Über die vorzeitige Lösung der normal sitzenden Plazenta. Forsch. Praxis Fortbild. 18:231–237, 1967.

Lemtis, H., and Hörmann, G.: Über die sogenannten Plazentametastasen maligner Blastome der Mutter. In, Fortschritte der Krebsforschung. C.G. Schmidt and O. Wetter, eds., pp. 521–527. Schattauer Verlag, Stuttgart, 1969.

Leone, G., Monetta, E., Paparatti, G., and Boni, P.: Von Willebrand's disease in pregnancy. N. Engl. J. Med. 293: 456, 1975.

Levine, M.G., and Esser, D.: Total parenteral nutrition for the treatment of severe hyperemesis gravidarum: maternal nutritional effects and fetal outcome. Obstet. Gynecol. 72: 102–107, 1988.

Li, M.C., Hertz, R., and Spencer, D.B.: Effects of methotrexate therapy upon choriocarcinomas and chorioadenomas. Proc. Soc. Exp. Biol. Med. 93:361–366, 1956.

Lichtig, C., Deutsch, M., and Brandes, J.: Vascular changes of endometrium in early pregnancy. Am. J. Clin. Pathol. 81:702–707, 1984.

Liebhardt, M.: Tkanka Laczna lozysk pochodzacych z ciaz powiklanych prdzez cukrzyce matki. Ginecol Pol. 39:1353–1362, 1968.

Lilford, R.J.: Classification of hypertensive disorders of pregnancy. Lancet 2:112–113, 1989.

Little, B.B., Snell, L.M., Klein, V.R., and Gilstrap III, L.C.: Cocaine abuse during pregnancy: maternal and fetal implications. Obstet. Gynecol. 73:157–160, 1989.

Lockshin, M.D., Druzin, M.L., and Qamar, T.: Prednisone does not prevent recurrent fetal death in women with antiphospholipid antibody. Am. J. Obstet. Gynecol. 160:439–443, 1989.

Lockwood, C.J., Reece, E.A., Romero, R., and Hobbins, J.C.: Anti-phospholipid antibody and pregnancy wastage. Lancet 2:742–743, 1986.

Lockwood, C.J., Romero, R., Feinberg, R.F., Clyne, L.P., Coster, B., and Hobbins, J.C.: The prevalence and biologic significance of lupus anticoagulant and anticardiolipin antibodies in a general obstetric population. Am. J. Obstet. Gynecol. 161:369–373, 1989.

Loizoll, S., Byron, M.A., Englert, H.J., David, J., Hughes, G.R.V., and Walport, M.J.: Association of quantitative anticardiolipin antibody levels with fetal loss and time of loss in systemic lupus erythematosus. Q. J. Med. 68:525–531, 1988.

Long, E.G., Tsin, T.Y., Reinarz, J.A., Schnadig, V.J., McLucas, E., and Kelly, R.T.: "Hydatoxi lualba" identified. Am. J. Obstet. Gynecol. 149:462–463, 1984.

Lopez-Zeno, J.A., Carlo, W.A., O'Grady, J.P., and Fanaroff, A.A.: Infant survival following delayed postmortem cesarean delivery. Obstet. Gynecol. 76:991–992, 1990.

Lotgering, F.K., Pijpers, L., Eijck, J.v., and Wallenburg, H.C.S.: Pregnancy in a patient with diffuse cavernous hemangioma of the uterus. Am. J. Obstet. Gynecol. 160: 628–630, 1989.

Lubbe, W.F., and Liggins, G.C.: Lupus anticoagulant and pregnancy. Am. J. Obstet. Gynecol. 153:322–327, 1985.

Lubbe, W.F., Butler, W.S., Palmer, S.J., and Liggins, G.C.: Fetal survival after prednisone suppression of maternal lupus-anticoagulant. Lancet 1:1361–1363, 1963.

Lueck, J., Brewer, J.I., Aladjem, S., and Novotny, M.: Observation of an organism found in patients with gestational trophoblastic disease and in patients with toxemia of pregnancy. Am. J. Obstet. Gynecol. 145:15–26, 1983

Lundberg, C., Marceau, F., Huey, R., and Hugli, T.E.: Anaphylatoxin C5a fails to promote prostacyclin release in cultured endothelial cells from human umbilical veins. Immunopharmacology 12:135–143, 1986.

Machin, G.A.: Maternal melanoma metastatic to the placenta. Pediatr. Pathol. 7:490, 1987.

MacLennan, A.H., Sharp, F., and Shaw-Dunn, J.: The ultrastructure of human trophoblast in spontaneous and induced hypoxia using a system of organ culture: a comparison with ultrastructural changes in pre-eclampsia and placental insufficiency. J. Obstet. Gynaecol. Br. Commonw. 79:113–121, 1972.

Mäkilä, U.-M., Viinikka, L., and Ylikorkala, O.: Evidence that prostacyclin deficiency is a specific feature in pree-clampsia. Am. J. Obstet. Gynecol. 148:772–774, 1984.

Mäkilä, U.-M., Jouppila, P., Kirkinen, P., Viinikka, L., and Ylikorkala, O.: Placental thromboxane and prostacyclin in the regulation of placental blood flow. Obstet. Gynecol. 68:537–540, 1986.

Maqueo, M., Azuela, J.C., Karchmer, S., and Arenas, J.C.: Placental morphology in pathologic gestations with or without toxemia: observations in cases of diabetes mellitus, hydrops fetalis, twin pregnancy, placenta previa, and hydatidiform mole. Obstet. Gynecol. 26:184–191, 1965.

Marais, W.D.: Human decidual spiral arterial studies. Part II. A universal thesis on the pathogenesis of intraplacental fibrin deposits, layered thrombosis, red and white infarcts and toxic and non-toxic abruptio placentae: a microscopic study. J. Obstet. Gynaecol. Br. Commonw. 69:213–224, 1962a.

Marais, W.D.: Human decidual spiral arterial studies. Part III. Histological patterns and some clinical implications of decidual spiral arteriosclerosis. J. Obstet. Gynaecol. Br. Commonw. 69:225–233, 1962b.

Marais, W.D.: Human decidual spiral arterial studies. Part V. Pathogenetic patterns of intraplacental lesions. J. Obstet. Gynaecol. Br. Commonw. 69:944–955, 1962c.

Marais, W.D.: Human decidual spiral arterial studies. Part VI: Postmortem circulation studies on an in situ placenta. S. Afr. Med. J. 36:678–681, 1962d.

Marais, W.D.: Human decidual spiral arterial studies. Part VII. The clinical evaluation of normal and abnormal spiral arterioles and of placental lesions: a statistical study. J. Obstet. Gynaecol. 70:777–786, 1963a.

Marais, W.D.: Human decidual spiral arterial studies. Part VIII. The aetiological relationship between toxaemia-hypertension of pregnancy and spiral arterial placental pathology. S. Afr. Med. J. 37:117–120, 1963b.

Marbury, M.C., Linn, S., Monson, R., Schoenbaum, S., Stubblefield, P.G., and Ryan, K.J.: The association of alcohol consumption with outcome of pregnancy. Am. J. Public Health 73:1165–1168, 1983.

Marcuse, P.M.: Pulmonary syncytial giant cell embolism: report of maternal death. Obstet. Gynecol. 3:210–213, 1954.

Marks, F., Ordorica, S., Hoskins, I., and Young, B.K.: Congenital hereditary fructose intolerance and pregnancy. Am. J. Obstet. Gynecol. 160:362–363, 1989.

Martinez, C.R.J.: Foetus in maternal renal failure. Lancet 1:504, 1967.

Massobrio, M., Benedetto, C., Bertini, E., Tetta, C., and Camussi, G.: Immune complexes in preeclampsia and normal pregnancy. Am. J. Obstet. Gynecol. 152:578–583, 1985.

Mayhew, T.M., Soerensen, F.B., Klebe, J.G., and Jackson, M.R.: Growth and maturation of villi in placentae from well-controlled diabetic women. Placenta 15:57–65, 1994.

Maymon, R., Bahari, C., and Moroz, C.: Placental isoferritin: a new serum marker in toxemia of pregnancy. Am. J. Obstet. Gynecol. 160:681–684, 1989.

McFaul, P.B., Dornan, J.C., Lamki, H., and Boyle, D.: Pregnancy complicated by maternal heart disease: a review of 519 women. Br. J. Obstet. Gynaecol. 95:861–867, 1988.

McFayden, I.R., Price, A.B., and Geirsson, R.T.: The relation of birthweight to histological appearances in vessels of the placental bed. Br. J. Obstet. Gynaecol. 93:476–481, 1986.

McGlothlin, W.H., Sparkes, R.S., and Arnold, D.O.: Effect of LSD on human pregnancy. J.A.M.A. 212:1483–1487, 1970.

McGowan, L.: Cancer and pregnancy. Obstet. Gynecol. Surv. 19:285–307, 1964.

McKay, D.G., Jewett, J.F., and Reid, D.E.: Endotoxin shock and the generalized Shwartzman reaction in pregnancy. Am. J. Obstet. Gynecol. 78:546–566, 1959.

McLaughlin, P.J., Stirrat, G.M., Redman, C.W.G., and Levinsky, R.J.: Immune complexes in normal and pre-eclamptic pregnancy. Lancet 1:934–935, 1979.

McVerry, B.A., Machin, S.J., Parry, H., and Goldstone, A.H.: Reduced prostacyclin activity in systemic lupus erythematosus. Ann. Rheum. Dis. 39:524–525, 1980.

Menon, R.K., Cohen, R.M., Sperling, M.A., Cutfield, W.S., Mimouni, F., and Khoury, J.C.: Transplacental passage of insulin in pregnant women with insulin-dependent diabetes mellitus: its role in fetal macrosomia. N. Engl. J. Med. 323:309–315, 1990.

Mercado, A., Johnson, G., Calver, D., and Sokol, R.J.: Cocaine, pregnancy, and postpartum intracerebral hemorrhage. Obstet. Gynecol. 73:467–468, 1989.

Mercer, B., Drouin, J., Jolly, E., and d'Anjou, G.: Primary thrombocythemia in pregnancy: a report of two cases. Am. J. Obstet. Gynecol. 159:127–128, 1988.

Messer, R.H.: Symposium on bleeding disorders in pregnancy: observations in pregnancy. Am. J. Obstet. Gynecol. 156: 1419–1425, 1987.

Metcalfe, J., Novy, M.J., and Peterson, E.N.: Reproduction at high altitude. In, Comparative Aspects of Reproductive Failure. K. Benirschke, ed., pp. 447–457. Springer-Verlag, New York, 1966.

Meyer, M.B., and Tonascia, J.A.: Maternal smoking, pregnancy complications, and perinatal mortality. Am. J. Obstet. Gynecol. 128:494–502, 1977.

Mijer, F., and Olsen, R.N.: Transplacental passage of L.E. factor. J. Pediatr. 52:690–693, 1958.

Mills, J.L., Simpson, J.L., Driscoll, S.G., Jovanovic-Peterson, L., Allen, M.V., Aarons, J.H., Metzger, B., Bieber, F.R., Knopp, R.H., Holmes, L.B., Peterson, C.M., Witham-Wilson, M., Brown, Z., Ober, C., Harley, E., MacPherson, T.A., Duckles, A., Mueller-Heubach, E., NICHD, and HD-DEPS: Incidence of spontaneous abortion among normal women and insulin-dependent diabetic women whose pregnancies were identified within 21 days of conception. N. Engl. J. Med. 319:1617–1623, 1988.

Milo, R., Neuman, M., Klein, C., Caspi, E., and Arlazoroff, A.: Acute intermittent porphyria in pregnancy. Obstet. Gynecol. 73:450–452, 1989.

Miodovnik, M., Skillman, C., Holroyde, J.C., Butler, J.B., Wendel, J.S., and Siddiqi, T.A.: Elevated maternal glycohemoglobin in early pregnancy and spontaneous abortion among insulin-dependent diabetic women. Am. J. Obstet. Gynecol. 153:439–442, 1985.

Mirro, R., and Brown, D.R.: Edema, proteinuria, thrombocytopenia, and leukopenia in infants of preeclamptic mothers. Am. J. Obstet. Gynecol. 144:851–852, 1982.

Moore, T.R., Sorg, J., Miller, L., Key, T.C., and Resnik, R.: Hemodynamic effects of intravenous cocaine on the pregnant ewe and fetus. Am. J. Obstet. Gynecol. 155:883–888, 1986.

Morales, W.J., and Stroup, M.: Intracranial hemorrhage in utero due to isoimmune neonatal thrombocytopenia. Obstet. Gynecol. 65:20S–24S, 1985.

Mordel, N., Birkenfeld, A., Goldfarb, A.N., and Rachmilewitz, E.A.: Successful full-term pregnancy in homozygous β-thalassemia major: case report and review of the literature. Obstet. Gynecol. 73:837–840, 1989.

Morrow, R.J., Ritchie, J.W.K., and Bull, S.B.: Maternal cigarette smoking: the effects on umbilical and uterine blood flow velocity. Am. J. Obstet. Gynecol. 159:1069–1071, 1988.

Mueller-Eckhardt, C., Kiefel, V., Jovanovic, V., Künzel, W., Becker, T., Wolf, H., and Zeh, K.: Prenatal treatment of alloimmune thrombocytopenia. Lancet 2:910, 1988.

Muller, G., Philippe, E., Lefakis, P., de Mot-Leclair, M., Dreyfus, J., Nusynowicz, G., Renaud, R., and Gandar, R.: Les lésions placentaires de la gestose: étude anatomo-clinique. Gynecol. Obstet. (Paris) 70:309–316, 1971.

Mund, A., Simson, J., and Rothfield, N.: Effect of pregnancy on course of systemic lupus erythematosus. J.A.M.A. 183:917–920, 1963.

Murphy, J.F., Mulcahy, R., and Drumm, J.E.: Smoking and the fetus. Lancet 2:36, 1977.

Musci, T.J., Roberts, J.M., Rodgers, G.M., and Taylor, R.N.: Mitogenic activity is increased in the sera of preeclamptic women before birth. Am. J. Obstet. Gynecol. 159:1446–1451, 1988.

Myers, R.E., and Fujikura, T.: Placental changes after experimental abruptio placentae and fetal vessel ligation of rhesus monkey placenta. Am. J. Obstet. Gynecol. 100:846–851, 1968.

Nadji, P., and Sommers, S.C.: Lesions of toxemia in first trimester pregnancies. Am. J. Clin. Pathol. 59:344–349, 1973.

Naeye, R.L.: Placental infarction leading to fetal or neonatal death. A prospective study. Obstetr. Gynecol. 50:583–588, 1977.

Naeye, R.L.: Relationship of cigarette smoking to congenital anomalies and perinatal death: a prospective study. Am. J. Pathol. 90:289–294, 1978.

Naeye, R.L., Blanc, W., Leblanc, W., and Khatamee, M.A.: Fetal complications of maternal heroin addiction: abnormal growth, infections, and episodes of stress. J. Pediatr. 83:1055–1061, 1973.

Naeye, R.L., Harkness, W.L., and Utts, J.: Abruptio placentae and perinatal death: a prospective study. Am. J. Obstet. Gynecol. 128:740–746, 1977.

Nagey, D.A., Fortier, K.J., and Linder, J.: Pregnancy complicated by periarteritis nodosa: induced abortion as an alternative. Am. J. Obstet. Gynecol. 147:103–105, 1983.

Ness, P.M., Budzynski, A.Z., Olexa, S.A., and Rodvien, R.: Congenital hypofibrinogenemia and recurrent placental abruption. Obstet. Gynecol. 61:519–523, 1983.

Nicholson, H.O.: Cytotoxic drugs in pregnancy. J. Obstet. Gynaecol. Br. Commonw. 75:307–312, 1968.

Nielsen, F.H., Jacobsen, B.B., and Rolschau, J.: Pregnancy complicated by extreme hyperlipaemia and foam-cell accumulation in placenta. Acta Obstet. Gynecol. Scand. 52:83–89, 1973.

Nilsson, I.M., Astedt, B., Hedner, U., and Berezin, D.: Intrauterine death and circulating anticoagulant, "antithromboplastin." Acta Med. Scand. 197:153–159, 1975.

Niswander, R.K., and Gordon, M.: The Women and their Pregnancies. p. 43. Saunders, Philadelphia, 1972.

Nordlund, J.J., DeVita, V.T., and Carbone, P.P.: Severe vinblastine-induced leukopenia during late pregnancy with delivery of normal infant. Ann. Intern. Med. 69:581–582, 1968.

Notelvitz, M., Bottoms, S.F., Dase, D.F., and Leichter, P.J.: Painless abruptio placentae. Obstet. Gynecol. 53:270–272, 1979.

Nummi, S., Koivisto, M., and Hakosalo, J.: Acute leukaemia in pregnancy with placental involvement. Ann. Chir. Gynaecol. Fenn. 62:394–398, 1973.

Nuñez, J.A.C.: La placenta de las cardiacas. Rev. Esp. Obstet. Ginecol. 22:129–134, 1963.

O'Brien, W.F., Knuppel, R.A., Saba, H.I., Angel, J.L., Benoit, R., and Bruce, A.: Platelet inhibitory activity in placentas from normal and abnormal pregnancies. Obstet. Gynecol. 70:597–600, 1987.

O'Brien, W.F., Knuppel, R.A., Saba, H.I., Angel, J.L., Benoit, R., and Bruce, A.: Serum prostacyclin binding and half-life in normal and hypertensive pregnant women. Obstet. Gynecol. 73:43–46, 1988.

Oga, M., Matsui, N., Anai, T., Yoshimatsu, J., Inoue, I., and Miyakawa, I.: Copper disposition of the fetus and placenta in a patient with untreated Wilson's disease. Am. J. Obstet. Gynecol. 169:196–198, 1993.

Ohba, T., Matsuo, I., Katabuchi, H., Nishimura, H., Fujisaki, S., and Okamura, H.: Adult T-cell leukemia/lymphoma in pregnancy. Obstet. Gynecol. 72:445–447, 1988.

Okudaira, Y., Hirota, K., Cohen, S., and Strauss, L.: Ultrastructure of the human placenta in maternal diabetes mellitus. Lab. Invest. 15:910–926, 1966.

O'Leary, J.A.: A continuing study of sarcoidosis and pregnancy. Am. J. Obstet. Gynecol. 101:610–613, 1968.

Ong, P.J.L., and Burton, G.J.: Thinning of the placental villous membrane during maintenance in hypoxic organ culture: structural adaptation or syncytial degeneration? Eur. J. Obstet. Gynecol. Reprod. Biol. 39:103–110, 1991.

Orr, J.W., Grizzle, W.E., and Huddleston, J.F.: Squamous cell carcinoma metastatic to placenta and ovary. Obstet. Gynecol. 59:81S–83S, 1982.

Out, H.J., Bruinse, H.W., Christiaens, G.C.M.L., Vliet, M.v., de Groot, P.G., Nieuwenhuis, H.K., and Derksen, R.H.W.M.: A prospective, controlled multicenter study on the obstetric risks of pregnant women with antiphospholipid antibodies. Am. J. Obstet. Gynecol. 167:26–32, 1992.

Owen, J., and Hauth, J.C.: Polyarteritis nodosa in pregnancy: a case report and brief literature review. Am. J. Obstet. Gynecol. 160:606–607, 1989.

Padmanabhan, R., Al-Zuhair, A.G.H., and Ali, A.H.: Histopathological changes of the placenta in diabetes induced by maternal administration of streptozotocin during pregnancy in the rat. Congen. Anom. (Jpn.) 28:1–15, 1988.

Page, D.V., Brady, K., Mitchell, J., Pehrson, J., and Wade, G.: The pathology of intrauterine thyrotoxicosis: two case reports. Obstet. Gynecol. 72:479–481, 1988.

Page, D.V., Brady, K., and Ward, S.: The placental pathology of substance abuse [abstract 410]. Mod. Pathol. 2(1):69A, 1989.

Palmer, A.E., London, W.T., Sly, D.L., and Rice, J.M.: Toxemia of pregnancy (preeclampsia, eclampsia, hypertensive disorders of pregnancy). In, Spontaneous Animal Models of Human Disease. Vol. I. E.J. Andrews, B.C. Ward, and N.H. Altman, eds., pp. 213–215. Academic Press, Orlando, FL, 1979.

Parker, C.R., Illingworth, D.R., Bissonette, J., and Carr, B.R.: Endocrine changes during pregnancy in a patient with homozygous familial hypobetalipoproteinemia. N. Engl. J. Med. 314:557–560, 1986.

Pavelka, M., Pavelka, R., and Gerstner, G.: Ultrastructure of the syncytiotrophoblast of the human term placenta in EPH-gestosis. Gynecol. Obstet. Invest. 10:177–185, 1979.

Payne, R.: Neonatal neutropenia and leukoagglutinins. Pediatrics 33:194–204, 1964.

Peaceman, A.M., and Rehnberg, K.A.: The effect of immunoglobulin G fractions from patients with lupus anticoagulant on placental prostacyclin and thromboxane production. Am. J. Obstet. Gynecol. 169:1403–1406, 1993.

Peaceman, A.M., Silver, R.K., MacGregor, S.N., and Socol, M.L.: Interlaboratory variation in antiphospholipid antibody testing. Am. J.. Obstet. Gynecol. 166:1780–1787, 1992.

Pearce, J.M., and McParland, P.: Doppler uteroplacental waveforms. Lancet 1:1287–1288, 1988.

Penn, I., Makowski, E.L., and Harris, P.: Parenthood following renal and hepatic transplantation. Transplantation 30:397–400, 1980.

Pestelek, B., and Kapor, M.: Pheochromocytoma and abruptio placentae. Am. J. Obstet. Gynecol. 85:538–540, 1963.

Pijnenborg, R., Anthony, J., Davari, D.A., Rees, A., Tiltman, A., Vercruysse, L., and van Assche, A.: Placental bed spiral arteries in hypertensive disorders of pregnancy. Br. J. Obstet. Gynaecol. 98:648–655, 1991.

Pinette, M.G., Loftus-Brault, K., Nardi, D.A., and Rodis, J.F.: Maternal smoking and accelerated placental maturation. Obstet. Gynecol. 73:379–382, 1989.

Pitkin, R.M., Plank, C.J., and Filer, L.J.: Fetal and placental composition in experimental maternal diabetes. Proc. Soc. Exp. Biol. Med. 138:163–166, 1971.

Pittard III, W.B., Schleich, D.M., Geddes, K.M., and Sorensen, R.U.: Newborn lymphocyte subpopulations: the influence of labor. Am. J. Obstet. Gynecol. 160:151–154, 1989.

Platt, H.S.: Effect of maternal sickle cell trait on perinatal mortality. B.M.J. 2:334–338, 1971.

Pober, J.S.: Cytokine-mediated activation of vascular endothelium: physiology and pathology. Am. J. Pathol. 133:426–433, 1988.

Pollack, R.N., Pollack, M., and Rochon, L.: Pregnancy complicated by medulloblastoma with metastases to the placenta. Obstet. Gynecol. 81:858–859, 1993.

Polzin, W.J., Kopelman, J.N., Robinson, R.D., Read, J.A., and Brady, K.: The association of antiphospholipid antibodies with pregnancies complicated by fetal growth restriction. Obstet. Gynecol. 78:1108–1111, 1991.

Potau, N., Riudor, E., and Ballabriga, A.: Insulin receptors in human placenta in relation to fetal weight and gestational age. Pediatr. Res. 15:798–802, 1981.

Potter, J.F., and Schoeneman, M.: Metastasis of maternal cancer to the placenta and fetus. Cancer 25:380–388, 1970.

Prentice, R.L., Gatenby, P.A., Loblay, R.H., Shearman, R.P., Kronenberg, H., and Basten, A.: Lupus anticoagulant in pregnancy. Lancet 2:464, 1984.

Priesel, A., and Winkelbauer, A.: Placentare Übertragung des Lymphogranuloms. Virchows Arch. [Pathol. Anat.] 262:749–765, 1926.

Pritchard, J.A., Scott, D.E., Whalley, P.J., and Haling, R.F.: Infants of mothers with megaloblastic anemia due to folate deficiency. J.A.M.A. 211:1982–1984, 1970.

Pritchard, M.H., Jessop, J.D., Trenchard, P.M., and Whiltaker, J.A.: Systemic lupus erythematosus, repeated abortions, and thrombocytopenia. Ann. Rheum. Dis. 37:476–478, 1978.

Provost, T.T., Watson, R., Gammon, W.R., Radowsky, M., Harley, J.B., and Reichlin, M.: The neonatal lupus syndrome associated with U_1RNP (nRNP) antibodies. N. Engl. J. Med. 316:1135–1138, 1987.

Pulitzer, D.R., Collins, P.C., and Gold, R.G.: Embryonic implantation in carcinoma of the endometrium. Arch. Pathol. Lab. Med. 109:1089–1092, 1985.

Ramahi, A.J., Lewkow, L.M., Dombrowski, M.P., and Bottoms, S.F.: Sickle cell E hemoglobinopathy and pregnancy. Obstet. Gynecol. 71:493–495, 1988.

Rauramo, I., and Forss, M.: Effect of exercise on placental blood flow in pregnancies complicated by hypertension, diabetes or intrahepatic cholestasis. Acta Obstet. Gynecol. Scand. 67:15–20, 1988.

Raymond, E.G., and Mills, J.L.: Placental abruption: maternal risk factors and associated fetal conditions. Acta Obstet. Gynecol. Scand. 72:633–639, 1993.

Read, E.J., and Platzer, P.B.: Placental metastasis from maternal carcinoma of the lung. Obstet. Gynecol. 58:387–391, 1981.

Redman, C.W.G., and Jefferies, M.: Revised definition of pre-eclampsia. Lancet 1:809–812, 1988.

Redman, C.W.G., Bodmer, J.G., Bodmer, W.F., Beilin, L.J., and Bonnar, J.: HLA antigens in severe pre-eclampsia. Lancet 2:397–399, 1978.

Reece, E.A., Romero, R., Clyne, L.P., Kriz, N.S., and Hobbins, J.C.: Lupus-like anticoagulant in pregnancy. Lancet 1:344–345, 1984.

Reece, E.A., Gabrielli, S., Cullen, M.T., Zheng, X.-Z., Hobbins, J.C., and Harris, E.N: Recurrent adverse pregnancy outcome and antiphospholipid antibodies. Am. J. Obstet. Gynecol. 163:162–169, 1990.

Reiss, R.E., Kuwabara, T., Smith, M.L., and Gahl, W.A.: Successful pregnancy despite placental cystine crystals in a woman with nephropathic cystinosis. N. Engl. J. Med. 319:223–226, 1988.

Reshetnikova, O.S., Burton, G.J., and Milovanov, A.P.: Hypoxia at altitude and villous vascularisation in the mature human placenta [abstract A]. Placenta 14:62, 1993.

Retik, A.B., Sabesin, S.M., Hume, R., Malmgren, R.A., and Ketcham, A.S.: The experimental transmission of malignant melanoma cells through the placenta. Surg. Gynecol. Obstet. 114:485–489, 1962.

Rewell, R.E., and Whitehouse, W.L.: Malignant metastasis to the placenta from carcinoma of the breast. J. Pathol. Bacteriol. 91:255–256, 1966.

Reynolds, A.G.: Placental metastasis from malignant melanoma: report of a case. Obstet. Gynecol. 6:205–209, 1955.

Rice, J.P., Kay, H.H., and Mahony, B.S.: The clinical significance of uterine leiomyomas in pregnancy. Am. J. Obstet. Gynecol. 160:1212–1216, 1989.

Richards, D.S., Wagman, A.J., and Cabaniss, M.L.: Ascites not due to congestive heart failure in a fetus with lupus-induced heart block. Obstet. Gynecol. 76:957–959, 1990.

Rigby, P.G., Hanson, T.A., and Smith, R.S.: Passage of leukemic cells across the placenta. N. Engl. J. Med. 271:124–127, 1964.

Robb, S.A., and Hytten, F.E.: Placental glycogen. Br. J. Obstet. Gynaecol. 83:43–53, 1976.

Robbins, P.G., Gorbach, A.G., and Reid, D.E.: Neurologic abnormalities at one year in infants delivered after late-pregnancy hemorrhage. Obstet. Gynecol. 29:358–361, 1967.

Roberts, J.M.: Classification of hypertensive disorders of pregnancy. Lancet 2:112, 1989.

Robertson, W.B., Brosens, I., and Dixon, H.G.: The pathological response of the vessels of the placental bed to hypertensive pregnancy. J. Pathol. Bacteriol. 93:581–592, 1967.

Robertson, W.B., Khong, T.Y., Brosens, I., DeWolff, F., Sheppard, B.L., and Bonnar, J.: The placental bed biopsy: review from three European centers. Am. J. Obstet. Gynecol. 155:401–412, 1986.

Robinson, M.: Salt in pregnancy. Lancet 1:178–181, 1958.

Rodriguez, S.U., Leikin, S.L., and Hiller, M.C.: Neonatal thrombocytopenia associated with ante-partum administration of thiazide drugs. N. Engl. J. Med. 270:881–884, 1964.

Roe, D.A., Little, B.B., Bawdon, R.E., and Gilstrap, L.C.: Metabolism of cocaine by human placentas: implications for fetal exposure. Am. J. Obstet. Gynecol. 163:715–718, 1990.

Roffman, B.Y., and Simons, M.: Syncytial trophoblastic embolism associated with placenta increta and preeclampsia. Am. J. Obstet. Gynecol. 104:1218–1220, 1969.

Rosenberg, A.M., Bingham, M.C., and Fong, K.C.: Antinuclear antibodies during pregnancy. Obstet. Gynecol. 68:560–562, 1986.

Rosenfeld, C.R.: Preeclampsia: a review of the role of prostaglandins. Obstet. Gynecol. 72:284–285, 1988.

Rosenow, E.C., and Lee, R.A.: Cystic fibrosis and pregnancy. J.A.M.A. 203:227–230, 1968.

Rosner, F., Soong, B.C., Krim, M., and Miller, S.P.: Normal pregnancy in a patient with multiple myeloma. Obstet. Gynecol. 31:811–820, 1968.

Rosove, M.H., Tabsh, K., Wasserstrum, N., Howard, P., Hahn, B.H., and Kalunian, K.C.: Heparin therapy for pregnant women with lupus anticoagulant or anticardiolipin andtibodies. Obstet. Gynecol. 75:630–634, 1990.

Rote, N.S., and Caudle, M.R.: Circulating immune complexes in pregnancy, preeclampsia, and autoimmune diseases: evaluation of Raji cell enzyme-linked immunosorbent assay and polyethylene glycol precipitation methods. Am. J. Obstet. Gynecol. 147:267–273, 1983.

Rothman, L.A., Cohen, C.J., and Astarloa, J.: Placental and fetal involvement by maternal malignancy: a report of rectal carcinoma and review of the literature. Am. J. Obstet. Gynecol. 116:1023–1034, 1973.

Rouget, J.P., Goudemand, J., Montreuil, G., Cosson, A., and Jaillard, J.: Lupus anticoagulant: a familial observation. Lancet 2:105, 1982.

Rubin, D.H., Krasilikoff, P.A., Leventhal, J.M., Weile, B., and Berget, A.: Effect of passive smoking on birthweight. Lancet 2:415–417, 1986.

Rushton, D.I.: Trophoblast cells in peripheral blood. Lancet 2:1153–1154, 1984.

Salafia, C.M., and Silberman, L.: Placental pathology and abnormal fetal heart rate patterns in gestational diabetes. Pediatr. Pathol. 9:513–520, 1989.

Samaan, N.A., Gallager, H.S., McRoberts, W.A., and Holt, B.: Differential evaluation of the fetoplacental unit in patients with diabetes. Am. J. Obstet. Gynecol. 120:825–832, 1974.

Sanerkin, N.G., and Evans, D.M.D.: Bilateral renal cortical necrosis in infants, associated with maternal antepartum haemorrhage. J. Pathol. Bacteriol. 90:269–274, 1965.

Sanyal, M.K., Li, Y.-L., Biggers, W., Satish, J., and Barnea, E.R.: Augmentation of polynuclear aromatic hydrocarbon metabolism of human placental tissues of first-trimester pregnancy by cigarette smoke exposure. Am. J. Obstet. Gynecol. 168:1587–1597, 1993.

Sasseville, D., Wilkinson, R.D., and Schnader, J.Y.: Dermatoses of pregnancy. Int. J. Dermatol. 20:223–241, 1981.

Schaffner, T., Taylor, K., Bartucci, E.J., Fischer-Dzoga, K., Beeson, J.H., Glasgo, S., and Wissler, R.W.: Arterial foam cells with distinctive immunomorphologic and histochemical features of macrophages. Am. J. Pathol. 100:57–80, 1980.

Schenker, J.G., and Polishuk, W.Z.: Idiopathic thrombocytopenia in pregnancy. Gynaecologia 165:271–283, 1968.

Schenker, J.G., Segal, S., and Polishuk, W.Z.: Systemic lupus erythematosus in pregnancy. Harefuah 82:1–4, 1972.

Schiff, E., Peleg, E., Goldenberg, M., Rosenthal, T., Ruppin, E., Tamarkin, M., Barkal, G., Ben-Baruch, G., Yahal, I., Blankstein, J., Goldman, B., and Mashiach, S.: The use of aspirin to prevent pregnancy-induced hypertension and lower the ratio of thromboxane A_2 to prostacyclin in relatively high risk pregnancies. N. Engl. J. Med. 321:351–356, 1989.

Schmidt, B.K., Muraji, T., and Zipursky, A.: Low antithrombin III in neonatal shock: DIC or non-specific protein depletion? Eur. J. Pediatr. 145:500–503, 1986.

Schmorl, G.: Pathologisch-Anatomische Untersuchungen Über Puerperale Eklampsie. Vogel, Leipzig, 1893.

Schneider, C.L.: "Fibrin embolism" (disseminated intravascular coagulation) with defibrination as one of the end results during placenta abruptio. Surg. Gynecol. Obstet. 92:27–34, 1951.

Schneider, C.L.: Abruptio placentae after fetal death in utero. Obstet. Gynecol. 1:321–326, 1953.

Schuhmann, R., and Geier, G.: Histomorphologische Placentabefunde bei EPH-Gestose: ein Beitrag zur Morphologie der insuffizienten Placenta. Arch. Gynecol. 213:31–47, 1972.

Schuhmann, R., and Lehmann, W.D.: Beziehungen zwischen Placentamorphologie und biochemischen Befunden bei EPH-Gestose und Diabetes mellitus: dehydroandrosteronbelastungstest, in vitro Umwandlungsrate von 4-^{14}C-Dehydroepiandrosteron in Oestrogene, Oestrogenausscheidung im 24 Std-Urin. Arch. Gynecol. 215:72–84, 1973.

Scott, J.R., and Beer, A.A.: Immunologic aspects of pre-eclampsia. Am. J. Obstet. Gynecol. 125:418–427, 1976.

Scott, J.R., Branch, D.W., Kochenour, N.K., and Ward, K.: Intravenous immunoglobulin treatment of pregnant patients with recurrent pregnancy loss caused by antiphospholipid antibodies and Rh immunization. Am. J. Obstet. Gynecol. 159:1055–1056, 1988.

Scott, J.S.: Immunological diseases and pregnancy. B.M.J. 1:1559–1568, 1966.

Scott, J.S., and Jenkins, D.M.: Review article: immunogenetic factors in aetiology of pre-eclampsia/eclampsia (gestosis). J. Med. Genet. 13:200–207, 1976.

Scott, J.S., Jenkins, D.M., and Need, J.A.: Immunology of pre-eclampsia. Lancet 1:704–706, 1978.

Scully, R.E., Galdabini, J.J., and McNeely, B.U.: Cabot Case # 37-1976. N. Engl. J. Med. 295:608–614, 1976.

Seip, M.: Systemic lupus erythematosus in pregnancy with haemolytic anaemia, leucopenia and thrombocytopenia in the mother and her newborn infant. Arch. Dis. Child. 35:364–366, 1960.

Shanklin, D.R.: The human placenta with especial reference to infarction and toxemia. Obstet. Gynecol. 13:325–336, 1959.

Shanklin, D.R.: Clinicopathologic correlates in placentas from women with sickle cell disease [abstract PPC-15]. Am. J. Pathol. 82:5A, 1976.

Shanklin, D.R., and Sibai, B.M.: Ultrastructural aspects of preeclampsia. I. Placental bed and uterine boundary vessels. Am. J. Obstet. Gynecol. 161:735–741, 1989.

Sharon, R., and Amar, A.: Maternal anti-HLA antibodies and neonatal thrombocytopenia. Lancet 1:1313, 1981.

Shaw, E.B., and Rees, E.L.: Fetal damage due to aminopterin ingestion: follow-up at 17½ years of age. Am. J. Dis. Child. 134:1172, 1980.

Sheridan-Pereira, M., Porreco, R., Hays, T., and Burke, M.S.: Neonatal aortic thrombosis associated with the lupus anticoagulant. Obstet. Gynecol. 71:1016–1018, 1988.

Sholl, J.S.: Abruptio placentae: clinical management in nonacute cases. Am. J. Obstet. Gynecol. 156:40–51, 1987.

Siegel, P.: Beziehungen zwischen eklamptischen Placentarveränderungen und intrauterinem Fruchttod. Fortschr. Med. 80:75–82, 1962.

Silver, M.M.: Massive placental infarction due to the lupus anticoagulant [abstract 508]. Mod. Pathol. 1:85A, 1988.

Silver, M.M., Laxer, R.M., Laskin, C.A., Smallhorn, J.F., and Gare, D.J.: Association of fetal heart block and massive placental infarction due to maternal autoantibodies. Pediatr. Pathol. 12:131–139, 1992a.

Silver, R.K., MacGregor, S.N., Pasternak, J.F., and Neely, S.E.: Fetal stroke associated with elevated maternal anticardiolipin antibodies. Obstet. Gynecol. 80:497–499, 1992b.

Silverstein, M.N., Aaro, L.A., and Kempers, R.D.: Evans' syndrome and pregnancy. Am. J. Med. Sci. 252:206–211, 1966.

Slate, W.G., and Graham, A.R.: Scleroderma and pregnancy. Am. J. Obstet. Gynecol. 101:335–341, 1968.

Sletnes, K.E., Wisloff, F., Moe, N., and Dale, P.O.: Antiphospholipid antibodies in pre-eclamptic women: relation to growth retardation and neonatal outcome. Acta Obstet. Gynecol. Scand. 71:112–117, 1992.

Smith, M.L., Clark, K.F., Davis, S.E., Greene, A.A., Marcusson, E.G., Chen, Y.-J., and Schneider, J.A.: Diagnosis of cystinosis with use of placenta. N. Engl. J. Med. 321:397, 1989.

Smythe, A.R., Underwood, P.B., and Kreutner, A.: Metastatic placental tumors: report of three cases. Am. J. Obstet. Gynecol. 125:1149–1151, 1976.

Sokol, R.J., Hutchison, P., Cowan, D., and Reed, G.B.: Amelanotic melanoma metastatic to the placenta. Am. J. Obstet. Gynecol. 124:431–432, 1976.

Sokol, R.J., Miller, S.I., and Reed, G.: Alcohol abuse during pregnancy: an epidemiologic study: alcoholism. Clin. Exp. Res. 4:135–145, 1980.

Soma, H., Yoshida, K., Mukaida, T., and Tabuchi, Y.: Morphologic changes in the hypertensive placenta. Contrib. Gynecol. Obstet. 9:58–75, 1982.

Sophian, J.: Antibodies to trophoblast post partum and toxemia. Am. J. Obstet. Gynecol. 88:280–281, 1964.

Sørensen, P.G., Mickley, H., Diederichsen, H., and Grunnert, N.: Maternal antibodies and neonatal thrombocytopenia. Lancet 1:452, 1982.

Soyannwo, M.A.O., Armstrong, M.J., and McGeown, M.G.: Survival of the foetus in a patient in acute renal failure. Lancet 2:1009–1011, 1966.

Spellacy, W.N.: Scleroderma and pregnancy: report of a case. Obstet. Gynecol. 23:297–300, 1964.

Sridama, V., Yang, S.L., Moawad, A., and De Groot, L.J.: T-cell subsets in patients with preeclampsia. Am. J. Obstet. Gynecol. 147:566–569, 1983.

Stark, J., and Kaufmann, P.: Infarktgenese in der Placenta. Arch. Gynecol. 217:189–208, 1974.

Steigrad, K.: Über die Beziehung von Plazentarinfarkten zur Schwangerschafts-Nephropathie: Zugleich ein Beitrag zur Pathologie der Plazenta. Gynaecologia 134:273–322, 1952.

Steinke, J., and Driscoll, S.G.: The extractable insulin content of pancreas from fetuses and infants of diabetic and control mothers. Diabetes 14:573–578, 1965.

Stephenson, H.E., Terry, C.W., Lukens, J.N., Shively, J.A., Busby, W.E., Stoeckle, H.E., and Esterly, J.A.: Immunologic factors in human melanoma "metastatic" to products of gestation (with exchange transfusion to mother). Surgery 69:515–522, 1971.

Stormorken, H., Gjemdal, T., and Njoro, K.: Lupus anticoagulant: A unique case with lupus anticoagulant and habitual abortion together with antifactor II antibody and bleeding tendency. Gynecol. Obstet. Invest. 26:83–88, 1988.

Streiff, R.R., and Little, A.B.: Folic acid deficiency in pregnancy. N. Engl. J. Med. 276:776–779, 1967.

Stuart, M.J., Clark, D.A., Sunderji, S.G., Allen, J.B., Yambo, T., Elrad, H., and Slott, J.H.: Decreased prostacyclin production: a characteristic of chronic placental insufficiency syndromes. Lancet 1:1126–1128, 1981.

Tatum, H.J.: Placental abruption. Obstet. Gynecol. 2:447–453, 1953.

Teasdale, F.: Histomorphometry of the placenta of the diabetic woman: class A diabetes mellitus. Placenta 2:241–252, 1981.

Teasdale, F.: Histomorphometry of human placenta in class B diabetes mellitus. Placenta 4:1–12, 1983.

Teasdale, F.: Histomorphometry of the human placenta in class C diabetes mellitus. Placenta 5:69–86, 1984.

Teasdale, F.: Histomorphometry of the human placenta in maternal preeclampsia. Am. J. Obstet. Gynecol. 152: 25–31, 1985.

Teasdale, F., and Ghislaine, J.-J.: Morphological changes in the placentas of smoking mothers: a histomorphometric study. Biol. Neonate 55:251–259, 1989.

Tedeschi, L.G., and Tedeschi, C.G.: Experimental trophoblastic embolism and hyperplasminemia. Arch. Pathol. 76:387–397, 1963.

Tenney, B., and Parker, F.: The placenta in toxemia of pregnancy. Am. J. Obstet. Gynecol. 39:1000–1005, 1940.

Thomas, K., de Gasparo, M., and Hoet, J.J.: Insulin levels in the umbilical vein and in the umbilical artery of newborns of normal and gestational diabetic mothers. Diabetes 3: 299–304, 1967.

Thomsen, K., and Lieschke, G.: Untersuchungen zur Placentamorphologie bei Diabetes mellitus. Acta Endocrinol. (Copenh.) 29:602–614, 1958.

Thornton, J.G., and Sampson, J.: Genetics of pre-eclampsia. Lancet 336:1319–1320, 1990.

Thornton, Y.S., Birnbaum, S.J., and Lebowitz, N.: A viable pregnancy in a patient with myositis ossificans. Am. J. Obstet. Gynecol. 156:577–578, 1987.

Thorp, J.A., Walsh, S.W., and Brath, P.C.: Low-dose aspirin inhibits thromboxane, but not prostacyclin, production by human placental arteries. Am. J. Obstet. Gynecol. 159: 1381–1384, 1988.

Toder, V., Blank, M., Gleicher, N., Voljovich, I., Mashiah, S., and Nebel, L.: Activity of natural killer cells in normal pregnancy and edema-proteinuria-hypertension gestosis. Am. J. Obstet. Gynecol. 145:7–10, 1983.

Tominaga, T., and Page, E.W.: Accommodation of the human placenta to hypoxia. Am. J. Obstet. Gynecol. 84:679–691, 1966.

Torpin, R., and Swain, B.: Placental infarction in 1,000 cases correlated with the clinical findings. Am. J. Obstet. Gynecol. 94:284–285, 1966.

Trauscht-VanHorn, J., Capeless, E., Bovill, E.G., Easterling, T.R., and Hermanson, B.: Pregnancy loss and thrombosis with protein C deficiency in pregnancy [abstract 114]. Am. J. Obstet. Gynecol. 166:311, 1992.

Triplett, D.A.: Antiphospholipid antibodies and recurrent pregnancy loss. Am. J. Reprod. Immunol. 20:52–67, 1989.

Triplett, D.A.: Antiphospholipid antibodies and thrombosis: a consequence, coincidence, or cause? Arch. Pathol. Lab. Med. 117:78–88, 1993.

Triplett, D.A., Brandt, J.T., and Maas, R.L.: The laboratory heterogeneity of lupus anticoagulant. Arch. Pathol. Lab. Med. 109:946–951, 1985.

Trudinger, B.J., Stewart, G.J., Cook, C.M., Connelly, A., and Exner, T.: Monitoring lupus anticoagulant-positive pregnancies with umbilical artery flow velocity waveforms. Obstet. Gynecol. 72:215–218, 1988.

Tsujimura, T., Matsumoto, K., and Aozasa, K.: Placental involvement by maternal non-Hodgkin's lymphoma. Arch. Pathol. Lab. Med. 117:325–327, 1993.

Unander, A.M., Norberg, R., Hahn, L., and Årfors, L.: Anticardiolipin antibodies and complement in ninety-nine women with habitual abortion. Am. J. Obstet. Gynecol. 156:114–119, 1987.

Uzan, S., Beaufils, M., Breart G., Bazin, B., Capitant, C., and Paris, J.: Prevention of fetal growth retardation with low-dose aspirin: findings of the EPREDA trial. Lancet 337:1427–1431, 1991.

Vasquez-Escobosa, C., Perez-Medina, R., and Gomez-Estrada, H.: Circulating immune complexes in hypertensive disease of pregnancy. Obstet. Gynecol. 62:45–48, 1982.

Vassalli, P., Morris, R.H., and McCluskey, R.T.: The pathogenic role of fibrin deposition in the glomerular lesions of toxemia of pregnancy. J. Exp. Med. 118:467–478, 1963.

Vintzileos, A.M., Campbell, W.A., Nochimson, D.J., and Weinbaum, P.J.: Preterm premature rupture of the membranes: a risk factor for the development of abruptio placentae. Am. J. Obstet. Gynecol. 156:1235–1238, 1987.

Vogel, M.: Plakopathia diabetica. Virchows Arch. [Pathol. Anat.] 343:51–63, 1967.

Vogel, J.J., de Moerloose, P.A., and Bounameaux, H.: Protein C deficiency and pregnancy: a case report. Obstet. Gynecol. 73:455–456, 1989.

Voigt, L.F., Hollenbach, K.A., Krohn, M.A., Daling, J.R., and Hickok, D.E.: The relationship of abruptio placentae with maternal smoking and small for gestational age infants. Obstet. Gynecol. 75:771–774, 1990.

Vulsma, T., Gons, M.H., and de Vijlder, J.J.M.: Maternal-fetal transfer of thyroxine in congenital hypothyroidism due to a total organification defect or thyroid agenesis. N. Engl. J. Med. 321:13–16, 1989.

Waddington, H.K.: Fetal salvage in abruptio placentae. Am. J. Obstet. Gynecol. 73:812–816, 1957.

Wagner, D.: Trophoblastic cells in the blood stream in normal and abnormal pregnancy. Acta Cytol. 12:137–139, 1968.

Wagner, D., Schunck, R., and Isebarth, H.: Der Nachweis von Trophoblastzellen im strömenden Blut der Frau bei normaler und gestörter Gravidität. Gynaecologia 158: 175–192, 1964.

Wallenburg, H.C.S.: Über den Zusammenhang zwischen Spätgestose und Placentarinfarkt. Arch. Gynecol. 208: 80–90, 1969.

Wallenburg, H.C.S., Hutchinson, D.L., Schuler, H.M., Stolte, L.A.M., and Janssens, J.: The pathogenesis of placental infarction. II. An experimental study in the rhesus monkey placenta. Am. J. Obstet. Gynecol. 116:841–846, 1973a.

Wallenburg, H.C.S., Stolte, L.A.M., and Janssens, J.: The pathogenesis of placental infarction. I. A morphologic study in the human placenta. Am. J. Obstet. Gynecol. 116: 835–840, 1973b.

Walsh, S.W.: Preeclampsia: an imbalance in placental prostacyclin and thromboxane production. Am. J. Obstet. Gynecol. 152:335–340, 1985.

Walsh, S.W., Behr, M.J., and Allen, N.H.: Placental prostacyclin production in normal and toxemic pregnancies. Am. J. Obstet. Gynecol. 151:110–115, 1985.

Wapner, R.J., Cowchock, F.S., and Shapiro, S.S.: Successful treatment in two women with antiphospholipid antibodies and refractory pregnancy losses with intravenous immunoglobulin infusions. Am. J. Obstet. Gynecol. 161:1271–1272, 1989.

Warrell, D.W., and Taylor, R.: Outcome for the foetus of mothers receiving prednisolone during pregnancy. Lancet 1:117–118, 1968.

Warren, R.J., Rimoin, D.L., and Sly, W.S.: LSD exposure in utero. Pediatrics 45:466–469, 1970.

Watov, S.E., and de Sandre, R.: Gaucher's disease and pregnancy: report of one case involving four pregnancies. Obstet. Gynecol. 23:247–250, 1964.

Weathers, W.T., Crane, M.M., Sauvain, K.J., and Blackhurst, D.W.: Cocaine use in women from a defined population: prevalence at delivery and effects on growth in infants. Pediatrics 91:350–354, 1993.

Weiner, C., and Keller, S.: Preeclampsia is not associated with excess fetal clotting. Obstet. Gynecol. 68:871–872, 1986.

Weir, P.E.: Immunofluorescent studies of the uteroplacental arteries in normal pregnancy. Br. J. Obstet. Gynaecol. 88:301–307, 1981.

Wells, M., and Bulmer, J.N.: The human placental bed: histology, immunohistochemistry and pathology. Histopathology 13:483–498, 1988.

Wen, S.W., Goldenberg, R.L., Cutter, G.R., Hoffman, H.J., Cliver, S.P., Davis, R.O., and DuBard, M.B.: Smoking, maternal age, fetal growth, and gestational age at delivery. Am. J. Obstet. Gynecol. 162:53–58, 1990.

Wentworth, P.: Placental infarction and toxemia of pregnancy. Am. J. Obstet. Gynecol. 99:318–326, 1967.

Whalley, P.J., Pritchard, J.A., and Richards, J.R.: Sickle cell trait and pregnancy. J.A.M.A. 186:1132–1135, 1963.

White, P.: Classification of obstetric diabetes. Am. J. Obstet. Gynecol. 130:228–230, 1978.

White, B.M., and Beischer, N.A.: Perinatal mortality in the infants of diabetic women. Aust. N.Z. J. Obstet. Gynaecol. 30:323–326, 1990.

Widmaier, G.: Zur Ultrastruktur menschlicher Placentazotten beim Diabetes mellitus. Arch. Gynecol. 208:396–409, 1970.

Wieland, R.G., Shaffer, M.B., and Glove, R.P.: Cushing's syndrome complicating pregnancy: a case report. Obstet. Gynecol. 38:841–843, 1971.

Wielenga, G., and Willighagen, R.G.J.: Histochemical investigation of ischemic villi in the placenta. Am. J. Obstet. Gynecol. 96:956–968, 1966.

Willems, J.: The etiology of preeclampsia: a hypothesis. Obstet. Gynecol. 50:495–499, 1977.

Wingerd, J., Christianson, R., Lovitt, W.V., and Schoen, E.J.: Placental ratio in white and black women: relation to smoking and anemia. Am. J. Obstet. Gynecol. 124: 671–675, 1976.

Winick, M., and Noble, A.: Cellular growth in human placenta. II. Diabetes mellitus. Am. J. Obstet. Gynecol. 71:216–219, 1967.

Winn, H.N., Setaro, J.F., Mazor, M., Reece, E.A., Black, H.R., and Hobbins, J.C.: Severe Takayasu's arteritis in pregnancy: the role of central hemodynamic monitoring. Am. J. Obstet. Gynecol. 159:1135–1136, 1988.

Winston, H.G., and Mastroianni, L.: Sickle cell disease in pregnancy. Obstet. Gynecol. 2:73–77, 1953.

Wisot, A.L.: Silent abruptio placentae with marked hypofibrinogenemia. J.A.M.A. 207:557–558, 1969.

Wladimiroff, J.W., Barentsen, R., Wallenburg, H.C.S., and Drogendijk, A.C.: Fetal urine production in a case of diabetes associated with polyhydramnios. Obstet. Gynecol. 46:100–102, 1975.

Wolf, H., Šabata, V., Frerichs, H., and Stubbe, P.: Evidence for the impermeability of the human placenta for insulin. Horm. Metab. Res. 1:274–275, 1969.

Woodhouse, S.: The lupus anticoagulant and the dilute Russell viper venom test. Pathologist July: 432–433, 1984.

Woods, J.R., Plessinger, M.A., and Clark, K.E.: Effect of cocaine on uterine blood flow and fetal oxygenation. J.A.M.A. 257:857–961, 1987.

Wurzel, J.M.: TTP lesions in placenta but not fetus. N. Engl. J. Med. 301:503–504, 1979.

Wynn, R.M.: The placenta in preeclampsia. Obstet. Gynecol. Annu. 6:191–196, 1977.

Xu, L., Chang, V., Murphy, A., Rock, J.A., Damewood, M., Schlaff, W., and Zacur, H.A.: Antinuclear antibodies in sera of patients with recurrent pregnancy wastage. Am. J. Obstet. Gynecol. 163:1493–1497, 1990. (For discussion see Am. J. Obstet. Gynecol. 166:1021–1022, 1992.)

Ylikorkala, O., and Mkil, U.-M.: Prostacyclin and thromboxane in gynecology and obstetrics. Am. J. Obstet. Gynecol. 152:318–329, 1985.

Zacks, S., and Blazar, A.S.: Chorionic villi in normal pregnancy, pre-eclamptic toxemia, erythroblastosis, and diabetes mellitus: a light- and electron-microscope study. Obstet. Gynecol. 22:149–167, 1963.

Zeek, P.M., and Assali, N.S.: Vascular changes in the decidua associated with eclamptogenic toxemia of pregnancy. Am. J. Clin. Pathol. 20:1099–1109, 1950.

Zhou, Y., Chiu, K., Brescia, R.J., Combs, C.A., Katz, M.A., Kitzmiller, J.L., Heilbron, D.C., and Fisher, S.J.: Increased depth of trophoblast invasion after chronic constriction of the lower aorta in rhesus monkeys. Am. J. Obstet. Gynecol. 169:224–229, 1993.

Zugaib, M., de Barros, A.C.S.D., Bittar, R.E., Burdmann, E.deA., and Neme, B.: Abruptio placentae following snake bite. Am. J. Obstet. Gynecol. 151:754–755, 1985.

20
Infectious Diseases

Prenatal infections are an important aspect of placental pathology. They are common and varied. Their pathogenesis and related circumstances must be understood if the pathological lesions are to be interpreted correctly. Many types of infection cause placental changes, but for some types the infection may be difficult to prove from placental examination. Ultrastructural studies are especially lacking in this area and might be helpful, particularly when virus infection is suspected. Infections may ascend from the endocervical canal, or they may reach the placenta hematogenously through the maternal blood. Rarely are they acquired by amniocentesis, chorionic villous sampling, amnioscopy (Horky & Amon, 1967), percutaneous umbilical blood sampling (Wilkins et al., 1989), or intrauterine fetal transfusion (Goodlin, 1965; Scott & Henderson, 1972). Many infections cause gross and microscopic changes of the placenta, whereas others (e.g., Coxsackie virus infection) leave few characteristic or specifically recognizable traces. This point is also the case with parvovirus B19 infection, which often leads to fetal hydrops but has no specific placental alteration other than perhaps intranuclear inclusions in nucleated red blood cell precursors and endothelium, as a report by Hartwick et al. (1989) showed. Samra et al. (1989) described villous necrosis and calcification in the placenta from a 20 weeks' gestation with hydrops due to this infection (see Chapter 16).

This chapter first covers chorioamnionitis, followed by infections with specific organisms that correlate with chorioamnionitis. Syphilis and necrotizing funisitis (inflammation of the umbilical cord) are next discussed followed by virus infections and villitides. Finally, rare infectious diseases such as malaria and parasitic infections are covered. A complete review of the early literature, especially the European references, may be found in the work of Flamm (1959). The comprehensive text on infections of the fetus and newborn infant by Remington and Klein (1983) may also be consulted. Excellent and complete reviews of fetal and placental infections have been provided by Blanc (1981) and Altshuler (1984).

Chorioamnionitis

Macroscopic Appearance

Typically, the placenta of the amnionic sac infection syndrome is a premature placenta. It lacks the blue sheen of the normal immature organ, and the membranes are obscured by an inflammatory exudate of polymorphonuclear leukocytes (neutrophils, PMNLs) (Figures 373–375). The surface becomes yellow when much leukocytic exudate has accumulated and when the process has been of long duration. The amnion may be roughened or may have lost the luster it normally possesses. The placenta is also frequently malodorous, and the astute observer may identify the prevailing organism by the odor. Thus the fecal odor of fusobacterial and *Bacteroides* infections, and the sweet odor of *Clostridium* and *Listeria* infections are useful identifiers. The membranes are typically friable, and the decidua capsularis is frequently detached and hemorrhagic. These prematurely delivered placentas are often accompanied by an acute marginal hemorrhage that undermines the edge of the placenta and originates from deciduitis. Although the picture mimics that of abruptio placentae, this hemorrhagic process (Figures 376, 377) markedly differs from that of typical abruptio placentae of preeclampsia. Vintzileos et al. (1987) believed that true abruptio occurs after premature rupture of the membranes. They found an incidence of 6.3% (2.7% in controls) of normally implanted placentas with "indentations in the placental substance." Unfortunately, they did not discuss inflammatory reactions. Gonen et al. (1989) also provided evidence that abruptio (loosely defined) is frequently preceded by prolonged rupture of membranes. Darby et al. (1989) compared women with severe preterm abruptions with control women requiring preterm delivery. The former group had significantly more frequently chorioamnionitis and funisitis (41% versus 4%). Darby et al. believed that infection preceded the abruptio.

Touch preparations made from the fetal surface of placentas from women with prenatal infection may be used to identify the inflammatory exudate as well as the bacteria quickly, especially when the infection is due to *Listeria monocytogenes*. When chorioamnionitis is found in twin placentas, it is nearly invariably twin A whose cavity has inflammation or that has the more

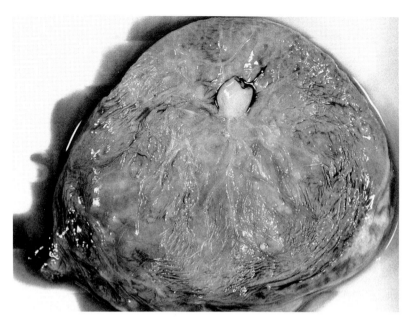

FIGURE 373. Near-term placenta with severe chorioamnionitis. Note the marginal hemorrhage at left caused by deciduitis. The surface of the placenta is obscured by a whitish exudate that obscures the normal underlying blue color; the vasculature is also indistinct. Neonatal death resulted.

severely inflamed portion (Benirschke, 1960) (Figure 378). We have considered this situation to mean that the amnionic sac infection is always ascending through the cervical canal. This correlation was questioned by Thiery et al. (1970), however, who found umbilical phlebitis in twin B as often as in twin A. These authors did not state how their twins were delivered, though, or how the twins were positively identified as to their intrauterine location. These specifications are crucial to the interpretation of such data.

Microscopic Appearance

Perhaps the earliest investigators to delineate chorioamnionitis were Wohlwill and Bock (1929). They described nine cases of "coccal" infection, some of

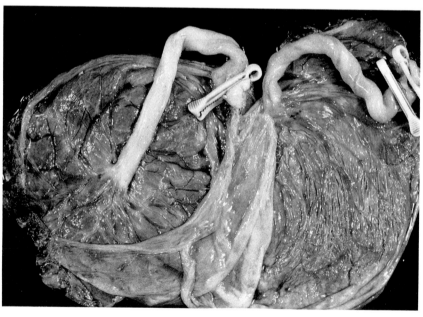

FIGURE 374. Immature diamnionic dichorionic twin placenta from a cesarean section. Twin A (left, one cord clamp) was located higher in the uterus; twin B (right), with a marginally inserted cord, was near the lower uterine segment and exhibited significant chorioamnionitis. Compare the luster of the normal placenta (left) with the indistinct features of the abnormal placenta (right), which are due to inflammation. Neonatal deaths resulted.

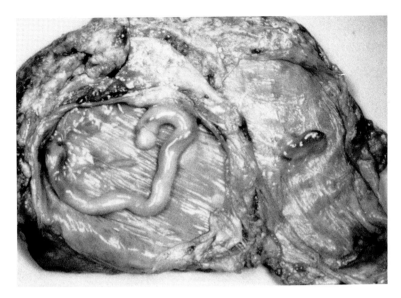

FIGURE 375. Immature twin placenta (19 weeks' gestation) from which twin A (right) had been delivered 1 week prior to twin B (left). Both twins had severe chorioamnionitis and fatal aspiration pneumonia. The placental surface was yellow, purulent, and malodorous.

which clearly followed attempted ("criminal") abortion. Reviews of Kückens (1938) and Müller (1956) made it clear that "round cell infiltration of the placenta" had been known before then. These authors suggested that infection of the fetus had caused the sepsis and then led to the placental inflammation. Wohlwill and Bock (1929) reviewed the placental inflammations that had been reported before their studies of chorioamnionitis (largely syphilis, tuberculosis, and leprosy) and decided that the coccal infection they found was of a different character.

As indicated, an extensive description of chorioamnionitis ("round cell infiltration") was authored by Kückens (1938). He found the literature to be contradictory and came to the following conclusions: The decidua has some round cell infiltration in 60% to 70% of normal placentas; villi never have such cellular infiltrates or abscesses; chorioamnionitis, with leukocytic

origin from the intervillous space, and funisitis are common perinatal phenomena. Kückens suggested that an ascending origin of the infection was the most likely pathway, an idea supported by Knox and Hoerner (1950). Kückens found that with funisitis the umbilical vein is the first vessel to be involved, with arterial inflammation to follow. He identified cocci in the lesions and found a 20.4% incidence of chorioamnionitis, relating it to the length of labor and rupture of membranes. Interestingly, a correlation with ophthalmia neonatorum due to gonorrheal infection had already been suggested.

Blanc (1953, 1957, 1959, 1961a) described chorioamnionitis in many important contributions and in great detail; he also coined the descriptive term "amnionic sac infection syndrome," which is now widely used. Blanc indicated methods for early diagnosis (gastric aspiration of the neonate, touch preparation from

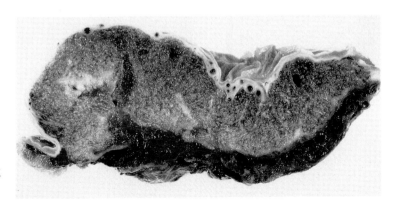

FIGURE 376. Placenta at 23 weeks' gestation with massive chorioamnionitis and marked marginal/retroplacental hemorrhage caused by deciduitis.

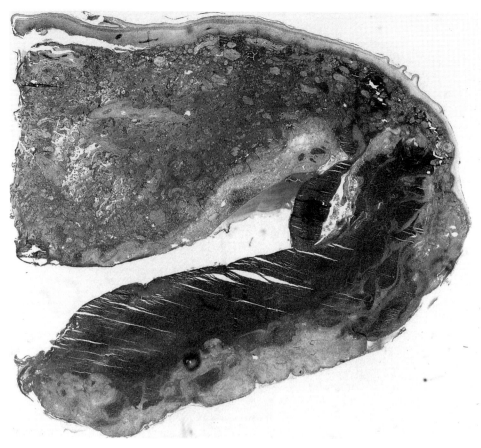

FIGURE 377. Margin of immature placenta at 23 weeks' gestation with marked chorioamnionitis and abruptio. The abruption is represented by the dark marginal retromembranous hematoma, which orginates from marked deciduitis and its disrupted vessels. H&E. ×3.5.

amnion), and he clearly explained that this disorder was an ascending infection of the amnionic sac. See also Müller (1956) and Pisarski et al. (1963) for references to the early European literature. There have been numerous pathological and clinical studies of this important entity since (reviewed by Altshuler, 1989).

Hallman et al. (1989) have shown that high concentrations of ceramide lactoside are contained in the amnionic fluid of patients with chorioamnionitis. They suggested that the lipid derives from phagocytosing granulocytes. Kirshon et al. (1991) found that patients with prenatal infection had amnionic fluid glucose levels

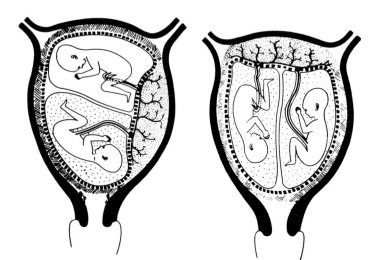

FIGURE 378. Twin placentation with inflammation (stippling), explaining the ascending nature of the infection.

of less than 10 mg/dl. Romero et al. (1987b) showed that arachidonate lipoxygenase products are much elevated in this infection. In a later study, these authors (Romero et al., 1989b) identified that infected amnionic fluid contained cachectin-tumor necrosis factor as evidence of macrophage activation. Many other intensive investigations have been published that attempt to clarify the role of amnionic sac infection in premature delivery.

In our opinion, chorioamnionitis is always due to infection, and the work of Gibbs et al. (1992) and many others cited below support this notion. The speculations of Dominguez et al. (1960) are nearly completely unfounded. These authors described umbilical cord inflammation (funisitis) in 10% of 1,000 consecutively studied placentas and portrayed it as being "lymphocytic" (which it practically never is); they related funisitis to prolonged labor and meconium discharge. The complete absence of inflammation in most meconium-stained umbilical cords, the published negative findings of Fox and Langley (1971), and the personal experience of most placental pathologists negate the notion that the common funisitis is caused by hypoxia, as was suggested. Widholm et al. (1963) stated summarily that

meconium causes funisitis. It is granted that meconium discharge and funisitis are often combined, but meconium per se is not an inflammatory agent. Maudsley et al. (1966), who presented a good description of the amnionic sac infection syndrome, also insisted that the term be reserved for cases with verified infection. Some other authors have neglected the consideration that fastidious organisms may cause chorioamnionitis (e.g., Olding, 1970). There is thus still lingering doubt and confusion as to the nature of chorioamnionitis (Anonymous, 1989a), but when Arias and colleagues (1993) studied the problem of preterm labor in 105 women they found that essentially two distinct subgroups exist: those with infection (n = 63) and those with decidual vasculopathy (n = 42).

Chorioamnionitis is an acute inflammatory reaction in which PMNLs principally participate. Eosinophils are found at times but only after protracted infections; and macrophages may participate to a variable extent. Plasma cells are generally absent in the membranes, however, except in some of the chronic infections discussed below. The leukocytes come from two sources: the intervillous space (and are then maternal) and fetal surface blood vessels (Figure 379). The emigration of

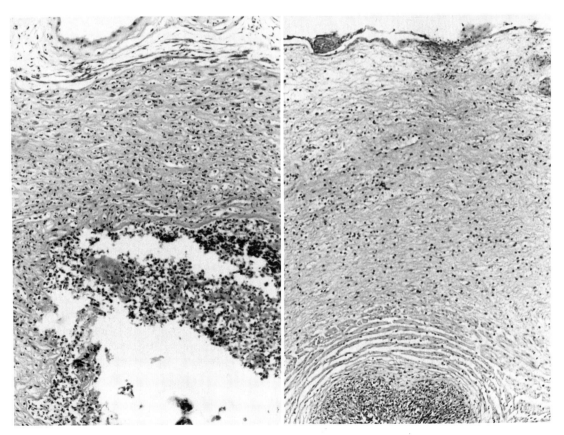

FIGURE 379. Placental surface from a 30 weeks' gestation delivery. The patient had gonorrhea, and her membranes had been ruptured for 40 hours. A 1,200 g infant with pneumonia was delivered. Note the exudation of PMNLs from the intervillous space (left), minimal vascular involvement (right), and amnion necrosis. H&E. Left ×240; right ×160.

leukocytes is always directional, toward the amnionic cavity, presumably toward an antigenic source. Pankuch and his colleagues (1989) studied this "amniotropism" of infected amnionic fluid. They found it to be a better indicator of infection than the Gram stain, culture, or chromatography.

In young gestations, especially those prior to the 20th week of gestation, the PMNLs are mainly of maternal origin. By midtrimester, the fetus begins to be capable of producing leukocytes that participate in the inflammatory response to leukotaxins (Müller, 1956). Neonates, when compared to adults, still have reduced leukocyte counts, and their PMNLs are less capable of ingesting microbes. Premature infants may therefore be prone to develop sepsis (Cairo, 1989). The maturation of the fetal lymphocyte system was studied by Berry et al. (1992), who found that fetuses had significantly fewer CD57[+] natural killer T cells. Other age-dependent changes are summarized in this study as well.

With funisitis, the inflammatory cells emigrate first from the umbilical vein and later from the arteries. They also migrate toward the amnionic surface and only rarely toward the center of the cord. Many die during the migration. It has been suggested that they rarely reach the amnionic fluid, but we believe that this suggestion is incorrect (Anonymous, 1989a). It is common, for instance, to find aspirated PMNLs in the lung and stomach of neonates with chorioamnionitis intermixed with squames. Moreover, pus can at times be aspirated at amniocentesis. The dead inflammatory cells of the placental surface frequently accumulate in large quantities underneath the amnion in the potential space that exists between amnion and chorion (Figure 380).

Experiments designed to identify the reason for the relatively slow permeation of the amnion by leukocytes have suggested that the type V collagen composition of the amnionic basal membrane prevents the ready transgression by PMNLs (Azzarelli & Lafuze, 1987). Some experimental evidence indicates that this amnionic sac infection reduces the strength of the chorion laeve (McGregor et al., 1987; Sbarra et al., 1987; Schoonmaker et al., 1989). Sbarra et al. (1985) demonstrated that when membranes are incubated with lysolecithin or phospholipase A_2, their bursting pressure decreases. Membrane "stripping" alone causes the release of this enzyme (McColgin et al., 1993). Parenthetically, it might be pointed out that the term amnionitis is, strictly speaking, erroneous. The amnion has no blood vessels; thus inflammation (a vascular phenomenon) can take place in the amnion only passively, by transmigration of leukocytes that originate elsewhere. Gleicher et al. (1979) have identified a "blocking factor" in the amnionic fluid that enhances leukocyte migration, presumably similar to the material that was studied by Schoonmaker et al. (1989).

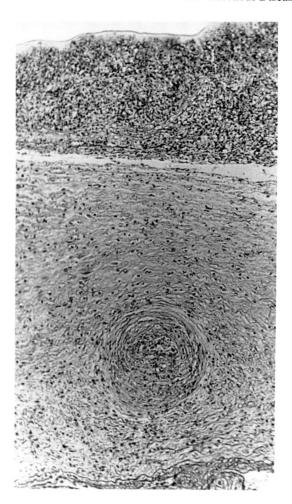

FIGURE 380. Massive chorioamnionitis in a stillborn at 23 weeks' gestation. The exudate is mostly necrotic and has accumulated in the amnion. The placenta had a purulent surface and marked funisitis. H&E. ×60.

The pus may reach the lung, stomach, and middle ears (Figure 381). When chronic aspiration pneumonia occurs, the lung contains lymphocyte and plasma cell infiltrations. They result from immunological recognition of the antigen (Figure 382). Benner (1940) found that 26% of stillborns had middle ear aspiration of pus. Moreover, a strong correlation exists between chorioamnionitis and otitis. McLellan et al. (1962) found purulent exudate in 19 of 28 temporal bones of neonates weighing between 1,000 and 1,500 g. The widely patent eustachian tube of premature infants is believed to be a possible portal of entry of this aspirated infected amnionic fluid. Congenital pneumonia has been documented in numerous publications following Ballantyne's (1904) first description. It is correlated with chorioamnionitis and funisitis. Barter (1962) argued in favor of Dominguez' hypothesis of hypoxia as the cause of the inflammation (see letter from Osborn, 1962; see

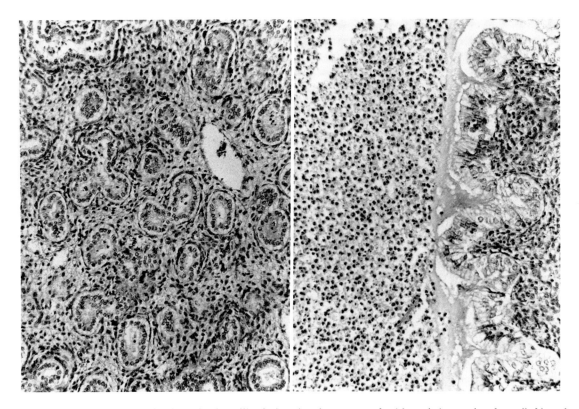

FIGURE 381. Aspiration of amnionic fluid pus in the still tubular alveolar spaces of a 16 weeks' gestation fetus (left) and stomach (right). H&E. ×120.

also Aherne & Davies, 1962; Browne, 1962). Anderson et al. (1962), Fujikura and Froehlich (1967), and Steiner et al. (1961), among the many authors who studied the phenomenon, found that "the drowning in pus" correlates with chorioamnionitis, prematurity, and premature rupture of the membranes; and in long-standing infections some plasma cell component may be found (Figure 383). Some of the necrotic exudate underneath the amnion may ultimately calcify, but the fetus is usually delivered before it happens. Simon et al.

(1989) undertook bacteriological studies of infants born after premature rupture of membranes. They found that 26% had the same bacteria in placental arterial blood, ear swabs, and meconium, the predominant organisms being *Escherichia coli*, *Bacteroides fragilis*, and streptococci. A significant study of the nature of organisms that cause chorioamnionitis comes from Hillier et al. (1991). The organisms most frequently associated with preterm delivery *and* chorioamnionitis were group B streptococci and *Fusobacterium*; *Pepto-*

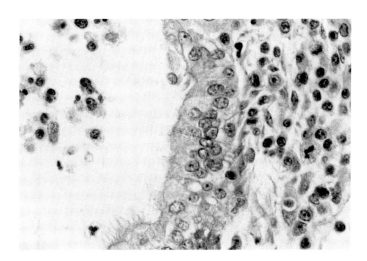

FIGURE 382. Chronic aspiration pneumonia in a stillborn. Note the pus in the bronchial lumen and plasma cells in the interstitial parenchyma. H&E. ×160.

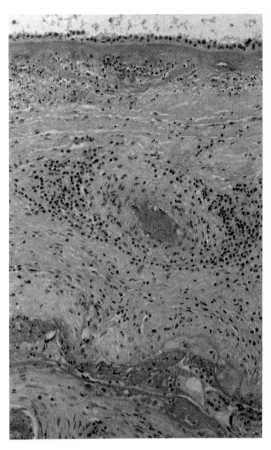

FIGURE 383. Placental surface at 28 weeks' gestation with chronic inflammation (plasma cells). H&E. ×60.

streptococcus was related only to preterm delivery, whereas *E. coli*, *Bacteroides*, and *Ureaplasma* were significantly related only to chorioamnionitis.

The fetal surface vessels partake in the inflammatory response to the leukotaxin, but generally little happens here before the 20th week of gestation. The maternal component of the leukocytic reaction originates in the intervillous space and in the maternal vessels of the decidua in the free membranes (Figure 384). Even in dichorionic twin placentas, some exudate may be found in the dividing membranes, where it originates from persisting maternal vessels (Figure 385). In this maternal response to amnionic sac infection, leukocytes first marginate underneath the fibrin under the chorionic plate. They then infiltrate the chorion and eventually the amnion. The subchorial accumulation has been designated intervillositis, an unfortunate term. Infectious organisms are rarely seen in the intervillous space, although toxins may accumulate here. The leukocytes merely react to the leukotactic signal that has permeated through the placental surface; they then accumulate in the subchorial space and finally migrate. Abscess formation underneath the chorionic plate and dissemination of exudate between villous trunks are rare (Vernon & Gauthier, 1971). When it is present, one must consider congenital listeriosis and *Campylobacter* infection first; other infections are much less frequently the cause. With listeriosis, villous and intervillous abscesses occur frequently (see below). Intervillous abscesses occur occasionally in maternal septicemias. We have seen them with maternal staphylococcal and *E. coli* infections. The mothers are usually so ill that labor and delivery occur before abscesses develop. Levy (1981) believed that a placental abscess he discovered could be the cause of the maternal fever. This abscess occupied 25% to 39% of the placental surface in a term pregnancy, but no bacteria were isolated, and listeriosis was not ruled out. Another placental abscess was due to *Proteus mirabilis* infection in a febrile patient, gram-negative bacilli being present in sections (Ravid & Toaff, 1976). In another pregnant

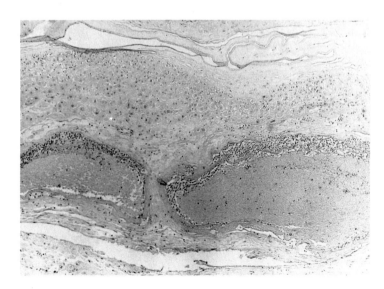

FIGURE 384. Placental membranes at term with early inflammation. Leukocytes are accumulating in maternal vessels, with direction toward the amnionic surface. Mural thrombosis is beginning. The patient was febrile, and funisitis was present. H&E. ×60.

FIGURE 385. Dividing membranes of a DiDi twin placenta with inflammation in the right sac. H&E. ×25. (Courtesy Dr. S.G. Driscoll, Boston.)

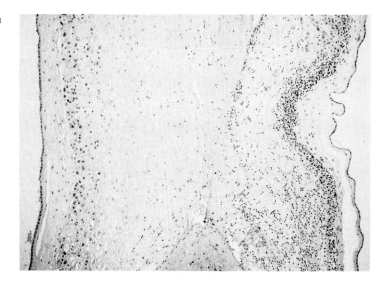

woman an intravenous line had been placed at 12 weeks' gestation as treatment for hyperemesis. She developed *Serratia* sepsis and was appropriately treated. When she delivered at 34 weeks, an old abscess without organisms was identified in the placenta. Villous abscesses do occur, as was reported, after intrauterine transfusion with infected blood (Scott & Henderson, 1972). The villi are otherwise almost never involved in common cases of chorioamnionitis, however severe that process may be. Subchorionic fibrin deposits are excellent sites from which to culture bacterial organisms, according to Aquino et al. (1984). These authors preferred to sample this site because it is not contaminated with vaginal organisms and because they experienced good recovery of bacteria from these specimens. They isolated group B hemolytic streptococci, anaerobic cocci, and rods, organisms that commonly cause endometritis, pelvic infection, and neonatal sepsis.

The exudate in funisitis is occasionally visible macroscopically (Figure 386). It must be emphasized, however, that funisitis (umbilical vasculitis) does *not* signify the existence of fetal sepsis, as is often believed. Blanc (1961a) has specified the possible means by which fetal sepsis can take place. It is a relatively late event in the course of prenatal infection with bacteria. Blanc opined that fetal sepsis may result from invasion of organisms through the lung and intestinal tract. Prior to delineation of the amnionic sac infection syndrome, funisitis was thought to be primarily related to congenital syphilis, and spirochetes were usually sought from endothelial scrapings by darkfield examination. This association is now no longer held to be firm (reviewed by Beckmann & Zimmer, 1931). With funisitis, the leukocytes marginate first at the vascular intima and then begin to dissect among the muscle bundles of the umbilical vein and arteries, finally infiltrating Wharton's

jelly (Figure 387). They also reach the cord's surface and may accumulate there in substantial numbers. The fetal PMNLs have the same fine-structural features as those from adults. When they emigrate through the umbilical vein wall, degeneration of its inner elastic components is observed (Figure 388). With some infections, notably that with *Candida albicans*, small accumulations of PMNLs are seen on the cord surface. Often visible macroscopically, they have a typical, granular appearance. Old exudate in the cord may accumulate in concentric perivascular rings, giving the appearance of Ouchterlony immunodiffusion plates (Figure 389). This old exudate is more prone to develop mineralization than the exudate of the fetal surface of

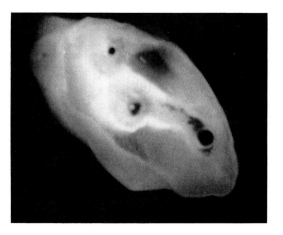

FIGURE 386. Cross section of an umbilical cord at 30 weeks' gestation. The patient had no fever. There was a velamentous insertion of the cord. A yellow streak was seen along the umbilical vein, and the cord appeared brownish. There is a prominent white ring of acute inflammatory exudate around the umbilical vein.

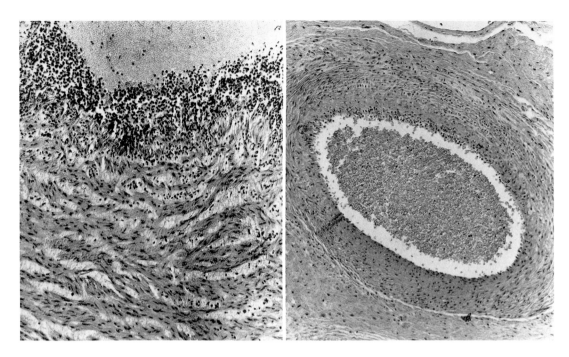

FIGURE 387. Umbilical phlebitis (left) and arteritis (right). Leukocytes are penetrating between muscle bundles toward the cord surface. H&E. ×260.

the placenta. In fact, this calcification reaches extraordinary proportions at times, so the cord cannot be clamped readily (see below).

The microorganisms that have caused the inflammatory response may be seen in many infected placentas, particularly in cases of listeriosis, candidiasis, fusobacterial infection, and some of the infections with common cocci. Most cases of chorioamnionitis, however, result from infection with organisms that are not so readily demonstrated histologically or that are not commonly considered. Examples include *Chlamydia* and *Mycoplasma*. Mural thrombosis in chorionic vessels is frequently present when the infection has been of longer duration. It begins at the intima of veins, usually toward the amnionic surface, and gradually increases (Figure 390). The thrombi may be grossly apparent as yellow-white streaks. In the umbilical cord, thrombi have a less characteristic macroscopic appearance but may also involve arteries (Figure 391). It is true, though, that most thromboses of large placental vessels have another etiology, mostly being secondary to obstructions. Finally, in the amnionic infection syndrome, the amnionic epithelium is frequently degenerated, especially in areas of severe inflammation (Figure 392).

Chorioamnionitis is common. Fox and Langley (1971), for instance, found it in 24.4% of 1,000 consecutive livebirths. A study of Salafia et al. (1989) showed that some degree of chorionitis was present in 4% of uncomplicated term deliveries; in 1.2% the

chorioamnionitis was "clinically silent." Inflammation of the membranes and cord is commoner still in the immature organs of spontaneous, premature births and in patients with premature rupture of membranes. Hillier et al. (1988) found infection in 67% of preterm deliveries, compared with 21% of term gestations. Guzick and Winn (1985) did a prospective study of 2,774 women and found the overall incidence of prematurity to be 5.4%. It was 11.0% when chorioamnionitis was present without membrane rupture but 56.7% when premature rupture of membranes and chorioamnionitis coexisted. The authors concluded that 25% of premature deliveries were attributable to chorioamnionitis. Newton et al. (1989) reported in a large study that "duration of membrane rupture [were] significant risk factors for intra-amniotic infection." The outcome of pregnancy in 59 patients with rupture of membranes before 26 weeks' gestation was studied by Bengtson et al. (1989). They ascertained chorioamnionitis in 45.8% (49.1% perinatal mortality) but also found that "there was a tendency for patients with extremely long latent periods to have lower rates of infection."

The ascending nature of this infection is signaled by three pathological findings and is supported by culture of intact sacs: (1) There is usually severe, acute necrotizing deciduitis associated with the membranitis, and it often exceeds the degree of chorioamnionitis (Figure 393). (2) When the intrauterine position of twins is known, including the partition of their amnionic sacs, it

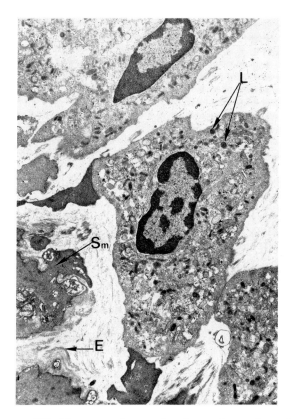

FIGURE 388. Electron micrograph of a polymorphonuclear leukocyte in the process of emigrating through an umbilical vein. The patient had a mature pregnancy with prolonged rupture of membranes. L = lysosomes; Sm = smooth muscle cell; E = degenerating elastic membrane. ×9,000. (Courtesy Dr. G. Altshuler, Oklahoma City.)

is invariably twin A that has chorioamnionitis or whose membranes are more severely inflamed (Figures 374, 375). (3) When membranes are rolled in such a manner as to have the point of spontaneous rupture on the inside, the degree of inflammation is most significant in that inner portions of the roll, that is, in the proximity of membrane rupture (Figure 394) (Benirschke & Altshuler, 1971).

It is well known that attempted abortion with non-sterile instruments is frequently followed by sepsis and chorioamnionitis (Studdiford & Douglas, 1956), but chorioamnionitis has also repeatedly been found with unruptured membranes (e.g., Miller et al., 1980b). A good example is the case of amnionic fluid infection ("chorioamnionitis" according to the authors) with the uncommon organism *Eikenella corrodens* (Jeppson & Reimer, 1991). Their 31-week gestation infant remained uninfected, perhaps because of prenatal antibiotic therapy when the gram-negative rods were identified by culture from amniocentesis. The association of prenatal infection with intact membranes is easiest to demonstrate with the relatively common *Candida albicans* infection of the amnionic sac. Gyr et al. (1994) showed that, experimentally, *E. coli* organisms could penetrate viable intact placental membranes, with simultaneous changes in glucose and lactate concentrations. Also, many cases have been described in which chorioamnionitis, with or without fetal pneumonia, existed in the presence of intact membranous sacs (en caul). Although it is an uncommon occurrence, it is an important finding to our understanding of the pathogenesis (Royston & Geoghegan, 1985). The general experience that inflamed membranes usually rupture prior to delivery does not argue against the fact that chorioamnionitis can exist with an intact sac. The loss of membrane integrity, resulting from inflammation, makes rupture a probability (Schoonmaker et al., 1989). Numerous reviews exist on this topic (Altshuler, 1984).

The predominant opinion now is that amnionic sac infection is a primary cause of premature rupture of membranes and premature labor, at least in those

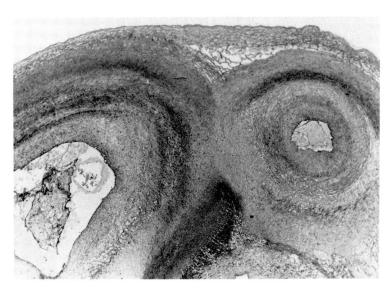

FIGURE 389. Chronic funisitis with rings of exudate (some of which are degenerated) around cord vessels. This small-for-gestational-age (SGA) infant was born near term; no villitis was present. H&E. ×40.

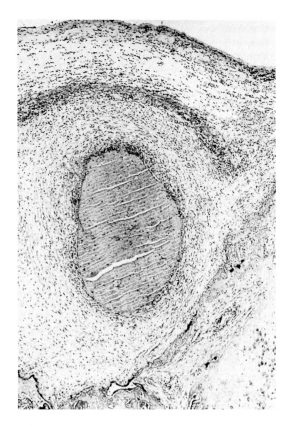

FIGURE 390. Long-standing chorioamnionitis and vasculitis of chorionic vessels at 26 weeks' pregnancy. The darker ring of exudate is degenerating, as is the amnionic epithelium. Early mural thrombosis is present at the surface of the vein. The placenta was malodorous. At 4 days after premature rupture of membranes, the woman gave birth to a 900 g infant. H&E. ×20.

pregnancies that terminate spontaneously before 30 weeks' gestation (Garite & Freeman, 1982; Toth et al., 1988). There is also evidence that these infections have an important role in the causation of stillbirths and neonatal deaths (Quinn et al., 1985). The commonly held idea that chorioamnionitis might "protect" the neonate against developing hyaline membrane disease by the attending "stress" was invalidated by the controlled clinicopathological study of Dimmick et al. (1976).

The clinical diagnosis of chorioamnionitis may pose problems for the clinician, as only some gravidas experience fever, uterine tenderness, or fetal tachycardia with amnionic sac infection. Bobitt et al. (1981) aspirated amnionic fluid for culture from women in premature labor and found microorganisms in 25%. Seven of eight went into labor within 48 hours, and 75% of positive women had no fever. These authors also advocated Gram stains for rapid diagnosis of organisms, a method found to be helpful in the management of patients with premature rupture of membranes and chorioamnionitis (Broekhuizen et al., 1985). Others (Gravett et al., 1982; Wagner et al., 1985; Romero, et al., 1988b) have advocated the use of gas-liquid chromatography for the early diagnosis of the amnionic sac infection syndrome. This rationale is based on the detection of short-chain organic acids, which are the by-products of bacterial metabolism. Romero et al. (1989e) found that this method is insensitive, especially when gram-negative organisms cause the infection, which is why Pankuch et al. (1989) suggested the use of leukotaxis studies. Maternal pyrexia and leukocytosis are also unreliable predictors, as has been found in numerous studies.

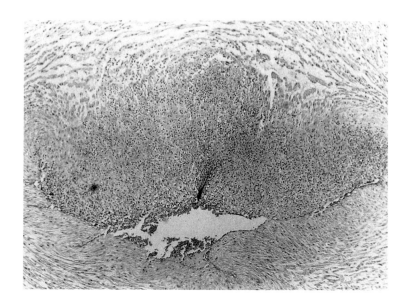

FIGURE 391. Organized, partially occlusive arterial thrombus in an umbilical artery associated with arteritis. Infant developed cerebral palsy. H&E. ×20.

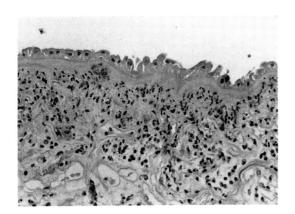

FIGURE 392. Chorioamnionitis associated with amnion necrosis. H&E. ×160.

Hawrylyshyn et al. (1983) found that elevated C-reactive protein (CRP) levels correlated better with infection than did maternal fever. Elevation of CRP levels in maternal serum, advocated by Evans et al. (1980) as a means to predict chorioamnionitis, has not been universally helpful. Farb et al. (1983) identified two patients with verified infection and normal levels; false-positive results were also obtained. Ernest et al. (1987) reported problems of both false-positive and false-negative levels. Watts and her colleagues (1993) found that elevated CRP levels were useful for deciding when to do cultures of amnionic fluid, but they found poor correlation with chorioamnionitis. Other investigators, however, have found excellent correlation with CRP levels and chorioamnionitis and have advocated its use in the clinical setting (Romem & Artal, 1984; Ismail et al., 1985; Potkul et al., 1985).

Because of the importance of this infection, investigators have sought new means of predicting the existence of chorioamnionitis before birth. Egley et al. (1988) suggested that amnionic fluid esterase levels (derived from PMNLs) have high specificity (100%) and sensitivity (81%). However, as with bacterial studies of cerebrospinal fluid, lactate, esterase, and so on are no more sensitive than looking for PMNLs from which they are derived. A Gram stain takes 5 minutes to perform and may be more useful. Ohlsson and Wang (1990) reviewed 39 studies and concluded that "an ideal test to predict chorioamnionitis or neonatal sepsis was not found."

Romero et al. (1987a, 1988a) and Cox et al. (1988) found that quantitation of the lipopolysaccharide component of gram-negative organisms (endotoxin) could be used for identification of these infections. Both groups of investigators found elevated levels of endotoxin in specific infections with the *Limulus* test; and when the test was combined with Gram stains, a more adequate means of prenatal diagnosis seemed possible. A variety of kinins, especially interleukin-1 and tumor necrosis factor, are currently being investigated as possible prime movers in initiating uterine contraction (Romero et al., 1989a,b; review by Mitchell et al., 1993). In one of the few studies of cervical mucus (that we consider to be of great importance in uterine defense mechanisms), Platz-Christensen et al. (1993) found that concentrations of endotoxin and interleukin-1α are significantly increased in vaginal fluid and cervical mucus of women with bacterial vaginosis. We found markedly increased amounts of interleukin-1 and its receptor in several areas of placentas with chorioamnionitis (Baergen et al., 1994).

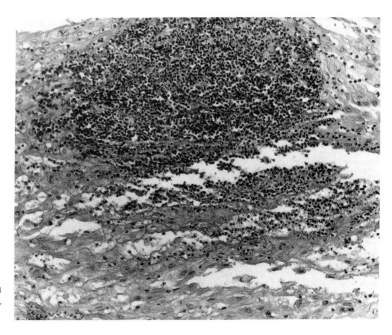

FIGURE 393. Acute and chronic deciduitis (decidua capsularis) in an immature placenta with chorioamnionitis. H&E. ×160.

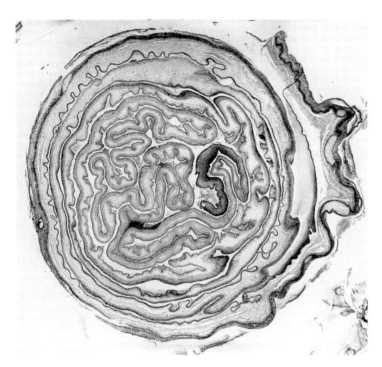

FIGURE 394. Membrane roll of placenta with marked chorioamnionitis. The edge of the spontaneous membrane rupture is in the center. Note the dark exudate in the decidua and chorion in the center. H&E. ×12. (From Benirschke & Altshuler, 1971, with permission.)

Because labor is readily induced with prostaglandins, their presence has been studied as the possible main mediators of the preterm labor associated with chorioamnionitis. Although prostaglandins are well known mediators of many aspects of disease, and they are also the chemicals that have proved to be useful for initiating labor, reservations exist as to their primacy in the initiation of normal labor. While seeking a possible link between premature labor and placental inflammation, we found that arachidonic acid was consumed during the process of labor (Curbelo et al., 1981). The testing was done by chromatography of phospholipids from placental membrane extracts obtained from various types of delivery. Arachidonic acid appeared to be electively stored in the amnion. Later, a large number of microorganisms were tested for phospholipase activity because initiation of labor was believed to result from phospholipase A_2 activity and because of its association with infection. It was then found that many organisms contain this enzyme in considerable quantities (Bejar et al., 1981; McGregor et al., 1991). This observation led to the hypothesis that bacterially mediated enzymatic conversion of arachidonic acid may signal the onset of premature labor in pregnancies complicated by chorioamnionitis. Others have since studied many more organisms and found that phospholipase is liberated from a large number of microorganisms, with release of prostaglandin from amnion (Lamont et al., 1990). Bennett and Elder (1992) found that bacterial infection cannot initiate labor from "intrinsic biosynthesis and release of prostaglandins . . . by the bacteria themselves."

We now believe that there is an insufficient quantity of lipase from the usually small number of bacteria to initiate and maintain labor. Rather, the enzyme is more likely provided by the large number of leukocytes, which are also known to possess phospholipase (Victor et al., 1981) and whose enzyme is activated by chemotactic peptides (Galbraith, 1988). The lipase also occurs in high concentrations in the placental membranes (review by Vadas & Pruzanski, 1986). Okita et al. (1983) identified substantial stores of arachidonic acid in human amnion and concluded that it originates from amnionic fluid.

Lamont et al. (1985) exposed amnion cells in culture to bacterial products and found prostaglandin E to rise markedly as a result. They thus affirmed that chorioamnionitis may cause premature labor. This finding was amplified by Bennett et al. (1987), who performed similar experiments. A correlation between chorioamnionitis and premature labor is additionally supported by findings of significantly elevated prostaglandin levels in infected amnionic fluid (Romero et al., 1986) and by the demonstration of markedly increased prostaglandin production in infected amnion (Lopez Bernal et al., 1987).

Despite these attractive findings of prostaglandin metabolism, attention has more recently been paid to the increase of amnionic leukotriene concentrations during labor (Romero et al., 1988c) and to the decidual interleukin-1 production during premature labor (Romero et al., 1989a,f) as well as many other proteins. Deciduitis, decidual macrophage activation, and PMNL exudation, in particular, play an important role in the initiation of premature labor. It must be admitted, however, that although the evidence of infection as a primary cause of chorioamnionitis and of premature labor is no longer in doubt the precise chemical cascade that ultimately leads to myometrial contractions is not yet elucidated.

Many investigators have graded the inflammatory infiltration (e.g., Thiery et al., 1970; Naeye et al., 1983) so as to perhaps correlate it with clinical findings (e.g., rupture of membranes and maternal fever). We have found this practice to be impractical for several reasons. For instance, there are severe prenatal infections with some types of organism, in particular the group B streptococcus, that elicit little placental inflammatory reaction but can produce devastating disease in the newborn. It is also likely that different organisms have differing ability to penetrate the membranes. This point was shown experimentally by Galask et al. (1984), who exposed membranes to bacterial cultures. They found that group B streptococci penetrated membranes more readily than did coliform bacilli and gonococci. We believe that the intensity of inflammation is more closely related to the nature of the organism than to the chronicity of the infection. It seems also difficult to estimate how long the infection has been active. This uncertainty has hindered acceptance of the opinion that membrane rupture *follows* membranitis, rather than *causes* it (see Naeye & Peters, 1980). The prevailing view certainly is that membranes rupture first, followed by amnionitis.

The preponderance of chorioamnionitis in immature pregnancies is striking. It has often been linked to the less effective bacteriostatic nature of amnionic fluid in immature pregnancies (Anonymous, 1989a). Thadepalli et al. (1978) showed that amnionic fluid of the first trimester is least inhibitory against anaerobic organisms. Schlievert et al. (1975, 1976a,b, 1977) had similar results using various organisms for analysis. Their studies showed that the inhibitory moiety of the amnionic fluid contains a zinc-dependent special peptide that develops mostly after 20 weeks' gestation. Others had identified immunoglobulins in amnionic fluid (Galask & Snyder, 1970) and that the fluid from patients with chorioamnionitis had elevated immunoglobulin levels (Blanco et al., 1983). Specific inhibition against *Mycoplasma* and *Chlamydia* was demonstrated in amnionic fluid by Thomas et al. (1988); and Gray et al. (1987) concluded that even the small quantities of type-specific streptococcal antibodies in amnionic fluid that they demonstrated may protect the fetus against this infection. All of these points may explain why chorioamnionitis is much more common during early pregnancy than toward term. It is our view that the more important aspect of labor initiation resides with the decidua, and that the bacteriostatic

activity of amnionic fluid is not the primary event preventing labor and chorioamnionitis during later gestation.

General Considerations of Chorioamnionitis

The amnionic sac infection syndrome develops from infection that commences in the endocervix and vagina and then ascends (Figure 395). Abundant evidence supports this opinion, and there is also much evidence that prematurity is often caused by prenatal infection. Premature rupture of the membranes (PROM) is a common antecedent of infection. Garite (1985) labeled it the "enigma of the obstetrician" because of the controversial aspects of diagnosis and management. A further problem is the difficulty of predicting rupture of membranes and premature delivery. It has been suggested that vaginal fibronectin may provide such a clue (Lockwood et al., 1991), but Feinberg and Kliman (1992), and others have taken exception to this approach. Gibbs and Blanco (1982) found that PROM complicates 4.5% to 7.6% of all deliveries, and that 1.0% of all gestations have preterm delivery with PROM. This study reviewed the evidence favoring the notion that PROM is often the consequence of subclinical vaginal infection. They also gave detailed protocols for management. McDuffie et al. (1992) showed in an experimental model that intracervical administration of coliform bacilli in rabbits leads to rapid and marked elevation of the various mediators that are usually associated with labor. Elst et al. (1991) found elevated prostaglandins and leukocytes in amniotic fluids aspirated by fetuses from spontaneous premature labor and concluded that chorioamnionitis may initiate preterm labor. Lettieri and her colleagues (1993) suggested that "idiopathic" preterm labor can be explained in 96%. They incriminated faulty implantation in one-half of cases, infection in 38%, immunological factors in 30%, cervical incompetence in 16%, uterine factors in 14%, maternal factors in 10%, trauma (surgery) in 8%, and fetal anomalies in 6%. It is our impression

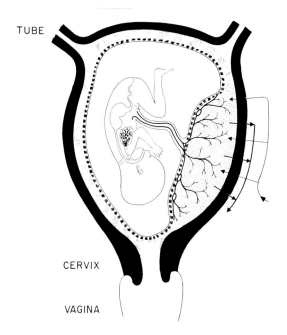

FIGURE 395. Intrauterine position of fetus and placenta. Infectious organisms ascend through an opened endocervical canal. They first infect the membranes that cover the internal os and then penetrate the amnionic cavity.

that ascending infection is the most important cause of preterm labor and PROM, certainly so in the 20- to 30-weeks' gestation group. There are now numerous studies that support this contention. Romero et al. (1989e) examined the amnionic fluid aspirated from 264 women with preterm labor and with intact membranes. They found positive cultures in 91.0%; 42% delivered preterm neonates, 21.6% of which had positive amnionic fluid cultures. Preterm delivery was especially frequent when endotoxins were detected with the *Limulus* amebocyte lysate assay. The commonest organisms isolated were *Ureaplasma urealyticum, Fusobacterium* sp., and *Mycoplasma hominis*; but later studies have indicated a spectrum of other organisms (Romero et al., 1992c). Inflammatory lesions (chorioamnionitis, funisitis) are essentially present only when microbacterial contamination can be shown to exist in the amnionic cavity (Harger et al., 1991). This study also emphasized that antimicrobial therapy failed to prolong pregnancy when chorioamnionitis was extant.

There is now a large number of investigation that incriminate all sorts of mediators in the initiation of labor during the process of ascending infection. Interleukin-1 (IL-1) was found elevated and championed by Taniguchi et al. (1991); but no elevation of levels of IL-1-receptor antagonists were identified (Romero et al., 1992d). In addition to IL-1, IL-6 was found to be increased in the presence of infections studied by Matsuzaki et al. (1993) but not during normal labor. Kelly et al. (1992) suggested that the "final common step of prostaglandin (PG) and antiprogestagen action in parturition was decidual release of IL-8." Hillier et al. (1993) found several cytokines and PGE_2 to be elevated in amnionic fluid during preterm labor and suggested their usefulness for predicting labor. Tumor necrosis factor (TNF) activates the cytokine machinery and may well be at the starting point of labor initiation by stimulating prostaglandin production from the decidua (Romero et al., 1992b; Norwitz et al., 1992a,b). Suffice it to say that the cytokine system is intimately involved in premature labor when it is caused by infection; absent inflammation, the kinin levels are not significantly elevated (Romero et al., 1993).

When membranes are ruptured and the endocervical mucous plug has disappeared, the amnionic cavity may be quickly colonized by organisms of the cervicovaginal tract (Miller et al., 1980a,b). Wahbeh et al. (1984) found that anaerobic organisms play an important role in PROM similar to the results of a study by Bobitt and Ledger (1977). When Pankuch et al. (1984) attempted the isolation of bacterial and chlamydial organisms from 75 placentas, they found that 72% of placentas with chorioamnionitis had bacteria (82% with clinical chorioamnionitis), whereas only 15% of uninflamed placentas contained organisms. Almost 50% were anaerobes. Johnson et al. (1981b) found in their large study of PROM that unless chorioamnionitis intervened rapid delivery was not necessary. They cautioned that, with modern management, the risk to the fetus is primarily one of prematurity. Earlier studies of the same group had shown that neonatal infections were much more common in preterm than term infants but that the risk of PROM alone was insignificant (Daikoku et al., 1981). Many authors have suggested that bacteriuria is specifically related to PROM and to prematurity (Naeye, 1979a), but it has not been confirmed by some well controlled studies of maternal bacteriuria (Bryant et al., 1964). The relation of asymptomatic maternal bacteriuria to low birth weight and preterm delivery has been reaffirmed by a "meta-analysis" of Romero et al. (1989d). They also believed that ascending infection was the mode for infection. An anamnestic lymphocyte response to the organism of maternal infection was demonstrated in some infants judged to be at high risk of dying (Wallach et al., 1969). Still controversial is whether ascending infection can truly be prevented by antibiotics and also whether treatment is beneficial (Christmas et al., 1992; Seo et al., 1992; Kirschbaum, 1993).

Another presumed cause of PROM, abortion, and premature delivery has been the syndrome of incompetent cervix, thought to have a congenital origin (review by Borglin, 1962). It has been suggested that 0.1% to 1.0% of pregnancies are thus complicated, and that up to 20% of midtrimester abortions result from an incompetent cervix (Anonymous, 1977b). Gans et al. (1966) suggested that trauma is the most common antecedent of an incompetent cervix, a notion with which we agree, especially when prior surgery is considered. They reported favorable surgical repairs of the defect. The alleged etiology of trauma is well supported by a review of the topic (Anonymous, 1983a). Hagen and Skjeldestad (1993) studied the outcome of cervical laser conization with a case control approach. They reported an increased frequency (38% versus 6%) of premature births in the operated cases and recommended that conization be done only in the presence of high grade in situ neoplasia. Barford and Rosen (1984) were more cautious in their assessment of diagnosis and therapy, and Charles and Edwards (1981) listed the many serious infectious complications (e.g., puerperal sepsis, chorioamnionitis) that may ensue, particularly when the Shirodkar stitch is undertaken during the second trimester of pregnancy. Heinemann et al. (1977) and others (e.g., Dunn et al., 1959) have reported maternal sepsis after intraamnionic *E. coli* infection in such cases. Abundant bacillary growth was present in placental capillaries, but there was only minimal inflammation in the case reported by Heinemann et al. (1977). Romero et al. (1992a) advocated that amniocentesis with culture should be undertaken before a cerclage is placed during the midtrimester; they found a high frequency of bacterial invasion. In our opinion, it is not likely that incompetent cervix is frequently an inherited defect; rather, we believe that trauma and infection are more probable antecedents. The cervix, affected by severe chronic cervicitis, is often patulous and prone to premature dilatation, which may be the origin of many of the 20% incompetent cervices cited to be associated with PROM. Leveno et al. (1986) published a study of gravid cervical dilatation that supported this assumption. They found that dilated cervices tend to lead to premature delivery; recurrent PROM and premature delivery are then serious problems. Asrat et al. (1991) studied 255 pregnancies and identified a recurrence rate of PROM in about one-third. Interestingly, Salafia et al. (1991) found about the same frequency of the amnionic sac infection syndrome in premature births.

The presence of an intrauterine device (IUD) has been correlated with pelvic inflammatory disease (PID) in some studies (Lee et al., 1988). Other studies have been less convincing, and the large cooperative study published by Kessel (1989) asserted that the relation is mostly due to the increased frequency of pelvic infections in general, noted since 1973, and not to IUD insertions. Generally, the device prevents pregnancy, but when it fails to do so (2–4%) premature labor and chorioamnionitis frequently ensue. The correlation of septic abortion and presence of an IUD has also been confirmed in the large study by Kessel (1989). In this context, Jewett (1973) reported a maternal death following *E. coli* infection at 22 weeks' gestation. Fatal maternal sepsis has also been reported as a complication of chorioamnionitis without an IUD (Webb, 1967). With cesarean section patients, myometritis is present in one-third of asymptomatic patients whose inflamed membranes had been ruptured for more than 6 hours (Azziz et al., 1988). An interesting association also exists between the occurrence of ectopic pregnancy and recurrent abortion (Fedele et al., 1989). It is likely that its basis is infection. Of parenthetical interest is the suggestion by Polunin (1958) that vaginal infection and birth practices in a North Bornean tribe (the Murut) cause sterility, and that it is the result of vaginal infection. In subsequent studies an anaerobic coccal (probably streptococcal) infection was found to cause vaginitis and PID in this tribe (Hare & Polunin, 1960).

Dinsmoor and Gibbs (1989) found that previous amnionic sac infection is not a risk factor for subsequent infection of the uterus.

Another topic of concern among the causes of premature labor, PROM, and fetal infections relates to the hypothesis that intercourse during late pregnancy may initiate premature delivery (Naeye, 1979b, 1980). Herbst (1979), in an editorial, reviewed evidence that meconium staining and risk of prematurity were greater when orgasm had been experienced during pregnancy. Naeye (1982) suggested that other causes of prematurity are smoking, parity, prior cervical surgery, and prior chorioamnionitis. There has been much criticism of these studies on coitus-related prematurity (e.g., Berg, 1980; Mills et al., 1981; Perkins, 1983), some of which has been answered by Naeye (1981, 1983, 1986). His finding of modal peaks of deliveries on certain days of presumed peak coital activity were used to further support a relation between coitus, infection, and premature labor. Klebanoff et al. (1984) could not accept this relation in their analysis of the same data, a study to which Naeye (1986) took exception. When Ekwo et al. (1993) studied coitus during late pregnancy to ascertain if it bears risks for preterm rupture of membranes, they found that "most sexual positions and activities during late pregnancy are not associated with adverse outcomes." Neilson and Mutambira (1989) found no relation between twin deliveries and coitus. Similarly, there was no relation to premature labor when frequent intercourse occurred among the patients studied by Read et al. (1993). This finding held true except some women who were already colonized with some specific organisms. Similarly, Kurki and Ylikorkala (1993) found that "in healthy nulliparous women, coitus during pregnancy is not related to bacterial vaginosis and does not predispose to preterm birth. The issue is currently not definitively decided, but additional data suggest that some relation may exist between coitus and premature deliveries (Anonymous, 1984; Naeye, 1988a).

Specific Microorganisms

1. *Neisseria gonorrhoeae* is the organism responsible for gonorrhea, which occasionally complicates pregnancy. In a cervical culture study of 1,309 antepartum patients, Kraus and Yen (1968) found a 5.73% asymptomatic infection rate during pregnancy, with 32% puerperal morbidity. They were primarily concerned with ophthalmia neonatorum and did not address the possible risk posed by chorioamnionitis. This study and others indicated that active cervical infection with this organism does not necessarily lead to chorioamnionitis. Baddeley and Shardlow (1973) saw two patients with normal deliveries after gonococcal arthritis during pregnancy. Infection of the amnionic sac with gonococci has been reported by Nickerson (1973) and Rothbard et al. (1975). We have seen several cases as well; and they were similar to other types of acute chorioamnionitis. In Nickerson's case, the infection was not recognized until the gastric aspirate was cultured. The febrile patient was near term and had spontaneous rupture of membranes and a tender abdomen. The placenta was not studied.

Rothbard and colleagues (1975) probably reported the first case of antenatally diagnosed and treated gonorrheal chorioamnionitis. The aspirated amnionic fluid was purulent, and gram-negative diplococci (gonococci) were identified at 35 weeks' gestation. Cesarean section, performed after ampicillin therapy, led to the birth of a normal infant whose neonatal course was uneventful. The placenta was not described. Smith et al. (1989) reported a case of acute gonococcal chorioamnionitis with sepsis. Their patient had a dark red vaginal discharge at 32 weeks, emesis, chills, migratory arthralgia, and abdominal pain. The membranes were intact, and at amniocentesis gonococci were demonstrated. The 1,960-g infant did well. The placenta exhibited acute chorioamnionitis.

Acute gonococcal salpingitis has even been described to complicate pregnancy (Genardy et al., 1976). Their patient was operated on for presumed appendicitis at 14 weeks' gestation; the fallopian tube had pus with gonococci identified therein, and the patient was successfully treated with cephalothin and kanamycin. At 37 weeks she delivered a normal infant and a normal placenta. This event is rare, however; and when present, ascending infections involve the tube only early during gestation, before the decidua capsularis makes contact with the opposing uterine wall. We have seen only one placenta of a patient with a history of ruptured membranes for 4 weeks who, in addition to marked *E. coli* chorioamnionitis, had developed sepsis from acute unilateral salpingitis at 32 weeks' gestation. The inference in this patient is that the salpingitis developed after the chorioamnionitis, also by ascending means.

Edwards and colleagues (1978) studied 178 patients with gonorrhea during pregnancy (2.75%) and reviewed the literature. They found chorioamnionitis in 26% (5% in controls). Premature rupture of membranes occurred significantly more often (63% versus 29%), a point that was denied by Amstey (1982).

2. Infections with *group B streptococci* are now important and frequent complications of the perinatal period, and we now differentiate between early- and late-onset neonatal infections because of their significant differences in outcome. This streptococcus is recognized to be one of the most virulent organisms during the perinatal period. Sepsis, pneumonia, and meningitis are common sequelae of this infection (Baker, 1977), and the organism has emerged as the number two cause of neonatal meningitis (Anonymous, 1977a). Prematurity and premature rupture of membranes are strongly correlated with group B streptococcal infections. The diagnosis is often difficult unless it is actively pursued. Occult streptococcal infection is an important cause of fetal asphyxia, and stillbirths frequently occur with unruptured membranes (Naeye & Peters, 1978; Peevy & Chalhub, 1983).

Novak and Platt (1985) described the placentas of 22 cases of early-onset group B streptococcal sepsis. They found that chorioamnionitis was present in 64%, 27% of patients had funisitis; and in 41% of these patients gram-positive organisms were found in the amnionic fluid. Importantly, though, some placentas showed no pathological changes or only villous edema. The authors were disappointed that, except for neutropenia, the placental findings did not correlate well with fetal outcome. They also emphasized that the extensive colonization of amnion and the leukocytic response argued strongly against late acquisition of the organism by the fetus during fetal descent. They reviewed other studies that gave similar incidence figures and concluded that an important part of the fetal response is related to the specific enzymatic types of the individual organisms.

Altshuler (1984) stated that "there is no inflammation in the placentas of at least 75% of newborns in whom group B β-hemolytic streptococcus has been cultured." Our experience also indicates that many placentas of infected babies, even those with neonatal sepsis, have no inflammation. Only careful search for bacteria can identify the cocci on the amnion. Vigorita and Parmley (1979), on the other hand, described focal abscesses underneath the amnion, areas of epithelial necrosis, and found an accumulation of bacterial colonies in a relevant case. Although we have also seen such abscesses, we have wondered if double infection may have been the cause, as this observation differs so much from previous reports.

Group B streptococci may actively grow in amnionic fluid alone. Abbasi and colleagues (1987) showed that virulent strains of streptococci grew as well in amnionic fluid as in optimal bacterial culture media, although some differences were found among various strains. The authors believed that this point is clinically signifi-cant. However, when the clinical manifestations of patients in whom amnionic contamination was proved are compared with those without positive cultures, no differences of clinical risk factors were ascertained (Silver et al., 1990). The differentiation and designation of the many streptococcal bacteria may not be widely appreciated; Table 20 summarizes their designation and features.

Numerous studies have addressed the need for early diagnosis and rapid therapy of perinatal group B streptococcal infection. The most modern studies employ a DNA probe for rapid detection (Yancey et al., 1993), in part because previous methods (enzyme-linked immunosorbent assay and Gram stain) were inefficient for screening tests (Hagay et al., 1993). Thus there is by no means agreement on how best to screen for the colonization, or how to deal with it when infection is recognized. Gibbs and Blanco (1981) investigated 48 patients with bacteremia, 31 of which infections were due to group B organisms. Endometritis and chorioamnionitis were the most commonly diagnosed clinical features. Although fever was often present, few localizing signs appeared. The authors also discussed effective therapy, but other studies show that even intrapartum administration of antibiotics often does not prevent neonatal sepsis (Ascher et al., 1993).

A prospective study of colonization with this organism was undertaken by Regan et al. (1981). They found a significant increase in PROM and an association with prematurity. That was not the case in the study reported by Amstey (1982). Singer and Campognone (1983) found organisms in the blood of immature stillborns associated with villous edema and mild chorioamnionitis. Two placentas showed acute and chronic villitis,

TABLE 20. Classification of aerobic streptococci.

Group	Species	Blood agar reaction[a]
A	*S. pyogenes*	β-hemolytic
B	*S. agalactiae*	Usually β-hemolytic
C[b]	Several species	β-hemolytic
D (enterococci)	*S. faecalis, S. faecium*	α-, β-, or nonhemolytic
E (non-enterococci)	*S. bovis*	α- or nonhemolytic
F	*S. anginosus*	Small colony β[c]
G[b]	Many species	Usually β-hemolytic[c]
Viridans hemolytic species		α-hemolytic
Pneumococci	*S. pneumoniae*	α-hemolytic

Modified from Gibbs and Blanco (1981).

[a] The β reaction is clear, complete hemolysis; the α reaction is green discoloration, partial hemolysis.

[b] Groups C and G are β-hemolytic streptococci.

[c] The British classify minute colonies of groups C, F, and G β-hemolytic streptococci and Lancefield-groupable, and the capnophilic strains of α-hemolytic and nonhemolytic *S. intermedius* and *S. constellatus* as *S. milleri*. The Center for Disease Control uses the designation *S. anginosus* for minute colonies of β-streptococci and retains the designations *S. intermedius* and *S. constellatus* (C. Davies, personal communication, 1989).

which suggested to them a transplacental (hematogenous) infection. It may well have been a dual infection also. They emphasized the high risk of colonization, particularly during the second trimester of pregnancy. Matorras et al. (1989) showed that maternal colonization (rectal or vaginal) carried a significant risk for PROM. Cervical colonization was especially deleterious. Fetal death due to streptococcal sepsis has even been described after intrauterine funipuncture for karyotyping (McColgin et al., 1989).

That the organism does not necessarily arrive in the fetus via hematogenous means, though, was shown by Pass et al. (1980a). They found a severely colonized dichorionic twin A whose co-twin (B) did not have the infection. They believed that twin pregnancies are particularly vulnerable. Iams and O'Shaughnessy (1982), who evaluated antenatal versus intrapartum screening, found no advantage in the former method, whereas Pass et al. (1982) correlated infection with puerperal fever and the finding of frequent chorioamnionitis in cases of perinatal infection. The attack rate in their study was 2 per 1,000 deliveries. They recommended intrapartum antibiotic prophylaxis, as did Boyer and Gotoff (1986). Strickland et al. (1990) also suggested a frequency of two early-onset infections per 1,000 births and found intrapartum screening for this infection to be cost-effective because of the severe handicaps that can result. Thomsen and colleagues (1987) found that urinary group B streptococcal infection correlated with preterm labor, and they also reported a beneficial effect from penicillin therapy. Dykes et al. (1985) investigated women who gave birth to infected babies. Chronic carriage in the urinary tract, without immunological response, was therein apparent. Similar findings were reported by Moller et al. (1984). They also found an increased risk of ruptured membranes. Matorras et al. (1989) found that PROM was significantly correlated with vaginal or rectal carrier status. It has also been shown that successive group B streptococcal infection, with early-onset disease of neonates, can occur despite proper antibiotic therapy (Carstensen et al., 1988).

For all these reasons, rapid diagnosis of infection with group B streptococci is urgent, a point addressed in several studies (e.g., Morales et al., 1986; Morales & Lim, 1987). Morales et al. used co-agglutination methods for identification; Sandy et al. (1988) tested Gram staining of cervicovaginal swabs; they found it to be an unreliable means for diagnosis. Of alternative methods explored in an editorial, most were considered to be unsatisfactory for routine use (Anonymous, 1986). Latex agglutination tests prepared from swabs may be a useful means of rapid identification (Howe et al., 1987; Stiller et al., 1989). Baker et al. (1988) obtained promising results after immunization of pregnant women.

In a large review of the possibility of immunization, Coleman et al. (1992) suggested that such vaccination is "attainable" and that studies in that direction showed be pursued; antigens such as cell wall polysaccharides and protein C are the most promising to be investigated.

The effect of this infection can be devastating to the newborn (and fetus), and its onset may be rapid. The neonatal diagnosis, manifestations, and therapy were lucidly discussed by McCracken (1976). Contrary to one's hopes, immediate penicillin therapy to the immature neonate does not prevent early-onset disease, nor does it reduce the excessive associated mortality (Pyati et al., 1983).

Of interest to the pathologist is the study of Katzenstein et al. (1976). Dissatisfied with the frequency of autopsy diagnosis of hyaline membrane disease in pregnancies at risk, they used immunofluorescence (on formalin-fixed tissue) to reexamine eight appropriate cases. They identified streptococci in the pulmonary hyaline membranes of five neonatal deaths. These structures were so numerous in one case that they appeared to make up the bulk of the "fibrinous" membrane. The deaths had previously been assigned to "routine" hyaline membrane disease at routine autopsy.

Hyde et al. (1989) have shown experimentally that extracts from cultures of this organism may cause isolated portions of umbilical vein wall to contract severely. They suggested that such effects may occur in vivo during intraamnionic infections, and that it may lead to reduced venous return from the placenta, causing fetal damage. Clinical investigations of this phenomenon are now commencing. Fleming et al. (1991) found a correlation of S/D ratios and biophysical profiles with chorioamnionitis, but Leo et al. (1992) did not. It must be pointed out, however, that the latter group did not study the placentas, and other problems exist with the protocol. It is too early to make decisions as to the possible value of predicting chorioamnionitis/funisitis with this methodology.

3. *Group A β-hemolytic streptococci* pose serious problems for mother and fetus (Swingler et al., 1988). Antenatal acquisition was demonstrated by Monif (1975) in a febrile patient with a tender uterus at 34 weeks' gestation. The membranes were unruptured, and the cervix was closed. A depressed infant was born with leukocytosis, left shift of white blood cells, and positive cord blood culture. Placental histological study was not undertaken. Other cases were reviewed by Lehtonen et al. (1984). The infection responds readily to penicillin or ampicillin, and the umbilical stump may be a reservoir for the organism. Puerperal infection with this organism, however, may pose serious risks (Silver et al., 1992). Both of their seriously ill patients required hysterectomy but their pregnancies had ended uneventfully.

4. Fatal maternal and fetal infection with *Strepto-coccus pneumoniae* (type III) was reported by Tarpay et al. (1980), but the placenta was not studied. Duff and Gibbs (1983) identified two similar infections with *S. pneumoniae* demonstrable in amnionic fluid. They thought that ascending infection was unlikely because of the stringent pH requirements (pH 6.5–8.3) of the organism. They did not identify the source of infection and did not report on the placenta. Andreu et al. (1989), however, did report chorioamnionitis in the placentas of several infants prenatally infected with this organism and having pneumonia.

5. *Hemophilus influenzae* was contracted prenatally in a premature infant reported by Barton et al. (1982). It had septicemia and recovered after ampicillin therapy. The membranes had ruptured 15 hours before delivery. The placenta was not described. Gibson and Williams (1978) observed this infection in a 28-week gestation complicated by leukorrhea, abdominal pain, and fever. The amnionic fluid was opaque and contained the organisms on smears. The placenta had chorioamni-onitis and funisitis. The infant died from hyaline mem-brane disease. There was no pneumonia. A study of 19 patients with this infection by Campognone and Singer (1986) drew attention to the serious nature of this disease. All of their cases had chorioamnionitis, and three had acute villitis in addition. Winn and Egley (1987) added another case with chorioamnionitis and funisitis. The patient had intact membranes. The or-ganisms may be readily identified as gram-negative rods in smears. Rusan and her colleagues (1991) agreed that this infection poses serious problems; they undertook a retrospective review and found 13 cases with chorio-amnionitis, endometritis, or both over a 10-year span. Of 23 infected neonates, 15 presented with sepsis, pneumonia, or both.

6. *Diplococcus pneumoniae* (*Streptococcus pneu-moniae*) was the cause of neonatal laryngitis in a term infant delivered to a febrile patient with positive amnion and cervical cultures (Hazard et al., 1964). It may here be mentioned that smears of the placental surface have been usefully employed by Nessmann-Emmanuelli et al. (1983) in establishing prenatal infection. Positive smears were obtained in 9% of a high-risk group (63% gram-positive, 17% gram-negative, and 20% mixed). It was especially useful for group B streptococcal and *E. coli* infections.

7. Gram-negative bacilli, in particular *E. coli*, fre-quently cause chorioamnionitis. Their association with neonatal meningitis is well known (Kagan et al., 1949; Watson, 1957; McCracken and Sarff, 1974). That this organism, especially the K1 type, is transmitted ver-tically has been firmly established by the large coopera-tive study of Sarff et al. (1975). These authors found a strong association with maternal rectal colonization of

the organism and likened the acquisition to that of streptococcal infection. The investigators did not examine placentas. Their concept of pathogenesis in-cluded lung infection, intestinal infection, sepsis, and meningitis. We believe that the mode of transmission for neonatal meningitis is often through the aspirated amnionic fluid via the middle ear. De Sa (1974) has shown that squames, admixed with pus and organisms, are often found in the middle ears of stillborns and neonatal deaths.

8. *Salmonella typhi* and other salmonella organisms may cause meningitis of neonates. They may be trans-mitted vaginally. Pugh and Vakil (1952), Watson (1958), and Scialli and Rarick (1992) reported cases of congenital infection and some fetal deaths, and they also reviewed the literature. Infection by symptomatic women or carriers was also shown by Luder and Tomson (1963) and Freedman et al. (1970). The pla-centa is usually not mentioned. An exception is the case reported by Awadalla et al. (1985): a patient with gastroenteritis at 26 weeks' gestation. A foul-smelling intact gestational sac containing cloudy amnionic fluid was delivered. Blood, stool, cervical specimens, and amnionic fluid yielded the organism. Despite these findings, the authors were of the opinion that tran-splacental, rather than ascending, infection took place. Seoud et al. (1988) recorded the occurrence of typhoid fever during pregnancy in 13 patients. One infant died with pneumonia. The mothers were treated with chloramphenicol and did well.

9. Infection with *Shigella sonnei* caused septicemia and enterocolitis in a term infant reported by Kraybill and Controni (1968). Prenatal infection of this infant seemed likely, but the placenta was not studied.

10. *Clostridium perfringens* infection occasionally complicates pregnancy. Among anaerobic infections, this type has been particularly feared because of the postabortal sepsis and uterine gas gangrene that may be life-threatening for the gravida (Ramsey, 1949). Nash et al. (1963) described a patient at 35 weeks' gestation who had had ruptured membranes for 5 days, a tender uterus, fetal death, and abdominal crepitation due to gas infiltration. They carefully described the placenta: It had a greenish amnionic surface and a putrefactive odor. The purulent exudate covered the membranes and fetal placental surface; it contained gram-positive rods. The maternal surface and villous tissue were not involved. A similar case is shown in Figure 396. Several cases of abortion due to *C. perfringens* infection have been reported (Decker & Hall, 1966; Pritchard & Whalley, 1971) that emphasized the severity of this infection and the frequent lethal outcome. Decker and Hall (1966) demonstrated that inflammatory exudate and necrosis of villous tissue may be found in septic cases, and the fetus may be invaded by organisms.

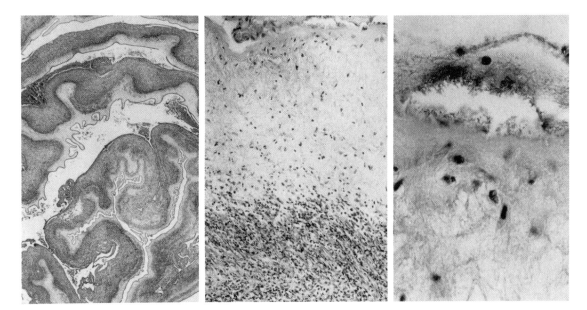

FIGURE 396. Clostridial chorioamnionitis at term. The membranes were friable and meconium-stained. The infant survived with antibiotic therapy. Membrane roll (left) shows intensive deciduitis and chorionitis. Note the umbilical arteritis (center, right) with a pocket of gram-positive rods underneath the amnion. Touch preparations were strongly positive. H&E. Left ×16; center ×160; right ×640.

11. Diphtheroids or corynebacteria are frequent normal vaginal inhabitants and can often be cultured from placental surfaces. However, they occasionally have been shown to cause chorioamnionitis. Fitter et al. (1979) described a case of funisitis and chorioamnionitis due to *Corynebacterium kutscheri*. It occurred at 26 weeks of pregnancy in a grand multipara who delivered 24 hours after rupture of membranes. Gram-positive organisms were demonstrated and were grown in pure culture from cord, membranes, rectum, nose, throat, eye, and external ear. There was no sepsis in the 980-g premature infant who survived after ampicillin and gentamicin therapy. The placental surface was discolored and had gray-brown plaques. Similar plaques were present on the umbilical cord. The plaques were comprised of organisms that also invaded the underlying tissue. Funisitis and chorioamnionitis were pronounced. The case proves that not all "diphtheroids" isolated from the placenta or amnionic fluid are due to vaginal contamination at delivery. In this case, the infection must have occurred prior to membrane rupture.

12. Altshuler and Hyde (1985, 1988) have drawn attention to the importance of *Fusobacterium necrophorum* and *F. nucleatum* infections as important complications of pregnancy. These pleomorphic, filamentous, gram-negative, anaerobic organisms were isolated from 3 of 297 placentas examined for various indications. These authors described in detail the fluorescent antibody identification, chromatography, and usefulness of the Warthin-Starry stain for identifica-

tion on slides. Brown-Brenn stains were not so useful for demonstrating the bacteria, and in hematoxylin and eosin (H&E) preparations the organisms were even more difficult to identify microscopically. It is also important to note that Bouin's fixative makes their demonstration particularly difficult. Of 92 prematurely delivered placentas, 62 had chorioamnionitis; and of the latter, 11 (18%) had filamentous organisms in the membranes.

In the rat animal model developed by Altshuler and Hyde, inflammation similar to chorioamnionitis was consistently produced. In a subsequent contribution (Altshuler & Hyde, 1988), these investigators reaffirmed the association of fusobacterial infection and prematurity. Among 586 placentas examined, they identified 14 with fusobacteria; and from their literature review it is evident that as many as 30% of patients with "occult" chorioamnionitis may be infected with a *Fusobacterium* species.

A typical case of fusobacterial chorioamnionitis is shown in Figure 397. It was associated with the scattered villous edema (Figure 398) that Naeye et al. (1983) considered to be so important for causing prenatal hypoxia in association with chorioamnionitis and prematurity. Easterling and Garite (1985), for instance, reported three cases of fusobacterial infection and emphasized the importance of this rarely recognized organism as a cause of premature labor. Romero et al. (1989e) found it commonly in prenatally obtained amnionic fluid with intact membranes. Cox et al. (1988)

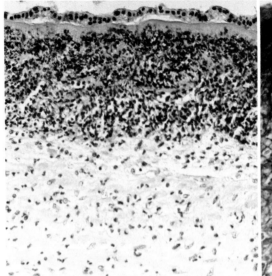 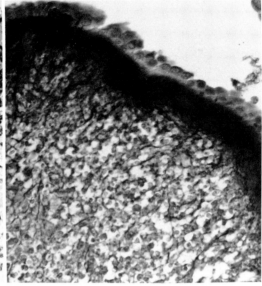

FIGURE 397. Chorioamnionitis due to fusobacteria in the placenta at 23 weeks' gestation. The placental surface was opaque. Fusobacteria were also found in the fetal lung. At left are Bouin-fixed membranes with inflammation; few indications exist of the massive bacterial growth seen with the silver stain at right. The dark filaments radiating from the amnionic basement membrane are easily identified as the filamentous organisms. Left: H&E, ×160. Right: Gomori methenamine silver, ×240.

found bacterial endotoxin in the amnionic fluid of a patient with fusobacterial infection of a preterm delivery, reaffirming the suggestion by Altshuler and Hyde (1988) that these organisms are rich in lipopolysaccharide.

13. *Bacteroides fragilis* was found to be the cause of ascending infection in 5 of 15 patients with premature rupture of membranes reported by Evaldson et al. (1982). *Campylobacter (Vibrio) fetus*, a common enteric pathogen in humans and a common cause of venereally transmitted abortion in hoofed animals, has been

described to cause placentitis, infarcts, and fetal death (Gribble et al., 1981). Their patient had fever for 3 weeks, and fetal death occurred at 19 weeks of pregnancy. The amnionic fluid and placental surface were normal, but histologically there were areas of villous necrosis and "acute inflammation in the villous tissue." The organism was isolated from maternal blood, placenta, and fetal spleen. These authors reviewed the few other cases reported with pregnancy; when described, the placentas were similar to their case. The route or

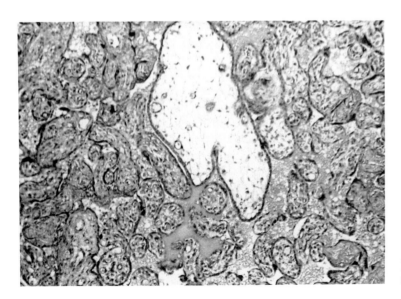

FIGURE 398. Villi of placenta in Figure 397, showing scattered villous edema. H&E. ×160.

source of infection was not identified in any of the cases, nor was venereal transmission verified. Some patients had recurrent abortions. Placental tropism has been suggested to exist in sheep. The earlier literature of infection with this organism was reviewed by White (1967).

14. Chorioamnionitis due to *Streptobacillus moniliformis*, the cause of rat bite fever, was reported by Faro et al. (1980). The patient had cervical cerclage for repeated abortions; and with unruptured membranes, amniocentesis yielded pus and gram-negative rods. The placenta had a fetid odor. The patient's house was infested with rats. The organism also causes the Haverhill (milk) fever.

15. Gibbs et al. (1987) isolated the gram-variable organism *Gardnerella* (*Hemophilus*, *Corynebacterium*) *vaginalis* from 28% of 86 patients who had intra-amnionic infection. Because controls had a similar frequency of isolation (21%), the authors considered that this common vaginal organism is part of a microbial spectrum that does not cause PROM. We have isolated it occasionally from maternal and neonatal blood; it causes mild disease. Hillier et al. (1988), in a case-control study of chorioamnionitis, isolated *G. vaginalis* in 26% and *Ureaplasma urealyticum* in 47% of cases of prematurely delivered infants. They considered that these organisms are etiologically important.

16. Tularemia is an uncommon disease, but the responsible organism (*Francisella tularensis*) has once been described to infect placenta and fetus (Lide, 1947). The placenta of the macerated fetus showed granulomatous lesions with frequent central necrosis, and similar granulomas were found in the fetus. The patient had become infected while preparing rabbits for eating.

17. Brucellosis is caused by a variety of organisms belonging to the genus *Brucella*. Malta and Bang fevers in humans are due to infection with these organisms, but a wide variety of animal diseases are frequently caused by host-specific species of these organisms (Moore & Schnurrenberger, 1981). Among the animal diseases, abortion and placentitis are prominent findings. The lesions are frequently characteristic (Molello et al., 1963). Human infection with several of the *Brucella* species has been well documented. It may be a fatal or protracted disease; often it is self-limited, and the organism appears to be acquired from contact with animals or their products, especially raw milk and unpasteurized cheese (Anonymous, 1983b). Although abortions have been described due to *Brucella abortus* and the organism has been isolated from the fetus (Carpenter & Boak, 1931), it is an uncommon event. In cattle the organisms are much enriched in placental cotyledons and allantoic fluid, and in mice this infection has provided an important model (Tobias et al., 1993). Meador and Deyoe (1989) depicted large numbers of

these bacteria in the trophoblast of infected bovine placentas. Sarram et al. (1974) isolated *Brucella melitensis* from the placenta of abortion in a highly endemic area; and they suggested a causal relation to the abortion. The placentas were not described. The topic was completely reviewed by Porreco and Haverkamp (1974). They found little evidence of an increased abortion rate with this infection and cited only a few cases with positive isolation from the placenta or fetus. The patient they described had verified infection from fresh goat cheese during the 32nd week of gestation. She was treated with kanamycin and delivered a healthy infant at term. The placenta was normal. No characteristic lesions have been described in the human placenta with this disease. Salpingitis has often been reported with brucellosis, and sexual transmission was suggested in several studies (see Ruben et al., 1991).

Leprosy

Leprosy is due to *Mycobacterium leprae*. It is now relatively uncommon in the United States, but pregnancy complicating leprosy has been investigated on many occasions. It has been reported that vertical transmission is usually either uncommon or that it does not occur. Duncan et al. (1985), however, described two young children (12 and 17 months of age) with leprosy. Whether these children acquired the disease transplacentally or shortly after birth remains unknown. The authors examined sections of the placenta and failed to identify acid-fast bacilli. When they made concentrates of the 10 most "bacilliferous" patients' placentas, they found only scanty organisms or cell debris.

Maurus (1978) found no organisms in one placenta and gave up searching for organisms in the placenta following a report by King and Marks (1958), who said they were unable to identify placental organisms in patients with treated leprosy. This statement contrasts with earlier reports, summarized by Duncan (1983), in which frequent abortion with bacterial isolation of organisms from placenta and cord blood was alleged.

For this reason, the detailed study of the human placenta in leprosy patients by Duncan et al. (1984) is of great value. In their review of the literature, there was one reported placenta with a granulomatous lepromatous lesion in villi; *M. leprae* was present in 66 of 172 placentas studied in the past. Duncan and colleagues (1984) reported a detailed investigation of 81 placentas from leprous women. No lepromatous lesions were detected histologically in the placentas by electron microscopy or immunological study. Homogenates of placentas from two patients with active lepromatous leprosy yielded a few acid-fast bacilli. The previously recognized relatively small size of placentas in leprosy patients (Duncan, 1980) was reaffirmed. This "hypoplasia," however, was now held to be due to smaller placental cell sizes (rather than cell numbers) and not to an altered immune status. Patients with leprosy have depressed T cell reactivity that is allegedly worse during pregnancy. For unknown reasons, these mothers excrete reduced amounts of estriol during pregnancy (Duncan & Oakey, 1982).

Nine-banded armadillos suffer leprosy spontaneously, and they can be infected with the human organism. When Job et al. (1987) studied the placentas of three pregnant armadillos, they found acid-fast organisms in decidua, trophoblast, and villous cores, as well as in the spleens of some fetuses. Although focal villous necrosis was found, no granulomas were seen in the placentas. One animal had thrombosed cord vessels. In light of the occasional finding of organisms in placentas from leprous women, and because of some degree of similarity between armadillo and human placentas, vertical transmission remains a good possibility, even though it may be uncommon.

Tuberculosis

In contrast to leprosy, congenital tuberculosis has been repeatedly demonstrated to occur, despite the fact that generalized tuberculosis is a frequent cause of sterility. In some cases there is doubt as to the timing of infection. Neonatal disease may have been acquired postpartum from milk or sputum of an infected mother. No epidemiological doubt, however, exists about the disease in the macerated stillborn with the extrauterine pregnancy described by Nokes et al. (1957). This 23 cm crown-rump (CR) fetus, removed from an abdominal implantation, had multiple caseating pulmonary nodules and acid-fast bacilli in the liver, spleen, and kidneys. The placenta had many hard, white plaques that represented tubercles and contained acid-fast organisms. The patient had a partially tubally implanted pregnancy, and tuberculous salpingitis and miliary tuberculosis existed in most organs. The authors reviewed briefly 68 previously reported cases of extrauterine pregnancies complicated by tuberculosis.

Beitzke (1935) established criteria for the acceptance of congenital tuberculosis, which is now a rare and preventable disease of infants. These criteria included evidence of hematogenous infection via the umbilical vein. Beitzke also emphasized the need to separate infant from mother at birth.

Nemir and O'Hare (1986) reviewed diagnostic criteria, reported the longest follow-up of a severely infected child, and gathered more than 200 cases from the literature. Their own case was criticized by Corrall (1986) as

not fulfilling all of the established criteria. The discussion further elaborated on the difficulties of distinguishing truly transplacentally acquired tuberculosis from infection transmitted by inhalation of infected amnionic fluid and from neonatal disease acquired nosocomially.

The placenta has rarely been examined in putative cases of congenital tuberculosis. Schmorl and Kockel (1894) examined three patients who died with tuberculosis during pregnancy. The placentas appeared grossly normal. The fetuses were near term; all three associated placentas contained typical but rare granulomas with giant cells in the villous tissue. In two fetuses, tuberculous lesions were also found; the placental membranes were uniformly negative. Schmorl and Geipel (1904) found nine additional cases of placental tuberculosis among 20 new specimens. For some of these specimens, more than 2,000 sections had to be prepared before tubercles were found. They insisted that acid-fast stains must be made lest early lesions be overlooked. Bacilli were frequently found in fetal vessels, intervillous fibrin, and septa.

Warthin (1907) provided additional detailed descriptions of placental tuberculosis, with numerous tubercles and acid-fast bacilli identified. He found that the decidua contained areas of necrosis but no giant cells; there were many intervillous and villous granulomas, and the chorion was involved only sparsely. In a previous case, he also made thousands of sections to verify tuberculous infection. His initial opinion that the syncytium was resistant to infection was subsequently modified because he saw necrosis of trophoblast.

Boesaart (1959) also found tubercles in the placenta of an infected patient whose infant remained well. We saw a placenta membranacea at 35 weeks' gestation from a patient with tuberculous peritonitis. The placental floor had several tuberculous granulomas. The neonate was well and was treated prophylactically (Kaplan et al., 1980). In the same report, we demonstrated numerous acid-fast bacilli in the therapeutically aborted villous tissue of a patient who had cavitary tuberculosis for which she was taking appropriate medication. There was neither necrosis nor a granulomatous reaction. Finding the organisms was unexpected.

Listeriosis

Listeriosis is caused by a gram-positive bacillus that is occasionally confused with diphtheroids. The disease occurs in a wide variety of mammals and birds, as well as in humans (Dennis, 1968). The literature suggests that the human disease is underdiagnosed (Bowmer et al., 1973). Most adults successfully eliminate the causative organism, *Listeria monocytogenes*. Immunodeficiency of adults (Nieman & Lorber, 1980; Wetli et al., 1983), various chronic disease states (Boucher et al., 1984), and characteristically pregnancy may be complicated by significant disease (Gantz et al., 1975). Transmission from mother's milk has been recorded in neonates (Svabic-Vlahovic et al., 1988). Nosocomial infection occurs in nurseries (Nelson et al., 1985), and direct contact with infected animals has also caused infection (Anonymous, 1980).

Food-borne acquisition of the organism is the most common mode of infection (Gill, 1988; Lamont et al., 1988; Jones, 1990). Numerous epidemics have been reported, and the source of bacteria has been defined in some (Anonymous, 1985). Some of these epidemics have originated from pasteurized milk (Fleming et al., 1985b), Mexican-style cheese (Linnan et al., 1988), cabbage contaminated by sheep feces and made into coleslaw (Schlech et al., 1983), poorly cooked sausage and chicken (Schwartz et al., 1988), pâté (37 of 73 examined contained the organisms) (Morris & Ribeiro, 1989), and other sources. At times the precise source of an infection could not be defined despite intensive search (Filice et al., 1978), but a gastrointestinal route appears to be the most likely mode of infection (Breer & Schopfer, 1988). The organism may survive moderate heat, and it thrives in chilled food (Kerr et al., 1988; Gilbert et al., 1989). Guidelines have thus been established for the food industry in order to avoid wide dissemination of this ubiquitous agent to susceptible people (Update, 1988).

The implication that livestock are the cause of transmission of this infection has been challenged, as the organism also occurs in the stool of many normal people and in the soil (Low & Donachie, 1989). Ortel (1975) investigated stools from a large population of "normal" people after a devastating outbreak occurred in Halle during 1968. Pregnant patients had a 24% rate of contamination (6.5% after delivery), meatpackers 3.6%, and nurse-midwives 9%; finally, the personnel of a laboratory had a 91.6% (!) rate of carriage.

The organism is a danger principally to pregnant women, newborns, and immunocompromised individuals. A 60% perinatal mortality has been ascribed to this infection (Barresi, 1980). We have seen congenital listeriosis in the offspring of a microbiology laboratory technician, suggesting that special vigilance is needed when such personnel are pregnant. Fortunately, the neonate was promptly treated and survived.

In infants, listeriosis is known as granulomatosis infantiseptica. Granulomatosis is a misnomer because the visible lesions are truly abscesses, not granulomas (Seeliger, 1955). An autopsy report of seven children with perinatal listeriosis indicates that grossly visible microabscesses are relatively uncommon (Klatt et al., 1986). During an outbreak in Los Angeles, which originated from infected cheese, maternal pyrexia and a

high index of suspicion were the most essential factors for the early diagnosis (Boucher & Yonekura, 1986). Neonatal meningitis is a serious complication of fetal infection with this organism (Ahlfors et al., 1977; Visintine et al., 1977; Laugier et al., 1978). A rash is often present in the neonate, and gastric aspirates as well as Gram stains (and culture) of skin rashes are helpful for identifying the organism (Halliday & Hirata, 1979). One case of nonimmune fetal hydrops has been attributed to listeriosis; the placenta and stillborn fetus had numerous abscesses (Gembruch et al., 1987). The diagnosis is easily established from cultures, when the infection is suspected. Berche et al. (1990) found that anti-listeriolysin 0 titers quickly develop after infection, and that they are useful for diagnosis.

The placenta in listeriosis has the following characteristic lesions: villous abscesses, villous necrosis, necrotizing villitis, and an abundance of bacterial growth on the amnionic surface, usually accompanied by chorioamnionitis. Case reports with good descriptions of these lesions have been provided by Olding and Philipson (1960), Driscoll et al. (1962), Soma (1979), and many other pathologists. Yamazaki et al. (1977) found abscesses, chorioamnionitis, and funisitis in a stillborn with proved granulomatosis infantiseptica, but they were unable to demonstrate the organisms in the placenta. They referred to other authors with a similar experience. The development of unusual "macroabscesses" in congenital listeriosis was described by Steele and Jacobs (1979), and Topalovski et al. (1993) thought that the diagnosis could be made solely from a placental examination. They depicted the macroabscesses in the placenta and suggested that silver impregnation is a better means to demonstrate the organisms than a Gram stain. The diagnosis of listeriosis complicating pregnancy is important because prompt therapy with ampicillin rapidly cures the maternal and fetal infection. There is also good evidence that listeriosis is a common cause of abortion in France (Lallemand et al., 1992) and produces similar pathological lesions.

Aside from the usually opaque surface of the placenta, which is occasionally described as greenish, there are often typical abscesses visible in cross sections of the fresh placenta (Figures 399, 400). When smears of these yellowish lesions are stained with Gram solution, the organisms are often readily apparent. Microscopically, the abscess frequently has a central area of necrosis and is composed of a massive PMNL infiltration (Figure 401). The chorioamnionitis is usually severe and often extends into the villous tissue; the amnion commonly contains a large number of organisms. There is no doubt that some of them have proliferated during cold storage of the placenta prior to examination (Figure 402). The amnionic colonization is so prominent in utero, however, that amniocentesis for the differential

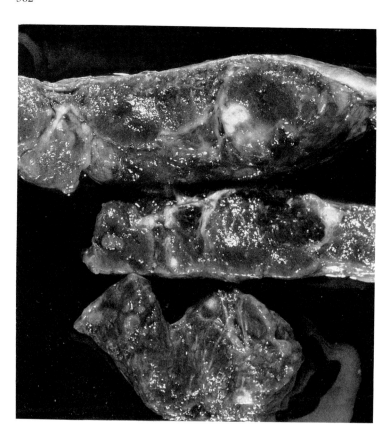

FIGURE 399. Numerous placental abscesses (white nodules) due to *Listeria* infection. A premature infant was born. Immediate therapy was applied, and the infant survived.

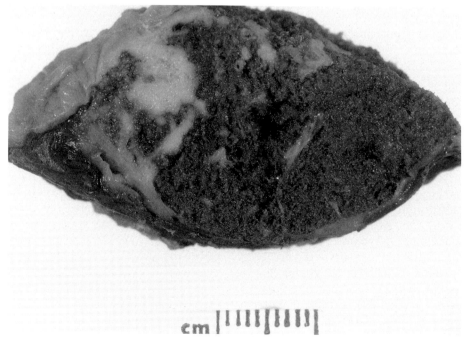

FIGURE 400. *Listeria* abscess in the placenta underneath the discolored chorionic plate at 37 weeks' gestation. Maternal fever was immediately diagnosed as due to listeriosis by examining smears of the abscess. Ampicillin therapy of the neonate cured the infant, who had a diffuse rash at birth.

FIGURE 401. *Listeria* abscess in an immature placenta of stillborn twins. There is much necrosis of villi, fibrin deposition, and infiltration with PMNLs. Numerous organisms were found on Gram stain. H&E. Left ×60; right ×240.

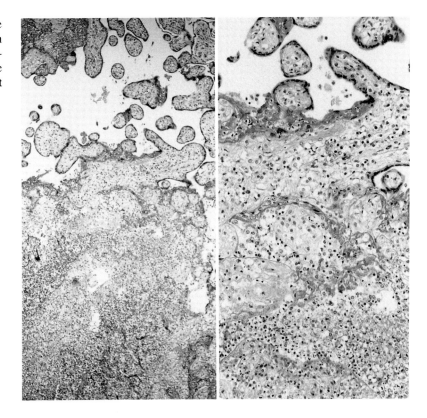

diagnosis of febrile patients has been advocated (Petrilli et al., 1980).

When listeriosis is recognized during pregnancy and adequately treated, the placental abscesses undergo scarring. They are then sometimes still recognizable histologically as a former abscess. One must assume that abscesses in the fetus have a similar fate. Effective therapy during pregnancy has been described by Zervoudakis and Cederqvist (1977) and Fleming et al. (1985a). The latter authors presented another case and described meconium staining and chorioamnionitis. Koh et al. (1980) also saw meconium discharge and found many placental abscesses in a newborn who was severely ill; the infant recovered after ampicillin therapy, which had been commenced prenatally. A similar sporadic occurrence was related by Barresi (1980). The organisms were present in gastric aspirate and on body surfaces. Placental abscesses were present. In another case, treated at 13 weeks' gestation, the placenta and infant were normal when the patient delivered at term (Cruikshank & Warenski, 1989). Identical lesions of placenta and fetus have been described in nonhuman primates (McClure & Strozier, 1975).

Recurrence of listeriosis during subsequent pregnancies has occasionally been described (Rappaport et al., 1960; Dungal, 1961; Ruffolo et al., 1962). Such events and the unexplained reason for the unusual frequency of severe listeriosis during pregnancy and in newborns have raised questions about the pathogenesis

of this disease. Flamm (1959) experimented with rabbits and was of the opinion that septic transplacental infection causes the placental and fetal infection. This opinion is partly supported by the findings of typical abscesses in the placenta and the occasional finding of organisms within intact amnionic sacs. The presence of organisms in the vagina and in stool, and the typically severe chorioamnionitis, however, suggest that an ascending mode of infection also occurs. Perhaps the placental abscesses form after fetal septicemia has taken place, similar to the abscesses in the fetus. Whether one or both of these modes of infection is the predominant way of fetal infection with listerial organisms is currently not known.

The susceptibility of immunodeficient and pregnant patients may result from their altered T cell function. Schaffner et al. (1983) addressed this question experimentally by treating mice with cyclosporin A and cortisone and by infecting nude mice. Their conclusion was that *Listeria* infection is biphasic: "Bacterial multiplication is controlled by nonspecific defense mechanisms in the early phase, and by acquired T-cell-dependent immunity in the second." This question was further explored in the work of Redline and Lu (1987), who found that local, decidual immune response regulated infection of the fetoplacental unit. They suggested an analogy to the nonrejection of the placental graft in regard to this immunological interaction of *Listeria* and the decidua. In later studies, Redline et al. (1988) found

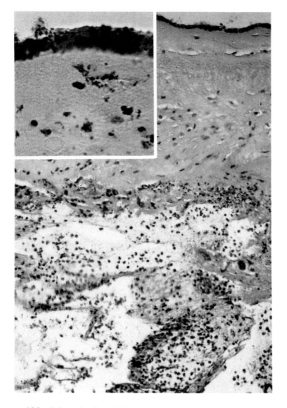

FIGURE 402. Listeriosis of the placenta in a stillborn. There is extensive subchorial infiltration with leukocytes, edema of membranes, and massive bacterial growth in amnion. H&E. ×160. Inset: Gram stain. ×640.

that hormonal induction of deciduomas allows bacterial proliferation in the uterus, but that this endocrine manipulation does not influence the infection of peripheral organs of mice. It was also true when the mice were preimmunized. The investigators then studied the composition of the immune cells in the decidua and found that "increased bacterial titers were correlated with an inability of macrophages and T lymphocytes to reach tissue *Listeria* in discrete regions of deciduoma-bearing uteri." They further suggested that an antifetal (placental) immune response of the host was hindered by the same decidual mechanism that allows uncontrolled listerial growth locally (Redline & Lu, 1988). These findings suggested that the lack of recurrent listeriosis transmission by 74 women who had once delivered an infected child (Degen et al., 1970) is *not* the result of immunization. Bortolussi et al. (1989) found in rat experiments that neonatal interferon deficiency may be responsible for the susceptibility of infants.

Bacterial Vaginosis

Bacterial vaginosis has been defined by Westrom et al. (1985) as the "replacement of the lactobacilli of the vagina by characteristic groups of bacteria accompanied by changed properties of the vaginal fluid." The "other bacterial species" include *Bacteroides*, *Gardnerella vaginalis*, *Mycoplasma hominis*, *Ureaplasma urealyticum*, and perhaps others. A relation to PROM and amnionic sac infection has been reported to exist (Gravett et al., 1986). Silver et al. (1989) also suggested that bacterial vaginosis is a common cause of intra-amnionic infection. Consideration of this entity, however, is beyond the scope of this chapter. An extensive review has been provided by Martius and Eschenbach (1990) that considers the relation of vaginosis to chorioamnionitis.

Mycoplasma hominis and *Ureaplasma urealyticum*

Mycoplasmas are a well recognized group of pathogens of many animals. They cause infections of the urogenital tract, are responsible for respiratory and joint diseases, and are a frequent cause of epidemics in laboratory animal colonies (Tully & Whitcomb, 1979). Two organisms, *Mycoplasma hominis* and *Ureaplasma urealyticum* (also known as the T strain because the colonies are so *tiny*) are known urogenital pathogens for humans (Cassel & Cole, 1981); other *Mycoplasma* species affect different organ systems. *M. hominis* is a known cause of pelvic inflammatory disease (PID), febrile conditions during the postpartum period (Naessens et al., 1989), and possibly urinary tract infections. *U. urealyticum* (as well as *Chlamydia trachomatis*) is known to cause nongonococcal urethritis in men (Shepard, 1970; Taylor-Robinson & McCormack, 1980). The organism attaches itself to spermatozoa and may thus more readily penetrate the endocervical mucous barrier. It is also likely that combined infection with these two organisms is a cause of mucopurulent cervicitis in women (Paavonen et al., 1986). The available evidence suggests that these organisms are sexually transmitted (McCormack et al., 1972). Sterility in women is often secondary to PID, and much direct evidence exists that *U. urealyticum* infection of fallopian tubes is an important cause (e.g., Friberg, 1978). On the other hand, Gump et al. (1984) found that there is no relation between involuntary infertility and *Mycoplasma* infection.

Kundsin et al. (1967) first suggested that infection with the T strain of *Mycoplasma* may cause chorio-amnionitis and repeated abortion. They observed this new strain in cultures from decidua and aborted fetal membranes of a patient who had had four previous unsuccessful pregnancies. The fetal lung contained aspirated pus. Microorganisms were not identified histologically in the inflamed tissues. Additional specimens gave similar results. These observations suggested that this new strain (*U. urealyticum*) may be the cause of repetitive abortions as well as of sterility. A case similar to that described by these investigators is depicted in Figure 403; it is a patient with four previous abortions. Severe chorioamnionitis in this abortus is evident from the opacity of the fetal surface. Subsequent treatment of this patient and her husband with antibiotics resulted in a healthy term pregnancy (Quinn et al., 1983).

Since the initial description of placental infection with *Mycoplasma*, there have been numerous clinical and pathological studies that aimed to define the roles of these pathogens in reproductive failure of women, specifically attempting to relate them to PROM and chorioamnionitis. Some conflicting results have been obtained. The studies are hampered by the facts that these organisms have specific culture requirements and cannot be identified by routine microscopic examination of tissues. Prenatal infection of fetal tissues has been demonstrated microbiologically in many studies, but positive antepartum cultures do not predict outcome effectively (Carey et al., 1991). Furthermore, erythromycin treatment of infected women does not apparently prevent premature delivery (Eschenbach et al., 1991). Both organisms are a cause of neonatal meningitis (Waites et al., 1988); *M. hominis* has been the cause of neonatal lung abscess (Sacker et al., 1970); and *U. urealyticum* infection has been associated with chronic neonatal lung disease (Cassell et al., 1988; Sanchez & Regan, 1988; Wang et al., 1988).

Madan et al. (1988, 1989) made detailed microbiological studies of autopsy and placental material; they found that "genital *Mycoplasma* were isolated from 36 cases (8.3%), and acute chorioamnionitis and funisitis were present significantly more often in cases with genital mycoplasmas." In their detailed study of perinatal deaths, including isolation of various pathogens from placenta and neonatal lung, they came to similar conclusions. One of their stillborns had myocardial calcifications, and some had not only aspirated pus in the lung but also an interstitial chronic inflammatory response, suggesting prolonged exposure to this mycoplasmal antigen. In this decisive pathological study of perinatal infection with this organism, the authors were much impressed with the attending villous edema in the placenta.

The disease caused by these organisms is similar to that of other acute infections, except for the absence of demonstrable bacteria. The chorioamnionitis is similar as well. There have been some other suggestions that mycoplasmal infection causes villous alterations. Kundsin et al. (1967) found "unusual sclerosis of villi." and Romano et al. (1971), who described aspiration bronchopneumonia in an aborted 19-week fetus with isolation of T strain organisms, described degenerative changes of villous vessels, thrombosis, and villous edema. The illustration accompanying their article, however, depicted normal architecture. This study, as many others, was hampered by our current inability to demonstrate the organism microscopically in tissue sections. In the future it will require special techniques, such as study with immunofluorescence.

The relation of *Mycoplasma* to PROM, premature labor, and chorioamnionitis is still in dispute. Romero et al. (1989c,d; Romero, 1989) have critically reviewed

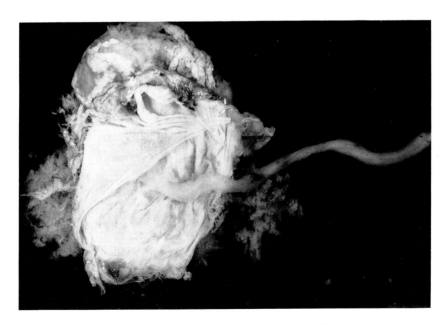

FIGURE 403. Placenta of spontaneous abortion due to *U. urealyticum* infection. The patient had had four previous abortions with similar morphology. Note the creamy pus underneath the amnionic surface and fresh marginal hemorrhage.

12 published studies to assess this relation. They criticized several of them as being indecisive and poorly designed. It is their opinion that the association of cultured organisms and PROM "does not prove a cause-and-effect relationship"; and when all studies were analyzed in detail, "it seems unlikely that genital colonization with *Mycoplasma* species without a failure of the host defense (fetal and/or maternal) leads to preterm delivery." This report was criticized by Kundsin and Horne (1989), and the reply must be read to appreciate the current controversies, especially with respect to effective therapy.

In a prospective cohort study of 6,500 women, no association of *U. urealyticum* infection with premature labor was found by Nugent (1988). Pathological and microbiological studies on neonates from patients with and without chorioamnionitis by Quinn et al. (1987) established a strong correlation between *U. urealyticum* colonization and chorioamnionitis. When maternal antibody response was taken into consideration, Gibbs et al. (1986) found a strong correlation of a pathogenic role of *M. hominis* infection. Considering the frequently mixed nature of infection, the high prevalence of some of these organisms, and the differences in the composition of the populations studied, it is presently impossible to come to a clear-cut decision. Our impression is that the genital mycoplasmas are pathogenic organisms, and that they are a frequent cause of chorioamnionitis and premature birth. In fact, several studies have shown that they are the principal organisms isolated from the placental surface and amnionic fluid of patients with PROM.

Chlamydia trachomatis

The genus *Chlamydia* has two species: *Chlamydia psittaci*, responsible for parrot fever (psittacosis), and *Chlamydia trachomatis*, responsible for the most common sexually transmitted disease in the United States. It also causes trachoma, lymphogranuloma venereum, nongonococcal urethritis in men, and the diseases in women to be discussed next. It is estimated that between 10% and 20% of sexually active men and women are infected with this organism (Saxer, 1989). Ryan et al. (1990) surveyed a large population of women by cervical culture and found that 21.08% were positive. They recommended routine culture for this organism. Approximately one-half of infants born to infected mothers develop ophthalmia neonatorum (inclusion body blennorrhea). Others develop pneumonitis. It is estimated that 3% to 4% of neonates have ophthalmia, and 1% to 2% have pneumonitis due to infection with this organism (Harrison et al., 1978; Harrison, 1985).

The bacterium-like intracellular microbe can be visualized in the cytoplasm of infected cells by direct immunofluorescence study. *Chlamydia* has also been isolated from neonates, even from the pneumonia of stillborns infected through intact membranes (Thorpe et al., 1989). Other than by culture, the infection can be diagnosed in infected tissues and amnionic fluid with the immunoperoxidase technique, as employed by Shurbaji et al. (1988), and by DNA sequences following polymerase chain reaction amplification (Pao et al., 1991). The direct immunofluorescence technique has a sensitivity of approximately 89% (Binns et al., 1988), and "fine tuning" allows some additional improvement (Pastorek et al., 1988). Livengood et al. (1988) investigated various staining methods and emphasized the diagnostic importance of having experience when reading the slides. An enzyme immunoassay was advocated by Binns et al. (1988) as being highly sensitive and therefore a good diagnostic test. Reports on the prevalence of the disease must thus be interpreted with these limitations in mind.

Chlamydia trachomatis infection of the cervix, where it causes mucopurulent cervicitis (Brunham et al., 1984), is relatively easily demonstrated by the use of the direct fluorescence method (Graber et al., 1985). Brunham et al. (1984) provided impressive color photographs of the stained organisms. *C. trachomatis* is responsible for a significant number of cases of acute salpingitis (Magnusson et al., 1986); and it also causes chronic salpingitis and sterility (Guderian & Trobough, 1986; Moss et al., 1986). The effect of a *C. trachomatis* infection on pregnancy is still controversial. Sweet et al. (1987) reported that PROM was more likely to occur when infection had caused a maternal antibody response, but statistical significance was not reached. Alger et al. (1988) found that the organism was isolated from 44% of patients with PROM and in only 16% of controls. There are suggestions that PROM and perhaps chorioamnionitis are linked to this infection, but much more direct evidence is needed before such a conclusion can be affirmed. The organism has not been isolated from the placenta but has been demonstrated in amnionic fluid and in the eye and nasopharynx of neonates (Thomas et al., 1990). It has also not yet been demonstrated conclusively to be a direct cause of chorioamnionitis, except in rat models (Rettig & Altshuler, 1981). Ryan and his colleagues (1990), however accumulated data on the infection during pregnancy that suggested premature rupture of membranes to be much more likely when the infection was not treated. Other investigators support the notion that chlamydial infection during pregnancy should be treated with antibiotics (Crombleholme et al., 1990; Foster et al., 1991).

Chlamydia psittaci infection is uncommon. Reports by Johnson et al. (1985) and Wong et al. (1985) indicated that sheep farmers have high exposure. A pregnant wife of a farmer became infected and aborted at 28 weeks' gestation. Acute intervillositis was found in the grossly normal-appearing placenta. Syncytiotrophoblastic inclusions were present that showed numerous organisms by ultrastructural study and positive immunofluorescence testing. The fetus was also infected, with organisms recovered from various organs.

Syphilis

Infection with *Treponema pallidum* may occur at any time during pregnancy. The organism may pass to the fetus through the placenta during all stages of maternal syphilis infection. The responsible organism is a 4 to 10 μm long and 0.5 μm wide spirochete. According to Grossman (1977), "most frequently, dissemination is associated with a placentitis arising from hematogenous spread of the spirochetes between the first and second stages of infection of the mother." The commonly held notion that the placenta is impermeable to spirochetes before the 20th week of pregnancy because of the thickness of Langhans' cytotrophoblast layer (Fiumara, 1975) can no longer be accepted. Braunstein (1978) described a spontaneous abortus (12.8 cm CR length, approximately 4.5 months' gestation) with an abundance of spirochetes in the liver and other organs and marked placental changes. We had shown, by immunofluorescence and electron microscopic studies, that spirochetes can be demonstrated in fetuses as early as at 9 to 10 weeks' gestation (Harter & Benirschke, 1976). One reason prior studies had failed to identify fetal syphilis is because the expression of the disease's features depends on the fetus's ability to react with antibody production to the spirochetal antigen. Histopathological changes cannot be seen before that developmental time, and the disease is thus not diagnosed. Ohyama et al. (1990) have since demonstrated spirochetes in syphilitic placentas by the immunoperoxidase technique.

The relation of infection to disease was first clearly demonstrated by Silverstein (1962) and Silverstein and Lukes (1962). They found congenital syphilis with attendant fetal plasma cell infiltration and reasoned that the inflammatory response was the cause of illness. Another reason for lack of recognition of early fetal infections is that it is often difficult to demonstrate spirochetes histologically. Fetuses from such infections are often macerated, and radiographic study of long bones, often diagnostic of the infection, is frequently neglected. They may also appear as hydrops fetalis (Barton et al., 1992). The treponemes in macerated fetuses are most abundant in the liver; they are rare in the placenta and umbilical cord. Wendel et al. (1989, 1991) have shown that in such gestations, with fetal death due to syphilis, darkfield examination of amnionic fluid always readily allows demonstration of treponemes.

In addition to the conventional silver stains, it has been demonstrated that spirochetes may be stained with immunofluorescence in formalin-fixed tissue (Hunter et al., 1984). Thus Epstein and King (1985) demonstrated spirochetes in macerated liver tissue by immunofluorescence. Nevertheless, improved Warthin-Starry silver stains are probably the best means of identifying spirochetes in tissues (Kerr, 1938). It has now been established also that the organism can be identified in macerated fetuses with the Warthin-Starry stain (Young & Crocker, 1994).

A classic paper of the neonatal pathology in congenital syphilis was written by Oppenheimer and Hardy (1971). They confined their report to 16 neonatal deaths and did not consider the 31 macerated fetuses they saw during the same time. Hepatosplenomegaly was found in all, but after penicillin therapy spirochetes were not demonstrable with the Levaditi stain. The report does not include a consideration of placental lesions. Judge (1988) also provided an excellent review of congenital syphilis, with emphasis on the stage of pregnancy when the disease was acquired.

Many morphological changes are found in the placenta and umbilical cord with congenital syphilis (Russell & Altshuler, 1974; Horn et al., 1992a). By and large, the more severely the fetus is affected, the greater are the pathological changes in the placenta. A macerated fetus with congenital syphilis may have a massively enlarged placenta with numerous pathological features; a general increase in placental weight has been demonstrated by Malan et al. (1990). Most authors who have studied the placenta of congenital syphilis have concluded that there are no absolutely characteristic pathological findings, but bulky villi and some other changes to be discussed should raise the suspicion. When suspicion of fetal syphilis exists, silver preparations for spirochetes are indicated. They may ultimately prove that lesions are due to syphilis when other means such as serology and radiographs of the fetus are not available. It must be cautioned, however, that the stains are not always easy to execute and that incomplete treatment with antibiotics may prevent identification of spirochetes. Fojaco et al. (1989) have claimed that necrotizing funisitis is a specific lesion of congenital syphilis, and Knowles and Frost (1989) have expressed a similar view. Discussion of this fallacy is included in the next section of the present chapter. Because much of the informative literature on placental syphilis comes from an era when the other causes of banal types of chorioamnionitis and funisitis were not recognized, the early literature must be interpreted with caution.

When congenital syphilis was suspected in the past, physicians made scrapings of the umbilical venous intima for darkfield examination; and in the discussion of congenital syphilis by Ricci et al. (1989), beautiful silver preparations of this type were illustrated. They also showed the plasma cell villitis in such a case. Hörmann (1954) has reviewed this and other aspects of syphilis in great detail. Baniecki (1928) is one of many authors who sought treponemes in umbilical cords. He found inflammation in 5 of 14 living infants with syphilis; 12 of 17 stillborns had such inflammation, and 5 of 40 non-luetic infants had umbilical phlebitis. During the same year, Kaufmann (1928) found no placental lesions in two-thirds of children with positive spirochetal infection. Beckmann and Zimmer (1931) made another detailed study of umbilical cords in syphilis. They had 420 cases, of which 392 were at term gestation, including 9 still-borns; 28 were premature, including 5 stillborns. They found inflammation in 18.3% (77 cases, 25 of which were mild). Of these cases, only three infants had con-genital syphilis. Conversely, 13 infants with congenital syphilis had no inflammation. These authors concluded that funisitis was not characteristic of syphilis but, rather, was a nonspecific inflammation that was perhaps caused "mechanically." Organisms are also readily identified in amnionic fluid (Wendel et al., 1989, 1991). The spirochetes may be identified in formalin-fixed sections of infected placentas using fluroescent anti-bodies, in addition to the more difficult silver stains.

The villous tissue has somewhat more characteristic changes with congenital syphilis. In Braunstein's (1978) 4 months' gestation fetus, the placenta had enlarged villi with endothelial and fibroblastic proliferation. Few mononuclear cells were present. The cellularity of the villi demonstrated in his photomicrographs, however, is impressive and is similar to that shown in Figure 405. McCord (1934) had described these features of villous "crowding" and enlargement of the placenta. Russell and Altshuler (1974) were also impressed with the pla-cental enlargement, a feature already commented on by Hörmann (1954), who had referred to a case with a placental weight of 2,500 g accompanied by a fetus weighing 2,600 g. Russell and Altshuler's diagnostic features included relative villous immaturity, decidual plasma cell infiltration, perivascular fibrous tissue pro-liferation, and alterations of capillary endothelium. They also found plasma cell infiltrations in the enlarged villi of syphilitic placentas, a finding made repeatedly by us. These changes are all nonspecific. Gummas or gran-ulomas have never been reported in the placenta, but Hörmann (1954) depicted villous abscesses that had also been seen in earlier studies. In our experience, the villous enlargement is often striking, and there are fre-quent decidual infiltrations with plasma cells; foci of decidual necrosis are common (Figure 404). Abscesses or villous necroses are frequent in severe infections, and chorioamnionitis may be present, but it is also often absent. When it is found, it may include plasma cells, which is an otherwise unusual finding in banal

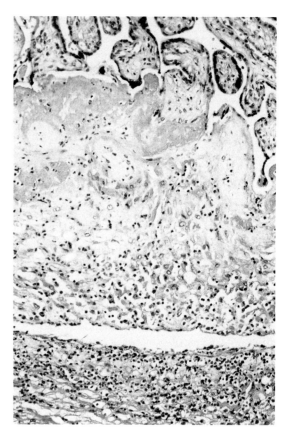

FIGURE 404. Plasma cell infiltration of decidua basalis in a placenta of 28 weeks' gestation and an infant afflicted with typical congenital syphilis. The placenta was large (580 g). H&E. ×160.

chorioamnionitis (Figure 406). Spirochetes can be found, but often it requires a prolonged search (Figure 407) unless one uses fluorecent antibodies. Regrettably, though, the art of silver-staining spirochetes in tissues is gradually being forgotten by histologists. There is a reported decrease of estriol production by the placenta in syphilis (Parker & Wendel, 1988), perhaps due to a decrease in fetal adrenal androgen precursors, rather than to a placental inability to aromatize androgens.

Samson and colleagues (1994) have shown that the syphilis-involved placenta has specific deposits of immune complexes (C3), IgM, and rheumatoid factor along small villous capillaries. They likened the pla-cental results of this infection to an "immunopathy."

Necrotizing Funisitis

The term subacute necrotizing funisitis was introduced by Navarro and Blanc (1974) in a report of 16 cases. In the earlier literature this condition had been referred to as phlegmonous funisitis (see Hörmann, 1954). It is an

FIGURE 405. Villi of placenta in congenital syphilis (same case as in Figure 407). Villi are hypercellular, infiltrated with mononuclear cells. Note the focal necrosis and vascular obliteration. H&E. ×240.

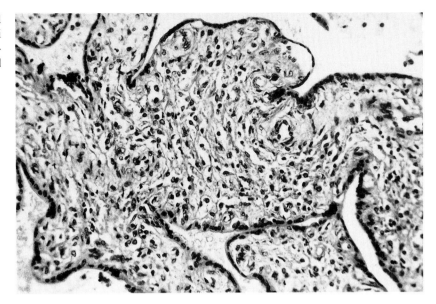

unusual type of chronic inflammation of the umbilical cord in which calcification of the old exudate may even occur. Calcifications of the umbilical cord had only rarely been reported before the descriptions by Navarro and Blanc. Eight of their cases were stillborn infants. With the exception of two isolations of *Candida* species, no pathogen was identified. Syphilis and other specific agents were carefully excluded by serology in that study.

The umbilical cords of these infants had severe inflammation deposited in "successive waves." It was present in a ring-like fashion around the umbilical cord vessels. The exudate was often degenerated and had become calcific. Mural thrombosis was present in several vessels. Two infants had an uncommon presence of plasma cells in their umbilical cord. The nature of the exudate indicated that it is a chronic infection, as did similar inflammatory changes in the lungs of several stillborns. Other signs of chronic infection were found in the stillbirths, and they occurred during the neonatal life of survivors. Chorioamnionitis with frequent surface necrosis was invariably additionally present. In the opinion of Navarro and Blanc, the funisitis differed in severity and chronicity from the usual type of funisitis found in the amnionic sac infection syndrome.

Perrin and Bel (1965) had previously described three cases of cord calcification, one of which, however, may

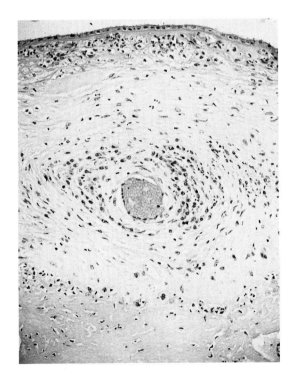

FIGURE 406. Perivascular plasma cell infiltration of chorion in congenital syphilis at 30 weeks' gestation. Mild chorioamnionitis is also present. H&E. ×160.

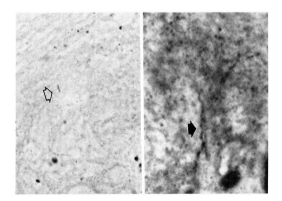

FIGURE 407. Spirochete (arrow) in the placenta of a stillborn infant with congenital syphilis. Levaditi stain. ×1,600.

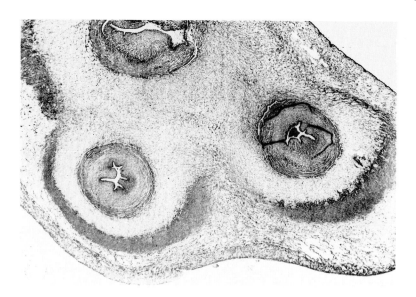

FIGURE 408. Umbilical cord at 31 weeks' gestation with chronic inflammatory exudate (necrotizing funisitis). The exudate is concentrically deposited around the vessels; much of the old exudate is necrotic and beginning to calcify. A partially organized mural thrombus is present in the umbilical vein. The patient had rupture of the membranes for more than 12 hours, a circumvallate placenta, and massive chorioamnionitis. von Gieson. ×12.

have originated in a hematoma. In one of these cases, there was difficulty clamping the cord at delivery. An interesting aspect of this inflammation was the "neovascularization" of the exudate, with the origin of these capillaries being unknown. Schiff et al. (1976) described calcification of all three vessels in the cord and had even visualized it sonographically before birth. As in other cases, the calcifications followed the cord vessels, but they stopped before entering the abdomen of the infant. This observation is important, as it further clarifies the pathogenesis of chorioamnionitis and funisitis. It indicates the presence of antigen within the amnionic sac and negates the opinion that the umbilical vasculitis results from a systemic infection. No inflammation was described in their case, but the fetal growth retardation was thought to be secondary to the restriction of blood flow. Gille (1977) described a similar case and drew

attention to the fact that granulation tissue was present in the vessels. The patient was a premature infant who did well. The exudate accompanied the vessels for the length of the cord, and a fresh thrombus was present within the vein. The accompanying photographs showed an impressive and uncommon amount of inflammation and "organization," which is otherwise rare in the placental vasculature. Knowles and Frost (1989) have added a case report of necrotizing funisitis in congenital syphilis, with organisms plentiful in this lesion but sparse elsewhere.

Numerous cases of chronic, necrotizing funisitis have been seen in our experience. Some had calcifications, others did not. In our view, they represent different stages in the evolution of funisitis. Figure 408 shows a cross section of umbilical cord in an immature placenta with necrotizing funisitis. Figure 409 shows the con-

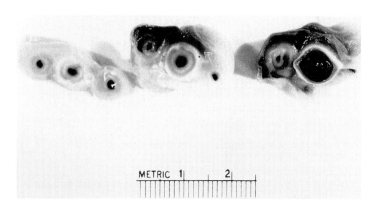

FIGURE 409. Concentric rings of perivascular exudate in necrotizing funisitis. There was marked chorioamnionitis in this 31-week pregnancy.

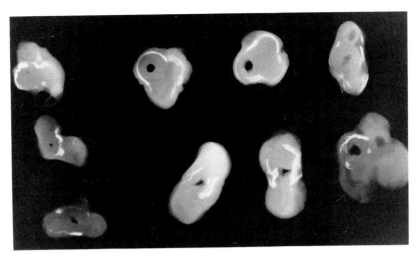

FIGURE 410. Radiographic appearance of calcific rings in a cord with necrotizing funisitis. A normal infant was delivered at term. There was no history of maternal problems except a febrile illness during the first trimester. (Courtesy Dr. R.R. Oldham, Nashville, TN.)

centric rings of white exudate in a growth-retarded infant at 31 weeks; in contrast to the previous case, here the inflammatory reaction totally surrounds the vessels. In Figure 410, a radiograph shows the peripheral calcification that has formed in the old exudate. Numerous plasma cells were found in the inflammatory debris, but electron microscopic search for organisms was unrewarding. The mother had had a febrile illness during the first trimester, but otherwise mother and infant were entirely normal. In other cases, herpes virus 2 antigen could be localized to such cords with specific antibodies (Robb et al., 1986b).

Craver and Baldwin (1992) reviewed 60 cases of this necrotizing funisitis, 45 of which had clinical information. This report is clearly the largest case collection of this lesion. It occurred in 0.1% of deliveries of more than 20 weeks' gestation. Growth retardation (28%), stillbirths (18%), and necrotizing enterocolitis (22%) were prominently associated problems. These investigators did not find any single agent or maternal condition that caused chronic funisitis. Calcification was present in 47% of their cases and chorioamnionitis in 98%. The investigators considered that a diffusible toxin in the amnionic cavity might cause this lesion because of its similarity to an Ouchterlony immunodiffusion plate. As stated earlier, Fojaco et al. (1989) suggested that necrotizing funisitis "permits a presumptive diagnosis of congenital syphilis at birth." They referred to the gross appearance as a "barber-pole cord" and found 16 cases of this association with congenital syphilis. All their cases of necrotizing funisitis were in luetic pregnancies, and spirochetes were found in 4 of 10 patients. Fojaco and her colleagues stated that information in the early literature suggests that necrotizing funisitis is diagnostic of syphilis. In fact, however, Hörmann (1954) had extensively studied syphilis and funisitis, and he did not find an absolute relation between these conditions. It is true that funisitis often occurs with syphilis, but not as regularly as suggested. Hörmann and other authors have often found necrotizing funisitis in nonsyphilitic pregnancies. This point was well made by Craver and Baldwin (1992), with whom we agree. In some umbilical cords with necrotizing funisitis, we have identified herpes antigen, to be discussed below. Thus necrotizing funisitis is a chronic, severe inflammation of the cord, frequently associated with calcification and caused by immune reaction to presumably several antigens. Likewise, Jacques and Qureshi (1992) found it not be a strong association when they studied 45 cases. Like other investigators, they found *Candida*, streptococci, and other bacteria to be responsible. The necrotizing funisitis is merely the manner by which the umbilical cord can express its chronic inflammatory damage, not being able to remove efficiently the debris that accumulates with chronic exudation.

Other Spirochetal Diseases

Leptospirosis, an infection due to one of several species of *Leptospira*, has rarely been reported during pregnancy. Coghlan and Bain (1969) have gathered the few reports of abortion that were presumed to result from this infection; they described the pregnancy of a patient who was infected with *Leptospira canicola*, acquired from a pig. The mother delivered a macerated fetus. Organisms were not recovered from the fetus or from the placenta. Moreover, there were no histopathological lesions. Abortion due to leptospirosis is said to be a common disease in China, with organisms having been recovered from the affected fetuses.

Borrelia, the spirochetal organism that causes relapsing fever, has been isolated from the blood of a febrile mother and her newborn infant who died shortly after birth (Fuchs & Oyama, 1969). The placenta was not described. The infection follows the bite of an infected tick. The disease is geographically widespread, for example, in Oregon (the case just cited) and in Israel (Yagupsky & Moses, 1985). Shirts et al. (1983) reported a nonfatal case of congenital borreliosis in a febrile patient from Colorado. The spirochetes were depicted in the neonate's blood smear, placental villous capillaries, and umbilical artery. Placental lesions were not described.

Lyme disease (erythema migrans) is an emerging borreliosis of epidemic proportion in the northeastern United States (Eichenfield & Athreya, 1989; Lastavica et al., 1989; Steere, 1989). This infection, caused by *Borrelia burgdorferi*, has been encountered in other parts of the United States and Europe as well. Transplacental infection has been reported in Wisconsin by Schlesinger et al. (1985) and in Utah by MacDonald et al. (1987). In the macerated stillborn of the latter case, the placenta was not enlarged and had "rare plasma cells in isolated villi." Grossly, the specimen was unremarkable. Spirochetes were identified in the fetus and placenta by special stains. The placental histology showed such excess of erythrocyte precursors (in the fetal circulation) that it could easily have been mistaken for erythroblastosis fetalis. In these two cases, the fetuses had congenital anomalies. Hemminki and Kyyrönen (1989) found an overrepresentation of gastrointestinal atresias in offspring from animal caretakers and forestry and agricultural workers. They suggested that infection with *B. burgdorferi* may be an etiological factor. The review of Steere (1989), however, suggested that there is no causal relation between this infection and anomalies. The same assertion was made by Strobino et al. (1993), who undertook a prospective study and found neither a definite increase of fetal anomalies nor adverse pregnancy outcomes.

Abramowsky et al. (1991) found nontreponemal spirochetes primarily in the intestines of four spontaneously aborted fetuses, with chorioamnionitis, severe chronic villitis, and villous vasculitis in some. It was possible to rule out *Treponema*, *Borrelia*, *Leptospira* and *Campylobacter*, but the precise nature of the spirochete remains to be determined.

Fungus Infections

Candida albicans infection of the vagina is common during pregnancy. Oriel and colleagues (1972) estimated that 26% of women harbored yeast: *C. albicans* in 81% and *Torulopsis (Candida) glabrata* in 16%. The use of oral contraceptives increased the frequency. Peeters et al. (1972) reported similar results. They opined that an increased use of antibiotics, contraceptives, and trichomonacides may be responsible for this frequency. Bret and Coupe (1958) demonstrated that neonatal fungal infection (mostly candidiasis) can be traced to maternal vaginal infection in most cases. The organisms usually then disappear spontaneously for unknown reasons.

Prenatal infection of placenta, cord, and fetus has been reported in well over 50 cases since its first description (Benirschke & Raphael, 1958; Whyte et al., 1982). Figure 411 illustrates a classical case. The patient was a gravida 6, para 1, who had had five consecutive abortions. The pregnancy terminated at 25 weeks with severe chorioamnionitis. The umbilical cord had numerous tiny white-yellow plaques. Histologically, these nodules consisted of infiltrates with acute inflammatory cells underneath areas of epithelial necrosis (Figure 412).

Fungal hyphae are readily demonstrated with silver stains but may be difficult to identify in H&E preparations. Touch preparations from scraping cord lesions are diagnostic. Relative to the severity of the chorio-

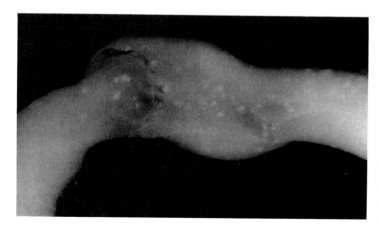

FIGURE 411. Umbilical cord from a patient with congenital candidiasis at 25 weeks' gestation. Note the numerous small, white plaques, representing abscesses (granulomas). Gravida 6, para 1, abortus 5.

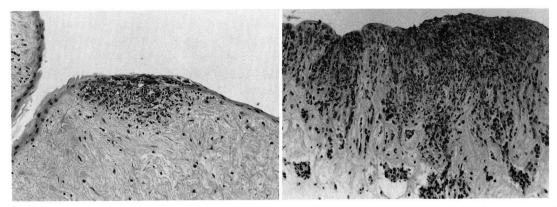

FIGURE 412. Candidiasis of umbilical cord. The lesions shown in Figure 411 are accumulations of inflammatory cells, debris, and hyphal organisms of *Candida albicans*. Epithelial necrosis is striking at the right. H&E. Left ×60; right ×240.

amnionitis, the funisitis is slight. It is often remarkably focal. The umbilical cord finding of surface granules with inflammatory cells and fungi is characteristic of congenital candidiasis. Although *C. albicans* is the most common candidal organism, infection with *C. parapsilosis*, a common skin inhabitant, has also been reported (Kellogg et al., 1974). We have seen two cases of infection with *C. tropicalis*. Other than a lack of hyphae, the findings were generally similar (Figure 413).

A remarkable feature of congenital candidiasis is the frequency of its occurrence with unruptured membranes. We had postulated a "silent, healed" rupture in our original report. Our subsequent experience was that the organisms may readily penetrate intact membranes. Why the placental infection is so uncommon, in comparison with the frequency of the vaginal infection, is unknown. It had been speculated that it results from fetal immunodeficiency, but findings of good plasma cell response to the congenital pulmonary infection

negates this hypothesis (Hood et al., 1985). More likely is the efficiency of the endocervical mucus plug in preventing ascension. Neonatal candidiasis may be widespread, with skin rash, dark red skin appearance, pneumonia (Emanuel et al., 1962), meningitis (Levin et al., 1978), sepsis, and frequent intestinal contamination (Taschdjian & Kozinn, 1957). It may cause death but has also been treated successfully on several occasions. Abortions have also been due to *Candida* infection (Buchanan & Sworn, 1979; Smith et al., 1988). We have seen elevations of neonatal white blood cell counts to $80,000/\text{m}^3$ in congenital infection of a premature infant. There had been rupture of membranes for 3 days.

A well-studied case showed convincing evidence of antenatal septicemia (Bittencourt et al., 1984). In this case, a large fungal invasion into an umbilical vein was shown; Moreover, there were many fetal and villous candidal lesions. The latter showed focal necrosis,

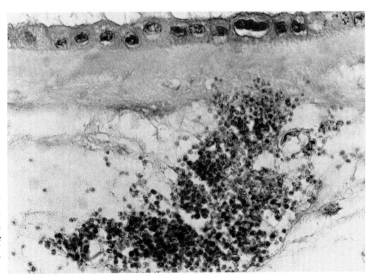

FIGURE 413. Subamnionic cluster of *Candida parapsilosis* in an infant with cutaneous congenital candidiasis (blisters) after prolonged rupture of membranes. The infant did well. Note the absence of hyphae and the intact amnionic epithelium. Chorioamnionitis was prominent at other sites H&E. ×600.

chronic villitis, and intervillous abscesses. Congenital infection has been associated with a retained IUD on several occasions (Schweid & Hopkins, 1968; Ho & Aterman, 1970; Bittencourt et al., 1984; Spaun & Klünder, 1986; Smith et al., 1988; Elliott, 1989). Delaplane et al. (1983) believed that in their case the fungus may have been introduced by amniocentesis. Whyte et al. (1982) suggested that at least 30 cases had been reported, and they added 18 of their own. At least 10 additional cases can be added to this list, bringing the total to well over 50 congenital candidal infections. Bader (1966) reported its occurrence in an anencephalic fetus and depicted the extent of placental involvement. Rhatigan (1968) and Franciosi and Jarzynski (1970) each added a case. Nagata et al. (1981), described a fatal case of pulmonary mycosis and cited some cases from the Japanese literature. Johnson et al. (1981a) reported two cases and gave suggestions for therapy. Delprado et al. (1982) provided excellent illustrations in their report of three cases; they highlighted the association with unruptured membranes and a retained IUD.

The case report by Levin et al. (1978) is of particular interest. It involved a set of diamnionic monochorionic (DiMo) twins delivered vaginally at approximately 30 weeks' gestation. The mother was febrile. The amniotomy of twin A resulted in meconium-stained fluid, but this infant did not have fungal infection at autopsy. Twin B, whose membranes had ruptured 9 days prior to delivery and whose amnionic sac was found to be dry at delivery, had cerebral candidiasis. In the placenta, a focus of candidal hyphae was found near the insertion of the umbilical cord from twin B, and chorioamnionitis was more severe.

A case of *Torulopsis (Candida) glabrata* infection of placenta and fetus in a patient with sickle cell anemia was illustrated by Sander et al. (1983). They assumed that the maternal immune compromise may have rendered this infection more possible. The only previously described case was in a patient with a retained IUD. This widely distributed yeast has now been placed

in the *Candida* genus; it lacks hyphae. In the two reported cases there was chorioamnionitis, but the umbilical cords had no lesions. In Sander's case the patient had had cerclage for repeated abortions; the stillborn twins had a fungal aspiration pneumonia. Infection had occurred before rupture of membranes, and marked deciduitis was present. The most remarkable feature of the lesion in the umbilical cord are the peripheral nodules with invading fungi. These nodules contain fungi but are compressed Wharton's jelly, perhaps from digestion of the mucopolysaccharides by the yeast. Few white blood cells are present in these nodules. Other comprehensive reviews are those by Johnson et al. (1981a), Gerberding et al. (1989), and Schwartz and Reef (1990).

Approximately 65 pregnant patients with coccidioidomycosis had been reported when VanBergen et al. (1976) reported a fatal case. The placenta had numerous infarcts with spherules of *Coccidioides immitis*, accompanied by inflammation, necrosis, and fibrin deposits. Figure 414 shows a cross section of a placenta with coccidioidomycosis. Figure 415 is a representative microscopic appearance of the lesions and the organisms. An acute inflammatory response around the fungal spherules is common, as is extensive fibrin deposition. Smale and Waechter (1970), in an analysis of 15 cases with disseminated infection, mentioned three with placental involvement and one presumed fetal infection. Most commonly, the organism remains confined to the placenta, where it produces infarctive necroses. This picture was first described by Vaughan and Ramirez (1951), who saw 33 cases of coccidioidomycosis complicating pregnancy. Only one had lesions in the placenta. They were infarctive, necrotic lesions with "purulent filled centers, full of spherules." The premature infant delivered to that mother died at the age of 6 months but was free of the disease. The other infants also did not contract the infection transplacentally. Shafai (1978) described disseminated infection in a set of premature twins whose mother died soon

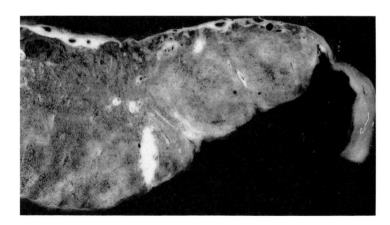

FIGURE 414. Section of mature placenta from a mother with coccidioidal meningitis. The coccidioidomycosis lesions are the white infarct and the punctate fibrin deposits. The mother was treated with amphotericin B. The neonate was normal.

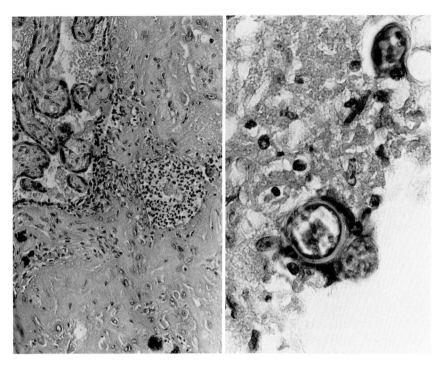

FIGURE 415. Coccidioidomycosis of the placenta (case in Figure 414). (Left) Note the spherule in the X cell deposit with fibrin and an acute inflammatory reaction. (Right) Several large spherules are engulfed in macrophages (at right). H&E. Left ×250; right ×640.

after giving birth. He found no lesions in the placenta but still assumed that transplacental infection must have occurred. Bernstein et al. (1981) described another presumptive congenital infection, but they did not describe the placenta. Spark (1981) critically reviewed all cases of "congenital" coccidioidomycosis and came to the conclusion that transplacental dissemination was unlikely for any of them. The mode of neonatal infection, he believed, was inhalation of infected material (decidua) during delivery.

We have seen massive placental involvement with *Coccidioides* lesions unaccompanied by neonatal illness (McCaffree et al., 1978). In one patient in whom the disease was treated with amphotericin B during the entire gestation, the fetus was normal and the placenta merely showed old infarcts and fibrin deposits, without stainable organisms. Peterson et al. (1989) also described a patient with coccidioidal meningitis treated with amphotericin during two pregnancies in whose placentas there were no organisms. Walker et al. (1992) described maternal reactivation of coccidioidomycosis during pregnancy, positive neonatal cord titers, but a negative placenta.

Cryptococcosis of the placenta was found in a patient with acquired immunodeficiency syndrome (AIDS) by Kida et al. (1989). It had not invaded villi, and the infant did not develop lesions. The mother developed widespread cryptococcosis. Through the courtesy of G.

Altshuler we examined placental sections with cryptococcal abscesses from a patient with systemic lupus erythematosus (SLE). She suffered cryptococcal meningitis, presumably because of steroid therapy for SLE. In the intervillous spaces of the immature placenta there were large colonies of cryptococcal organisms; inflammation was scant, and no invasion of the villi was found. The neonate (850 g) died and had no evidence of disease (Molnar-Nadasdy et al., in press). We have also had the good fortune to see the slides from a patient who had been treated with ketoconazole for pulmonary *blastomycosis* 4 years earlier (Dr. E.G. Chadwick, Chicago, personal communication). The patient had been free of apparent disease but was initially infertile. A healthy term infant was eventually delivered. The placenta then appeared grossly peculiar. It had a nodular consistency, numerous granulomas, and chronic villitis at the maternal floor. Organisms were not identified. It remains unknown whether the lesions were due to endometrial blastomycosis or if this is a case of villitis of unknown etiology.

Virus Infections and Villitides

Cytomegalovirus Infection

Congenital cytomegalovirus (CMV) infection is a common disease. Yow (1989) stated that 3,000 to 4,000 infants are born in the United States with symptomatic disease, and a large number of children suffer late-onset manifestations of the infection, including hearing loss, blindness, and retardation. Stagno et al. (1986) found that 1.6% of seronegative women of high-income groups converted CMV titers during pregnancy, whereas 3.7% of low-income group women did so. An editorial (Anonymous, 1989c) has found that the rate of transmission to the fetus after recent maternal infection is between 20% and 50%. Moreover, infection during the first half of pregnancy is more destructive to the fetus.

It is now recognized that the virus is often acquired by sexual contact (Chretien et al., 1977). The widespread nature of this infection was first appreciated by Weller (1971), who had emphasized its protean clinical manifestations. Many virus infections are accompanied by severe inflammation of the placental villi (villitis). An excellent review of these lesions is found in the contribution by Altshuler and Russell (1975). Schwartz and his colleagues (1992) have characterized the inflammatory response in this villous infection. They found marked "hyperplasia of fetal-derived placental macrophages . . . lymphocytic villitis . . . characterized by positive staining with T-cell antibodies." Plasma cells staining for IgG and IgM secretion were present during the second trimester, but no IgA positivity was found.

Infection with CMV is a major cause of chronic villitis. The fetal and neonatal disease has many manifestations, ranging from hydrops fetalis (Quagliarello et al., 1978; Fadel & Riedrich, 1988), obstructive uropathy (Symonds & Driscoll, 1974), meconium peritonitis (Pletcher et al., 1991), macerated stillbirth, cerebral palsy, to minimal hearing loss (Saigal et al., 1982b). Moreover, some of these manifestations may be ascertained only years later (Pass et al., 1980b; Williamson et al., 1982, 1990). Details of congenital CMV infection have been reported on many occasions (Embil et al., 1970; Krech et al., 1971).

Ahlfors and colleagues (1988) reviewed the literature of the infection in twins and reported two of their own cases that were discordant for manifestations of CMV infection. They postulated that monochorionic (MZ) twins were more likely to be concordant for CMV infection but lamented that the information on placental and genetic status is too often missing from case reports to draw definitive conclusions. It was their suggestion that the fetal (as well as the maternal) immunological response may be of importance in the expression of the prenatally acquired infection. They ruled out that a CMV endocervicitis caused ascending fetal infection from knowing the location of the twin placentas.

Congenital infection is perhaps also occasionally acquired from infected endometrium. The presence of CMV in endometrial glands was demonstrated in 5 of 59 spontaneous abortions by Dehner and Askin (1975).

CMV inclusions have also been found in the endocervix (Wenckebach & Curry, 1976). The virus has often been cultured from seminal fluid (Lang & Kummer, 1972) and amnionic fluid (Weiner & Grose, 1990). Stagno et al. (1982) showed that fetal infection is more serious when it occurs during a primary maternal infection than when it follows recurrent maternal disease. These cases are reasons to consider the benefit of a vaccine (Medearis, 1982). Neonates with this infection may excrete virus for years and thus become a major source for infection of pregnant mothers and toddlers in day-care centers (Pass et al., 1987). In twin pregnancies, CMV infections have been seen in both twins (Saigal et al., 1982a) or in only one (Eachempati & Woods, 1976; Stagno et al., 1982).

Fetal intracranial calcifications have been seen sonographically (Ghidini et al., 1989), and neonatal perivascular echogenic signals were demonstrated in their basal ganglia (Teele et al., 1988); the involvement of vessels is a hallmark of this infection. It has been suggested that it may be the cause of cerebral microgyria and other lesions (Dias et al., 1984).

Fetal infection is undoubtedly most often acquired during primary maternal infection from maternal viremia and by the passage of virions through the destroyed trophoblast. This ability of CMV to infect and destroy the trophoblast has been shown in placental explants by Amirhessami-Aghili et al. (1987). Despite this placental infection, no uniform macroscopic findings can identify CMV infection of the placenta, so the selection of histological material is difficult. Small placentas with growth-retarded fetuses are common, and thromboses may exist. A significant problem in understanding this infection is that some known prenatal infections (positive culture from amnionic fluid) may be followed by normal outcome (Weiner & Grose, 1990). We have also seen many cases of unsuspected CMV infection histologically when the placenta was sectioned for other reasons. For instance, in one case of "maternal porphyria," typical CMV inclusions were found in the placenta, and the neonate had "hepatitis." The maternal disease was a manifestation of a primary infection with this virus and was misinterpreted as porphyria. In another case of a spontaneous abortus at 15 weeks' gestation with an unremarkable macerated fetus, there were widespread cytomegalic cells in the lung, spleen, skeletal muscle, and placenta. The mother had had only a minor sore throat 1 week prior. Remarkably, the placenta had extensive destructive villitis. Ultimately, either the virus must be cultured, or inclusion body cells must be identified. Although the classical histological features are not mistakable, they are often so widely scattered through the villous tissue that only extreme scrutiny of many sections allows the diagnosis from placental sections.

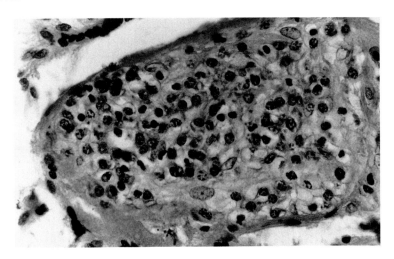

FIGURE 416. Congenital CMV infection. Marked chronic villitis, composed almost entirely of plasma cells, is evident, as is focal necrosis of the trophoblast and capillary walls. The specimen is from a term gestation, and the mother reportedly had porphyria. H&E. ×650.

The histological hallmark of CMV infection in the placenta are chronic lymphoplasmacytic villitis (Figure 416), thrombosis of villous capillaries often with adjacent hemosiderin deposits, necrosis of villous tissue and trophoblast (Figure 417), fibrosis of villous stroma (Figure 418), and inclusion-bearing cytomegalic cells (Figure 419). The inclusion bodies may be characteristic nuclear owl-eye cells but are often also of cytoplasmic nature. They are commonly seen in villous capillary endothelium but are also found in the stromal cells of villi. Garcia et al. (1989), who provided an excellent study of placental changes in CMV infection, found owl-eye cells in decidua and amnion as well. They employed the fluorescent antibody technique for diagnosis (see also McCaffree & Altshuler, 1979) and suggested that some types of gross morphological abnormalities are frequent. Mostoufi-Zadeh et al. (1984) depicted owl-eye cells in the epithelium of the umbilical cord. Saito et al. (1977) described an abortion with a large number of villous inclusion bodies typical of CMV infection. They diagnosed it as herpes simplex infection, however. We believe they made an incorrect diagnosis caused by error in the interpretation of the serological results. The CMV titers were also rising. Their analysis included an excellent electron microscopic demonstration of the virus packets, typical of a herpes-type virus (see also Donnellan et al., 1966, for electron microscopy). Vasculitis of chorionic vessels (Figure 420) may lead to thrombosis and calcification. Huikeshoven et al. (1982) and Grose and Weiner (1990) made the diagnosis of CMV infection by recovering the virus from amnionic fluid at amniocentesis, undoubtedly because of fetal renal involvement. The placental and neonatal features in the former study were typical of CMV infection. The virus can now be detected in histological sections by in situ hybridization (Wolber & Lloyd, 1989). Sachdev et al. (1990) have used the hybridization technique to identify CMV infection in cases of chronic villitis. They

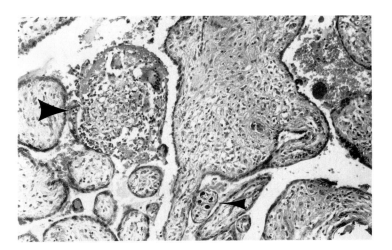

FIGURE 417. Destructive villitis (large arrowhead) in congenital CMV infection. Inclusion bodies, or owl-eye cells (small arrowhead), are also present in this 14 weeks' gestation. H&E. ×150.

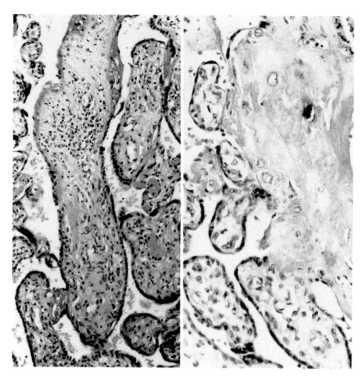

FIGURE 418. Evolution of fibrosis of the villi with a CMV infection. (Left) A villus has plasma cell infiltration, trophoblast necrosis, vascular obliteration, and early fibrosis. (Right) A completely hyalinized villus contains a focus of calcification and hemosiderin but no trace of CMV infection. H&E. Left ×160; right ×260.

found typical inclusions in three of eight cases of villitis and were able to diagnose three additional cases of CMV infection using this technique. Mühlemann and her colleagues (1992) have provided an excellent immunocytochemical study of six CMV-infected placentas. They suggested that histological features are often inconclusive in this congenital infection and found inclusion bodies in only one of six cases. Immunocytochemistry, on the other hand, revealed viral antigen in five of the six placentas. The antigen was found to be mostly in the villous stroma, once in the syncytiotrophoblast, and sometimes in endothelial cells as demonstrated by double-staining these cells.

The cellular response to this infection is characteristic. It is mononuclear; during the second half of gestation, it is typically accompanied by fetal plasma cells, but we have seen it as early as at 15 weeks' gestation in the placental villi. Here it is then a question of whether the plasma cells are of fetal or maternal origin. This question has not yet been satisfactorily answered. Plasma

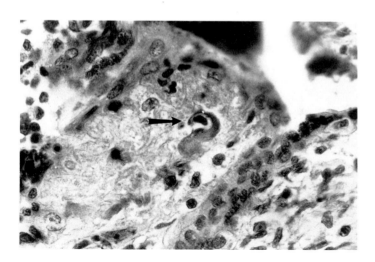

FIGURE 419. Owl-eye nucleus (arrow) of a cytomegalic cell in the villus of a patient with CMV-induced placentitis. This cell also contains many cytoplasmic virus particles. H&E. ×650.

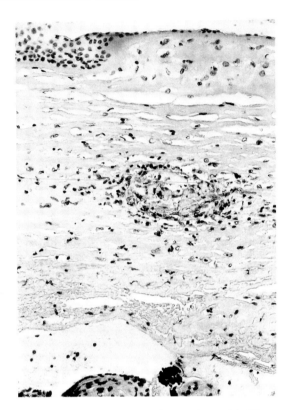

FIGURE 420. Chorionic vasculitis in a patient with CMV infection at term. There is more necrosis than inflammation. The placenta had marked chronic villitis. The fetus was stillborn. H&E. ×160.

macroscopic lesions were seen at dissection, but viral inclusions were found in many organs histologically (Figure 421). There was only a sparse inflammatory response. The villous infection and focal thrombosis in pulmonary vessels were particularly striking. A case of presumed double infection was described by De Zegher et al. (1988), in which *Toxoplasma* was definitely identified, and saliva and urine cultures yielded CMV. The alleged double infection illustrated by Demian et al. (1973), however, was not correctly identified. Only CMV was shown, the cytoplasmic granules representing virus—not *Toxoplasma* as had been presumed.

It has often been asked just when the first fetal plasma cell response to CMV can be seen. This question is not yet resolved. Altshuler and McAdams (1971) clearly identified plasma cell villitis at 19 weeks' gestation, but it *may* commence as early as at 10 weeks, judging from Altshuler's second case, seen at 13 weeks' gestation (Altshuler, 1973a) (Figure 422). The owl-eye inclusions are characteristic of CMV infection, and the diagnosis can be made confidently on that basis alone. When only enlarged cells with cytoplasmic inclusions are present, however, the diagnosis of CMV infection is less secure. Serological studies, virus isolation, and

cells are not expected to be produced by fetuses at 13 weeks' gestation. Hybridization studies with Y probes in appropriate cases are indicated to rule out maternal B cell immigration. Mostoufi-Zadeh et al. (1984) opined that the fetal infection is more severe when a plasmacellular, rather than a lymphocytic, response is found in the villi. The plasma cell infiltration and the cytomegalic cells in the placenta were first described by LePage and Schramm (1958) and subsequently by LeLong et al. (1960). Since then there have been numerous observations substantiating and expanding on these findings (e.g., Rosenstein & Navarrete-Reyna, 1964; Monif & Dische, 1972). Blanc (1961b), in a thorough review of the placenta of prenatal infections, described the villous necrosis; Quan and Strauss (1962) discussed the differential diagnosis of CMV infection from erythroblastosis.

The findings of many other authors are summarized in our previous review (Benirschke et al., 1974). In that paper we described five cases, one of which is of particular interest. It was a therapeutic abortion at approximately 15 weeks' gestation. The patient had fever of unknown origin and antibody titers to CMV and *Toxoplasma*. A double infection was suspected, but no toxoplasmosis was found in the abortus. No

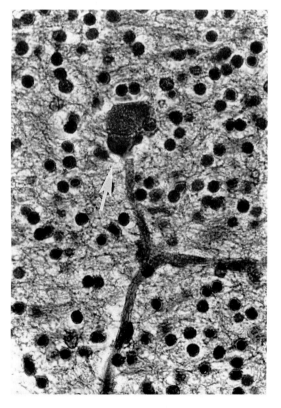

FIGURE 421. Fetal brain at 15 weeks' gestation with a CMV cell at the terminus of the capillary. There is no inflammation or destruction. The placenta had numerous CMV cells. H&E. ×150. (From Benirschke et al., 1974, with permission.)

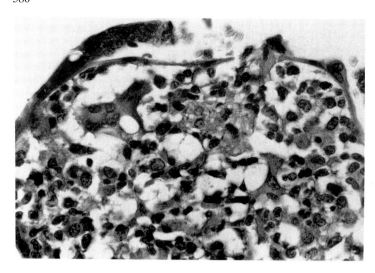

FIGURE 422. Cytomegalovirus infection of the placenta at 13 weeks' gestation, with plasma cell infiltration, edema, and trophoblast necrosis. H&E. ×520. (Courtesy Dr. G. Altshuler, Oklahoma City.)

modern techniques of demonstrating the viral genome by hybridization are then needed. When different strains of the virus were thus identified with endonuclease cleavage of viral DNA, "no common pattern could be associated with these eight strains (of congenitally acquired virus) in comparison with strains from postnatally infected children" (Grillner et al., 1987). Borisch et al. (1988) successfully identified the antigen in the nucleus and cytoplasm by in situ hybridization, and Chehab et al. (1989) were able to do so with the polymerase chain reaction from DNA obtained from paraffin-embedded tissues. One can only hope that in the future the nature of such placental lesions, as depicted in Figures 423 and 424, will be resolved by these methods.

Herpes Simplex Virus Infection

Transplacental infection with herpes simplex virus (HSV) does occasionally occur. It is more serious for the fetus when the primary (rather than recurrent) infection occurs during pregnancy (Brown et al., 1987). Transplacental infection is uncommon, presumably because of the protective nature of transplacentally acquired maternal antibodies; most women become immune to HSV before reaching child-bearing age (Nahmias et al., 1970). "The major problem in newborn infection then is one of natal transmission of HVH ('herpesvirus hominis') through recurrent type 2 infections of the maternal genital tract" (Alford et al., 1975). Why it is that fatal infections occur sometimes in utero and not at other times and what the reason is for recurrent and latent infections remain unresolved questions. Ideas about the latency of HSV were discussed in an editorial (Anonymous, 1989b), and a succinct review of the fetal infection with HSV has been provided by Baldwin and Whitley (1990). Johnson et al. (1989)

found in a survey of 4,201 serum samples that 16.4% of the U.S. population from 15 to 74 years of age was infected with HSV-2.

Herpes virus is "silently" shed by 2.3% of pregnant women (Wittek et al., 1984). Yen et al. (1965) succinctly described and depicted the cervical and vaginal lesions of herpes virus infection and presented three infants with symptomatic mothers. Two newborns had an

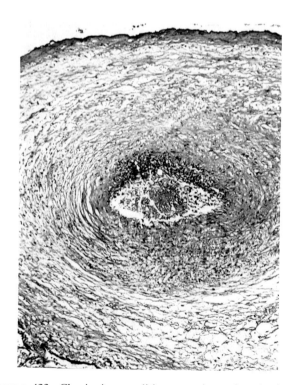

FIGURE 423. Chorionic vasculitis, necrosis, and early thrombosis with a congenital infection, presumably due to CMV, at 20 weeks' gestation. Outcome was a stillborn fetus. See Figure 424. H&E. ×100.

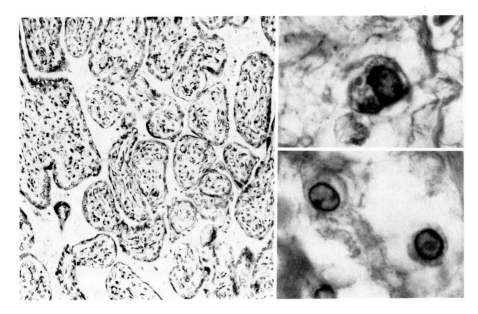

FIGURE 424. Same case as in Figure 423. Chronic villitis (left) is present, with enlarged cells that have some of the qualities of CMV cells. The inclusions are not typical, however. H&E. Left ×160; right ×1,600.

apparently congenital infection. Herpes virus has also been detected before delivery (of a healthy child) from aspirated amnionic fluid (Zervoudakis et al., 1980). Herpetic endometritis has been demonstrated with and without an IUD (Abraham, 1978; Schneider et al., 1982), and Altshuler (1974) presented evidence for prenatal infection with an involved placenta (see below). Another case of presumed ascending infection was presented by Hain et al. (1980). They described the premature birth of a 590-g infant with a rash; there was necrosis in various organs at autopsy. The placenta showed cloudy membranes due to "extensive necrosis of amnion without inflammation." Necrotic areas were also present in chorion, and a lymphoplasmacellular infiltration was evident, as in Altshuler's case. In their case, however, chorionic vessel thrombosis and many inclusion bodies as well as "ground-glass nuclei" were present. The mother had primary herpetic vulvitis 4 weeks before delivery. Hyde and Giacoia (1993) have described an important case of severe, destructive congenital HSV infection, with the infant delivered by cesarean section from a cervically infected patient. At those portions of the intact membranes that were closest to the cervix, they found immunologically HSV-positive cells in the subamnionic connective tissue, in addition to a mild chronic funisitis. This case strongly supports the idea of an ascending infection, occurring even with intact membranes.

The review of Baldwin and Whitley (1990) summarized 71 cases of presumed prenatal herpes virus infection. Many of these cases were not fully studied, and the placentas were examined in only a few. The

early reports of fetal infection by Mitchell and McCall (1963), Zavoral et al. (1970), Torphy et al. (1970), and Monif et al. (1985) had no placental studies. Witzleben and Driscoll (1965) were the first investigators to describe the placental changes in proved congenital HSV infection, and they reviewed other fatal cases of neonatal herpes infections. The mother in their case suffered a primary disseminated infection 1 month before delivery. The neonate remained well until day 6 and then died from generalized disease. The placenta was grossly unremarkable but had many areas of villous necrosis. It included trophoblast and stroma. An inflammatory reaction was absent, but inclusions were found in the placenta and fetus. Nakamura et al. (1985) demonstrated immunological staining and, by electron microcopy, typical herpes particles in stromal cells of villi in a presumably hematogenously transplacental infection.

Another excellent description of the placenta in herpetic infection came from Altshuler (1974, 1984), who summarized the earlier-mentioned case in the context of other placental inflammations. There were no complications in the term pregnancy he described, and no herpetic lesions had been known or noted. The infant developed blisters on day 4, with isolation of herpes virus hominis (HVH). He was treated and discharged but continued having skin lesions. The meconium-stained placenta had many areas of necrotizing deciduitis and amnionitis; chorionic vasculitis and funisitis were attended by superficial amnion necrosis. The exudate contained leukocytic and extensive plasmacellular infiltrates (Figure 425). The villous tissue was not altered, and inclusion bodies were absent, but the prenatal

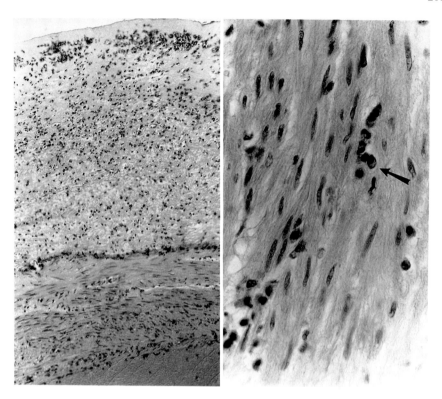

FIGURE 425. Congenital herpes virus infection of the placenta. Note the necrosis of the amnion, thickening of membranes, and intense plasma cell (arrow) infiltration. H&E. Left ×160; right ×640. (Courtesy Dr. G. Altshuler, Oklahoma City.)

acquisition of the infection is evident from the unusual plasmacellular funisitis, not known in banal infections.

The role of molecular pathology in the diagnosis of transplacental herpes infection was described by Schwartz and Caldwell (1991). They reported the delivery of a neonate who remained well from a patient with suspicious genital lesions. Previously, HSV had been confirmed by culture. Microscopic sections of the placenta were grossly and microscopically normal. In situ "hybridization" with a biotinylated DNA probe was undertaken for HSV and counterstained. Subchorionic ("maternal-derived tissue of the decidua capsularis") tissue stained positively for the antigen. It is our opinion that these findings are not specific for herpes antigen but that they reflect the biotin content that was so well later defined in endometrium by Yokoyama et al. (1993). These investigators were conscious of the similarity of apparent inclusions in endometrium to those of herpes infection; they showed, however, that these vacuoles contained biotin. Thus extreme care should be exercised in the interpretation of such immunological localizations employing biotinylated probes in the immunological reaction.

Bendon et al. (1987) emphasized deciduitis associated with their two cases of intrauterine HVH infection. One was a stillborn 300-g abortus with macular skin lesions and the other a 3,200-g neonate with blisters who was

treated and survived. The authors were unable to detect antigen in cord or amnionic sac by immunohistochemical reaction but found it at the decidual base of the placentas. For this reason, they suggested that infection may have been disseminated via neural fibers or through endometrial channels, rather than in an ascending manner. Berger et al. (1986) described a mother with herpetic encephalitis during pregnancy; a meconium-stained placenta and fetal infection occurred, despite acyclovir therapy. Gagnon (1968) recovered virus from the placenta but did not describe the organ. Dublin and Merten (1977) showed the severe cerebral necroses that occurred in discordantly affected DiMo twins at 29 weeks' gestation. They stated that the placenta was affected with hemorrhagic and fibrotic changes.

The differences in severity and types of placental and fetal reactions in prenatal herpes infection suggest that transplacental and ascending infection may both occur. Boué and Loffredo (1970) isolated HSV-2 from abortion material and suggested that this infection may play a causal role in abortion. Naib et al. (1970) studied the outcome of pregnancy in women with herpes infection. When infection occurred during the first 4 months of pregnancy, abortions occurred significantly more frequently, suggesting a causal relation.

Two cases with undisputed congenital herpes infection have been seen by us. One was a stillborn without

FIGURE 426. Congenital HSV-2 infection with still-birth outcome. Note the subamnionic blister filled with plasma cells. Also present are chorionitis and amnion necrosis. H&E. ×64.

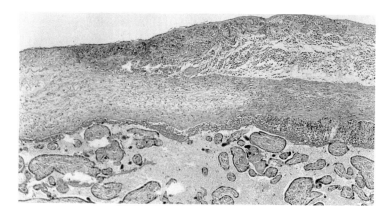

maternal illness or herpetic lesions. The placenta had necrotizing chorioamnionitis with true blisters (Figures 426, 427). Plasma cells were the most abundant cell type in the exudate. The unusual occurrence of plasma cells at this site cannot be overemphasized. The other case was reported by Herzen and Benirschke (1977). A cesarean section had been done for breech presentation;

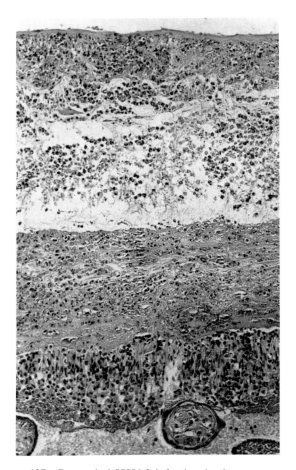

FIGURE 427. Congenital HSV-2 infection in the same case as in Figure 426. The large collection of subamnionic plasma cells is unusual. H&E. ×160.

the membranes were intact. There was no maternal history of herpetic lesions, nor was the virus cultured from the mother. She had a titer of 1:32 that rose to 1:64 after birth, perhaps an insufficient criterion. The infant had severe disease and died. The placenta was circumvallate and had an unusually adherent amnion, and there were infarcts but no villitis. Inclusion bodies were found in the chorion. Severe plasma cell infiltration was present in the decidua; HSV-2 was isolated from fetal skin vesicles and the placental surface. Because of the absent villitis and the presence of chorioamnionitis, we speculated that it was an ascending infection. That opinion is supported by the absence of genital lesions in a large number of mothers with infected offspring.

This case raised further questions. In addition to the characteristic necrotic lesions found in neonatal herpes deaths (Hass, 1935), the autopsy findings included ocular, renal, and cerebral anomalies. The occasional association of congenital anomalies with HSV infection was discussed by Baldwin and Whitley (1989); some of these anomalies surely are the result of the virus infection. When this infant died at 21 days of age, he had massive destructive disease of the brain, resembling hydranencephaly. Virus recovery was attempted by culture and electron microscopy. Because of this failure and the proved HSV-2 disease, we searched for antigen by immunohistological procedures (Robb et al., 1986a). Characteristic staining was found with this technique in a variety of tissues from this infant. We then studied abortion specimens and other conditions with unresolved etiology for the presence of herpes antigens. In some of these cases, herpes viral DNA could be detected by hybridization study. The brain and placenta of the neonatal death just discussed also had a strong staining reaction (Robb et al., 1986b). Although we are aware that this method cannot *prove* the existence of local residual HSV antigen, it is presumptive evidence for this correlation. In the placenta the antigen was prominently found in a subamnionic location, as were the herpetic lesions. Strong antigen reactivity was seen in other cases as well, such as in necrotizing funisitis and many cases of maternal floor infarction. Future studies must to be undertaken to interpret these findings. Finally, Altshuler (personal communication, 1992) has sent us the placenta of a child with congenital herpes infection whose umbilical cord surface showed only extensive acellular necrosis, without any attending inflammatory response. Herman and Siegel (1994), who described another case of congenital HSV-2 infection, emphasized the many calcifications in the newborn's organs but did not discuss the placenta.

Varicella (Chickenpox)

Pregnancy complicated by chickenpox is fairly uncommon. Despite the fact that most cases of adult chickenpox occur beyond the reproductive period (Stagno & Whitley, 1985), presumptive transplacental infection has been described several times. In a review of 18 maternal varicella pneumonias, Pickard (1968) noted that only three infants were without the disease; 38 neonatal cases of chickenpox had been described by then, with a 21% mortality. Purtilo et al. (1977) described numerous placental infarcts, without viral inclusions, in their report of a case of fatal varicella in a pregnant woman and newborn. Balducci and his colleagues (1992) identified in a prospective study 40 patients with first trimester varicella. Three aborted, one was terminated, the other 36 went to term. One had an omphalocele, the others were normal. From this information the authors concluded that the risk of the congenital varicella syndrome is small.

The congenital varicella syndrome of cutaneous scars, limb hypoplasia, chorioretinitis, and cataracts (see Williamson, 1975; Alkalay et al., 1987) was found in only 1 of 11 infants of women with first trimester varicella infection (Paryani & Arvin, 1986). According to these authors, who comprehensively reviewed the topic, infection later in gestation rarely has these fetal sequelae. Magliocco et al. (1992) reported a severely malformed child with numerous destructive lesions that are superbly illustrated. The fetal infection dated from the 12th week of gestation. The placenta showed only old infarcts and calcification. Jones and his colleagues (1994) also found only a small risk to the fetus from first trimester varicella infection in their prospective study. Paryani and Arvin (1986) and Brazin et al. (1979) reported that herpes zoster complicating pregnancy usually has a benign prognosis. The fetus and placenta are typically not affected, although some cases of fetal growth retardation and blindness have occurred. A comprehensive review of varicella infection during pregnancy and the resulting fetal pathology, especially of the nervous system, has been provided by Grose and Itani (1989). Regrettably, they did not address possible placental pathology of this infection. In fact, the placenta of varicella infection during pregnancy has rarely been described. Garcia (1963), who reported two congenital cases, found scattered "firm areas, rice seed-like." He depicted focal necroses. Garcia likened these lesions to granulomas, with epithelioid cells and a giant cell component. Decidual cells contained inclusion bodies.

No specific changes were encountered by Saito et al. (1989). They described giant cell pneumonia in a small, prematurely delivered fetus who probably had varicella infection. Immunohistochemical staining of varicella antigens was present on the giant cells in the neonatal lung, but no such antigen was detected in the placenta. It showed merely mild chorioamnionitis.

Epstein-Barr Virus

Infection with the Epstein-Barr virus is uncommon during pregnancy. In a few instances, however, congenital infection is believed to have produced congenital anomalies in fetuses. The topic has been reviewed by Ornoy et al. (1982), who studied the induced abortuses of five such pregnancies. They found lesions in all, consisting of deciduitis, villitis with lymphoplasmacellular infiltration, trophoblastic necrosis, and endothelial damage to capillaries. Myocarditis was seen in two fetuses. The cases are circumstantial in that the virus was not shown to be present, but lesions as described are otherwise uncommon at that gestational age. Thus at present one must assume that the virus can affect placenta and fetus.

Transplacental transfer of the Epstein-Barr virus to the fetus has rarely been proved. In the few cases where it was shown (Joncas et al., 1981), the placenta was not described. The child described by these authors died from apparently simultaneous CMV infection.

Smallpox, Vaccinia, Alastrim, Parvovirus B19

Fetal infection with smallpox virus has often been depicted in early obstetrics texts. This virus can readily pass the placenta and cause fetal death and abortion. Prior to the eradication of smallpox, fetal and placental vaccinia occurred occasionally, primarily with primary vaccinations. Wentworth (1966) examined 65 placentas of women who were vaccinated during pregnancy; those mothers did not have an increased abortion rate. Histological examination and search for virus inclusions were negative.

Intrauterine infection was well described by Wielenga et al. (1961). The neonate died within a short time and had extensive skin lesions. There were numerous areas of villous and membrane necrosis, and a leukocytic response was present. The lesions were similar to a case we have seen (Figure 428) in which extensive necrosis of trophoblast, intervillous fibrin deposits, and focal calcification, but no plasma cells, were found. Killpack (1963) also found necrotic foci "resembling miliary tubercles" and scanty eosinophilic inclusions. Other descriptions came from Hood and McKinnon (1963)

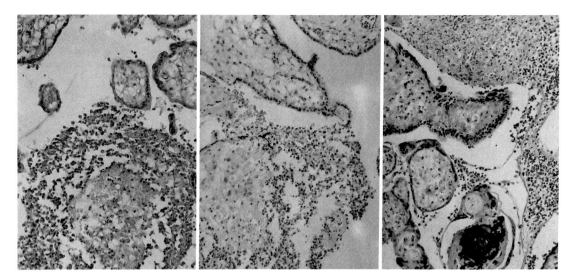

FIGURE 428. Vaccinia during pregnancy. Many villi are necrotic, and an intense inflammatory reaction is seen around their remnants. Note the focal calcification of the necrotic area at bottom right. H&E. ×160. (Courtesy Dr. B. Ivemark, Stockholm.)

and Naidoo and Hirsch (1963). Garcia (1963) reported macerated stillborns affected with cutaneous alastrim (variola minor). Similar "granulomatous" areas of necrosis were depicted in the placentas accompanying these two fetuses. Guarnieri bodies were present in the decidua.

Infection with parvovirus B19 is covered in Chapter 16. It is an apparently frequent cause of fetal anemia because of the preferential infection of erythrocyte precursors by this virus. Hartwick et al. (1989) demonstrated parvovirus B19 in a dot-blot hybridization study of a 9 weeks' gestation fetus. Considerable vascular endothelial damage was present in the embryo and placenta. In a portion of one umbilical artery the endothelium and muscle were partially destroyed, and in main stem vessels perivascular lymphocytic infiltration was seen. The lymphocytic infiltration was composed of cells belonging to the cytotoxic or suppressor T cell variety. There is a provocative discussion of the origin of these inflammatory cells that bears relevance to the topic of villitis of unknown origin (see below). Despite the fact that heretofore the embryo was not believed to be capable of mounting an immunological response at this stage of development, the authors gave cogent reasons for assuming that the T cells they identified were not of maternal origin. Interestingly, inclusions were absent in the red blood cell precursors of this embryo but were found in skeletal muscle cells.

Samra et al. (1989) reviewed all reports on parvovirus infection of the fetus and concluded that the virus passes the placenta readily. They described a stillborn, hydropic fetus in whose placenta were villous necrosis and calcifications. Infection with different species of parvoviruses

has been shown to cause a wide spectrum of diseases in various animals, including congenital anomalies. The subject has been reviewed in detail by Margolis and Kilham (1975), who make reference to human conditions.

Enteroviruses

Transplacental poliomyelitis infection has been described, and the virus was isolated from the placenta in some of these cases (Barsky & Beale, 1957). No pathological lesions of the placenta are known.

Infection with ECHO and Coxsackie viruses occurs commonly during the neonatal period and may have serious consequences in neonates. When infection occurs during pregnancy, the fetus is usually spared, perhaps protected by maternal antibody transfer (Amstey et al., 1988). Amstey et al. also perfused two placentas with a mixture of viruses and found them not to transfer. Nevertheless, transplacental passage and fetal infection have occasionally been shown for ECHO viruses (Hughes et al., 1972; Modlin, 1986; C. Davis, personal communication, 1985) and Coxsackie B virus (Kibrick & Benirschke, 1958). There is also speculation that such prenatal infection may be a cause of juvenile diabetes. The placentas of the few cases proved to have caused prenatal Coxsackie virus infection have shown occasional meconium staining, but other meaningful changes were usually absent. Fetal hydrops secondary to myocarditis has occurred with Coxsackie virus infection; placental lesions were not apparent in that abortus (Benirschke et al., 1986). Garcia et al. (1990) described three perinatal deaths from ECHO 33 and ECHO 27 infections, with isolation of virus from placentas and fetal tissues. They described villitis and intervillositis in the placentas.

Batcup et al. (1985) reported villous necrosis and severe intervillositis in the placenta of a patient who had Coxsackie virus A9 meningitis at 33 weeks' gestation. A stillborn, macerated fetus was delivered 5 days later, and the virus was recovered from the placenta. Moreover, mild myocarditis and early meningitis were seen in the fetus. Remarkably, the placenta had massive intervillous fibrin deposits, much as one sees in the *gitterinfarcts* discussed in Chapter 11. Villous stem vessels had mural thrombi, and many aspects of the placenta showed features that are usually designated villitis of unknown etiology (see below). It is difficult to believe that the extensive placental alterations depicted in their report could have arisen within this short time span, but further observations to investigate this possibility are clearly mandated.

Ogilvie and Tearne (1980) described three abortions during episodes of infection with Coxsackie virus A16 virus (hand, foot, and mouth disease) and recovered the virus from one placenta. The pathological features of the placenta, however, were not discussed.

Influenza, Mumps, Rabies

Transplacental influenza A2 (Hong Kong) infection was reported by Yawn et al. (1971). The virus was recovered from the fetus and amnionic fluid in the fatally ill gravida. Fetal tissues and placenta were found to be structurally normal. In an abortus delivered during the febrile period of parainfluenza 1 virus infection, Lavergne et al. (1969) observed a normal placenta. McGregor et al. (1984) recovered influenza A/Bangkok virus from maternal secretions and the amnionic fluid of an acutely ill patient who appeared to have amnionic fluid infection syndrome. The pregnancy continued, and a normal birth ensued. The placenta was not described, but transplacental infection was inferred. Conover and Roesmann (1990) reported the autopsy findings of a malformed infant in whose brain influenza virus was identified immunohistochemically. The placenta was not described.

Fetal mumps virus infection may occur, and it has been suggested that some congenital anomalies are due to this agent. Virus has been recovered from the placenta, but no histopathological change has been described (Yamauchi et al., 1974). Herbst et al. (1970) found only ultrastructural changes in the placenta of a patient with mumps. Severe villous necrosis, simulating that of herpes simplex virus, was found in three cases of intrauterine mumps infection described by Garcia et al. (1980). They also reviewed the sparse and contradictory literature. Small cytoplasmic inclusion bodies were depicted in the decidua.

Transplacental rabies infection is not known to occur in women. Spence et al. (1975) observed two normal fetuses after maternal rabies complicated pregnancy. The placenta was not described.

Hepatitis

Transplacental infection with hepatitis viruses has been reported; the topic was reviewed by Altshuler and Russell (1975) and Snydman (1985). Because hepatitis A viremia is short and a carrier state does not occur, fetal infection with this virus is rare. Asymptomatic hepatitis B infection, however, was found to occur in 0.66% of a low-risk population (Christian & Duff, 1989). Transmission of hepatitis C virus from chronically infected mothers to fetuses occurs but appears to be uncommon (Thaler et al., 1991; Wejstal et al., 1992; Silverman et al., 1993). Placentas have not been described.

In contrast to hepatitis A, the high carrier state of hepatitis B virus in adults is a potential hazard to many fetuses. It is generally agreed, however, that this virus is usually acquired enterically during birth or thereafter; nevertheless, the transplacental acquisition of hepatitis B virus has occasionally been verified (Fawaz et al., 1975; Mulligan & Stiehm, 1994). Mitsuda et al. (1989) found positive cord blood once in 10 patients but showed that the antigen was present in colostrum of eight patients using the sensitive polymerase chain reaction method. Prospective studies of aborted fetuses from virus-carrying mothers showed that 4 of 48 fetuses (8%) were thus infected (Li et al., 1986).

The placenta has rarely been examined by pathologists. Altshuler and Russell (1975) stated that the placenta shows "relative immaturity." Buchholz et al. (1974) described the placenta of an infected infant delivered by cesarean section as showing "placental insufficiency." Studies with direct and indirect immunofluorescence indicated the presence of antigen, confined to "the basement membranes of the (infantile part) of cells." The authors were uncertain that the placental insufficiency was caused by the infection.

Lucifora et al. (1988) studied the placentas of three asymptomatic hepatitis B surface antigen (HBsAg) carriers with immunohistochemistry. All showed strong reactivity of the Hofbauer cells and villous endothelium, but no pathological changes were noted. More recently, Lucifora et al. (1990) have detected the antigen (HBcAg) histochemically in all placentas of symptom-free carriers. It was again primarily localized in trophoblast and Hofbauer cells but was also found in fetal endothelium and fibroblasts. They suggested minor pathological changes (edema, congestion) but were not convincing. We described the placentas of two patients with active hepatitis (Khudr & Benirschke, 1972). The only abnormal finding was the presence of large amounts of bilirubin in Hofbauer cells and chorionic membrane macrophages. There was neither degeneration nor inflammation. The pigment bleached readily when slides were exposed to light. We have seen the placenta and fetus of a patient who had a therapeutic abortion for hepatitis B. The patient was still icteric when the procedure was done. The fetus, umbilical cord, and membranes were entirely unstained and normal; however, the villous tissue were the color of marmalade, a deep yellow-green. Histologically, numerous deeply bilirubin-stained macrophages were present as villous Hofbauer cells (Figure 429). Some syncytial trophoblastic cells and the membranes had relatively few stained cells. Focal syncytial cell necrosis was present, but there was no inflammation or obvious villous necrosis. There was intense enteritis of the fetus, with meconium deposits and eosinophilic leukocyte infiltration in the submucosa. Several intestinal ulcers were present, and in some areas the bowel was nearly perforated. We assumed that the fetus may have become infected by swallowing amnionic fluid. The case further indicates that bilirubin

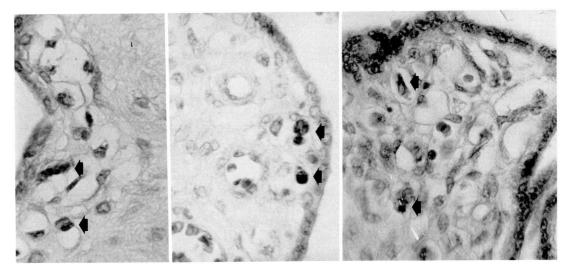

Figure 429. Placenta with hepatitis B. Pregnancy was interrupted at 20 weeks' gestation. Hofbauer cells are filled with bilirubin (arrows), but there was no inflammation. H&E. Left & center ×240; right ×640. Red filter.

may traverse the placental "barrier" but that it then becomes trapped by villous Hofbauer cells.

Rubella (German Measles)

The fetal rubella syndrome exemplifies transplacental fetal virus infection; but because of vaccination rubella is now uncommon. A variety of characteristic anomalies are produced in the fetus when infection occurs early, and the precise mechanism by which the degenerative changes responsible for the fetal rubella syndrome (e.g., cataracts) are generated has been a matter of intense investigation in the past. Many investigators have detected the virus in the placenta, amnionic fluid, and abortus by virological means (Alford et al., 1964; Thompson & Tobin, 1970; Catalano et al., 1971). When they isolated the virus from products of conception, Monif et al. (1965) suggested that many macerated fetuses died from placental, rather than fetal, infection. Töndury, in numerous contributions (1951, 1952a,b, 1964), has championed the idea that the fetal damage resulted from embolism of virus-damaged fetal (placental) endothelial cells. Others have suggested that the damage is due to chromosomal breakage.

Endothelial damage in villi of infected products of conception was confirmed in the large study conducted by Driscoll (1969) and more recently by the finding of "endangitis obliterans" in about 40% of the stem villous vessels of infected cases by Horn et al. (1992b, 1993). Driscoll further described sclerosing villous inflammation, which she interpreted as possibly responsible for the growth retardation. Töndury and Smith (1966) observed focal trophoblastic necrosis and elaborated on their idea of extensive damage to the villous capillary endothelium in early embryos with rubella infection. Selzer (1963, 1964) described basophilic inclusion bodies, but these structures have not been reported in other descriptions of placental lesions. Similar lesions have been described in a report of 45 cases interrupted because of gestational rubella infection (Ornoy et al., 1973). Ornoy et al. discovered some placental lesions in all cases that resulted in malformed fetuses. Decidual perivascular round cell infiltration was prominent; necrosis and fibrosis were found, and swollen Hofbauer cells were prominent, in villi of early gestations. Vascular inflammation was also a prominent finding, similar to that reported earlier. These authors described inclusions in trophoblast and villous stroma but did not depict them; and other authors (Horn et al., 1992b, 1993) were unable to identify inclusion bodies. It must be pointed out also that the endothelial abnormalities described are neither diagnostic nor present in all cases of virologically confirmed cases of rubella. Moreover, some of these changes are also observed in stillbirths unrelated to virus infections; thus a degree of skepticism is needed in their interpretation.

The attenuated strain of rubella vaccine virus has been isolated from placentas and fetuses, but villous lesions have not been observed (Phillips et al., 1970; Vaheri et al., 1972). Only Larson et al. (1971) described "histologic changes in placenta or decidua consistent with rubella infection." The fetuses were normal, and apparently only decidual changes were detected.

Rubeola (Measles)

Measles during pregnancy has been uncommon, and its consequences have been described only rarely. There is, however, an extensive database from the 1951 Greenland and the recent U.S. epidemics as to the effects of measles on pregnancy. The infection is apparently not teratogenic, and a significantly increased fetal mortality may relate primarily to fever. Access to this literature is readily provided by Stein and Greenspoon (1991). Placental disease has not been described, and congenital measles does not apparently exist (Eberhart-Phillips et al., 1993). The only report with identification of the antigen in the placenta is the case of Moroi et al. (1991). Their patient suffered fetal demise at 25 weeks after an acute infection, and the virus was detected in the decidua and syncytiotrophoblast by immunohistochemistry. It was not found in the fetus. The placenta was firm and infiltrated with an excessive amount of fibrin and mononuclear cells. Stein and Greenspoon (1991) described three cases; one had an unexplained intrauterine fetal demise (true knot of cord, 30% placental infarct), the other two did well. Placental lesions were not described, and fetal infection was not apparent.

Human Immunodeficiency Virus Infection

Infection of the fetus with the human immunodeficiency virus (HIV) has frequently been reported (Berrebi et al., 1987; European Collaborative Study, 1988; Sperling et al., 1989). The prevalence of HIV infection was studied in an obstetrical population by Barton et al. (1989). They found antibodies only in patients with risk factors (7.1%), whereas those without risk factors were negative. AIDS has occurred in some of the offspring, and the vertical transmission rate of HIV is estimated to be 24% (European Collaborative Study, 1988). Nevertheless, Katz and Wilfert (1989) were uncertain that the infection occurred transplacentally, rather than during delivery. Their editorial discussed at length the reports of neonatal AIDS presented in the same journal issue. On the other hand, the high titers of HIV DNA within 48 hours after birth suggests prenatal transmission (Brandt et al., 1994). Fetal deaths and prematurity have also been seen in women infected with HIV, but many of these patients had other problems that may have been responsible (Gloeb et al., 1988). Monozygotic twins discordant for HIV infection and with a single placenta were reported by Menez-Bautista et al. (1986). These twins had presumably been exposed to the agent only during fetal life. Alger et al. (1993) found no adverse effect on pregnancy performance in women who are infected with the HIV and showed that an HIV embryopathy does not exist.

The virus has been isolated from amnionic fluid (Mundy et al., 1987) and perhaps from the placenta (Hill et al., 1987). In the latter report, HIV was ob-

tained from placenta but not from lochia, the infant, or cord blood. The infant was well; an electron micrograph of an infected T cell accompanied the report, presumably infected with virus from this placenta's culture, but the authors suggested that the isolation may reflect maternal blood infection. The report was criticized by Peuchmaur et al. (1989) who, subsequent to this report, failed to isolate HIV from placental samples. Greenspoon and Settlage (1989) also believed that the virus of this placenta was more likely contained within the maternal blood of the placenta; the child, now age 3 years, has remained well.

Brady et al. (1989) used immunoperoxidase stains on placentas of HIV-infected patients. They found positive staining, particularly in Hofbauer cells, and suggested that this presence of viral protein in placental macrophages might present a reservoir for perinatal infection.

A morphological study of the placentas of 49 HIV-infected patients was undertaken by Jauniaux et al. (1988). The light microscopic findings were unremarkable. No significant alterations were seen, and the lesions were nonspecific. An ultrastructural study showed "retrovirus-like particles" in the syncytiotrophoblast of one induced abortus's placenta. Five other mature placentas showed isolated virus particles. They were similar to the C-type particles described formerly in many human placentas. More recently, Lewis et al. (1990) have demonstrated the presence of HIV by immunocytochemistry and in situ hybridization in maternal decidual leukocytes, trophoblast, Hofbauer cells, and embryonic blood cell precursors of aborted specimens (Figure 430). Although the specific CD4 receptors were not identified on the trophoblastic surface, the authors refer to experiments with trophoblast culture that have demonstrated CD4 presence. It is suggested that transmission (±30%) occurs directly, without transfer of maternal leukocytes being a prerequisite, as had been postulated. On the other hand, in a sizable prospective study of 44 patients with viremia, Ehrnst et al. (1991) found no transplacental HIV transmission to the 27 infants born. In only one of seven placentas was the virus identified. Andiman et al. (1990) similarly reported a low vertical transmission rate but also did not examine the placentas. That placental explants can support growth of HIV was shown by Amirhessami-Aghili and Spector (1991). They cultured first trimester villous tissue, infected it, and demonstrated the presence of the CD4 and HIV antigens; surprisingly, human chorionic gonadotropin (hCG) and progesterone production increased in infected cultures. We have not been able to detect histopathological placental changes in patients with the infection. It has also been pointed out that unusual tumors metastatic to the placenta may signal HIV infection. Pollack et al. (1993) described a patient

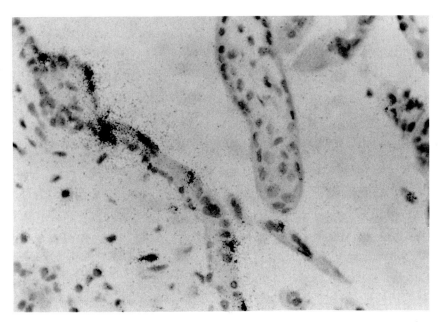

FIGURE 430. Villi at 8 weeks' gestation in an HIV-1-infected mother. Specimen was hybridized with a ^{35}S-labeled probe. Syncytium, Langhans cells, and Hofbauer cells are labeled. Hematoxylin. ×312. (Courtesy Dr. S.H. Lewis, New York.)

who had abdominal delivery for fetal distress. The grossly normal placenta (it had white granular areas on the maternal surface) had intervillous infiltrates by "sheets of small noncohesive, round tumor cells." It was diagnosed as non-Hodgkin lymphoma. The mother developed further signs of AIDS, but the infant remained normal.

Kalter et al. (1973) had found C-type particles in four of six normal human placentas at the junction of syncytiotrophoblast and basement membrane. Their "budding" was more common in premature placentas. Other investigators have shown cross-reactivity of these particles to certain retroviruses (Sawyer et al., 1978; Maeda et al., 1983), and similar organisms have been detected in many nonhuman primate placentas (Panem, 1979). C-type particles are ubiquitous RNA viruses, parasites, whose functions are presently unknown. Imamura et al. (1976) detected these RNA virus-like structures in the placenta of a patient with lupus but also in normal placentas, albeit in smaller numbers. They also described "tubuloreticular inclusions" in villous endothelium from patients with lupus erythematosus. Similar structures have been induced in Hofbauer cells by maternal interferon therapy in rhesus monkeys (Feldman et al., 1986).

The significance of all of these findings with respect to true viral infections remains uncertain, but congenital HIV infection occurs with certainty (see Goedert et al., 1989). Indeed, the neonatal mortality is significant, and most cases manifest during the first year of life (Scott et al., 1989).

Toxoplasmosis

Toxoplasmosis is caused by the coccidian *Toxoplasma gondii*, a panglobal parasite of cats and other felids. In cats a well-explored life cycle for *T. gondii* exists in the intestinal epithelium. Oocysts are shed in the stools of infected animals. Rodents and other animals ingest these oocysts and acquire the disease. Cats, preying on infected rodents, complete the cycle. The disease is also widespread in domestic animals.

There are several excellent reviews on congenital toxoplasmosis (Kirchhoff & Kräubig, 1966; Frenkel, 1973, 1974; Dubey, 1977; Dubey & Beattie, 1988; Sever et al., 1988). Frenkel (1971) presented a particularly good consideration of all aspects of this disease. The human infection is acquired in adults by two means: (1) contamination with oocysts from feces of infected cats; and (2) ingestion of cysts and tachyzoites in raw, infected meat, largely pork and mutton (Kean et al., 1969). Pregnant women should not eat undercooked or raw meat, and they should also avoid having contact with "wild" (hunting) cats. Heating to 150°F kills the organism. Cats raised solely on commercial diets are not infected; cats that hunt and are given raw meat may become infected. Emptying their litter box daily to prevent drying and dust-producing feces is recommended (Kimball et al., 1974). A thoughtful review of these aspects has been written by Swartzberg and Remington (1975). Of the Parisian human adult population, 84% have antibodies because of the frequency of raw meat consumption in France.

Transplacental toxoplasmosis is not uncommon. It has been well described to cause severe destructive disease in the offspring, who are infected during early gestation. Minor degrees of damage are incurred when infection develops later during pregnancy. Chorioretinitis, encephalitis, and other organ involvement may nevertheless cause crippling disease. Wilson and Remington (1980) estimated that the lifetime support for the 3,300 children born annually in the United States with toxoplasmosis is the staggering sum of more than $200 million.

It is generally assumed that almost all, if not all, congenital *Toxoplasma* infections occur when a woman has her primary infection during pregnancy. There are few reports that congenital toxoplasmosis occurs in successive pregnancies. It has also been assumed that the presence of maternal antibodies prevents fetal infection. That it is not so was shown by the important case detailed by Forther et al. (1991). They found a *Toxoplasma* cyst in an abortion specimen from an immune patient who had had contact with an infected cat that caused acute toxoplasmosis in her brother. Feldman (1963) has doubted that recurrent infection ever occurs. Desmonts and Couvreur (1974) have provided the most conclusive prospective study of toxoplasmosis during pregnancy. Almost 45% of Parisian women with primary infection during pregnancy had infants with congenital toxoplasmosis. The rate of infection increased with the gestational trimesters (17%, 25%, 65%, respectively). Fetal destruction was the most severe during early, rather than late, gestation. The authors were skeptical that toxoplasmosis causes abortion and denied the occurrence of repeated congenital toxoplasmosis. Others have found *Toxoplasma* organisms in the placenta and uterus of infected, macerated fetuses (Mellgren et al., 1952) or have isolated it from spontaneously aborted products of conception (Remington et al., 1964; Forther et al., 1991). Stray-Pedersen and Lorentzen-Styr (1977) studied endometrial biopsies of women with habitual abortion; 6 of 96 women had tachyzoites in endometrium and menstrual blood, demonstrated by fluorescent antibody studies, but none was isolated in mouse inoculations. Treatment of these women abolished the organisms.

The method by which the organism is identified in tissues appears to be of great importance. It is easiest to demonstrate *Toxoplasma* by placing ground tissue samples into the peritoneal cavity of young mice or into appropriate tissue culture cell lines (Kaufman & Maloney, 1962). Handling this organism, however, is often avoided because of the hazards of infection. Immunological means are generally preferred, although the results are often dubious. For positive identification in tissues, Dallenbach and Piekarski (1960) have advocated the fluorescence antibody technique. A similar methodology was used by Foulon et al. (1990a) to identify the antigen from tissue cultures infected with chorionic villous sampling (CVS) specimens. The electron microscopic appearance of *Toxoplasma* cysts (pseudocysts) is characteristic and has been well shown by Callaway et al. (1968). Detailed considerations of modern diagnostic tests for toxoplasmosis have been outlined in a review of all aspects of this disease by Koskiniemi et al. (1989). Savva and Holliman (1990) reviewed the polymerase chain reaction methodology that allows unequivocal detection of the toxoplasma DNA (see also Hohlfeld et al., 1994). The problems of prenatal diagnosis were considered by Foulon et al. (1990b) who had much success with amnionic fluid culture and funipuncture.

The organism has been isolated from amnionic fluid and placentas of infected pregnancies (Stray-Pedersen, 1980; Teutsch et al., 1980). More recently, the diagnosis of congenital infection has been made by fetal blood sampling, which has led to beneficial prenatal therapy in some cases (Desmonts et al., 1985; Daffos et al., 1988). Couvreur et al. (1976) described congenital toxoplasmosis in 14 twins. In two of these pairs, only one twin was affected. Although it is stated that these twins were dizygotic, one of the two had a DiMo placenta, and they must thus have been "identical" twins. The authors reviewed previous reports of discordant DZ twins, whereas all MZ twins had been similarly affected. Cox et al. (1987) also reported two discordant twins when they assayed fetal blood during pregnancy for antibodies.

Evidence of congenital disease is at times difficult. It may require a long follow-up. Thus the MZ twins reported by Glasser and Delta (1965) were judged to be normal at birth. Their placenta had many cysts in the membranes but no other pathological features. The children first became symptomatic at 7 months of age. Another set of twins, described by Miller et al. (1971), also had late onset, and toxoplasmosis was not suspected until hydrocephaly developed. The mother had eaten ground beef during the pregnancy, the presumed source of infection. Late onset of symptomatology was further explored by Koppe et al. (1986), who showed that in children with congenital toxoplasmosis "new lesions continue to appear well after the age of 5 years, and the impairment can be severe." In other cases of apparent fetal well-being despite maternal infection during pregnancy, the maternal therapy may have prevented fetal disease (e.g., Hammer & Wegmann, 1966).

Placental infection with *Toxoplasma* has been well documented. It is presumably always produced by organisms circulating in the maternal blood, although the isolation of cysts from endometrium in chronic aborters makes direct infection from the endometrium possible (Werner et al., 1963). Altshuler (1973c), who described a fatal case with placental study, bemoaned that the placenta is not studied more often in this disease and suggested rapid means for identification of the organism. The case he studied was typical. The infant had hydranencephaly, a frequent feature of this disease (Larsen, 1977), hepatosplenomegaly, and hydrops. (Hydrops in congenital toxoplasmosis has been described repeatedly.) Typical cysts were present in the subamnionic/chorionic tissues, and they were unaccompanied by inflammation. It is only when the cysts rupture that a local plasmacellular reaction and necrosis take place. Altshuler found a marked increase in villous Hofbauer cells, erythroblasts in the fetal circulation, and vascular proliferation in placental villi. He also depicted a lymphocytic-plasmacellular villitis (Figure 431).

Similar villitis, including necrosis and villous *Toxoplasma* cysts, were found by Elliott (1970) in the placenta of a 3-month macerated abortus. He described the placenta as being "shaggy." Becket and Flynn (1953) found the placenta in toxoplasmosis to be as pale as it is in cases of erythroblastosis. They depicted the cysts in villi in both of their cases. Driscoll noted that in most of her cases marked plasmacellular deciduitis was a pronounced feature (Benirschke & Driscoll, 1967). Excellent illustrations of cysts within villi, occurring apparently even within trophoblast, were provided by Werner et al. (1963). They considered it to be the result of transmission from infected endometrium. Popek

(1992) described granulomatous villitis in an 18-week stillbirth with intensive chronic villitis; she also reviewed the literature on placental *Toxoplasma* infection in this contribution. Popek found organisms in every section of her case and was able to stain them immunologically. Nevertheless, careful study identified the organisms without additional aid. There were no plasma cells in the villi.

Although the cysts depicted by these authors are classical, care must be taken with the interpretation of *Toxoplasma* cysts in other publications. In consultation, we have seen several cases where cysts had been suspected; they were, however, degenerating syncytium. The photographs shown by Sarto et al. (1982) of syncytial nuclei in "endomitosis" simulate *Toxoplasma* cysts. They must not be mistaken for the organism. Janssen et al. (1970) have discussed these difficulties and urged that these problems must be borne in mind when toxoplasmosis is diagnosed from slides. As difficult as cyst identification is the diagnosis of tachyzoites in histological sections. Without fluorescent antibody staining or smears of infected tissue, they usually cannot be recognized with certainty. Dr. Jean Hustin (Belgium) has made available to us a case of primary infection at 24 weeks' gestation that was treated with spiramycin. Despite this therapy, the fetus developed hydrocephaly and was aborted at 31 weeks. Numerous cysts were found in the chorion (Figure 432), and plasmacellular

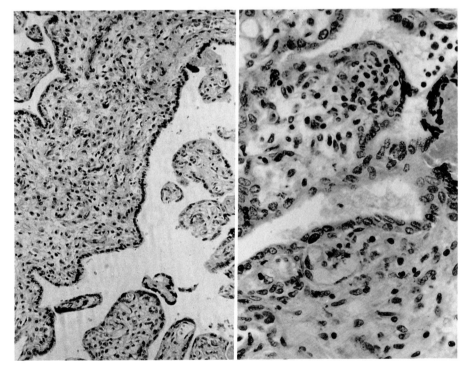

FIGURE 431. Villi in a patient with congenital toxoplasmosis. (Left) Same case as in Figure 433. (Right) Same case as in Figure 432. There is a diffuse lymphoplasmacytic infiltration, with sclerosis of the villi. H&E. Left ×125; right ×240. (Courtesy Dr. G. Khodr, San Antonio, and Dr. J. Hustin, Loverval, Belgium.)

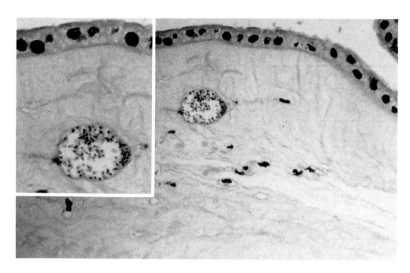

FIGURE 432. *Toxoplasma* cysts in the amnion/chorion of a child with congenital infection and hydrocephaly at 31 weeks' gestation. H&E. ×640. (Inset) Enlargement of a cyst. H&E. ×1,200. (Case courtesy of Dr. J. Hustin, Loverval, Belgium.)

infiltration, with necrosis and fibrosis, was found in villi. This maternal therapy is thus ineffective in combating the infection.

In toxoplasmosis, as in CMV infection, thrombosis of chorionic vessels occurs. The thrombi and vessel walls may be calcified, as is illustrated in the case of Figure 433; even vessels of the umbilical cord have been thus calcified (Khodr & Matossian, 1978). Pathologists are frequently challenged to provide a specific diagnosis when chronic villitis is found. They must then find cysts, proceed with antibody staining, or, ideally, isolate the organism by injecting tissue homogenate into the peritoneal cavity of mice. Tissue culture methods of identification may also be used.

The questions of whether recurrent toxoplasmosis occurs and with what frequency are not resolved. Kimball et al. (1971) conducted a prospective study of 5,000 obstetrical patients and came to the conclusion that abortion is significantly associated with antibodies to *Toxoplasma*, but in none of their 260 abortion specimens could they demonstrate the organism. Moreover, habitual abortion was not due to toxoplasmosis in the mother. Feldman (1963) thought that recurrent toxoplasmosis does not occur. Others are dubious or believe that recurrent infection is most likely associated with immune suppression.

Langer (1963a,b) first suggested that toxoplasmosis may be a cause of spontaneous abortion. He inoculated

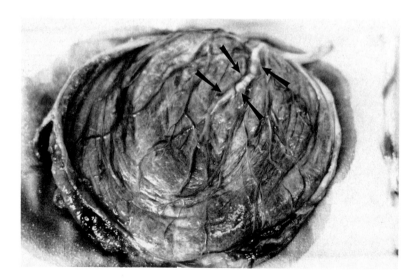

FIGURE 433. Placenta of a stillborn with hydranencephaly and other destructive features due to toxoplasmosis. Note the calcified venous thrombus at (arrows). (Courtesy Dr. G. Khodr, San Antonio.)

mice with material from 70 repeat aborters and isolated organisms from 23 of them. He also obtained organisms from nine control specimens. Only 19 of the 23 patients had a positive serological reaction. He isolated *Toxoplasma* from the brain of two successive abortuses. He also described another case with probable toxoplasmosis. In several cases, however, he required several passages for identification, an important aspect of his work.

Garcia (1968) observed a similar patient. This woman delivered a severely affected child who died within a day. Aside from many areas of typical destruction, organisms were shown to exist in several organs. The placenta had many cysts and villitis with conglutination of villi. Cysts were also found around the umbilical vein. A second pregnancy ended with a macerated abortus, also with typical histopathological changes. Again *Toxoplasma* organisms were identified; they were also present within the decidua, but they were much less well depicted there. Thus some doubt of recurrent disease lingers.

Chagas' Disease

Chagas' disease (American trypanosomiasis) is caused by infection with *Trypanosoma cruzi*, an organism that is transmitted by the bite of an infected triatomid, the "kissing bug." The disease is largely limited to Brazil, Paraguay, Chile, and Argentina, but rare cases (also of organism and vector) have come from the United States (Woody & Woody, 1974). Chagas' disease produces a wide variety of symptoms and is characterized by a frequently long latent period. Best known are myocarditis and esophagitis, but encephalitis, hepatosplenomegaly, and many other manifestations are well recorded. It is an important and frequent disease in northeastern Brazil. The disease is also known in Venezuela, from which the first congenitally acquired cases were described (de Gavaller, 1953). Since then, numerous instances of congenital Chagas' disease have been reported. Most have been from Salvador (Bahia, Brazil).

The extensive Brazilian literature on congenital and placental Chagas' disease has been reviewed in English by Bittencourt (1976), who is the major contributor to our knowledge of this disease in newborns. Her paper also described, in detail, the placental pathology. The (maternal) disease was often first identified by the autopsy of stillborn infants, whose organs contained large numbers of the organisms. When parasitemia exists in the mother, the trypanosomes gain access from the intervillous space by traversing the trophoblast as trypomastigotes. This step may occur during an acute infection but is most common during the chronic phase of the disease. In the villi the organisms change character, becoming amastigotes, and remain phagocytosed by Hofbauer cells. When they are released from these cells, they enter the fetal circulation as trypomastigotes. Not all placentas with Hofbauer cell infection cause congenital disease in the fetus. Most of the placentas studied by Bittencourt showed a massive parasitic load, chronic destructive villitis, and intervillous accumulation of fibrin and inflammatory cells (Figure 434). Fibrosis and an occasional villous granuloma-like reaction were also seen. The amnionic epithelium and Hofbauer cells were the commonest place for amastigotes to be located, although in one case a massive accumulation was found in the syncytium (Figure 435). In a later contribution, Bittencourt et al. (1981) beautifully depicted the amnionic amastigote infection and showed that the umbilical cord also had surface and internal amastigote aggregates; she speculated that an important route of amnionic epithelial infection may be from infected fetal lung. The chorion also occasionally contained organisms. The placentas of many affected fetuses were markedly enlarged, pale, and disrupted.

BABESIOSIS, TRICHOMONIASIS

Transplacental babesiosis has been described, but the placenta was not studied (Esernio-Jenssen et al., 1987). The mother had been bitten by a tick 1 week before delivery; the infant was treated successfully. The organism, *Babesia microti*, was identified in 5% of the child's red blood cells.

Trichomoniasis of the vagina, caused by *Trichomonas vaginalis*, has frequently complicated pregnancy, and it has been speculated that it may be a cause of premature delivery, especially as it may be associated with bacterial vaginosis (James et al., 1992). Mason and Brown (1980), who studied 70 infected parturients and a control group of patients, found that there was no relation of premature delivery and vaginal trichomoniasis. Neonatal infection of respiratory passages and pneumonia, presumably acquired at delivery, have been reported in a few newborns (Al-Salihi et al., 1974; McLaren et al., 1983). They were delivered vaginally; the placentas were not described. The organisms are difficult to identify histologically, and they would most likely be overlooked in routine examinations (see Lossick & Kent, 1991). Fetal and placental inflammatory lesions have been well delineated in bovine abortions due to a related flagellate (Rhyan et al., 1988).

Malaria

Infection with one of the four species of malaria plasmodia is the commonest infectious disease in the world, but truly congenital infection has been described only rarely. Naeye (1988b) made the point that it is important to differentiate between malaria in endemic regions and malaria in areas where the disease is sporadic. The former have continuously new antigen presentation and different, enhanced immune reactions. He believed that this point may be important in the

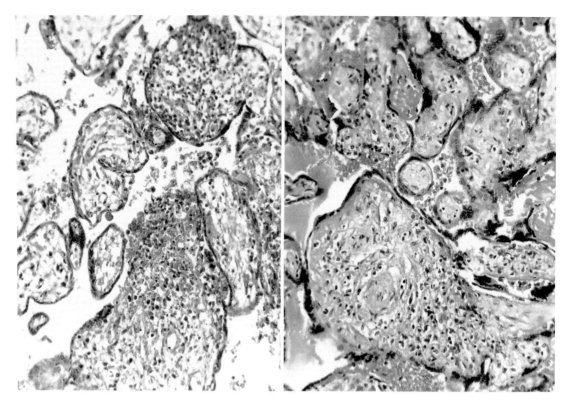

FIGURE 434. Chronic, destructive villitis due to Chagas' disease. Although many organisms are present, they cannot be seen at this magnification. The villi at top right are agglutinated; they have long been fibrosed and are functionless. H&E. ×250. (Courtesy Dr. Achiléa Lisboa Bittencourt, Bahia, Brazil.)

outcome of the disease and its possible transmission to the fetus. The mechanism of fetal/neonatal infection is still uncertain, however, despite the prevalence of malaria.

Most authors have found that pregnancy substantially increases the severity of malaria. The disease is associated with premature birth, and it reduces the weight of the fetus and placenta (references in Bruce-Chwatt,

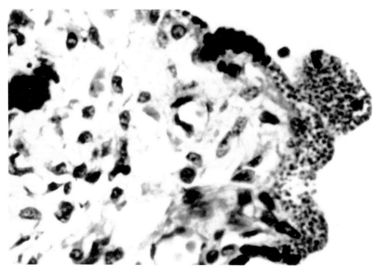

FIGURE 435. Placenta of a mother with Chagas' disease, showing amastigotes in the syncytiotrophoblast. This newborn was without overt disease, even though the placenta was infected during the acute phase of the maternal disease. H&E. ×400. (Courtesy Dr. Achiléa Lisboa Bittencourt, Bahia, Brazil.)

1966; Wyler, 1983). There is also some evidence that malaria-infected erythrocytes may be "sequestered" in the intervillous space of pregnant patients (Bray & Sinden, 1979). The organisms have often been identified in the blood of the intervillous space (e.g., Jelliffe, 1968). It is also stated that the placenta may be "diagnostically black at parturition" owing to malaria pigment (Anonymous, 1983c).

Congenital infection with malarial organisms occurred in only one of twins reported by Tanner and Hewlett (1935). Following an epidemic, Wickramasuriya (1935) described six cases of congenital malaria. He believed that congenital infection is much more common than was believed prior to his report. It included a review of previous statements that denied or assumed congenital infection to occur. The patients in his study were severely infected, and several died undelivered with fetus in utero. Parasites were found in umbilical cord blood of one patient and in the brain and spleen of two. Five fetuses had malaria-pigmented spleens, and one placenta had many infarcts and an abruptio. Other reports of congenital malaria have been reviewed in case reports by Woods et al. (1974) and Thompson et al. (1977). A frequently cited report of Quinn et al. (1982) described four children who had their first febrile episode at 3 to 4 weeks of life. Their mothers had come to the United States from abroad, and new infection is unlikely to have occurred in Seattle. The mothers had been febrile during labor or before; the placentas were not studied, and the mechanism of fetal infection is only surmised. It was suggested that perhaps antibodies or other proteins suppressed fever before the children finally became ill. In general, perhaps because of transferred immunity, symptomatic disease becomes evident only after several weeks in the neonate, as in the four infants just described. The disease is virtually never recognized at birth. That the transmission was prenatal (or occurred during delivery) in some of these cases is evidenced by reports of neonatal malaria in patients returning from abroad to the United States and delivering their infants there.

When it is stated in the literature that the "placenta was infected," it usually refers to the demonstration of organisms in blood smears made from the placenta. Such organisms could have originated from the intervillous space. Histological studies have usually not been done or have been reported only infrequently. One such report, including ultrastructural study, came from Gabon (Walter et al., 1982). Walter et al. found placental parasites in smears from 33% of cases in an unselected population collected in an endemic area. Infected erythrocytes were frequent in the intervillous space, and there was an accumulation of associated macrophages. An increased amount of intervillous fibrin was present; thickening of trophoblastic lamina was interpreted as possibly representing the results of an immune reaction. The authors considered that syncytial damage may have occurred, and they found ample malaria pigment (a hemoglobin breakdown product) in fibrinoid and macrophages, and "free" in the intervillous space. In the authors' opinion, plasmodia cross the placenta infrequently, and in their study the event was not demonstrable. This opinion is different from that of Naeye (1988b). He quoted Reinhardt as having found parasites in the fetus as frequently as in 55% of cases.

The discrepancy is not resolved. The workers who have looked at the placentas histologically have not identified organisms in the fetal circulation. This is also our observation, based on studies of infected Vietnamese patients who have delivered at our hospital. Our present view is that the plasmodium does not cross by itself. When transplacental infection does occur, the parasites are probably transferred within red blood cells. Although maternal to fetal transfer of red blood cells is rare, it does occasionally happen (see Chapter 17). This concept accords with the original observations made by Wickramasuriya (1935) as well. He demonstrated organisms in some stillborns and in the umbilical cord blood of one fetus. His patients had unusually severe pregnancy complications, several having died before delivery. These complications may well have contributed to the enhanced transfer of infected red blood cells.

Coxiella burnetii is the organism that causes Q fever, a zoonosis commonly contracted from domestic animals. Congenital infection with intrauterine fetal death was reported by Friedland et al. (1994). The placenta had a 40% involvement with severe necrotizing villitis with many organisms in the villi. Raoult and Stein (1994) reported another case and reviewed other cases from the abortion literature.

OTHER PARASITIC INFECTIONS

Kain and Keystone (1988) reported a patient with recurrent hydatid disease (*Echinococcus granulosus*) during pregnancy. A normal child was born; the placenta was not described. Invasion of the embryo by *Enterobius vermicularis* was described by Mendoza et al. (1987). They depicted a 2 cm embryo, with placenta, and showed the worm to reside within the abdomen of the embryo. The pregnancy was surgically aborted because of the presence of a dead embryo. There was no inflammatory reaction in the embryo or placenta. When Cort (1921) reviewed the topic of fetal worm infestation, he found only indisputable evidence for transmission of hookworm and *Schistosoma japonicum*. In dogs, sheep, and other animals, prenatal transmission of lung worm is well known. Sutherland et al. (1965) depicted placental infection with *Schistosoma haematobium* from a normal delivery. The organisms were located within decidua and villi, but no inflammatory reaction was described. In an addendum, additional cases were discovered. Several other references were made to a case of placental infection with different species of schistosomes.

Bittencourt et al. (1980) found placental infection with *Schistosoma mansoni* in four cases. The gross morphology of the placenta showed no characteristic features, but microscopically granulomas around schistosome eggs were present in fibrin and villi; occasional worms were also present and are illustrated. Although all four fetuses died, they had no evidence of infection by the worms. Presumably the rarity of this description relates to the paucity of placental studies. Pregnant women also suffer occasionally from disseminated strongyloidiasis, but we are not aware of a report of placental pathology in this disease.

Villitis of Unknown Etiology

Chronic villitis occurs frequently. Labarrere et al. (1990), who referred to it as villitis of unestablished origin, reviewed the incidence and found it to vary in studies from 6% to 33.8%; and Altshuler (personal communication, 1993) estimated a frequency of 5% to 10% in consecutive placentas. At times the etiology is apparent from the history (rubella) or the pathological features (CMV infection). At other times, despite much effort, no specific etiology is elicited, often even when there are severe clinical abnormalities and autopsies are performed. The entity has then been termed villitis of unknown etiology (VUE) (Altshuler, 1973b). VUE remains a significant challenge to perinatal pathologists because of its frequency, its high recurrence rate, and the associated poor pregnancy outcome. Sporadic cases such as one we saw with maternal granulomatous disease do not ensure a causal relation. No conclusive information on the etiology of VUE has been gained since it was first mentioned by Gershon and Strauss (1961). It is unfortunate that these authors misused the term placental insufficiency in this context, a designation to which we do not subscribe. In the literal sense, that term should be used only to represent a pathophysiological state; it is not synonymous with morphological abnormalities. In our view, few well defined lesions of the placenta exist for which a fetal or maternal cause cannot be assigned; the term placental insufficiency subtly implies that there is an intrinsic defect in placental function or its development. We believe this concept to be misleading and one that diverts attention from a search for pathogenetic mechanisms.

The pathological findings of VUE have often been depicted since the initial emphasis of this entity's importance (Benirschke & Altshuler, 1971), but there is evidence that interpathologist diagnostic error in this diagnosis is considerable (Khong et al., 1993). The constituent lesions have a wide spectrum of appearance, from occasional villous involvement to extreme involvement wherein all villi have some pathological reaction (Russell, 1980). Altshuler (1973b, 1984) has summarized the salient features of VUE as follows: proliferative villitis, necrotizing villitis, granulomatous, cicatricial, reparative, evanescent villitis; fetal vasculopathy, avas-

cular villi, placental dysmaturity, increase in nucleated red blood cells, hemosiderin, hemorrhagic vasculitis, necrotizing deciduitis, basal villitis, chorangiosis, and ischemia or infarction. All of these abnormalities may be found in cases of placental VUE, or only some of them may be present.

The similarity to known infectious causes of villitis, such as seen with CMV and rubella, is striking. Even though no infectious cause has been delineated for VUE, this entity is discussed here because of its presumed relation to congenital infection. It may well be proved in the future that VUE is not a single or uniform infection, independent of host immune factors, but that it is comprised of several etiologically distinct variants. It is a challenge for future investigation.

One should also note that degenerative lesions, somewhat simulating VUE, occur peripheral to infarcts (subinfarctive villous degenerations). These lesions are not to be confused with typical VUE as here discussed. VUE is often associated with fetal growth retardation. Altshuler (1984) saw it in 33% of his cases. Dollmann and Schmitz-Moormann (1972) described it in their patient with recurrent abortions, and others found similar effects (Russell et al., 1980; Labarrere et al., 1982; Salafia et al., 1988). Rüschoff et al. (1985) described the placentas of VUE as "stiff," but a macroscopic delineation of VUE has not yet been possible. The placentas are occasionally smaller and have more fibrin content, but no other change allows macroscopic identification.

The frequency of VUE varies with the nature of the investigation (i.e., the selection of the material). In general, one may expect VUE in approximately 5% to 8% of consecutively studied placentas. When the placentas of complicated pregnancies, growth-retarded infants, or fetal deaths are studied, the incidence is much higher.

There is little doubt that VUE eliminates a considerable amount of placental parenchyma from nutrient transfer. Fetal growth retardation is thus not surprising. One must emphasize, however, that there is no absolute relation between the severity of VUE and the severity of fetal growth retardation. Attempts to show a relation to elevated fetal IgM levels have not been successful (Mortimer et al., 1985), nor have numerous attempts to identify specific organisms with a variety of serological, cultural, or structural tools.

Of greatest interest to us is the frequently recurrent nature of this lesion, so well described in the contribution by Dollmann and Schmitz-Moormann (1972). They saw a patient with two growth-retarded infants followed by three abortions, all with VUE as probable cause. They found that in some instances there was a marked intervillous accumulation of macrophages (intervillositis). These cells they determined to be of maternal

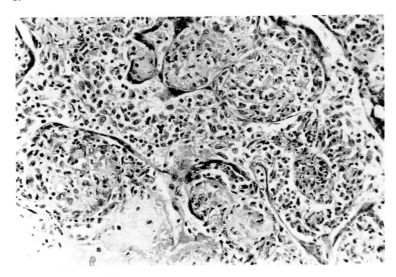

FIGURE 436. Placenta of a 36 weeks' gestation stillborn with VUE. It was the second of three successive such events. Note the intense "intervillositis" with histiocytes and lymphocytes, villous infiltration, villous necroses, and vascular obliteration. H&E. ×250.

origin, whereas most of the intravillous inflammatory cells could not be "typed" with sex chromatin but were thought to be of fetal origin. Jacques and Qureshi (1993) observed six cases of "chronic intervillositis" and determined the cells to be primarily histiocytes. They were unable to rule out infection, found an association with increased fibrin deposition, and identified some other pathological features. The lesion had a poor prognosis, but they were unable to define it more precisely, let alone identify an etiology. They favored an immunological determination.

The only attempt at determining the precise nature of the inflammatory cells in villitis was by Hartwick et al. (1989) in a case of fetal parvovirus B19 infection. They found the cells to have a T cell derivation and provided some support for the fetal origin in this admittedly different disease. Although most of the inflammation in VUE is apparently histiocytic/lymphocytic, plasma cells (B cell-derived) occur as well. We have reason to believe that in CMV infection they are fetal in origin. Histological considerations lead us also to believe that most inflammatory cells of VUE are of fetal origin.

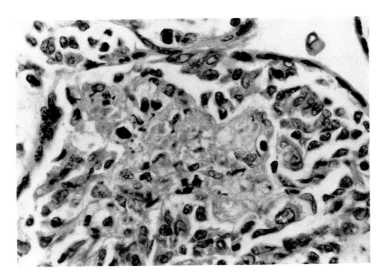

FIGURE 437. Same case of VUE as in Figure 436. The villous destruction and cellular infiltration are pronounced; occasional plasma cells are present. H&E. ×640.

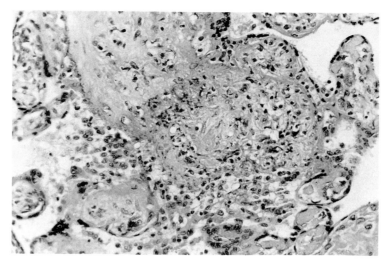

FIGURE 438. Placenta of the third pregnancy of a patient with recurrent losses and VUE (same woman as in Figures 436 and 437). The patient was also hypothyroid and on medication for this problem. When the amnionic fluid lecithin/sphingomyelin (L/S) ratio became more than 3:1, a cesarean section produced a viable fetus. Ten years later the infant was well. Despite the extensive necrosis and inflammation, this infant weighed 2,500 g at 37 weeks' gestation. The placenta weighed 510 g and had massive VUE with destruction of villi and trophoblast. H&E. ×250.

Nevertheless, many cases have a major inflammatory component in the anchoring villi, often with maternal plasma cell infiltration of the decidua. Indeed, chronic villitis may be limited to anchoring villi. Here, the cellular components have a maternal origin, and a dual derivation of the histiocytes can therefore not be excluded. Labarrere et al. (1982) and Russell (1980) have also emphasized the frequent decidual involvement with lymphocytic inflammation and suggested that VUE may have a relation to chronic endometritis. Whether the recurrent VUE in a patient with recurrent herpes gestationis described by Baxi et al. (1991) has a causal relation will remain unknown until more cases are studied.

The possibility of chronic brucellosis was entertained in a patient of ours with three consecutive pregnancy failures and histological VUE (Figures 436, 437). Detailed study, however, was negative. In a later pregnancy, the progress was monitored with estriol levels; and when they declined, an elective cesarean section was performed. The growth-retarded infant did well and has remained healthy during the 10 years since this

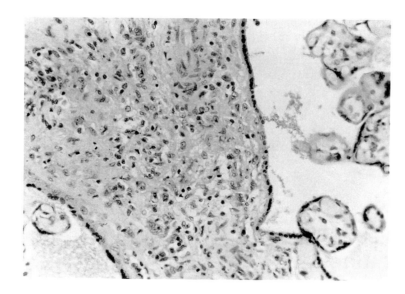

FIGURE 439. Same case as in Figure 438. Note the degeneration of the villous vessels. There is no trophoblast necrosis at this site, so the inflammatory cells are likely of fetal origin. H&E. ×250.

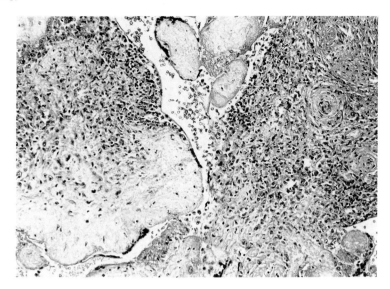

FIGURE 440. This placenta comes from the first stillborn (at 37 weeks' gestation) of the patient with recurrent VUE (see Figures 300, 436–439). There is even more necrosis and inflammation of villi than in the other pregnancies depicted. H&E. ×100.

occurrence. The placenta was so severely involved with villitis that one wonders how this infant could have been born alive (Figure 438, 439). The lesion of the first pregnancy was identical (Figure 440). The severity and destructive nature of VUE is further exemplified in Figure 441, a stillborn, growth-retarded fetus. In yet another case, it was our opinion that the increased frequency of late decelerations during monitoring was caused by the placental lesions shown in Figure 442 (Benirschke, 1975). These inexplicable areas of villitis were scattered throughout the placenta. In the case of a severely compromised newborn, the placenta had many vascular occlusions and surface thrombi (Figures 443–446). No virus infection was diagnosed. This picture is substantially different from the hemorrhagic endovasculitis (HEV) of Sander et al. (1986), which is further discussed in Chapter 13.

The etiology of VUE is unknown. Infants can survive severe placental villitis without subsequent impairment. Their long-term outcome requires much additional investigation. Three suggestions have been made with respect to its possible etiology.

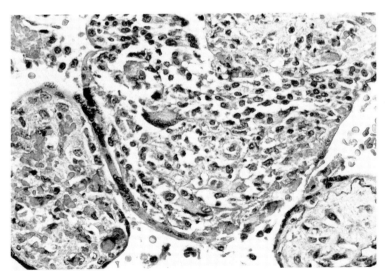

FIGURE 441. Villitis of unknown etiology in a stillborn fetus. Intense infiltration with lymphocytes, plasma cells, and histiocytes is widespread. Mineralization of the villous basement membrane is seen at bottom right. Several histiocytic giant cells are present in the central villus, whose trophoblast is degenerating focally. Vessels are obliterated. H&E. ×640.

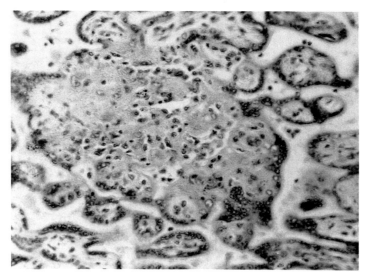

FIGURE 442. Mild chronic villitis in a 39-week pregnancy with good outcome. Late decelerations during labor were believed to be secondary to VUE. H&E. ×250.

1. It is a viral disease due to an as yet unrecognized agent. That this concept has some merit derives from the great histological similarity of VUE to rubella and other known virus disorders that affect the placenta. Moreover, the discovery of parvovirus B19 infection and the similarity of placental response suggest that a viral agent must be sought in future studies.

2. It is an immune reaction akin to placental "rejection" or even graft-versus-host disease. Several investigators have raised this possibility, in particular because of the histiocytic predominance of the inflammatory reaction and the frequently recurrent episodes. At present, no new studies have conclusively shown or rejected this possibility. It is necessary to have more information on the "normal" fetomaternal immune interactions before this hypothesis can be rejected or

affirmed. Redline and Abramowsky (1984) have commented on this possibility. They found a 60% reproductive loss in patients with recurrent chronic villitis in contrast to a 37% loss in nonrecurrent villitis (Redline & Abramovsky, 1985). They suggested that VUE is much more common than heretofore believed; perhaps as many as 4% to 10% of placentas have some degree of VUE. They also suggested that "immunological and structural abnormalities (uterine) in the host may play a role in its pathogenesis." Several of their patients had autoimmune diseases. Importantly, Redline and Patterson (1993) found with X-specific markers in male conceptuses' placentas that approximately 60% of the infiltrating immunocytes of VUE represent maternal

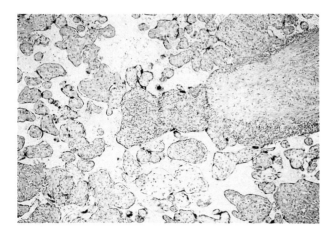

FIGURE 443. Severe chronic villitis in a premature infant with meconium aspiration. Note the extensive areas of villous destruction and inflammation. H&E. ×64.

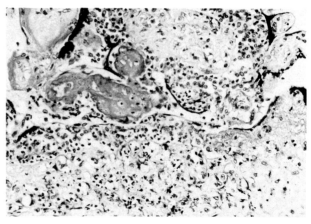

FIGURE 444. Same case as in Figure 443, showing the subtrophoblastic accumulation of lymphocytic infiltrate and villous necrosis. There were also chorionic vessel thrombi in this placenta. CMV and herpes infections were ruled out. H&E. ×250.

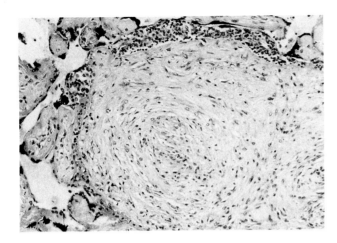

FIGURE 445. Same case as in Figures 443 and 444, again showing subtrophoblastic inflammatory cells and obliteration of villous stem vessel. H&E. ×640.

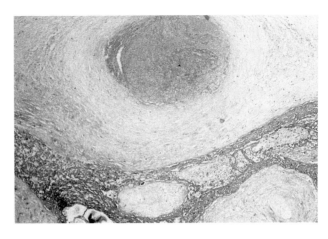

FIGURE 446. Same case as in Figures 443, 444, and 445, showing an old thrombosis of a chorionic surface vessel in VUE. H&E. ×64.

CD3$^+$ T cells that have infiltrated from the intervillous space. The reason for this response is presently unknown but is speculated on in that contribution. Greco and colleagues (1992) had also investigated the nature of villous stromal cells in VUE, syphilis, and CMV infection with a battery of antibodies and in situ hybridization. They concluded that these infiltrating elements had often markedly different phenotypes, and that this expression was somewhat dependent on the nature of the underlying disease. They expressed an inability to decide about a possible immune reaction portrayed by this villitis (e.g., maternal cell invasion) but pointed out that "the expression of certain cellular markers for villous stromal cells is identical in both CMV and nonspecific villitis."

3. The disease has a relation to preeclampsia and infarcts. Most of the patients we have seen do not have signs of pregnancy toxemia, and the "villitis" that is associated with preeclampsia is different. It has much less inflammation and is mostly degenerative in nature. Therefore we prefer to reject this hypothesis.

At this time the only certain and common finding is that VUE is not the result of infection with common pathogens. No virus or other agent has been consistently identified. Moreover, the children who are born from such pregnancies develop normally. The efforts of several laboratories to identify the origin and nature of the inflammatory infiltrate suggests that most of the infiltrating cells are of maternal origin. Whether it is tantamount to an immune "rejection" phenomenon mounted by the mother against the placenta requires further investigation. The fact that the surviving infants of VUE placentas remain well and that the disease frequently recurs in families point in that direction.

References

Abbasi, I.A., Hemming, V.G., Eglinton, G.S., and Johnson, T.R.B.: Proliferation of group B streptococci in human amniotic fluid in vitro. Am. J. Obstet. Gynecol. 156:95–99, 1987.

Abraham, A.A.: Herpesvirus hominis endometritis in a young woman wearing an intrauterine contraceptive device. Am. J. Obstet. Gynecol. 131:340–342, 1978.

Abramowsky, C., Beyer-Patterson, P., and Cortinas, E.: Nonsyphilitic spirochetosis in second trimester fetuses. Pediatr. Pathol. 11:827–838, 1991.

Aherne, W., and Davies, P.A.: Congenital pneumonia. Lancet 1:275, 1962.

Ahlfors, C.E., Goetzman, B.W., Halsted, C.C., Sherman, M.P., and Wennberg, R.P.: Neonatal listeriosis. Am. J. Dis. Child. 131:405–408, 1977.

Ahlfors, K., Ivarsson, S.-A., and Nilsson, H.: On the unpredictable development of congenital cytomegalovirus infection: a study of twins. Early Hum. Dev. 18:125–135, 1988.

Alford, C.A., Neva, F.A., and Weller, T.H.: Virologic and serologic studies on human products of conception after maternal rubella. N. Engl. J. Med. 271:1275–1281, 1964.

Alford, C.A., Stagno, S., and Reynolds, D.W.: Diagnosis of chronic perinatal infections. Am. J. Dis. Child. 129:455–463, 1975.

Alger, L.S., Lovchik, J.C., Hebel, J.R., Blackmon, L.R., and Crenshaw, M.C.: The association of Chlamydia trachomatis, Neisseria gonorrhoeae, and group B streptococci with premature rupture of the membranes and pregnancy outcome. Am. J. Obstet. Gynecol. 159:397–404, 1988.

Alger, L.S., Farley, J.J., Robinson, B.A., Hines, S.E., Berchin, J.M., and Johnson, J.P.: Interactions of human immunodeficiency virus infection and pregnancy. Obstet. Gynecol. 82:787–796, 1993.

Alkalay, A.L., Pomerance, J.J., and Rimoin, D.L.: Fetal varicella syndrome. J. Pediatr. 111:320–323, 1987.

Al-Salihi, F.L., Curran, J.P., and Wang, J.-S.: Neonatal Trichomonas vaginalis: report of three cases and review of the literature. Pediatrics 53:196–200, 1974.

Altshuler, G.: Implications of two cases of human placental plasma cells? Reports of cytomegalic inclusion disease in a thirteen week's fetus and of ascending herpes infection of the newborn. Am. J. Pathol. 70:18a, 1973a.

Altshuler, G.: Placental villitis of unknown etiology: harbinger of serious disease? A four months' experience of nine cases. J. Reprod. Med. 11:215–222, 1973b.

Altshuler, G.: Toxoplasmosis as a cause of hydranencephaly. Am. J. Dis. Child. 125:251–252, 1973c.

Altshuler, G.: Pathogenesis of congenital herpesvirus infection: case report including a description of the placenta. Am. J. Dis. Child. 127:427–429, 1974.

Altshuler, G.: Placental infection, and inflammation. In, Pathology of the Placenta. E.V.D.K. Perrin, ed., pp. 141–163. Churchill Livingstone, New York, 1984.

Altshuler, G.: The placenta. In, Diagnostic Surgical Pathology. S.S. Sternberg, ed., pp. 1503–1522. Raven Press, New York, 1989.

Altshuler, G., and Hyde, S.: Fusobacteria: an important cause of chorioamnionitis. Arch. Pathol. Lab. Med. 109:739–743, 1985.

Altshuler, G., and Hyde, S.: Clinicopathologic considerations of fusobacteria chorioamnionitis. Acta Obstet. Gynecol. Scand. 67:513–517, 1988.

Altshuler, G., and McAdams, A.J.: Cytomegalic inclusion disease of a nineteen-week fetus: case report including a study of the placenta. Am. J. Obstet. Gynecol. 111:295–298, 1971.

Altshuler, G., and Russell, P.: The human villitides: a review of chronic intrauterine infection. Curr. Top. Pathol. 60:63–112, 1975.

Amirhessami-Aghili, N., and Spector, S.A.: Human immunodeficiency virus type 1 infection of human placenta: potential route for fetal infection. J. Virol. 65:2231–2236, 1991.

Amirhessami-Aghili, N., Manalo, P., Hall, M.R., Tibbitts, F.D., Ort, C.A., and Afsari, A.: Human cytomegalovirus infection of human placental explants in culture: histologic and immunohistochemical studies. Am. J. Obstet. Gynecol. 156:1365–1374, 1987.

Amstey, M.S.: Group B streptococcus and premature rupture of membranes. Am. J. Obstet. Gynecol. 143:607–608, 1982.

Amstey, M.S., Miller, R.K., Menegus, M.A., and di Sant'Agnese, P.A.: Enterovirus in pregnant women and the perfused placenta. Am. J. Obstet. Gynecol. 158:775–782, 1988.

Anderson, G.S., Green, C.A., Neligan, G.A., Newell, D.J., and Russell, J.K.: Congenital bacterial pneumonia. Lancet 2:585–587, 1962.

Andiman, W.A., Simpson, J., Olson, B., Dember, L., Silva, T.J., and Miller, G.: Rate of transmission of human immunodeficiency virus type 1 infection from mother to child and short-term outcome of neonatal infection. Am. J. Dis. Child. 144:758–766, 1990.

Andreu, A., Genover, E., Coira, A., and Farran, I.: Antepartum infection as a result of Streptococcus pneumoniae and sepsis in neonate. Am. J. Obstet. Gynecol. 161:1424–1425, 1989.

Anonymous: Group-B streptococci in the newborn. Lancet 1:520–521, 1977a.

Anonymous: The Shirodkar stitch. Lancet 2:691–692, 1977b.

Anonymous: Perinatal listeriosis. Lancet 1:911, 1980.

Anonymous: Avoiding damage to the cervix. Lancet 2:552–553, 1983a.

Anonymous: How does Brucella abortus infect human beings? Lancet 2:1180, 1983b.

Anonymous: Malaria in pregnancy. Lancet 2:84–85, 1983c.

Anonymous: Does coitus embarrass the fetus? Lancet 1:374–375, 1984.

Anonymous: Listeriosis. Lancet 2:364–365, 1985.

Anonymous: Rapid detection of beta haemolytic streptococci. Lancet 1:247–248, 1986.

Anonymous: Chorioamnionitis: cause or effect? Lancet 1:362, 1989a.

Anonymous: Herpes simplex virus latency. Lancet 1:194–195, 1989b.

Anonymous: Screening for congenital CMV. Lancet 2:599–600, 1989c.

Aquino, T.I., Zhang, J., Kraus, F.T., Knefel, R., and Taff, T.: Subchorionic fibrin cultures for bacteriologic study of the placenta. Am. J. Clin. Pathol. 81:482–486, 1984.

Arias, F., Rodriguez, L., Rayne, S.C., and Kraus, F.T.: Maternal placental vasculopathy and infection: two distinct subgroups among patients with preterm labor and preterm ruptured membranes. Am. J. Obstet. Gynecol. 168:585–591, 1993.

Ascher, D.P., Becker, J.A., Yoder, B.A., Weisse, M., Waecker, N.J., Heroman, W.M., Davis, C., Fajardo, J.E., and Fischer, G.W.: Failure of intrapartum antibiotics to prevent culture-proved neonatal group B streptococcal sepsis. J. Perinatol. 13:212–216, 1993.

Asrat, T., Lewis, D.F., Garite, T.J., Major, C.A., Nageotte, M.P., Towers, C.V., Montgomery, D.M., and Dorchester, W.A.: Rate of recurrence of preterm premature rupture of membranes in consecutive pregnancies. Am. J. Obstet. Gynecol. 165:1111–1115, 1991.

Awadalla, S.G., Mercer, L.J., and Brown, L.G.: Pregnancy complicated by intraamniotic infection by Salmonella typhi. Obstet. Gynecol. 65:30S-31S, 1985.

Azzarelli, B., and Lafuze, J.: Amniotic basement membrane: a barrier to neutrophil invasion. Am. J. Obstet. Gynecol. 156:1130–1136, 1987.

Azziz, R., Cummings, J., and Naeye, R.: Acute myometritis and chorioamnionitis during cesarean section of asymptomatic women. Am. J. Obstet. Gynecol. 159:1137–1139, 1988.

Baddeley, P., and Shardlow, J.P.: Antenatal gonococcal arthritis. J. Obstet. Gynaecol. Br. Commonw. 80:186–187, 1973.

Bader, G.: Beitrag zur Chorioamnionitis mycotica. Arch. Gynecol. 203:251–225, 1966.

Baergen, R., Benirschke, K., and Ulich, T.R.: Cytokine expression in the placenta: the role of interleukin 1 and interleukin 1 receptor antagonist expression in chorioamnionitis and parturition. Arch. Pathol. Lab. Med. 118:52–55, 1994.

Baker, C.J.: Summary of workshop on perinatal infections due to group B streptococcus. J. Infect. Dis. 136:137–152, 1977.

Baker, C.J., Rench, M.A., Edwards, M.S., Carpenter, R.J., Hays, B.M., and Kasper, D.L.: Immunization of pregnant women with a polysaccharide vaccine of group B streptococcus. N. Engl. J. Med. 319:1180–1185, 1988.

Balducci, J., Rodis, J.F., Rosengren, S., Vintzileos, A.M., Spivey, G., and Vosseller, C.: Pregnancy outcome following first-trimester varicella infection. Obstet. Gynecol. 79:5–6, 1992.

Baldwin, V. and Whitley, R.J.: Teratogen update: intrauterine herpes simplex virus infection. Teratology 39:1–10, 1989.

Ballantyne, J.W.: Manual of Antenatal Pathology and Hygiene. The Embryo. Wm. Greene & Sons, Edinburgh, 1904.

Baniecki, H.: Über den Wert der histologischen Luesdiagnose der Nabelschnur. Z. Geburtshilfe Gynakol. 93:313–315, 1928.

Barford, D.A.G., and Rosen, M.G.: Cervical incompetence: diagnosis and outcome. Obstet. Gynecol. 64:159–163, 1984.

Barresi, J.A.: Listeria monocytogenes: a cause of premature labor and neonatal sepsis. Am. J. Obstet. Gynecol. 136:410–411, 1980.

Barsky, P., and Beale, A.J.: The transplacental transmission of poliomyelitis. J. Pediatr. 51:207–211, 1957.

Barter, R.A.: Congenital pneumonia. Lancet 1:165, 1962.

Barton, J.J., O'Connor, T.M., Cannon, M.J., and Weldon-Linne, C.M.: Prevalence of human immunodeficiency virus in a general prenatal population. Am. J. Obstet. Gynecol. 160:1316–1324, 1989.

Barton, J.R., Thorpe, E.M., Shaver, D.C., Hager, W.D., and Sibai, B.M.: Nonimmune hydrops fetalis associated with maternal infection with syphilis. Am. J. Obstet. Gynecol. 167:56–58, 1992.

Barton, L.L., Cruz, R.D., and Walentik, C.: Neonatal Haemophilus influenzae type C sepsis. Am. J. Dis. Child. 136:463–464, 1982.

Batcup, G., Holt, P., Hambling, M.H., Gerlis, L.M., and Glass, M.R.: Placental and fetal pathology in Coxsackie virus A9 infection: a case report. Histopathology 9:1227–1235, 1985.

Baxi, L.V., Kovilam, O.P., Collins, M.H., and Walther, R.R.: Recurrent herpes gestationis with postpartum flare: a case report. Am. J. Obstet. Gynecol. 164:778–780, 1991.

Becket, R.S., and Flynn, F.J.: Toxoplasmosis: report of two new cases, with a classification and with a demonstration of the organisms in human placenta. N. Engl. J. Med. 249:345–350, 1953.

Beckmann, S., and Zimmer, E.: Über die Bedeutung der "Nabelschnurentzündung." Arch. Gynecol. 145:194–218, 1931.

Beitzke, H.: Über die angeborene tuberkulöse Infection. Ergebn. Ges. Tuberk. Forsch. 7:1–30, 1935.

Bejar, R., Curbelo, V., Davis, C., and Gluck, L.: Premature labor. II. Bacterial sources of phospholipase. Obstet. Gynecol. 57:479–482, 1981.

Bendon, R.W., Perez, F., and Ray, M.B.: Herpes simplex virus: fetal and decidual infection. Pediatr. Pathol. 7:63–70, 1987.

Bengtson, J.M., VanMarter, L.J., Barss, V.A., Greene, M.F., Tuomala, R.E., and Epstein, M.F.: Pregnancy outcome after premature rupture of the membranes at or before 26 weeks' gestation. Obstet. Gynecol. 73:921–927, 1989.

Benirschke, K.: Routes and types of infection in the fetus and the newborn. Am. J. Dis. Child. 99:714–721, 1960.

Benirschke, K.: Diseases of the placenta. Contemp. Obstet. Gynecol. 6:17–20, 1975.

Benirschke, K., and Altshuler, G.: The future of perinatal physiopathology. In, Symposium on the Functional Physiopathology of the Fetus and Neonate. H. Abramson ed., pp. 158–168. Mosby, St. Louis, 1971.

Benirschke, K., and Driscoll, S.G.: The Pathology of the Human Placenta. Springer-Verlag, New York, 1967.

Benirschke, K., and Raphael, S.I.: Candida albicans infection of the amniotic sac. Am. J. Obstet. Gynecol. 75:200–202, 1958.

Benirschke, K., Mendoza, G.R., and Bazeley, P.L.: Placental and fetal manifestations of cytomegalovirus infection. Virchows Arch. [B] 16:121–139, 1974.

Benirschke, K., Swartz, W.H., Leopold, G., and Sahn, D.: Hydrops due to myocarditis in a fetus. Am. J. Cardiovasc. Pathol. 1:131–133, 1986.

Benner, M.C.: Congenital infection of the lungs, middle ears and nasal accessory sinuses. Arch. Pathol. 29:455–472, 1940.

Bennett, P.R., and Elder, M.G.: The mechanisms of preterm labor: Common genital tract pathogens do not metabolize arachidonic acid to prostaglandins or to other eicosanoids. Am. J. Obstet. Gynecol. 166:1541–1545, 1992.

Bennett, P.R., Rose, M.P., Myatt, L., and Elder, M.G.: Preterm labor: stimulation of arachidonic acid metabolism in human amnion cells by bacterial products. Am. J. Obstet. Gynecol. 156:649–655, 1987.

Berche, P., Reich, K.A., Bonnichon, M., Beretti, J.-L., Geoffroy, C., Raveneau, J., Cossart, P., Gaillard, J.-L., Geslin, P., Kreis, H., and Veron, M.: Detection of anti-listeriolysin O for serodiagnosis of human listeriosis. Lancet 335:624–627, 1990.

Berg, B.J. v.d.: Coitus and amniotic-fluid infections. N. Engl. J. Med. 302:632, 1980.

Berger, S.A., Weinberg, M., Treves, T., Sorkin, P., Geller, E., Yedwab, G., Tomer, A., Rabey, M., and Michaeli, D.: Herpes encephalitis during pregnancy: failure of acyclovir and adenine arabinoside to prevent neonatal herpes. Isr. J. Med. Sci. 22:41–44, 1986.

Bernstein, D.I., Tipton, J.R., Schott, S.F., and Cherry, J.D.: Coccidioidomycosis in a neonate: maternal-infant transmission. J. Pediatr. 99:752–754, 1981.

Berrebi, A., Puel, J., Federlin, M., Gayet, C., Kobuch, W.E., Monrozies, X., and Watrigant, M.P.: Transmission du HIV (human immunodeficiency virus) de la mère à l'enfant. Rev. Fr. Gynecol. Obstet. 82:25–28, 1987.

Berry, S.M., Fine, N., Bichalski, J.A., Cotton, D.B., Dombrowski, M.P., and Kaplan, J.: Circulating lymphocyte subsets in second- and third-trimester fetuses: comparison with newborns and adults. Am. J. Obstet. Gynecol. 167: 895–900, 1992.

Binns, B., Williams, T., McDowell, J., and Brunham, R.C.: Screening for Chlamydia trachomatis infection in a pregnancy counseling clinic. Am. J. Obstet. Gynecol. 159:1144–1149, 1988.

Bittencourt, A.L.: Congenital Chagas disease. Am. J. Dis. Child. 130:97–103, 1976.

Bittencourt, A.L., Cardoso de Almeida, M.A., Iunes, M.A.F., and Casulari da Motta, L.D.C.: Placental involvement in schistosomiasis mansoni: report of four cases. Am. J. Trop. Med. Hyg. 29:571–575, 1980.

Bittencourt, A.L., de Freitas, L.A.R., Galvao, M.O., and Jacomo, K.: Pneumonitis in congenital Chagas' disease: a study of ten cases. Am. J. Trop. Med. Hyg. 30:38–42, 1981.

Bittencourt, A.L., dos Santos, W.L.C., and de Oliveira, C.H.: Placental and fetal candidiasis: presentation of a case of an abortus. Mycopathologia 87:181–187, 1984.

Blanc, W.A.: Infection amniotique et néonatale: diagnostic cytologique rapide. Gynaecologia 136:101–110, 1953.

Blanc, W.A.: Role of the amniotic infection syndrome in perinatal pathology. Bull. Sloane Hosp. 3:79–85, 1957.

Blanc, W.A.: Amniotic sac infection syndrome: pathogenesis, morphology and significance in circumnatal mortality. Clin. Obstet. Gynecol. 2:705–734, 1959.

Blanc, W.A.: Amniotic infection syndrome: practical significance and quick diagnostic test. N.Y. State J. Med. 61:1487–1492, 1961a.

Blanc, W.A.: Pathways of fetal and early neonatal infection: viral placentitis, bacterial and fungal chorioamnionitis. J. Pediatr. 59:473–496, 1961b.

Blanc, W.A.: Pathology of the placenta, membranes, and umbilical cord in bacterial, fungal, and viral infections in man. In, Perinatal Diseases. R.L. Naeye, J.M. Kissane, and N. Kaufman, eds., pp. 67–132. Williams & Wilkins, Baltimore, 1981.

Blanco, J.D., Gibbs, R.S., and Krebs, L.F.: A controlled study of amniotic fluid immunoglobulin levels in intra-amniotic infection. Obstet. Gynecol. 61:450–453, 1983.

Bobitt, J.R., and Ledger, W.J.: Unrecognized amnionitis and prematurity: a preliminary report. J. Reprod. Med. 19:8–12, 1977.

Bobitt, J.R., Hayslip, C.C., and Damato, J.D.: Amniotic fluid infection as determined by transabdominal amniocentesis in patients with intact membranes in premature labor. Am. J. Obstet. Gynecol. 140:947–952, 1981.

Boesaart, J.W.: Een geval van placenta-tuberculose. Nederl. Tijdschr. Geneesk. 103:1849–1852, 1959.

Borglin, N.E.: Placental function in incompetence of the internal os of the cervix. Fertil. Steril. 13:575–582, 1962.

Borisch, B., Jahn, G., Scholl, B.-C., Filger-Brillinger, J., Heymer, B., Fleckenstein, B., and Müller-Hermelink, H.K.: Detection of human cytomegalovirus DNA and viral antigens in tissues of different manifestations of CMV infection. Virchows Arch. [B] 55:93–99, 1988.

Bortolussi, R., Issekutz, T., Burbridge, S., and Schellekens, H.: Neonatal host defense mechanisms against Listeria monocytogenes infection: the role of lipopolysaccharides and interferons. Pediatr. Res. 25:311–315, 1989.

Boucher, M., and Yonekura, M.L.: Perinatal listeriosis (early-onset): correlation of antenatal manifestations and neonatal outcome. Obstet. Gynecol. 68:593–597, 1986.

Boucher, M., Yonekura, M.L., Wallace, R.J., and Phelan, J.P.: Adult respiratory distress syndrome: a rare manifestation of Listeria monocytogenes infection in pregnancy. Am. J. Obstet. Gynecol. 149:686–688, 1984.

Boué, A., and Loffredo, V.: Avortement causé par le virus de l'herpès type II: isolement du virus à partir de tissus zygotiques. Presse Med. 78:103–106, 1970.

Bowmer, E.J., McKiel, J.A., Cockcroft, W.H., Schmitt, N., and Rappay, D.E.: Listeria monocytogenes infections in Canada. Can. Med. Assoc. J. 109:125–135, 1973.

Boyer, K.M., and Gotoff, S.P.: Prevention of early-onset neonatal group B streptococcal disease with selective intrapartum chemoprophylaxis. N. Engl. J. Med. 314:1665–1669, 1986.

Brady, K., Martin, A., Page, D., Purdy, S., and Neiman, R.S.: Localization of human immunodeficiency virus in placental tissue [abstract 63]. Mod. Pathol. 2:11A, 1989.

Brandt, C.D., Rakusan, T.A., Sison, A.V., Saxena, E.S., Ellaurie, M., and Sever, J.L.: Human immunodeficiency virus infection in infants during the first 2 months of life: reliable detection and evidence of in utero transmission. Arch. Pediatr. Adolesc. Med. 148:250–254, 1994.

Braunstein, H.: Congenital syphilis in aborted second trimester fetus: diagnosis by histological study. J. Clin. Pathol. 31:265–267, 1978.

Bray, R.S., and Sinden, R.E.: The sequestration of Plasmodium falciparum infected erythrocytes in the placenta. Trans. R. Soc. Trop. Med. Hyg. 73:716–719, 1979.

Brazin, S.A., Simkovich, J.W., and Johnson, W.T.: Herpes zoster during pregnancy. Obstet. Gynecol. 53:175–181, 1979.

Breer, C., and Schopfer, K.: Listeria and food. Lancet 2:1022, 1988.

Bret, J., and Coupe, C.: Vaginites et infection neo-natale: étiologie des mycoses du nouveau-né. Presse Med. 66:937–938, 1958.

Broekhuizen, F.F., Gilman, M., and Hamilton, P.R.: Amniocentesis for Gram stain and culture in preterm premature rupture of the membranes. Obstet. Gynecol. 66:316–321, 1985.

Brown, Z.A., Vontver, L.A., Benedetti, J., Critchlow, C.W., Sells, C.J., Berry, S., and Corey, L.: Effects on infants of a first episode of genital herpes during pregnancy. N. Engl. J. Med. 317:1246–1251, 1987.

Browne, F.J.: Congenital pneumonia. Lancet 1:748, 1962.

Bruce-Chwatt, L.J.: Low birthweight. Lancet 1:1161, 1966.

Brunham, R.C., Paavonen, J., Stevens, C.E., Kiviat, N., Kuo, C.-C., Critchlow, C.W., and Holmes, K.K.: Mucopurulent cervicitis—the ignored counterpart in women of urethritis in men. N. Engl. J. Med. 311:1–6, 1984.

Bryant, R.E., Windom, R.E., Vineyard, J.P., Sanford, J.P., and Mays, B.A.: Asymptomatic bacteriuria in pregnancy and its association with prematurity. J. Lab. Clin. Med. 63:224–231, 1964.

Buchanan, R., and Sworn, M.J.: Abortion associated with intrauterine infection by Candida albicans: case report. Br. J. Obstet. Gynaecol. 86:741–744, 1979.

Buchholz, H.M., Frösner, G.G., and Ziegler, G.B.: HBAg carrier state in an infant delivered by cesarean section. Lancet 2:343, 1974.

Cairo, M.S.: Neonatal neutrophil host defense: prospects for immunologic enhancement during neonatal sepsis. Am. J. Dis. Child. 143:40–46, 1989.

Callaway, C.S., Walls, K.W., and Hicklin, M.D.: Electron microscopic studies of Toxoplasma gondii in fresh and frozen tissue. Arch. Pathol. 86:484–491, 1968.

Campognone, P., and Singer, D.B.: Neonatal sepsis due to nontypable Haemophilus influenzae. Am. J. Dis. Child. 140:117–121, 1986.

Carey, J.C., Blackwelder, W.C., Nugent, R.P., Matteson, M.A., Rao, A.V., Eschenbach, D.A., Lee, M.L.F., Rettig, P.J., Regan, J.A., Geromanos, K.L., Martin, D.H., Pastorek, J.G., Gibbs, R.S., Lipscomb, K.A., and the Vaginal Infections and Prematurity Study Group: Antepartum cultures for Ureaplasma urealyticum are not useful in predicting pregnancy outcome. Am. J. Obstet. Gynecol. 164:728–733, 1991.

Carpenter, C.M., and Boak, R.: Isolation of Brucella abortus from a human fetus. J.A.M.A. 96:1212–1216, 1931.

Carstensen, H., Christensen, K.K., Grennert, L., Persson, K., and Polberger, S.: Early-onset neonatal group B streptococcal septicaemia in siblings. J. Infect. Dis. 17:201–204, 1988.

Cassell, G.H., and Cole, B.C.: Mycoplasmas as agents of human disease. N. Engl. J. Med. 304:80–89, 1981.

Cassell, G.H., Waites, K.B., Crouse, D.T., Rudd, P.T., Canupp, K.C., Stagno, S., and Cutter, G.R.: Association of Ureaplasma urealyticum infection of lower respiratory tract with chronic lung disease and death in very-low-birthweight infants. Lancet 2:240–244, 1988.

Catalano, L.W., Fuccilo, D.A., Traub, R.G., and Sever, J.L.: Isolation of rubella virus from placentas and throat cultures of infants: a prospective study after the 1964–1965 epidemic. Obstet. Gynecol. 38:6–14, 1971.

Charles, D., and Edwards, W.R.: Infectious complications of cervical cerclage. Am. J. Obstet. Gynecol. 141:1065–1071, 1981.

Chehab, F.F., Xiao, X., Kan, Y.W., and Yen, T.S.B.: Detection of cytomegalovirus infection in paraffin-embedded tissue specimens with the polymerase chain reaction. Mod. Pathol. 2:75–78, 1989.

Chretien, J.H., McGinnis, C.G., and Muller, A.: Venereal causes of cytomegalovirus mononucleosis. J.A.M.A. 238:1644–1645, 1977.

Christian, S.S., and Duff, P.: Is universal screening for hepatitis B infection warranted in all prenatal populations? Obstet. Gynecol. 74:259–261, 1989.

Christmas, J.T., Cox, S.M., Andrews, W., Dax, J., Leveno, K.J., and Gilstrap, L.C.: Expectant management of preterm ruptured membranes: effects of antimicrobial therapy. Obstet. Gynecol. 80:759–762, 1992.

Coghlan, J.D., and Bain, A.D.: Leptospirosis in human pregnancy followed by death of the foetus. B.M.J. 1:228–230, 1969.

Coleman, R.T., Sherer, D.M., and Maniscalco, W.M.: Prevention of neonatal group B streptococcal infections: advances in maternal vaccine development. Obstet. Gynecol. 80:301–309, 1992.

Conover, P.T., and Roesmann, U.: Malformed complex in an infant with intrauterine viral infection. Arch. Pathol. Lab. Med. 114:535–538, 1990.

Corrall, C.J.: Diagnostic criteria of congenital tuberculosis. Am. J. Dis. Child. 140:739–740, 1986.

Cort, W.W.: Prenatal infestation with parasitic worm. J.A.M.A. 76:170–171, 1921.

Couvreur, J., Desmonts, G., and Girre, J.Y.: Congenital toxoplasmosis in twins: a series of 14 pairs of twins: absence of infection in one twin in two. J. Pediatr. 89:235–240, 1976.

Cox, W.L., Forestier, F., Capella-Pavlovsky, M., and Daffos, F.: Fetal blood sampling in twin pregnancies: prenatal diagnosis and management of 19 cases. Fetal Ther. 2:101–108, 1987.

Cox, S.M., MacDonald, P.C., and Casey, M.L.: Assay of bacterial endotoxin (lipopolysaccharide) in human amniotic fluid: potential usefulness in diagnosis and management of preterm labor. Am. J. Obstet. Gynecol. 159:99–106, 1988.

Craver, R.D., and Baldwin, V.: Necrotizing funisitis. Obstet. Gynecol. 79:64–70, 1992.

Crombleholme, W.R., Schachter, J., Grossman, M., Landers, D.V., and Sweet, R.L.: Amoxicillin therapy for Chlamydia trachomatis in pregnancy. Obstet. Gynecol. 75:752–756, 1990.

Cruikshank, D.P., and Warenski, J.C.: First-trimester maternal Listeria monocytogenes sepsis and chorioamnionitis with normal neonatal outcome. Obstet. Gynecol. 73:469–471, 1989.

Curbelo, V., Bejar, R., Benirschke, K., and Gluck, L.: Premature labor. I. Prostaglandin precursors in human placental membranes. Obstet. Gynecol. 57:473–478, 1981.

Daffos, F., Forester, F., Capella-Pavlovsky, M., Thulliez, P., Aufrant, C., Valenti, D., and Cox, W.L.: Prenatal management of 746 pregnancies at risk for congenital toxoplasmosis. N. Engl. J. Med. 318:271–275, 1988.

Daikoku, N.H., Kaltreider, D.F., Johnson, T.R.B., Johnson, J.W.C., and Simmons, M.A.: Premature rupture of membranes and preterm labor: neonatal infection and perinatal mortality risks. Obstet. Gynecol. 58:417–425, 1981.

Dallenbach, F., and Piekarski, G.: Über den Nachweis von Toxoplasma gondii im Gewebe mit Hilfe markierter fluorescierender Antikörper (Methode nach Coons). Virchows Arch. [Pathol. Anat.] 333:607–618, 1960.

Darby, M.J., Caritis, S.N., and Shen-Schwarz, S.: Placental abruption in the preterm gestation: an association with chorioamnionitis. Obstet. Gynecol. 74:88–92, 1989.

Decker, W.H., and Hall, W.: Treatment of abortions infected with Clostridium welchii. Am. J. Obstet. Gynecol. 95:394–399, 1966.

De Gavaller, B.: Enfermedad de Chagas congénita: observacion anatomo-patologica en gemelos. Bol. Matern. Concepcion Palacios (Caracas) 4:59–64, 1953.

Degen, R., Stimpel, E., and Morawietz, I.: Katamnestische Untersuchungen von 74 Frauen nach Geburt eines listeriosekranken Kindes. Wien. Klin. Wochenschr. 82:875–880, 1970.

Dehner, L.P., and Askin, F.B.: Cytomegalovirus endometritis: report of a case associated with spontaneous abortion. Obstet. Gynecol. 45:211–214, 1975.

Delaplane, D., Wiringa, K.S., Shulman, S.T., and Yogev, R.: Congenital mucocutaneous candidiasis following diagnostic amniocentesis. Am. J. Obstet. Gynecol. 147:342–343, 1983.

Delprado, W.J., Baird, P.J., and Russell, P.: Placental candidiasis: report of three cases with a review of the literature. Pathology 14:191–195, 1982.

Demian, S.D.E., Donnelly, W.H., and Monif, G.R.G.: Coexistent congenital cytomegalovirus and toxoplasmosis in a stillborn. Am. J. Dis. Child. 125:420–421, 1973.

Dennis, S.M.: Comparative aspects of infectious abortion: diseases common to animals and man. Int. J. Fertil. 13: 191–197, 1968.

DeSa, D.J.: Infection and amniotic aspiration in the middle ears of stillbirths and newborn infants [abstract 29]. Am. J. Pathol. 74:7a, 1974.

Desmonts, G., and Couvreur, J.: Congenital toxoplasmosis: a prospective study of 378 pregnancies. N. Engl. J. Med. 290:1110–1116, 1974.

Desmonts, G., Daffos, F., Forestier, F., Capella-Pavlovsky, M., Thulliez, P., and Chartier, M.: Prenatal diagnosis of congenital toxoplasmosis. Lancet 1:500–504, 1985.

De Zegher, F., Sluiters, J.F., Stuurman, P.M., van der Voort, E., Bos, A.P., and Neijens, H.J.: Concomitant cytomegalovirus infection and congenital toxoplasmosis in a newborn. Eur. J. Pediatr. 147:424–425, 1988.

Dias, M.J.M., van Rijckevorsel, G.H., Landrieu, P., and Lyon, G.: Prenatal cytomegalovirus disease and cerebral microgyria: evidence for perfusion failure, not disturbance of histogenesis, as the major cause of fetal cytomegalovirus encephalopathy. Neuropediatrics 15:18–24, 1984.

Dimmick, J., Mahmood, K., and Altshuler, G.: Antenatal infection: adequate protection against hyaline membrane disease? Obstet. Gynecol. 47:56–62, 1976.

Dinsmoor, M.J., and Gibbs, R.S.: Previous intra-amniotic infection as a risk factor for subsequent peripartal uterine infections. Obstet. Gynecol. 74:299–301, 1989.

Dollmann, A., and Schmitz-Moormann, P.: Rekurriende Plazentainsuffizienz durch villöse Plazentitis mit extremer fetaler Hypotrophie. (Geburtsgewicht 1,030 g und 1,000 g am Termin). Geburtshilfe Frauenheilkd. 32:795–801, 1972.

Dominguez, R., Segal, A.J., and O'Sullivan, J.A.: Leukocytic infiltration of the umbilical cord: manifestation of fetal hypoxia due to reduction of blood flow in the cord. J.A.M.A. 173:346–349, 1960.

Donnellan, W.L., Chantra-Umporn, S., and Kidd, J.M.: The cytomegalic inclusion cell: an electron microscopic study. Arch. Pathol. 82:336–348, 1966.

Driscoll, S.G.: Histopathology of gestational rubella. Am. J. Dis. Child. 118:49–53, 1969.

Driscoll, S.G., Gorbach, A., and Feldman, D.: Congenital listeriosis: diagnosis from placental studies. Obstet. Gynecol. 20:216–220, 1962.

Dubey, J.P.: Toxoplasma, Hammondia, Besnoitia, Sarcocystis, and other tissue cyst-forming coccidia of man and animals. In, Parasitic Protozoa. Vol. III. J.P. Kreier, ed., pp. 101–237. Academic Press, Orlando, FL, 1977.

Dubey, J.P., and Beattie, C.P.: Toxoplasmosis of Animals and Man. CRC Press, Boca Raton, 1988.

Dublin, A.B., and Merten, D.F.: Computed tomography in the evaluation of herpes simplex encephalitis. Radiology 125:133–134, 1977.

Duff, P., and Gibbs, R.S.: Acute intraamniotic infection due to Streptococcus pneumoniae. Obstet. Gynecol. 61:25S–27S, 1983.

Duncan, M.E.: Babies of mothers with leprosy have small placentae, low birth weights and grow slowly. Br. J. Obstet. Gynaecol. 87:471–479, 1980.

Duncan, M.E.: Perspectives in leprosy in mothers and children. In, Advances in International Maternal and Child Health. D.B. Jelliffe and E. Jelliffe, eds., Clarendon Press, Oxford. 5:122–143, 1985.

Duncan, M.E., and Oakey, R.E.: Estrogen excretion in pregnant women with leprosy: evidence of diminished fetoplacental function. Obstet. Gynecol. 60:82–86, 1982.

Duncan, M., Melsom, R., Pearson, J.M.H., Menzel, S., and Barnetson, R.St.C.: A clinical and immunological study of four babies of mothers with lepromatous leprosy, two of whom developed leprosy in infancy. Int. J. Leprosy 51:7–17, 1983.

Duncan, M.E., Fox, H., Harkness, R.A., and Rees, R.J.W.: The placenta in leprosy. Placenta 5:189–198, 1984.

Dungal, N.: Listeriosis in four siblings. Lancet 2:513–516, 1961.

Dunn, L.J., Robinson, J.C., and Steer, C.M.: Maternal death following suture of incompetent cervix during pregnancy. Am. J. Obstet. Gynecol. 78:335–339, 1959.

Dykes, A.-K., Christensen, K.K., and Christensen, P.: Chronic carrier state in mothers of infants with group B streptococcus infections. Obstet. Gynecol. 66:84–88, 1985.

Eachempati, U., and Woods, R.E.: Cytomegalic virus disease in pregnancy. Obstet. Gynecol. 47:615–618, 1976.

Easterling, T.R., and Garite, T.J.: Fusobacterium: anaerobic occult amnionitis and premature labor. Obstet. Gynecol. 66:825–828, 1985.

Eberhart-Phillips, J.E., Frederick, P.D., Baron, R.C., and Mascola, L.: Measles in pregnancy: a descriptive study of 58 cases. Obstet. Gynecol. 82:797–801, 1993.

Edwards, L.E., Barrada, M.I., Hamann, A.A., and Hakanson, E.Y.: Gonorrhea in pregnancy. Am. J. Obstet. Gynecol. 132:637–641, 1978.

Egley, C.C., Katz, V.L., and Herbert, W.N.P.: Leukocyte esterase: a simple bedside test for the detection of bacterial colonization of amniotic fluid. Am. J. Obstet. Gynecol. 159:120–122, 1988.

Ehrnst, A., Lindgren, S., Dictor, M., Johannson, B., Sönnborg, A., Czajkowski, J., Sundin, G., and Bohlin, A.-B.: HIV in pregnant women and their offspring: evidence for late transmission. Lancet 338:203–207, 1991.

Eichenfield, A.H., and Athreya, B.H.: Lyme disease: of ticks and titers. J. Pediatr. 114:328–333, 1989.

Ekwo, E.E., Gosselink, C.A., Woolson, R., Moawad, A., and Long, C.R.: Coitus late in pregnancy: risk of preterm rupture of amniotic sac membranes. Am. J. Obstet. Gynecol. 168:22–31, 1993.

Elliott, W.G.: Placental toxoplasmosis: report of a case. Am. J. Clin. Pathol. 53:413–417, 1970.

Elliott, J.P.: Candida warrants concern. Am. J. Obstet. Gynecol. 161:503, 1989.

Elst, C.W. van der, Bernal, A.L., and Sinclair-Smith, C.C.: The role of chorioamnionitis and prostaglandins in preterm labor. Obstet. Gynecol. 77:672–676, 1991.

Emanuel, B., Lieberman, A.D., Goldin, M., and Sanson, J.: Pulmonary candidiasis in the neonatal period. J. Pediatr. 61:44–52, 1962.

Embil, J.A., Ozere, R.L., and Haldane, E.V.: Congenital cytomegalovirus infection in two siblings from consecutive pregnancies. J. Pediatr. 77:417–421, 1970.

Epstein, H., and King, C.R.: Diagnosis of congenital syphilis by immunofluorescence following fetal death in utero. Am. J. Obstet. Gynecol. 152:689–690, 1985.

Ernest, J.M., Swain, M., Block, S.M., Nelson, L.H., Hatjis, C.G., and Meis, P.J.: C-reactive protein: a limited test for managing patients with preterm labor or preterm rupture of membranes? Am. J. Obstet. Gynecol. 156:449–454, 1987.

Eschenbach, D.A., Nugent, R.P., Rao, A.V., Cotch, M.F., Gibbs, R.S., Lipscomb, K.A., Martin, D.H., Pastorek, J.G., Rettig, P.J., Carey, J.C., Regan, J.A., Geromanos, K.L., Lee, M.L.F., Poole, W.K., Edelman, R., and the Vaginal Infections and Prematurity Study Group: A randomized placebo-controlled trial of erythromycin for the treatment of Ureaplasma urealyticum to prevent premature delivery. Am. J. Obstet. Gynecol. 164:734–742, 1991.

Esernio-Jenssen, D., Scimeca, P.G., Benach, J.L., and Tenenbaum, M.J.: Transplacental/perinatal babesiosis. J. Pediatr. 110:570–572, 1987.

European Collaborative Study: Mother-to-child transmission of HIV infection. Lancet 2:1039–1045, 1988.

Evaldson, G.R., Malmborg, A.S., and Nord, C.E.: Premature rupture of the membranes and ascending infection. Br. J. Obstet. Gynaecol. 89:793–801, 1982.

Evans, M.I., Hajj, S.N., Devoe, L.D., Angerman, N.S., and Moawad, A.H.: C-reactive protein as a predictor of infectious morbidity with premature rupture of membranes and premature labor. Am. J. Obstet. Gynecol. 138:648–652, 1980.

Fadel, H.E., and Riedrich, D.A.: Intrauterine resolution of nonimmune hydrops associated with cytomegalovirus infection. Obstet. Gynecol. 71:1003–1005, 1988.

Farb, H.F., Arnesen, M., Geistler, P., and Knox, G.E.: C-reactive protein with premature rupture of membranes and premature labor. Obstet. Gynecol. 62:49–51, 1983.

Faro, S., Walker, C., and Pierson, R.L.: Amnionitis with intact amniotic membranes involving Streptobacillus moniliformis. Obstet. Gynecol. 55:9S–11S, 1980.

Fawaz, K.A., Grady, G.F., Kaplan, M.M., and Gellis, S.S.: Repetitive maternal-fetal transmission of fatal hepatitis B. N. Engl. J. Med. 293:1357–1359, 1975.

Fedele, L., Acaia, B., Parazzini, F., Ricciardiello, O., and Candiani, G.B.: Ectopic pregnancy and recurrent spontaneous abortion: two associated reproductive failures. Obstet. Gynecol. 73:206–208, 1989.

Feinberg, R.F., and Kliman, H.J.: Fetal fibronectin and preterm labor. N. Engl. J. Med. 326:708–709, 1992.

Feldman, H.A.: Congenital toxoplasmosis. N. Engl. J. Med. 269:1212, 1963.

Feldman, D., Hoar, R.M., Niemann, W.H., Valentine, T., Cukierski, M., and Hendrickx, A.G.: Tubuloreticular inclusions in placental chorionic villi of rhesus monkeys after maternal treatment with interferon. Am. J. Obstet. Gynecol. 155:413–424, 1986.

Filice, G.A., Cantrell, F., Smith, A.B., Hayes, P.S., Feeley, J.C., and Fraser, D.W.: Listeria monocytogenes infection in neonates: investigation of an epidemic. J. Infect. Dis. 138:17–23, 1978.

Fitter, W.F., De Sa, D.J., and Richardson, H.: Chorioamnionitis and funisitis due to Corynebacterium kutscheri. Arch. Dis. Child. 54:710–712, 1979.

Fiumara, N.J.: Syphilis in newborn children. Clin. Obstet. Gynecol. 18:183–189, 1975.

Flamm, H.: Die pränatalen Infektionen des Menschen. Unter besonderer Berücksichtigung von Pathogenese und Immunologie. Georg Thieme, Stuttgart, 1959.

Fleming, A.D., Ehrlich, D.W., Miller, N.A., and Monif, G.R.G.: Successful treatment of maternal septicemia due to Listeria monocytogenes at 26 weeks' gestation. Obstet. Gynecol. 66:52S–53S, 1985a.

Fleming, A.D., Salafia, C.M., Vintzileos, A.M., Rodis, J.F., Campbell, W.A., and Bantham, K.F.: The relationship among umbilical artery velocimetry, fetal biophysical profile, and placental inflammation in preterm premature rupture of the membranes. Am. J. Obstet. Gynecol. 164:38–41, 1991.

Fleming, D.W., Cochi, S.L., MacDonald, K.L., Brondum, J., Hayes, P.S., Plikaytis, B.D., Holmes, M.B., Audurier, A., Broome, C.V., and Reingold, A.L.: Pasteurized milk as a vehicle of infection in an outbreak of listeriosis. N. Engl. J. Med. 312:404–407, 1985b.

Fojaco, R.M., Hensley, G.T., and Moskowitz, L.: Congenital syphilis and necrotizing funisitis. J.A.M.A. 261:1788–1790, 1989.

Forther, B., Aissi, E., Ajana, F., Dieusart, P., Denis, P., de Lassalle, E.M., Lecomte-Houcke, M., and Vinatier, D.: Spontaneous abortion and reinfection by Toxoplasma gondii. Lancet 338:444, 1991.

Foster, G.E., Estreich, S., and Hooi, Y.S.: Chlamydial infection and pregnancy outcome. Am. J. Obstet. Gynecol. 164:234, 1991.

Foulon, W., Naessens, A., de Catte, L., and Amy, J.-J.: Detection of congenital toxoplasmosis by chorionic villus sampling and early amniocentesis. Am. J. Obstet. Gynecol. 163:1511–1513, 1990a.

Foulon, W., Naessens, A., Mahler, T., de Waele, M., de Catte, L., and de Meuter, F.: Prenatal diagnosis of congenital toxoplasmosis. Obstet. Gynecol. 76:769–772, 1990b.

Fox, H., and Langley, F.A.: Leukocytic infiltration of the placenta and umbilical cord: a clinico-pathologic study. Obstet. Gynecol. 37:451–458, 1971.

Franciosi, R.A., and Jarzynski, D.J.: Mycotic abortion in man: a case report. J. Reprod. Med. 4:48–51, 1970.

Freedman, M.L., Christopher, P., Boughton, C.R., Lucey, M., Freeman, R., and Hansman, D.: Typhoid carriage in pregnancy with infection of neonate. Lancet 1:310–311, 1970.

Frenkel, J.K.: Toxoplasmosis: mechanisms of infection, laboratory diagnosis and management. Curr. Top. Pathol. 54:28–75, 1971.

Frenkel, J.K.: Toxoplasmosis: parasite life cycle, pathology and immunology. In, The Coccidia. D.M. Hammond and

P.L. Long, eds., pp. 343–410. University Park Press, Baltimore, 1973.

Frenkel, J.K.: Pathology and pathogenesis of congenital toxoplasmosis. Bull. N.Y. Acad. Med. 50:182–191, 1974.

Friberg, J.: Genital mycoplasma infections. Am. J. Obstet. Gynecol. 132:573–578, 1978.

Friedland, J.S., Jeffrey, I., Griffin, G.E., Booker, M., and Courtenay-Evans, R.: Q fever and intrauterine death. Lancet 343:288–289, 1994.

Fuchs, P.C., and Oyama, A.A.: Neonatal relapsing fever due to transplacental transmission of Borrelia. J.A.M.A. 208: 690–692, 1969.

Fujikura, T., and Froehlich, L.A.: Intrauterine pneumonia in relation to birth weight and race. Am. J. Obstet. Gynecol. 97:81–84, 1967.

Gagnon, R.A.: Transplacental inoculation of fetal herpes simplex in the newborn. Obstet. Gynecol. 31:682–684, 1968.

Galask, R.P., and Snyder, I.S.: Antimicrobial factors in amniotic fluid. Am. J. Obstet. Gynecol. 106:59–65, 1970.

Galask, R.P., Varner, M.W., Petzold, C.R., and Wilbur, S.L.: Bacterial attachment to the chorioamniotic membranes. Am. J. Obstet. Gynecol. 148:915–928, 1984.

Galbraith, G.M.P.: Chemotactic peptide-induced arachidonic acid mobilization in human polymorphonuclear leukocytes. Am. J. Pathol. 133:347–354, 1988.

Gans, B., Eckerling, B., and Goldman, J.A.: Abortion due to incompetence of the internal os of the cervix: a report of 250 cases. Obstet. Gynecol. 27:875–879, 1966.

Gantz, N., Myerowitz, R.L., Medeiros, A.A., Carrera, G.F., Wilson, R.E., and O'Brien, T.F.: Listeriosis in immuno-suppressed patients. Am. J. Med. 58:637–643, 1975.

Garcia, A.G.P.: Fetal infection in chickenpox and alastrim, with histopathologic study of the placenta. Pediatrics 32: 895–901, 1963.

Garcia, A.G.P.: Congenital toxoplasmosis in two successive sibs. Arch. Dis. Child. 43:705–710, 1968.

Garcia, A.G.P., Pereira, J.M.S., Vidigal, N., Lobato, Y.Y., Pegado, C.S., and Branco, J.P.C.: Intrauterine infection with mumps virus. Obstet. Gynecol. 56:756–759, 1980.

Garcia, A.G.P., Fonseca, E.F., de Marques, R.L., and Lobato, Y.: Placental morphology in cytomegalovirus infection. Placenta 10:1–18, 1989.

Garcia, A.G.P., Basso, N.G.daS., Fonseca, M.E.F., and Outani, H.N.: Congenital ECHO virus infection—morphological and virological study of fetal and placental tissue. J. Pathol. 160:123–127, 1990.

Garite, T.J.: Premature rupture of the membranes: the enigma of the obstetrician. Am. J. Obstet. Gynecol. 151:1001–1005, 1985.

Garite, T.J., and Freeman, R.K.: Chorioamnionitis in the preterm gestation. Obstet. Gynecol. 59:539–545, 1982.

Gembruch, U., Niesen, M., Hansmann, M., and Knöpfle, G.: Listeriosis: a cause of non-immune hydrops fetalis. Prenat. Diagn. 7:277–282, 1987.

Genardy, R.R., Thompson, B.H., and Niebyl, J.R.: Gonococcal salpingitis in pregnancy. Am. J. Obstet. Gynecol. 126: 512–514, 1976.

Gerberding, K.M., Eisenhut, C.C., Engle, W.A., and Cohen, M.D.: Congenital candida pneumonia and sepsis: a case

report and review of the literature. J. Perinatol. 135:159–161, 1989.

Gershon, R., and Strauss, L.: Structural changes in human placentas associated with fetal inanition or growth arrest ("placental insufficiency syndrome"). Am. J. Dis. Child. 102:645–646, 1961.

Ghidini, A., Sirtori, M., Vergani, P., Mariani, S., Tucci, E., and Scola, G.C.: Fetal intracranial calcifications. Am. J. Obstet. Gynecol. 160:86–87, 1989.

Gibbs, R.S., and Blanco, J.D.: Streptococcal infections in pregnancy: a study of 48 bacteremias. Am. J. Obstet. Gynecol. 140:405–411, 1981.

Gibbs, R.S., and Blanco, J.D.: Premature rupture of the membranes. Obstet. Gynecol. 60:671–679, 1982.

Gibbs, R.S., Cassell, G.H., Davis, J.K., and St. Clair, P.J.: Further studies on genital mycoplasms in intraamniotic infection: blood cultures and serologic response. Am. J. Obstet. Gynecol. 154:717–726, 1986.

Gibbs, R.S., Weiner, M.H., Walmer, K., and St. Clair, P.J.: Microbiologic and serologic studies of Gardnerella vaginalis in intra-amniotic infection. Obstet. Gynecol. 70:187–190, 1987.

Gibbs, R.S., Romero, R.S., Hillier, S.L., Eschenbach, D.A., and Sweet, R.L.: A review of premature birth and sub-clinical infection. Am. J. Obstet. Gynecol. 166:1515–1528, 1992.

Gibson, M., and Williams, P.P.: Haemophilus influenzae amnionitis associated with prematurity and premature membrane rupture. Obstet. Gynecol. 52:70S–72S, 1978.

Gilbert, R.J., Miller, K.L., and Roberts, D.: Listeria monocytogenes and chilled foods. Lancet 1:383–384, 1989.

Gill, P.: Is listeriosis often a foodborne illness? J. Infect. 17:1–6, 1988.

Gille, J.: Granulation tissue in the umbilical cord. J. Reprod. Med. 18:35–37, 1977.

Glasser, L., and Delta, B.G.: Congenital toxoplasmosis with placental infection in monozygotic twins. Pediatrics 35:276–283, 1965.

Gleicher, N., Cohen, C.J., Kerenyi, T.D., and Gusberg, S.B.: A blocking factor in amniotic fluid causing leukocyte migration enhancement. Am. J. Obstet. Gynecol. 133:386–390, 1979.

Gloeb, D.J., O'Sullivan, M.J., and Efantis, J.: Human immunodeficiency virus infection in women. I. The effects of human immunodeficiency virus on pregnancy. Am. J. Obstet. Gynecol. 159:756–761, 1988.

Goedert, J.J., Mendez, H., Drummond, J.E., Robert-Guroff, M., Minkoff, H.L., Holman, S., Stevens, R., Rubinstein, A., Blattner, W.A., Willoughby, A., and Landesman, S.H.: Mother-to-infant transmission of human immunodeficiency virus type 1: association with prematurity or low anti-gp120. Lancet 2:1351–1354, 1989.

Gonen, R., Hannah, M.E., and Milligan, J.E.: Does prolonged preterm premature rupture of the membranes predispose to abruptio placentae? Obstet. Gynecol. 74:347–350, 1989.

Goodlin, R.C.: Intrauterine transfusion complicated by amnionitis and maternal peritonitis: report of a case. Obstet. Gynecol. 26:803, 1965.

Graber, C.D., Williamson, O., Pike, J., and Valicenti, J.: Detection of Chlamydia trachomatis infection in endocervical specimens using direct immunofluorescence. Obstet. Gynecol. 66:727–730, 1985.

Gravett, M.G., Eschenbach, D.A., Speigel-Brown, C.A., and Holmes, K.K.: Rapid diagnosis of amniotic-fluid infection by gas-liquid chromatography. N. Engl. J. Med. 306:725–728, 1982.

Gravett, M.G., Nelson, H.P., DeRouen, T., Critchlow, C., Eschenbach, D.A., and Holmes, K.K.: Independent association of bacterial vaginosis and Chlamydia trachomatis infection with adverse pregnancy outcome. J.A.M.A. 256:1899–1903, 1986.

Gray, B.M., Springfield, J.D., and Dillon, H.C.: Type-specific streptococcal antibodies in amniotic fluid. Am. J. Obstet. Gynecol. 156:666–669, 1987.

Greco, M.A., Wieczorek, R., Sachdev, R., Kaplan, C., Nuovo, G.J., and Demopoulos, R.I.: Phenotype of villous stromal cells in placentas with cytomegalovirus, syphilis, and nonspecific villitis. Am. J. Pathol. 141:835–842, 1992.

Greenspoon, J.S., and Settlage, R.H.: Isolation of human immunodeficiency virus from the placenta or from maternal blood contaminating the placenta? Am. J. Obstet. Gynecol. 161:501–502, 1989.

Gribble, M.J., Salit, I.E., Isaac-Renton, J., and Chow, A.W.: Campylobacter infections in pregnancy: case report and literature review. Am. J. Obstet. Gynecol. 140:423–426, 1981.

Grillner, L., Ahlfors, K., Ivarsson, S.-A., Harris, S., and Svanberg, L.: Endonuclease cleavage pattern of cytomegalovirus of strains isolated from congenitally infected infants with neurologic sequelae. Pediatrics 81:27–30, 1987.

Grose, C., and Itani, O.: Pathogenesis of congenital infection with three diverse viruses: varicella-zoster virus, human parvovirus, and human immunodeficiency virus. Semin. Perinatol. 13:278–293, 1989.

Grose, C., and Weiner, C.P.: Prenatal diagnosis of congenital cytomegalovirus infection: two decades later. Am. J. Obstet. Gynecol. 163:447–450, 1990.

Grossman, J.: Congenital syphilis. Teratology 16:217–224, 1977.

Guderian, A.M., and Trobough, G.E.: Residues of pelvic inflammatory disease in intrauterine device users: a result of the intrauterine device of Chlamydia trachomatis infection? Am. J. Obstet. Gynecol. 154:497–503, 1986.

Gump, D.W., Gibson, M., and Ashikaga, T.: Lack of association between genital mycoplasmas and infertility. N. Engl. J. Med. 310:937–941, 1984.

Guzick, D.S., and Winn, K.: The association of chorioamnionitis with preterm delivery. Obstet. Gynecol. 65:11–16, 1985.

Gyr, T.N., Malek, A., Mathez-Loic, F., Altermatt, H.J., Bodmer, T., Nicolaides, K., and Schneider, H.: Permeation of human chorioamniotic membranes by Escherichia coli in vitro. Am. J. Obstet. Gynecol. 170:223–227, 1994.

Hagay, Z.J., Miskin, A., Goldchmit, R., Federman, A., Matzkel, A., and Mogilner, B.M.: Evaluation of two rapid tests for detection of maternal endocervical group B streptococcus: enzyme-linked immunosorbent assay and Gram stain. Obstet. Gynecol. 82:84–87, 1993.

Hagen, B., and Skjeldestad, F.E.: The outcome of pregnancy after CO_2 laser conization of the cervix. Br. J. Obstet. Gynaecol. 100:717–720, 1993.

Hain, J., Doshi, N., and Harger, J.H.: Ascending transcervical herpes simplex infection with intact fetal membranes. Obstet. Gynecol. 56:106–109, 1980.

Halliday, H.L., and Hirata, T.: Perinatal listeriosis—a review of twelve patients. Am. J. Obstet. Gynecol. 133:405–410, 1979.

Hallman, M., Bry, K., and Pitkänen, O.: Ceramide lactoside in amniotic fluid: high concentration in chorioamnionitis and in preterm labor. Am. J. Obstet. Gynecol. 161:313–318, 1989.

Hammer, B., and Wegmann, T.: Toxoplasmose und Schwangerschaft. Geburt eines Kindes bei Lymphknotentoxoplasmose der Mutter in der Frühschwangerschaft. Schweiz. Med. Wochenschr. 96:37–44, 1966.

Hare, R., and Polunin, I.: Anaerobic cocci in the vagina of native women in British North Borneo. J. Obstet. Gynaecol. Br. Emp. 67:985–989, 1960.

Harger, J.H., Meyer, M.P., Amortegui, A., Macpherson, T., Kaplan, L., and Mueller-Heubach, E.: Low incidence of positive amnionic fluid cultures in preterm labor between 27–32 weeks in the absence of clinical evidence of chorioamnionitis. Obstet. Gynecol. 77:228–234, 1991.

Harrison, H.R.: Chlamydial ophthalmia neonatorum: the dilemma of diagnosis and treatment. Am. J. Dis. Child. 139:550–551, 1985.

Harrison, H.R., English, M.G., Lee, C.K., and Alexander, E.R.: Chlamydia trachomatis infant pneumonitis: comparison with matched controls and other infant pneumonitis. N. Engl. J. Med. 298:702–708, 1978.

Harter, C.A., and Benirschke, K.: Fetal syphilis in the first trimester. Am. J. Obstet. Gynecol. 124:705–711, 1976.

Hartwick, N.G., Vermeij-Keers, C., van Elsacker-Niele, A.M.W., and Fleuren, G.J.: Embryonic malformations in a case of intrauterine parvovirus B 19 infection. Teratology 39:295–302, 1989.

Hass, M.: Hepato-adrenal necrosis with intranuclear inclusion bodies; report of a case. Am. J. Pathol. 11:127–142, 1935.

Hawrylyshyn, P., Bernstein, P., Milligan, J.E., Soldin, S., Pollard, A., and Papsin, F.R.: Premature rupture of membranes: the role of C-reactive protein in the prediction of chorioamnionitis. Am. J. Obstet. Gynecol. 147:240–246, 1983.

Hazard, G.W., Porter, P.J., and Ingall, D.: Pneumococcal laryngitis in the newborn infant. N. Engl. J. Med. 271:361–362, 1964.

Heinemann, M.-H., Tang, C.-K., and Kramer, E.E.: Placental bacteremia and maternal Shirodkar procedure. Am. J. Obstet. Gynecol. 128:226–228, 1977.

Hemminki, K., and Kyyrönen, P.: Gastrointestinal atresias and borreliosis. Lancet 1:1395, 1989.

Herbst, A.L.: Coitus and the fetus. N. Engl. J. Med. 301:1235–1236, 1979.

Herbst, P., Multier, A.-M., and Jaluvka, V.: Morphologische Untersuchungen der Plazenta einer an Parotitis erkrankten Mutter. Z. Geburtshilfe Gynakol. 174:187–193, 1970.

Herman, T.E., and Siegel, M.J.: Special imaging casebook. J. Perinatol. 14:80–82, 1994.

Herzen, J.L.v., and Benirschke, K.: Unexpected disseminated herpes simplex infection in a newborn. Obstet. Gynecol. 50:728–730, 1977.

Hill, W.C., Bolton, V., and Carlson, J.R.: Isolation of acquired immunodeficiency syndrome virus from the placenta. Am. J. Obstet. Gynecol. 157:10–11, 1987.

Hillier, S.L., Martius, J., Krohn, M., Kiviat, N., Holmes, K.K., and Eschenbach, D.A.: A case-control study of chorioamnionic infection and histologic chorioamnionitis in prematurity. N. Engl. J. Med. 319:972–978, 1988.

Hillier, S.L., Krohn, M.A., Kiviat, N.B., Watts, D.H., and Eschenbach, D.A.: Microbiologic causes and neonatal outcomes associated with chorioamnion infection. Am. J. Obstet. Gynecol. 165:955–961, 1991.

Hillier, S.L., Witkin, S.S., Krohn, M.A., Watts, D.H., Kiviat, N.B., and Eschenbach, D.A.: The relationship of amniotic fluid cytokines and preterm delivery, amniotic fluid infection, histologic chorioamnionitis, and chorioamnion infection. Obstet. Gynecol. 81:941–948, 1993.

Ho, C.-Y., and Aterman, K.: Infection of the fetus by Candida in a spontaneous abortion. Am. J. Obstet. Gynecol. 106:705–710, 1970.

Hohlfeld, P., Daffos, F., Costa, J.M., Thulliez, P., Forester, F., and Vidaud, M.: Prenatal diagnosis of congenital toxoplasmosis with a polymerase-chain-reaction test on amniotic fluid. N. Engl. J. Med. 331:695–696, 1994.

Hood, C.K., and McKinnon, G.E.: Prenatal vaccinia. Am. J. Obstet. Gynecol. 85:238–240, 1963.

Hood, I.C., Browning, D., Desa, D.J., and Whyte, R.K.: Fetal inflammatory response in second trimester candidal chorioamnionitis. Early Hum. Dev. 11:1–10, 1985.

Horky, Z., and Amon, K.: Rundzelluläre Infiltrationen der Eihäute nach Amnioskopie. Geburtshilfe Frauenheilkd. 27:1065–1074, 1967.

Hörmann, G.: Placenta und Lues: ein Beitrag zur Diagnose und Prognose konnataler Syphilis. Arch. Gynecol. 184:481–521, 1954.

Horn, L.-C., and Becker, V.: Morphologische Plazentabefunde bei klinisch-serologisch gesicherter und vermuteter Rötelninfektion in der zweiten Schwangerschaftshälfte. Z. Geburtshilfe Perinatol. 196:199–204, 1992b.

Horn, L.-C., Emmrich, P., and Krugmann, J.: Plazentabefunde bei Lues connata. Pathologe 13:146–151, 1992a.

Horn, L.-C., Büttner, W., and Horn, E.: Rötelnbedingte Plazentaveränderungen. Perinat. Med. 5:5–10, 1993.

Howe, R.S., Voychehovski, T.H., Uraizee, F., Bentsen, C., and Spear, M.L.: Neonatal group B streptococcal disease. N. Engl. J. Med. 316:1163, 1987.

Hughes, J.R., Wilfert, C.M., Moore, M., Benirschke, K., and de Hoyos-Guevara, E.: Echovirus 14 infection associated with fatal neonatal hepatic necrosis. Am. J. Dis. Child. 123:61–67, 1972.

Huikeshoven, F.J.M., Wallenburg, H.C.S., and Jahoda, M.G.J.: Diagnosis of severe fetal cytomegalovirus infection from amniotic fluid in the third trimester of pregnancy. Am. J. Obstet. Gynecol. 142:1053–1054, 1982.

Hunter, E.F., Greer, P.W., Swisher, B.L., Simons, A.R., Farshy, C.E., Crawford, J.A., and Sulzer, K.R.: Immuno-fluorescent staining of Treponema in tissues fixed with formalin. Arch. Pathol. Lab. Med. 108:878–880, 1984.

Hyde, S.R., and Giacoia, G.P.: Congenital herpes infection: placental and umbilical cord findings. Obstet. Gynecol. 81:852–855, 1993.

Hyde, S., Smotherman, J., Moore, J.I., and Altshuler, G.: A model of bacterially induced umbilical vein spasm, relevant to fetal hypoperfusion. Obstet. Gynecol. 73:966–970, 1989.

Iams, J.D., and O'Shaughnessy, R.: Antepartum versus intrapartum selective screening for maternal group B streptococcal colonization. Am. J. Obstet. Gynecol. 143:153–156, 1982.

Imamura, M., Phillips, P.E., and Mellors, R.C.: The occurrence and frequency of type C virus-like particles in placentas from patients with systemic lupus erythematosus and from normal subjects. Am. J. Pathol. 83:383–394, 1976.

Ismail, M.A., Zinaman, M.J., Lowensohn, R.I., and Moawed, A.H.: The significance of C-reactive protein levels in women with premature rupture of membranes. Am. J. Obstet. Gynecol. 151:541–544, 1985.

Jacques, S.M., and Qureshi, F.: Necrotizing funisitis: a study of 45 cases. Hum. Pathol. 23:1278–1283, 1992.

Jacques, S.M., and Qureshi, F.: Chronic intervillositis of the placenta. Arch. Pathol. Lab. Med. 117:1032–1035, 1993.

James, J.A., Thomason, J.L., Gelbart, S.M., Osypowski, P., Kaiser, P., and Hanson, L.: Is trichomoniasis often associated with bacterial vaginosis in pregnant adolescents? Am. J. Obstet. Gynecol. 166:859–863, 1992.

Janssen, P., Piekarski, G., and Korte, W.: Zum Problem des Abortes bei latenter Toxoplasma-Infektion der Frau. Klin. Wochenschr. 48:25–30, 1970.

Jauniaux, E., Nessmann, C., Imbert, M.C., Meuris, S., Puissant, F., and Hustin, J.: Morphological aspects of the placenta in HIV pregnancies. Placenta 9:633–642, 1988.

Jelliffe, E.F.P.: Low birth-weight and malarial infection of the placenta. Bull. W.H.O. 38:69–78, 1968.

Jeppson, K.G., and Reimer, L.G.: Eikenella corrodens chorioamnionitis. Obstet. Gynecol. 78:503–505, 1991.

Jewett, J.F.: Chorioamnionitis complicated by an intrauterine device. N. Engl. J. Med. 289:1251–1252, 1973.

Job, C.K., Sanchez, R.M., and Hastings, R.C.: Lepromatous placentitis and intrauterine fetal infection in lepromatous nine-banded armadillos (Dasypus novemcinctus). Lab. Invest. 56:44–48, 1987.

Johnson, D.E., Thompson, T.R., and Ferrieri, P.: Congenital candidiasis. Am. J. Dis. Child. 135:273–275, 1981a.

Johnson, F.W.A., Matheson, B.A., Williams, H., Laing, A.G., Jandiel, V., Davidson-Lamb, R., Halliday, G.J., Hobson, D., Wong, S.Y., Hadley, K.M., Moffat, M.A.J., and Postlethwaite, R.: Abortion due to infection with Chlamydia psittaci in a sheep farmer's wife. B.M.J. 290:592–594, 1985.

Johnson, J.W., Daikoku, N.H., Niebyl, J.R., Johnson, T.R.B., Khouzami, V.A., and Witter, F.R.: Premature rupture of the membranes and prolonged latency. Obstet. Gynecol. 57:547–556, 1981b.

Johnson, R.E., Nahmias, A.J., Magder, L.S., Lee, F.K., Brooks, C.A., and Snowden, C.B.: A seroepidemiologic survey of the prevalence of herpes simplex virus type 2 infection in the United States. N. Engl. J. Med. 321:7–12, 1989.

Joncas, J.H., Alfieri, C., Leyritz-Wills, M., Brochu, P., Jasmin, G., Boldogh, I., and Huang, E.-S.: Simultaneous congenital infection with Epstein-Barr virus and cytomegalovirus. N. Engl. J. Med. 304:1399–1403, 1981.

Jones, D.: Foodborne listeriosis. Lancet 336:1171–1174, 1990.

Jones, K.L., Johnson, K.A., and Chambers, C.D.: Offspring of women infected with varicella during pregnancy: a prospective study. Teratology 49:29–32, 1994.

Judge, D.M.: Congenital syphilis. In, Transplacental Effects on Fetal Health. D.G. Scarpelli and G. Migaki, eds., pp. 87–106. Liss, New York, 1988.

Kagan, B.M., Hess, B., Mirman, B., and Lundeen, E.: Meningitis in premature infants. Pediatrics 4:479–483, 1949.

Kain, K.C., and Keystone, J.S.: Recurrent hydatid disease during pregnancy. Am. J. Obstet. Gynecol. 159:1216–1217, 1988.

Kalter, S.S., Helmke, R.J., Heberling, R.L., Panigel, M., Fowler, A.K., Strickland, J.E., and Hellman, A.: C-type particles in normal human placentas. J. Natl. Cancer Inst. 50:1081–1083, 1973.

Kaplan, C., Benirschke, K., and Tarzy, B.: Placental tuberculosis in early and late pregnancy. Am. J. Obstet. Gynecol. 137:858–860, 1980.

Katz, S.L., and Wilfert, C.M.: Human immunodeficiency virus infection of newborns. N. Engl. J. Med. 320:1687–1689, 1989.

Katzenstein, A.-L., Davis, C., and Braude, A: Pulmonary changes in neonatal sepsis due to group B β-hemolytic streptococcus: relation to hyaline membrane disease. J. Infect Dis. 133:430–435, 1976.

Kaufman, H.E., and Maloney, E.D.: Multiplication of three strains of Toxoplasma gondii in tissue culture. J. Parasitol. 48:358–361, 1962.

Kaufmann, K.: Zur histologischen Diagnostik luischer Plazenten. Z. Geburtshilfe Gynakol. 93:306–313, 1928.

Kean, B.H., Kimball, A.C., and Christenson, W.N.: An epidemic of acute toxoplasmosis. J.A.M.A. 208:1002–1004, 1969.

Kellogg, S.G., Davis, C., and Benirschke, K.: Candida parapsilosis: previously unknown cause of fetal infection: a report of two cases. J. Reprod. Med. 12:159–161, 1974.

Kelly, R.W., Leask, R., and Calder, A.A.: Choriodecidual production of interleukin-8 and mechanism of parturition. Lancet 339:776–777, 1992.

Kerr, D.A.: Improved Warthin-Starry method of staining spirochetes in tissue sections. Am. J. Clin. Pathol. 8:63–67, 1938.

Kerr, K., Dealler, S.F., and Lacey, R.W.: Listeria in cook-chill food. Lancet 2:37–38, 1988.

Kessel, E.: Pelvic inflammatory disease with intrauterine device use: a reassessment. Fertil. Steril. 51:1–11, 1989.

Khodr, G., and Matossian, R.: Hydrops fetales and congenital toxoplasmosis: value of direct immunofluorescence test. Obstet. Gynecol. 51:74S–77S, 1978.

Khong, T.Y., Staples, A., Moore, L., and Byard, R.W.: Observer reliability in assessing villitis of unknown aetiology. J. Clin. Pathol. 46:208–210, 1993.

Khudr, G., and Benirschke, K.: Placental lesion in viral hepatitis. Am. J. Obstet. Gynecol. 40:381–384, 1972.

Kibrick, S., and Benirschke, K.: Severe generalized disease (encephalohepatomyocarditis) occurring in the newborn period and due to infection with Coxsackie virus, group B: evidence of intrauterine infection with this agent. Pediatrics 22:857–875, 1958.

Kida, M., Abramowsky, C.R., and Santoscoy, C.: Cryptococcosis of the placenta in a woman with acquired immunodeficiency syndrome. Hum. Pathol. 20:920–921, 1989.

Killpack, W.S.: Prenatal vaccinia. Lancet 1:388, 1963.

Kimball, A.C., Kean, B.H., and Fuchs, F.: The role of toxoplasmosis in abortion. Am. J. Obstet. Gynecol. 111:219–226, 1971.

Kimball, A.C., Kean, B.H., and Fuchs, F.: Toxoplasmosis: risk variations in New York City obstetrics patients. Am. J. Obstet. Gynecol. 119:208–214, 1974.

King, J.A., and Marks, R.A.: Pregnancy and leprosy. Am. J. Obstet. Gynecol. 76:438–442, 1958.

Kirchhoff, H., and Kräubig, H., eds.: Toxoplasmose: Praktische Fragen und Ergebnisse. Thieme, Stuttgart, 1966.

Kirschbaum, T.: Antibiotics in the treatment of preterm labor. Am. J. Obstet. Gynecol. 168:1239–1246, 1993.

Kirshon, B., Rosenfeld, B., Mari, G., and Belfort, M.: Amniotic fluid glucose and intraamniotic infection. Am. J. Obstet. Gynecol. 164:818–820, 1991.

Klatt, E.C., Pavlova, Z., Teberg, A.J., and Yonekura, M.L.: Epidemic perinatal listeriosis at autopsy. Hum. Pathol. 17:1278–1281, 1986.

Klebanoff, M.A., Nugent, R.P., and Rhoads, G.G.: Coitus during pregnancy: is it safe? Lancet 2:914–917, 1984.

Knowles, S., and Frost, T.: Umbilical cord sclerosis as an indicator of congenital syphilis. J. Clin. Pathol. 42:1157–1159, 1989.

Knox, I.C., and Hoerner, J.K.: Role of infection in premature rupture of membranes. Am. J. Obstet. Gynecol. 59:190–194, 1950.

Koh, K.S., Cole, T.L., and Orkin, A.J.: Listeria amnionitis as a cause of fetal distress. Am. J. Obstet. Gynecol. 136:261–263, 1980.

Koppe, J.G., Loewer-Sieger, D.H., and de Roever-Bonnet, H.: Results of 20-year follow-up of congenital toxoplasmosis. Lancet 1:254–256, 1986.

Koskiniemi, M., Lappalainen, M., and Hedman, K.: Toxoplasmosis needs evaluation: an overview and proposals. Am. J. Dis. Child. 143:724–728, 1989.

Kraus, G.W., and Yen, S.S.C.: Gonorrhea during pregnancy. Obstet. Gynecol. 31:258–260, 1968.

Kraybill, E.N., and Controni, G.: Septicemia and enterocolitis due to Shigella sonnei in a newborn infant. Pediatrics 42:530–531, 1968.

Krech, U., Konjajev, Z., and Jung, M.: Congenital cytomegalovirus infection in siblings from consecutive pregnancies. Helv. Paediatr. Acta 26:355–362, 1971.

Kückens, H.: Über Rundzelleninfiltrate in reifer Placenta mit Anhängen, sowie ihre Beziehungen zum Geburts- und Wochenbettverlauf. Arch. Gynecol. 167:564–621, 1938.

Kundsin, R.B., and Horne, H.W.: Is genital colonization with Mycoplasma hominis or Ureaplasma urealyticum associated with prematurity/low birth weight? Obstet. Gynecol. 74:679, 1989.

Kundsin, R.B., Driscoll, S.G., and Ming, P.-M.L.: Strain of mycoplasma associated with human reproductive failure. Science 157:1573–1574, 1967.

Kurki, T., and Ylikorkala, O.: Coitus during pregnancy is not related to bacterial vaginosis or preterm birth. Am. J. Obstet. Gynecol. 169:1130–1134, 1993.

Labarrere, C., Althabe, O., and Telenta, M.: Chronic villitis of unknown aetiology in placentae of idiopathic small for gestational age infants. Placenta 3:309–318, 1982.

Labarrere, C.A., McIntyre, J.A., and Faulk, W.P.: Immunohistologic evidence that villitis in human normal term placentas is an immunologic lesion. Am. J. Obstet. Gynecol. 162:515–522, 1990.

Lallemand, A.V., Gaillard, D.A., Paradis, P.H., and Chippaux, C.G.: Fetal listeriosis during the second trimester of gestation. Pediatr. Pathol. 12:665–671, 1992.

Lamont, R.F., Rose, M., and Elder, M.G.: Effect of bacterial products on prostaglandin E production by amnion cells. Lancet 2:1331–1333, 1985.

Lamont, R.J., Postlethwhaite, R., and MacGowan, A.P.: Listeria monocytogenes and its role in human infection. J. Infect. 17:7–28, 1988.

Lamont, R.F., Anthony, F., Myatt, L., Booth, L., Furr, P.M., and Taylor-Robinson, D.: Production of prostaglandin E$_2$ by human amnion in vitro in response to addition of media conditioned by microorganisms associated with chorioamnionitis and preterm labor. Am. J. Obstet. Gynecol. 162:819–825, 1990.

Lang, D.J., and Kummer, J.F.: Demonstration of cytomegalovirus in semen. N. Engl. J. Med. 287:756–758, 1972.

Langer, H.: Intrauterine Toxoplasma-Infektion. Thieme, Stuttgart, 1963a.

Langer, H.: Repeated congenital infection with Toxoplasma gondii. Obstet. Gynecol. 21:318–329, 1963b.

Larsen, J.W.: Congenital toxoplasmosis. Teratology 15:213–218, 1977.

Larson, H.E., Parkman, P.D., Davis, W.J., Hopps, H.E., and Meyer, H.M.: Inadvertent rubella virus vaccination during pregnancy. N. Engl. J. Med. 284:870–873, 1971.

Lastavica, C.C., Wilson, M.L., Berardi, V.P., Spielman, A., and Deblinger, R.D.: Rapid emergence of a focal epidemic of Lyme disease in coastal Massachusetts. N. Engl. J. Med. 320:133–137, 1989.

Laugier, J., Borderon, J.-C., Chantepie, A., Tabarly, J.-L., and Gold, F.: Meningite du nouveau-né a Listeria monocytogenes et contamination en maternité. Arch. Fr. Pediatr. 35:168–171, 1978.

Lavergne, E. de, Olive, D., Maurin, J., and Feugier, J.: Isolement d'une souche de "myxovirus parainfluenzae 1" chez un embryon humain, expulse au cours d'un avortement fébrile. Arch. Fr. Pediatr. 26:179–183, 1969.

Lee, N.C., Rubin, G.L., and Borucki, R.: The intrauterine device and pelvic inflammatory disease revisited: new results from the Women's Health Study. Obstet. Gynecol. 72:1–6, 1988.

Lehtonen, O.-P., Ruuskanen, O., Kero, P., Hollo, O., Erkkola, R., and Salmi, T.: Group-A streptococcal infection in the newborn. Lancet 2:1473–1474, 1984.

LeLong, M., LePage, F., Vinh, L.T., Tournier, P., and Chany, C.: Le virus de la maladie des inclusions cytomégaliques. Arch. Fr. Pediatr. 17:1–14, 1960.

Leo, M.V., Skurnick, J.H., Ganesh, V.V., Adhate, A., and Apuzzio, J.J.: Clinical chorioamnionitis is not predicted by umbilical artery Doppler velocimetry in patients with premature rupture of the membranes. Obstet. Gynecol. 79: 916–918, 1992.

LePage, F., and Schramm, P.: Aspects histologiques du placenta et des membranes dans la maladies des inclusions cytomégaliques. Gynecol. Obstet. (Paris) 57:273–279, 1958.

Lettieri, L., Vintzileos, A.M., Rodis, J.F., Albini, S.M., and Salafia, C.M.: Does "idopathic" preterm labor resulting in preterm birth exist? Am. J. Obstet. Gynecol. 168:1480–1485, 1993.

Leveno, K.J., Cox, K., and Roark, M.L.: Cervical dilatation and prematurity revisited. Obstet. Gynecol. 68:434–435, 1986.

Levin, S., Zaidel, L., and Bernstein, D.: Intrauterine infection of fetal brain. Am. J. Obstet. Gynecol. 130:597–599, 1978.

Levy, D.L.: Placental abscess as a cause of fever of unknown origin. Am. J. Obstet. Gynecol. 140:338–339, 1981.

Lewis, S.H., Reynolds-Kohler, C., Fox, H.E., and Nelson, J.A.: HIV-1 in trophoblastic and villous Hofbauer cells, and haematological precursors in eight-week fetuses. Lancet 335:565–568, 1990.

Li, L., Sheng, M.-H., Tong, S.-P., Chen, H.-Z., and Wen, Y.-M.: Transplacental transmission of hepatitis B virus. Lancet 2:872, 1986.

Lide, T.N.: Congenital tularemia. Arch. Pathol. 43:165–169, 1947.

Linnan, M.J., Mascola, L., Lou, X.D., Goulet, V., May, S., Salminen, C., Hird, D.W., Yonekura, L., Hayes, P., Weaver, R., Audurier, A., Plikaytis, B., Fannin, S.L., Kleks, A., and Broome, C.V.: Epidemic listeriosis associated with Mexican-style cheese. N. Engl. J. Med. 319: 823–828, 1988.

Livengood, C.H., Schmitt, J.W., Addison, W.A., Wrenn, J.W., and MacGruder-Habib, K.: Direct fluorescent antibody testing for endocervical Chlamydia trachomatis: factors affecting accuracy. Obstet. Gynecol. 72:803–809, 1988.

Lockwood, C.J., Senyei, A.E., Dische, R., Casal, D., Shah, K.D., Thung, S.N., Jones, L., Deligdisch, L., and Garite, T.J.: Fetal fibronectin in cervical and vaginal secretions as a predictor of preterm delivery. N. Engl. J. Med. 325:669–674, 1991.

Lopez Bernal, A., Hansell, D.J., Canete Soler, R., Keeling, J.W., and Turnbull, A.C.: Prostaglandins, chorioamnionitis and preterm labor. Br. J. Obstet. Gynaecol. 94:1156–1158, 1987.

Lossick, J.G., and Kent, H.L.: Trichomoniasis: trends in diagnosis and management. Am. J. Obstet. Gynecol. 165: 1217–1222, 1991.

Low, J.C., and Donachie, W.: Listeria in food: a veterinary perspective. Lancet 1:322, 1989.

Lucifora, G., Calabro, S., Carroccio, G., and Brigandi, A.: Immunocytochemical HBsAg evidence in placentas of asymptomatic carrier mothers. Am. J. Obstet. Gynecol. 159:839–842, 1988.

Lucifora, G., Martines, F., Calabro, S., Carroccio, G., Brigandi, A., and de Pasquale, R.: HbcAg identification in the placental cytotypes of symptom-free HBsAg-carrier mothers: a study with the immunoperoxidase method. Am. J. Obstet. Gynecol. 163:235–239, 1990.

Luder, J., and Tomson, P.R.V.: Salmonella meningitis in the newborn. Postgrad. Med. J. 39:100–102, 1963.

MacDonald, A.B., Benach, J.L., and Birgdorfer, W.: Stillbirth following maternal Lyme disease. N.Y. State J. Med. 87:615–616, 1987.

Madan, E., Meyer, M.P., and Amortegui, A.J.: Isolation of genital mycoplasmas and Chlamydia trachomatis in stillborn and neonatal autopsy material. Arch. Pathol. Lab. Med. 112:749–751, 1988.

Madan, E., Meyers, M.P., and Amorgtegui, A.J.: Histologic manifestations of perinatal genital mycoplasmal infection. Arch. Pathol. Lab. Med. 113:465–469, 1989.

Maeda, S., Mellors, R.C., Mellors, J.W., Jerabek, L.B., and Zervoudakis, I.A.: Immunohistologic detection of antigen related to primate type C retrovirus p30 in normal human placentas. Am. J. Pathol. 112:347–356, 1983.

Magliocco, A.M., Demetrick, D.J., Sarnat, H.B., and Hwang, W.S.: Varicella embryopathy. Arch. Pathol. Lab. Med. 116:181–186, 1992.

Magnusson, S.S., Oskarsson, T., Geirsson, R.T., Sveinsson, B., Steingrimsson, O., and Thorarinsson, H.: Lower genital tract infection with Chlamydia trachomatis and Neisseria gonorrhoeae in Icelandic women with salpingitis. Am. J. Obstet. Gynecol. 155:602–607, 1986.

Malan, A.F., Woods, D.L., v.d. Elst, C.W., and Meyer, M.P.: Relative placental weight in congenital syphilis. Placenta 11:3–6, 1990.

Margolis, G., and Kilham, L.: Problems of human concern arising from animal models of intrauterine and neonatal infections due to viruses: a review. II. Pathological studies. Prog. Med. Virol. 20:144–179, 1975.

Martius, J., and Eschenbach, D.A.: The role of bacterial vaginosis as a cause of amniotic fluid infection, chorioamnionitis and prematurity—a review. Arch. Gynecol. Obstet. 247:1–13, 1990.

Mason, P.R., and Brown, I.McL.: Trichomoniasis in pregnancy. Lancet 2:1025–1026, 1980.

Matorras, R., Perea, A.G., Omenaca, F., Usandizaga, J.A., Nieto, A., and Herruzo, R.: Group B streptococcus and premature rupture of membranes and preterm delivery. Gynecol. Obstet. Invest. 27:14–18, 1989.

Matsuzaki, N., Taniguchi, T., Shimoya, K., Neki, R., Okada, T., Saji, F., Nakayama, M., Suehara, N., and Tanizawa, O.: Placental interleukin-6 production is enhanced in intrauterine infection but not in labor. Am. J. Obstet. Gynecol. 168:94–97, 1993.

Maudsley, R.F., Brix, G.A., Hinton, N.A., Robertson, E.M., Bryans, A.M., and Haust, M.D.: Placental inflammation and infection. Am. J. Obstet. Gynecol. 95:648–659, 1966.

Maurus, J.N.: Hansen's disease in pregnancy. Obstet. Gynecol. 52:22–25, 1978.

McCaffree, M.A., and Altshuler, G.: Placental fluorescent-antibody studies as test for congenital cytomegalovirus infection. Lancet 1:1029–1030, 1979.

McCaffree, M.A., Altshuler, G., and Benirschke, K.: Placental coccidioidomycosis without fetal disease. Arch. Pathol. Lab. Med. 102:512–514, 1978.

McClure, H.M., and Strozier, L.M.: Perinatal listeric septicemia in a Celebese black ape. J. Am. Vet. Med. Assoc. 167:637–638, 1975.

McColgin, S.W., Hess, L.W., Martin, R.W., Martin, J.N., and Morrison, J.C.: Group B streptococcal sepsis and death in utero following funipuncture. Obstet. Gynecol. 74:464–465, 1989.

McColgin, S.W., Bennett, W.A., Roach, H., Cowan, B.D., Martin, J.N., and Morrison, J.C.: Parturitional factors associated with membrane stripping. Am. J. Obstet. Gynecol. 169:71–77, 1993.

McCord, J.R.: Syphilis of the placenta: the histologic examination of 1,085 placentas of mothers with strongly positive blood Wassermann reactions. Am. J. Obstet. Gynecol. 28:743–750, 1934.

McCormack, W.M., Almeida, P.C., Bailey, P.E., Grady, E.M., and Lee, Y.-H.: Sexual activity and vaginal colonization with genital mycoplasmas. J.A.M.A. 221:1375–1377, 1972.

McCracken, G.H.: Neonatal septicemia and meningitis. Hosp. Pract. 11:89–97, 1976.

McCracken, G.H., and Sarff, L.D.: Current status and therapy of neonatal E. coli meningitis. Hosp. Pract. 9:57–64, 1974.

McDuffie, R.S., Sherman, M.P., and Gibbs, R.S.: Amniotic fluid tumor necrosis factor-α and interleukin-1 in a rabbit model of bacterially induced preterm pregnancy loss. Am. J. Obstet. Gynecol. 167:1538–1588, 1992.

McGregor, J.A., Burns, J.C., Levin, M.J., Burlington, B., and Meiklejohn, G.: Transplacental passage of influenza A/Bangkok (H_3N_2) mimicking amniotic fluid infection syndrome. Am. J. Obstet. Gynecol. 149:856–859, 1984.

McGregor, J.A., French, J.I., Lawellin, D., Franco-Buff, A., Smith, C., and Todd, J.K.: Bacterial protease-induced reduction of chorioamniotic membrane strength and elasticity. Obstet. Gynecol. 69:167–174, 1987.

McGregor, J.A., Lawellin, D., Franco-Buff, A., and Todd, J.K.: Phospholipase C activity in microorganisms associated with reproductive tract infection. Am. J. Obstet. Gynecol. 164:682–686, 1991.

McLaren, L.C., Davis, L.E., Healy, G.R., and James, C.G.: Isolation of Trichomonas vaginalis from the respiratory tract of infants with respiratory disease. Pediatrics 71:888–890, 1983.

McLellan, M.S., Strong, J.P., Johnson, Q.R., and Dent, J.H.: Otitis media in premature infants: a histopathologic study. J. Pediatr. 61:53–57, 1962.

Meador, V.P., and Deyoe, B.L.: Intracellular localization of Brucella abortus in bovine placenta. Vet. Pathol. 26:513–315, 1989.

Medearis, D.N.: CMV immunity: imperfect but protective. N. Engl. J. Med. 306:985–986, 1982.

Mellgren, J., Alm, L., and Kjessler, A.: The isolation of Toxoplasma from the human placenta and uterus. Acta Pathol. Microbiol. Scand. 30:59–67, 1952.

Mendoza, E., Jorda, M., Rafel, E., Simon, A., and Andrada, E.: Invasion of human embryo by Enterobius vermicularis. Arch. Pathol. Lab. Med. 111:761–762, 1987.

Menez-Bautista, R., Fikrig, S.M., Pahwa, S., Sarangadharan, M.G., and Stoneburner, R.L.: Monozygotic twins discordant for the acquired immunodeficiency syndrome. Am. J. Dis. Child. 140:678–679, 1986.

Miller, J.M., Hill, G.B., Welt, S.I., and Pupkin, M.J.: Bacterial colonization of amniotic fluid in the presence of ruptured membranes. Am. J. Obstet. Gynecol. 137:451–458, 1980a.

Miller, J.M., Pupkin, M.J., and Hill, G.B.: Bacterial colonization of premature labor. Am. J. Obstet. Gynecol. 136:796–804, 1980b.

Miller, L.H., Reifsnyder, D.N., and Martinez, S.A.: Late onset of disease in congenital toxoplasmosis. Clin. Pediatr. 10:78–80, 1971.

Mills, J.L., Harlap, S., and Harley, E.E.: Should coitus late in pregnancy be discouraged? Lancet 2:136–138, 1981.

Mitchell, J.E., and McCall, F.C.: Transplacental infection by herpes simplex virus. Am. J. Dis. Child. 106:207–209, 1963.

Mitchell, M.D., Trautman, M.S., and Dudley, D.J.: Cytokine networking in the placenta. Placenta 14:249–275, 1993.

Mitsuda, T., Yokota, S., Mori, T., Ibe, M., Ookawa, N., Shimizu, H., Aihara, Y., Yoshida, N., Kosuge, K., and Matsuyama, S.: Demonstration of mother-to-infant transmission of hepatitis B virus by means of polymerase chain reaction. Lancet 2:886–888, 1989.

Modlin, J.F.: Perinatal echovirus infection: insight from a literature review of 61 cases of serious infection and 16 outbreaks in nurseries. Rev. Infect. Dis. 8:918–926, 1986.

Molello, J.A., Jensen, R., Flint, J.C., and Collier, J.R.: Placental pathology. I. Placental lesions of sheep experimentally infected with Brucella ovis. Am. J. Vet. Res. 24:897–904, 905–911, 915–922, 1963.

Moller, M., Thomsen, A.C., Borch, K., Dinesen, K., and Zdravkovic, M.: Rupture of fetal membranes and premature delivery associated with group B streptococci in urine of pregnant women. Lancet 2:69–70, 1984.

Molnar-Nadasdy, G., Haesly, I., Reed, J., and Altshuler, G.: Placental cryptococcus in a mother with systemic lupus erythematosus. Arch. Pathol. Lab. Med. 118:757–759, 1994.

Monif, G.R.G.: Antenatal group A streptococcal infection. Am. J. Obstet. Gynecol. 123:213–214, 1975.

Monif, G.R.G., and Dische, R.: Viral placentitis in congenital cytomegalovirus infection. Am. J. Clin. Pathol. 58:445–449, 1972.

Monif, G.R.G., Sever, J.L., Schiff, G.M., and Traub, R.G.: Isolation of rubella virus from products of conception. Am. J. Obstet. Gynecol. 91:1143–1146, 1965.

Monif, G.R.G., Kellner, K.R., and Donnelly, W.H.: Congenital herpes simplex type II infection. Am. J. Obstet. Gynecol. 152:1000–1002, 1985.

Moore, C.G., and Schnurrenberger, P.R.: A review of naturally occurring Brucella abortus infections in wild mammals. J. Am. Vet. Med. Assoc. 179:1105–1122, 1981.

Morales, W.J., and Lim, D.: Reduction of group B streptococcal maternal and neonatal infections in preterm pregnancies with premature rupture of membranes through a rapid identification test. Am. J. Obstet. Gynecol. 157:13–16, 1987.

Morales, W.J., Lim, D.V., and Walsh, A.F.: Prevention of neonatal group B streptococcal sepsis by use of rapid screening test and selective intrapartum chemoprophylaxis. Am. J. Obstet. Gynecol. 155:979–983, 1986.

Moroi, K., Saito, S., Kurata, T., Sata, T., and Yanagida, M.: Fetal death associated with measles virus infection of the placenta. Am. J. Obstet. Gynecol. 164:1107–1108, 1991.

Morris, I.J., and Ribeiro, C.D.: Listeria monocytogenes and pate. Lancet 2:1285–1286, 1989.

Mortimer, G., MacDonald, D.J., and Smeeth, A.: A pilot study of the frequency and significance of placental villitis. Br. J. Obstet. Gynaecol. 92:629–633, 1985.

Moss, T.R., Nicholls, A., Viercant, P., Gregson, S., and Hawkswell, J.: Chlamydia trachomatis and infertility. Lancet 2:281, 1986.

Mostoufi-Zadeh, M., Driscoll, S.G., Biano, S.A., and Kundsin, R.B.: Placental evidence of cytomegalovirus infection of the fetus and neonate. Arch. Pathol. Lab. Med. 108:403–406, 1984.

Mühlemann, K., Miller, R.K., Metlay, L., and Menegus, M.A.: Cytomegalovirus infection of the human placenta: an immunocytochemical study. Hum. Pathol. 23:1234–1237, 1992.

Müller, G.: Die primäre Fruchtwasserinfektion und die Möglichkeiten ihrer Entstehung. Virchows Arch. 328:68–97, 1956.

Mulligan, M.J., and Stiehm, E.R.: Neonatal hepatitis B infection: clinical and immunological considerations. J. Perinatol. 14:2–9, 1994.

Mundy, D.C., Schinazi, R.F., Gerber, A.R., Nahmias, A.J., and Randall, H.W.: Human immunodeficiency virus isolated from amniotic fluid. Lancet 2:459–460, 1987.

Naessens, A., Foulon, W., Breynart, J., and Lauwers, S.: Postpartum bacteremia and placental colonization with genital mycoplasmas and pregnancy outcome. Am. J. Obstet. Gynecol. 160:647–650, 1989.

Naeye, R.L.: Causes of the excessive rates of perinatal mortality and prematurity in pregnancies complicated by maternal urinary-tract infections. N. Engl. J. Med. 300:819–823, 1979a.

Naeye, R.L.: Coitus and associated amniotic-fluid infections. N. Engl. J. Med. 301:1198–1200, 1979b.

Naeye, R.L.: Coitus and amniotic-fluid infections. N. Engl. J. Med. 302:633, 1980.

Naeye, R.L.: Safety of coitus in pregnancy. Lancet 2:686, 1981.

Naeye, R.L.: Factors that predispose to premature rupture of fetal membranes. Obstet. Gynecol. 60:93–98, 1982.

Naeye, R.L.: Adverse pregnancy outcome and coitus. Obstet. Gynecol. 62:400, 1983.

Naeye, R.L.: Coitus and preterm delivery. Pediatr. Pathol. 5:106–197, 1986.

Naeye, R.L.: Acute bacterial chorioamnionitis. In, Transplacental Effects on Fetal Health. D.G. Scarpelli and G. Migaki, eds., pp. 73–86. Liss, New York, 1988a.

Naeye, R.L.: Antenatal malarial infection. In, Transplacental Effects on Fetal Health. D.G. Scarpelli and G. Migaki, eds., pp. 165–173. Liss, New York, 1988b.

Naeye, R.L., and Peters, E.C.: Amniotic fluid infections with intact membranes leading to perinatal death: a prospective study. Pediatrics 61:171–177, 1978.

Naeye, R.L., and Peters, E.C.: Causes and consequences of premature rupture of fetal membranes. Lancet 1:192–194, 1980.

Naeye, R.L., Maisels, M.J., Lorenz, R.P., and Botti, J.J.: The clinical significance of placental villous edema. Pediatrics 71:588–594, 1983.

Nagata, K., Nakamura, Y., Hosokawa, Y., Nakashima, T., Nagasue, N., Kabashima, K., and Hidaka, S.: Intrauterine Candida infection in premature baby. Acta Pathol. Jpn. 31:695–699, 1981.

Nahmias, A.J., Alford, C.A., and Korones, S.B.: Infection of the newborn with herpes-virus. Adv. Pediatr. 17:185–226, 1970.

Naib, Z.M., Nahmias, A.J., Josey, W.E., and Wheeler, J.H.: Association of maternal genital herpetic infection with spontaneous abortion. Obstet. Gynecol. 35:260–263, 1970.

Naidoo, P., and Hirsch, H.: Prenatal vaccinia. Lancet 1: 196–197, 1963.

Nakamura, Y., Yamamoto, S., Tanaka, S., Yano, H., Nishimura, G., Saito, Y., Tanaka, T., Tanimura, A., Hirose, F., Fukuda, S., Shingu, M., and Hashimoto, T.: Herpes simplex viral infection in human neonates: an immunohistochemical and electron microscopic study. Hum. Pathol. 16:1091–1097, 1985.

Nash, L., Janovski, N.A., and Bysshe, S.M.: Localized clostridial chorioamnionitis. Obstet. Gynecol. 21:481–485, 1963.

Navarro, C., and Blanc, W.A.: Subacute necrotizing funisitis: a variant of cord inflammation with a high rate of perinatal infection. J. Pediatr. 85:689–697, 1974.

Neilson, J.P., and Mutambira, M.: Coitus, twin pregnancy, and preterm labor. Am. J. Obstet. Gynecol. 160:416–418, 1989.

Nelson, K.E., Warren, D., Tomasi, A.M., Raju, T.N., and Vidyasagar, D.: Transmission of neonatal listeriosis in a delivery room. Am. J. Dis. Child. 139:903–905, 1985.

Nemir, R.L., and O'Hare, D.: Congenital tuberculosis: review and diagnostic criteria. Am. J. Dis. Child. 139: 284–287, 1985; 140:740–741, 1986.

Nessmann-Emmanuelli, C., Paul, G., Amiel-Tison, C., Goujard, J., Firtion, G., Henrion, R., and Sureau, C.: Frottis placentaires en maternité: intérêt pour le diagnostic précoce des infections bactériennes néonatales par contamination materno-foetale. J. Gynecol. Obstet. Biol. Reprod. (Paris) 12:373–380, 1983.

Newton, E.R., Prihoda, T.J., and Gibbs, R.S.: Logistic regression analysis of risk factors for intra-amniotic infection. Obstet. Gynecol. 73:571–575, 1989.

Nickerson, C.W.: Gonorrhea amnionitis. Obstet. Gynecol. 42:815–817, 1973.

Nieman, R.E., and Lorber, B.: Listeriosis in adults: a changing pattern; report of eight cases and review of the literature, 1968–1978. Rev. Infect. Dis. 2:207–227, 1980.

Nokes, J.M., Claiborne, H.A., Thornton, W.N., and Yiu-Tang, H.: Extrauterine pregnancy associated with tuberculous salpingitis and congenital tuberculosis in the fetus. Obstet. Gynecol. 9:206–211, 1957.

Norwitz, E.R., Bernal, A.L., and Starkey, P.M.: Tumor necrosis factor-α selectively stimulates prostaglandin $F_{2\alpha}$ production by macrophages in human term decidua. Am. J. Obstet. Gynecol. 167:815–820, 1992a.

Norwitz, E.R., Starkey, P.M., and Bernal, A.L.: Prostaglandin D_2 production by term human decidua: cellular origins defined using flow cytometry. Obstet. Gynecol. 80:440–445, 1992b.

Novak, R.W., and Platt, M.S.: Significance of placental findings in early-onset group B streptococcal neonatal sepsis. Clin. Pediatr. 24:256–258, 1985.

Nugent, R.P [for the vaginal infection and pregnancy study]: Ureaplasma urealyticum and pregnancy outcome: results of an observational study and clinical trial. Am. J. Epidemiol. 128:929–930, 1988.

Ogilvie, M.M., and Tearne, C.F.: Spontaneous abortion after hand-foot-and-mouth disease caused by Coxsackie virus A 16. B.M.J. 281:1527–1528, 1980.

Ohlsson, A., and Wang, E.: An analysis of antenatal tests to detect infection in preterm premature rupture of the membranes. Am. J. Obstet. Gynecol. 162:809–818, 1990.

Ohyama, M., Itani, Y., Tanaka, Y., Goto, A., and Sasaki, Y.: Syphilitic placentitis: demonstration of Treponema pallidum by immunoperoxidase staining. Virchows Arch. A Pathol. Anat. Histopathol. 417:343–345, 1990.

Okita, J.R., Johnston, J.M., and MacDonald, P.C.: Source of prostaglandin precursor in human fetal membranes: arachidonic acid content of amnion and chorion laeve in diamnionic-dichorionic twin placentas. Am. J. Obstet. Gynecol. 147:477–482, 1983.

Olding, L.: Value of placentitis as a sign of intrauterine infection in human subjects. Acta Pathol. Microbiol. Scand. [A] 78:256–264, 1970.

Olding, L., and Philipson, L.: Two cases of listeriosis in the newborn, associated with placental infection. Acta Pathol. Microbiol. Scand. 48:24–30, 1960.

Oppenheimer, E.H., and Hardy, J.B.: Congenital syphilis in the newborn infant: clinical and pathological observations in recent cases. Johns Hopkins Med. J. 129:63–82, 1971.

Oriel, J.D., Partridge, B.M., Denny, M.J., and Coleman, J.C.: Genital yeast infections. B.M.J. 4:761–764, 1972.

Ornoy, A., Segal, S., Nishmi, M., Simcha, A., and Polishuk, W.Z.: Fetal and placental pathology in gestational rubella. Am. J. Obstet. Gynecol. 116:949–956, 1973.

Ornoy, A., Dudai, M., and Sadovsky, E.: Placental and fetal pathology in infectious mononucleosis: a possible indicator for Epstein-Barr virus teratogenicity. Diagn. Gynecol. Obstet. 4:11–16, 1982.

Ortel, S.: Listerienausscheider und ihre epidemiologische Bedeutung. Munchen Med. Wochenschr. 117:1145–1148, 1975.

Osborn, G.R.: Congenital pneumonia. Lancet 1:275, 1962.

Paavonen, J., Critchlow, C.W., DeRouen, T., Stevens, C.E., Kiviat, N., Brunham, R.C., Stamm, W.E., Kuo, C.-C., Hyde, K.E., Corey, L., Eschenbach, D.A., and Holmes, K.K.: Etiology of cervical inflammation. Am. J. Obstet. Gynecol. 154:556–564, 1986.

Panem, S.: C-type virus expression in the placenta. Curr. Top. Pathol. 66:175–189, 1979.

Pankuch, G.A., Appelbaum, P.C., Lorenz, R.P., Botti, J.J., Schachter, J., and Naeye, R.L.: Placental microbiology and histology and the pathogenesis of chorioamnionitis. Obstet. Gynecol. 64:802–806, 1984.

Pankuch, G.A., Cherouny, P.H., Botti, J.J., and Appelbaum, P.C.: Amniotic fluid leukotaxis assay as an early indicator of chorioamnionitis. Am. J. Obstet. Gynecol. 161:802–807, 1989.

Pao, C.C., Kao, S.-M., Wang, H.-C., and Lee, C.C.: Intraamniotic detection of Chlamydia trachomatis deoxyribonucleic acid sequences by polymerase chain reaction. Am. J. Obstet. Gynecol. 164:1295–1299, 1991.

Parker, C.R., and Wendel, G.D.: The effects of syphilis on endocrine function of the fetoplacental unit. Am. J. Obstet. Gynecol. 159:1327–1331, 1988.

Paryani, S.G., and Arvin, A.M.: Intrauterine infection with varicella-zoster virus after maternal varicella. N. Engl. J. Med. 314:1542–1546, 1986.

Pass, M.A., Khare, S., and Dillon, H.C.: Twin pregnancies: incidence of group B streptococcal colonization and disease. J. Pediatr. 97:635–637, 1980a.

Pass, M.A., Gray, B.M., and Dillon, H.C.: Puerperal and perinatal infections with group B streptococci. Am. J. Obstet. Gynecol. 143:147–152, 1982.

Pass, R.F., Stagno, S., Myers, G.J., and Alford, C.A.: Outcome of symptomatic congenital cytomegalovirus infection: results of long-term longitudinal follow-up. Pediatrics 66:758–762, 1980b.

Pass, R.F., Little, E.A., Stagno, S., Britt, W.J., and Alford, C.A.: Young children as a probable source of maternal and congenital cytomegalovirus infection. N. Engl. J. Med. 316:1366–1370, 1987.

Pastorek, J.G., Mroczkowski, T.F., and Martin, D.H.: Finetuning the fluorescent antibody test for chlamydial infections in pregnancy. Obstet. Gynecol. 72:957–960, 1988.

Peeters, F., Snauwaert, R., Segers, J., van Cutsem, J., and Amery, W.: Observations on candidal vaginitis: vaginal pH, microbiology, and cytology. Am. J. Obstet. Gynecol. 112:80–86, 1972.

Peevy, K.J., and Chalhub, E.G.: Occult group B streptococcal infection: an important cause of intrauterine asphyxia. Am. J. Obstet. Gynecol. 146:989–990, 1983.

Perkins, R.P.: Adverse pregnancy outcome and coitus. Obstet. Gynecol. 62:399–400, 1983.

Perrin, E.V.D., and Bel, J.K.-V.: Degeneration and calcification of the umbilical cord. Obstet. Gynecol. 26:371–373, 1965.

Peterson, C.M., Johnson, S.L., Kelly, J.V., and Kelly, P.C.: Coccidial meningitis and pregnancy: a case report. Obstet. Gynecol. 73:835–836, 1989.

Petrilli, E.S., D'Ablaing, G., and Ledger, W.J.: Listeria monocytogenes chorioamnionitis: diagnosis by transabdominal amniocentesis. Obstet. Gynecol. 55:5S–8S, 1980.

Peuchmaur, M., Pons, J.C., Papiernik, E., and Delfraissy, J.F.: Isolation of acquired immunodeficiency syndrome virus from the placenta. Am. J. Obstet. Gynecol. 160:765, 1989.

Phillips, C.A., Maeck, J.V.S., Rogers, W.A., and Savel, H.: Intrauterine rubella infection following immunization with rubella vaccine. J.A.M.A. 213:624–625, 1970.

Pickard, R.E.: Varicella pneumonia in pregnancy. Am. J. Obstet. Gynecol. 101:504–508, 1968.

Pisarski, T., Breborowicz, H., and Prybora, L.A.: Leucocytic infiltration in the placenta and membranes. Biol. Neonate 5:129–150, 1963.

Platz-Christensen, J.J., Mattsby-Baltzer, I., Thomsen, P., and Wiqvist, N.: Endotoxin and interleukin-1α in the cervical mucus and vaginal fluid of pregnant women with bacterial vaginosis. Am. J. Obstet. Gynecol. 169:1161–1166, 1993.

Pletcher, B.A., Williams, M.K., Mulivor, R.A., Barth, D., Linder, C., and Rawlinson, K.: Intrauterine cytomegalovirus infection presenting as fetal meconium peritonitis. Obstet. Gynecol. 78:903–905, 1991.

Pollack, R.N., Sklarin, N.T., Rao, S., and Divon, M.Y.: Metastatic placental lymphoma associated with maternal human immunodeficiency virus infection. Obstet. Gynecol. 81:856–857, 1993.

Polunin, I.: Infertility and depopulation: a study of the Murut tribes of North Borneo. Lancet 2:1005–1008, 1958.

Popek, E.J.: Granulomatous villitis due to Toxoplasma gondii. Pediatr. Pathol. 12:281–288, 1992.

Porreco, R.P., and Haverkamp, A.D.: Brucellosis in pregnancy. Obstet. Gynecol. 44:597–602, 1974.

Potkul, R.K., Moawad, A.H., and Ponto, K.L.: The association of subclinical infection with preterm labor: the role of C-reactive protein. Am. J. Obstet. Gynecol. 153:642–645, 1985.

Pritchard, J.A., and Whalley, P.J.: Abortion complicated by Clostridium perfringens infection. Am. J. Obstet. Gynecol. 111:484–490, 1971.

Pugh, V.W., and Vakil, S.: Salmonella typhimurium meningitis in a premature infant during the neonatal period. Arch. Dis. Child. 27:473–474, 1952.

Purtilo, D.T., Bhawan, J., Liao, S., Brutus, A., Yang, J.P.S., and Balogh, K.: Fatal varicella in a pregnant woman and a baby. Am. J. Obstet. Gynecol. 127:208–209, 1977.

Pyati, S.P., Pildes, R.S., Jacobs, N.M., Ramamurthy, R.S., Yeh, T.F., Raval, D.S., Lilien, L.D., Amma, P., and Metzger, W.I.: Penicillin in infants weighing two kilograms or less with early-onset group B streptococcal disease. N. Engl. J. Med. 308:1383–1389, 1983.

Quagliarello, J.R., Passalaqua, A.M., Greco, M.A., Zinberg, S., and Young, B.K.: Ballantyne's triple edema syndrome: prenatal diagnosis with ultrasound and maternal renal biopsy findings. Am. J. Obstet. Gynecol. 132:580–581, 1978.

Quan, A., and Strauss, L.: Congenital cytomegalic inclusion disease: observations in a macerated fetus with congenital defect, including study of the placenta. Am. J. Obstet. Gynecol. 83:1240–1247, 1962.

Quinn, P.A., Shewchuk, A.B., Shuber, J., Lie, K.I., Ryan, E., Chipman, M.L., and Bocilla, D.M.: Efficacy of antibiotic therapy in preventing spontaneous pregnancy loss among couples colonized with genital mycoplasmas. Am. J. Obstet. Gynecol. 145:239–250, 1983.

Quinn, P.A., Butany, J., Chipman, M., Taylor, J., and Hannah, W.: A prospective study of microbial infection in stillbirths and neonatal death. Am. J. Obstet. Gynecol. 151:238–249, 1985.

Quinn, P.A., Butany, J., Taylor, J., and Hannah, W.: Chorioamnionitis: its association with pregnancy outcome and microbial infection. Am. J. Obstet. Gynecol. 156:379–387, 1987.

Quinn, T.C., Jacobs, R.F., Mertz, G.J., Hook, E.W., and Locksley, R.M.: Congenital malaria: a report of four cases and a review. J. Pediatr. 101:229–232, 1982.

Ramsey, A.M.: The significance of Clostridium welchii in the cervical swab and blood stream in post partum and post abortum sepsis. J. Obstet. Gynaecol. Br. Emp. 56:247–258, 1949.

Raoult, D., and Stein, A.: Q fever during pregnancy—a risk for women, fetuses, and obstetricians. N. Engl. J. Med. 330:371, 1994.

Rappaport, F., Rabinovitz, M., Toaff, R., and Krochik, N.: Genital listeriosis as a cause of recurrent abortion. Lancet 1:1273–1275, 1960.

Ravid, R., and Toaff, R.: Solitary abscess of the placenta in a pregnancy treated with cerclage. Int. Surg. 61:553–554, 1976.

Read, J.S., and Klebanoff, M.A., for the Vaginal Infection and Prematurity Study Group: Sexual intercourse during pregnancy and preterm delivery: effects of vaginal microorganisms. Am. J. Obstet. Gynecol. 168:514–519, 1993.

Redline, R.W., and Abramowsky, C.R.: Clinical and pathological aspects of recurrent villitis [abstract]. Lab. Invest. 50:10P, 1984.

Redline, R.W., and Abramowsky, C.R.: Clinical and pathological aspects of recurrent villitis. Hum. Pathol. 16:727–731, 1985.

Redline, R.W., and Lu, C.Y.: Role of local immunosuppression in murine fetoplacental listeriosis. J. Clin. Invest. 79:1234–1241, 1987.

Redline, R.W., and Lu, C.Y.: Specific defects in the anti-listerial immune response in discrete regions of the murine uterus and placenta account for susceptibility to infection. J. Immunol. 140:3947–3955, 1988.

Redline, R.W., and Patterson, P.: Villitis of unknown etiology is associated with major infiltration of fetal tissues by maternal inflammatory cells. Am. J. Pathol. 143:473–479, 1993.

Redline, R.W., Shea, C.M., Papaionnou, V.E., and Lu, C.Y.: Defective anti-listerial responses in deciduoma of pseudopregnant mice. Am. J. Pathol. 133:485–497, 1988.

Regan, J.A., Chao, S., and James, L.S.: Premature rupture of membranes, preterm delivery, and group B streptococcal colonization of mothers. Am. J. Obstet. Gynecol. 141:184–186, 1981.

Remington, J.S., and Klein, J.O., eds.: Infectious Diseases of the Fetus and Newborn Infant. 2nd Ed. Saunders, Philadelphia, 1983.

Remington, J.S., Newell, J.W., and Cavanaugh, E.: Spontaneous abortion and chronic toxoplasmosis: report of a case, with isolation of the parasite. Obstet. Gynecol. 24:25–31, 1964.

Rettig, P.J., and Altshuler, G.: Rat model of prenatal Chlamydial trachomatis (Ct) infection. In, Proceedings 21st Interscience Conference on Antimicrobial Agents and Chemotherapy. American Society of Microbiologists. Abstract 517, 1981.

Rhatigan, R.M.: Congenital cutaneous candidiasis. Am. J. Dis. Child. 116:545–546, 1968.

Rhyan, J.C., Stackhouse, L.L., and Quinn, W.J.: Fetal and placental lesions in bovine abortion due to Tritrichomonas foetus. Vet. Pathol. 25:350–355, 1988.

Ricci, J.M., Fojaco, R.M., and O'Sullivan, M.J.: Congenital syphilis: the University of Miami/Jackson Memorial Medical Center experience, 1986–1988. Obstet. Gynecol. 74:687–693, 1989.

Robb, J.A., Benirschke, K., and Barmeyer, R.: Intrauterine latent herpes simplex virus infection. I. Spontaneous abortion. Hum. Pathol. 17:1196–1209, 1986a.

Robb, J.A., Benirschke, K., Mannino, F., and Voland, J.: Intrauterine latent herpes simplex virus infection. II. Latent neonatal infection. Hum. Pathol. 17:1210–1217, 1986b.

Romano, N., Romano, F., and Carollo, F.: T-strain of mycoplasma in bronchopneumonic lungs of an aborted fetus. N. Engl. J. Med. 285:950–952, 1971.

Romem, Y., and Artal, R.: C-reactive protein as a predictor for chorioamnionitis in cases of premature rupture of the membranes. Am. J. Obstet. Gynecol. 150:546–550, 1984.

Romero, R.: Is genital colonization with Mycoplasma hominis or Ureaplasma urealyticum associated with prematurity/low birth weight? Obstet. Gynecol. 74:679–680, 1989.

Romero, R., Emamian, M., Quintero, R., Wan, M., Hobbins, J.C., and Mitchell, M.D.: Amniotic fluid prostaglandin levels and intra-amniotic infections. Lancet 1:1380, 1986.

Romero, R., Kadar, N., Hobbins, J.C., and Duff, G.W.: Infection and labor: the detection of endotoxin in amniotic fluid. Am. J. Obstet. Gynecol. 157:815–819, 1987a.

Romero, R., Quintero, R., Emamiam, M., Wan, M., Grzyboski, C.L.T., Hobbins, J.C., and Mitchell, M.D.: Arachidonate lipoxygenase metabolites in amniotic fluid of women with intra-amniotic infection and preterm labor. Am. J. Obstet. Gynecol. 157:1457–1460, 1987b.

Romero, R., Roslansky, P., Oyarzun, E., Wan, M., Emamian, M., Novitsky, T.J., Gould, M.J., and Hobbins, J.C.: II. Bacterial endotoxin in amniotic fluid and its relationship to the onset of preterm labor. Am. J. Obstet. Gynecol. 158:1044–1049, 1988a.

Romero, R., Scharf, K., Mazor, M., Emamian, M., Hobbins, J.C., and Ryan, J.L.: The clinical value of gas-liquid chromatography in the detection of intra-amniotic microbial invasion. Obstet. Gynecol. 72:44–50, 1988b.

Romero, R., Wu, Y.K., Mazor, M., Hobbins, J.C., and Mitchell, M.D.: Increased amniotic fluid leukotriene C_4 concentration in term human parturition. Am. J. Obstet. Gynecol. 159:655–657, 1988c.

Romero, R., Brody, D.T., Oyarzun, E., Mazor, M., Wu, Y.K., Hobbins, J.C., and Durum, S.K.: Infection and labor. III. Interleukin-1: a signal for the onset of parturition. Am. J. Obstet. Gynecol. 160:1117–1123, 1989a.

Romero, R., Manogue, K.R., Mitchell, M.D., Wu, Y.K., Oyarzun, E., Hobbins, J.C., and Cerami, A.: Infection and labor. IV. Cachectin-tumor necrosis factor in the amniotic fluid of women with intraamniotic infection and preterm labor. Am. J. Obstet. Gynecol. 161:336–341, 1989b.

Romero, R., Mazor, M., Oyarzun, E., Sirtori, M., Wu, Y.K., and Hobbins, J.C.: Is genital colonization with Mycoplasma hominis or Ureaplasma urealyticum associated with prematurity/low birth weight? Obstet. Gynecol. 73:532–536, 1989c.

Romero, R., Oyarzun, E., Mazor, M., Sirtori, M., Hobbins, J.C., and Bracken, M.: Meta-analysis of the relationship between asymptomatic bacteriuria and preterm delivery/low birth weight. Obstet. Gynecol. 73:576–582, 1989d. Romero, R., Sirtori, M., Oyarzun, E., Avila, C., Mazor, M., Callahan, R., Sabo, V., Athanassiadis, A.P., and Hobbins, J.C.: Infection and labor. V. Prevalence, microbiology, and clinical significance of intraamniotic infection in women with preterm labor and intact membranes. Am. J. Obstet. Gynecol. 161:817–824, 1989e.

Romero, R., Wu, Y.K., Brody, D.T., Oyarzun, E., Duff, G.W., and Durum, S.K.: Human decidua: a source of interleukin-1. Obstet. Gynecol. 73:31–34, 1989f.

Romero, R., Gonzalez, R., Sepulveda, W., Brandt, F., Ramirez, M., Sorokin, Y., Mazor, M., Treadwell, M.C., and Cotton, D.B.: Infection and labor. VIII. Microbial invasion of the amniotic cavity in patients with suspected cervical incompetence: prevalence and clinical significance. Am. J. Obstet. Gynecol. 167:1086–1091, 1992a.

Romero, R., Mazor, M., Sepulveda, W., Avila, C., Copeland, D., and Williams, J.: Tumor necrosis factor in preterm and term labor. Am. J. Obstet. Gynecol. 166:1576–1587, 1992b.

Romero, R., Salafia, C.M., Athanassiadis, A.P., Hanaoka, S., Mazor, M., Sepulveda, W., and Bracken, M.B.: The relationship between acute inflammatory lesions of the preterm placenta and amniotic fluid microbiology. Am. J. Obstet. Gynecol. 166:1382–1388, 1992c.

Romero, R., Sepulveda, W., Mazor, M., Brandt, F., Cotton, D.B., Dinarello, C.A., and Mitchell, M.D.: The natural interleukin-1 receptor antagonist in term and preterm parturition. Am. J. Obstet. Gynecol. 167:863–872, 1992d.

Romero, R., Baumann, P., Gomez, R., Salafia, C., Rittenhouse, L., Barberio, D., Behnke, E., Cotton, D.B., and Mitchell, M.D.: The relationship between spontaneous rupture of membranes, labor, and microbial invasion of the amniotic cavity and amniotic fluid concentrations of prostaglandins and thromboxane B$_2$ in term pregnancy. Am. J. Obstet. Gynecol. 168:1654–1668, 1993.

Rosenstein, D.L., and Navarrete-Reyna, A.: Cytomegalic inclusion disease. Am. J. Obstet. Gynecol. 89:220–224, 1964.

Rothbard, M.J., Gregory, T., and Salerno, L.J.: Intrapartum gonococcal amnionitis. Am. J. Obstet. Gynecol. 121:565–566, 1975.

Royston, D., and Geoghegan, F.: Amniotic fluid infection with intact membranes in relation to stillborns. Obstet. Gynecol. 65:745–746, 1985.

Ruben, B., Band, J.D., Wong, P., and Colville, J.: Person-to-person transmission of Brucella melitensis. Lancet 337:14–15, 1991.

Ruffolo, E.H., Wilson, R.B., and Lyle, W.A.: Listeria monocytogenes as a cause of pregnancy wastage. Obstet. Gynecol. 19:533–536, 1962.

Rusan, P., Adam, R.D., Petersen, E.A., Ryan, K.J., Sinclair, N.A., and Weinstein, L.: Haemophilus influenzae: an important cause of maternal and neonatal infections. Obstet. Gynecol. 77:92–96, 1991.

Rüschoff, J., Böger, A., and Zwiens, G.: Chronic placentitis —a clinicopathological study. Arch. Gynecol. 237:19–25, 1985.

Russell, P.: Inflammatory lesions of the human placenta. III. The histopathology of villitis of unknown aetiology. Placenta 1:227–244, 1980

Russell, P., and Altshuler, G.: Placental abnormalities of congenital syphilis: a neglected aid to diagnosis. Am. J. Dis. Child. 128:160–163, 1974.

Russell, P., Atkinson, K., and Krishnan, L.: Recurrent reproductive failure due to severe placental villitis of unknown etiology. J. Reprod. Med. 24:93–98, 1980.

Ryan Jr., G.M., Abdella, T.N., McNeeley, S.G., Baselski, V.S., and Drummond, D.E.: Chlamydia trachomatis infection in pregnancy and effect of treatment on outcome. Am. J. Obstet. Gynecol. 162:34–39, 1990.

Sachdev, R., Nuovo, G.J., Kaplan, C., and Greco, M.A.: In situ hybridization analysis for cytomegalovirus in chronic villitis. Pediatr. Pathol. 10:909–917, 1990.

Sacker, I., Walker, M., and Brunell, P.A.: Abscess in newborn infants caused by mycoplasma. Pediatrics 46:303–304, 1970.

Saigal, S., Eisele, W.A., and Chernesky, M.A.:Congenital cytomegalovirus infection in a pair of dizygotic twins. Am. J. Dis. Child. 136:1094–1095, 1982a.

Saigal, S., Lunyk, O., Bryce-Larhe, R.P., and Chernesky, M.A.: The outcome of children with congenital cytomegalovirus infection: a longitudinal follow-up study. Am. J. Dis. Child. 136:896–901, 1982b.

Saito, K., Koizumi, F., and Sumiyoshi, Y.: Viral placentitis— a case report. Acta Pathol. Jpn. 27:275–282, 1977.

Saito, F., Yutani, C., Imakita, M., Ishibashi-Veda, H., Kanzaki, T., and Chiba, Y.: Giant cell pneumonia caused by varicella zoster virus in a neonate. Arch. Pathol. Lab. Med. 113:201–203, 1989.

Salafia, C.M., Silberman, L., Herrera, N.E., and Mahoney, M.J.: Placental pathology at term associated with elevated midtrimester maternal serum α-fetoprotein concentration. Am. J. Obstet. Gynecol. 158:1064–1066, 1988.

Salafia, C.M., Weigl, C., and Silberman, L.: The prevalence and distribution of acute placental inflammation in uncomplicated term pregnancies. Obstet. Gynecol. 73:383–389, 1989.

Salafia, C.M., Vogel, C.A., Vintzileos, A.M., Bantham, K.F., Pezzullo, J., and Silberman, L.: Placental pathologic findings in preterm birth. Am. J. Obstet. Gynecol. 165:934–938, 1991.

Samra, J.S., Obhrai, M.S., and Constantine, G.: Parvovirus infection in pregnancy. Obstet. Gynecol. 73:832–834, 1989.

Samson, G.R., Meyer, M.P., Blake, D.R.B., Cohen, M.C., and Mouton, S.C.E.: Syphilitic placentitis: an immunopathy. Placenta 15:67–77, 1994.

Sanchez, P.J., and Regan, J.A.: Ureaplasma urealyticum colonization and chronic lung disease in low birth weight infants. Pediatr. Infect. Dis. J. 7:542–546, 1988.

Sander, C.H., Martin, J.N., Rogers, A.L., Barr, M., and Heidelberger, K.P.: Perinatal infection with Torulopsis glabrata: a case associated with maternal sickle cell anemia. Obstet. Gynecol. 61:21S–24S, 1983.

Sander, C.H., Kinnane, L., Stevens, N.G., and Echt, R.: Haemorrhagic endovasculitis of the placenta: a review with clinical correlation. Placenta 7:551–574, 1986.

Sandy, E.A., Blumenfeld, M.L., and Iams, J.D.: Gram stain in the rapid determination of maternal colonization with group B beta-streptococcus. Obstet. Gynecol. 71:796–798, 1988.

Sarff, L.D., McCracken, G.H., Schiffer, M.S., Glode, M.P., Robbins, J.B., Orskov, I., and Orskov, F.: Epidemiology of Escherichia coli K1 in healthy and diseased newborns. Lancet 1:1099–1104, 1975.

Sarram, M., Feiz, J., Foruzandeh, M., and Gazanfarpour, P.: Intrauterine fetal infection with Brucella melitensis as a possible cause of second-trimester abortion. Am. J. Obstet. Gynecol. 119:657–660, 1974.

Sarto, G.E., Stubblefield, P.A., and Therman, E.: Endomitosis in human trophoblast. Hum. Genet. 62:228–232, 1982.

Savva, D., and Holliman, R.E.: PCR to detect toxoplasma. Lancet 336:1325, 1990.

Sawyer, M.H., Nachlas, N.E., and Panem, S.: C-type viral antigen expression in human placenta. Nature 275:62–64, 1978.

Saxer, J.J.: Chlamydia trachomatis genital infections in a community-based family practice clinic. J. Fam. Pract. 28:41–47, 1989.

Sbarra, A.J., Selvaraj, R.J., Cetrulo, C.L., Feingold, M., Newton, E., and Thomas, G.B.: Infection and phagocytosis as possible mechanisms of rupture in premature rupture of the membranes. Am. J. Obstet. Gynecol. 153:38–43, 1985.

Sbarra, A.J., Thomas, G.B., Cetrulo, C.L., Shakr, C., Chaudhury, A., and Paul, B.: Effect of bacterial growth on the bursting pressure of fetal membranes in vitro. Obstet. Gynecol. 70:107–110, 1987.

Schaffner, A., Douglas, H., and Davis, C.E.: Models of T cell deficiency in listeriosis: the effects of cortisone and cyclosporin A on normal and nude Balb/c mice. J. Immunol. 131:450–453, 1983.

Schiff, I., Driscoll, S.G., and Naftolin, F.: Calcification of the umbilical cord. Am. J. Obstet. Gynecol. 126:1046–1048, 1976.

Schlech, W.F., Lavigne, P.M., Bortolussi, R.A., Allen, A.C., Haldane, E.V., Wort, A.J., Hightower, A.W., Johnson, S.E., King, S.H., Nicholls, E.S., and Broome, C.V.: Epidemic listeriosis—evidence for transmission by food. N. Engl. J. Med. 308:203–206, 1983.

Schlesinger, P.A., Duray, P.H., Burke, B.A., Steere, A.C., and Stillman, M.T.: Maternal-fetal transmission of a Lyme disease spirochete Borrelia burgdorferi. Ann. Intern. Med. 103:67–68, 1985.

Schlievert, P., Larsen, B., Johnson, W., and Galsk, R.P.: Bacterial growth inhibition by amniotic fluid. III. Demonstration of the variability of bacterial growth inhibition by amniotic fluid with a new plate-count technique. Am. J. Obstet. Gynecol. 122:809–813, 1975.

Schlievert, P., Johnson, W., and Galsk, R.P.: Bacterial growth inhibition by amniotic fluid. V. Phosphate-to-zinc ratio as a predictor of bacterial growth-inhibitory activity. Am. J. Obstet. Gynecol. 125:899–906, 1976a.

Schlievert, P., Johnson, W., and Galsk, R.P.: Bacterial growth inhibition by amniotic fluid. VI. Evidence for a zinc-peptide antibacterial system. Am. J. Obstet. Gynecol. 125:906–910, 1976b.

Schlievert, P., Johnson, W., and Galsk, R.P.: Bacterial growth inhibition by amniotic fluid. VII. The effect of zinc supplementation on bacterial inhibitory activity of amniotic fluids from gestation of 20 weeks. Am. J. Obstet. Gynecol. 127:603–608, 1977.

Schmorl, G., and Geipel, P.: Ueber die Tuberkulose der menschlichen Plazenta. Munchen Med. Wochenschr. 51:1676–1679, 1904.

Schmorl, G., and Kockel: Die Tuberkulose der menschlichen Placenta und ihre Beziehung zur congenitalen Infection mit Tuberkulose. Beitr. Pathol. Anat. Pathol. 16:313–339, 1894.

Schneider, V., Behm, F.G., and Mumaw, V.R.: Ascending herpetic endometritis. Obstet. Gynecol. 59:259–262, 1982.

Schoonmaker, J.N., Lawellin, D.W., Lunt, B., and McGregor, J.A.: Bacteria and inflammatory cells reduce chorioamniotic membranes integrity and tensile strength. Obstet. Gynecol. 74:590–596, 1989.

Schwartz, B., Ciesielski, C.A., Broome, C.V., Gaventa, S., Brown, G.R., Gellin, B.G., Hightower, A.W., Mascola, L., and the Listeriosis Study Group: Association of sporadic listeriosis with consumption of uncooked hot dogs and undercooked chicken. Lancet 2:779–782, 1988.

Schwartz, D.A., and Caldwell, E.: Herpes simplex virus infection of the placenta. Arch. Pathol. Lab. Med. 115:1141–1144, 1991.

Schwartz, D.A., and Reef, S.: Candida albicans placentitis and funisitis: early diagnosis of congenital candidemia by histopathologic examination of umbilical cord vessel. Pediatr. Infect. Dis. J. 9:661–665, 1990.

Schwartz, D.A., Khan, R., and Stoll, B.: Characterization of the fetal inflammatory response to cytomegalovirus placentitis: an immunohistochemical study. Arch. Pathol. Lab. Med. 116:21–27, 1992.

Schweid, A.I., and Hopkins, G.B.: Monilial chorionitis associated with an intrauterine contraceptive device. Obstet. Gynecol. 31:719–721, 1968.

Scialli, A.R., and Rarick, T.L.: Salmonella sepsis and second-trimester pregnancy loss. Obstet. Gynecol. 79:820–821, 1992.

Scott, J.M., and Henderson, A.: Acute villous inflammation in the placenta following intrauterine transfusion. J. Clin. Pathol. 25:872–875, 1972.

Scott, G.B., Hutto, C., Makuch, R.W., Mastrucci, M.T., O'Connor, T., Mitchell, C.D., Trapido, E.J., and Parks, W.P.: Survival of children with perinatally acquired human immunodeficiency virus type 1 infection. N. Engl. J. Med. 321:1791–1796, 1989.

Seeliger, H.: Listeriose. Barth, Leipzig, 1955.

Selzer, G.: Virus isolation, inclusion bodies, and chromosomes in a rubella-infected human embryo. Lancet 2:336–337, 1963.

Selzer, G.: Rubella in pregnancy: virus isolation and inclusion bodies. S. Afr. J. Obstet. Gynaecol. 2:5–9, 1964.

Seo, K., McGregor, J.A., and French, J.I.: Preterm birth is associated with increased risk of maternal and neonatal infection. Obstet. Gynecol. 79:75–80, 1992.

Seoud, M., Saade, G., Uwaydah, M., and Azoury, R.: Typhoid fever in pregnancy. Obstet. Gynecol. 71:711–714, 1988.

Sever, J.L., Ellenberg, J.H., Ley, A.C., Madden, D.L., Fuccillo, D.A., Tzan, N.R., and Edmonds, D.M.: Toxoplasmosis: maternal and pediatric findings in 23,000 pregnancies. Pediatrics 82:181–192, 1988.

Shafai, T.: Neonatal coccidioidomycosis in premature twins. Am. J. Dis. Child. 132:634, 1978.

Shepard, M.C.: Nongonococcal urethritis associated with human strains of "T" mycoplasmas. J.A.M.A. 211:1335–1340, 1970.

Shirts, S.R., Brown, M.S., and Bobitt, J.R.: Listeriosis and borreliosis as causes of antepartum fever. Obstet. Gynecol. 62:256–261, 1983.

Shurbaji, M.S., Gupta, P.K., and Myers, J.: Immunohistochemical demonstration of chlamydial antigens in association with prostatitis. Mod. Pathol. 1:348–351, 1988.

Silver, H.M., Sperling, R.S., St. Clair, P.J., and Gibbs, R.S.: Evidence relating bacterial vaginosis to intraamniotic infection. Am. J. Obstet. Gynecol. 161:808–812, 1989.

Silver, H.M., Gibbs, R.S., Gray, B.M., and Dillon, H.C.: Risk factors for perinatal group B streptococcal disease after amniotic fluid colonization. Am. J. Obstet. Gynecol. 163:19–25, 1990.

Silver, R.M., Heddleston, L.N., McGregor, J.A., and Gibbs, R.S.: Life-threatening puerperal infection due to group A streptococci. Obstet. Gynecol. 79:894–896, 1992.

Silverman, N.S., Jenkin, B.K., Wu, C., McGillin, P., and Knee, G.: Hepatitis C virus in pregnancy: seroprevalence and risk factors for infection. Am. J. Obstet. Gynecol. 169:583–587, 1993.

Silverstein, A.M.: Congenital syphilis and the timing of immunogenesis in the human foetus. Nature 194:196–197, 1962.

Silverstein, A.M., and Lukes, R.: Fetal response to antigenic stimulus. I. Plasma cellular and lymphoid reactions in the human fetus to intrauterine infection. Lab. Invest. 11:918–932, 1962.

Simon, C., Schröder, H., Weisner, D., Brück, M., and Krieg, U.: Bacteriological findings after premature rupture of the membranes. Arch. Gynecol. Obstet. 244:69–74, 1989.

Singer, D.B., and Campognone, P.: Group B streptococcus: a hazard in the second trimester. Lab. Invest. 48:13P–14P, 1983.

Smale, L.E., and Waechter, K.G.: Dissemination of coccidioidomycosis in pregnancy. Am. J. Obstet. Gynecol. 197:356–361, 1970.

Smith, C.V., Horenstein, J., and Platt, L.D.: Intrauterine infection with Candida albicans associated with a retained intrauterine contraceptive device: a case report. Am. J. Obstet. Gynecol. 159:123–124, 1988.

Smith, L.G., Summers, P.R., Miles, R.W., Biswas, M.K., and Pernoll, M.L.: Gonococcal chorioamnionitis associated with sepsis: a case report. Am. J. Obstet. Gynecol. 160:573–574, 1989.

Snydman, D.R.: Hepatitis in pregnancy. N. Engl. J. Med. 313:1398–1401, 1985.

Soma, H.: Feto-placental listeriosis as a model of intrauterine infection. Excerpta Med. Int. Cong. Ser. 512:1020–1024, 1979.

Spark, R.P.: Does transplacental spread of coccidioidomycosis occur? Report of a neonatal fatality and review of the literature. Arch. Pathol. Lab. Med. 105:347–350, 1981.

Spaun, E., and Klünder, K.: Candida chorioamnionitis and intra-uterine contraceptive device. Acta Obstet. Gynecol. Scand. 65:183–184, 1986.

Spence, M.R., Davidson, D.E., Dill, G.S., Boonthal, P., and Sagartz, J.W.: Rabies exposure during pregnancy. Am. J. Obstet. Gynecol. 123:655–656, 1975.

Sperling, R.S., Sacks, H.S., Mayer, L., Joyner, M., and Berkowitz, R.L.: Umbilical cord blood serosurvey for human immunodeficiency virus in parturient women in a voluntary hospital in New York City. Obstet. Gynecol. 73:179–181, 1989.

Stagno, S., and Whitley, R.J.: Herpesvirus infections of pregnancy. Part II. Herpes simplex virus and varicella-zoster virus infections. N. Engl. J. Med. 313:1327–1330, 1985.

Stagno, S., Pass, R.F., Dworsky, M.E., Henderson, R.E., Moore, E.G., Walton, P.D., and Alford, C.A.: Congenital cytomegalovirus infection: the relative importance of primary and recurrent maternal infection. N. Engl. J. Med. 306:945–949, 1982.

Stagno, S., Pass, R.F., Cloud, G., Britt, W.J., Henderson, R.E., Walton, P.D., Veren, D.A., Page, F., and Alford, C.A.: Primary cytomegalovirus infection in pregnancy: incidence, transmission to fetus, and clinical outcome. J.A.M.A. 256:1904–1908, 1986.

Steele, P.E., and Jacobs, D.S.: Listeria monocytogenes macroabscesses of placenta. Obstet. Gynecol. 53:124–127, 1979.

Steere, A.C.: Lyme disease. N. Engl. J. Med. 321:586–596, 1989.

Stein, S.J., and Greenspoon, J.S.: Rubeola during pregnancy. Obstet. Gynecol. 78:925–929, 1991.

Steiner, B., Putnoky, G., Kovacs, K., and Földes, G.: Pneumonia in newborn infants. Acta Paediatr. Hung. 2:227–236, 1961.

Stiller, R.J., Blair, E., Clark, P., and Tinghitella, T.: Rapid detection of vaginal colonization with group B streptococci by means of latex agglutination. Am. J. Obstet. Gynecol. 160:566–568, 1989.

Stray-Pedersen, B.: Infants potentially at risk for congenital toxoplasmosis: a prospective study. Am. J. Dis. Child. 134:638–642, 1980.

Stray-Pedersen, B., and Lorentzen-Styr, A.-M.: Uterine toxoplasma infections and repeated abortions. Am. J. Obstet. Gynecol. 128:716–721, 1977.

Strickland, D.M., Yeomans, E.R., and Hankins, G.D.V.: Cost-effectiveness of intrapartum screening and treatment for maternal group B streptococci colonization. Am. J. Obstet. Gynecol. 163:4–8, 1990.

Strobino, B.A., Williams, C.L., Abid, S., Chalson, R., and Spierling, P.: Lyme disease and pregnancy outcome: a prospective study of two thousand prenatal patients. Am. J. Obstet. Gynecol. 169:367–374, 1993.

Studdiford, W.E., and Douglas, G.W.: Placental bacteremia: a significant finding in septic abortion accompanied by vascular collapse. Am. J. Obstet. Gynecol. 71:842–858, 1956.

Sutherland, J.C., Berry, A., Hynd, M., and Proctor, N.S.F.: Placental bilharziasis: report of a case. S. Afr. J. Obstet. Gynaecol. 3:76–80, 1965.

Svabic-Vlahovic, M., Pantic, D., Pavicic, M., and Bryner, J.H.: Transmission of Listeria monocytogenes from mother's milk to her baby and to puppies. Lancet 2:1201, 1988.

Swartzberg, J.E., and Remington, J.S.: Transmission of Toxoplasma. Am. J. Dis. Child. 129:777–779, 1975.

Sweet, R.L., Landers, D.V., Walker, C., and Schachter, J.: Chlamydia trachomatis infection and pregnancy outcome. Am. J. Obstet. Gynecol. 156:824–833, 1987.

Swingler, G.R., Bigrigg, M.A., Hewitt, B.G., and McNulty, C.A.M.: Disseminated intravascular coagulation associated with group A streptococcal infection in pregnancy. Lancet 1:1456–1457, 1988.

Symonds, D.A., and Driscoll, S.G.: Massive fetal ascites, urethral atresia, and cytomegalic inclusion disease. Am. J. Dis. Child. 127:895–897, 1974.

Taniguchi, T., Matsuzaki, N., Kameda, T., Shimoya, K., Jo, T., Saji, F., and Tanizawa, O.: The enhanced production of placental interleukin-1 during labor and intrauterine infection. Am. J. Obstet. Gynecol. 165:131–137, 1991.

Tanner, N.C., and Hewlett, R.F.L.: Congenital malaria with report in one of twins. Lancet 2:369–370, 1935.

Tarpay, M.M., Turbeville, D.F., and Krous, H.F.: Fatal Streptococcus pneumoniae type III sepsis in mother and infant. Am. J. Obstet. Gynecol. 136:257–258, 1980.

Taschdjan, C.T., and Kozinn, P.J.: Laboratory and clinical studies on candidiasis in the newborn infant. J. Pediatr. 50:426–433, 1957.

Taylor-Robinson, D., and McCormack, W.M.: The genital mycoplasmas. N. Engl. J. Med. 302:1003–1010, 1063–1067, 1980.

Teele, R.L., Hernanz-Schulman, M., and Sotrel, A.: Echogenic vasculature in the basal ganglia of neonates: a sonographic sign of vasculopathy. Radiology 169:423–427, 1988.

Teutsch, S.M., Sulzer, A.J., Ramsey, J.E., Murray, W.A., and Juranek, D.D.: Toxoplasma gondii isolated from amniotic fluid. Obstet. Gynecol. 55:2S–4S, 1980.

Thadepalli, H., Bach, V.T., and Davidson, E.C.: Antimicrobial effect of amniotic fluid. Obstet. Gynecol. 52:198–204, 1978.

Thaler, M.M., Park, C.-K., Landers, D.V., Wara, D.W., Houghton, M., Veereman-Wauters, G., Sweet, R.L., and Han, J.H.: Vertical transmission of hepatitis C virus. Lancet 338:17–18, 1991.

Thiery, M., le Sian, A.Y., Derom, R., and Boelaert, R.: Leukocytic infiltration of the umbilical cord in twins. Acta Genet. Med. Gemellol. 19:92–95, 1970.

Thomas, G.B., Sbarra, A.J., Feingold, M., Cetrulo, C.L., Shakr, C., Newton, E., and Selvaraj, R.J.: Antimicrobial activity of amniotic fluid against Chlamydia trachomatis, Mycoplasma hominis, and Ureaplasma urealyticum. Am. J. Obstet. Gynecol. 158:16–22, 1988.

Thomas, G.B., Jones, J., Sbarra, A.J., Cetrulo, C., and Reisner, D.: Isolation of Chlamydia trachomatis from amniotic fluid. Obstet. Gynecol. 76:519–520, 1990.

Thompson, D., Pegelow, C., Underman, A., and Powars, D.: Congenital malaria: a rare cause of splenomegaly and anemia in an American infant. Pediatrics 60:209–212, 1977.

Thompson, K.M., and Tobin, J.O'H.: Isolation of rubella virus from abortion material. B.M.J. 2:264–266, 1970.

Thomsen, A.C., Morup, L., and Hansen, K.B.: Antibiotic elimination of group-B streptococci in urine in prevention of preterm labour. Lancet 1:591–593, 1987.

Thorpe, J.M., Katz, V.L., Fowler, L.J., Kurtzman, J.T., and Bowles, W.A.: Fetal death from chlamydial infection across intact amniotic membranes. Am. J. Obstet. Gynecol. 161:1245–1246, 1989.

Tobias, L., Cordes, D.O., and Schurig, G.G.: Placental pathology of the pregnant mouse inoculated with Brucella abortus strain 2308. Vet. Pathol. 30:119–129, 1993.

Töndury, G.: Zum Problem der Embryopathia rubeolosa: untersuchungen an menschlichen Keimlingen verschiedener Entwicklungsstadien. Bull. Schweiz. Akad. Med. Wiss. 7:307–325, 1951.

Töndury, G.: Zur Kenntnis der Embryopathia rubeolica, nebst Bemerkungen über die Wirkung anderer Viren auf den Keimling. Geburtshilfe Frauenheilkd. 12:865–888, 1952a.

Töndury, G.: Zur Wirkung des Erregers der Rubeolen auf den menschlichen Keimling. Helv. Paediatr. Acta 7:105–135, 1952b.

Töndury, G.: Über den Infektionsweg und die Pathogenese von Virusschädigung beim menschlichen Keimling. Bull. Schweiz. Akad. Med. Wiss. 20:379–396, 1964.

Töndury, G., and Smith, D.W.: Fetal rubella pathology. J. Pediatr. 68:867–879, 1966.

Topalovski, M., Yang, S.S., and Boonpasat, Y.: Listeriosis of the placenta: clinicopathologic study of seven cases. Am. J. Obstet. Gynecol. 169:616–620, 1993.

Torphy, D.E., Ray, C.G., McAlister, R., and Du, J.N.H.: Herpes simplex virus infection in infants: a spectrum of disease. J. Pediatr. 76:405–408, 1970.

Toth, M., Witkin, S.S., Ledger, W., and Thaler, H.: The role of infection in the etiology of preterm birth. Obstet. Gynecol. 71:723–736, 1988; 73:142–1444, 1989.

Tully, J.G., and Whitcomb, R.F., eds.: The Mycoplasmas. Academic Press, Orlando, FL, 1979.

Update: Foodborne listeriosis. Bull. W.H.O. 66:421–428, 1988.

Vadas, P., and Pruzanski, W.: Role of secretory phospholipases A_2 in the pathobiology of disease. Lab. Invest. 55:391–404, 1986.

Vaheri, A., Vesikari, T., Oker-Bloom, N., Seppala, M., Parkman, P.D., Veronelli, J., and Robbins, F.C.: Isolation of attenuated rubella-vaccine virus from human products of conception and uterine cervix. N. Engl. J. Med. 286:1071–1074, 1972.

VanBergen, W.S., Fleury, F.J., and Cheatle, E.L.: Fatal maternal disseminated coccidioidomycosis in a nonendemic area. Am. J. Obstet. Gynecol. 124:661–664, 1976.

Vaughan, J.E., and Ramirez, H.: Coccidioidomycosis as a complication of pregnancy. Calif. Med. 74:121–125, 1951.

Vernon, M., and Gauthier, C.: L'infection bactérienne du placenta dans les cas d'interruption spontanée de la grossesse: corrélation avec les lésions histologiques. Pathol. Biol. 19:129–138, 1971.

Victor, M., Weiss, J., Klempner, M.S., and Elsbach, P.: Phospholipase A$_2$ activity in the plasma membrane of human polymorphonuclear leukocytes. FEBS Lett. 136: 298–300, 1981.

Vigorita, V.J., and Parmley, T.H.: Intramembranous localization of bacteria in β-hemolytic group B streptococcal chorioamnionitis. Obstet. Gynecol. 53:13S–15S, 1979.

Vintzileos, A.M., Campbell, W.A., Nochimson, D.J., and Weinbaum, P.J.: Preterm premature rupture of the membranes: a risk factor for the development of abruptio placentae. Am. J. Obstet. Gynecol. 156:1235–1238, 1987.

Visintine, A.M., Oleske, J.M., and Nahmias, A.J.: Listeria monocytogenes infection in infants and children. Am. J. Dis. Child. 131:393–397, 1977.

Wagner, G.P., Hanley, L.S., Farb, H.F., and Knox, G.E.: Evaluation of gas-liquid chromatography for the rapid diagnosis of amniotic fluid infection: a preliminary report. Am. J. Obstet. Gynecol. 152:51–56, 1985.

Wahbeh, C.J., Hill, G.B., Eden, R.D., and Gall, S.A.: Intra-amniotic bacterial colonization in premature labor. Am. J. Obstet. Gynecol. 148:739–743, 1984.

Waites, K.B., Rudd, P.T., Crouse, D.T., Canupp, K.C., Nelson, K.G., Ramsey, C., and Cassell, G.H.: Chronic Ureaplasma urealyticum and Mycoplasma hominis infections of central nervous system in preterm infants. Lancet 1:17–21, 1988.

Walker, M.P.R., Brody, C.Z., and Resnik, R.: Reactivation of coccidioidomycosis in pregnancy. Obstet. Gynecol. 79:815–817, 1992.

Wallach, E.E., Brody, J.I., and Oski, F.A.: Fetal immunization as a consequence of bacilluria during pregnancy. Obstet. Gynecol. 33:100–105, 1969.

Walter, P.R., Garin, Y., and Blot, P.: Placental pathologic changes in malaria: a histologic and ultrastructural study. Am. J. Pathol. 109:330–342, 1982.

Wang, E.E.L., Frayha, H., Watts, J., Hammerberg, O., Chernesky, M.A., Mahony, J.B., and Cassell, G.H.: Role of Ureaplasma urealyticum and other pathogens in the development of chronic lung disease of prematurity. Pediatr. Infect. Dis. J. 7:547–551, 1988.

Warthin, A.S.: Tuberculosis of the placenta: a histological study with especial reference to the nature of the earliest lesions produced by the tubercle bacillus. J. Infect. Dis. 4:347–398, 1907.

Watson, D.G.: Purulent neonatal meningitis: a study of forty-five cases. J. Pediatr. 50:352–360, 1957.

Watson, K.C.: Salmonella meningitis. Arch. Dis. Child. 33:171–175, 1958.

Watts, D.H., Krohn, M.A., Hillier, S.L., Wener, M.H., Kiviat, N.B., and Eschenbach, D.A.: Characteristics of women in preterm labor associated with elevated C-reactive protein levels. Obstet. Gynecol. 82:509–514, 1993.

Webb, G.A.: Maternal death associated with premature rupture of the membranes. Am. J. Obstet. Gynecol. 98: 594–601, 1967.

Weiner, C.P., and Grose, C.: Prenatal diagnosis of congenital cytomegalovirus infection by virus isolation from amniotic fluid. Am. J. Obstet. Gynecol. 163:1253–1255, 1990.

Wejstal, R., Widell, A., Mansson, A.-S., Hermodsson, S., and Norkrans, G.: Mother-to-infant transmission of hepatitis C virus. Ann. Intern. Med. 117:887–890, 1992.

Weller, T.H.: The cytomegaloviruses: ubiquitous agents with protean manifestations. N. Engl. J. Med. 285:203–214, 262–274, 1971.

Wenckebach, G.F.C., and Curry, B.: Cytomegalovirus infection of the female genital tract: histologic findings in three cases and review of the literature. Arch. Pathol. Lab. Med. 100:609–612, 1976.

Wendel, G.D., Maberry, M.C., Christmas, J.T., Goldberg, M.S., and Norgard, M.V.: Examination of amniotic fluid in diagnosing congenital syphilis with fetal death. Obstet. Gynecol. 74:967–970, 1989.

Wendel, G.D., Sanchez, P.J., Peters, M.T., Harstad, T.W., Potter, L.L., and Norgard, M.V.: Identification of Treponema pallidum in amniotic fluid and fetal blood from pregnancies complicated by congenital syphilis. Obstet. Gynecol. 78:890–895, 1991.

Wentworth, P.: Studies on placentae and infants from women vaccinated for smallpox during pregnancy. J. Clin. Pathol. 19:328–330, 1966.

Werner, H., Schmidtke, L., and Thomascheck, G.: Toxoplasmose-Infektion und Schwangerschaft: der histologische Nachweis des intrauterinen Infektionsweges. Klin. Wochenschr. 41:96–101, 1963.

Westrom, L., Evaldson, G., Holmes, K.K., Meijden, W.v.d., Rylander, E., and Fredricksson, B.: Taxonomy of vaginosis; bacterial vaginosis—a definition. In, Bacterial Vaginosis. P.A. Mardh and D. Taylor-Robinson, eds., pp. 259–260. Almqvist & Wiksell, Stockholm, 1985.

Wetli, C.V., Roldan, E.O., and Fojaco, R.M.: Listeriosis as a cause of maternal death: an obstetric complication of the acquired immunodeficiency syndrome (AIDS). Am. J. Obstet. Gynecol. 147:7–9, 1983.

White, W.D.: Human vibriosis: indigenous cases in England. B.M.J. 1:283–287, 1967.

Whyte, R.K., Hussain, Z., and Desa, D.: Antenatal infections with Candida species. Arch. Dis. Child. 57:528–535, 1982.

Wickramasuriya, G.A.W.: Some observations on malaria occurring in association with pregnancy: with special reference to the transplacental passage of parasites from the maternal to the fetal circulation. J. Obstet. Gynaecol. Br. Emp. 42:816–834, 1935.

Widholm, O., Meyer, B., and Numers, C.v.: Inflammation of the umbilical cord in cases of foetal asphyxia of unknown clinical etiology. Gynaecologia 155:385–399, 1963.

Wielenga, G., van Tongeren, H.A.E., Ferguson, A.H., and van Rijssel, T.G.: Prenatal infection with vaccinia virus. Lancet 1:258–260, 1961.

Wilkins, I., Mezrow, G., Lynch, L., Bottone, E.J., and Berkowitz, R.L.: Amnionitis and life-threatening respiratory distress after percutaneous umbilical blood sampling. Am. J. Obstet. Gynecol. 160:427–428, 1989.

Williamson, A.: The varicella zoster virus in the etiology of severe congenital defects. Clin. Pediatr. 14:553–559, 1975.

Williamson, W.D., Desmond, M.M., LaFevers, N., Taber, L.H., Catlin, F.I., and Weaver, Y.G.: Symptomatic congenital cytomegalovirus: disorders of language, learning, and hearing. Am. J. Dis. Child. 136:902–905, 1982.

Williamson, W.D., Percy, A.K., Yow, M.D., Gerson, P., Catlin, F.I., Koppelman, M.L., and Thurber, S.: Asymptomatic congenital cytomegalovirus infection: audiologic, neuroradiologic, and neurodevelopmental abnormalities during the first year. Am. J. Dis. Child. 144:1365–1368, 1990.

Wilson, C.B., and Remington, J.S.: What can be done to prevent congenital toxoplasmosis? Am. J. Obstet. Gynecol. 138:357–363, 1980.

Winn, H.N., and Egley, C.C.: Acute Haemophilus influenzae chorioamnionitis associated with intact amniotic membranes. Am. J. Obstet. Gynecol. 156:458–459, 1987.

Wittek, A.E., Yeager, A.S., Au, D.S., and Hensleigh, P.A.: Asymptomatic shedding of herpes simplex virus from the cervix and lesion site during pregnancy: correlation of antepartum shedding with shedding at delivery. Am. J. Dis. Child. 138:439–442, 1984.

Witzleben, C.L., and Driscoll, S.G.: Possible transplacental transmission of herpes simplex infection. Pediatrics 36:192–199, 1965.

Wohlwill, F., and Bock, H.E.: Über Entzündungen der Placenta und fetale Sepsis. Arch. Gynecol. 135:271–319, 1929.

Wolber, R.A., and Lloyd, R.V.: Cytomegalovirus detection by nonisotopic in situ DNA hybridization and viral antigen immunostaining using a two-color technique. Hum. Pathol. 19:736–741, 1989.

Wong, S.Y., Gray, E.S., Buxton, D., Finlayson, J., and Johnson, F.A.H.: Acute placentitis and spontaneous abortion caused by Chlamydia psittaci in sheep origin: a histopathologic and ultrastructural study. J. Clin. Pathol. 38:707–711, 1985.

Woods, W.G., Mills, E., and Ferrieri, P.: Neonatal malaria due to Plasmodium vivax. J. Pediatr. 85:669–671, 1974.

Woody, N.C., and Woody, H.B.: Possible Chagas's disease in United States. N. Engl. J. Med. 290:750–751, 1974.

Wyler, D.J.: Malaria—resurgence, resistance, and research. N. Engl. J. Med. 308:875–879, 1983.

Yagupsky, P., and Moses, S.: Neonatal Borrelia species infection (relapsing fever). Am. J. Dis. Child. 139:74–76, 1985.

Yamauchi, T., Wilson, C., and St. Geme, J.W.: Transmission of live, attenuated mumps virus to the human placenta. N. Engl. J. Med. 290:710–712, 1974.

Yamazaki, K., Price, J.T., and Altshuler, G.: A placental view of the diagnosis and pathogenesis of congenital listeriosis. Am. J. Obstet. Gynecol. 129:703–705, 1977.

Yancey, M.K., Clark, P., Armer, T., and Duff, P.: Use of a DNA probe for the rapid detection of group B streptococci in obstetric patients. Obstet. Gynecol. 81:635–640, 1993.

Yawn, D.H., Pyeatte, J.C., Joseph, J.M., Eichler, S.L., and Garcia-Bunuel, R.: Transplacental transfer of influenza virus. J.A.M.A. 216:1022–1023, 1971.

Yen, S.S.C., Reagan, J.W., and Rosenthal, M.S.: Herpes simplex infection in female genital tract. Obstet. Gynecol. 25:479–492, 1965.

Yokoyama, S., Kashima, K., Inoue, S., Daa, T., Nakayama, I., and Moriuchi, A.: Biotin-containing intranuclear inclusions in endometrial glands during gestation and puerperium. Am. J. Clin. Pathol. 99:13–17, 1993.

Young, S.A., and Crocker, D.W.: Occult congenital syphilis in macerated stillborn fetuses. Arch. Pathol. Lab. Med. 118:44–47, 1994.

Yow, M.D.: Congenital cytomegalovirus disease: a NOW problem. J. Infect. Dis. 159:163–167, 1989.

Zavoral, J.H., Ray, W.L., Kinnard, P.G., and Nahmias, A.J.: Neonatal herpetic infection: a fatal consequence of penile herpes in a serviceman. J.A.M.A. 213:1492–1493, 1970.

Zervoudakis, I.A., and Cederqvist, L.L.: Effect of Listeria monocytogenes septicemia during pregnancy on the offspring. Am. J. Obstet. Gynecol. 129:465–467, 1977.

Zervoudakis, I.A., Silverman, F., Senterfit, L.B., Strongin, M.J., Read, S., and Cederquist, L.L.: Herpes simplex in the amniotic fluid of an unaffected fetus. Obstet. Gynecol. 55:16S–17S, 1980.

21
Abortion, Placentas of Trisomies, and Immunological Considerations of Recurrent Reproductive Failure

For the present discussions, an abortion or miscarriage is designated a conceptus that is expelled before the 20th week of gestation. That is important to state at the outset, as the pathological features of failed pregnancies differ markedly in specimens obtained later during gestation. In the United States terminations before 20 weeks constitute abortions; later gestations are premature deliveries. A pregnancy of 20 weeks is legally at the dividing line; it is considered a gestation either with an embryo (that may be treated as a surgical specimen) or a fetus, whose examination constitutes an autopsy. The terminology employed in publications and statistics differs widely and is not the same in different countries. For instance, Vogel (1969, 1992) considered an abortion an expelled fetus of less than 1,000 g. He differentiated between embryonic and fetal (15–28 weeks) abortion. Legal viability is frequently considered to be attained only at 28 weeks' gestation when the fetus has attained approximately 1,000 g in weight; but that is not so in the United States. Byrne et al. (1985), in a study of early fetal deaths, considered all specimens less than 28 weeks' gestation. For these reasons it is difficult to place in context with current terminology the studies of Vogel (1969, 1992). Most spontaneous abortions occur before 12 weeks' gestation, and most are due to chromosomal errors in the conceptus. Relatively few truly spontaneous abortions take place between 12 and 20 weeks' gestation. Thereafter, between 20 and 30 weeks, another type of premature spontaneous termination becomes prevalent—that due to ascending infection. These are fundamentally different processes with vastly different pathological findings.

There are terms other than spontaneous abortion as well, and they have often confused the issue of abortion. We speak of spontaneous (involuntary), therapeutic (electively terminated; TAB), missed (retained for more than 8 weeks after embryonic death), criminal (illegally instrumented), habitual, and recurrent abortions; and

we use other terms as well as to designate specific entities. Not all of these definitions are universally acceptable, and there is for instance cogent argument that the term missed abortion should be abandoned (Pridjian & Moawad, 1989). It is best to clarify the specific nomenclature before one compares data from different institutions and countries. A useful method for categorization of abortion specimens was provided by Fujikura et al. (1966). They divided specimens into groups with and without embryos, those with ruptured and unruptured sacs, and the degree of their completeness. In their experience, 22% were classified as incomplete, and most (35.8%) had a normal embryo or fetus. An "embryo" may be considered to be specimens with a crown-rump (CR) length of up to 30 mm (less than 9 weeks), and a "fetus" as an unborn conceptus greater than 30 mm CR (Moore, 1982). When only incomplete specimens are available, it has been practical to determine fetal age from measurements of fetal foot length. Other extensive considerations of classification and specimen examination have been laid out in detail by Kalousek et al. (1990). Hern (1984) correlated various fetal measurements with gestational age in 1,000 specimens and provided excellent tables from which reasonably exact age determination is possible.

Spontaneous abortions are common. The exact frequency with which pregnancy failure occurs spontaneously has been debated, and our understanding of its pathogenesis has undergone marked changes in recent years. Trauma is no longer considered to be a common cause of abortion. Hertig and Sheldon (1943) found only one set of twins whose abortion was probably caused by external trauma among the 1,000 miscarriages they studied. "Internal trauma" was incriminated in 22 cases. Published figures on the incidence of abortion depend largely on the method of sampling a population. When prospective studies of complete populations are done so as to include also all those pregnancies that give few or no clinical symptoms of pregnancy, it is found that nearly 50% of conceptions terminate in abortion spontaneously. For example, Miller et al. (1980) collected urine from 197 women who were wishing to conceive. They began the collection at ovulation to obtain the earliest evidence of pregnancy and investigated 623 menstrual cycles. Their diagnoses of pregnancy was made with sensitive radioimmunoassays for beta human chorionic gonadotropin (β-hCG). There were 152 conceptions, with a pregnancy loss of 43%; but only 14 of the abortions were recognized clinically as pregnancies. The other 50 patients merely had a rise of urinary hCG level. McLean (1987) reviewed other studies that arrived at similar figures: Approximately 50% of implanted pregnancies aborted spontaneously, and most of them were clinically unrecognized. Additionally, there are probably conceptuses that vanish even before implantation. Wilcox et al. (1988) identified 31% spontaneous abortions of 707 cycles collected from 221 women. Mills et al. (1988) found that diabetic women in good control may expect similar rates of abortion and cited an incidence of 16% of clinically recognized gestations. Hertz-Picciotto and Samuels (1988) have criticized some of these results and gathered the following figures from four studies.

Losses (no.)		Recognized pregnancies (no.)	Risk of loss in recognized pregnancies
Subclinical	Clinical		
43	18	154	11.7
7	11	85	12.9
50	14	102	13.7
67	6	41	14.6

Most spontaneous abortions occur before 12 weeks of pregnancy, and chromosomal errors are their most prominent cause. The exact mechanism of the abortion event is still disputed. Stern and Coulam (1992) found in a study of recurrent abortions that the reduction in sonographic size of the "fetal pole" and differences in fetal heart rate activity at 6 weeks allowed great accuracy in anticipating abortion. The hypoplasia of the placenta, so often observed and which presumably correlates with decreased hCG secretion and hence progesterone support of the decidua, is an accepted possibility. A specific inquiry into the small gestational sac (sonographically) and other gestational parameters was undertaken by Dickey et al. (1992). They found small gestational sacs more often in chromosomally normal abortuses. It has been suggested that "illegal" blood flow into the intervillous space at an early gestational age may equally be of importance in causing spontaneous abortions. Schaaps and Hustin (1988) and Hustin et al. (1988) reviewed the interesting evidence of early trophoblast invasion. From

this evidence they concluded that massive trophoblastic infiltration of uteroplacental arteries essentially occludes these vessels before 12 weeks' gestation. This trophoblastic proliferation permits only plasma filtrate to circulate in the intervillous space, at least during early gestation. It is apparently for this reason that chorionic villous sampling specimens are usually bloodless. Sonographic and pathological evidence suggest, on the other hand, that in spontaneous abortuses blood circulates in the intervillous space before the interruption of pregnancy. It is thus speculated that it may come about as the result of inadequate trophoblastic proliferation into the decidual arteries and that it affects normal nidation.

Increasing maternal age considerably increases the risk of spontaneous abortion, especially at age 35 years or older (Stein, 1985), and it correlates with a risk of fetal trisomies. No such association could be made with respect to paternal age (Hatch et al., 1990). Moreover, Neuber et al. (1993) found that the frequency of monosomy X and of triploidy decreases with advancing maternal age. When triploids are observed in abortuses of older women, they tend to be more often the result of digyny. Abortions due to chromosomal nondisjunction were lucidly detailed by Magenis (1988), who summarized especially well the paternal versus maternal nondisjunctional events in trisomies and X monosomy. Also, numerous investigators have commented on the apparent excess of male conceptuses among abortion specimens (reviewed by Shettles, 1964). Contradictory reports have been examined by Kellokumpu-Lehtinen and Pelliniemi (1984). They studied the sex ratio of 551 induced abortions by histological examination of gonads or by sex chromatin. Early embryos had a sex ratio of 1.64, which became 1.17 during later fetal stages, presumably because of losses in early gestation. There is no convincing explanation for the disproportionately high loss of male embryos. Embryos also are often improperly sexed. It has been our experience that male gender is often inaccurately assigned because of misinterpretation of a normally large clitoris in young female embryos. Kirby et al. (1967) have suggested immunological reasons for the excess male wastage.

Carr (1965) was the first investigator to establish that spontaneous abortions principally result from chromosomal errors of the conceptus. Subsequent investigations from many countries have confirmed and extended these observations. Boué and Boué (1969) reported that 70% of spontaneous abortions occurring during the first 6 weeks of pregnancy had chromosomal errors and 50% during the first 10 weeks. Trisomies constituted 56% of the errors, triploidy 18%, and monosomy X 15%; the remainder were double trisomies, tetraploidies, and individual chromosome errors, such as rings, translocations, and mosaics. Hassold et al. (1980), in a detailed study of 1,000 spontaneous abortions, found 44.5% trisomies, 24.2% monosomy X, and 15.1% triploidy. Kajii et al. (1980) found 53% of their specimens to be chromosomally aberrant. Other studies, largely from cultured material, have produced approximately similar results (Kuliev, 1971; Creasy et al., 1976). Eiben and colleagues (1990) studied 750 spontaneous abortions with direct chromosome preparations. Roughly similar error rates were detected, but it was striking that there was a considerable excess of females in chromosomally normal abortions (sex ratio 0.71). The use of "postmortem" villus sampling after the specimen is delivered was advocated by Johnson et al. (1990). They found it not only to be more successful than skin biopsy and amniocentesis but also discovered an unusually high error rate.

The pathologist is occasionally asked to provide material for chromosomal study from fetuses and placentas. In our experience, embryonic tissue (or tissue from the chorionic surface when an embryo is not available) is best. Although general sterile techniques are desirable when obtaining the material, Boué used tap-water-washed specimens with good results. Absolute sterility may not be needed, but it is preferable. When sampling the placenta, it is best to cleanse the fetal surface, peel the amnion away, and obtain chorionic tissue with sterile instruments, ideally including some chorionic surface vessels. Geisler and Gropp (1967) have provided more detailed instructions for the explantation of this material.

Anatomical Findings

The evaluation of specimens from spontaneously aborted conceptions has greatly changed. The *Windei* (blighted ovum) noted by early authors, the pathological ovum (with its many subgroups), and many other designations used in the past have now become obsolete. Likewise, terms such as nodular, cylindrical, stunted, and disorganized embryo have little specific use when describing the nature of the embryonic abnormality (Figure 447). For better understanding the pathogenesis of the many defects in aborted specimens, it is necessary to know their chromosomal constitution. It is not reasonable to undertake complex cytogenetic studies of spontaneous abortion specimens on a routine basis, however, because of the expense and because it adds little to management. Understanding the principles is sufficient; an excellent pictorial guide is found in Kalousek et al. (1990). Salafia and her colleagues (1993) undertook a study to ascertain how the histopathological findings can be used to diagnose chromosomally caused abortions. They devised scoring criteria and concluded that an intact fetal circulation, villous infarcts, decidual arteriopathy, and

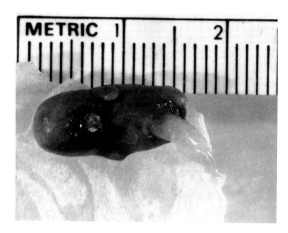

FIGURE 447. Cylindrical embryo of a spontaneous abortion at 9 weeks' gestation. The embryo is growth-retarded (should be 2.5 cm) and hemorrhagic. It was undergoing autolysis on microscopic study, undoubtedly due to a chromosomal error.

chronic "intervillositis" argued against cytogenetic error as the cause of abortion. Methodology is now evolving that will make it feasible to describe the genetic defects more accurately, including DNA studies, the polymerase chain reaction (PCR), and other techniques. Such tests are feasible even using fixed and paraffin-embedded tissues (for reviews see Antonarakis, 1989; Kovacs et al., 1989). Horn and his colleagues (1991) suggested that abortion material be examined with a lens so as to identify hydropic swelling and hypoplasia; histologically, there are few additional findings of importance.

Because hydropic villi are such a frequent finding in many placentas of spontaneous abortions, the differential diagnosis from moles and partial moles is often required. To do so, we will probably see much wider use of flow cytometry, the most rapid means for this differentiation. The ploidy (2n versus 3n) of aborted specimens, particularly triploid partial moles, will thus be differentiated from true hydatidiform moles much more quickly (see Chapter 22). We also recommend that a miniautopsy be performed on embryos when they are present, as its findings are often startling.

The youngest described abnormal specimens originated from systematic studies of early human implantations. Hertig et al. (1959) summarized their extensive search for early conceptuses, which they conducted in 210 women. They described 34 early ova, 10 of which were abnormal. Histological abnormalities included multinucleated blastomeres, necrotic blastomeres, lack of cavitation, hemorrhage, and deficient trophoblastic proliferation. Harrison et al. (1966) depicted an abnormal 13-day ovum with unbranched villi and abnormal amnionic budding.

Most of the descriptions of aborted specimens, however, come from systematic studies of spontaneous abortion. Kaeser (1949) presented an extensive study of

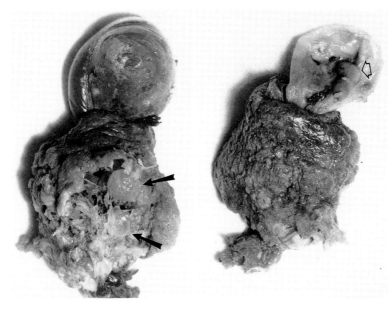

FIGURE 448. Spontaneous abortus at approximately 8 weeks' gestation. Note the opened sac (at right) with the nodular embryo at the open arrow. The hypoplastic placenta with focal marked villous edema (hydatid degeneration) is seen at the arrows (left). Decidua basalis is hemorrhagic.

the frequency, nature, and pathological features of abortions, highlighting the hydatidiform degeneration of villi (Figure 448). Huber et al. (1957) found that in 76% of their specimens the embryo was abnormal; 40% of the specimens had hydatid changes of villi. Sadovsky and Laufer (1961) emphasized the extensive decidual hemorrhage that is often regarded as being one cause of early abortions, especially those with intact villi (Figure 449). Eckman and Carrow (1962) described the presence of extensive villous stromal collagenization as a prominent feature of their abortion specimens and found

29% to possess hydatid changes. The fibrosis of villi was considered to be secondary by Abaci and Aterman (1968), who studied 237 abortion specimens. They found changes of hydatidiform mole in 41.3% and subchorionic hematomas (Breus mole) in 20.2% (Figure 450).

The hydropic degeneration (hydatid change) of villi is a recurrent finding in all studies of abortion specimens (Figure 451). This feature was reviewed by Ladefoged (1980), who compared 100 spontaneously aborted specimens with 160 therapeutic abortions. Whereas hydropic change was noted in as many as 81% of instru-

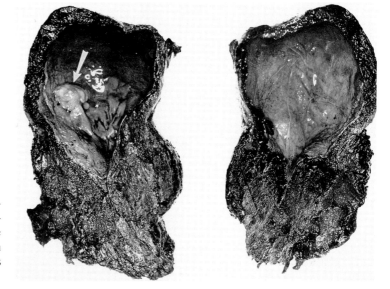

FIGURE 449. Spontaneous abortus with a fragmented, macerated embryo (arrow). It would previously have been described as a hematoma mole (carneous mole). The specimen exhibits a common feature of many early abortions: The amnion is prematurely attached to the chorionic sac.

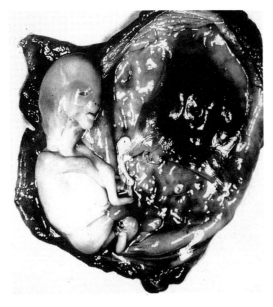

FIGURE 450. Breus subchorionic tuberous hematoma in a missed abortion at 6 months' gestation. Note the large hematoma to the right of the macerated fetus.

mented specimens (representing probably the normally edematous appearance of these villi), in only 6.9% was the hydatid change excessive, in contrast to the 41.0% found in spontaneously aborted specimens. Jurkovic and Muzelak (1970) observed focal hydatid changes in 21% of legal abortions, and in 2% it was diffusely distributed. Fibrosis was seen in 4.4%; other, nonspecific changes were less frequently identified. These authors emphasized that the frequency of pathological findings demands more careful scrutiny of these specimens than is usually done. Abortions with hydatid changes had

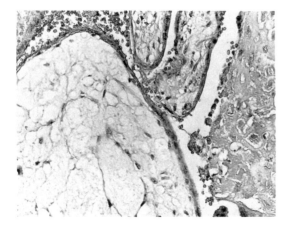

FIGURE 451. Hydatidiform swelling of a villus in a spontaneous abortus. Microcystic spaces develop in the distended villus. Note the trophoblastic hypoplasia and focal necrosis. H&E. ×160.

significantly more DNA aneuploidies, as identified by flow cytometry, than nonhydropic abortuses (Fukunaga et al., 1993).

Fujikura et al. (1971) also compared spontaneous with induced abortion specimens. They pointed out that the hydropic changes found in normal (induced) abortuses is primarily a feature of villi in the chorion laeve, where the villi are expected to undergo degenerative changes. Thus the sampling site is of importance when such specimens are compared. In their analysis, the number of villi also did not differ in the two groups, and so reduced villous growth cannot be held responsible for abortion. The first ultrastructural studies of aborted specimens were presented by Herbst and Multier (1971). They depicted microvillous hypoplasia, lacunar spaces, and enlarged endoplasmic reticulum of the syncytium, as well as villous fibrosis. No specific and constant changes were described that characterized abortion specimens.

All of the placental alterations described so far are relatively nonspecific. They are also not uniformly present, and many (e.g., the hydatid changes) may be the sequelae of embryonic death. The reason for the preponderance of hydatid change in aborted specimens is not fully understood. It is generally believed that following fetal death the trophoblast continues to transport water from the intervillous space into the villi, from where it cannot be removed by an absent fetal circulation; hence the villi enlarge. This explanation is probably too facile for a complex process.

The comparison of chromosomally abnormal tissues with euploid abortion material produced more insight. Singh and Carr (1967) made the first efforts to identify morphological features of the aborted specimens and related them to cytogenetic findings, but Philippe (1986), collaborating with Boué (Philippe & Boué, 1969), has probably investigated this issue in more detail than most pathologists. Their observations and those by some other investigators (Honoré et al., 1976; Ornoy et al., 1981; Byrne et al., 1985; Göcke et al., 1985) allowed some subdivision of abortion specimens into major categories. Indeed, some of these investigators have gone so far as to suggest that many of these pathological changes are so characteristic that they enable chromosomal diagnosis from the morphological findings in the villous tissue alone. Others who have studied these specimens could not find a good correlation between cytogenetic findings and morphology (Rehder et al., 1989; Horn et al., 1991). Much the same applies to molar or hydatid abortion material. A group of investigators from Europe and Australia have analyzed the potential error in the diagnosis of molar (hydatid) specimens by several observers (Howat et al., 1993). They obtained 50 molar abortion specimens of different types and sent them for independent assessment to seven colleagues, two with a special interest in gynecological pathology. The details will have to be read by the interested pathologist. Suffice it to say here that these experts and regular diagnostic pathologists were unable to specifically label a given microscopic appearance with confidence. Especially, they were not able to reliably distinguish complete moles from partial moles. Partial moles could not be reliably differentiated from nonmolar abortion material. Howat et al. found that reliable histopathological criteria do not exist for this differential diagnosis. We agree with this interpretation of the pathological findings. Indeed, Rehder and her colleagues were unable to differentiate structural findings of aneuploid abortuses from those of euploid material. It is true that generally the placentas of spontaneous abortions are too small and too thin. When examined by dissecting microscopy, their villous ramification is decreased, and hydropic degeneration is visible in some (Honoré et al., 1989; Shepard et al., 1989b). More extensive data provided by Shepard et al. (1989c) showed that placentas of trisomy 18 fetuses were small, and some of trisomy 13 placentas were of low weight. In the placentas with triploidy the placental weights were determined, in part at least, by their chromosomal contribution. In conformity with the findings of Jacobs et al. (1982), those triploid fetuses whose extra chromosome set was acquired from the mother were smaller; and when two paternal sets were present, the placentas were larger or hydropic. One might have postulated that anembryonic, but nonmolar, spontaneous abortion specimens have a genetic similarity to complete hydatidiform moles. A specific study directed to elucidate this point comes from Henderson et al. (1991). They studied 14 such specimens with locus-specific minisatellite probes and showed that these anembryonic placentas possessed both maternal and paternal genomes. They were thus not androgenetic as are the hydatidiform moles. A succinct appraisal of the current dilemma in the differential diagnosis of general abortion material for histopathologists was provided by Fox (1993). He reviewed all the relevant publications and concluded that precise histopathological classification is a "valueless exercise." Cytogenetic study and flow cytometry are needed for more precision.

Summary of Placental Findings in Chromosomally Defined Abortions

Trisomies

For historical purposes the usage trisomy C, D, E, and so on is used here. Because usually the exact chromosome involved is not identified, we employ this grouping as merely indicating that these elements belong to the major subgroups of chromosomes so designated.

Trisomy E (16–18)

Trisomy 16 is one of the commonest cytogenetic anomalies found in spontaneous abortion material (Figure 452). Generally, the embryo is absent, and the chorionic cavity is empty and small. Anembryonic gestations may be confused with other abnormal gestational products, and it is for that reason that, as mentioned earlier, Henderson et al. (1991) had examined the genetic makeup of anembryonic specimens. Trisomy 16 was one of the results. Importantly, these embryo-deficient abortuses had maternal and paternal genetic contributions. Most trisomy 16 abortuses constitute the typical blighted ovum, the *windei*. The villous growth is reduced, trophoblast is hypoplastic, villi are usually avascular, and some are hydropic (Vernof et al., 1992). Enlarged cytotrophoblastic giant cells (see below) are found in the stroma of up to 30% of villi.

Trisomy C (6–12)

Abortions with the trisomy C genotype have a variable morphology, and the placenta is less matured than expected. Giant villous trophoblast cells are found in 40%

Trisomy D (13–15)

The trisomy D chromosome anomaly exhibits variable placental maturation, reduced villous vasculature, and giant cytotrophoblast in 50% of villi. Occasionally, hydropic villi exist. The embryo frequently has facial and other anomalies.

Other Trisomies

There are no characteristic patterns of the placentas of other trisomies, although Zerres et al. (1988) described hydatid swelling of villi in four cases of trisomy 22; the villi also had vascularization. One of their cases was terminated at 36 weeks' gestation; it had fewer villous abnormalities. Honoré et al. (1974) described significant molar changes, including atypical trophoblastic proliferation in the placenta of trisomy 2, and trisomy 22 was found in the placenta of a severely growth-retarded infant by Stioui et al. (1989).

Polyploidies

Triploidy

The triploidy category is discussed in greater detail under partial moles in Chapter 22. Macroscopically, the placentas of triploids are frequently partially molar (Figures 453, 454), but it depends largely on the origin of the extra set of chromosomes in triploid conceptuses. It is generally the finding that when an extra paternal

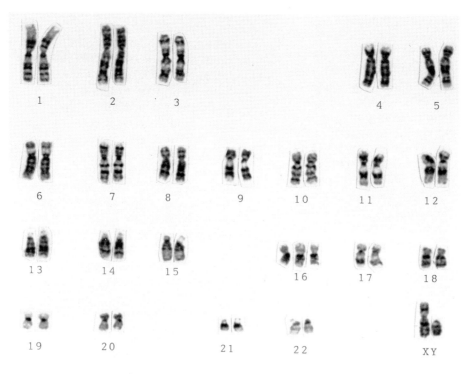

FIGURE 452. Trisomy 16, the commonest trisomy of spontaneous abortions. Giemsa-banded karyotype. (Courtesy Dr. M. Bogart, San Diego.)

set is present the placenta has molar change and a severely abnormal or absent embryo; when an extra maternal set is involved, the embryo is better formed and has some characteristic anomalous features such as digital fusion, and the placenta is less molar or not at all involved. Also, the embryos, when present, are small for expected age. Some villi have microscopic cavities (lacunae) (Figure 455), and others may be broken or are compacted, with increased cellularity (Figure 456); the trophoblast is variably hypoplastic or moderately proliferated. There is characteristic "infolding" (scal-

loping) of trophoblast into the villi, with trophoblastic nests occurring seemingly isolated in the villous stroma (Figure 455). A Breus' mole is occasionally found with triploid abortuses as well. It is important for the pathologist to recognize that the villous edema disappears quickly when the specimen is stored. Numerous abnormalities, such as fusion of some digits or toes, have been described in the fetus of triploid conceptuses (Rehder & Gropp, 1971; Ornoy et al., 1978; Moen et al., 1984), but frequently the embryos are nodular and degenerating (Geisler et al., 1972). They may have a

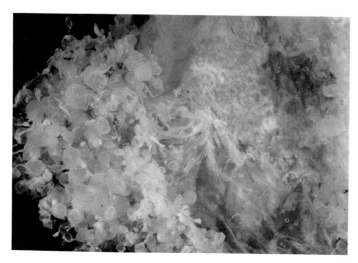

FIGURE 453. Partial hydatidiform mole associated with triploidy (69,XXX). Most villi have hydatid enlargement but are attached to a chorionic sac. A chorionic cavity would not be expected in a true mole.

FIGURE 454. Partial molar degeneration associated with triploidy (69,XXY). Many villi are not hydropic.

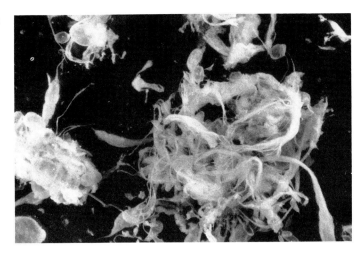

single umbilical artery (Kulazenko & Kulazenko, 1976), as is the case of many other spontaneous abortus specimens. Triploid fetuses rarely survive as long as the 10-month-old child described by Sherard et al. (1986). As expected, the extra set of chromosomes was of maternal origin. Digyny is much commoner in triploids than diandry (McFadden et al., 1994).

Tetraploidy

Tetraploid abortuses have an empty cavity and voluminous, poorly vascularized villi. They frequently have severe decidual and villous hemorrhages, and their villi are invariably somewhat cystic.

Monosomy

Frequently, only a cord remnant is found in a cavity that is small for gestational age (Figure 457). There are well developed villous vessels. Intervillous thrombi of the Breus' mole type are often present (Figure 458). Occasionally, these specimens have a form of amnion nodosum (Figure 459) that may be accompanied by hemosiderin deposits in the membranes. Often these specimens appear to be relatively normal; there are no cystic villi, but villous fibrosis may exist. The embryo may have nuchal hygroma and severe hydrops (Figure 460). Mostello et al. (1989) have reported spontaneous resolution of a hygroma and hydrops in serial sono-

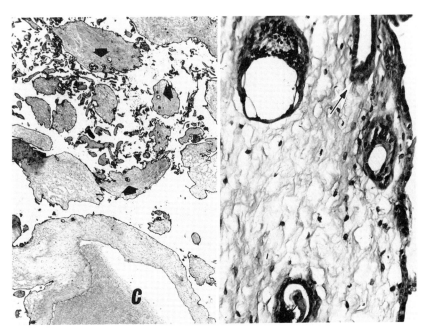

FIGURE 455. Triploid abortus with macrocystic villous hydropic change at bottom left (C) intermixed with small villi above. This picture is typical of a partial mole. Numerous trophoblastic inclusions are seen at arrows and at right. They come about by infolding, as seen at the white arrow. H&E. Left ×64; right ×240.

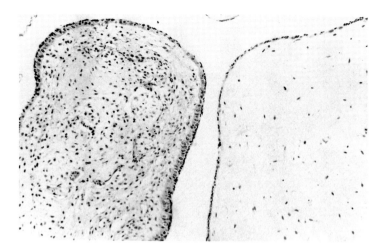

FIGURE 456. Two enlarged villi in a triploid abortus. One villus (left) is hypercellular, with faintly visible remnants of former fetal vessels; the other is hydropic. H&E. ×160.

grams. Microscopic examination of the ovaries shows that they are nearly normal up to the second trimester, whereafter they become depopulated of germinal cells.

The "giant cytotrophoblastic cells" in villi discussed above were initially described by Philippe and Boué (1969). Honoré et al. (1976) suggested that they were internally "delaminating" from the cytotrophoblast. Ornoy et al. (1981) were cautious in their interpretation of the origin of this cell type but apparently leaned toward the view that the cells are swollen (edematous) stromal cells; they suggested that the origin be clarified by ultrastructural study. We also believe that these cells are enlarged Hofbauer cells (Figure 461).

Philippe (1986) considered that a hallmark of many chromosomally aborted specimens is their growth retardation. Byrne et al. (1985) have provided the most comprehensive correlation of fetal phenotype with chromosome findings. Other studies of fetal morphology in spontaneous abortuses have been reported by Bruyere et al. (1987) and Kalousek (1987). The latter investigator correlated chromosomal findings with embryonic phenotype. Ornoy et al. (1981) and Novak et al. (1988) found frequent inflammatory changes of the membranes and villi in their studies, a finding not made by ourselves or other investigators and one that is probably unrelated to the chromosomal aberrations. Shepard et al. (1989a) undertook a 20-year analysis of aborted specimens and found that 19% of fetuses had a localized defect. Neural tube defects existed in 3.6%, and recognizable abnormal phenotypes due to chromosomal errors were present in 2.7%. Shepard et al. encountered amnionic bands in 4 specimens, renal agenesis in 2, and facial clefts in 30 of 214 abnormal embryos.

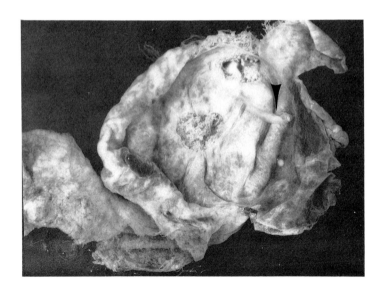

FIGURE 457. Monosomy X abortus, with only a cord remnant (arrow) present. A small yolk sac remnant is also found. The defects in the chorionic membranes are due to cytogenetic sampling. This site is convenient for tissue culture material.

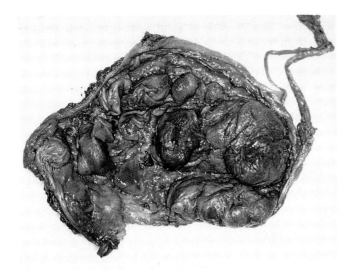

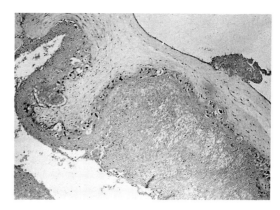

FIGURE 458. Breus mole (subchorionic tuberous hematoma). No embryo is present. This finding occurs frequently with monosomy X.

FIGURE 459. Microscopic appearance of the specimen shown in Figure 458. There is old subchorionic, intervillous thrombus in a pocket of bulging membranes. The amnion is focally defective and has attached debris. It has been considered to be amnion nodosum, but the debris is not squames, as there is no embryo. It is often seen with monosomy X. H&E. ×40.

INDUCED ABORTION

Pregnancies may be terminated legally (therapeutic or induced abortion) or illegally (criminal abortion). There is little difference between the two from a pathologist's point of view, except that the latter is frequently followed by uterine infection. Induced abortion has been a common cause of maternal mortality in the past, but since the introduction of legalized abortion approximately one-fourth of pregnancies in the United States are aborted. The safety of the procedure has increased dramatically, with markedly reduced maternal mortality (approximately 1.5 in 100,000). A succinct review of legal abortion and its history was provided in an

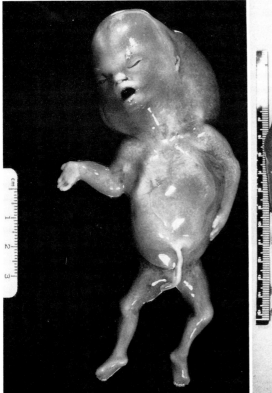

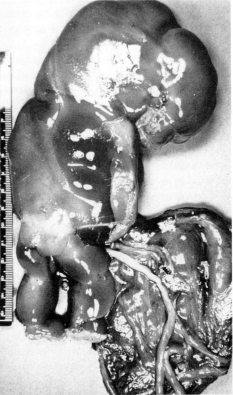

FIGURE 460. Two abortuses with monosomy X. The left embryo (10 weeks) has pronounced hygroma; that on the right is edematous and has hygroma as well. Note the hypoplastic placenta.

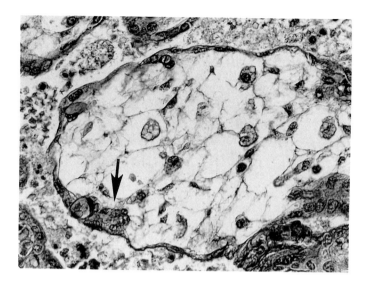

FIGURE 461. Villus with cytotrophoblastic giant cells from a spontaneous abortion. The much enlarged cells in the villous core represent enlarged Hofbauer cells, although a suggestion of cytotrophoblast proliferation is seen at the arrow. Cystic lacunae are developing in the villus. H&E. ×400.

editorial (Anonymous, 1989). Induced abortions are performed by dilatation and curettage (D&C), use of prostaglandins (with or without the use of cervical laminaria), intraamnionic injection of hypertonic saline or urea solutions, and other means (Palomaki & Little, 1972). The pathological findings in the aborted fetal/placental specimen differ somewhat for each procedure. The study of therapeutic abortion material is often helpful for understanding normal placental relations. A superb electron microscopic study was performed on an 11-day-old previllous ovum that had recently implanted (Knoth & Larsen, 1972). In such material, pathologists may also find microscopic structures with which they are not familiar, particularly the early yolk sac. This normal feature of early gestation is shown in Figures 462 to 464. It is the probable initial site of α-fetoprotein production and hematopoiesis and may serve in early fetal nutrition (Luckett, 1972).

When D&C or suction curettage is performed, instrumentation of the cervix and uterus has occasionally led to misplacement of fetal tissues and to sporadic uterine perforation (Kaali et al., 1989). Ayers et al. (1971) reported a 3 cm paracervical bony mass containing a fetal skeleton. The original suction curettage had been done 3 months earlier, when the mother was 10 weeks pregnant. (She had suffered symptoms of pulmonary embolism.) Placental

and various other fetal tissues were present, including bone. Incompletely removed fetal tissues have been incriminated in causing infertility. Dawood and Jarrett (1982) reported uterine retention of fetal bones for 6 years; the authors suggested that this material acted similar to an intrauterine device (IUD), perhaps by inducing endometrial synechiae. Melius and colleagues (1991) found bones in the uterus 13 years and 14 months, respectively, after abortion. A similar case is shown in Figure 465. We have seen a case with maternal death following TAB at 20 weeks' gestation. The uterus was inadvertently perforated, and massive intraabdominal hemorrhage occurred. The patient survived for 2 days and died with disseminated intravascular coagulation (DIC) and adult respiratory distress syndrome. Pulmonary emboli contained deported placental villi enmeshed in fibrin coagulum (Figure 466). Uterine perforations were the topic of a review by Darney et al. (1990). They suggested that errors when estimating the gestational age were common in such cases. Lawson et al. (1990) reviewed fatal pulmonary embolism after legal abortion. They found that 45 patients among 231 maternal deaths were caused by embolism with air, clot, or amnionic fluid. DIC occurred in 11 patients.

When bougies are used for termination of midtrimester pregnancies, the placentas were found to be entirely normal (Manabe

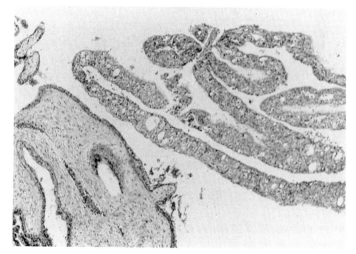

FIGURE 462. Yolk sac at 5 weeks' gestation intermixed with primitive villi (left). The specimen is from a therapeutic abortion. H&E. ×64.

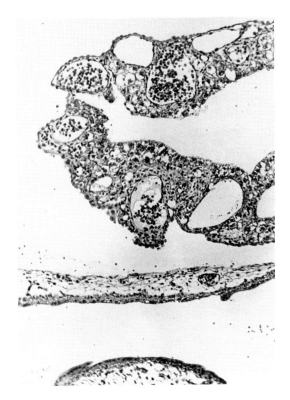

FIGURE 463. Yolk sac at 6 weeks' gestation with chorionic membrane, carrying a fetal vessel (below). Note the large sinusoids in the yolk sac epithelium filled with erythropoietic cells. H&E. ×240.

et al., 1971). Suter et al. (1970) found that suction curettage in infected pregnancies was more difficult to complete; the reason was a presumably more adherent placenta.

There are severe placental changes when pregnancies are terminated with intrauterine installation of hypertonic saline, as extensive fetal ion fluxes occur (Anderson & Turnbull, 1968; Frigoletto & Pokoly, 1971). When these changes are also reflected in the maternal circulation because of accidental injection into the maternal sinusoids, maternal hypernatremia and death have ensued

(Schulman et al., 1971; Gustavii, 1972). Clostridial infection is another feared complication (Sehgal et al., 1972). Saline-induced terminations are now rare; they are performed without general anesthesia. Associated pathological changes include amnion necrosis and fluid accumulation underneath the amnion. Most importantly, coagulation of intervillous blood and focal necrosis underneath the chorionic plate occur.

These changes were well illustrated in the study of Christie et al. (1966). A placenta from such a termination is shown in Figure 467. It has the characteristic band of hemorrhagic necrosis and coagulation underneath the chorionic plate. The tissue is typically pale owing to hemolysis of fetal blood. Another detailed study of the placental changes in saline terminations was reported in the dissertation of Gustavii (1973; see also Gustavii & Brunk, 1972). Other authors who have examined the effect of saline installation into the amnionic cavity are Bengtsson and Stormby (1962) and Jaffin et al. (1962). Gustavii found that saline installation into the extramembranous space quickly stripped the membranes from the uterine wall and led to marked sodium fluxes into the amnionic fluid. It caused decidual necrosis and lysis, whereas the trophoblast remained normal. Gustavii regarded the decidua as the "target" in the procedure. Steinberg et al. (1972) observed a febrile reaction after saline termination in about 20% of cases. From negative placental cultures, they deduced that it was rarely caused by infection.

Hospital admissions for septic abortion have decreased significantly since abortion became legal (Stewart & Goldstein, 1971; Seward et al., 1973). In the large Yugoslavian experience with legal abortion (D&C or suction), the maternal mortality was 0.02% and the morbidity 4.29% (Jurukovski, 1969). Similar reports have come from other countries. Kubatova and Trnka (1967) histologically examined the specimens of 100 legal abortions and found that myometrial admixture was more common with D&C (22%) than with suction curettage. Decidual necrosis and inflammation were common, but the villous tissue was usually normal.

The intentional termination of early pregnancies allows an insight into embryogenesis. Nishimura et al. (1968) thus studied the phenotype of 1,213 "undamaged" fetuses from therapeutic terminations undertaken by D&C for psychosocial reasons. Fetal death had occurred in 2.39%, most commonly in women with genital bleeding and of slightly older age. The investigators found macroscopic anomalies in 1.15% of these embryos. It is also important to note that no hydatidiform moles were encountered by these investigators in this survey, even though this disease is more common in Japan than in the United States. Singh and Carr (1968) also

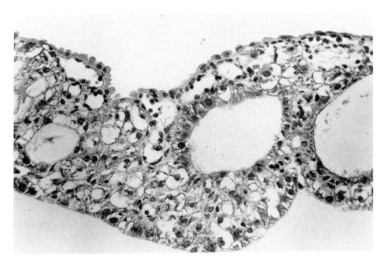

FIGURE 464. Same case as in Figure 463. The tissue of this yolk sac at 6 weeks' abortion is rich in glycogen and has glandular spaces. Endodermal epithelium is seen inside (above). H&E. ×640.

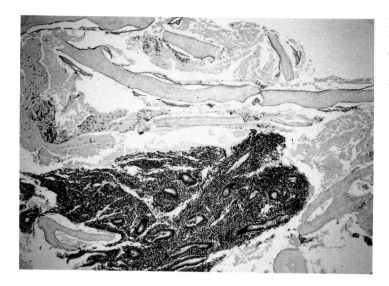

FIGURE 465. Retained, necrotic fetal bony lamellae in inactive endometrium that also shows mild chronic endometritis. They are remains of an abortion that took place several years ago. These fragments presumably acted as a contraceptive device; they were removed in 1987, and term delivery ensued in 1989. H&E. ×60. (Courtesy Dr. W. Tench, San Diego.)

described fetal specimens with anomalies but normal karyotypes; most commonly these were omphaloceles. Several large studies have been undertaken to assess the karyotypes of legally aborted embryos. For instance, Sasaki et al. (1967) examined the chromosomes of 140 such abortion specimens, terminated at an average gestational age of 9.6 weeks of pregnancy. Of the 140 specimens, 133 were normal, 3 were mosaic, and 4 had other chromosomal errors (5%). The investigators additionally cited other published surveys. Yamamoto and Watanabe (1979) found a 6.4% incidence of chromosomal errors among 1,661 legal abortions before the 12th week of gestation. Of interest again is the therein reported absence of hydatidiform moles, despite the prevalence of moles in this population.

Jewett (1973) reported maternal deaths when saline had been instilled illicitly; and Monrozies (1971), who studied 426 "criminal" abortions, found that 55 (13%) had serious complications, including uterine hemorrhages, perforations, DIC, and life-threatening infections. In placentas of septic abortions, Studdiford and Douglas (1956) found acute villitis, intervillositis, and bacterial colonies filling the fetal villous capillaries. Because they had elicited no inflammatory reaction in some of the cases, the colonies doubtless grew postmortem, although sepsis must have preceded the deaths.

Segal et al. (1976) studied the placental changes associated with infusion of hypertonic urea solution. They examined 52 placentas and found subchorionic fibrin deposits (similar to those of saline infusion) and swollen Hofbauer cells. These authors indicated that no placental changes occur with hypertonic glucose instillation. In our experience, the changes seen in the subchorionic space following urea termination are usually much less severe than when hypertonic saline solutions are used. Accumulations of polymorphonuclear leukocytes are frequent in the subchorionic space as well but not in the fetal vasculature. In other cases there is chorionic vascular obliteration and much the same subchorionic thrombosis as is seen with hypertonic saline (Figure 468). A detailed study of these changes was reported by Babaknia and colleagues (1979).

Incomplete Abortion

Pathologists are often required to make the diagnosis of intrauterine pregnancy from curettings of women who are presumed to have sustained an abortion. When villi

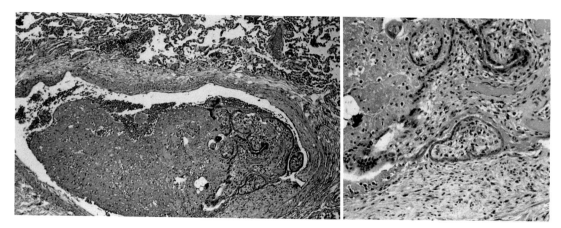

FIGURE 466. Pulmonary embolus following a therapeutic abortion complicated by fatal uterine perforation, abdominal hemorrhage, and disseminated intravascular coagulation. Immature villi are engulfed in a fibrin coagulum. H&E. Left ×160; right ×240.

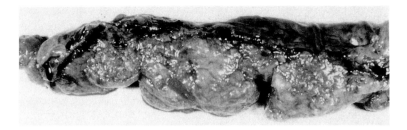

FIGURE 467. Macroscopic appearance of an immature placenta from a saline-induced abortion. Note the subchorionic hemorrhage, fibrin deposit, and pallor of the placenta. The superficial villi are necrotic; fetal blood is hemolyzed.

or syncytiotrophoblast are seen the diagnosis is obvious, but frequently these elements are not present in the decidual debris that is intermixed with fibrin and hemorrhagic material. The diagnosis of pregnancy is then more difficult. It then depends on the pathologist's ability to differentiate degenerating decidual changes (which could result from an ectopic pregnancy) from those of intrauterine implantation sites. The decidua basalis at the placental implantation site undergoes characteristic

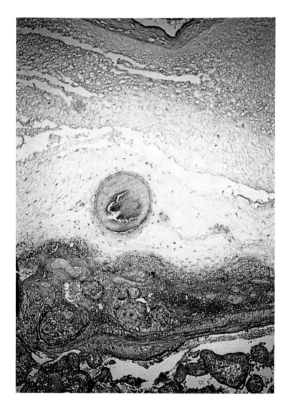

FIGURE 468. Placental surface in urea termination at 19 weeks' gestation. The large chorionic, fetal vessel is thrombosed. There is much edema in the membranes, and underneath the chorionic plate is a dense accumulation of fibrin, blood clot, and some polymorphonuclear leukocytes. H&E. ×40.

morphological changes that should be identified in curettings, even in the absence of villi and syncytium, and serve as a diagnostic clue. These changes include infiltration with fibrin and alterations of decidual blood vessels (physiological changes, see Chapter 11); most characteristically the decidua basalis contains X cells at the implantation site. These cells are usually easily recognized in spontaneous abortions, and their presence establishes the presence of placentation at this site. In addition, there are frequently some decidual degeneration and inflammatory cell infiltration. The principal microscopic indicators of a placental site are shown in Figures 469 and 470.

Lichtig et al. (1988) have described the vascular component of this decidual change. They believed that it is a pathological change and thus differ from the many authors who have considered the vascular invasion by trophoblast as "physiological." They cited these authors but still preferred a different interpretation. What is important in their contribution is that they addressed the dilemma often faced by the practicing pathologist, and they provided valuable and practical suggestions for the differential diagnosis.

The term placental polyp is occasionally applied. It refers to the residuum of placental tissue from abortion or more often term pregnancy. A placental polyp is frequently embedded in degenerating blood clot. Its cause may be placenta accreta or incompletely aborted placental tissue. It is more fully discussed in Chapter 26.

Placenta in Chorionic Villous Sampling

Alvarez (1966) first used placental biopsy for differential diagnosis of hydatidiform mole and later for assessment of villous morphology in erythroblastosis, syphilis, and other disorders. Chorionic villous sampling (CVS) was subsequently used to determine fetal sex (Anonymous, 1975). Kazy et al. (1982) applied CVS to the determination of fetal genetic disorders. CVS is now widely used for the prenatal diagnosis of chromosomal and genetic

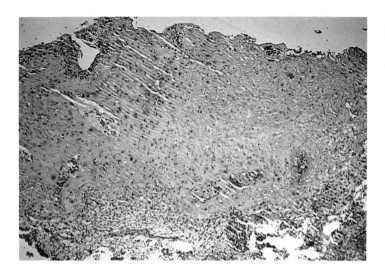

FIGURE 469. Curettings from a placental site of an incomplete spontaneous abortion. There are foci of decidual necrosis, lymphocyte and macrophage infiltration, and fibrin deposition throughout this former placental implantation site. H&E. ×64.

disorders and is undertaken during the first trimester. Some clinicians prefer this method because it allows access to the fetal genotype before the feasibility of amniocentesis. Chieri and Aldini (1989) used CVS also during the second trimester, encountering one abortion in 220 patients.

Although the method is generally safe, it has caused placental complications, including fetal bleeding (Shulman et al., 1990). Cashner et al. (1987) suggested that great difficulties exist in the precise risk evaluation from CVS because of the general risk of spontaneous abortion in this gestational age group. With a live fetus from an 8- to 12-week gestation, the risk of spontaneous abortion was 2% in their analysis, and it was greater in the older women, who are more likely to be sampled. Lippman et al. (1984) also estimated spontaneous abortion rates. They were not convinced that CVS is a significant cause of fetal loss. The complications of CVS were followed by sonographic surveillance in 714 patients studied by Wade and Young (1989); who reported a 4.1% "unintended" abortion, rate by 20 weeks' gestation; it was higher when repeated catheter insertion was necessary. Subchorionic bleeding was witnessed in one patient, with abortion following in 48 hours. Late abortions were "more likely to have in utero death or premature rupture of the membranes." During CVS, Pozniak et al. (1988) noted sonographically the rapid development of a retromembranous hematoma that

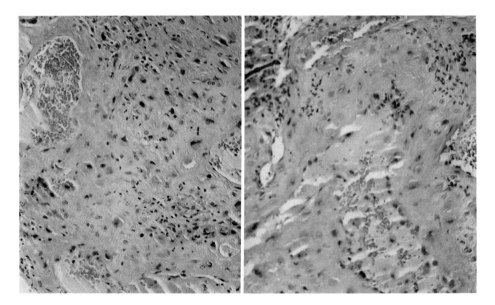

FIGURE 470. Curettings from a placental site of a spontaneous abortion. Note the infiltration with fibrinoid and large placental site giant cells. These X cells have infiltrated and altered the blood vessel wall at right. Despite the absence of villi and syncytium, this histological picture suffices for the diagnosis of placental site. H&E. ×260.

formed from a venous lake. Its expansion ceased spontaneously. Facial hemorrhages in the fetus were demonstrated by fetoscopy during CVS by Quintero et al. (1993).

Occasional cases of septic abortion have followed CVS. Brambati and Varotto (1985), who found bacterial cultures from the cervix of CVS patients to be positive in a large percentage of cases, performed 700 CVS procedures and found acute infection twice. Barela et al. (1986) reported septic shock and renal failure 4 days after CVS at 11.5 weeks' gestation. Associated endomyometritis ultimately necessitated hysterectomy. Muggah et al. (1987) found degenerated villi with transcervical CVS at 73 days' gestation. CVS was repeated 4 days later. The patient experienced fever that disappeared at 12 weeks' gestation. She miscarried at 16 weeks and was treated for septic shock. Coliform organisms were cultured from the placenta and fetal parts but not from amnionic fluid. Marini et al. (1988) reported septic abortion 10 weeks aften CVS. The placenta (at 20 weeks) showed acute chorioamnionitis, but it is doubtful that this event was causally related to the CVS.

The procedure does not usually have serious placental sequelae. When we have examined the placentas of patients who have had CVS during the first trimester, no abnormal findings were apparent. Similar results were reported from a large multicenter study of 2,278 CVS procedures; the findings were compared with the results of amniocentesis in 617 patients. There was only a 0.8% increase of fetal loss in the CVS group (Rhoads et al., 1989). Concern has been expressed over the finding that limb-reduction defects may follow CVS (Firth et al., 1991; Burton et al., 1992). Letters to the editor (1991) have subsequently examined the issue. Some of these letters noted that "organized thrombi" were found in fetal stem vessels (Scott, 1991); a vascular etiology was also suggested by Burton et al. (1992). It is currently thought that the relation may exist principally in the gestationally earlier CVS practiced in Europe. No limb-reduction defects were identified in the large series by Williams et al. (1992) when CVS was done after 9 weeks.

Most concern about prenatal diagnosis relates to discrepancies of chromosomal findings by the various methods used: CVS, amniocentesis, and fetal blood culture. Often the reason for these findings is real mosaicism; at other times, however, pseudomosaicism exists. Some authors have attributed it to the usage of Chang tissue culture medium (Krawczun et al., 1989), and contamination with maternal tissue is another possible cause. The finding of mosaic cell lines has caused much concern in the fetal prenatal assessment, and discrepant results are not always easy to explain. They may reflect the differing origin of cells from the inner cell mass (fetus) or its shell (placenta), as well as nondisjunctional events taking place in the sometimes prolonged tissue culture.

One of the most interesting cases in this respect was the finding of trisomy 16 confined to villi, with ultimately a normal fetal karyotype. Verp et al. (1989) reported such a case in which there was a grossly and histologically normal placenta associated with a growth-retarded fetus. They also referred to a report with a normal stillborn fetus described earlier. These investigators cautioned that the presence of a fetus with an otherwise lethal karyotype found by CVS should alert one to the possible confinement of aneuploidy to the placenta. Perhaps the aneuploid placenta functioned less efficiently than would a normal organ. It might have produced the fetal growth retardation they observed. Another interesting case addresses a similar problem. Nonmosaic trisomy 16 was observed by CVS in a pregnancy associated with an apparently normal fetus (Tharapel et al., 1989). Fetus and placenta were found to be normal 46,XX at delivery, but a "placental nodule" had 46,XX/47,XX,+16 mosaicism. The authors inferred that it represented a vanished twin gestation. Regrettably, a histological study of the nodule was not undertaken. A similar case of pure trisomy 16 in the placenta and a normal 46,XY fetus was observed in a severely preeclamptic woman by Vernof et al. (1992). The neonate was growth-retarded but otherwise normal. At other times, placenta and fetus were found chromosomally and structurally normal after a nonmosaic trisomy 16 diagnosis from CVS (Sundberg & Smidt-Jensen, 1991).

In the large study reported by Rhoads et al. (1989), 1.8% of the samples were correctly diagnosed as aneuploid. Reports of two specimens (tetraploidy and trisomy 22) were later proved to be false. Kalousek and Dill (1983) have produced evidence that chromosomal mosaicism is often confined to the placenta (confined placental mosaicism, or CPM); they have expanded this concept in many subsequent contributions to the literature. In a relevant review, Kalousek and Barrett (1994) found it most likely that in many cases the embryo had originally been trisomic as well. Regrettably, there is not yet any direct correlation with placental phenotype (e.g., pathological features) in the various types of CPM that have been described by the authors. DeLozier-Blanchet et al. (1993) suggested that the chromosomally abnormal areas of villous biopsies show structural pathological features but have not elaborated further. It appears, however, that this condition is also found more frequently in stillbirths that are otherwise unexplained. Its elucidation has certainly made the interpretation of some chromosomal errors in CVS more difficult. Breed et al. (1986) found a deletion of chromosome 16 in a CVS specimen but a normal fetal karyotype. The chorionic tissue was later found to be mosaic. Verjaal et al. (1987) reported six discrepant results and cited many other such inconsistencies from the literature. Schulze et al. (1987) found two cases of CVS with mosaic trisomic cells in which the aborted fetuses were euploid, and Vernof et al. (1992) had another. Cheung et al. (1987) suggested that direct preparations of extended chromosomes be made from multiple villi in order to ascertain mosaicism that is confined to the placenta. Some investigators have argued that such mosaicism, detected at CVS and amnionic fluid study, should be followed by fetal blood karyotyping. They have suggested that it usually would reveal fetal euploidy, but Kaffe et al. (1988) confirmed the mosaicism found earlier in amnionic fluid cells. Thus mosaicism is not always confined to the placenta. It is of interest here that Kalousek and McGillivray (1987) found that all surviving fetuses with trisomy 13 and trisomy 18 had placental karyotype mosaicism. Subsequently, this finding was extended to terminated pregnancies with these trisomies (Kalousek et al., 1989). The mosaicism was confined to cytotrophoblast and was not found in villous stroma, chorion, or amnion. Moreover, no such mosaicism was found in fetuses with trisomy 21. The suggestion is that trisomics with mosaic (aneuploid/diploid) placentas have a better chance of reaching maturity than those with truly trisomic placentas.

Villous tissue is useful for structural and genetic studies. Besley et al. (1988) diagnosed Gaucher's disease (and trisomy 21) from β-glucosidase deficiency in aspirated villi. We had the opportunity to examine tissues of a fetus who was diagnosed as having Hunter syndrome (mucopolysaccharidosis II, iduronate sulfatase deficiency) by amnionic fluid analysis. Although some inclusions were present in the liver, the spinal cord showed striking abnormalities. Ultrastructural analysis of the placenta was normal. Further consideration of the identification of fetal storage disorders with CVS is undertaken in Chapter 18.

Fetal cells may enter in sufficient numbers to allow chromosomal diagnosis by aspiration of maternal blood. Lo et al. (1990) identified Y-specific sequences, but Holzgreve et al. (1990) and Gänshirt-Ahlert et al. (1992) were not convinced. Kao et al. (1992) were more successful in positively identifying Y chromosome-specific genes; Elias et al. (1992) used hybridization with 21-specific probes to identify fetal trisomy 21. Fetal cells in the maternal circulation were tentatively also identified by Suzumori et al. (1992) from fetal blood cells in the maternal circulation, and Adinolfi et al. (1993) diagnosed trisomy 18 in nucleated cells from cervical flushes. Thus methods are currently under study to enhance fetal diagnosis using less invasive techniques. They rely on sorting fetal cells with flow cytometry, using antibodies, and enriching the DNA with PCR.

Trisomic Placentas

There are few specific findings that truly characterize a placenta with trisomy, but many types of abnormality have been found sporadically. For example, the incidence of single umbilical artery (SUA) is higher than normal. Hecht (1963) reported five cases of trisomy 18 and found that the associated placentas were unusually small. Histologically, one of his specimens showed markedly increased fibrin deposits, syncytial knotting, and infarcts. Similar findings were reported by Matayoshi et al. (1977). Rochelson and colleagues (1990) studied the placentas of 18 trisomic fetuses with quantitative morphometry, using appropriate controls. Doppler analysis of umbilical arterial blood flow had been performed in 10 of them. They found that the placentas had a "significant reduction in small muscular artery count and small muscular artery/villus ratio," which correlated with abnormal Doppler waveforms. A quantitative study of normal and chromosomally abnormal placentas between 18 and 23 weeks' gestation was reported by Kuhlmann et al. (1990). They found no differences in fetal and placental weights, but a significant decrease in small muscular arteries and total vessel counts was seen in the aneuploids. Aside from smaller size, we have noted an increase in syncytial knots associated with trisomy 18 (Figure 471), increased cellularity of villous stroma (Figure 472), and vascular abnormalities. The latter were either old occlusions or fresh thromboses of surface and umbilical cord vessels (Figure 473). Villitis of unknown etiology was found in another case, but its relation to trisomy 18 may be spurious. In one case of trisomy 18 associated with many abnormalities of fetal development, the small placenta had numerous cysts scattered throughout. They were composed of large villi with cisternae (Figure 474). Although this appearance was different from that of the partial moles in triploidy, this morphology certainly is not characteristic for or diagnostic of trisomy 18. With trisomy 13, the placenta is also frequently smaller and more often has SUA; the villi are frequently dysmature (Figure 475). We have the impression that the villi have deficient capillarization. The relation of SUA to chromosome errors has been explored by Saller et al. (1990) in 109 chromosomally abnormal pregnancies, with 53 cords identified. Six single umbilical arteries were found (two of 9 trisomy 18; two of 6 with trisomy 13; two of other cytogenetic errors). Quantitative studies, especially combined with assessment of SUA, have not been done. Trisomy 21 is not accompanied by characteristic pathological changes in the placenta. Kouvalainen and Österlund (1967) found a somewhat enlarged placental weight in a trisomy 21 pregnancy and suggested that it may "be a reflection of an immunological reaction of the mother against her

FIGURE 471. Villi of a immature placenta (28 weeks' gestation) from a growth-retarded (370 g) stillborn fetus with trisomy 18. There is markedly increased syncytial knotting despite the absence of preeclampsia. Villi lack fetal vessels because of fetal demise, but many have hyalinized centers. H&E. ×64.

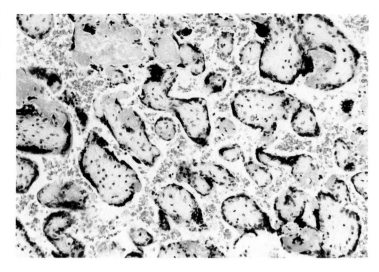

incompatible fetus." Qureshi et al. (1994) found an increased number of irregular villi (dysmature villi) and some villous hypovascularity in trisomy 21 placentas.

Chemical Markers and Trisomy

Steier et al. (1986) evaluated the amount of hCG in the blood and uterine contents of women with legal abortions, spontaneous abortions, and ectopic pregnancies. They found identical values in the first group, but in the other two groups the uterine levels were significantly higher than those obtained from the peripheral circulation. When Bogart et al. (1987) measured hCG, α-subunit levels of hCG, and α-feto protein in serum of pregnancies with chromosomally normal and abnormal conceptuses, they found that 56% of the abnormal gestations had elevated gonadotropin levels beyond 18 weeks' gestation (1.35% of normals). Elevated α-subunit levels were found in 28% of abnormal pregnancies and in none of the normals. The authors suggested that these findings may be useful for screening procedures, but they had no explanation for them. In a later study, Bogart et al. (1989) examined maternal sera for these hormones in earlier pregnancies and found that aneuploid fetuses did not deviate from the normal controls, and their earlier

findings were confirmed. The importance of adequate monitoring was highlighted by the danger of overlooking an ectopic abortion when a therapeutic abortion is undertaken; three fatal cases of this complication were reported by Li and Smialek (1993).

OTHER FINDINGS

There are many causes of spontaneous abortion in addition to the genetic abnormalities just described. Among them are amnionic adhesions (see Chapter 12), infections (see Chapter 20), knots in the umbilical cord (Figure 476), and umbilical cord twists (see Chapter 13). The pathologist is urged to undertake microscopic study of even macerated fetuses. Frequently unexpected features are found (e.g., cytomegalovirus infection) that cannot be anticipated from the history or gross morphology. Fetal and maternal deaths are more likely to occur in women using IUDs, especially the formerly used Dalkon Shield (Cates et al., 1976). We have found in the placenta of a spontaneous abortion specimen large numbers of Hofbauer cells whose cytoplasm contained granular accumulations that resembled Russell bodies, but they were not plasma cells (Figure 477). Their presence remains an unresolved mystery.

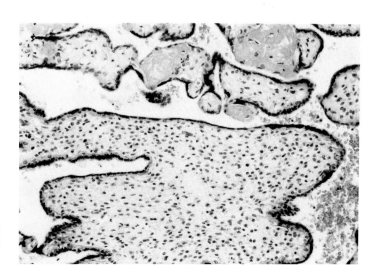

FIGURE 472. Other areas of the trisomy 18 premature placenta shown in Figure 464. Note the marked increase in villous stromal cells. H&E. ×160.

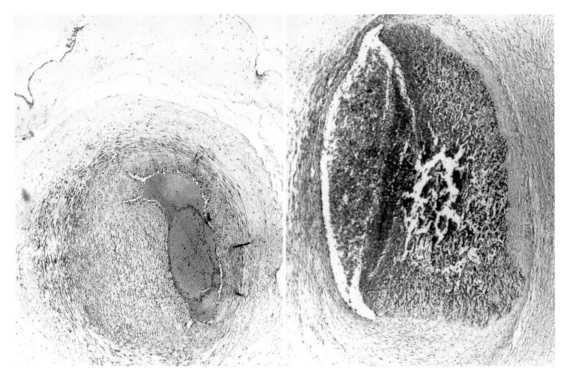

FIGURE 473. Umbilical vessels of a placenta with trisomy 18 showing thrombosis, hemorrhage into the vascular wall, and irregular thickening of the vessel wall. H&E. ×60.

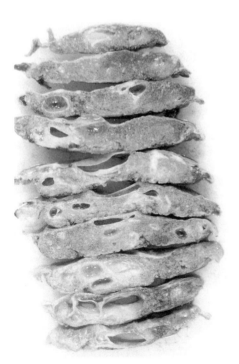

FIGURE 474. Cross sections through the placenta from a trisomy 18 stillbirth. The cysts are composed of enlarged villi; the fetus had numerous anomalies and growth retardation.

Recurrent or Habitual Abortion

Habitual abortion has been variously defined. Wall and Hertig (1948) considered it a "condition in which a woman had two or more consecutive abortions." They examined 100 such patients and found that the same pathological findings were observed in 58% of their cases. Of these abnormalities, 43% were considered to result from "ovular factors" and 15% from other maternal factors. This topic has been comprehensively reviewed by Gant (1989). He lamented that this entity has not only been differently defined but that other aspects of nomenclature hinder precise analysis. Stirrat (1990a), in an extensive analysis of recurrent abortion, thought that the definition should be three or more spontaneous abortions, because after two mishaps the chance of successful pregnancy was 80%.

Several distinct types of recurrent abortion exist, the known etiologies vary widely, and many causes are either poorly understood or overrated (Stirrat, 1990b). Infectious causes are discussed in Chapter 20; chronic debilitating disease (e.g., lupus erythematosus, maternal heart disease, endocrine disorders, and nephritis) are discussed in Chapter 19; recurrent villitis of unknown etiology (see Chapter 20) and maternal floor infarction (see Chapter 11), constitute another sizable group. The relation of substance abuse to spontaneous abortion

FIGURE 475. Placental villi in a trisomy 13 pregnancy at 27 weeks' gestation. Villi are irregularly matured. Some are edematous with capillary ectasia, and others are excessively small with deficient vascularization. H&E. ×160.

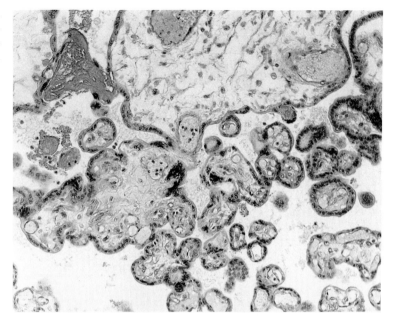

and to abruptio placentae is difficult to evaluate, especially the possible contribution of maternal smoking. Many patients who smoke or use various toxic substances additionally consume alcohol, have various infections, and are prone to suffer misuse and trauma. Although they probably do not make up a large segment

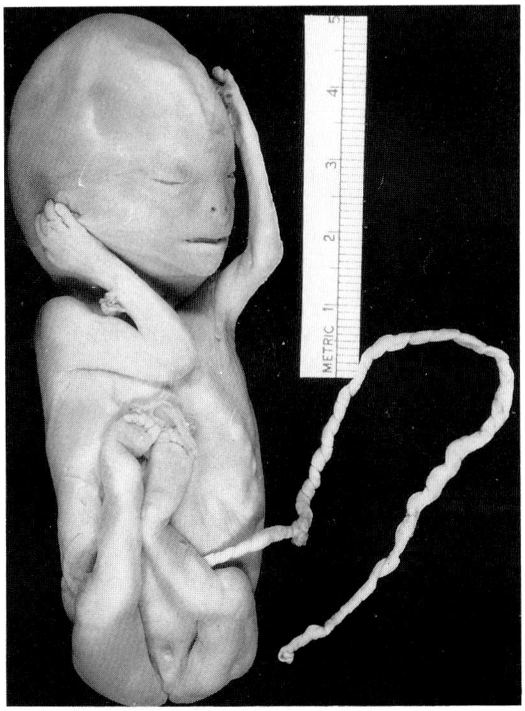

FIGURE 476. Fetal demise due to a tight, true knot in the umbilical cord, followed by abortion at 10 weeks' gestation.

of this entity of repetitive abortion, they form a substantial aspect of polemics in medicine. Direct studies are few; most are epidemiological correlations that seem to establish a connection between these agencies and abortion.

Parental chromosome aberrations and some immunological errors associated with placentation are other well studied causes of recurrent abortion, and they need special consideration here. Occasionally, a balanced chromosomal translocation of one parent has been the cause of habitual abortion. Granat et al. (1981) described a 22/22 translocation in a man whose wife had had six consecutive abortions. All of the specimens had been early, "partially necrotic, and incomplete missed abortions." As is usual, the presumably aneuploid conceptuses were not studied chromosomally. The authors reviewed previous studies of similar case material but with different cytogenetic errors. Their experience led them to urge physicians that for couples with recurrent abortions the mother *and* her husband be examined cytogenetically. Simpson et al. (1989), who studied 342 women and 297 men with more than one first-trimester miscarriage, found that parental translocations were not a common cause of recurrent spontaneous abortions. Such chromosomal errors were more frequent only when anomalies and other reproductive failures were combined. Smith and Gaha (1990) found an appreciable incidence of translocation carriers in a large study of recurrent abortion families. There were 15 balanced reciprocal translocations and 9 Robertsonian fusions in that population. Table 21 reviews some of the large cytogenetic studies of recurrent abortions. There are a number of reasons studies of this kind are difficult to

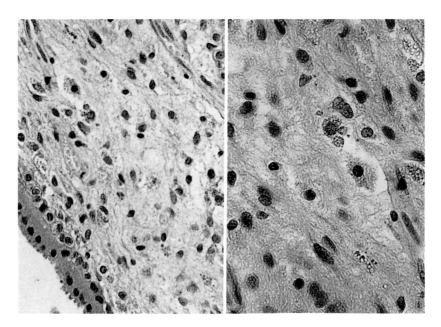

FIGURE 477. Villi from a spontaneous abortion. Note the accumulation of a large number of granular, proteinaceous Hofbauer cell inclusions, whose origin remained obscure. H&E. Left ×160; right ×600.

compare: The methods of analysis differ, the interpretation of chromosomal "variants" is problematical, and aneuploidy is usually only inferred to be the reason for spontaneous abortion as the aborted specimen is virtually never karyotyped. Some recurrent abortions then are caused by parental chromosomal errors, and others are due to increasing maternal age with its increased chance of aneuploidy. The morphology of the specimens does not differ from those of other spontaneous abortions. The pathologist can make a contribution to a better understanding of the etiology by requesting cytogenetic evaluation of aborted specimens from recurrent aborters.

There is not only considerable disagreement as to whether immunological disturbances cause abortion, there is even more controversy as to the management of such mothers. Because autoimmune diseases, such as lupus erythematosus, have a deleterious effect on preg-

nancy (Scott et al., 1987), it has been suggested that an immunological mechanism may also be responsible for "rejection" of the fetal genotype. These considerations could involve specific antibodies, whose actions may be evident in arterial lesions; but such has not often been shown to be the case with the "usual" habitual abortions. That there are changes in a variety of immune parameters with pregnancy, and especially with abortion, has been shown by MacLean et al. (1991) who described alterations in T cell counts (decreased), white blood cell counts (increased), mitogen response (increased), and interleukin-2 receptors (marked increase in abortion). Parazzini and colleagues (1991) studied 220 women with recurrent abortion and found lupus anticoagulant in 17 but none in the controls. Increased anti-cardiolipin antibodies were present in 19, and the authors suggested that in at least a portion of such patients immunological causes may be operative.

TABLE 21. Cytogenetic studies of recurrent abortions.

Source	Year	Families (no.)	Error rate (%)	Types of error
Rosenmann et al.	1977	12	38.4	Variants
Mennuti et al.	1978	34	14.7	Translocations (T)
Heritage et al.	1978	37	8.1	2 T; 1 XXX
Neu et al.	1979	30	3.3	Translocation
Turleau et al.	1979	413	2.3	T, inversion (i), others
Ward et al.	1980	100	6.0	i, variants
Sachs et al.	1985	500	10.0	20 T, mosaics, i, deletions
Castle & Bernstein	1988	688	6.83	XXX, XYY, mosaics, T, i
Portnoi et al.	1988	1,142	4.8	T, i, others

They did not describe the associated placentas. Kwak et al. (1992) made similar observations but warned that "what constitutes an autoimmune abnormality in women with recurrent spontaneous abortion is not yet defined or agreed on." Bahar et al. (1993) studied 103 patients with unexplained recurrent abortions in Kuwait and found anti-cardiolipin antibodies significantly more frequently in this population. The complexity of the problem and the lack of our understanding of feto-maternal immunological interactions is further discussed extensively in letters to the editor (Letters, 1992) that address the case-control study of Infante-Rivard et al. (1992). It can also be illustrated by the existence of several large texts that attempt to summarize relevant data (Edwards et al., 1975; Beer & Billingham, 1976; Wegmann et al., 1983; Gill et al., 1987). Despite the large body of investigative data, there are still many areas of uncertainty. It would be inappropriate to attempt to itemize all of these findings in a text of placental pathology. Central to the problem is our deficient understanding of the failure by the mother to reject the placental "graft." The physiology of this adaptation has been a topic of intense study for many years. This paradox has yet to be resolved. Of the many approaches, the following main positions have been investigated.

1. The mother does not "recognize" the placenta as a foreign genotype perhaps because the trophoblast does not present histocompatibility antigens. Study has suggested, however, that some HLA-G antigens are expressed by young human trophoblast (Kovats et al., 1990), but that recurrent abortion is not influenced by HLA antigens (Eroglu et al., 1992).
2. Maternal immune recognition (and rejection) may be intact but thwarted by local (decidual) regulators.
3. Maternal immune cells, normally endowed with properties to reject allogeneic grafts (T lymphocytes, macrophages) cannot reach the target (because of decidual barriers). Michel et al. (1989) have suggested that the decidual "granular cells" contain smaller granules in repetitive abortion material. For further consideration, see Chapter 11.

Cogent evidence has been provided by immunological studies that placentation proceeds more advantageously when fetus and mother have maximal histocompatibility differences. It is admitted, however, that inbred lines of mice, having no such dissimilarity, have successful gestations. These studies showed that the circulation of maternal blocking antibodies to paternal (placenta present) antigens prevent rejection. These antibodies can be assayed; they are present in normal pregnancies. Other antibodies (against fetal leukocytes, for instance) can also be detected in maternal sera. That fetal proteins interact with maternal lymphocytes in vitro (suppressing their proliferation) has long been recognized (Olding et al., 1974). Whether this interaction has sequelae in vivo is undecided. Proteins from embryos (early pregnancy factor) have been shown to modulate immunosuppressive properties (Bose et al., 1989). Extensive studies on 300 couples with recurrent abortion and 30 control women have shown that a large proportion of the former possess factors in their circulation that are directly toxic to trophoblast or embryonic tissues. These authors suggested that this newly recognized cause of recurrent abortion may "involve the 18 kd, heat-labile, T-lymphocyte cytokinin interferon gamma" (Hill et al., 1992).

Because of the desperate wish for children, couples with habitual abortions have tried many immunological therapeutic interventions, including transfusion and immunization with paternal cells (e.g., Mowbray et al., 1985; McIntyre et al., 1986; Cauchi et al., 1987). Fraser et al. (1993), who reviewed the topic in some detail, thought that immunization for recurrent pregnancy loss should be abandoned. Treatment with "polyvalent intravenous immunoglobin" has been advocated with some seemingly good result by Mueller-Eckhardt et al. (1991), and intravenous infusion of trophoblast plasma membranes isolated from term placentas was undertaken by Johnson et al. (1988). Some of the many studies have been summarized in the cited reference texts and by Stirrat (1990b). In an effort to circumvent possible cryptic endometrial herpes virus infection, Kundsin et al. (1987) have used acyclovir to treat women with habitual abortions. It was moderately successful in the small number of these cases treated.

Other than the placentas of lupus patients, those of habitual aborters have no distinctive pathological features. Most emphatically, they do not possess histological changes of "rejection," as seen in other transplanted tissues. Salafia and Burns (1989) have found "decidual vasculitis" in some such specimens and suggested that it may signal pregnancy loss on an immunological basis. Still, it is sobering to read that, despite all these new insights, the study of Plouffe et al. (1992) failed to show any improvement of outcome with varied therapy when they compared recurrent abortions in two widely separated time zones (1968–1977 and 1987–1991). Aksel (1992), who reviewed all aspects of reproductive immunological disease, is also cautious about advocating immunotherapy for recurrent abortion.

References

Abaci, F., and Aterman, K.: Changes of the placenta and embryo in early spontaneous abortion. Am. J. Obstet. Gynecol. 102:252–263, 1968.

Adinolfi, M., Davies, A., Sharif, S., Soothill, P., and Rodeck, C.: Detection of trisomy 18 and Y-derived sequences in fetal nucleated cells obtained by transcervical flushing. Lancet 342:403–404, 1993.

Aksel, S.: Immunologic aspects of reproductive disease. J.A.M.A. 268:2930–2934, 1992.

Alvarez, H.: Diagnosis of hydatidiform mole by transabdominal placental biopsy. Am. J. Obstet. Gynecol. 95:538–541, 1966.

Anderson, A.B.M., and Turnbull, A.C.: Changes in amniotic fluid, serum and urine following the intra-amniotic injection of hypertonic saline. Acta Obstet. Gynecol. Scand. 47:1–21, 1968.

Anonymous: Anshan department of obstetrics and gynecology: fetal sex prediction by sex chromatin of chorionic villi cells during early pregnancy. Chin. Med. J. 1:117–126, 1975.

Anonymous: Abortion USA. Lancet 1:879–880, 1989.

Antonarakis, S.E.: Diagnosis of genetic disorders at the DNA level. N. Engl. J. Med. 320:153–163, 1989.

Ayers, L.R., Drosman, S., and Saltzstein, S.L.: Iatrogenic paracervical implantation of fetal tissue during therapeutic abortion: a case report. Obstet. Gynecol. 37:755–760, 1971.

Babaknia, A., Parmley, T.H., Burkman, R.T., Atienza, M.F., and King, T.M.: Placental histopathology of midtrimester termination. Obstet. Gynecol. 53:583–586, 1979.

Bahar, A.M., Alkarmi, T., Kamel, A.S., and Sljivic, V.: Anticardiolipin and antinuclear antibodies in patients with unexplained recurrent abortions. Ann. Saudi Med. 13:535–540, 1993.

Barela, A.I., Kleinman, G.E., Golditch, I.M., Menke, D.J., Hogge, W.A., and Golbus, M.S.: Septic shock with renal failure after chorionic villus sampling. Am. J. Obstet. Gynecol. 154:1100–1102, 1986.

Beer, A.E., and Billingham, R.E.: The Immunobiology of Mammalian Reproduction. Prentice Hall, Englewood Cliffs, NJ, 1976.

Bengtsson, L.P., and Stormby, N.: The effect of intraamniotic injection of hypertonic sodium chloride in human midpregnancy. Acta Obstet. Gynecol. Scand. 41:115–123, 1962.

Besley, G.T.N., Ferguson-Smith, M.E., Frew, C., Morris, A., and Gilmore, D.H.: First trimester diagnosis of Gaucher disease in a fetus with trisomy 21. Prenat. Diagn. 8:471–474, 1988.

Bogart, M.H., Pandian, M.R., and Jones, O.W.: Abnormal maternal serum chorionic gonadotropin levels in pregnancies with fetal chromosome abnormalities. Prenat. Diagn. 7:623–630, 1987.

Bogart, M.H., Golbus, M.S., Sorg, N.D., and Jones, O.W.: Human chorionic gonadotropin levels in pregnancies with aneuploid fetuses. Prenat. Diagn. 9:379–384, 1989.

Bose, R., Cheng, H., Sabbadini, E., McCoshen, J., Mahadevan, M.M., and Fleetham, J.: Purified human early pregnancy factor from preimplantation embryo possesses immunosuppressive properties. Am. J. Obstet. Gynecol. 160:954–960, 1989.

Boué, J.G., and Boué, A.: Fréquence des aberrations chromosomiques dans les avortements spontanés humains. C. R. Acad. Sci. Paris 269:283–288, 1969.

Brambati, B., and Varotto, F.: Infection and chorionic villus sampling. Lancet 2:609, 1985.

Breed, A., Mantingh, A., Govaerts, L., Booger, A., Anders, G., and Laurini, R.: Abnormal karyotype in the chorion, not confirmed in a subsequently aborted fetus. Prenat. Diagn. 6:375–377, 1986.

Bruyere, H.J., Arya, S., Kozel, J.S., Gilbert, E.F., Fitzgerald, J.M., Reynolds, J.F., Lewin, S.O., and Opitz, J.M.: The value of examining spontaneously aborted human embryos and placenta. Birth Defects 23:169–178, 1987.

Burton, B.K., Schulz, C.J., and Burd, L.I.: Limb anomalies associated with chorionic villus sampling. Obstet. Gynecol. 79:726–730, 1992.

Byrne, J., Warburton, D., Kline, J., Blanc, W., and Stein, Z.: Morphology of early fetal deaths and their chromosomal characteristics. Teratology 32:297–315, 1985.

Carr, D.H.: Chromosomal studies in spontaneous abortions. Obstet. Gynecol. 26:308–326, 1965.

Cashner, K.A., Christopher, C.R., and Dysert, G.A.: Spontaneous fetal loss after demonstration of a live fetus in the first trimester. Obstet. Gynecol. 70:827–830, 1987.

Castle, D., and Bernstein, R.: Cytogenetic analysis of 688 couples experiencing multiple spontaneous abortions. Am. J. Med. Genet. 29:549–556, 1988.

Cates, W., Ory, H.W., Rochat, R.W., and Tyler, C.W.: The intrauterine device and deaths from spontaneous abortion. N. Engl. J. Med. 295:1155–1159, 1976.

Cauchi, M.N., Koh, S.H., Tait, B., Mraz, G., Kloss, M., and Pepperell, R.J.: Immunogenetic studies in habitual abortion. Aust. N.Z. J. Obstet. Gynaecol. 27:52–54, 1987.

Cheung, S.W., Crane, J.P., Kyine, M., and Cui, M.Y.: Direct chromosome preparations from chorionic villi: a method for obtaining extended chromosomes and recognizing mosaicism confined to the placenta. Cytogenet. Cell Genet. 45:118–120, 1987.

Chieri, P.R., and Aldini, A.J.R.: Feasibility of placental biopsy in the second trimester for fetal diagnosis. Am. J. Obstet. Gynecol. 160:581–583, 1989.

Christie, J.L., Anderson, A.B.M., Turnbull, A.C., and Beck, J.S.: The human placenta and membranes: a histological and immunofluorescent study of the effects of intra-amniotic injection of hypertonic saline. J. Obstet. Gynaecol. Br. Commonw. 73:399–409, 1966.

Creasy, M.R., Crolla, J.A., and Alberman, E.D.: A cytogenetic study of human spontaneous abortions using banding techniques. Hum. Genet. 31:177–196, 1976.

Darney, P.D., Atkinson, E., and Hirabayashi, K.: Uterine perforation during second-trimester abortion by cervical dilation and instrumental extraction: a review of 15 cases. Obstet. Gynecol. 75:441–444, 1990.

Dawood, M.Y., and Jarrett, J.C.: Prolonged intrauterine retention of fetal bones after abortion causing infertility. Am. J. Obstet. Gynecol. 143:715–717, 1982.

DeLozier-Blanchet, C., Francipane, L., Ebener, J., Cox, J., and Extermann, P.: Cytogenetic discrepancies between fetus and placenta: a frequent cause of reproductive pathologies? [abstract A.14]. Placenta 14:A14, 1993.

Dickey, R.P., Olar, T.T., Taylor, S.N., Curole, D.N., and Matulich, E.M.: Relationship of small gestational sac–crown-rump length differences to abortion and abortus karyotypes. Obstet. Gynecol. 79:554–557, 1992.

Eckman, T.R., and Carrow, L.A.: Placental lesions in spontaneous abortion. Am. J. Obstet. Gynecol. 84:222–228, 1962.

Edwards, R.G., Howe, C.W.S., and Johnson, M.H.: Immunobiology of Trophoblast. Cambridge University Press, Cambridge, 1975.

Eiben, B., Bartels, I., Bähr-Porsch, S., Borgmann, S., Gatz, G., Gellert, G., Goebel, R., Hammans, W., Hentemann, M., Osmers, R., Rauskolb, R., and Hansmann, I.: Cytogenetic analysis of 750 spontaneous abortions with the direct-preparation method of chorionic villi and its implications for studying genetic causes of pregnancy wastage. Am. J. Hum. Genet. 47:656–663, 1990.

Elias, S., Price, J., Dockter, M., Wachtel, S., Tharapel, A., Simpson, J.L., and Klinger, K.W.: First trimester prenatal diagnosis of trisomy 21 in fetal cells from maternal blood. Lancet 340:1033, 1992.

Eroglu, G., Betz, G., and Torregano, C.: Impact of histocompatibility antigens on pregnancy outcome. Am. J. Obstet. Gynecol. 166:1364, 1369, 1992.

Firth, H.V., Boyd, P.A., Chamberlain, P., MacKenzie, I.Z., Lindenbaum, R.H., and Huson, S.M.: Severe limb abnormalities after chorion villus sampling at 56–66 days' gestation. Lancet 337:762–763, 1991.

Fox, H.: Histological classification of tissue from spontaneous abortions: a valueless exercise? Histopathology 22:599–600, 1993.

Fraser, E.J., Grimes, D.A., and Schulz, K.F.: Immunization as therapy for recurrent spontaneous abortion: a review and meta-analysis. Obstet. Gynecol. 82:854–859, 1993.

Frigoletto, F.D., and Pokoly, T.B.: Electrolyte dynamics in hypertonic saline-induced abortions. Obstet. Gynecol. 38:647–652, 1971.

Fujikura, T., Froehlich, L.A., and Driscoll, S.G.: A simplified anatomic classification of abortions. Am. J. Obstet. Gynecol. 95:902–905, 1966.

Fujikura, T., Ezaki, K., and Nishimura, H.: Chorionic villi and syncytial sprouts in spontaneous and induced abortions. Am. J. Obstet. Gynecol. 110:547–555, 1971.

Fukunaga, M., Ushigome, S., and Fukunaga, M.: Spontaneous abortions and DNA ploidy: an application of flow cytometric DNA analysis in detection of non-diploidy in early abortions. Mod. Pathol. 6:619–624, 1993.

Gänshirt-Ahlert, D., Burschyk, M., Garritsen, H.S.P., Helmer, L., Miny, P., Horst, J., Schneider, H.P.G., and Holzgreve, W.: Magnetic cell sorting and the transferrin receptor as potential means of prenatal diagnosis from maternal blood. Am. J. Obstet. Gynecol. 166:1350–1355, 1992.

Gant, N.F.: Recurrent spontaneous abortion. Supplement 21 to Williams Obstetrics. J.A. Pritchard, P.C. MacDonald, and N.F. Gant, eds., pp. 1–11. Appleton & Lange, East Norwalk, CT, 1989.

Geisler, M., and Gropp, A.: Zur Methode der Züchtung von Abortmaterial für Chromosomenuntersuchungen (Zugleich Mitteilung über die Beobachtung einer B-Trisomie bei Abortus). Geburtshilfe Frauenheilkd. 27:113–126, 1967.

Geisler, M., Kleinebrecht, J., and Degenhardt, K.-H.: Histologische Analysen von triploiden Spontanaborten. Humangenetik 16:283–294, 1972.

Gill, T.J., Wegmann, T.G., and Nisbet-Brown, E.: Immunoregulation and Fetal Survival. Oxford University Press, New York, 1987.

Göcke, H., Schwanitz, G., Muradow, I., and Zerres, K.: Pathomorphologie und Genetik in der Frühschwangerschaft. Pathologe 6:249–259, 1985.

Granat, M., Aloni, T., Makler, A., and Dar, H.: Autosomal translocation in an apparently normospermic male as a cause of habitual abortion. J. Reprod. Med. 26:52–55, 1981.

Gustavii, B.: Studies on accidental intravascular injection in extra-amniotic saline induced abortion and a method for reducing this risk. J. Reprod. Med. 8:70–74, 1972.

Gustavii, B.: Studies on the mode of action of intra-amniotically and extra-amniotically injected hypertonic saline in therapeutic abortion. Acta Obstet. Gynecol. Scand. Suppl. 25:1–22, 1973.

Gustavii, B., and Brunk, U.: A histological study of the effect on the placenta of intra-amniotically and extra-amniotically injected hypertonic saline in therapeutic abortion. Acta Obstet. Gynecol. Scand. 51:121–125, 1972.

Harrison, R.G., Jones, C.H., and Jones, E.P.: A pathological presomite human embryo. J. Pathol. Bacteriol. 92:583–584, 1966.

Hassold, T., Chen, N., Funkhouser, J., Jooss, T., Manuel, B., Matsuura, J., Matsuyama, A., Wilson, C., Yamana, J.A., and Jacobs, P.A.: A cytogenetic study of 1,000 spontaneous abortions. Ann. Hum. Genet. 44:151–178, 1980.

Hatch, M., Kline, J., Levin, B., Hutzler, M., and Warburton, D.: Paternal age and trisomy among spontaneous abortions. Hum. Genet. 85:355–361, 1990.

Hecht, F.: The placenta in trisomy 18 syndrome: report of 2 cases. Obstet. Gynecol. 22:147–148, 1963.

Henderson, D.J., Bennett, P.R., Rodeck, C.H., Gau, G.S., Blunt, S., and Moore, G.E.: Trophoblast from anembryonic pregnancy has both a maternal and paternal contribution to its genome. Am. J. Obstet. Gynecol. 165:98–102, 1991.

Herbst, R., and Multier, A.-M.: Structures pathologiques du placenta examinées au microscope électronique: premiéres observations des villosités de l'oef abortif humain. Gynecol. Obstet. (Paris) 70:369–376, 1971.

Heritage, D.W., English, S.C., Young, R.B., and Chen, A.T.L.: Cytogenetics of recurrent abortions. Fertil. Steril. 29:414–417, 1978.

Hern, W.M.: Correlation of fetal age and measurements between 10 and 26 weeks of gestation. Obstet. Gynecol. 63:26–32, 1984.

Hertig, A.T., and Sheldon, W.H.: Minimal criteria required to prove prima facie case of traumatic abortion or miscarriage: an analysis of 1,000 spontaneous abortions. Ann. Surg. 117:596–606, 1943.

Hertig, A.T., Rock, J., Adams, E.C., and Menkin, M.C.: Thirty-four fertilized human ova, good, bad and indifferent, recovered from 210 women of known fertility: a study of biologic wastage in early human pregnancy. Pediatrics 23:202–211, 1959.

Hertz-Picciotto, I., and Samuels, S.J.: Incidence of early loss of pregnancy. N. Engl. J. Med. 319:1483–1484, 1988.

Hill, J.A., Polgar, K., Harlow, B.L., and Anderson, D.J.: Evidence of embryo- and trophoblast-toxic cellular immune response(s) in women with recurrent spontaneous abortion. Am. J. Obstet. Gäynecol. 166:1044–1052, 1992.

Holzgreve, W., Gänshirt-Ahlert, D., Burschyk, M., Horst, J., Miny, P., Gal, A., and Pohlschmidt, M.: Detection of fetal DNA in maternal blood by PCR. Lancet 335:1220–1221, 1990.

Honoré, L.H., Dill, F.J., and Poland, B.J.: The association of hydatidiform mole and trisomy 2. Obstet. Gynecol. 43: 232–237, 1974.

Honoré, L.H., Dill, F.J., and Poland, B.J.: Placental morphology in spontaneous humans abortuses with normal and abnormal karyotypes. Teratology 14:151–166, 1976.

Honoré, L.H., Lin, C.C., and Bamforth, J.S.: Spontaneous abortion with uncommon Five cases of trisomy 15 in first trimester spontaneous abortion: gross and microscopic pathology [abstract P42]. Teratology 37:458–459, 1989.

Horn, L.-C., Rosenkranz, M., and Bilek, K.: Wertigkeit der Plazentahistologie für die Erkennung genetisch bedingter Aborte. Z. Geburtshilfe Perinatol. 195:47–53, 1991.

Howat, A.J., Beck, S., Fox, H., Harris, S.C., Hill, A.S., Nicholson, C.M., and Williams, R.A.: Can histopathologists reliably diagnose molar pregnancy? J. Clin. Pathol. 46:599–602, 1993.

Huber, C.P., Melin, J.R., and Vellios, F.: Changes in chorionic tissue of aborted pregnancy. Am. J. Obstet. Gynecol. 73:569–578, 1957.

Hustin, J., Schaaps, J.P., and Lambotte, R.: Anatomical studies of the utero-placental vascularization in the first trimester of pregnancy. Trophoblast Res. 3:49–67, 1988.

Infante-Rivard, C., David, M., Gauthier, R., and Rivard, G.-E.: Lupus anticoagulants, anticardiolipin antibodies, and fetal loss. N. Engl. J. Med. 325:1063–1066, 1992.

Human triploidy: relationship between parental origin of the additional haploid complement and development of partial hydatidiform mole. Ann. Hum. Genet. 46:223–231, 1982.

Jaffin, H., Kerenyi, T., and Wood, E.C.: Termination of missed abortion and the induction of labor in midtrimester pregnancy. Am. J. Obstet. Gynecol. 84:602–608, 1962.

Jewett, J.F.: Two deaths from mid-trimester abortion. N. Engl. J. Med. 288:47–48, 1973.

Johnson, M.P., Drugan, A., Koppitch, F.C., Uhlmann, W.R., and Evans, M.I.: Postmortem chorionic villus sampling is a better method for cytogenetic evaluation of early fetal loss than culture of abortus material. Am. J. Obstet. Gynecol. 163:1505–1510, 1990.

Johnson, P.M., Chia, K.V., Hart, C.A., Griffith, H.B., and Francis, W.J.A.: Trophoblast membrane infusion for unexplained recurrent miscarriage. Br. J. Obstet. Gynaecol. 95:342–347, 1988.

Jurkovic, I., and Muzelak, R.: Frequency of pathologic changes in the young cases studied histologically. Am. J. Obstet. Gynecol. 108:382–386, 1970.

Jurukovski, J.N.: Complications following legal abortions. Proc. R. Soc. Med. 62:830–831, 1969.

Kaali, S.G., Szigetvari, I.A., and Bartfai, G.S.: The frequency and management of uterine perforations during first-trimester abortions. Am. J. Obstet. Gynecol. 161: 406–408, 1989.

Kaeser, O.: Studien an menschlichen Aborteiern mit besonderer Berücksichtigung der frühen Fehlbildungen und ihrer Ursachen. Schweiz. Med. Wochenschr. 79:509–515, 780–785, 803–805, 1050–1056, 1979–1084, 1949.

Kaffe, S., Benn, P.A., and Hsu, L.Y.F.: Fetal blood sampling in investigation of chromosome mosaicism in amniotic fluid cell culture. Lancet 2:284, 1988.

Kajii, T., Ferrier, A., Niikawa, N., Takahara, H., Ohama, K., and Avirachan, S.: Anatomic and chromosomal anomalies in 639 spontaneous abortuses. Hum. Genet. 55:87–98, 1980.

Kalousek, D.K.: Anatomic and chromosome anomalies in specimens of early spontaneous abortion: 7 year experience. Birth Defects 23:153–168, 1987.

Kalousek, D.K., and Barrett, I.: Confined placental mosaicism and stillbirth. Pediatr. Pathol. 14:151–159, 1994.

Kalousek, D.K., and Dill, F.J.: Chromosomal mosaicism confined to the placenta in human conceptions. Science 221:665–667, 1983.

Kalousek, D., and McGillivray, B.: Confined placental mosaicism and intrauterine survival of trisomy 13 and 18. [abstract 828]. Am. J. Hum. Genet. 41:A278, 1987.

Kalousek, D.K., Barrett, I.J., and McGillivray, B.C.: Placental mosaicism and intrauterine survival of trisomies 13 and 18. Am. J. Hum. Genet. 44:338–343, 1989.

Kalousek, D.K., Fitch, N., and Paradice, B.A.: Pathology of the Human Embryo and Previable Fetus. An Atlas. Springer-Verlag, New York, 1990.

Kao, S.-M., Tang, G.-C., Hsieh, T.-T., Young, K.-C., Wang, H.-C., and Pao, C.C.: Analysis of peripheral blood of pregnant women for the presence of fetal Y chromosome-specific ZFY gene deoxyribonucleic acid sequences. Am. J. Obstet. Gynecol. 166:1013–1019, 1992.

Kazy, Z., Rozovsky, I.S., and Bakharev, V.A.: Chorion biopsy in early pregnancy: a method for early prenatal diagnosis for inherited disorders. Prenat. Diagn. 2:39–45, 1982.

Kellokumpu-Lehtinen, P., and Pelliniemi, L.J.: Sex ratio of human conceptuses. Obstet. Gynecol. 64:220–222, 1984.

Kirby, D.R.S., McWhirter, K.G., Teitelbaum, M.S., and Darlington, C.D.: A possible immunological influence on sex ratio. Lancet 2:139–140, 1967.

Knoth, M., and Larsen, J.F.: Ultrastructure of a human implantation site. Acta Obstet. Gynecol. Scand. 51:385–393, 1972.

Kouvalainen, K., and Österlund, K.: Placental weights in Down's syndrome. Ann. Med. Exp. Fenn. 45:320–322, 1967.

Kovacs, B.W., Shahbahrami, B., and Comings, D.E.: Studies of human germinal mutations by deoxyribonucleic acid hybridization. Am. J. Obstet. Gynecol. 160:798–804, 1989.

Kovats, S., Main, E.K., Librach, C., Stubblebine, M., Fisher, S.J., and DeMars, R.: A class I antigen, HLA-G, expressed in human trophoblast. Science 248:220–223, 1990.

Krawczun, M.S., Jenkins, E.C., Masia, A., Kunaporn, S., Stark, S.L., Duncan, C.J., Sklower, S.L., and Rudelli, R.D.: Chromosomal abnormalities in amniotic fluid cell cultures: a comparison of apparent pseudomosaicism in Chang and RPMI-1640 media. Clin. Genet. 35:139–145, 1989.

Kubatova, A., and Trnka, V.: Induced abortions of 8 to 12 weeks pregnancy: evaluation of methods and histological findings in decidua and chorionic villi. Acta Univ. Carol. Med. (Prague) 13:483–491, 1967.

Kuhlmann, R.S., Werner, A.L., Abramowicz, J., Warsof, S.L., Arrington, J., and Levy, D.L.: Placental histology in fetuses between 18 and 23 weeks' gestation with abnormal karyotype. Am. J. Obstet. Gynecol. 163:1264–1270, 1990.

Kulazenko, V.P., and Kulazenko, L.G.: Pathomorphological changes in an early spontaneous abortus with triploidy (69,XXX). Hum. Genet. 32:211–215, 1976.

Kuliev, A.M.: Cytogenetic investigation of spontaneous abortions. Humangenetik 12:275–283, 1971.

Kundsin, R.B., Falk, L., Hertig, A.T., and Horne, H.W.: Acyclovir treatment of twelve unexplained infertile couples. Int. J. Fertil. 32:200–204, 1987.

Kwak, J.Y.H., Gilman-Sachs, A., and Beaman, K.D.: Reproductive outcome in women with recurrent spontaneous abortions of alloimmune and autoimmune causes: preconception versus postconception treatment. Am. J. Obstet. Gynecol. 166:1787–1798, 1992.

Ladefoged, C.: Hydrop degeneration: a histopathological investigation of 260 early abortions. Acta Obstet. Gynecol. Scand. 59:509–512, 1980.

Lawson, H.W., Atrash, H.K., and Franks, A.L.: Fatal pulmonary embolism during legal induced abortion in the United States from 1972 to 1985. Am. J. Obstet. Gynecol. 162:986–990, 1990.

Letters to the editor: Lancet 337:1091–1092, 1991.

Letters to the Editor: Antiphospholipid antibodies and fetal loss. N. Engl. J. Med. 326:951–954, 1992.

Li, L., and Smialek, J.E.: Sudden death due to rupture of ectopic pregnancy concurrent with therapeutic abortion. Arch. Pathol. Lab. Med. 117:698–700, 1993.

Lichtig, C., Korat, A., Deutch, M., and Brandes, J.M.: Decidual vascular changes in early pregnancy as a marker for intrauterine pregnancy. Am. J. Clin. Pathol. 90:284–288, 1988.

Lippman, A., Vekemans, M.J.J., and Perry, T.B.: Fetal mortality at the time of chorionic villi sampling. Hum. Genet. 68:337–339, 1984.

Lo, Y.-M.D., Patel, P., Sampietro, M., Gillmer, M.D.G., Fleming, K.A., and Wainscoat, J.S.: Detection of single-copy fetal DNA sequence from maternal blood. Lancet 335:1463–1464, 1990.

Luckett, W.P.: The development of the yolk sac during the first three weeks of gestation in the human and rhesus monkey. Anat. Rec. 172:358, 1972.

MacLean, M.A., Wilson, R., Thomson, J.A., Krishnamurthy, S., and Walker, J.J.: Changes in immunologic parameters in normal pregnancy and spontaneous abortion. Am. J. Obstet. Gynecol. 165:890–895, 1991.

Magenis, R.E.: On the origin of chromosomal anomaly. Am. J. Hum. Genet. 42:529–533, 1988.

Manabe, Y., Okamura, H., and Yoshida, Y.: Bougie-induced abortion at mid-pregnancy and placental function: histo-

logical and histochemical study of the placenta. Endokrinologie 57:389–394, 1971.

Marini, A., Suma, V., Baccichetti, C., and Lenzini, E.: A case of septic miscarriage, a probable complication of chorion villus sampling. Prenat. Diagn. 8:399–400, 1988.

Matayoshi, K., Yoshida, K., Soma, H., Miyabara, S., and Okamoto, N.: Placental pathology associated with chromosomal anomalies of the human neonate: a survey of seven cases. Congen. Anom. (Japan) 17:507–512, 1977.

McFadden, D.E., Pantzer, J.T., and Langlois, S.: Parental origin of triploidy: digyny, not diandry [abstract 28]. Mod. Pathol. 7:5P, 1994.

McIntyre, J.A., Faulk, W.P., Nichols-Johnson, V.R., and Taylor, C.G.: Immunologic testing and immunotherapy in recurrent spontaneous abortion. Obstet. Gynecol. 67:169–174, 1986.

McLean, J.M.: Early embryo loss. Lancet 1:1033–1034, 1987.

Melius, F.A., Julian, T.M., and Nagel, T.C.: Prolonged retention of intrauterine bones. Obstet. Gynecol. 78:919–921, 1991.

Mennuti, M.T., Jingeleski, S., Schwarz, R.H., and Mellman, W.J.: An evaluation of cytogenetic analysis as a primary tool in the assessment of recurrent pregnancy wastage. Obstet. Gynecol. 52:308–313, 1978.

Michel, M., Underwood, J., Clark, D.A., Mowbray, J.F., and Beard, R.W.: Histologic and immunologic study of uterine biopsy tissue of women with incipient abortion. Am. J. Obstet. Gynecol. 161:409–414, 1989.

Miller, J.F., Williamson, E., Glue, J., Gordon, Y.B., Grudzinskas, J.G., and Sykes, A.: Fetal loss after implantation: a prospective study. Lancet 2:554–556, 1980.

Mills, J.L., Simpson, J.L., Driscoll, S.G., Jovanovic-Peterson, L., van Allen, M., Aarons, J.H., Metzger, B., Bieber, F.R., Knopp, R.H., Holmes, L.B., Peterson, C.M., Witham-Wilson, M., Brown, Z., Ober, C., Harley, E., MacPherson, T.A., Duckles, A., Mueller-Heubach, E., and National Institute of Child Health: Incidence of spontaneous abortion among normal women and insulin-dependent diabetic women whose pregnancies were identified within 21 days of conception. N. Engl. J. Med. 319:1617–1623, 1988.

Moen, D.W., Werner, J.K., and Bersu, E.T.: Analysis of gross anatomical variations in human triploidy. Am. J. Med. Genet. 18:345–356, 1984.

Monrozies, M.: La gravité actuelle de l'avortement provoqué. Gynecol. Obstet. (Paris) 70:79–94, 1971.

Moore, K.L.: The Developing Human: Clinically Oriented Embryology. 3rd Ed. Saunders, Philadelphia, 1982.

Mostello, D.J., Bofinger, M.K., and Siddiqi, T.A.: Spontaneous resolution of fetal cystic hygroma and hydrops in Turner syndrome. Obstet. Gynecol. 73:862–865, 1989.

Mowbray, J.F., Gibbings, C., Liddell, H., Reginald, P.W., Underwood, J.L., and Beard, R.W.: Controlled trial of treatment of recurrent spontaneous abortion by immunisation with paternal cells. Lancet 1:941–944, 1985.

Mueller-Eckhardt, G., Heine, O., and Polten, B.: IVIG to prevent recurrent spontaneous abortion. Lancet 337:424–425, 1991.

Muggah, H.F., D'Alton, M.E., and Hunter, A.G.W.: Chorionic villus sampling followed by genetic amniocentesis and septic shock. Lancet 1:867–868, 1987.

Neu, R.L., Entes, K., and Bannerman, R.M.: Chromosome analysis in cases with repeated spontaneous abortions. Obstet. Gynecol. 53:373–375, 1979.

Neuber, M., Rehder, H., Zuther, C., Lettau, R., and Schwinger, E.: Polyploidies in abortion material decreases with maternal age. Hum. Genet. 41:563–566, 1993.

Nishimura, H., Takano, K., Tanimura, T., and Yasuda, M.: Normal and abnormal development of human embryos: first report of the analysis of 1,213 intact embryos. Teratology 1:281–290, 1968.

Novak, R., Agamanolis, D., Dasu, S., Igel, H., Platt, M., Robinson, H., and Shehata, B.: Histologic analysis of placental tissue in first trimester abortions. Pediatr. Pathol. 8:477–482, 1988.

Olding, L., Benirschke, K., and Oldstone, M.B.A.: Inhibition of mitosis of lymphocytes from human adults by lymphocytes from newborns. Clin. Immun. Immunopathol. 3:79–89, 1974.

Ornoy, A., Kohn, G., Zur, Z.B., Weinstein, D., and Cohen, M.M.: Triploidy in human abortions. Teratology 18:315–320, 1978.

Ornoy, A., Salamon-Arnon, J., Ben-Zur, Z., and Kohn, G.: Placental findings in spontaneous abortions and stillbirths. Teratology 24:243–252, 1981.

Palomaki, J.F., and Little, A.B.: Surgical management of abortion. N. Engl. J. Med. 287:752–754, 1972.

Parazzini, F., Acacia, B., Faden, D., Lovotti, M., Marelli, G., and Cortelazzo, S.: Antiphospholipid antibodies and recurrent abortion. Obstet. Gynecol. 77:854–858, 1991.

Philippe, E.: Pathologie Foeto-Placentaire. Masson, Paris, 1986.

Philippe, E., and Boué, E.: Le placenta des aberrations chromosomiques létales. Ann. Anat. Pathol. (Paris) 14:249–266, 1969.

Plouffe, L., White, E.W., Tho, S.P., Sweet, C.S., Layman, L.C., Whitman, G.F., and McDonough, P.G.: Etiologic factors of recurrent abortion and subsequent reproductive performance of couples: have we made any progress in the past 10 years? Am. J. Obstet. Gynecol. 167:313–321, 1992.

Portnoi, M.-F., Joye, N., van den Akker, J., Morlier, G., and Taillemite, J.-L.: Karyotypes of 1,142 couples with recurrent abortion. Obstet. Gynecol. 72:31–34, 1988.

Pozniak, M.A., Cullenward, M.J., Zickuhr, D., and Curet, L.B.: Venous lake bleeding: a complication of chorionic villous sampling. J. Ultrasound Med. 7:297–299, 1988.

Pridjian, G., and Moawad, A.H.: Missed abortion: still appropriate terminology? Am. J. Obstet. Gynecol. 161:261–262, 1989.

Quintero, R.A., Romero, R., Mahoney, M.J., Abuhamad, A., Vecchio, M., Holden, J., and Hobbins, J.C.: Embryoscopic demonstration of hemorrhagic lesions on the human embryo after placental trauma. Am. J. Obstet. Gynecol. 168:756–759, 1993.

Qureshi, F., Jacques, S.M., Johnson, M.P., and Evans, M.I.: Histopathologic and growth characteristics of trisomy 21 placentas [abstract 40]. Mod. Pathol. 7:7P, 1994.

Rehder, H., and Gropp, A.: Triploidie als Ursache föto-placentarer Fehlbildung bei Abortus. Verh. Dtsch. Ges. Pathol. 55:525–529, 1971.

Rehder, H., Coerdt, W., Eggers, R., Klink, F., and Schwinger, E.: Is there a correlation between morphological and cytogenetic findings in placental tissue from early missed abortions? Hum. Genet. 82:377–385, 1989.

Rhoads, G.G., Jackson, L.G., Schlesselman, S.E., de la Cruz, F.F., Desnick, R.J., Golbus, M.S., Ledbetter, D.H., Lubs, H.A., Mahoney, M.J., Pergament, E., Simpson, J.L., Carpenter, R.J., Elias, S., Ginsberg, N.A., Goldberg, J.D., Hobbins, J.C., Lynch, L., Shiono, P.H., Wapner, R.J., and Zachary, J.M.: The safety and efficacy of chorionic villus sampling for early prenatal diagnosis of cytogenetic abnormalities. N. Engl. J. Med. 320:609–617, 1989.

Rochelson, B., Kaplan, C., Guzman, E., Arato, M., Hansen, K., and Trunca, C.: A quantitative analysis of placental vasculature in the third-trimester fetus with autosomal trisomy. Obstet. Gynecol. 75:59–63, 1990.

Rosenmann, A., Palti, Z., Segal, S., and Cohen, M.M.: Chromosomes in familial primary sterility and in couples with recurrent abortions and stillbirths. Isr. J. Med. Sci. 13:1131–1133, 1977.

Sachs, E.S., Jahoda, M.G.J., van Hemel, J.O., Hoogeboom, A.J.M., and Sandkuyl, L.A.: Chromosome studies of 500 couples with two or more abortions. Obstet. Gynecol. 65:375–378, 1985.

Sadovsky, A., and Laufer, A.: Placental changes in early spontaneous abortion. Obstet. Gynecol. 17:678–683, 1961.

Salafia, C.M., and Burns, J.P.: The correlation of placental and decidual histology with karyotype and fetal viability. Teratology 39:478 (P37), 1989.

Salafia, C., Maier, D., Vogel, C., Pezzullo, J., Burns, J., and Silberman, L.: Placental and decidual histology in spontaneous abortion: detailed description and correlations with chromosome number. Obstet. Gynecol. 82:295–303, 1993.

Saller, D.N., Keene, C.L., Sun, C.-C.J., and Schwartz, S.: The association of single umbilical artery with cytogenetically abnormal pregnancies. Am. J. Obstet. Gynecol. 163:922–925, 1990.

Sasaki, M., Makino, S., Muramoto, J.-I., Ikeuchi, T., and Shimba, H.: A chromosome survey of induced abortuses in a Japanese population. Chromosoma 20:267–283, 1967.

Schaaps, J.P., and Hustin, J.: In vivo aspect of the maternal-trophoblastic border during the first trimester of gestation. Trophoblast Res. 3:39–48, 1988.

Schulman, H., Kaiser, I.H., and Randolph, G.: Outpatient saline abortion. Obstet. Gynecol. 37:521–526, 1971.

Schulze, B., Schlesinger, C., and Miller, K.: Chromosomal mosaicism confined to chorionic tissue. Prenat. Diagn. 7:451–453, 1987.

Scott, J.R., Rote, N.S., and Branch, D.W.: Immunologic aspects of recurrent abortion and fetal death. Obstet. Gynecol. 70:645–656, 1987.

Scott, R.: Limb abnormalities after chorionic villus sampling. Lancet 337:1038–1039, 1991.

Segal, S., Ornoy, A., Bercovici, B., Antebi, S.O., and Polishuk, W.Z.: Placental pathology in midtrimester pregnancies interrupted by intra-amniotic injection of hypertonic urea. Br. J. Obstet. Gynaecol. 83:156–159, 1976.

Sehgal, N., Parr, M., and Haslett, E.: Clostridium infection after intra-amniotic hypertonic saline injection for induced abortion. J. Reprod. Med. 8:67–69, 1972.

Seward, P.N., Ballard, C.A., and Ulene, A.L.: The effect of legal abortion on the rate of septic abortion at a large county hospital. Am. J. Obstet. Gynecol. 115:335–338, 1973.

Shepard, T.H., Fantel, A.G., and Fitzsimmons, J.: Congenital defect rates among spontaneous abortuses: twenty years of monitoring. Teratology 39:325–331, 1989a.

Shepard, T.H., Fitzsimmons, J.M., Fantel, A.G., and Pascoe-Mason, J.: Placental weights of normal and aneuploid early human fetuses. Teratology 39:481 (P54), 1989b.

Shepard, T.H., Fitzsimmons, J.M., Fantel, A.G., and Pascoe-Mason, J.: Placental weights of normal and aneuploid early human fetuses. Pediatr. Pathol. 9:425–431, 1989c.

Sherard, J., Bean, C., Bove, B., DelDuca, V., Esterly, K.L., Karcsh, H.J., Munshi, G., Reamer, J.F., Suazo, G., Wilmoth, D., Dahlke, M.B., Weiss, C., and Borgaonkar, S.: Long survival in a 69,XXY triploid male. Am. J. Med. Genet. 25:307–312, 1986.

Shettles, L.: The great preponderance of human males conceived. Am. J. Obstet. Gynecol. 89:130–133, 1964.

Shulman, L.P., Meyers, C.M., Simpson, J.L., Andersen, R.N., Tolley, E.A., and Elias, S.: Fetomaternal transfusion depends on amount of chorionic villi aspirated but not on method of chorionic villus sampling. Am. J. Obstet. Gynecol. 162:1185–1188, 1990.

Simpson, J.L., Meyers, C.M., Martin, A.O., Elias, S., and Ober, C.: Translocations are infrequent among couples having repeated spontaneous abortions but no other abnormal pregnancies. Fertil. Steril. 51:811–814, 1989.

Singh, R.P., and Carr, D.H.: Anatomic findings in human abortions of known chromosomal constitution. Obstet. Gynecol. 29:806–818, 1967.

Singh, R.P., and Carr, D.H.: Congenital anomalies in embryos with normal chromosomes. Biol. Neonat. 13:121–128, 1968.

Smith, A., and Gaha, T.J.: Data on families of chromosome translocation carriers ascertained because of habitual abortion. Austr. N.Z. J. Obstet. Gynaecol. 30:57–62, 1990.

Steier, J.A., Sandvei, R., and Myking, O.L.: Human chorionic gonadotropin in early normal and pathological pregnancy: discordant levels in peripheral maternal blood and blood from the uterine and abdominal cavities. Am. J. Obstet. Gynecol. 154:1091–1094, 1986.

Stein, Z.A.: A woman's age: childbearing and child rearing. Am. J. Epidemiol. 121:327–342, 1985.

Steinberg, C.R., Berkowitz, R.L., Merkatz, I.R., and Roberts, R.B.: Fever and bacteremia associated with hypertonic saline abortion. Obstet. Gynecol. 39:673–678, 1972.

Stern, J.J., and Coulam, C.B.: Mechanism of recurrent spontaneous abortion. I. Ultrasonographic findings. Am. J. Obstet. Gynecol. 166:1844–1852, 1992.

Stewart, G.K., and Goldstein, P.J.: Therapeutic abortion in California: effects on septic abortion and maternal mortality. Obstet. Gynecol. 37:510–514, 1971.

Stioui, S., de Silvestris, M., Molinari, A., Stripparo, L., Ghisoni, L., and Simoni, G.: Trisomic 22 placenta in a case of severe intrauterine growth retardation. Prenat. Diagn. 9:673–676, 1989.

Stirrat, G.M.: Recurrent miscarriage. I. Definition and epidemiology. Lancet 336:673–675, 1990a.

Stirrat, G.M.: Recurrent miscarriage. II. Clinical associations, causes, and management. Lancet 336:728–733, 1990b.

Studdiford, W.E., and Douglas, G.W.: Placental bacteremia: a significant finding in septic abortion accompanied by vascular collapse. Am. J. Obstet. Gynecol. 71:842–858, 1956.

Sundberg, K., and Smidt-Jensen, S.: Non-mosaic trisomy 16 on chorionic villus sampling but normal placenta and fetus after termination. Lancet 337:1233–1234, 1991.

Suter, P.E.N., Chatfield, W.R., and Kotonya, A.O.: The use of suction curettage in incomplete abortion. J. Obstet. Gynaecol. Br. Commonw. 77:464–466, 1970.

Suzumori, K., Adachi, R., Okada, S., Narukawa, T., Yagami, Y., and Sonta, S.: Fetal cells in the maternal circulation: detection of Y-sequence by gene amplification. Obstet. Gynecol. 80:150–154, 1992.

Tharapel, A.T., Elias, S., Shulman, L.P., Seely, L., Emerson, D.S., and Simpson, J.L.: Resorbed co-twin as an explanation for discrepant chorionic villus results: non-mosaic 47,XX, +16 in villi (direct and culture) with normal (46,XX) amniotic fluid and neonatal blood. Prenat. Diagn. 9: 467–472, 1989.

Turleau, C., Chavin-Colin, F., and de Grouchy, J.: Cytogenetic investigation in 413 couples with spontaneous abortions. Eur. J. Obstet. Gynecol. Reprod. Biol. 9:65–74, 1979.

Verjaal, M., Leschot, N.J., Wolf, H., and Treffers, P.E.: Karyotypic differences between cells from placenta and other fetal tissues. Prenat. Diagn. 7:343–348, 1987.

Vernof, K.K., Ney, J.A., and Dewald, G.W.: Pure placental trisomy 16 associated with a 46,XY infant and severe preeclampsia: a case report [abstract]. Am. J. Obstet. Gynecol. 166:434, 1992.

Verp, M.S., Rosinsky, B., Sheikh, Z., and Amarose, A.P.: Non-mosaic trisomy 16 confined to villi. Lancet 2:915–916, 1989.

Vogel, M.: Placentabefunde beim Abort: ein Beitrag zur Patho-Morphologie placentarer Entwicklungsstörungen. Virchows Arch. [A] 346:212–223, 1969.

Vogel, M.: Atlas der Morphologischen Plazentadiagnostik. Springer-Verlag, Berlin, 1992.

Wade, R.V., and Young, S.R.: Analysis of fetal loss after transcervical chorionic villus sampling: a review of 719 patients. Am. J. Obstet. Gynecol. 161:513–519, 1989.

Wall, R.L., and Hertig, A.T.: Habitual abortion. Am. J. Obstet. Gynecol. 56:1127–1133, 1948.

Ward, B.E., Henry, G.P., and Robinson, A.: Cytogenetic studies in 100 couples with recurrent spontaneous abortions. Am. J. Hum. Genet. 32:549–554, 1980.

Wegmann, T.G., Gill, T.J., Cumming, C.D., and Nisbet-Brown, E., eds.: Immunology of Reproduction. Oxford University Press, New York, 1983.

Wilcox, A.J., Weinberg, C.R., O'Connor, J.F., Baird, D.D., Schlatterer, J.P., Canfield, R.E., Armstrong, E.G., and Nisula, B.C.: Incidence of early loss of pregnancy. N. Engl. J. Med. 319:189–194, 1988.

Williams, J., Wang, B.T., Rubin, C.H., and Aiken-Hunting, D.: Chorionic villus sampling: experience with 3016 cases performed by a single operator. Obstet. Gynecol. 80: 1023–1029, 1992.

Yamamoto, M., and Watanabe, G.: Epidemiology of gross chromosomal anomalies at early embryonic stage of pregnancy. Contrib. Epidemiol. Biostatist. 1:101–106, 1979.

Zerres, K., Niesen, M., Schwanitz, G., and Hansmann, M.: Trisomie 22—Pränatale Befunde unterschiedlicher Entwicklungsstadien. Geburtshilfe Frauenheilkd. 48: 720–723, 1988.

22
Molar Pregnancies

The term "gestational trophoblastic neoplasia" has become popular in recent years, although it comprises entities that are clearly not neoplastic, such as triploid partial moles. Driscoll (1981), in an excellent review of the morphology of these diseases, strongly favored abandonment of the time-honored term hydatidiform mole. Fox (1989) has added fuel to the fire by suggesting the following: "Is it, in fact, justifiable to continue distinguishing complete from partial moles in routine histopathological practice?" He based this opinion primarily on the exceptional finding of a single case of choriocarcinoma said to have followed a partial mole (Looi & Sivanesaratnam, 1981). This view is not ours. After all, choriocarcinoma is also an occasional sequela of an apparently normal gestation, as Fox readily conceded, and there may have been a choriocarcinomatous cell line ab initio. The typical hydatidiform mole (complete mole), syncytial endometritis, invasive moles (chorioadenoma destruens), benign metastasizing mole, the partial hydatidiform mole with or without fetus, and ectopic moles are discussed in this chapter. Their terminology is often confusing and imprecisely used. Choriocarcinoma is covered in Chapter 23.

Hydatidiform moles are excessively edematous placentas characterized by massive fluid accumulation within the villous parenchyma, the formation of microcysts within the villi, and an absence of fetal blood vessels. When *all* villi are so changed, we speak of a true, or complete, mole. When only some villi are involved, with large portions of the placenta being grossly more normal, the process is called a partial mole. The distinction is often difficult, however, and strict morphological guidelines are not easily established. Moreover, the distinction is often blurred at early gestational ages during the evolution of the altered placenta. Because choriocarcinoma (chorionepithelioma) so frequently follows the occurrence of a hydatidiform mole, all of these entities are now often encompassed by the term gestational trophoblastic disease. Several comprehensive books have treated this group of placental diseases (Smalbraak, 1957; Holland & Hreshchyshyn, 1967; Park, 1971; Goldstein & Berkowitz, 1982; Szulman & Buchsbaum, 1987). These volumes consider the evolution of our understanding of the genetic derivation of moles, the frequently confusing terminology, the clinical features, and therapy of these entities.

Hydatidiform Mole

Complete hydatidiform mole (CHM) is a diffusely edematous placenta in which the macroscopically enlarged villi lack blood vessels and have cistern-like fluid-filled cavities. The villi are connected to one another by thin strands of connective tissue, the former mainstem villi. Intervillous thrombi occur frequently. Although there is usually no embryo or identifiable chorionic cavity in CHM, a few exceptions have been described. CHM occasionally coexists with a normal twin pregnancy. This situation, however does not make a partial mole. It can be differentiated genetically as well as macroscopically. The partial hydatidiform mole (PHM) is composed of normal and distended villi, and it is also more often associated with an embryo or remnants thereof. The trophoblast of complete moles is usually more abundant in CHM than it is in PHM and normal placentas. In the CHM there is also frequently much nuclear pleomorphism and anaplasia. These cellular abnormalities have given rise to several classifications, some of which have endeavored to assign prognostic values. Thus it was considered that a hydatidiform mole grade V was at one time believed to have greater malignant potential than one to which a grade II designation was attached. Hydatidiform moles usually occur as uterine pregnancies, but they are occasionally also present as ectopic pregnancies in the fallopian tube (Depypere et al., 1993) and ovary. The trophoblast of moles invades the uterus, much as it does in a placenta increta. When hydatid villi and its trophoblast invade the uterus and destroy portions of it in the process, this entity is designated an invasive mole or a chorioadenoma destruens.

Moles have occasionally been observed to occur repetitively, and Parazzini et al. (1991) found that this situation was much more likely to occur in patients with CHM. Sand et al. (1984), who reviewed this literature, suggested that it occurred in 0.60% to 2.57% of patients. There were no differences in outcome. Hsu et al. (1963) described five cases of two moles in the same patient; one patient suffered three moles. Johnson (1966) observed a patient with four consecutive moles. We have seen a young black patient who had three consecutive complete moles; the last developed into a fatal choriocarcinoma. It is of interest that this patient conceived these moles with two different husbands. Kronfol et al. (1969) described five patients with repetitive moles and commented on the greater frequency of the condition in the Lebanese population. Patek and Johnson (1978) and Endres (1961) each had a patient with five consecutive hydatidiform moles and no children. Wu (1973) observed a patient with nine consecutive molar pregnancies. Remarkably, all of the moles in the last case lacked Barr bodies, and one was karyotyped as being 46,XY. Although the author speculated on a paternal cause for this repetitive event, normal paternal and maternal karyotypes were found. Semen analysis was refused. Ambrani et al. (1980) reported familial moles in three family trees, but the possible genetic cause was not determined. Parazzini et al. (1984) reported on two sisters, one with three CHMs and the other with one. La Vecchia et al. (1982) described monozygotic twins, each with a molar pregnancy. An important genetic study of the origin of two choriocarcinomas was undertaken by Osada et al. (1991). They examined the restriction fragment length polymorphism of the moles and preceding pregnancies in two patients. In one family the choriocarcinoma could be traced to a previous complete, androgenetic, hydatidiform mole, not the two normal pregnancies. In the other patient, however, the tumor derived from the third of three normal pregnancies and carried both parental chromosomal markers. The publication does not provide details about whether one or the other genome had a better prognosis. The few similar studies in the literature are referred to by these authors. Studies of this kind can now be employed to correlate choriocarcinoma with putative precursors; such an effort is especially important when long time spans occur between such pregnancy and tumor, or when primary choriocarcinomas of presumably nongestational types are observed, for example the cervical lesion reported by Ben-Chetrit et al. (1990).

The natural history of recurrent molar disease was discussed by Federschneider et al. (1980) in their presentation of seven patients. They also reviewed the literature and stated that their recurrent cases were more malignant and more often required treatment for residual disease than nonrecurrent moles (see also Rice et al., 1989). Mor-Joseph and his colleagues (1985) reported four recurrent moles following three spontaneous abortions. The moles occurred after clomiphene therapy, as was previously described by Schneider and Waxman (1972). These experiences support the finding by Parazzini et al. (1985) that moles are significantly more common with increasing numbers of spontaneous abortion.

Not only is the genetic derivation of moles unusual (most have only paternal chromosomes), but there is great variation in the prevalence of moles in different populations. Oriental women, especially Japanese and Filipinas, suffer an increased frequency of molar pregnancies. Hydatidiform moles have been observed only in human pregnancies; no other primate has exhibited this pathology, although choriocarcinoma has been reported (see Chapter 23). There are rare reports of "moles" in cows (Folger, 1934), and Drieux and Thiéy (1948) reviewed rare cases described in a cat and dog. They are truly exceptional circumstances, and their analogy to human CHM is uncertain. Choriocarcinoma is also exceptionally uncommon in animals.

Incidence

The prevalence of hydatidiform moles varies in different populations, and it is impossible to ascertain exactly. An estimate of 1 per 2,000 pregnancies is generally cited for the United States (Hertig, 1950), and Grimes (1984) undertook an extensive epidemiological study of many populations. The incidence of CHM he found was 1 in 1,000 pregnancies for the general U.S. population. Regrettably, clear etiological factors were not obtained from his investigation. In part, the inability to ascertain a precise prevalence is due to the probable confusion of CHM with PHMs and presumed triploid conceptuses. Undoubtedly, PHMs have often been counted as CHMs (presumed androgenetic moles), especially when one considers the early literature; and we know that this is still the case. The methodological problems in ascertaining a true incidence have been dealt with particularly well by Buckley (1987). There is little doubt that vast differences in frequency of CHM exist; it is especially common in Hawaiian, Philippine, and Japanese populations. Table 22 summarizes incidence figures derived from several relevant studies. Other tables may be found in these publications and the books cited. Several authors have provided additional reviews of early incidence figures that add little important information.

TABLE 22. Incidence of complete hydatidiform moles in various populations.

Country	Author	Year	Time span of the study	Incidence/term gestations
India	Das	1938	108,951 gestations	1:502
Mexico	Márquez-Monter et al.	1963	1961 gestations	1:200
Hong Kong	Chun et al.	1964	1953–1961	1:242
Sweden	Ringertz	1970	1958–1965	1:1,560
Singapore	Teoh et al.	1971	1963–1965	1:823
Israel	Matalon & Modan	1972	1950–1965	1:1,300
Hawaii	Natoli & Rashad	1972	1950–1970	1:977
Paraguay	Rolon & de Lopez	1977	1960–1969	1:4,369
Paraguay	Rolon et al.	1990	1970–1982	1:3,906
The Netherlands	Franke et al.	1983b	1978–1980	1:2,270
Italy	Mazzanti et al.	1986	1979–1982	1:1,510
England	Bagshawe et al.	1986	1973–1983	1:1,000 to 1.54:1,000

There is general agreement that the incidence of moles is, at least partially, racially influenced. This phenomenon is not completely explicable by the higher parity and older age of Asian gravidas (Iverson et al., 1959). Das (1938) found moles more commonly in the Indian than the Caucasian population. In an inquiry that distinguishes environmental from racial causes, Natoli and Rashad (1972) observed moles much more often in the Japanese and Hawaiian stock than in Chinese and Caucasians resident of Hawaii; many other examples can be found in the cited publications.

These reports all found that the incidence of CHM correlated with race, rather than with geography. Bracken (1987) undertook a special study of these features and identified that the incidence of CHM in Japanese was inexplicably twofold higher than that of Caucasians and Chinese. He stated that "maternal age is the most consistently demonstrated risk factor; teenagers and, especially, women over age 35 being at increased risk" (see also Bandy et al., 1984).

Maudsley and Robertson (1965) described the development of a mole in a 52-year-old woman. They reviewed the literature of approximately 60 similar cases in older women. Mathieu (1939), who made a thorough review of moles and choriocarcinomas, found a 55-year-old patient and emphasized the dependence on maternal age. The possible influence of the father's age has also been studied. No relation was ascertained in most studies, except in that undertaken by La Vecchia et al. (1984), who found a higher incidence of fathers over 45 years, and this predilection was compounded by smoking. Other investigators have not identified smoking as a risk factor. The possible and disputed etiological role of herbicides is unlikely to be resolved, according to Bracken (1987).

McCorriston (1968) evaluated possible reasons for the higher incidence in particular racial groups of Hawaii and stated that their different food preferences are unlikely antecedents. This point was further examined in a case-control study from China; no relation to diet was identified (Brinton et al., 1989). Berkowitz et al. (1985a) suggested that vitamin A deficiency may be causally related to molar gestations and suggested carotene supplements for prevention. There have been no other meaningful concepts that explain the racial differences.

The possibility that the marked ethnic differences in molar incidence reflect different diets and possible other environmental factors and so might disappear upon immigration to other countries has been studied. A key question thus is whether the incidence of CHM in Orientals who emigrated to San Francisco and live Western life styles differs from that of Caucasians. Overstreet (personal communication, 1963) ascertained that in the immigrant Oriental population of San Francisco the incidence of CHM is 1 per 2,000 deliveries, much the same as in Caucasian women. Atrash et al. (1986) similarly identified molar pregnancies among 84,18 abortions from different institutions. The incidence of moles was 7.5 per 10,000 pregnancies (1 per 1,333). Bracken (1988), however, has criticized this result on methodological grounds and as being a gross underestimate. Although more moles were found in Chinese, this difference was not significant. Blacks had the same incidence as Whites. The only significant correlation occurred with maternal age.

Genetics

Ever since Park's early studies (1957), cytogeneticists have known that "sexing" of trophoblastic tumors is impossible. Shorofsky (1960), applying cytometrics, found that nuclei of molar trophoblast had the same parameters as normal trophoblast. Márquez-Monter (1966), using radioautography, showed that the syncytium of molar trophoblast originates from cytotrophoblastic precursors, just as it does in normal villi. With the discovery of sex chromatin, it became known that most moles were known to possess a Barr body (sex chromatin—the inactivated X chromosome of females) (see Tominaga & Page, 1966; Baggish et al., 1968; Loke, 1969). Early systematic studies by Sasaki et al. (1962) had shown that most hydatidiform moles possessed an apparently normal female or occasionally male diploid complement. Bourgoin et al. (1965a,b) also found male and female karyotypes but further observed some aneuploidy in their specimens. They encountered methodological difficulties in making cell preparations, however. The late Sajiri Makino and his colleagues (1964, 1965) ascertained that some apparent moles, the partial moles, have a triploid chromosomal constitution, an observation that was soon confirmed by Carr (1969). It is now known that triploidy is the karyotype of most partial hydatidiform moles.

The major breakthrough in our understanding of molar pregnancies came when Kajii and Ohama (1977)

showed that moles are "androgenetic"; that is, all molar chromosomes are paternally derived. It is easiest to envisage that it occurs as the result of fertilization of an "empty egg," with subsequent duplication of the haploid spermatozoal complement. That mechanism also explains why moles are almost always $2n = 46,XX$. If a male-determining spermatozoon with Y chromosome were to fertilize an empty egg, a karyotype of 46,YY would result from such sperm duplication, which is apparently a lethal condition. Kajii and Ohama karyotyped 20 moles and determined the disposition of the chromosomal Q- and R-band polymorphism. There is sufficient heterogeneity in the normal human chromosomal structure that this polymorphism allows one to ascertain with confidence that in CHM these markers were exclusively paternal (Figure 478). These findings were quickly confirmed by Wake et al. (1978b) and Jacobs et al. (1978). Many markers are available now on chromosomes. They extend from the Q and R bands

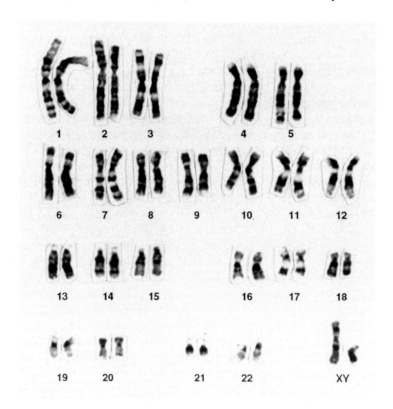

FIGURE 478. Normal human diploid karyotype, 46,XY, Q-banded (Q = quinacrine). In the normal karyotype chromosomes may be banded by different techniques. Here a normal male set is banded with quinacrine stain (Q bands), which allows precise comparison between elements (maternal and paternal). Note that in this male there are differences between the banding pattern of several elements. Various segments do not "match"; they represent normal variations in our chromosomes that are inherited. The following chromosomes differ in this karyotype: no. 1, the right element has additional heterochromatin at the centromere; no. 9, the left element has additional centromeric heterochromatin, and the right chromosome has an inversion; no. 14, there are prominent satellites; no. 15, the right chromosome has a centromeric variant; no. 16, the right chromosome has additional centromeric material; no. 22: the left chromosome has prominent satellites, and the right chromosome has a centromeric variant. It has been possible to show that in the typical CHM there is only the banding profile of the paternal chromosome set; both elements are exactly alike (Kajii & Ohama, 1977). (Courtesy Dr. Mark Bogart, San Diego.)

to C bands, inversions, translocations, and other minor varieties, as shown in Figure 478. Since this original description, not only has the concept been amply confirmed but androgenesis has also been verified by genetic markers, such as polymorphic enzymes (Jacobs et al., 1980) and HLA markers (Wake et al., 1978a; Couillin et al., 1985). Interestingly, two of the mothers studied by Kajii and Ohama (1977) had reciprocal translocations of different chromosomes. Similar findings were then made in the later studies of Lawler et al. (1979) and Vejerslev et al. (1987d). This apparent frequency of translocations might initially be assumed to have possible etiological significance for the creation of an "empty egg." Subsequent studies have negated this possibility. Vejerslev et al. (1987d) karyotyped 237 mothers and 217 fathers of CHM as well as 125 mothers and 106 fathers of PHM. "No significant increase in the frequency of translocations . . . was found."

To explain the genesis of moles, it is further hypothesized that molar transformation of the conceptus results from the homozygous concentration of some lethal genes. It is currently estimated that four or five lethal genes are regularly carried (in the heterozygous state) in normal individuals. When they are homozygous (as they would be in CHM), they cause embryonic death; only the placenta survives, to transform to molar vesicles. The notion of an "empty egg" with fertilization by a 23,X sperm and subsequent chromosomal duplication was supported by the genetic studies of Jacobs et al. (1980). Moreover, experimental investigations in mice indicated that maternal *and* paternal genomes are essential for normal embryonic and placental development. Paternal genes are apparently especially important for normal placenta formation. It was found that embryos from two female pronuclei (gynogenesis) developed poorly, and particularly their placental membranes were abnormal. Those derived from two male pronuclei died early, but their placentas were reasonably well formed (Surani & Barton, 1983; Barton et al., 1984; Ho et al., 1984). Irregular X chromosome inactivation inexplicably also occurs in placental membranes of female conceptuses. There is preferential female X chromosome activity in a variety of cells of the placenta of female fetuses (Takagi & Sasaki, 1975; Roper et al., 1978; Harrison & Warburton, 1986; Harrison, 1989).

After this definition of androgenesis as the cause of molar development was clarified, many cytogenetic studies have been performed on CHMs and PHMs to further delineate the possible relations of chromosome sets and the possible impact on the prognosis of the various molar conceptions. Tsuji et al. (1981) determined that there is a higher frequency of aneuploidy ($2n = >6$) in the moles from older women and in invasive moles and choriocarcinomas. They suggested that it may have

prognostic significance. Jacobs et al. (1978) had also observed an apparently "malignant" mole with aneuploidy and hypotetraploidy but with a paternal origin of all chromosomes. When trophoblastic cells are separated from molar tissue and then cultured, Habibian and Surti (1987) found that these cells exhibit a 2.8 times greater frequency of polyploidy compared to normal trophoblast. Chromosomal breakage was also much more common. The X chromosomal replication pattern of diploid, androgenetic molar cells, however, was found to be normal (Tsukahara & Kajii, 1985). A useful review may be found in the paper of Lindor et al. (1992).

As more moles were investigated by genetic study, exceptions to these findings have come to light. The existence of 46,XY moles was then first recognized (Surti et al., 1979, 1982; Ohama et al., 1981; Pattillo et al., 1981). Fisher and Lawler (1984) found three 46,XY moles and determined that they derived from dispermy. It now appears that about 8% of CHMs are the result of fusion of two male pronuclei following dispermic fertilization (Ford et al., 1986). In addition to the XY moles, occasional heterozygous 46,XX moles were found (approximately 5–10% of moles are now known to be heterozygous *and* androgenetic). Wake et al. (1981) suggested that these moles may have a greater malignant potential. Kajii et al. (1984) studied nine XY moles and compared the clinical outcome with 16 "normal" XX moles. Their study showed dispermy as the causal mechanism in the XY moles. Three of eight XY moles and five of fifteen XX moles had a delayed decrease in human chorionic gonadotropin (hCG) titers. Mutter et al. (1993) were unable to show that an increased risk for metastasis exists in the XY moles they studied with the polymerase chain reaction (PCR). They found 7.7% of the moles with metastatic consequence and 9.1% of the metastatic group in their large sample of moles studied to possess a Y chromosome. In the experience of Fisher and Lawler (1984), 31% of patients with heterozygous moles needed further treatment for trophoblastic tumor. In a subsequent study of this important observation, Lawler and Fisher (1987) examined 163 moles, 38 (23%) of which were PMHs and 125 were CHMs. All of the PHMs were either triploid or hypertriploid, with most having arisen by dispermic fertilization; they had no untoward sequelae. Of the CHM, whose genetic study was informative, 10% were heterozygous diploid moles. Of these heterozygous moles, 25% required subsequent chemotherapy, in contrast to 17.6% of the CHMs with homozygous constitution (a result that was not statistically significant). Hitchcock et al. (1991) addressed the difficult differential diagnosis between CHM and PHM when they undertook an important retrospective flow cytometric study of molar specimens diagnosed at the Armed

Forces Institute of Pathology (AFIP). Their diagnosis of CHM differed from that of the submitting pathologist in 78%, in the diagnosis of PHM in 57% of cases. Fukunaga et al. (1993) found by employing flow cytometry that of 129 cases originally diagnosed as CHM 91 were diploid, 25 tetraploid, 1 triploid, and 12 aneuploid. Of five invasive moles, two were diploid and three tetraploid. When the 49 PHMs were analyzed, 34 were found to be triploid and 13 diploid. These authors highlighted the problems attending the simple histopathological differentiation of the two entities and strongly advocated the use of DNA determination of moles. They found that no residual disease followed PHM, whereas 18% of CHMs were associated with persistent trophoblastic disease. Lage et al. (1991) found that with one course of single-agent chemotherapy all triploid PHMs underwent complete remission; more courses were required for the two diploid PHMs they studied. Later these authors studied 142 hydropic placentas (Lage et al., 1992) and found 38% CHM, 35% PHM, and 26% hydropic abortuses, most of the latter being near diploid; only 11% were triploid. "Persistent tumor" was seen in 33% of CHMs and 12% of PHMs. Finally, Howat et al. (1993) evaluated the pathologist's ability to reliably distinguish between these conditions and provided specific criteria. The findings of an evaluation of 50 molar pregnancies by seven competent pathologists gave no assurance of a correct diagnosis.

From these studies, then, it appears that it is not yet possible to reliably diagnose the molar pregnancies by histological study alone, let alone assign a prognosis on the basis of a CHM karyotype. The most important decision when encountering a mole is to differentiate between triploidy and diploidy; flow cytometry is an important methodology whose usage should be more widely employed. The former group of patients (with PHMs) *never* experienced metastatic disease. Only rarely have such patients required chemotherapy, and there I have grave doubt that it was needed; moreover, the diagnosis may have been in error or was poorly supported, as for the patient recorded by Gardener and Lage (1992).

Although the morphology alone of PHM is often decisive, difficult cases do arise, especially when twin pregnancies are admixed with moles. In addition, the existence of "confined placental mosaicism" has been evoked to explain unusual cases. Thus Sarno et al. (1993) described a partial mole (69,XXX) associated with a surviving diploid premature girl. Because cytogenetic studies are not feasible for all laboratories, it has been strongly advocated that ploidy of moles be determined by the rapid method of flow cytometry (Anonymous, 1987; Benirschke, 1989). Fisher et al. (1987) showed that this technique unequivocally distinguishes the two entities. The same method was employed by Hemming et al. (1987), who demonstrated that CHMs more often had hyperdiploid cells. Lage et al. (1988) also produced similarly good results in distinguishing CHMs from PHMs with this method (Figure 479). It is noteworthy that paraffin-embedded material can be used for retrospective flow cytometric studies. Bell et al. (1989) have recommended such studies for difficult cases. Moreover, because flow cytometry easily distinguishes diploid complete moles from the triploid partial moles, it is important to note that occasional and unexpected findings occur that further mandate employment of this methodology. As an example, Lage et al. (1989) found three tetraploid moles. One of them, a 92,XXXX mole, was a CHM. Another specimen had a complement of 92,XXYY (two paternal and two maternal genomes), and one was diploid/triploid mosaic (69,XXY/90,XXXY). After evacuation, none of these moles recurred. Martin et al. (1989) have determined the ploidy of various moles from paraffin blocks, as in the study of Hitchcock et al. (1991), reviewed above.

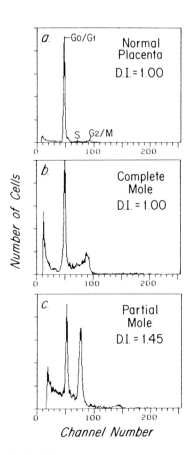

FIGURE 479. DNA histogram of normal placenta, a complete mole, and a triploid partial mole. The vertical axis is the number of cells; the horizontal axis is fluorescence and indicates DNA content. There is a single diploid peak in the normal placenta, a large diploid peak in the CHM with a minor peak at tetraploidy, and a large peak of triploid cells in the partial mole. (From Lage et al., 1988, with permission.)

The outcome for the patients following delivery of the moles was known. It was found that moles with an aneuploid population of cells had a significantly higher incidence of gestational neoplastic sequelae than did those with diploid (euploid) moles. Although these "malignant" moles also had a higher "proliferative index," it was not statistically significant. Newer technology employs DNA fingerprinting from small samples to differentiate these conditions (Nobunaga et al., 1990; Ko et al., 1991) or advocate the PCR technique for rapid diagnosis (Fisher & Newlands, 1993).

Mixed populations of cells with different karyotypes occur in the occasional, the "exceptional" CHM. Takagi et al. (1969) described a triploid/diploid "mosaic" XX mole without providing further relevant information. Ford et al. (1986) found an avascular, androgenetic diploid CHM (608 g) that was mosaic for normally fertilized cells. Interestingly, there was a reciprocal translocation in one population that enhanced the ease of analysis of the chromosomal origins. To explain their finding, the authors suggested that the fusion of DZ twins was unlikely and favored an origin from the abnormal fertilization of a single egg. In our interpretation, fusion of two dizygotic twins (a chimera) remains a strong possibility. The case also argues strongly against the simplistic notion that moles result from fertilization of an "empty egg." The authors urged that other diploid moles be examined for possible mosaicism/chimerism. Vejerslev et al. (1987a) found two homozygous moles with second cell lines, which also suggested twin gestations. Other possible admixtures of fraternal twins, one a mole and the other normal, are discussed below. Vejerslev et al. (1987c) have summarized all unusual karyotypes of CHM, diploid PHM, and the hyperdiploid CHM.

Other exceptional karyotypes include the tetraploids. Vejerslev et al. (1987b) found one tetraploid mole with

three paternal and one maternal contributions among 29 molar conceptuses, 24 of which were dispermic triploids. This tetraploid specimen was, in principle, similar to the PHM but did not have the clinical presentation of that entity. Lage et al. (1989) identified three tetraploid moles. One of them, a CHM, had 92, XXXX; the two PHMs had 92,XXYY and 90,XXXY,-11,-13/69,XXY, respectively. These authors strongly advocated the use of flow cytometry for identification of unusual specimens. It now appears that most diploid moles also have tetraploid peaks; those with diploid genomes occurred in younger women (Frankforter et al., 1994). The diagnostic methods of genetic analysis already referred to may be just as rapid in appropriately equipped laboratories, and they are decisive. Saji et al. (1989) elegantly showed by DNA fingerprinting that CHMs have only paternal genes. The advantage of such a study with restriction fragment length polymorphism (RFLP) is that only minute samples are required. When RFLP studies of trophoblast and corresponding fetuses were compared in 50 samples, four pairs showed differences in DNA content (Butler et al., 1988). This unexpected finding has not yet been fully explained, but it is likely to be important.

Morphology

A "hydatidiform mole is defined as a conceptus, usually devoid of an intact fetus, in which all or many of the chorionic villi show (1) gross nodular swelling culminating in cyst formation, (2) disintegration of blood vessels, and (3) variable proliferation of trophoblast" (Edmonds, 1959). It must be regarded as the swelling of most or all of the villi in a placenta that may once have been more normal. When usually diagnosed, the molar tissue fills most of the uterine cavity (Figure 480). Intervillous coagula are common because of the aberrant

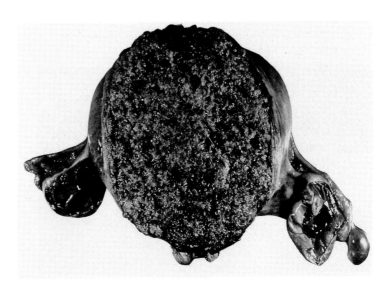

FIGURE 480. Hydatidiform mole in situ. Note the distension of the uterus and the bilateral theca lutein cysts in the ovaries. The vesicular nature of molar villi is apparent.

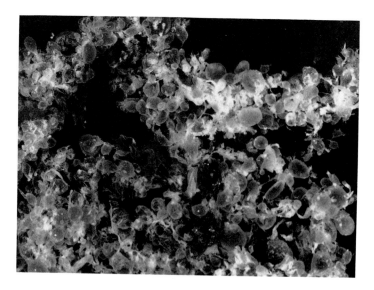

FIGURE 481. Hydatidiform molar villi photographed under water. Note the bulbous swelling of the terminal villi and the slender nature of the mainstem villi.

intervillous circulation, and it may cause vaginal bleeding. Moles occasionally present with the clinical picture of abruptio placentae, according to Sauter (1965). The uterus may be markedly distended and may rupture, especially when it is stimulated to contract (Lee & Siegel, 1965). Ovarian theca lutein cysts are often present (Figure 480) because of the stimulation by the excessive hCG production. Because the cysts regress spontaneously after evacuation of the mole, the ovaries need not be removed when hysterectomy is performed for molar sequelae.

The molar villi are fairly uniformly distended by fluid. McKay et al. (1955a,b) have analyzed this fluid biochemically and found its osmolality to be lower than that of maternal serum. The authors suggested that later gestational trophoblast has different capacities, which explains why villi atrophy rather than expand when fetal death occurs during later fetal life. When molar tissue is floated in water (Figure 481), the translucent nature of the distended terminal villi is evident. The protein content of the fluid is apparent when such villi are first fixed and then floated (Figure 482). The connections to a possible former chorionic sac also become evident. The swelling is primarily one of the terminal villi and can be construed to result from the continued water transport by trophoblast. The syncytium has this singular transport function. In the absence of fetal vessels to remove the transported fluid, the villi expand. The absence of a fetus, a chorionic cavity, and chorionic vasculature are characteristic of CHM. Nevertheless, two cases with tiny embryos have been described.

Hertig (1968) depicted a chorionic cavity in the center of an apparently complete mole that was fixed in situ within a uterus (his Figure 196). This chorionic sac contained a deformed, stunted embryo with this mole (his Figure 199). Because an embryo was associated with the specimen, it may be argued in retrospect that the specimens were PHMs. This consideration is invalidated by the case shown in Figure 483. In this patient, a tiny embryo was present within a typical hydatidiform mole (the patient's third). This pregnancy was followed by fatal, disseminated choriocarcinoma.

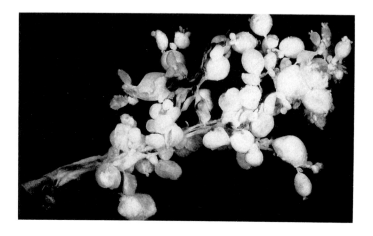

FIGURE 482. Same villi as in Figure 481 but after fixation in Bouin's fixative. The protein has precipitated, making the villi opaque. The connecting stalks are obvious.

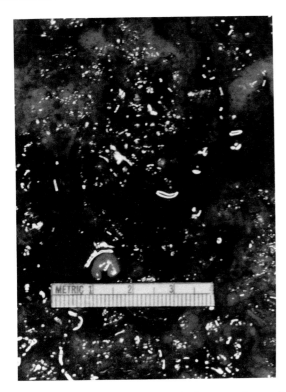

FIGURE 483. Hydatidiform mole with degenerating embryo. There were no vessels in this "malignant" mole. It was the third consecutive CHM and was followed by fatal choriocarcinoma. The tiny embryo is visible above the 1.0 to 1.5 cm portion of the ruler. The choriocarcinoma of this pregnancy is shown in Chapter 23.

Thus occasional embryos accompany moles, especially perhaps during their early development. Moles are now typically removed by suction curettage. Because the specimens are usually markedly disrupted and accompanied by much clot, it is not surprising that possible chorionic sacs and embryos are not found more often.

The stalks from which the hydatid villi emanate indicate that such a more normal structure must have preceded the typical CHM configuration. Also, in "younger" CHMs there is generally less villous swelling, and the connections to a possible chorionic sac by stem villi are more visible (Figure 484). Kajii et al. (1984), moreover, found that "younger" moles had smaller, elliptical or club-shaped villi and poorly delineated cisternae, whereas "older" moles had more globular villi. The latter also had more trophoblastic hyperplasia and fewer remnants of capillaries; no significant morphological differences were found between XY and XX moles.

It is of historical interest to cite the invasive mole described by Jarotzky and Waldeyer (1868). They observed a chorionic cavity in the center of this typical invasive mole, from where all the hydropic villi emanated. One may thus ask: What would a CHM, usually delivered between 15 and 20 weeks' gestation, have looked like at 6 week's gestation? The answer is unknown, but the observations by Sasaki et al. (1967) and Nishimura et al. (1968) suggested that typical hydatidiform moles might not be recognized in such age groups. These investigators examined a large number of therapeutic abortions in Japan and found no CHMs, although many would have been expected in that population. Early CHMs might even contain fetal blood vessels, similar to the occasional embryos that have been seen with CHM. Blood vessels in the placenta disappear rapidly after fetal death. Their absence from a CHM does not ensure that there never were villous capillaries. We suggest then that during transitional stages the differential diagnosis may be difficult to make by morphology alone. It is here that flow cytometry and DNA fingerprinting become useful adjuncts.

Edmonds (1959) employed the term transitional mole. Whether it applied to the transition from a more normal young placenta or to what is now known as partial mole

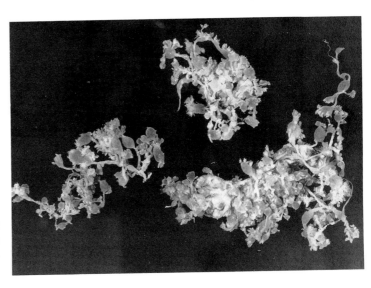

FIGURE 484. Hydropic villi of "early" CHM at 10 weeks' gestation. Note that only some villi are bulbous and that the connecting mainstem villi are still prominent. (From Benirschke, 1981, with permission.)

remains unknown. For these reasons, we prefer not to use this terminology. It would be much better if we identified these abortions as diploid androgenetic, triploid, or diploid-triploid moles, if distinctions are needed. The availability of more precise techniques will demand this precision from future pathologists.

Cohen et al. (1979) suggested that 8 of their 4,829 elective first-trimester abortion specimens were molar. In our opinion, however, the criteria for their diagnosis of CHM and their photomicrographs are not convincing.

Microscopically, moles are characterized by swollen villi with apparently empty cisternae. The cisternae result from the dissociation of loose villous connective tissue; transitional stages are frequently observed (Figure 485). There are no blood vessels or recognizable vascular remnants. An abundance of Hofbauer cells is frequent, as in PHMs. The trophoblastic covering of CHMs varies enormously from mole to mole. It may even vary within a mole (Figure 486). Occasionally, the trophoblast is degenerated or enmeshed in fibrin. Hertig and Sheldon (1947) paid particular attention to the nature and abundance of trophoblast. They subdivided moles into groups I to VI (later revised to three groups), from benign to malignant, and sought a correlation with subsequent development of choriocarcinoma and other sequelae. Hertig (1950) later stated, however, that "it is well nigh impossible to predict accurately which mole will be followed by this most rapidly malignant of all cancers." Although Douglas (1962) affirmed this relation between graded moles and choriocarcinoma, most other pathologists have had difficulty with so rigorously classifying moles, and their results have not allowed a perfect correlation with outcome (Novak, 1950; Hunt et al., 1953; Javey et al., 1979; Genest et al., 1991). A detailed study by Messerli et al. (1987) showed that the classi-

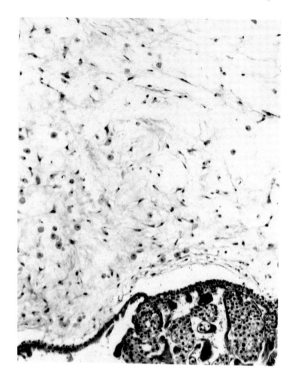

FIGURE 485. Microscopic appearance of the villous surface in CHM. The villous core lacks fetal capillaries; it shows marked edema and early cisterna formation at right. There are many Hofbauer cells. The villous surface has normal epithelium at left and markedly hyperplastic trophoblast on the right. H&E. ×100.

fication of moles and related entities had poor correlation among observers. A quantitative study of nuclear dimensions of trophoblastic cells in CHM by Franke et al. (1985) also failed to use such parameters as predictors of outcome. "Benign" moles are said to have

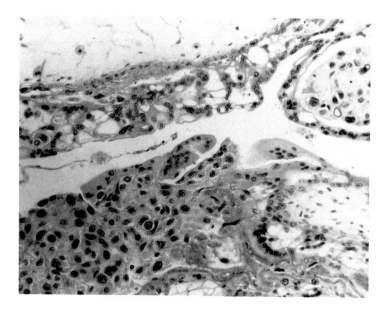

FIGURE 486. Surface of a molar villus with a greater degree of trophoblastic proliferation than that seen in Figure 485. Note the aneuploidy of many syncytial nuclei and the syncytial cisternae (dilated transport vesicles) at top. H&E. ×160.

been followed by pulmonary metastases of choriocarcinoma (e.g., Bonnar & Tennent, 1962), and choriocarcinoma has followed normal pregnancy and abortion. For these reasons and because clinical follow-up with hCG titers is efficient, this scheme of classifying moles into groups with histological differences is no longer followed. A variety of histochemical studies on molar villi have added little useful information regarding pathogenesis (Bur et al., 1962; Lauslahti, 1969).

Several ultrastructural studies of CHM have been undertaken. They have yielded little additional information to our understanding of the biology of these placental errors. Wynn and Davies (1964) showed especially clearly the spectrum of cells that are transitional between cytotrophoblast and syncytium. They also pointed to the fluid imbibition by the syncytium, which is often clearly seen light microscopically as empty spaces in syncytial cytoplasm (Figure 486; see also Figure 502). Wynn and Davies found a correlation between hCG levels and the abundance of syncytium but not with that of cytotrophoblast. Essentially similar findings were reported by González-Angulo et al. (1966) and Okudaira and Strauss (1967). Merkow et al. (1971), who studied a mole that progressed to choriocarcinoma, were impressed by the lipid inclusions in the syncytiotrophoblast. Ockleford et al. (1989) undertook a scanning electron microscopic study of 31 CHMs and 12 placentas. They observed peculiar and novel surface organelles in several moles. These structures are absent from normal trophoblast, especially the reticular organization of the surface that betrays the underlying cytoskeletal architecture of villi.

Several studies have attempted to localize various markers and antigens to molar trophoblast. Thus to better understand possible immunological interactions with the mother, HLA antigen characterization of moles has been done. Lawler et al. (1974) found HLA antibodies against the husband's antigens in women with persistent trophoblastic disease, and Berkowitz et al. (1983) showed that monoclonal anti-HLA antibodies stained villous stroma but not the trophoblast of CHM. Using the peroxidase antibody technique, Sunderland et al. (1985) showed that class II antigens are not present on molar trophoblast. They detected class I antigens, however, on "proliferating extravillous trophoblast and on villous stromal cells, but not on quiescent villous trophoblast." This finding is similar to those in normal first trimester placentas. When Yamashita et al. (1979) compared the HLA types of parents with those of the molar tissue, they identified the molar antigen as paternal. Berkowitz et al. (1985b) also detected transferrin receptors in the villous trophoblastic surface, similar to those that occur in normal tissue. These investigators localized trophoblast-leukocyte common antigens on normal and molar villous surfaces (Berkowitz

et al., 1983, 1986). $Rh_0(D)$ antigens were demonstrated on the malignant trophoblast of a d-negative patient who became sensitized by a choriocarcinoma that had developed after the delivery of a D-positive child (Fischer et al., 1985). Goto et al. (1980) had previously demonstrated that trophoblast may contain the D antigen, and Tomoda et al. (1981) subsequently suggested that the racial disparity of incidence in gestational neoplastic disease may be secondary to the irregular distribution of the D antigen. Sarkar et al. (1986) found an expression of c-*myc* and c-*ras* oncogenes in early trophoblast, CHM, and malignant trophoblast cell lines. This pattern was absent from an 11-week conceptus. The expression of merosin, a novel basement membrane protein, was found in normal and malignant trophoblast (Leivo et al., 1989). Remarkably, this antigen was present only in intermediate trophoblast (X cells). It was not in the syncytium or in Langhans cells. This observation further suggests that the X cells represent a distinct and separate lineage of chorionic cells. Minami et al. (1993) demonstrated with antibody staining methodology that molar trophoblast contains inhibin-activin subunits after having shown earlier their presence in normal placentas. Certain moieties are found in syncytium and cytotrophoblast, others in extravillous trophoblast. However, like the localization of various other placental hormones to different trophoblastic components (Sasagawa et al., 1987), the immunological localization does not necessarily prove that these cells are the production sites.

The prenatal diagnosis of CHM moles is now usually possible with sonography. Ultrasonography identifies the lack of fetus and displays the multiple echogenic signals, the "speckled" appearance of the molar placental tissue. Additionally, in PHMs a fetus may be visualized (Harper & MacVicar, 1963). Despite general knowledge of molar gestations, physicians make the diagnosis infrequently at the first antenatal visit (Ringertz, 1970), probably because during early gestation the villous swelling is minimal. Other physicians who have made similar observations have also pointed to the frequent difficulty of early diagnosis (e.g., Stroup, 1956). The sonographic differentiation from missed abortions was further refined by the studies of Fine et al. (1989). Gynecologists have had the experience, however, that sonography during early pregnancy fails to make the diagnosis consistently (e.g., Woodward et al., 1980). Romero et al. (1985) therefore correlated hCG levels with sonography. They set the hCG level of 82,350 mIU/ml as a diagnostic criterion, in addition to absent heart movement seen by ultrasonography. The diagnostic accuracy of recognizing moles thereby increased from 41.6% to 88.8%. Amniography has also been utilized (Gerber, 1970), as has arteriography (Hendrickse et al., 1964; Borell et al., 1966; Breit &

Schedel, 1970). It is of special interest that ultrasono-graphic examination of first trimester pregnancies that eventuated in CHM did not show alterations that could be used to anticipate molar development (Woodward et al., 1980).

Other Characteristics

Maternal hyperthyroidism often accompanies hydatidiform moles (Hershman & Higgins, 1971), and sometimes it causes pulmonary edema. Both disappear promptly after evacuation. The nature of the thyroid-stimulating agent that is presumably released from the placental tissue is controversial. Some findings have suggested that it is identical with placental hCG (Nisula & Taliafouros, 1980). Amir et al. (1984) conducted a detailed study to identify this agent and concluded that it was unlikely to be hCG, but that it must represent another protein moiety released from the trophoblast of moles. Gunasegaram et al. (1986) suggested that it was a thyroid-stimulating hormone (TSH)-like protein, distinct from the hCG and the luteinizing hormone (LH) which they identified in molar vesicles. Other alterations of enzymes and proteins have been described in molar gestations. α-Fetoprotein is consistently absent in choriocarcinoma patients. It is rarely found in moles and then only in low concentration (Ishiguro, 1975). Yoshimatsu et al. (1987) immunologically examined tissues of various types of abortuses for the presence of α-fetoprotein. Molar fluid and trophoblast were consistently negative, but the protein was found in villi of PHM. Elevated serum glutamic oxaloacetic transaminase (SGOT) levels, found in some moles by Tobin (1963), were believed to result from cellular degeneration. Borek et al. (1983) suggested that urinary levels of DNA breakdown products after molar evacuation may be a useful adjunctive measure to indicate successful therapy. They found nucleosides and some DNA-derived enzymes to be elevated when active trophoblast remained after therapy. The disappearance especially of β-aminoisobutyric acid from the urine, even in the presence of persisting hCG levels, forecast a good prognosis. Lee et al. (1981) found that circulating levels of the pregnancy-specific β₁-glycoprotein (SP-1) and placental protein 5 (PP5) were markedly reduced in patients with untreated CHM and choriocarcinoma. They suggested that this measurement was a decisive means for differentiating benign and malignant trophoblast.

The usual means for following patients with CHM, of course, is the serial determination of serum hCG levels or its β-subunits. This hormone is concentrated in molar villi, according to the studies of Sciarra (1970). He found mean values of 1,524 mIU/ml in the fluid of small vesicles and 1,202 mIU/ml in the larger villi. Normal values of all hormones and secretory products of neoplastic trophoblast have been able summarized by Clayton et al. (1981). Yedema and colleagues (1993) have constructed a gonadotropin regression curve from 130 patients with no trophoblastic sequelae after evacuation of a molar pregnancy. They found that 71 of 77 patients with persistent trophoblastic disease could be identified from their elevated hCG levels, and in more than 50% it was possible to achieve this diagnosis within 6 weeks of operation. Khazaeli et al. (1986) suggested that the determination of a ratio between β-hCG and hCG has prognostic significance. The more "malignant" moles apparently produce significantly more free β-hCG units (Khazaeli et al., 1989). Ozturk et al. (1988) found that the of β-hCG/hCG ratio fairly reliably distinguishes between normal pregnancy and CHM and between CHM and choriocarcinoma. Presumably the hCG secretion, known to be of syncytial origin (Yorde et al., 1979; Bonduelle et al., 1988), reflects the increased quantity of syncytium in moles, rather than a qualitative change in its secretion pattern. Abnormal trophoblast

appears to produce an excessive amount of β-hCG subunits. The rate of decline in β-hCG levels following delivery of moles has also been summarized by Yuen (1983), a study that also included data of prolactin and estradiol secretion. In general, the β-hCG levels fall rapidly to zero within 8 weeks after evacuation. Bagshawe et al. (1986) stated that in 42% of women with CHM serum hCG was undetectable 56 days after evacuation; none of the patients required chemotherapy. Franke et al. (1983a) determined that the average disappearance time of serum hCG after CHM was 99.3 days, after PHM 58.9 days, and after hydatid degeneration in abortuses 50.7 days. They recommended that, provided there is a continued decrease in the levels, therapy not commence before day 100 after evacuation. Human placental lactogen (hPL) levels correlated poorly with hCG levels of moles and choriocarcinomas; they were generally low (Ehnholm et al., 1967). This finding suggests that chorionepithelium is not the principal source of hPL and that its cellular source, the X cell, has undergone little proliferation during molar development, which is borne out histologically. The interpretation of enhanced hCG secretion by moles because of increased villous (and hence trophoblastic) surface may be an oversimplification. A suggestion has been made that it relates to the expression of paternal genes. Goshen and Hochberg (1994), commenting on a paper by Fejgin et al. (1993) that studied placental hormone secretion, made these interesting comments: They suggested that high hCG values are expected in CHM because of paternal disomy 19 (the hCG locus is on that chromosome); low levels are expected (and found) in triploid PHM with maternal contribution of the extra haploid set.

Numerous studies have examined how the implantation site of moles might differ from that of normal gestation. The reader is referred to the section on X cells (see Chapter 11). In complete hydatidiform moles (CHM) the site of implantation often shows exuberant trophoblast and, especially, "placental site giant cells." They are mostly X cells (called intermediate trophoblast by some authors), but syncytiotrophoblast is also present. The amount of trophoblast at the placental site may be confusing, and there may be difficulty differentiating it from invasive choriocarcinoma. King (1956) has paid special attention to the "borderline" lesions of gestational trophoblastic neoplasia. These lesions encompass (1) residual mole and syncytial endometritis, and (2) invasive mole (chorioadenoma destruens). To minimize the problem of recurrent disease, King advocated routine curettage after removal of a CHM.

Syncytial endometritis is not a neoplasm. It represents "a residuum of trophoblastic cells after a normal pregnancy, abortion, or hydatidiform mole" (Novak & Seah, 1954). Strictly speaking, syncytial endometritis does not contain molar villi. Also, there are no solid areas of pure trophoblast that might indicate the presence of choriocarcinoma. The placental floor in syncytial endometritis is composed of trophoblast intermingled with decidual cells, with a few inflammatory cells also admixed. Its cellular composition is highly variable. Berkowitz et al. (1982) examined the composition of the "maternal floor" in 11 CHM cases, specifically looking for deposits of immunoglobulins (Igs) and complement. Immunofluorescent deposits of IgG, IgM, and C3 were confined to the spiral arterioles. The authors thus concluded that CHM does not evoke a "a vigorous host humoral immune response." In a later study this same group of investigators (Kabawat et al., 1985) demonstrated the presence of increased numbers of inflammatory cells at molar implantation sites, especially T cells with predominance of T4$^+$ cells. They speculated that this infiltrate relates to the development of a delayed hypersensitivity reaction, participating in "rejection." In the peripheral circulation of patients with trophoblastic tumors, however, there is a significant reduction of T cells and other immunocytes (Ho et al., 1986). Ho and his colleagues discussed the immunological significance of these findings.

Because there is no accompanying fetus in CHM, moles lack the fetal adrenal precursors for estriol formation. They therefore have an extremely low E3 content (Chamberlain et al., 1968). Incubation studies with dehydroisoandrosterone and other androgenic precursors indicate that moles and choriocarcinoma do possess the ability to convert this steroid to estriol (MacDonald and Siiteri, 1966; Houtzager et al., 1970). From their in vivo studies with the appropriate precursors, Barlow et al. (1967) suggested that the low E3 production may be useful for differentiating moles from normal early pregnancies.

Moles and partial moles are also frequently associated with preeclampsia. Llewellyn-Jones (1967) related it to uterine size. Eclampsia was seen at 17 weeks in a triploid pregnancy with partial molar transformation of the placenta by Slattery et al. (1993). The existence of pregnancy-induced hypertension (PIH), however, is not a useful differential diagnostic feature for clinical differentiation between CHM and PHM. Scott (1958) reviewed this subject in context with the frequent PIH that is found in hydrops and hydramnios. He concluded that similar hormonal disturbances must exist to evoke PIH. Fatal eclampsia has occurred with molar pregnancy. Lee (1965) described a mother with a mole and severe PIH at 13 weeks' gestation. Sicuranza and Tisdall (1976) found eclampsia associated with what was apparently a PHM and with a live fetus of 125 g. Their report was similar to the case earlier described by Lloyd (1921). An increase of syncytiotrophoblastic glycogen content was observed by Arkwright et al. (1993) to exist in molar and PIH-related trophoblast. Choriocarcinomatous cells contain the most glycogen. The authors suggested that this accumulation may be a marker of "immaturity" of this cell. The relation to PIH was one of increased syncytial turnover in PIH that was observed by them (Chua et al., 1991).

Deportation

Molar tissue, as the normal syncytium, may be transported to the lung. This deportation may occur spontaneously and during the evacuation of a molar uterus. It may cause acute pulmonary hypertension, edema, and even death. In other cases, such vascular deportation has been associated with disseminated intravascular coagulation (DIC). "Benign" molar tissue has even been observed to grow in the lung—hence the term benign metastasizing mole. This term was coined by Ring (1972), who observed two patients with isolated pulmonary nodules associated with invasive moles. Both lesions pursued a benign course. Leeder (1964) had previously described a molar pregnancy with metastatic molar tissue in lung, vagina, and vulva. All regressed spontaneously. The patient described by Johnson et al. (1979) suffered hemothorax from a pleural mole that improved only after chemotherapy. Meyer (1966) also reported a pulmonary nodule composed of molar tissue. The patient had a typical CHM with considerable trophoblastic pleomorphism. She developed the lung lesion and had persistent uterine trophoblast 7 weeks after delivery of the mole. There was an intense lymphoplasmacellular reaction at the pulmonary site. Reed et al. (1959) reported similar cases, and Bardawil et al. (1957) described a case with spontaneous regression of pulmonary metastases developing months after evacuation of a mole. They considered immunological rejection to have been the most likely mechanism for this regression. Mark and Moel (1961) discussed the radiological differential diagnosis, and Hsu et al. (1962) found that deported molar metastases occurred most commonly in the pudendal tissues. These entities all fall into the broader category of invasive mole.

Clinical follow-up and therapy do not differ from those of CHM that remains confined to the uterus. Although deportation of complete molar villous tissue can readily produce radiological pulmonary lesions, the events described by Cohle and Petty (1985) and Lipp et al. (1962) are more difficult to understand. They found extensive pulmonary capillary plugging by syncytial cells and suggested that it was the cause of fatal embolism. Syncytium normally reaches the lung of pregnant patients (Schmorl, 1905; Lee et al., 1986; see also discussion by Pool et al., 1987; Chua et al., 1991); presumably this dissemination occurs even more readily with molar gestations (Figures 487, 488). Hankins et al. (1987) studied this problem with pulmonary artery catheters during mole evacuation. They found multinucleated giant cells (probable syncytium) but no villi. Moreover, there was no change in pulmonary arterial pressures or lung perfusion. Tanimura et al. (1985) identified deported trophoblast in pulmonary capillaries in nine of ten patients who died after abortion or delivery. That this deportation of cells can be massive enough to occlude the pulmonary circulation remains to be shown. It is more likely that DIC occurred in these cases, as similar instances have been observed repeatedly (Beyth, 1973; Egley et al., 1975; Orr et al., 1980). Parenthetically, it might be mentioned that intrauterine instillation of hypertonic saline (for attempted

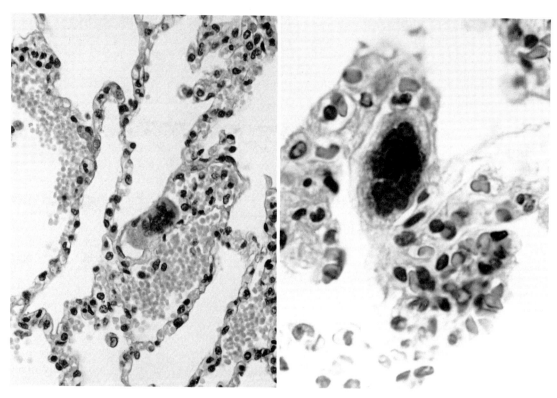

FIGURE 487. Syncytial trophoblast in pulmonary capillaries after maternal death at 16 weeks' gestation. H&E. Left ×100; right ×260.

pregnancy termination) may be fatal to patients with hydatidiform mole (Frost, 1968). Even normal villi are deported on occasion. Figure 489 shows the presence of immature villi, enmeshed in coagulum, within a pulmonary artery. They were discovered at autopsy of a woman who died after traumatic disruption of the uterus during therapeutic abortion.

Chorioadenoma Destruens (Invasive Mole)

Invasive mole is a malignant neoplasm composed of infiltrating trophoblast and molar villi. The tumor invades the uterus and often the adjacent structures. It overlaps the aforementioned condition of benign

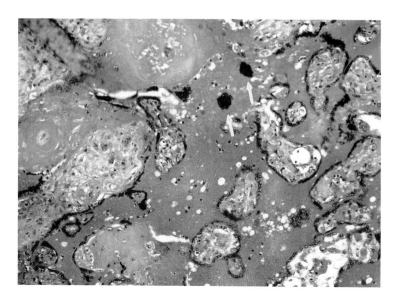

FIGURE 488. Term placenta with syncytial knots (arrows) that have detached and are being swept into the maternal intervillous circulation, from where they reach the maternal lung. H&E. ×160.

FIGURE 489. Pulmonary artery filled with thrombus and immature villi, which had been deported during therapeutic abortion, when the uterus was perforated. H&E. ×60.

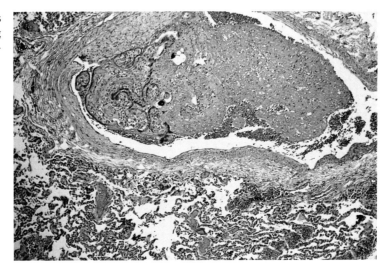

metastasizing mole and the pseudotumor, later renamed placental site tumor (discussed in Chapter 23). Invasive mole is differentiated from true choriocarcinoma only by the presence of villi scattered among the trophoblast. Its behavior often is similar to that of choriocarcinoma, and usually it requires similar therapy. Perhaps it is unwise to retain this category. King (1956) placed it into his category of borderline conditions. An invasive mole is nothing more than the molar equivalent of placenta increta, and it may be as destructive. The term was coined by Ewing (1910). King distinguished three types: simple invasive mole, invasive mole with regression, and invasive mole with signs of progression. The terms speak for themselves. The prognosis is conditional on the initial nature of the mole and the efficacy of its primary removal.

Figure 490 shows a typical invasive mole. The molar villi, including exuberant trophoblast, have deeply invaded the myometrium. Often this picture is combined with much more hemorrhage than is demonstrated by this particular case. Invasive moles often present challenging diagnostic and therapeutic problems. The following case illustrates it well.

A 34-year-old gravida 3 had vaginal bleeding at 3 months; sonograms at 14 weeks were suspicious but not diagnostic of mole. An amniogram at 16 weeks showed CHM, which was evacuated by suction after a single dose of methotrexate (5 mg) had been administered. The molar tissue showed much trophoblastic exuberance (Figures 491, 492). Methotrexate was continued for another 5 days, causing the development of oral lesions and leukopenia. The patient had the serial hCG titers shown in Figure 493. Two pulmonary metastases were diagnosed radiologically 2.5 months after evacuation. After five additional courses of methotrexate and two courses of actinomycin D therapy, the lung lesions faded. Six months after evacuation, the hCG levels had still not returned to normal. Three additional courses of actinomycin D were given. Arteriography was performed and found to be negative. Hysterectomy was done at this time. Serial slicing of the uterus showed a single hemorrhagic cavity (Figure 494) that contained a small group

of degenerated villi (Figure 495), adjacent to which was intramuscular viable trophoblast with fluorescence to anti-hCG antibodies. The patient remained well thereafter.

Similar cases abound in the literature. Invasive moles are also known to produce late pulmonary metastases. Such cases have been well illustrated and discussed by Spademan and Tuttle (1964) and many other authors. Conservative therapy was advocated by Rubin (1964) because many of these "tumors" have an innate benign

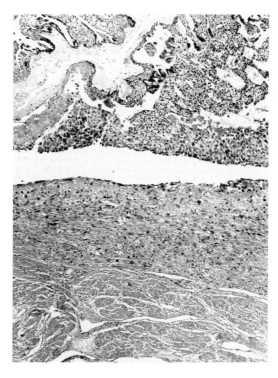

FIGURE 490. Invasive mole (chorioadenoma destruens) in the myometrial wall (below), showing marked trophoblastic hyperplasia. H&E. ×40.

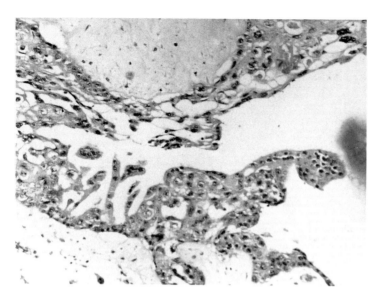

FIGURE 491. Molar villous surface of a patient with the invasive mole shown in Figures 492 to 494. There is moderate trophoblastic hyperplasia in an otherwise typical CHM. H&E. ×100.

potential. There is even a report of uterine perforation by a "destructive mole" (Kyodo et al., 1988), but this patient also had an apparently normal fetus. It is not clear from the report, however, whether the mole was a partial, triploid pregnancy or a twin gestation. Thiele and de Alvarez (1962) described two patients with CHM and metastases. They reviewed the literature on invasive moles and secondary, implants, and Thatcher et al. (1989) described the tubal equivalent of such a lesion. Most tubal pregnancies are accretas; and when they rupture they resemble placenta percreta. The implantation of trophoblast outside the tube is therefore not surprising. These authors saw secondary peritoneal implants of trophoblast after laparoscopic salpingostomy (see also Cataldo et al., 1990). The nodules were excised and proved to be normal trophoblast; the patient recovered. Ultrastructurally, invasive moles are similar to normal placenta, CHM, and choriocarcinoma (Wynn & Harris, 1967), but the chromosomes of invasive chorionic lesions have rarely been studied. Makino et al. (1963) found invasive moles to have hyperdiploid and aneuploid chromosome numbers more frequently than CHM; choriocarcinoma was even more aneuploid.

Therapy

The treatment of trophoblastic neoplasms has changed drastically with the introduction of methotrexate therapy in 1956 (Li et al., 1956). Li et al. recognized the specific toxicity of this agent to trophoblastic and embryonic cells because of its folic acid-inhibiting quality. It has effects in vitro as well (Sand et al., 1986), including the well known leucovorin rescue that is often needed during therapy. Detailed protocols for the various trophoblastic disorders have been provided in the contributions to the Symposium on Gestational Trophoblastic Neoplasms (Goldstein & Berkowitz,

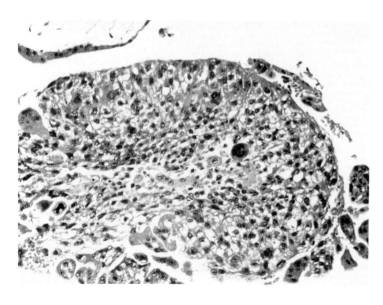

FIGURE 492. Invasive mole (same case as in Figure 491). Note the markedly anaplastic area of trophoblast. H&E. ×100.

Course of Invasive Mole
HCG Levels mIU/ml

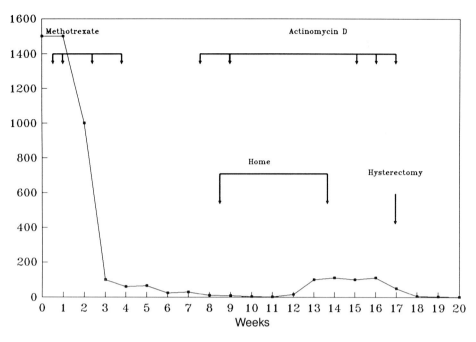

FIGURE 493. Course of a patient who developed pulmonary metastases and invasive mole after evacuation of an intrauterine mole (see text). The mole is shown in Figures 491 and 492 and the chorioadenoma destruens in Figures 494 and 495.

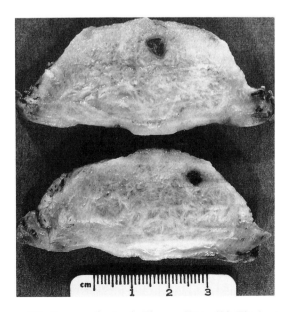

FIGURE 494. Same patient as in Figures 491 to 493. The hysterectomy specimen shown here had a small subendometrial hemorrhagic cavity containing molar tissue.

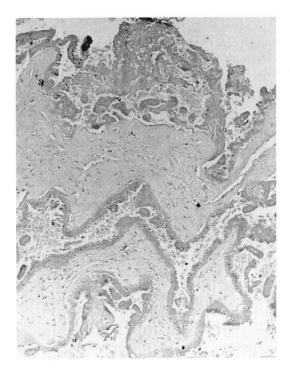

FIGURE 495. Invasive mole of the patient in Figures 491 to 494. Note the largely degenerated villi and trophoblast. H&E. ×40.

1981). This area is beyond the scope of the present book. As Acosta-Sison (1964) has so aptly stated already, there are changing attitudes to the management of moles. Early and complete evacuation is perhaps the most important aspect of successful therapy (Mathieu, 1939). When properly done, the new therapeutic regimens are nearly uniformly effective (Lurain et al., 1983; Schlaerth et al., 1988). Some patients require no therapy, and it has repeatedly been noted that metastatic lesions may disappear spontaneously. There is continued controversy as to the wisdom of "prophylactic therapy" for all patients with CHM (Goldstein, 1971; Kim et al., 1986). Hertz et al. (1963) showed that rigorous treatment with methotrexate and actinomycin D is generally completely successful when metastases develop. Kashimura et al. (1986) suggested that the recurrence rate of trophoblastic disease is between 5.7% and 26.0%. These investigators followed 420 patients with CHM, 293 of whom were given prophylactic methotrexate (10 mg for 7 days). There was significant improvement of those receiving therapy (7.5% versus 18.1%), and it was more marked in older patients.

The surveillance of molar cases after evacuation with serial hCG levels is a convenient way to ensure success. It must be reemphasized, however, that the exclusion of PHM cases from therapeutic regimens is mandatory. Such patients are most easily identified with routine flow cytometry on the initial specimen. Hysterectomy is now rarely necessary. Moreover, appropriate chemotherapy is compatible with future fertility (Song et al., 1988).

Ectopic Moles

The occurrence of moles in the tube and ovary has been described, including tubal rupture (Westerhout, 1964). Data from the older literature are not necessarily convincing, however, because of the possible presence of a PHM in these reports. Pettit (1941) reviewed 42 cases of tubal moles and choriocarcinomas and reported a new case with good outcome. Sze et al. (1988) described a patient who had an intrauterine "molar" pregnancy 2 months after salpingostomy for tubal ectopic pregnancy. The "mole" was accompanied by a malformed fetus. It was a partial mole, most likely a triploid conceptus. The authors believed this report to be the first description of such a combination of implantations. The case is important because it highlights the care one must exercise when reviewing the topic. Although listed as "molar" pregnancy, the text clearly described it to be a PHM. It is also acknowledged that the excessive levels of hCG in this patient (467,000 mIU/ml) are not helpful in the differential diagnosis between CHM and PHM. Other examples of triploid PHM in the tube abound in the literature, as for instance the case of Montgomery et al. (1993).

On rare occasions, a hydatidiform mole is believed to have originated in the ovary. Jock et al. (1981) described the sixth such reported case and estimated that this condition occurs perhaps only once in 50 million pregnancies. They also reviewed the literature. Their patient, a 27-year-old primigravida, was admitted for evacuation of a sonographically evident intrauterine mole at 12 weeks' gestation. The uterus, however, was found to be empty. The mole was present within a 14-cm ovarian mass. No postoperative chemotherapy was needed. Of interest was the extensive decidual change found on the omental surface. The case described by Stanhope et al. (1983) resulted in a benign outcome following local resection. Yenen et al. (1965), who described and illustrated a similar case, removed the uterus. In retrospect, this surgery seems to have been unnecessary.

Partial Hydatidiform Mole

The usual CHM has an almost uniform distribution of hydatid villi, and remnants of fetal capillaries are exceptionally rare. There are, however, hydatidiform moles in which only a portion of the placenta is hydropically altered. These moles are also more often associated with fetuses. Atkin and Klinger (1962) were the first to correlate triploidy with molar change. Sporadic reports followed (Schlegel et al., 1966). It was Carr (1971), however, who first established that "85% of triploid and hypertriploid embryos showed hydatidiform degeneration or mole." Subsequently, Vassilakos et al. (1977) drew sharp attention to the entity that we now know as partial hydatidiform mole. They clearly distinguished it from the CHM. In a series of 811 spontaneous and 1,097 induced abortions, they found 75 placentas with gross villous swelling. Most of them showed chromosomal anomalies, primarily triploidy and trisomy 16. None had marked trophoblastic anaplasia, and all had a good outcome. The diagnosis of PHM is not always correctly established by pathological criteria, as the studies with flow cytometry and DNA fingerprinting have shown (see Takahashi et al., 1990). Therefore one must be cautious when interpreting the data from many series that have been published in the past.

Vassilakos and Kajii (1976) coined the phrase "hydatidiform mole, two entities." This observation was immediately confirmed, and PHM is now well established as a distinct entity. Szulman and Surti (1978a,b) have made many contributions to delineate this placental abnormality. All but three of their initial 12 cases had an associated fetus. There was often striking elevation of hCG levels, but these levels dropped rapidly after delivery. The authors emphatically stated that there is no transition between mole types, and that the older term transitional mole is inappropriate. One of their cases of PHM with 46,XX and fetal parts is of interest. Its true nature remains unknown, but it served to caution that these designations are not "water-tight" syndromes. It should be pointed out that not all triploid conceptuses have elevated hCG titers. Fejgin et al. (1992) suggested that placental insufficiency may be one cause of such

FIGURE 496. Histological appearance of villi of triploid PHM at 12 weeks' gestation. Note the irregular size of the villi and the small amount of trophoblast. Remnants of atrophying fetal capillaries are present (arrows). There is early cisterna formation of villi between the arrows and prominent infolding (scalloping) of villi. H&E. ×65.

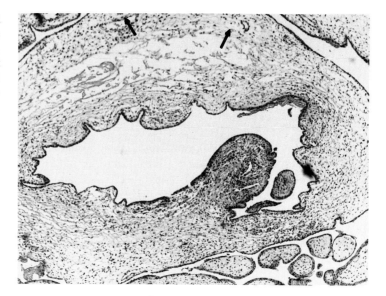

low levels, and Morrish et al. (1992) thought that PHMs have an impaired facility of hormone production in response to stimulants.

The **morphology** of PHM is variable and dependent on the genotype. The villi of PHM are much more irregularly swollen than those of CHM, and many normal villi may intervene among grossly molar tissue. Cisternae may be present, but they are also generally less common than is true for CHM. The more important feature for the differential diagnosis is the frequent presence of villous capillary remnants (Figure 496). Many of these contain fetal red blood cells, even though the fetus may have died or was not recognized in the specimen received. There is generally much less, and usually only focal, trophoblastic hyperplasia. The villous covering is frequently scalloped, and villous inclusions of trophoblast (tangentially cut surfaces) are

common (Figure 497). Most investigators have suggested that these trophoblastic inclusions are found only in triploid moles, but that is somewhat contrary to our experience. We find trophoblastic inclusions occasionally even in normal immature placentas and certainly in other chromosomally abnormal abortuses (Novak et al., 1988). Therefore, we do no use this criterion as important feature for the diagnosis of PHM. Szulman et al. (1981) reviewed cytogenetically verified triploid abortuses and found that 86% of them had placentas that could be classified as PHM. Their fetuses tended to have died by the eighth week of pregnancy, but uterine retention tended to be longer than for other chromosomally aberrant conceptuses.

Szulman and Surti (1982) estimated, from a hospital population, that CHM occurs in 1 of 1,330 pregnancies and PHM in 1 of 1,730 pregnancies. Triploidy arises in

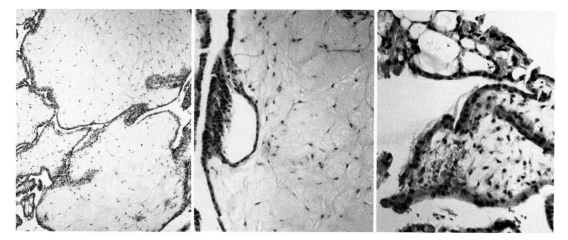

FIGURE 497. Partial (triploid) hydatidiform mole with extensive edema and prominent infolding (scalloping) of the minimally hyperplastic trophoblast. This infolding leads to the histo-logical appearance of trophoblast islands within edematous villi. There is much syncytial cisterna dilatation at right. H&E. Left ×60; center ×120; right ×260.

approximately 1% of recognized human pregnancies. Jacobs et al. (1982) reported that most triploids are due to fertilization with two paternal genomes (dispermy). Only 1% to 3% eventuate in a molar pregnancy (Lawler et al., 1979). The analysis of 106 triploid specimens by Jacobs et al. (1982) is especially interesting. The extra haploid set of chromosomes was of paternal origin (androgenetic) in 51 cases; it was maternally derived (gynogenetic) in 15. The former gestations lasted longer (122 days) than the latter (74 days). This difference may in part explain why paternally derived triploid conceptuses are concentrated among the PHMs, as it takes time for grossly visible swelling to come about. The studies of Uchida and Freeman (1985) gave similar results. Ohama and his collaborators (1986) investigated the chromosome status of 56 partial moles. They found that 46 were triploid, and 9 were diploid. The diploid moles lacked trophoblastic hyperplasia and stromal inclusions (Figure 498). Importantly, four of these nine diploid PHMs had chromosomal heteromorphisms. In other words, they were *not* androgenetic, as is typical for the diploid CHM. Although most partial moles are triploid, a few are not. McFadden et al. (1994) found different origins of the extra set of chromosomes. They found more cases of digyni rather than the former prevalent diandry. All PHMs were diandric triploids, and one of four diandrics developed PHM.

The important question arises if there is a possibly different prognosis for these groups. Davis et al. (1987), who analyzed ploidy by flow cytometry in 35 PHMs, unexpectedly found that 17% ($n = 6$) were triploid and 83% ($n = 29$) were diploid. The investigators did not find any complications in the triploid group, but 20% ($n = 5$) of the diploid cases had nonfatal sequelae. Examples of these complications included the need for recurettage and chemotherapy. Teng and Ballon (1984) described three patients with moles and a coexisting fetus. The patients had persistent hCG, elevations, and two required chemotherapy. This report has been criticized by Szulman and Surti (1985), who considered these cases to be dizygotic twin gestations and urged that stricter criteria be employed in reports of these conditions.

Some reports have emphasized the existence of preeclampsia with PHM, and that theca lutein cysts of the ovaries may complicate PHM (Lewis & Cefalo, 1979). These cystic changes of molar and partial molar placentas have been recognized sonographically (Harper & MacVicar, 1963; Bendon et al., 1988). Several investigators have studied hCG levels in CHMs and compared them with those in PHMs. Smith et al. (1984) found that after evacuation of the uterus the hCG levels disappeared similarly quickly, but that the levels immediately after evacuation were significantly higher

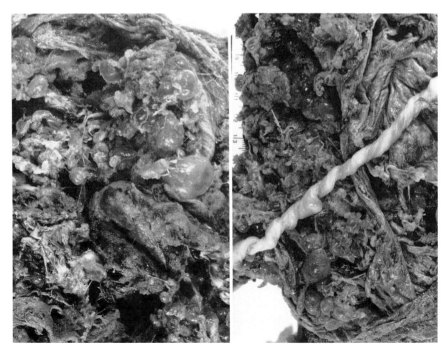

FIGURE 498. Possible partial hydatidiform mole with diploid, 46,XX, homozygous karyotype on C banding. A 720 g, 24 weeks' gestation, female infant with renal dysplasia resulted in neonatal death. The placenta weighed 1,460 g and had scattered molar vesicles throughout. The umbilical cord was normal, and there was virtually no trophoblastic proliferation. Maternal outcome was good.

with CHMs. Berkowitz et al. (1989), in a detailed analysis of the various gonadotropin moieties, found the following in maternal serum: CHMs had higher levels of β-hCG than PHMs, but the latter had higher α-hCG levels; both moles had higher levels of both subunit levels than did comparable normal pregnancies (see also Khazaeli et al., 1986). Markedly elevated α-fetoprotein levels were present in two patients with PHM and triploidy (Kazazian et al., 1989), something that does not happen in CHM.

The **natural history** of PHM has been evaluated by several authors, especially with emphasis on possible malignant sequelae. Czernobilsky et al. (1982) found no untoward outcome in 25 PHMs. Berkowitz et al. (1983) followed 81 patients with PHM. Serum hCG levels exceeded 100,000 mIU/ml in only two patients. Eight of their patients (9.9%) developed *nonmetastatic* trophoblastic disease that was successfully treated with methotrexate. In six of eight patients, residual molar tissue was found on curettage; there were no choriocarcinomas. The only possible exception in the large experience with partial moles is the case of Looi and Sivanesaratnam (1981). The patient in their study was said to have developed a choriocarcinoma following a partial mole. Kohorn (1986) has questioned the need for this (premature) intervention with chemotherapy. There are few reports that have verified true trophoblastic neoplasia following partial moles, an important point made in the report by Heifetz and Czaja (1992). Their 69,XXX gestation with fetus had a nodule of what appeared to be choriocarcinoma in situ, but the postpartum course was entirely benign. Szulman et al. (1981) did a retrospective study of 13 PHM patients from Hong Kong. One, a case of "invasive (partial) mole, required chemotherapy." In our opinion, the case was one of placenta increta of a triploid specimen, not

trophoblastic neoplasia. Gaber et al. (1986) reported a similar case. PHM may of course recur (Honoré, 1987; Honoré et al., 1988). We believe that when the diagnosis of triploidy is truly established for a PHM, *complete evacuation* cures the patient. Bagshawe and his colleagues (1990) undertook a study of 11 patients whose condition had been originally diagnosed as PHM and whose course was complicated by gestational trophoblastic tumor (GTD). DNA analysis led to revision of PHM to CHM in four cases, and two cases had been incorrectly diagnosed as moles. These authors suggested that four patients required chemotherapy, although their last pregnancy was a triploid PHM. No proof is provided, however, that these lesions were choriocarcinomas, and it was also not discussed how far the GTD had spread. Lawler et al. (1991), who studied 202 molar specimens (51 PHMs with 44 triploid; 149 CHMs with 105 diploid; 1 haploid[!]; 1 triploid) saw no need for chemotherapy in any of their PHMs.

Mole and Fetus

There have been numerous reports of molar pregnancies with associated fetuses. Popek (1994), who studied 10 cases of CHM with a twin fetus, indicated the incidence to be 1 per 10,000 gestations, most being triploid specimens. Although CHMs with a twin fetus also exist, he estimated their occurrence to be as uncommon as 1 per 250,000. Such fetuses occasionally survive, and the situation warrants answers to the following precise questions: Are these triploid gestations, or are they dizygotic twins with one a CHM or PHM and the other a normal conceptus (Figure 499)? The differential diagnosis of these cases is often uncertain, and frequently it cannot be reconstructed from the published

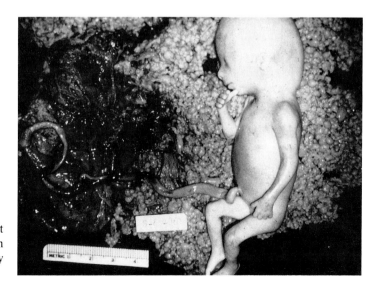

FIGURE 499. Mole with a living coexisting fetus. It is most likely a triploid conceptus: male fetus, 9 cm crown–rump length. There was nearly completely molar change of the placenta.

TABLE 23. Twin pregnancies, one a molar gestation.

Author	Year	Fetus	Mole	Outcome
Krone	1955	3,200 g, ♀, live	Separate	Twin family; good; review
Logan	1957	16 weeks	Separate	Good
Beischer	1961	36 weeks, ♂, live	Separate	Good
		39 weeks, ♀, live	Separate	Good; 13 cases diffuse
Chamberlain	1963	18 weeks, ♂	Separate, ♀	Good
Hohe et al.	1971	1,975 g, ♂, live	Attached, separate	Choriocarcinoma
Jones & Lauersen	1975	2,900 g, ♀	Fused	Good
		13 weeks, ♀	?Fused	Needed chemotherapy
Suzuki et al.	1980	1,425 g, ♀	Separate	Good; review of cases
Yee et al.	1982	910 g, ♂ died	Separate	Needed chemotherapy
Block & Merrill	1982	1,850 g, ♂, live	Separate	Barr body-negative mole
		2,020 g, ♂, live	Fused	Barr body-negative mole
Sande & Eyjolfsson	1985	22 weeks, ♂	Separate	Good
		Dead fetus	Separate	Good
Khoo et al.	1986	2,000 g, ♂, live	Fused	Review of 23 cases
Vejerslev et al.	1986	22 weeks, ♀, dead	Separate	Mole androgenetic; review

reports. The natural history of eight "well documented cases" of apparent CHM and coexisting fetus was described by Steller et al. (1994). These authors also analyzed the literature on this topic and found that the presence of a fetus often led to the sonographic (mis)diagnosis of PHM. They performed flow cytometry and found that five of eight patients developed persistent trophoblastic disease that required chemotherapy. In other cases, the characteristic pattern of fetal anomalies allows identification of triploidy, especially the digital fusions. There is not only a rich literature on the frequency of triploidy in spontaneous abortuses, but numerous cases have delineated the various anomalies occurring in live-born infants with triploidy (e.g., Uher et al., 1963; Beischer et al., 1967; Goecke, 1967; Butler et al., 1969; Schmickel et al., 1971; deGrouchy et al., 1974; Niebuhr, 1974; Fraikor et al., 1980; Graham et al., 1989). In some of these cases, the infant was living (Crooij et al., 1985), and the outcome was otherwise not complicated by trophoblastic sequelae. It is noteworthy that the placenta of some large triploid fetuses has not included hydatid changes. Fetus and placenta are also often growth-retarded, and single umbilical artery is common. Absent umbilical artery diastolic flow has been reported in them (Sherer et al., 1993). It would be interesting to correlate the phenotypes of

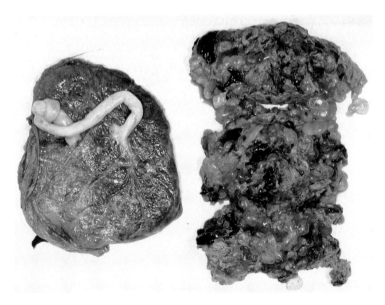

FIGURE 500. Twin with mole. The patient was a 24-year-old woman who had had three pregnancies, one ending in abortion. Her course was benign until 32 weeks, when she delivered a 1,900 g male infant who did well. There was a normal 330 g placenta and a separate 780 g complete, Barr body-positive hydatidiform mole (see Figure 501).

FIGURE 501. Molar villi of the pregnancy shown in Figure 500. Note the typical, uniform villous swelling.

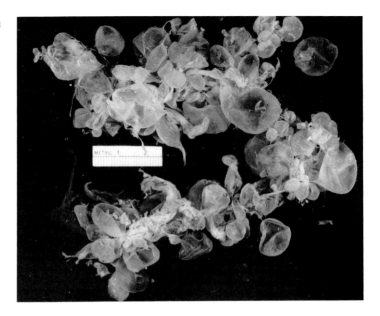

placentas with paternal/maternal sets of chromosomal contributions. The present belief is that, with triploidy, two paternal chromosome sets more often lead to PHM than do two maternal sets of chromosomes, which is more often characterized by malformed fetuses. Some cases of PHM with fetus have been diploid, with a normal, heterozygotic, chromosome set (Kubo et al., 1986). Feinberg et al. (1988) reported such a case (46,XX) that was diagnosed sonographically. The fetus was hydropic but did not have any congenital anomalies.

PHM with Twin Gestation

The occurrence of a PHM with a fetus raises the question of triploidy; alternately, there is a possibility of a twin pregnancy when less than the entire placenta shows hydatidiform changes. The complex topic is discussed in some detail by Vejerslev et al. (1991) who describe five pregnancies in a woman who had four consecutive molar pregnancies. The one that was associated with the fetus was a biparental diploid mole that they considered to constitute a distinct and separate entity. Most cases turn out to be singleton pregnancies. There are many reports, however, in which one normal placenta and fetus was present with a molar placenta. The assumption is often made that all of the cases were dizygotic gestations. The fact that some of them were later complicated by choriocarcinoma (Hohe et al., 1971) indicates that at least some of the moles may have been typical CHMs. Table 23 provides a summary of the major reports describing such twin gestations. A typical case is shown in Figures 500 to 502. Beischer and Fortune (1968) used the sex chromatin method (Barr bodies) to approach the nature of karyotypes in their early studies of this phenomenon. They delineated a number of twin gestations where one was normal and the other molar. Important summaries of large series of moles with coexisting fetuses are those by Beischer

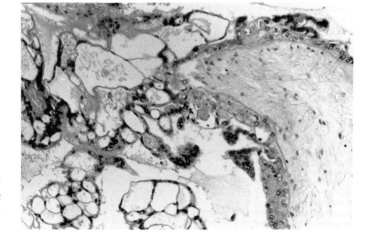

FIGURE 502. Histological appearance of the twin's mole in Figures 500 and 501. There is moderate trophoblastic hyperplasia and especially proliferation of cytotrophoblast, which is rarely seen in PHMs. H&E. ×400.

(1966) and Vejerslev et al. (1986). They contain several cases of verified twin gestations and can be consulted for details.

References

Acosta-Sison, H.: Changing attitudes in the management of hydatidiform mole. Am. J. Obstet. Gynecol. 88:634–636, 1964.

Ambrani, L.M., Vaidya, R.A., Rao, C.S., Daftary, S.D., and Motashaw, N.D.: Familial occurrence of trophoblastic disease—report of recurrent molar pregnancies in sisters in three families. Clin. Genet. 18:27–29, 1980.

Amir, S.M., Osathanondh, R., Berkowitz, R.S., and Goldstein, D.P.: Human chorionic gonadotropin and thyroid function in patients with hydatidiform mole. Am. J. Obstet. Gynecol. 150:723–728, 1984.

Anonymous: Editorial: flow cytometry and gestational trophoblastic disease. Lancet 2:950, 1987.

Arkwright, P.D., Rademacher, T.W., Dwek, R.A., and Redman, C.W.G.: Pre-eclampsia is associated with an increase in trophoblast glycogen content and glycogen synthase activity, similar to that found in hydatidiform moles. J. Clin. Invest. 91:2744–2753, 1993.

Atkin, N.B., and Klinger, H.P.: The superfemale mole. Lancet 2:727, 1962.

Atrash, H.K., Hogue, C.J.R., and Grimes, D.A.: Epidemiology of hydatidiform mole during early gestation. Am. J. Obstet. Gynecol. 154:906–909, 1986.

Baggish, M.S., Woodruff, J.D., Tow, S.H., and Jones, H.W.: Sex chromatin pattern in hydatidiform mole. Am. J. Obstet. Gynecol. 102:362–370, 1968.

Bagshawe, K.D., Dent, J., and Webb, J.: Hydatidiform mole in England and Wales 1973–1983. Lancet 2:673–677, 1986.

Bagshawe, K.D., Lawler, S.D., Paradinas, F.J., Dent, J., Brown, P., and Boxer, G.M.: Gestational trophoblastic tumours following initial diagnosis of partial hydatidiform mole. Lancet 335:1074–1076, 1990.

Bandy, L.C., Clarke-Pearson, D.L., and Hammond, C.B.: Malignant potential of gestational trophoblastic disease at the extreme ages of reproductive life. Obstet. Gynecol. 64:395–399, 1984.

Bardawil, W.A., Hertig, A.T., and Velardo, J.T.: Regression of trophoblast. I. Hydatidiform mole; a case of unusual features, possibly metastasis and regression; review of literature. Obstet. Gynecol. 10:614–625, 1957.

Barlow, J.J., Goldstein, D.P., and Reid, D.E.: A study of in vivo estrogen biosynthesis and production rates in normal pregnancy, hydatidiform mole and choriocarcinoma. J. Clin. Endocrinol. Metab. 27:1028–1034, 1967.

Barton, S.C., Surani, M.A.H., and Norris, M.L.: Role of paternal and maternal genomes in mouse development. Nature 311:374–376, 1984.

Beischer, N.A.: Hydatidiform mole with co-existent foetus. J. Obstet. Gynaecol. Br. Commonw. 68:231–237, 1961.

Beischer, N.A.: Hydatidiform mole with coexistent foetus. Aust. N.Z. J. Obstet. Gynaecol. 6:127–141, 1966.

Beischer, N.A., and Fortune, D.W.: Significance of chromatin patterns in cases of hydatidiform mole with an associated fetus. Am. J. Obstet. Gynecol. 100:276–282, 1968.

Beischer, N.A., Fortune, D.W., and Fitzgerald, M.G.: Hydatidiform mole and coexisting foetus, both with triploid chromosome constitution. B.M.J. 2:476–478, 1967.

Bell, D.A., Flotte, T.J., Pastel-Levy, C., Ware, A., Preffer, F., and Colvin, R.B.: Flow cytometric analysis of DNA-ploidy in partial hydatidiform moles (PHM) utilizing paraffin-embedded material [abstract 44]. Mod. Pathol. 2:8A, 1989.

Ben-Chetrit, A., Yagel, S., Ariel, I., Zacut, D., Shimonovitz, S., and Celnikier-Hochner, D.: Successful conservative management of primary nonmetastatic cervical choriocarcinoma. Am. J. Obstet. Gynecol. 163:1161–1163, 1990.

Bendon, R.W., Siddiqi, T., Soukup, S., and Srivastava, A.: Prenatal detection of triploidy. J. Pediatr. 112:149–153, 1988.

Benirschke, K.: Abortions and moles. In, Perinatal Diseases. R.L. Naeye, J.M. Kissane, and N. Kaufman, eds., pp. 23–48. Williams & Wilkins, Baltimore, 1981.

Benirschke, K.: Editorial: flow cytometry for ALL mole-like abortion specimens. Hum. Pathol. 20:403–404, 1989.

Berkowitz, R.S., Anderson, D.J., Hunter, N.J., and Goldstein, D.P.: Distribution of major histocompatibility (HLA) antigens in chorionic villi of molar pregnancy. Am. J. Obstet. Gynecol. 146:221–220, 1983.

Berkowitz, R.S., Mostoufizadeh, M., Kabawat, S.E., Goldstein, D.P., and Driscoll, S.G.: Immunopathologic study of the implantation site in molar pregnancy. Am. J. Obstet. Gynecol. 144:925–930, 1982.

Berkowitz, R.S., Goldstein, D.P., and Bernstein, M.R.: Natural history of partial molar pregnancy. Obstet. Gynecol. 66:677–681, 1983.

Berkowitz, R.S., Cramer, D.W., Bernstein, M.R., Cassells, S., Driscoll, S.G., and Goldstein, D.P.: Risk factors for complete molar pregnancy from a case-control study. Am. J. Obstet. Gynecol. 152:1016–1020, 1985a.

Berkowitz, R.S., Dubey, D.P, Goldstein, D.P., and Anderson, D.J.: Localization of transferrin receptor in the chorionic villi of complete molar pregnancy. Am. J. Obstet. Gynecol. 151:128–129, 1985b.

Berkowitz, R.S., Umpierre, S.A., Johnson, P.M., McIntyre, J.A., and Anderson, D.J.: Expression of trophoblast-leukocyte common antigens and placental-type alkaline phosphatase in complete molar pregnancy. Am. J. Obstet. Gynecol. 155:443–446, 1986.

Berkowitz, R., Ozturk, M., Goldstein, D., Bernstein, M., Hill, L., and Wands, J.R.: Human chorionic gonadotropin and free subunits' serum levels in patients with partial and complete hydatidiform moles. Obstet. Gynecol. 74:212–216, 1989.

Beyth, Y.: Hypofibrinogenemia in hydatidiform mole. J. Reprod. Med. 11:223–224, 1973.

Block, M.F., and Merrill, J.A.: Hydatidiform mole with coexisting fetus. Obstet. Gynecol. 60:129–134, 1982.

Bonduelle, M.-L., Dodd, R., Liebaers, I., van Steirteghem, A., Williamson, R., and Akhurst, R.: Chorionic gonadotrophin-β mRNA, a trophoblast marker, is expressed in human 8-cell embryos derived from tripronucleate zygotes. Hum. Reprod. 3:909–914, 1988.

Bonnar, J., and Tennent, R.A.: Benign hydatidiform mole followed by late pulmonary choriocarcinoma. J. Obstet. Gynaecol. Br. Commonw. 69:999–1005, 1962.

Borek, E., Sharma, O.K., and Brewer, J.I.: Urinary nucleic acid breakdown products as markers for trophoblastic diseases. Am. J. Obstet. Gynecol. 146:906–910, 1983.

Borell, U., Fernström, I., Moberger, G., and Ohlson, L.: The Diagnosis of Hydatidiform Mole, Malignant Hydatidiform Mole and Choriocarcinoma with Special Reference to the Diagnostic Value of Pelvic Arteriography. Charles C Thomas, Springfield, IL, 1966.

Bourgoin, P., Baylet, R., and Ballon, C.: Études des chromosomes de la grossesse molaire. C. R. Soc. Biol. 159:957, 1965a.

Bourgoin, P., Baylet, R., and Grattepanche, H.: Exploration d'une hypothèse sur l'étiopathogénie des môles hydatiformes: étude chromosomique. Rev. Fr. Gynecol. Obstet. 60:673–684, 1965b.

Bracken, M.B.: Incidence and aetiology of hydatidiform mole: an epidemiological review. Br. J. Obstet. Gynaecol. 94:1123–1135, 1987.

Bracken, M.B.: Incidence of hydatidiform mole (letter to the editor). Am. J. Obstet. Gynecol. 158:1016–1017, 1988.

Breit, A., and Schedel, E.: Ergebnisse der Beckenarteriographie bei Plazentatumoren. Fortschr. Geb. Roentgenstr. Nuklearmed. 112:431–439, 1970.

Brinton, L.A., Wu, B.-Z., Wang, W., Ershow, A.G., Song, H.-Z., Li, J.-Y., Bracken, M.B., and Blot, W.J.: Gestational trophoblastic disease: a case-control study from the People's Republic of China. Am. J. Obstet. Gynecol. 161: 121–127, 1989.

Buckley, J.: Epidemiology of gestational trophoblastic diseases. In, Gestational Trophoblastic Disease. A.E. Szulman and H.J. Buchsbaum, eds., pp. 8–26. Springer-Verlag, New York, 1987.

Bur, G.E., Hertig, A.T., McKay, D.G., and Adams, E.C.: Histochemical aspects of hydatidiform mole and choriocarcinoma. Obstet. Gynecol. 19:156–182, 1962.

Butler, L.J., Chantler, C., France, N.E., and Keith, C.G.: A liveborn infant with complete triploidy (69,XXX). J. Med. Genet. 6:413–421, 1969.

Butler, W.J., Schwartz, C.E., Sauer, S.M., Wilson, J.T., and McDonough, P.G.: Discordance in deoxyribonucleic acid analysis of fetus and trophoblast. Am. J. Obstet. Gynecol. 158:642–645, 1988.

Carr, D.H.: Cytogenetics and the pathology of hydatidiform degeneration. Obstet. Gynecol. 33:333–342, 1969.

Carr, D.H.: Chromosome studies in selected spontaneous abortions: polyploidy in man. J. Med. Genet. 8:164–174, 1971.

Cataldo, N.A., Nicholson, M., and Bihrle, D.: Uterine serosal trophoblastic implant after linear salpingostomy for ectopic pregnancy at laparotomy. Obstet. Gynecol. 76:523–525, 1990.

Chamberlain, G.: Hydatidiform mole in twin pregnancy. Am. J. Obstet. Gynecol. 87:140–142, 1963.

Chamberlain, J., Morris, N.F., and Smith, N.C.: Steroids of hydatidiform moles. J. Endocrinol. 41:289–290, 1968.

Chua, S., Wilkins, T., Sargent, I., and Redman, C.: Trophoblast deportation in pre-eclamptic pregnancy. Br. J. Obstet. Gynaecol. 98:973–979, 1991.

Chun, D., Braga, C., Chow, C., and Lok, L: Clinical observations on some aspects of hydatidiform mole. J. Obstet. Gynaecol. Br. Commonw. 71:180–184, 1964.

Clayton, L.A., Tyrey, L., Weed, J.C., and Hammond, C.B.: Endocrine aspects of trophoblastic neoplasia. J. Reprod. Med. 26:192–199, 1981.

Cohen, B.A., Burkman, R.T., Rosenshein, N.B., Atienza, M.F., King, T.M., and Parmley, T.H.: Gestational trophoblastic disease within an elective abortion population. Am. J. Obstet. Gynecol. 135:452–454, 1979.

Cohle, S.D., and Petty, C.S.: Sudden death caused by embolization of trophoblast from hydatidiform mole. J. Forensic Sci. 30:1279–1283, 1985.

Couillin, P., Afoutou, J.M., Faye, O., Correa, P., and Boué, A.: Androgenetic origin of African complete hydatidiform moles demonstrated by HLA markers. Hum. Genet. 71: 113–116, 1985.

Crooij, M.J., van der Harten, J.J., Puyenbroek, J.I., van Geijn, H.P., and Arts, N.F.: A partial hydatidiform mole, dispersed throughout the placenta, coexisting with a normal living fetus: case report. Br. J. Obstet. Gynaecol. 92:104–106, 1985.

Czernobilsky, B., Barash, A., and Lancet, M.: Partial moles: a clinicopathologic study of 25 cases. Obstet. Gynecol. 59: 75–77, 1982.

Das, P.C.: Hydatidiform mole: a statistical and clinical study. J. Obstet. Gynaecol. Brit. Emp. 45:265–280, 1938.

Davis, J.R., Kerrigan, D.P., Way, D.L., and Weiner, S.A.: Partial hydatidiform moles: deoxyribonucleic acid content and course. Am. J. Obstet. Gynecol. 157:969–973, 1987.

De Grouchy, J., Roubin, M., Risse, J.-C., and Sarrut, S.: Enfant triploide (69,XXX) ayant vécu neuf jours. Ann. Gnt. (Paris) 17:283–286, 1974.

Depypere, H.T., Dhont, M., Verschraegen-Spae, M.R., and Coppens, M.: Tubal hydatidiform mole. Am. J. Obstet. Gynecol. 169:209–210, 1993.

Douglas, G.W.: Malignant changes in trophoblastic tumors. Am. J. Obstet. Gynecol. 84:884–894, 1962.

Drieux, H., and Thiéry, G.: Les tumeurs du placenta chez les animaux domestiques. Rev. Pathol. Comp. 48:445–451, 1948.

Driscoll, S.G.: Trophoblastic growths: morphologic aspects and taxonomy. J. Reprod. Med. 26:181–191, 1981.

Edmonds, H.W.: Genesis of hydatidiform mole: old and new concepts. Ann. N.Y. Acad. Sci. 80:86–104, 1959.

Egley, C.C., Simon, L.R., and Haddox, T.: Hydatidiform mole and disseminated intravascular coagulation. Am. J. Obstet. Gynecol. 121:1122–1123, 1975.

Ehnholm, C., Seppälä, M., Tallberg, T., and Widholm, O.: Immunological studies in human placental lactogen hormone in chorionepithelioma and hydatidiform mole. Ann. Med. Exp. Fenn. 45:318–319, 1967.

Endres, R.J.: Hydatidiform mole: report of a patient with 5 consecutive hydatidiform moles. Am. J. Obstet. Gynecol. 81:711–714, 1961.

Ewing, J.: Chorioma: a clinical and pathological study. Surg. Gynecol. Obstet. 10:366–392, 1910.

Federschneider, J.M., Goldstein, D.P., Berkowitz, R.S., Marean, A.R., and Bernstein, M.R.: Natural history of recurrent molar pregnancy. Obstet. Gynecol. 55:457–459, 1980.

Feinberg, R.F., Lockwood, C.J., Salafia, C., and Hobbins, J.C.: Sonographic diagnosis of a pregnancy with a diffuse hydatidiform mole and coexisting 46,XX fetus: a case report. Obstet. Gynecol. 72:485–488, 1988.

Fejgin, M.D., Amiel, A., Goldberger, S., Barnes, I., Zer, T., and Kohn, G.: Placental insufficiency as a possible cause of low maternal serum human gonadotropin and low maternal serum unconjugated estriol levels in triploidy. Am. J. Obstet. Gynecol. 167:766–767, 1992.

Fine, C., Bundy, A.L., Berkowitz, R.S., Boswell, S.B., Berezin, A.F., and Doubilet, P.M.: Sonographic diagnosis of partial hydatidiform mole. Obstet. Gynecol. 73:414–418, 1989.

Fischer, H.E., Lichtiger, B., and Cox, I.: Expression of $Rh_0(D)$ antigen in choriocarcinoma of the uterus in an $Rh_0(D)$-negative patient: report of a case. Hum. Pathol. 16:1165–1167, 1985.

Fisher, R.A., and Lawler, S.D.: Heterozygous complete hydatidiform moles: do they have a worse prognosis than homozygous complete moles? Lancet 2:51, 1984.

Fisher, R.A., and Newlands, E.S.: Rapid diagnosis and classification of hydatidiform moles with polymerase chain reaction. Am. J. Obstet. Gynecol. 168:563–569, 1993.

Fisher, R.A., Lawler, S.D., Ormerod, M.G., Imrie, P.R., and Povey, S.: Flow cytometry used to distinguish between complete and partial hydatidiform moles. Placenta 8:249–256, 1987.

Folger, A.F.: Über die Blasenmole beim Rinde. Acta Pathol. Microbiol. Scand. Suppl. 18:104–128, 1934.

Ford, J.H., Brown, J.K., Lew, W.Y., and Peters, G.B.: Diploid complete hydatidiform mole, mosaic for normally fertilized cells and androgenetic homozygous cells: case report. Br. J. Obstet. Gynaecol. 93:1181–1186, 1986.

Fox, H.: Hydatidiform moles: editorial. Virchows Arch. A 415:387–389, 1989.

Fraikor, A.L., Vigneswaran, R., and Honeyfield, P.: Liveborn triploid. Am. J. Dis. Child. 134:988–989, 1980.

Franke, H.R., Risse, E.K.J., Kenemans, P., Houx, P.C.W., Solk, J.G., and Vooijs, G.P.: Plasma human chorionic gonadotropin disappearance in hydatidiform mole: a central registry report from The Netherlands. Obstet. Gynecol. 62:467–473, 1983a.

Franke, H.R., Risse, E.K.J., Kenemans, P., Vooijs, G.P., and Stolk, J.G.: Epidemiologic features of hydatidiform mole in The Netherlands. Obstet. Gynecol. 62:613–616, 1983b.

Franke, H.R., Alons, C.L., Caron, F.J.M., Boog, M.C., Oort, J., and Stolk, J.G.: Quantitative morphology: a study of the trophoblast. Virchows Arch. [Pathol. Anat.] 406:323–331, 1985.

Frankforter, S., Marcus, J., Grant, D., and Bewtra, C.: Clinicopathologic differences between diploid and tetraploid complete hydatidiform moles. [abstract 506]. Mod. Pathol. 7:88A, 1994.

Frost, A.C.G.: Death following intrauterine injection of hypertonic saline solution with hydatidiform mole. Am. J. Obstet. Gynecol. 101:342–344, 1968.

Fukunaga, M., Ushigome, S., Fukunaga, M., and Sugishita, M.: Application of flow cytometry in diagnosis of hydatidiform moles. Mod. Pathol. 6:353–359, 1993.

Gaber, L.W., Redline, R.W., Mostoufi-Zadeh, M., and Driscoll, S.G.: Invasive partial mole. Am. J. Clin. Pathol. 85:722–724, 1986.

Gardener, H.A., and Lage, J.M.: Choriocarcinoma following a partial hydatidiform mole: a case report. Hum. Pathol. 23:468–471, 1992.

Genest, D.R., Laborde, O., Berkowitz, R.S., Goldstein, D.P., Bernstein, M.R., and Lage, J.: A clinicopathologic study of 153 cases of complete hydatidiform mole (1980–1990): histologic grade lacks prognostic significance. Obstet. Gynecol. 78:402–409, 1991.

Gerber, A.H.: Amniographic diagnosis of trophoblastic disease. J.A.M.A. 212:630, 1970.

Goecke, C.: Partielle Blasenmole und fötale Mißbildungen. Z. Geburtshilfe Gynäkol. 166:201–210, 1967.

Goldstein, D.P.: Prophylactic chemotherapy of patients with molar pregnancy. Obstet. Gynecol. 38:817–822, 1971.

Goldstein, D.P., and Berkowitz, R.S.: Gestational trophoblastic neoplasms: an invitational symposium. J. Reprod. Med. 26:179–229, 1981.

Goldstein, D.P., and Berkowitz, R.S.: Gestational Trophoblastic Neoplasms. Clinical Principles of Diagnosis and Management. Saunders, Philadelphia, 1982.

Gonzalez-Angulo, A., Marquez-Monter, H., Zavala, B.J., Yabur, E., and Salazar, H.: Electron microscopic observations in hydatidiform mole. Obstet. Gynecol. 27:455–467, 1966.

Goshen, R., and Hochberg, A.A.: The genomic basis of the β-subunit of human chorionic gonadotropin diversity in triploidy. Am. J. Obstet. Gynecol. 170:700–701, 1994.

Goto, S., Nishi, H., and Tomoda, Y.: Blood group Rh-D factor in human trophoblast determined by immunofluorescent method. Am. J. Obstet. Gynecol. 137:707–712, 1980.

Graham, J.M., Rawnsley, E.F., Simmons, G.M., Wurster-Hill, D.H., Park, J.P., Marin-Padilla, M., and Crow, H.C.: Triploidy: pregnancy complications and clinical findings. in seven cases. Prenat. Diagn. 9:409–419, 1989.

Grimes, D.A.: Epidemiology of gestational trophoblastic disease. Am. J. Obstet. Gynecol. 150:309–318, 1984.

Gunasegaram, R., Peh, K.L., Loganath, A., Kottegoda, S.R., and Ratnam, S.S.: Elevated intravesicular fluid thyroid-stimulating hormone concentration in hydatidiform mole. Int. J. Gynaecol. Obstet. 24:177–181, 1986.

Habibian, R., and Surti, U.: Cytogenetics of trophoblasts from complete hydatidiform moles. Cancer Genet. Cytogenet. 29:271–287, 1987.

Hankins, G.D.V., Wendel, G.D., Snyder, R.R., and Cunningham, F.G.: Trophoblastic embolization during molar evacuation—central hemodynamic observations. Obstet. Gynecol. 69:368–372, 1987.

Harper, W.F., and MacVicar, J.: Hydatidiform mole and pregnancy diagnosed by sonar. B.M.J. 2:1178–1179, 1963.

Harrison, K.B.: X-chromosome inactivation in the human cytotrophoblast. Cytogenet. Cell Genet. 52:37–41, 1989.

Harrison, K.B., and Warburton, D.: Preferential X-chromosome activity in human female placental tissues. Cytogenet. Cell Genet. 41:163–168, 1986.

Heifetz, S.A., and Czaja, J.: In situ choriocarcinoma arising in partial hydatidiform mole: implications for the risk of persistent trophoblastic disease. Pediatr. Pathol. 12:601–611, 1992.

Hemming, J.D., Quirke, P., Womack, C., Wells, M., Elston, C.W., and Bird, C.C.: Diagnosis of molar pregnancy and persistent trophoblastic disease by flow cytometry. J. Clin. Pathol. 40:615–620, 1987.

Hendrickse, J.P.deV., Cockshott, W.P., Evans, K.T.E., and Barton, C.J.: Pelvic angiography in the diagnosis of malignant trophoblastic disease. N. Engl. J. Med. 271:859–866, 1964.

Hershman, J.M., and Higgins, H.P.: Hydatidiform mole—a cause of clinical hyperthyroidism: report of two cases with evidence that molar tissue secreted a thyroid stimulator. N. Engl. J. Med. 284:573–577, 1971.

Hertig, A.T.: Hydatidiform mole and chorionepithelioma. In, Progress in Gynecology. Vol. II. J.V. Meigs and S.H. Sturgis, eds., pp. 372–394. Grune & Stratton, Orlando, FL, 1950.

Hertig, A.T.: Human Trophoblast. Charles C Thomas, Springfield, IL, 1968.

Hertig, A.T., and Sheldon, W.H.: Hydatidiform mole—a pathologico-clinical correlation of 200 cases. Am. J. Obstet. Gynecol. 53:1–36, 1947.

Hertz, R., Ross, G.T., and Lipsett, M.B.: Primary chemotherapy of nonmetastatic trophoblastic disease in women. Am. J. Obstet. Gynecol. 86:808–814, 1963.

Hitchcock, C.L., Conran, R.M., and Griffin, J.L.: Hydatidiform moles and the use of flow cytometry in their diagnosis. Perspect. Pediatr. Pathol. 15:117–141, 1991.

Ho, P.-C., Wong, L.C., Lawton, J.W.M., and Ma, H.K.: Mixed lymphocyte reaction in hydatidiform mole. Am. J. Reprod. Immunol. 6:25–27, 1984.

Ho, P.-C., Lawton, J.W.M., Wong, L.-C., and Ma, H.-K.: T-cell subsets and natural killer cell activity in patients with gestational trophoblastic neoplasia. Am. J. Obstet. Gynecol. 155:330–334, 1986.

Hohe, P.T., Cochrane, C.R., Gmelich, J.T., and Austin, J.A.: Coexisting trophoblastic tumor and viable pregnancy. Obstet. Gynecol. 38:899–904, 1971.

Holland, J.F., and Hreshchyshyn, M.M., eds.: Choriocarcinoma. Springer-Verlag, Heidelberg, 1967.

Honoré, L.H.: Recurrent partial hydatidiform mole: report of a case. Am. J. Obstet. Gynecol. 156:922–924, 1987.

Honoré, L.H., Lin, E.C., and Morrish, D.W.: Recurrent partial mole. Am. J. Obstet. Gynecol. 158:442, 1988.

Houtzager, H.L., van Leusden, H.A., and Siemerink, M.: Conversion of androgens into oestrogens by hydatidiform moles in vitro. Acta Endocrinol. (Copenh.) 64:17–37, 1970.

Howat, A.J., Beck, S., Fox, H., Harris, S.C., Hill, A.S., Nicholson, C.M., and Williams, R.A.: Can histopathologists reliably diagnose molar pregnancy? J. Clin. Pathol. 46:599–602, 1993.

Hsu, C.-T., Huang, L.-C., and Chen, T.-Y.: Metastases in benign hydatidiform mole and chorioadenoma destruens. Am. J. Obstet. Gynecol. 84:1412–1424, 1962.

Hsu, C.-T., Lai, C.H., Chanchien, C.L., and Changchien, B.-C.: Repeat hydatidiform moles. Am. J. Obstet. Gynecol. 87:543–547, 1963.

Hunt, W., Dockerty, M.B., and Randall, L.M.: Hydatidiform mole: a clinicopathologic study "grading" as a measure of possible malignant change. Obstet. Gynecol. 1:593–609, 1953.

Ishiguro, T.: Serum α-fetoprotein in hydatidiform mole, choriocarcinoma, and twin pregnancy. Am. J. Obstet. Gynecol. 12:539–541, 1975.

Iverson, L., and The Joint Project Investigators: Geographic variation in the occurrence of hydatidiform mole and choriocarcinoma. Ann. N.Y. Acad. Sci. 80:178–195, 1959.

Jacobs, P.A., Hassold, T.J., Matsuyama, A.M., and Newlands, I.M.: Chromosome constitution of gestational trophoblastic disease. Lancet 2:49, 1978.

Jacobs, P.A., Wilson, C.M., Sprenkle, J.A., Rosenheim, N.B., and Migeon, B.R.: Mechanism of complete hydatidiform moles. Nature 286:714–716, 1980.

Jacobs, P.A., Szulman, A.E., Funkhouser, J., Matsuura, J.S., and Wilson, C.C.: Human triploidy: relationship between parental origin of the additional haploid complement and development of partial hydatidiform mole. Ann. Hum. Genet. 46:223–231, 1982.

Jarotzky, V., and Waldeyer: Traubenmole in Verbindung mit dem Uterus: intraparietale und intravasculäre Weiterentwicklung der Chorionzotten. Arch. Pathol. Anat. Physiol. Klin. Med. 44:88–94, 1868.

Javey, H., Borazjani, G., Behnard, S., and Langley, F.A.: Discrepancies in the diagnosis of hydatidiform mole. Br. J. Obstet. Gynaecol. 86:480–483, 1979.

Jock, D.E., Schwartz, P.E., and Portnoy, L.: Primary ovarian hydatidiform mole: addition of a sixth case to the literature. Obstet. Gynecol. 58:657–660, 1981.

Johnson, F.L.: Recurrent hydatidiform mole. Can. Med. Assoc. J. 94:344, 1966.

Johnson, T.R., Comstock, C.H., and Anderson, D.G.: Benign gestational trophoblastic disease metastatic to pleura: unusual cause of hemothorax. Obstet. Gynecol. 53:509–511, 1979.

Jones, W.B., and Lauersen, N.H.: Hydatidiform mole with coexisting fetus. Am. J. Obstet. Gynecol. 122:267–272, 1975.

Kabawat, S.E., Mostoufi-Zadeh, M., Berkowitz, R.S., Driscoll, S.G., Goldstein, D.P., and Bhan, A.K.: Implantation site in complete molar pregnancy: a study of immunologically competent cells with monoclonal antibodies. Am. J. Obstet. Gynecol. 152:97–99, 1985.

Kajii, T., and Ohama, K.: Androgenetic origin of hydatidiform mole. Nature 268:633–634, 1977.

Kajii, T., Kurashige, H., Ohama, K., and Uchino, F.: XY and XX complete moles: clinical and morphological correlations. Am. J. Obstet. Gynecol. 150:57–64, 1984.

Kashimura, Y., Kashimura, M., Sugimori, H., Tsukamoto, N., Matsuyama, T., Matsukuma, K., Kamura, T., Saito, T., Kawano, D., Nose, R., Nose, Y., Nakano, H., and

Taki, I.: Prophylactic chemotherapy for hydatidiform mole: five to 15 years follow-up. Cancer 58:624–629, 1986.

Kazazian, L.C., Baramki, T.A., and Thomas, R.L.: Triploid fetus: an important consideration in the evaluation of very high maternal serum alpha-fetoprotein. Prenat. Diagn. 9:27–30, 1989.

Khazaeli, M.B., Hedayat, M.M., Hatch, K.D., To, A.C.W., Soong, S.-J., Shingleton, H.M., Boots, L.R., and LoBuglio, A.F.: Radioimmunoassay of free β-subunit of human chorionic gonadotropin as a prognostic test for persistent trophoblastic disease in molar pregnancy. Am. J. Obstet. Gynecol. 155:320–324, 1986.

Khazaeli, M.B., Buchina, E.S., Pattillo, R.A., Soon, S.-J., and Hatch, K.D.: Radioimmunoassay of free β-unit of human chorionic gonadotropin in diagnosis of high-risk and low-risk gestational trophoblastic disease. Am. J. Obstet. Gynecol. 160:444–449, 1989.

Khoo, S.K., Monks, P.L., and Davies, N.T.: Hydatidiform mole coexisting with a live fetus: a dilemma of management. Aust. N.Z. J. Obstet. Gynaecol. 26:129–135, 1986.

Kim, D.S., Moon, H., Kim, K.T., Moon, Y.J., and Hwang, Y.Y.: Effects of prophylactic chemotherapy for persistent trophoblastic disease in patients with complete hydatidiform mole. Obstet. Gynecol. 67:690–694, 1986.

King, G.: Hydatidiform mole and chorion-epithelioma—the problem of the borderline case. Proc. R. Soc. Med. 49:381–390, 1956.

Ko, T.-M., Hsieh, C.-Y., Ho, H.-N., Hsieh, F.-J., and Lee, T.-Y.: Restriction fragments length polymorphism analysis to study the genetic origin of complete hydatidiform mole. Am. J. Obstet. Gynecol. 164:901–906, 1991.

Kohorn, E.I.: Natural history of partial molar pregnancy. Obstet. Gynecol. 68:731–732, 1986.

Krone, H.A.: Blasenmole mit einem ausgetragenen lebenden Kind. Zentralbl. Gynäkol. 77:1391–1395, 1955.

Kronfol, N.M., Iliya, F.A., and Hajj, S.N.: Recurrent hydatidiform mole: a report of five cases with review of the literature. Lebanese Med. J. 22:507–520, 1969.

Kubo, H., Abe, Y., Shimada, M., Katayama, S., and Date, R.: Two cases of hydatidiform mole with a surviving coexisting fetus. Congen. Anomal. 26:256, 1986.

Kyodo, Y., Inatomi, K., Abe, T., and Kudo, K.: A case report of destructive mole after uterine rupture. Am. J. Obstet. Gynecol. 158:1182–1183, 1988.

Lage, J.M., Driscoll, S.G., Yavner, D.L., Olivier, A.P., Mark, S.D., and Weinberg, D.S.: Hydatidiform moles: application of flow cytometry in diagnosis. Am. J. Clin. Pathol. 89:596–600, 1988.

Lage, J.M., Weinberg, D.S., Yavner, D.L., and Bieber, F.R.: The biology of tetraploid hydatidiform moles: histopathology, cytogenetics, and flow cytometry. Hum. Pathol. 20:419–425, 1989.

Lage, J.M., Berkowitz, R.S., Rice, L.W., Goldstein, D.P., Bernstein, M.R., and Weinberg, D.S.: Flow cytometric analysis of DNA content in partial hydatidiform moles with persistent gestational trophoblastic tumor. Obstet. Gynecol. 77:111–115, 1991.

Lage, J.M., Mark, S.D., Roberts, D.J., Goldstein, D.P., Bernstein, M.R., and Berkowitz, R.S.: A flow cytometric study of 137 fresh hydropic placentas: correlation between types of hydatidiform moles and nuclear DNA ploidy. Obstet. Gynecol. 79:403–410, 1992.

Lauslahti, K.: A histological and histochemical study of trophoblastic disease in a Finnish material 1958–1962. Acta Pathol. Microbiol. Scand. Suppl. 201:1–71, 1969.

La Vecchia, C., Franceschi, S., Fasoli, M., and Mangioni, C.: Gestational trophoblastic neoplasms in homozygous twins. Obstet. Gynecol. 60:250–252, 1982.

La Vecchia, C.L., Parazzini, F., Decarli, A., Franceschi, S., Fasoli, M., Favalli, G., Negri, E., and Pampallona, S.: Age of parents and risk of gestational trophoblastic disease. J. Natl. Cancer Inst. 73:639–642, 1984.

Lawler, S.D., and Fisher, R.A.: Genetic studies in hydatidiform mole with clinical correlations. Placenta 8:77–88, 1987.

Lawler, S.D., Kloudas, P.T., and Bagshawe, K.D.: Immunogenicity of molar pregnancies in the HL-A system. Am. J. Obstet. Gynecol. 120:857–861, 1974.

Lawler, S.D., Pickthall, V.J., Fisher, R.A., Povey, S., Evans, M.W., and Szulman, A.E.: Genetic studies of complete and partial hydatidiform moles. Lancet 2:580, 1979.

Lawler, S.D., Fisher, R.A., and Dent, J.: A prospective genetic study of complete and partial hydatidiform moles. Am. J. Obstet. Gynecol. 164:1270–1277, 1991.

Lee, E.E.: Gross early enlargement of a hydatidiform mole with severe pre-eclampsia. Can. Med. Assoc. J. 93:79–80, 1965.

Lee, A.T.C., and Siegel, I.: Hydatidiform mole with rupture of the uterus: report of a case. Obstet. Gynecol. 26:133–134, 1965.

Lee, J.N., Salem, H.T., Al-4Ani, A.T.M., Huang, S.C., Ouyang, P.C., Wei, P.Y., and Seppälä, M.: Circulating concentrations of specific placental proteins (human chorionic gonadotropin, pregnancy-specific beta-1 glycoprotein, and placental protein 5) in untreated gestational trophoblastic tumors. Am. J. Obstet. Gynecol. 139:702–704, 1981.

Lee, W., Ginsburg, K.A., Cotton, D.B., and Kaufman, R.H.: Squamous and trophoblastic cells in the maternal pulmonary circulation identified by invasive hemodynamic monitoring during the peripartum period. Am. J. Obstet. Gynecol. 155:999–1001, 1986.

Leeder, J.R.: Metastasizing hydatidiform mole. Am. J. Obstet. Gynecol. 88:833–835, 1964.

Leivo, I., Laurila, P., Wahlström, T., and Engvall, E.: Expression of merosin, a tissue-specific basement membrane protein, in the intermediate trophoblast cells of choriocarcinoma and placenta. Lab. Invest. 60:783–790, 1989.

Lewis, P.E., and Cefalo, R.C.: Triploidy syndrome with theca lutein cysts and severe pre-eclampsia. Am. J. Obstet. Gynecol. 133:110–111, 1979.

Li, M.C., Hertz, R., and Spencer, D.B.: Effect of methotrexate therapy upon choriocarcinoma and chorioadenomas. Proc. Soc. Exp. Biol. Med. 93:361–366, 1956.

Lindor, N.M., Ney, J.A., Gaffey, T.A., Jenkins, R.B., Thibodeau, S.N., and Dewald, G.W.: A genetic review of complete and partial hydatidiform moles and nonmolar triploidy. Mayo Clin. Proc. 67:791–799, 1992.

Lipp, R.G., Kindshi, J.D., and Schmitz, R.: Death from pulmonary embolism associated with hydatidiform mole. Am. J. Obstet. Gynecol. 83:1644–1647, 1962.

Llewellyn-Jones, D.: Relation of pregnancy toxaemia to trophoblastic tumours. B.M.J. 2:720, 1967.

Lloyd, C.E.: A case of hydatidiform mole associated with toxaemia. J. Obstet. Gynaecol. Br. Emp. 28:307–310, 1921.

Logan, B.J.: Occurrence of a hydatidiform mole in twin pregnancy: case report. Am. J. Obstet. Gynecol. 73:911–913, 1957.

Loke, Y.W.: Sex chromatin of hydatidiform moles. J. Med. Genet. 6:22–25, 1969.

Looi, L.M., and Sivanesaratnam, V.: Malignant evolution with fatal outcome in a patient with partial hydatidiform mole. Aust. N.Z. J. Obstet. Gynaecol. 21:51–52, 1981.

Lurain, J.R., Brewer, J.I., Torok, E.E., and Halpern, B.: Natural history of hydatidiform mole after primary evacuation. Am. J. Obstet. Gynecol. 145:591–595, 1983.

MacDonald, P.C., and Siiteri, P.K.: The in vivo mechanisms of origin of estrogen in subjects with trophoblastic tumors. Steroids 8:589–603, 1966.

Makino, S., Sasaki, M.S., and Fukuschima, T.: Preliminary notes on the chromosomes of human chorionic lesions. Proc. Jpn. Acad. 39:54–58, 1963.

Makino, S., Sasaki, M.S., and Fukuschima, T.: Triploid chromosome constitution in human chorionic lesions. Lancet 2:1273–1275, 1964.

Makino, S., Sasaki, M.S., and Fukuschima, T.: Cytologic studies of tumors. XLI. Chromosomal instability in human chorionic lesions. Okajimas Fol. Anat. Jpn. 40:439–465, 1965.

Mark, L.K., and Moel, M.: Pulmonary metastasis from trophoblastic tumors. Radiology 76:601–605, 1961.

Marquez-Monter, H.: Deoxyribonucleic acid synthesis of hydatidiform moles in organ culture: an autoradiographic investigation. Nature 209:1037–1038, 1966.

Marquez-Monter, H., de la Vega, G.A., Robles, M., and Bolio-Cicero, A.: Epidemiology and pathology of hydatidiform mole in the general hospital in Mexico. Am. J. Obstet. Gynecol. 85:856–864, 1963.

Martin, D.A., Sutton, G.P., Ulbright, T.M., Sledge, G.W., Stehman, F.B., and Ehrlich, C.E.: DNA content as a prognostic index in gestational trophoblastic neoplasia. Gynecol. Oncol. 34:383–388, 1989.

Matalon, M., and Modan, B.: Epidemiologic aspects of hydatidiform mole in Israel. Am. J. Obstet. Gynecol. 112:107–112, 1972.

Mathieu, A.: Hydatidiform mole and chorio-epithelioma: collective review of the literature for the years 1935, 1936 and 1937. Surg. Gynecol. Obstet. 68:52–70, 181–198, 1939.

Maudsley, R.F., and Robertson, E.M.: Hydatidiform mole in a woman over 52 years old: report of a case. Obstet. Gynecol. 26:542–543, 1965.

Mazzanti, P., La Vecchia, C., Parazzini, F., and Bolis, G.: Frequency of hydatidiform mole in Lombardy, northern Italy. Gynecol. Oncol. 24:337–342, 1986.

McCorriston, C.C.: Racial incidence of hydatidiform mole. Am. J. Obstet. Gynecol. 101:377–382, 1968.

McFadden, D.E., Pantzer, J.T., and Langlois, S.: Parental origin of triploidy—digyny, not diandry [abstract 28]. Mod. Pathol. 7:5P, 1994.

McKay, D.G., Richardson, M.V., and Hertig, A.T.: Studies of the function of early human trophoblast. III. A study of the protein structure of mole fluid, chorionic and amniotic fluids by paper electrophoresis. Am. J. Obstet. Gynecol. 75:699–707, 1955a.

McKay, D.G., Roby, C.C., Hertig, A.T., and Richardson, M.V.: Studies of the function of early human trophoblast. I. Observations on the chemical composition of the fluid of hydatidiform moles. Am. J. Obstet. Gynecol. 69:722–734, 1955b.

Merkow, L.P., Acevedo, H.F., Gilmore, J., and Pardo, M.: Trophoblastic disease: a correlative ultrastructural and biochemical study. Obstet. Gynecol. 37:348–357, 1971.

Messerli, M.L., Parmley, T., Woodruff, J.D., Lilienfeld, A.M., Bevilacqua, L., and Rosenshein, N.B.: Inter- and intra-pathologist variability in the diagnosis of gestational trophoblastic neoplasia. Obstet. Gynecol. 69:622–626, 1987.

Meyer, J.S.: Benign pulmonary metastasis from hydatidiform mole: report of a case. Obstet. Gynecol. 28:826–829, 1966.

Minami, S., Yamoto, M., and Nakano R.: Immunohistochemical localization of inhibin-activin subunits in hydatidiform mole and invasive mole. Obstet. Gynecol. 82:414–418, 1993.

Montgomery, E.A., Roberts, E.F., Conran, R.M., and Hitchcock, C.L.: Triploid abortus presenting as an ectopic pregnancy. Arch. Pathol. Lab. Med. 117:652–653, 1993.

Mor-Joseph, S., Anteby, S.O., Granat, M., Brzezinsky, A., and Evron, S.: Recurrent molar pregnancies associated with clomiphene citrate and human gonadotropins. Am. J. Obstet. Gynecol. 151:1085–1086, 1985.

Morrish, D.W., Honoré, L.H., and Bhardwaj, D.: Partial hydatidiform moles have impaired differentiated function (human chorionic gonadotropin and human placental lactogen secretion) in response to epidermal growth factor and 8-bromo-cyclic adenosin monophosphate. Am. J. Obstet. Gynecol. 166:160–166, 1992.

Mutter, G.L., Pomponio, R.J., Berkowitz, R.S., and Genest, D.R.: Sex chromosome composition of complete hydatidiform moles: relationship to metastasis. Am. J. Obstet. Gynecol. 168:1547–1551, 1993.

Natoli, W.J., and Rashad, M.N.: Hawaiian moles. Am. J. Roentgenol. Radium Ther. Nucl. Med. 114:142–144, 1972.

Niebuhr, E.: Triploidy in man: cytogenetical and clinical aspects. Humangenetik 21:103–125, 1974.

Nishimura, H., Takano, K., Tanimura, T., and Yasuda, M.: Normal and abnormal development of human embryos: first report of an analysis of 1,213 intact embryos. Teratology 1:281–290, 1968.

Nisula, B.C., and Taliafouros, G.S.: Thyroid function in gestational trophoblastic neoplasia: evidence that the thyrotropic activity of chorionic gonadotropin mediates the thyrotoxicosis of choriocarcinoma. Am. J. Obstet. Gynecol. 138:77–85, 1980.

Nobunaga, T., Azuma, C., Kimura, T., Tokugawa, Y., Takemura, M., Kamiura, S., Saji, F., and Tanizawa, O.:

Differential diagnostic between complete mole and hydropic abortus by deoxyribonucleic acid fingerprint. Am. J. Obstet. Gynecol. 163:634–638, 1990.

Novak, E.: Pathological aspects of hydatidiform mole and choriocarcinoma. Am. J. Obstet. Gynecol. 59:1355–1372, 1950.

Novak, E., and Seah, C.S.: Benign trophoblastic lesions in the Mathieu Chorionepithelioma Registry (hydatidiform mole, syncytial endometritis). Am. J. Obstet. Gynecol. 68:376–390, 1954.

Novak, R., Agamanolis, D., Dasu, S., Igel, H., Platt, M., Robinson, H., and Shebata, B.: Utility of histologic analysis of 1st trimester abortions [abstract 36]. Mod. Pathol. 1:7p, 1988.

Ockleford, C., Barker, C., Griffiths, J., McTurk, G., Fisher, R., and Lawler, S.: Hydatidiform mole: an ultrastructural analysis of syncytiotrophoblast surface organization. Placenta 10:195–212, 1989.

Ohama, K., Kajii, T., Okamoto, E., Fukuda, Y., Imaizumi, K., Tsukahara, M., Kobayashi, K., and Hagiwara, K.: Dispermic origin of XY hydatidiform moles. Nature 292:551–552, 1981.

Ohama, K., Ueda, K., Okamoto, E., Takenaka, M., and Fujiwara, A.: Cytogenetic and clinicopathologic studies of partial moles. Obstet. Gynecol. 68:259–262, 1986.

Okudaira, Y., and Strauss, L.: Ultrastructure of molar trophoblast: observations on hydatidiform mole and choriocarcinoma destruens. Obstet. Gynecol. 30:172–187, 1967.

Orr, J.W., Austin, J.M., Hatch, K.D., Shingleton, H.M., Younger, J.B., and Boots, L.R.: Acute pulmonary edema associated with molar pregnancies: a high-risk factor for development of persistent trophoblastic disease. Am. J. Obstet. Gynecol. 136:412–415, 1980.

Osada, H., Kawata, M., Yamada, M., Okumura, K., and Takamizawa, H.: Genetic identification of pregnancies responsible for choriocarcinomas after multiple pregnancies by restriction fragment length polymorphism analysis. Am. J. Obstet. Gynecol. 165:682–688, 1991.

Ozturk, M., Berkowitz, R., Goldstein, D., Bellet, D., and Wands, J.R.: Differential production of human chorionic gonadotropin and free subunits in gestational trophoblastic disease. Am. J. Obstet. Gynecol. 158:193–198, 1988.

Parazzini, F., La Vecchia, C., Franceschi, S., and Mangili, G.: Familial trophoblastic disease: case report. Am. J. Obstet. Gynecol. 149:382–383, 1984.

Parazzini, F., La Vecchia, C., Pampallona, S., and Franceschi, S.: Reproductive patterns and the risk of gestational trophoblastic disease. Am. J. Obstet. Gynecol. 152:866–870, 1985.

Parazzini, F., Mangili, G., La Vecchia, C., Negri, E., Bocciolone, L., and Fasoli, M.: Risk factors for gestational trophoblastic disease: a separate analysis of complete and partial hydatidiform moles. Obstet. Gynecol. 78:1039–1045, 1991.

Park, W.W.: The occurrence of sex chromatin in chorionepitheliomas, and hydatidiform moles. J. Pathol. Bacteriol. 74:197–206, 1957.

Park, W.W.: Choriocarcinoma: a Study of Its Pathology. Davis, Philadelphia, 1971.

Patek, E., and Johnson, P.: Recurrent hydatidiform mole: report of a case with five recurrences. Acta Obstet. Gynecol. Scand. 57:381–383, 1978.

Pattillo, R.A., Sasaki, S., Katayama, K.P., Roesler, M., and Mattingly, R.F.: Genesis of 46,XY hydatidiform mole. Am. J. Obstet. Gynecol. 141:104–105, 1981.

Pettit, M.D.W.: Hydatidiform mole following tubal pregnancy. Am. J. Obstet. Gystet. Gynecol. 42:1057–1060, 1941.

Pool, C., Aplin, J.D., Taylor, G.M., and Boyd, R.D.H.: Trophoblast cells and maternal blood. Lancet 1:804–805, 1987.

Popek, E.J.: Complete hydatidiform mole with coexisting twin: 10 cases [abstract 39]. Mod. Pathol. 7:7P, 1994.

Reed, S., Coe, J.I., and Bergquist, J.: Invasive hydatidiform mole metastatic to the lung. Obstet. Gynecol. 13:749–753, 1959.

Rice, L.W., Lage, J.M., Berkowitz, R.S., Goldstein, D.P., and Bernstein, M.R.: Repetitive complete and partial hydatidiform mole. Obstet. Gynecol. 74:217–219, 1989.

Ring, A.M.: The concept of benign metastasizing hydatidiform moles. Am. J. Clin. Pathol. 58:111–117, 1972.

Ringertz, N.: Hydatidiform mole, invasive mole and choriocarcinoma in Sweden 1958–1965. Acta Obstet. Gynecol. Scand. 49:195–203, 1970.

Rolon, P.A., and de Lopez, B.H.: Epidemiological aspects of hydatidiform mole in the Republic of Paraguay (South America). Br. J. Obstet. Gynaecol. 84:862–864, 1977.

Rolon, P.A., Hochsztajn, B., and Llamosas, F.: Epidemiology of complete hydatidiform mole in Paraguay. J. Reprod. Med. 35:15–18, 1990.

Romero, R., Horgan, G., Kohorn, E.I., Kadar, N., Taylor, K.J.W., and Hobbins, J.C.: New criteria for the diagnosis of gestational trophoblastic disease. Obstet. Gynecol. 66:553–558, 1985.

Roper, H.H., Wolff, G., and Hitzeroth, H.W.: Preferential X-inactivation in human placenta membranes: is the paternal X-inactive in early embryonic development of female mammals? Hum. Genet. 43:265–273, 1978.

Rubin, N.W.: Chorioadenoma destruens—perforation, resection, and subsequent pregnancy. Am. J. Obstet. Gynecol. 89:536–538, 1964.

Saji, F., Tokugawa, Y., Kimura, T., Nobunaga, T., Azuma, C., and Tanizawa, O.: A new approach using DNA fingerprinting for the determination of androgenesis as a cause of hydatidiform mole. Placenta 10:399–405, 1989.

Sand, P.K., Lurain, J.R., and Brewer, J.I.: Repeat gestational trophoblastic disease. Obstet. Gynecol. 63:140–144, 1984.

Sand, P.K., Stubblefield, P.A., and Orvy, S.J.: Methotrexate inhibition of normal trophoblast in vitro. Am. J. Obstet. Gynecol. 155:324–329, 1986.

Sande, H.A., and Eyjolfsson, O.: Case report: hydatidiform mole with a coexisting fetus. Acta Obstet. Gynecol. Scand. 64:353–355, 1985.

Sarkar, S., Kacinski, B.M., Kohorn, E.I., Merino, M.J., Carter, D., and Blakemore, K.J.: Demonstration of myc and ras oncogene expression by hybridization in situ in hydatidiform mole and in the BeWo choriocarcinoma cell line. Am. J. Obstet. Gynecol. 154:390–393, 1986.

Sarno, A.P., Moorman, A.J., and Kalousek, D.K.: Partial molar pregnancy with fetal survival: an unusual example of confined placental mosaicism. Obstet. Gynecol. 82:716–719, 1993.

Sasagawa, M., Yamazaki, T., Sudo, Y., Kanazawa, K., and Takeuchi S.: Immunohistochemical localization of hCGα, hCGβ CTP, hPL and SP1 on villous and extravillous trophoblasts in normal human pregnancy. Acta Obstet. Gynaecol. Jpn. 39:1073–1079, 1987.

Sasaki, M., Fukushima, T., and Makino, S.: Some aspects of the chromosome constitution of hydatidiform moles and normal chorionic villi. Gann 53:101–106, 1962.

Sasaki, M., Makino, S., Muramoto, J.-I., Ikeuchi, T., and Shimba, H.: A chromosome survey of induced abortuses in a Japanese population. Chromosoma 20:267–283, 1967.

Sauter, H.: Uteroplazentare Apoplexie bei Blasenmole. Gynaecologia 159:296–300, 1965.

Schlaerth, J.B., Morrow, C.P., Montz, F.J., and d'Ablaing, G.: Initial management of hydatidiform mole. Am. J. Obstet. Gynecol. 158:1299–1306, 1988.

Schlegel, R.J., Neu, R.L., Leao, J.C., Farias, E., Aspillaga, M.J., and Gardner, L.I.: Observations on the chromosomal, cytological and anatomical characteristics of 75 conceptuses: including euploid, triploid XXX, triploid XYY and mosaic triploid XXY/diploid XY cases. Cytogenetics 5:430–446, 1966.

Schmickel, R.D., Silverman, E.M., Floyd, A.D., Payne, F.E., Pooley, J.M., and Beck, M.L.: A live-born infant with 69 chromosomes. J. Pediatr. 79:97–103, 1971.

Schmorl, G.: Über das Schicksal embolisch verschleppter Plazentarzellen. Verh. Dtsch. Pathol. Ges. 8:39–46, 1905.

Schneider, C.I., and Waxman, B.: Clomid therapy and subsequent hydatidiform mole formation: a case report. Obstet. Gynecol. 39:787–788, 1972.

Sciarra, N.: Human chorionic gonadotrophin in hydatidiform moles. J. Obstet. Gynaecol. Br. Commonw. 77:420–423, 1970.

Scott, J.S.: Pregnancy toxaemia associated with hydrops foetalis, hydatidiform mole and hydramnios. J. Obstet. Gynaecol. Br. Emp. 65:689–701, 1958.

Sherer, D.M., Glantz, J.C., Metlay, L.A., and Saller, D.N.: Absent umbilical artery diastolic flow in a fetus with a partial mole at 18 weeks' gestation. Am. J. Obstet. Gynecol. 169:1167–1168, 1993.

Shorofsky, M.: A karyometric comparison of the normal human chorion with that of the hydatidiform mole. Acta Anat. (Basel) 41:45–56, 1960.

Sicuranza, B.J., and Tisdall, L.H.: Hydatidiform mole and eclampsia with coexistent living fetus in the second trimester of pregnancy. Am. J. Obstet. Gynecol. 126:513–514, 1976.

Slattery, M.A., Khong, T.Y., Dawkins, R.R., Pridmore, B.R., and Hague, W.M.: Eclampsia in association with partial molar pregnancy and congenital abnormalities. Am. J. Obstet. Gynecol. 169:1625–1627, 1993.

Smalbraak, J.: Trophoblastic Growths. A Clinical, Hormonal and Histopathological Study of Hydatidiform Mole and Chorionepithelioma. Elsevier, Amsterdam, 1957.

Smith, E.B., Szulman, A.E., Hinshaw, W., Tyrey, L., Surti, U., and Hammond, C.B.: Human chorionic gonadotropin levels in complete and partial hydatidiform moles and in nonmolar abortuses. Am. J. Obstet. Gynecol. 149:129–132, 1984.

Song, H.-Z., Wu, P.-C., Wang, Y.-E., Yang, X.-Y., and Dong, S.-Y.: Pregnancy outcomes after successful chemotherapy for choriocarcinoma and invasive mole: long-term follow-up. Am. J. Obstet. Gynecol. 158:538–545, 1988.

Spademan, L.C., and Tuttle, W.M.: Chorioadenoma destruens. Am. J. Obstet. Gynecol. 88:549–550, 1964.

Stanhope, C.R., Stuart, G.C.E., and Curtis, K.L.: Primary ovarian hydatidiform mole: review of the literature and report of a case. Am. J. Obstet. Gynecol. 145:886–888, 1983.

Steller, M.A., Genest, D.R., Bernstein, M.R., Lage, J.M., Goldstein, D.P., and Berkowitz, R.S.: Natural history of twin pregnancy with complete hydatidiform mole and coexisting fetus. Obstet. Gynecol. 83:35–42, 1994.

Stroup, P.E.: A study of thirty-eight cases of hydatidiform mole at the Pennsylvania hospital. Am. J. Obstet. Gynecol. 72:294–303, 1956.

Sunderland, C.A., Redman, C.W.G., and Stirrat, G.M.: Characterization and localization of HLA antigens on hydatidiform mole. Am. J. Obstet. Gynecol. 151:130–135, 1985.

Surani, M.A.H., and Barton, S.C.: Development of gynogenetic eggs in the mouse: implications for parthenogenetic embryos. Science 222:1034–1036, 1983.

Surti, U., Szulman, A.E., and O'Brien, S.: Complete (classic) hydatidiform mole with 46,XY karyotype of paternal origin. Hum. Genet. 51:153–155, 1979.

Surti, U., Szulman, A.E., and O'Brien, S.: Dispermic origin and clinical outcome of three complete hydatidiform moles with 46,XY karyotype. Am. J. Obstet. Gynecol. 144:84–87, 1982.

Suzuki, M., Matsunobu, A., Wakita, K., Nishijima, M., and Osanai, K.: Hydatidiform mole with a surviving coexisting fetus. Obstet. Gynecol. 56:384–386, 1980.

Sze, E.H.M., Adelson, M.D., Baggish, M.S., and Contente, N.: Combined tubal and molar pregnancy: case report. Am. J. Obstet. Gynecol. 159:1217–1219, 1988.

Szulman, A.E., and Buchsbaum, H.J., eds.: Gestational Trophoblastic Disease. Springer-Verlag, New York, 1987.

Szulman, A.E., and Surti, U.: The syndromes of hydatidiform mole. I. Cytogenetic and morphologic correlations. Am. J. Obstet. Gynecol. 131:665–671, 1978a.

Szulman, A.E., and Surti, U.: The syndromes of hydatidiform mole. II. Morphologic evolution of the complete and partial mole. Am. J. Obstet. Gynecol. 132:20–27, 1978b.

Szulman, A.E., and Surti, U.: The clinicopathologic profile of the partial hydatidiform mole. Obstet. Gynecol. 59:597–602, 1982.

Szulman, A.E., and Surti, U.: Strict clinicopathologic criteria in the diagnosis of partial hydatidiform mole: a plea renewed. Am. J. Obstet. Gynecol. 152:1107–1108, 1985.

Szulman, A.E., Ma, H.-K., Wong, L.C., and Hsu, C.: Residual trophoblastic disease in association with partial hydatidiform mole. Obstet. Gynecol. 57:392–394, 1981.

Takagi, N., and Sasaki, M.: Preferential inactivation of the paternally derived X chromosome in the extraembryonic membranes of the mouse. Nature 256:640–652, 1975.

Takagi, N., Asano, S.-I., Fujisawa, M., and Ichinoe, K.: A possible triploid/diploid case of hydatidiform mole. Chromos. Inform. Serv. 10:21–22, 1969.

Takahashi, H., Kanazawa, K., Ikarashi, T., Sudo, N., and Tanaka, K.: Discrepancy in the diagnoses of hydatidiform mole by macroscopic and microscopic findings and the deoxyribonucleic acid fingerprint method. Am. J. Obstet. Gynecol. 163:112–113, 1990.

Tanimura, A., Natsuyama, H., Kawano, M., Tanimura, Y., Tanaka, T., and Kitazono, M.: Primary choriocarcinoma of the lung. Hum. Pathol. 16:1281–1284, 1985.

Teng, N.N.H., and Ballon, S.C.: Partial hydatidiform mole with diploid karyotype: report of three cases. Am. J. Obstet. Gynecol. 150:961–964, 1984.

Teoh, E.S., Dawood, M.Y., and Ratnam, S.S.: Epidemiology of hydatidiform mole in Singapore. Am. J. Obstet. Gynecol. 110:415–420, 1971.

Thatcher, S.S., Grainger, D.A., True, L.D., and de Cherney, A.H.: Pelvic trophoblastic implants after laparoscopic removal of a tubal pregnancy. Obstet. Gynecol. 74:514–515, 1989.

Thiele, R.A., and de Alvarez, R.R.: Metastasizing benign trophoblastic tumors. Am. J. Obstet. Gynecol. 84:1395–1406, 1962.

Tobin, S.M.: A further aid in the diagnosis of hydatidiform mole—the serum glutamic oxalacetic transaminase. Am. J. Obstet. Gynecol. 87:213–217, 1963.

Tominaga, T., and Page, E.W.: Sex chromatin of trophoblastic tumors. Am. J. Obstet. Gynecol. 96:305–309, 1966.

Tomoda, Y., Kaseki, S., Goto, S., Nishi, H., Hara, T., and Naruki, M.: Rh-D factor in trophoblastic tumors: a possible cause of the high incidence in Asia. Am. J. Obstet. Gynecol. 139:742–743, 1981.

Tsuji, K., Yagi, S., and Nakano, R.: Increased risk of malignant transformation of hydatidiform moles in older gravidas: a cytogenetic study. Obstet. Gynecol. 58:351–355, 1981.

Tsukahara, M., and Kajii, T.: Replication of X chromosomes in complete moles. Hum. Genet. 71:7–10, 1985.

Uchida, I.A., and Freeman, V.C.: Triploidy and chromosomes. Am. J. Obstet. Gynecol. 151:65–69, 1985.

Uher, J., Jirasek, J.E., and Sima, A.: Histochemische Studie von Blasenmole und Plazenta eines fünf Monate alten Fetus. Zentralbl. Gynäkol. 85:477–482, 1963.

Vassilakos, P., and Kajii, T.: Hydatidiform mole: two entities. Lancet 1:259, 1976. See Stone, M., and Bagshawe, K.D.: Lancet 1:535–536, 1976.

Vassilakos, P., Riotton, G., and Kajii, T.: Hydatidiform mole: two entities: a morphologic and cytogenetic study with some clinical considerations. Am. J. Obstet. Gynecol. 127:167–170, 1977.

Vejerslev, L.O., Dueholm, M., and Nielsen, F.H.: Hydatidiform mole: cytogenetic marker analysis in twin gestation. Am. J. Obstet. Gynecol. 155:614–617, 1986.

Vejerslev, L.O., Dissing, J., Hansen, H.E., and Poulsen, H.: Hydatidiform mole: genetic markers in diploid abortuses with macroscopic villous enlargement. Cancer Genet. Cytogenet. 26:143–155, 1987a.

Vejerslev, L.O., Dissing, J., Hansen, H.E., and Poulsen, H.: Hydatidiform mole: genetic origin in polyploid conceptuses. Hum. Genet. 76:11–19, 1987b.

Vejerslev, L.O., Fisher, R.A., Surti, U., and Wake, N.: Hydatidiform mole: cytogenetically unusual cases and their implications for the present classification. Am. J. Obstet. Gynecol. 157:180–184, 1987c.

Vejerslev, L.O., Fisher, R.A., Surti, U., and Wake, N.: Hydatidiform mole: parental chromosome aberrations in partial and complete moles. J. Med. Genet. 24:613–615, 1987d.

Vejerslev, L.O., Sunde, L., Hansen, B.F., Larsen, J.K., Christensen, I.J., and Larsen, G.: Hydatidiform mole and fetus with normal karyotype: support of a separate entity. Obstet. Gynecol. 77:868–874, 1991.

Wake, N., Shiina, Y., and Ichinoe, K.: A further cytogenetic study of hydatidiform mole, with reference to its androgenetic origin. Proc. Jpn. Acad. 54:533–537, 1978a.

Wake, N., Takagi, N., and Sasaki, M.: Androgenesis as a cause of hydatidiform mole. J. Natl. Cancer Inst. 60:51–57, 1978b.

Wake, N., Tanaka, K., Chapman, V., Matsui, S., and Sandberg, A.A.: Chromosomes and cellular origin of choriocarcinoma. Cancer Res. 41:3137–3143, 1981.

Westerhout, F.C.: Ruptured tubal hydatidiform mole: report of a case. Obstet. Gynecol. 23:138–139, 1964.

Woodward, R.M., Filly, R.A., and Callen, P.W.: First trimester molar pregnancy: nonspecific ultrasonographic appearance. Obstet. Gynecol. 55:31S–33S, 1980.

Wu, F.Y.W.: Recurrent hydatidiform mole: a case report of nine consecutive molar pregnancies. Obstet. Gynecol. 41:200–204, 1973.

Wynn, R.M., and Davies, J.: Ultrastructure of hydatidiform mole: correlative electron microscopic and functional aspects. Am. J. Obstet. Gynecol. 90:293–307, 1964.

Wynn, R.M., and Harris, J.A.: Ultrastructure of trophoblast and endometrium in invasive hydatidiform mole (chorioadenoma destruens). Am. J. Obstet. Gynecol. 99:1125–1135, 1967.

Yamashita, L., Wake, N., Araki, T., Ichinoe, K., and Makoto, K.: Human lymphocyte antigen expression in hydatidiform mole: androgenesis following fertilization by a haploid sperm. Am. J. Obstet. Gynecol. 135:597–600, 1979.

Yedema, K.A., Verheijen, R.H., Kenemans, P., Schijf, C.P., Borm, G.F., Segers, M.F., and Thomas, C.M.: Identification of patients with persistent trophoblastic disease by means of a normal human chorionic gonadotropin regression curve. Am. J. Obstet. Gynecol. 168:787–792, 1993.

Yee, B., Tu, B., and Platt, L.D.: Coexisting hydatidiform mole with a live fetus presenting as a placenta previa on ultrasound. Am. J. Obstet. Gynecol. 144:726–728, 1982.

Yenen, E., Inanc, F.A., and Babuna, C.: Primary ovarian hydatidiform mole: report of a case. Obstet. Gynecol. 26:721–724, 1965.

Yorde, D.E., Hussa, R.O., Garancis, J.C., and Pattillo, R.A.: Immunocytochemical localization of human choriogonadotropin in human malignant trophoblast: model for human choriogonadotropin secretion. Lab. Invest. 40: 391–398, 1979.

Yoshimatsu, N., Hoshi, K., Sato, A., Munakata, S., and Fukushima, T.: The significance of alpha-fetoprotein-negativity in the interstitial area of total hydatidiform mole

tissue. Nippon Sanka Fujinka Gakkai Zasshi 39:918–924, 1987 (Japanese).

Yuen, B.H.: Relationship of prolactin and estradiol to human chorionic gonadotropin following molar gestation. Am. J. Obstet. Gynecol. 145:618–620, 1983.

23
Choriocarcinoma

Choriocarcinoma is a malignant neoplasm composed exclusively of cytotrophoblast and syncytiotrophoblast. If villi are associated with such invasive tumors, the lesion is referred to as invasive mole or chorioadenoma destruens (see Chapter 22). In this discussion, only the choriocarcinoma of gestational trophoblastic neoplasia is covered. The nature of this tumor was first correctly identified by Marchand (1895). Teacher's detailed observations (1903) followed Marchand's description. The early history of this tumor, the deciduoma as it was first known, has been admirably recounted by Ober and Fass (1961). Until the neoplastic elements of choriocarcinoma were ultimately shown to be derived from the embryonic cells, not the maternal cells, their derivation had been in dispute. Ewing (1910) was the first investigator to differentiate between the various types of trophoblastic neoplasm. He introduced or used the terms invasive mole, syncytial endometritis, and syncytioma. Some of these terms are still in usage even though some should now be replaced as greater knowledge of their biology has been accumulating.

In the United States, gestation-related choriocarcinoma is said to occur with a frequency of about 1 per 40,000 pregnancies (Hertig & Mansell, 1956). In their oft-depicted diagram (Figure 503), Hertig and Mansell estimated that the lesion was preceded by a complete hydatidiform mole (CHM) in 50%, an abortion in 25%, a normal pregnancy in 22.5%, and an ectopic pregnancy in 2.5%. There is wide geographic variation in its incidence and in that of its precursors. In a study of choriocarcinoma from Japan, five of eight choriocarcinomas followed complete moles, one followed a term pregnancy (the only patient who died), and two followed abortions (Fukunaga & Ushigome, 1993a). All were diploid by flow cytometry.

The tumor consists of solid sheets of cytotrophoblast and syncytium. This tumor has a propensity of vascular invasion (Figure 504), and consequently many choriocarcinomas are hemorrhagic and friable (Figures 505, 506). So much blood may be present in some choriocarcinoma metastases that one may have to search for the tumor cells (Figure 507). Characteristically, broad sheets of cytotrophoblast form the central portion of the tumor, the periphery being syncytium. Nuclear pleomorphism is common, but mitoses are confined to the cytotrophoblast. Wolf and Michalopoulos (1992) studied the distribution of nuclear antigen in normal placentas and trophoblastic tumors. Its presence correlates with mitotic, reproductive activity, and in placentas it is confined to the cytotrophoblast, where it is strongly expressed. The same was true in CHM and choriocarcinomas; the cytotrophoblast and intermediate trophoblast (X cells) stained, but not the syncytium. Several studies have shown that many intermediate trophoblastic cells are present in choriocarcinoma. Those cells are truly intermediate between cytotrophoblast and syncytium. They are especially readily identified by electron microscopy (Pierce & Midgley, 1963; Wynn & Davies, 1964) (Figure 508). It is surprising that X cells, the other major line of trophoblastic elements, have only recently been identified with certainty in choriocarcinoma-like lesions; they are also not a striking feature of hydatidiform moles. These cells may be the principal cell types of the placental site tumor, discussed below. Because of its dilated cytoplasmic cisternae, the syncytium of choriocarcinomas is frequently vacuolated. This vacuolation may obscure the true nature of the cells. Much glycogen may be contained in this tissue (Arkwright et al., 1993).

It is usually difficult to assign a prognosis from the histological picture of a choriocarcinoma. Some choriocarcinomas (even metastatic lung lesions) have regressed spontaneously (see Bardawil & Toy, 1959; Rauter, 1968). Deligdisch and her co-workers (1978) suggested that solid tumor nests, with high pleomorphism and mitotic activity, have the worst prognosis. Fibrin deposits at the interface between tumor and host tissues are of good prognostic value. Another feature that

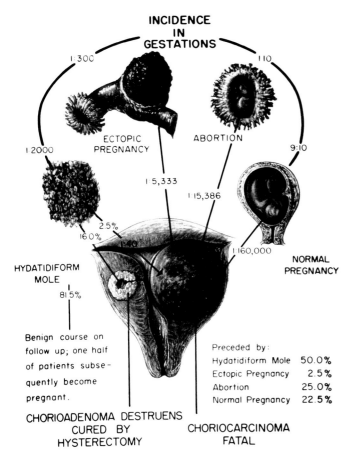

INCIDENCE IN GESTATIONS

FIGURE 503. Frequency of choriocarcinoma relative to its various precursors. (From Hertig and Mansell, 1956, with permission.)

bespeaks a better prognosis is a significant cellular "reaction" around the tumor (Elston, 1969).

Choriocarcinoma metastases occur most commonly in the lung and in the brain, but many other organs may be involved. The distribution of metastases was well recorded by Ober et al. (1971). That presentation also excelled in the description of the macroscopic lesions and in the microscopic appearance of choriocarcinoma. Vaginal secondaries and metastases to the cervix occur relatively frequently (Marquez-Monter & Velasco, 1967; Martin et al., 1983). Acosta-Sison (1958), who studied primary metastases in 32 patients, found the lung to be involved in 44% and the vagina in 31%. Eventually, the lungs were the site of metastases in 94% and the vagina in 44%; other organs were much less often involved. A relatively uncommon site is the kidney, although isolated cases have been reported (Jarrett & Pratt-Thomas, 1984; Soper et al., 1988). Some patients have been successfully treated, despite large tumor burdens. The patient whose third hydatidiform mole (Figure 483) proved fatal had extensive metastases in the liver but died from an exsanguinating hemorrhage that originated in an intestinal lesion. This location is otherwise a relatively uncommon site of metastasis.

Pulmonary dissemination of molar tissue occurs often, but such vascular tumor deportation may lie dormant for many years. Figures 509 to 511 illustrate the lung of a patient who died from pulmonary hypertension 4 years after delivery of a hydatidiform mole. Her pulmonary arteries had thrombi and numerous masses of pure trophoblast. Neoplastic tissue was present in many vessels, but it did not completely traverse the vascular wall. There was an intense chronic inflammatory reaction at these sites, simulating a barrier to invasion (Figure 512). Similar cases have been described by Seckl et al. (1991), but they were successfully treated. The hypertensive effects of tumor embolization to the lung in general have been discussed in detail by Veinot and colleagues (1992), who believe these effects to be an important and often unrecognized problem.

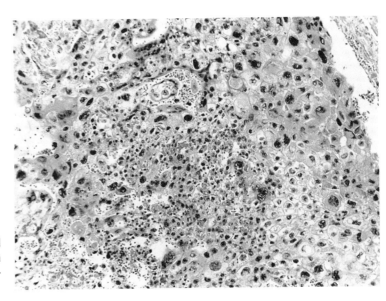

FIGURE 504. Choriocarcinoma of the uterus. Solid sheets of neoplastic cytotrophoblast with much nuclear pleomorphism and syncytium are intermixed with blood. H&E. ×160.

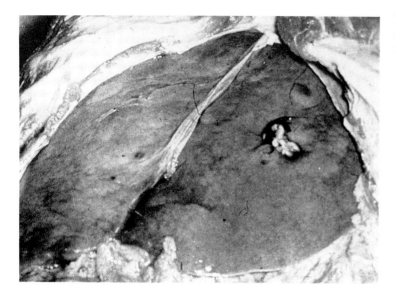

FIGURE 505. Liver metastases of choriocarcinoma after a third hydatidiform mole. There was no tumor in the uterus.

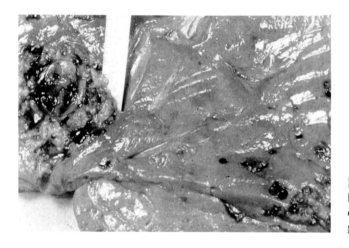

FIGURE 506. Same patient as in Figure 505. Numerous friable, hemorrhagic tumor nodules have caused massive enlargement of the liver. The ruler is placed underneath a large tumor growth within a hepatic vein.

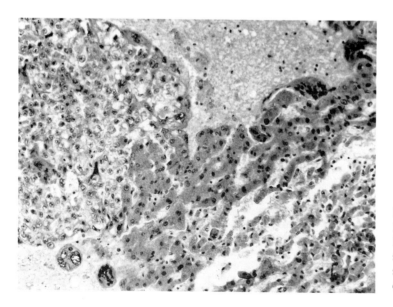

FIGURE 507. Same patient as Figures 505 and 506. Metastatic choriocarcinoma is in the liver following hydatidiform mole. Cords of disrupted liver cells are seen at right; a large tumor mass is at left and consists primarily of cytotrophoblast, with some syncytial surface. H&E. ×160.

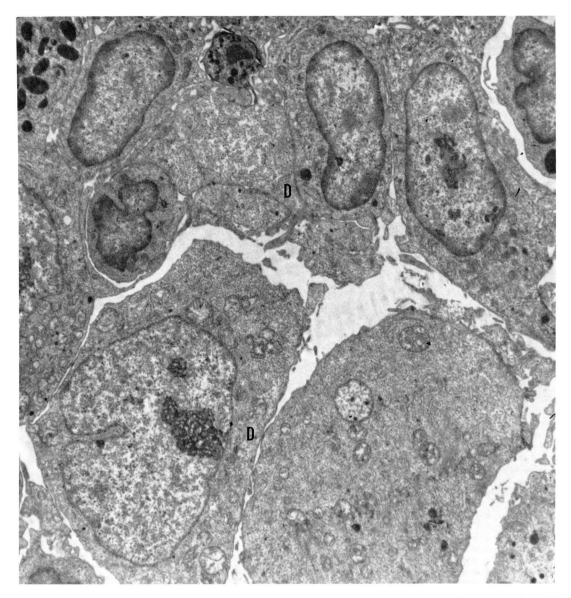

FIGURE 508. Electron micrograph of two types of cytotrophoblast. At top are uniform oval nuclei and abundant ribosomes but few other cytoplasmic constituents. Below are two large cells with irregular nuclei and many more mitochondria. Desmosomes (D) are seen in both of these cells. (From Wynn and Davies, 1964, with permission.)

This cellular response to trophoblastic tumors has been studied in some detail by Elston (1969). He found variable degrees of lymphocytic, histiocytic, and plasmacellular reactions in response to invading tumor cells and correlated it with outcome. Patients with tumors who had the most intense reaction fared best with chemotherapeutic treatment. Elston also saw in the maternal cellular response an attempt of the host to "reject" the neoplasm. This pulmonary complication of latent vascular tumor growth is apparently not uncommon. Fahrner et al. (1959) described a patient who died with cor pulmonale and end-arterial tumor growth 5 years after delivery of a mole. Spiegel (1964) described a similar case and reviewed 10 others from the literature. Excellent preservation of neoplastic tissue resulted from the ability of the neoplasm to grow within blood. Other cases came from Dyke and Fink (1967); and Bagshawe and Nobel (1966) described the various types of pulmonary metastasis in some detail. They paid special attention to the radiological and cardiac aspects. The latter authors and Evans and Hendrickse (1965) accumulated large series of cases with intraarterial pulmonary tumor spread; many were associated with acute pulmonary hypertension and cor pulmonale.

Diagnostic curettage for moles may be the mechanism of dissemination of malignant trophoblast with villous

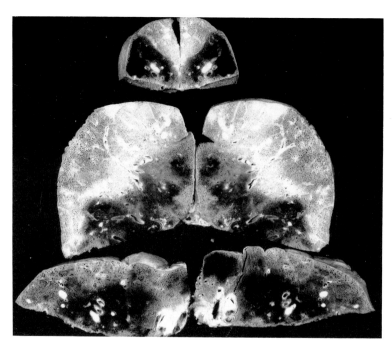

FIGURE 509. Lung sections from a patient with pulmonary hypertension and infarction 4 years after hydatidiform mole. Throughout this lung the arteries were obstructed by choriocarcinoma and thrombi. (Courtesy Dr. A.T. Hertig. Patient was discussed by Bardawil and Toy, 1959.)

tissue. Indeed, villi are occasionally present in such lesions. Bagshawe (1964) pointed out that the presence of villi in trophoblastic lesions "cannot be taken as a guarantee that it will remain benign indefinitely." We strongly agree with this statement but recognize the difficulty experienced by the practicing pathologist. Often an absolute diagnosis of chorionic malignancy cannot be made from curettings alone, especially when villi are present. Optimal care requires follow-up with gonadotropin levels. Carlson and his colleagues (1984) described a patient who developed fatal pulmonary lesions immediately after normal pregnancy, despite chemotherapy. Bagshawe (1988) is incorrect, however, to state that the pulmonary lesions occur only in London, and that they have not been recognized during life. They are rarely considered, to be sure, unless preceded by a recent CHM.

Choriocarcinoma most commonly follows CHM and invasive moles. Hertig and Mansell (1956) estimated that only 18.5% of CHMs terminate with choriocarcinoma. Most patients pursue a benign course, once the uterus has been evacuated. As Figure 503 shows,

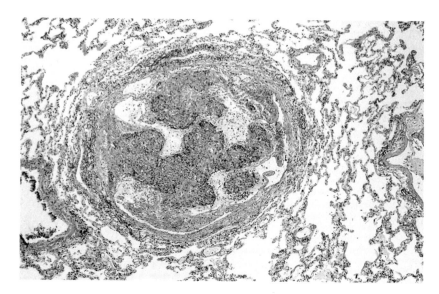

FIGURE 510. Same patient as in Figure 509. Pulmonary artery is filled with solid choriocarcinoma metastasis. There is an inflammatory reaction in the vascular wall at the point of invasion. H&E. ×40.

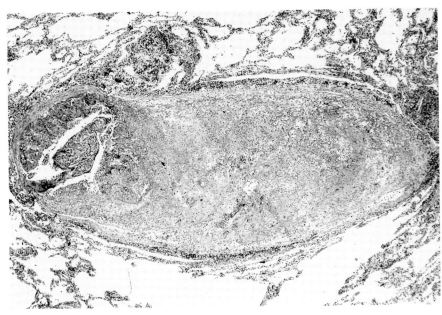

FIGURE 511. Same patient as in Figures 509 and 510. A small amount of viable tumor is present at left, and the remainder of the artery is filled with thrombus. H&E. ×40.

choriocarcinoma may also follow normal gestations. The neoplasm has been found within otherwise normal placentas and is then designated choriocarcinoma in situ. Other origins include gonadal teratomas and, rarely, teratomas at other sites. It is unusual for choriocarcinoma to arise without a known antecedent neoplasm. Suzuki et al. (1993) were able to determine the origin of their choriocarcinomas using DNA analysis. Two cases followed complete hydatidiform moles and had androgenetic profiles, and another had parental DNA and followed a term pregnancy. They concluded from nine cases that polymerase chain reaction (PCR) study of the DNA of these tumors allows determination of the androgenetic origin.

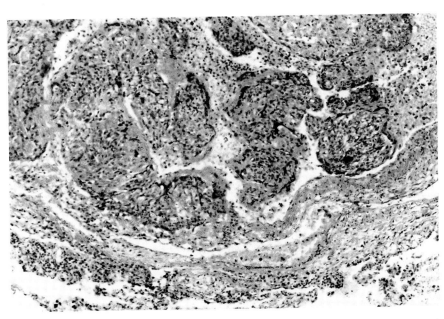

FIGURE 512. Same patient as Figures 509 to 511. Choriocarcinoma fills the artery and is enmeshed in thrombus. At points of invasion there is much chronic inflammation, including many plasma cells. No villous stroma is produced. H&E. ×100.

Choriocarcinoma has no villi, in contrast to chorio-adenoma destruens, in which villi are present. This arbitrary designation of the two lesions does not signify their biological behavior, as chorioadenoma destruens may be significantly invasive and destructive (Figure 513). Indeed, behaviorally the two lesions are essentially identical. Choriocarcinomas have also been reported in some experimental animals, but their commonest antecedent, the hydatidiform mole, has not been observed in nonhuman pregnancies. It is unknown if these animal tumors have the same unusual genetic background as some of the human gestational choriocarcinomas. There are several large reviews that discuss the major aspects of choriocarcinoma, including its historical perspectives, diagnosis, and treatment (Bagshawe, 1969; Ober et al., 1971; Park, 1971; Goldstein & Berkowitz, 1982; Silverberg & Kurman, 1992).

Choriocarcinoma In Situ and Choriocarcinoma with Pregnancy

Driscoll (1963) described an "incidental choriocarcinoma" in the mature, circumvallate placenta of a normal pregnancy (Figures 514, 515). The mother and child did well. A small "infarct"-like lesion was sampled for histology and found to be a typical choriocarcinoma. The tumor invaded adjacent villi but not their vessels. Brewer and Gerbie (1966) described two cases of choriocarcinoma developing within otherwise normal placentas. These authors paid special attention to the earliest formation of this proliferative lesion and described the degenerative changes that occur within it. The degenerative process, they thought, may lead to detachment and deportation of tumor fragments. We have seen two similar cases, one of which was the cause of massive transplacental fetal hemorrhage, hydrops, and fetal death (Santamaria et al., 1987) (Figure 516). Fox and Laurini (1988) found two additional cases of placental choriocarcinoma. In one the fetus was stillborn, but the other did well. The placental lesion had the macroscopic appearance of an infarct. It may be argued, of course, that these histologically identified lesions are not "malignant"; rather, in the sense used by Huber (1969), they represent benign lesions, which he described as "chorionepitheliosis interna." It may be so, except that not all such cases eventuate without causing metastases. The concept of carcinoma in situ is variably interpreted, and more must be learned from future biological studies of early lesions. The important case described by Heifetz and Czaja (1992) emphasizes this point. In their 69,XXX triploid partial hydatidiform mole (PHM) with fetus a small nodule of truly malignant-appearing trophoblastic growth was found. Despite

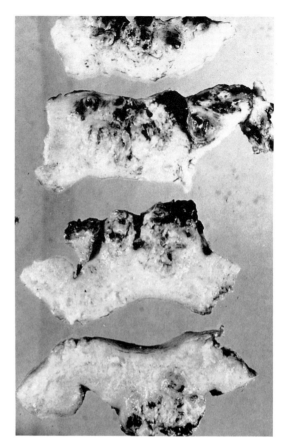

FIGURE 513. Invasive mole (chorioadenoma destruens). Slices of uterus show the invasive, hemorrhagic mass of tissue. It is composed mostly of solid trophoblast with a few villous remnants.

this finding the woman pursued a normal postpartum course; the report summarizes the 10 or so choriocarcinomas in situ reported to date. Additional cases with fetomaternal hemorrhage or rise in α-fetoprotein (AFP) levels and benign subsequent course were presented by Duleba et al. (1992) and Ollendorff et al. (1990). Duleba et al., as did several others, treated their patient "expectantly" and showed in photographs that the lesion appeared grossly as an infarct. Ollendorff's patient, with elevated maternal sersum AFP and a placental choriocarcinoma, had rising human chorionic gonadotropin (hCG) titers and developed a pulmonary nodule. The discussion following their paper (Hustin & Jauniaux, 1991) proves that the lesion differed from their "chorioangiocarcinoma."

Schopper and Pliess (1949) used the term chorionepitheliosis for borderline cases in a lengthy discussion of trophoblastic properties. They were especially concerned with spontaneous cures of alleged choriocarcinomas and with ectopic chorionepitheliomatous growths. They described a woman with a vulvar trophoblastic tumor that developed during normal pregnancy.

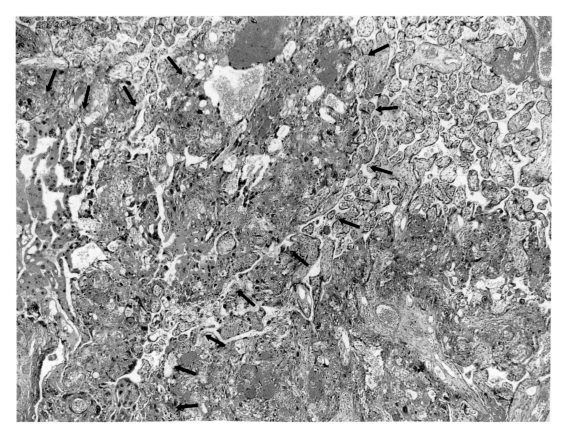

FIGURE 514. Mature placenta with choriocarcinoma in situ (arrows). This lesion was accidentally discovered and thought to be an infarct macroscopically. The patient did well. H&E. × 76. (Reprinted with permission from The American College of Obstetricians and Gynecologists (Obstetrics and Gynecology Driscoll 1963, 21:96–101).)

Benson et al. (1962) described massive fetomaternal hemorrhage in a patient who subsequently developed uterine choriocarcinoma with pulmonary metastases. Blackburn (1976) and Feldman (1977) reported similar cases. Disseminated maternal lesions were found in four additional patients with small placental choriocarcinomas reported by Brewer and Mazur (1981). The infants did not have tumors, but three were stillborn.

Hertig and Mansell (1956) indicated that choriocarcinoma follows normal pregnancies in a 1 per 160,000 incidence. It is thus not surprising that choriocarcinoma should also be found occasionally coincident with pregnancy and abortions (Figure 503). Relevant cases are those by Heller and Householder (1952), Driscoll (1983), Miller et al. (1979), and Olive et al. (1984). It is apparent from reviewing these reports that the choriocarcinoma that follows normal term pregnancy has a much poorer prognosis than that following CHM. Patients with this complication of pregnancy also have often much earlier metastatic disease (Hutchison et al., 1968; Greene & McCue, 1978; Miller et al., 1979). In occasional cases of neonates with tumors the placental choriocarcinoma was not detected or the placenta had not been examined. It was the case with cerebral choriocarcinoma metastases that caused death in a 1-month-old infant described by Chandra et al. (1990). The mother had no untoward sequelae and delivered another child with normal placenta.

There are many reports of choriocarcinoma that occurs simultaneously in mother and infant or fetus. Buckell and Owen (1954) described the death of a 7-week-old infant from chorionepitheliomatous metastases; the mother needed a hysterectomy because she suffered postpartum choriocarcinoma. The authors referred to a similar case described by Emery in 1952. Mercer et al. (1958) found a fatal choriocarcinoma in a 3-month-old infant whose mother died from disseminated disease. Another case, fatal for mother and infant, was reported by Daamen and Bloem (1961). Witzleben and Bruninga (1968), who reported a case, thought that these findings constituted a specific syndrome. In their case the mother had no obvious disease initially but later died from disseminated choriocarcinoma. Metastatic choriocarcinoma was the cause of fetal death in the report from Kruseman et al. (1977). The hydropic fetus had bled transplacentally. The mother developed metastatic disease and was successfully treated.

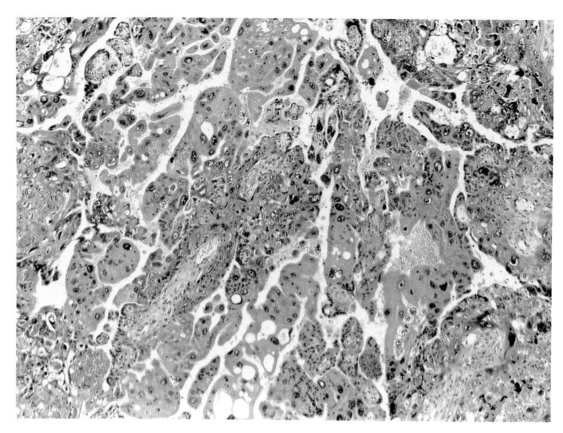

FIGURE 515. Same case as in Figure 514, but a higher power view of the tumorous elements. Note the obvious pleomorphism of tumor cells that surround the central villus. There is more syncytium than is usually present in choriocarcinoma. The dilated cisternae of the syncytium are obvious (bottom center). H&E. ×200. (Reprinted with permission from The American College of Obstetricians and Gynecologists (Obstetrics and Gynecology, Driscoll 1963, 21:96–101).)

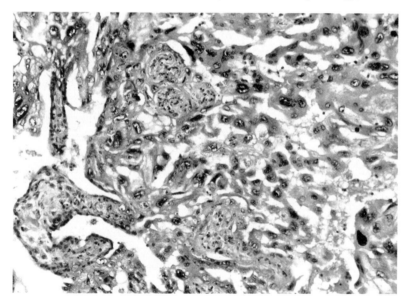

FIGURE 516. Choriocarcinoma in situ in an otherwise normal placenta. Solid nests of partially anaplastic tumor cells surround degenerating villi; note also the invaded villi (arrow). Fetus was hydropic and stillborn due to transplacental hemorrhage. H&E. ×125. (From Santamaria et al., 1987, with permission.)

Trophoblastic Pseudotumors

Kurman et al. (1976) introduced the term trophoblastic pseudotumor to designate an invasive trophoblastic lesions they saw in 12 patients but that behaved in a benign manner. The lesion tended to occur in young women, usually after pregnancy or abortion. The authors considered this entity to be "an exaggerated form of syncytial endometritis." This ancient term reflects the presence of many trophoblastic giant cells in the floor of the placenta, exaggerated in molar implantations. It has no relation to any inflammatory or infectious lesion and should be abandoned. In general, it is often impossible to distinguish this "lesion" from normal placental sites. It has usually been treated successfully by curettage, but the "pseudotumor" forms occasional hemorrhagic nodules in the myometrium. The entity is, we believe, equivalent to the concept of chorionepitheliosis, which was discussed at length by Schopper and Pliess (1949). It also probably encompasses the chorioma of Ewing (1910) and perhaps the syncytioma and other vague designations of borderline trophoblastic lesions. These entities are not uncommon but are infrequently reported. Their recognition depends much on the interpretation of individual pathologists. Trophoblastic pseudotumors are probably not true malignant tumors, but they must be differentiated from them. A cytogenetic NISH study done by Faul et al. (1994) in cases of exaggerated placental site trophoblast indicated that the often bizarre nuclei found in these lesions are polyploid/aneuploid, perhaps arising by cell fusion or by endoreduplication of chromosomes.

Figure 517 illustrates an exaggerated placental site. Others would use the term chorionepitheliosis or syncytial endometritis to describe this morphology. Similar elements are present in the invasive lesion of Figures 518 and 519. It is a nodule of trophoblast that had perforated the uterus 18 months after a normal term pregnancy. After hysterectomy, the patient thrived. There were no metastases. This lesion is classifiable as trophoblastic pseudotumor. Two cases of chorionepitheliosis were reported by van Bogaert and Staquet (1977), presumably representing the same entity. The authors also considered the lesion to be a benign proliferation of trophoblastic elements. Nickels et al. (1978) described such a lesion in a 52-year-old patient whose last pregnancy was 20 years earlier; they thought that the term syncytial endometritis should be abandoned, and we agree. According to them, the term represents "a normal anatomic event at the placental site after miscarriage or full-term pregnancy." Rosenheim et al. (1980), who described a patient with uterine hemorrhage after abortion, decided that this diagnosis can be made only on a hysterectomy specimen. The uterus they studied showed an "endometrial polyp" that was composed of clot, with masses of atypical trophoblast interspersed. Villi had earlier been obtained by curettage from this patient. The villous tissue was like that of a CHM. The trophoblast invaded 30% of the myometrium. After removal, the patient ex-

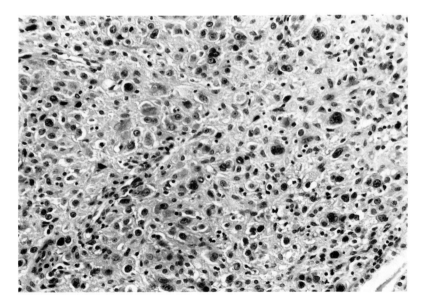

FIGURE 517. Curettings after normal pregnancy. There was postpartum bleeding by this 35-year-old woman who had had eight pregnancies with two live births. The lesion was interpreted as choriocarcinoma, but the patient had an uneventful course without chemotherapy. The lesion is best interpreted as exaggerated placental site. The cells are placental site giant cells (largely X cells). No solid sheets of cytotrophoblast are present, and there are no mitoses. H&E. ×260.

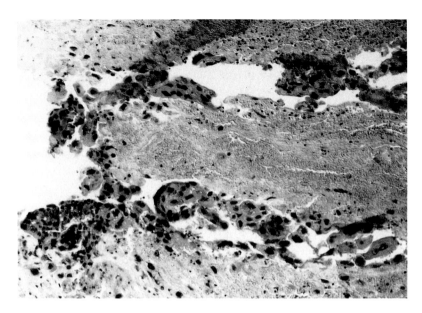

FIGURE 518. Invasive trophoblastic pseudotumor that had penetrated the uterus 18 months after a normal, term delivery. Hysterectomy alone cured this patient. The "malignant" cells are pleomorphic placental site giant cells (largely X-cells). There are no solid sheets of cytotrophoblast and few syncytial cells. There are no mitoses. H&E. ×100.

perienced full recovery. To clarify the differential diagnosis, these authors provided the scheme outlined in Table 24.

It is difficult to define this lesion precisely, especially when the diagnosis depends on tissue obtained at curettage. The trophoblastic pseudotumor may histologically blend with true choriocarcinoma, especially when newer information is considered. It thus came as no surprise that metastatic consequences were later observed, despite the earlier belief that the trophoblastic pseudotumor was a benign growth. Several patients

with apparently malignant lesions have since been identified, leading Scully and Young (1981) to introduce yet another term, the placental site trophoblastic tumor. This lesion is characterized by mononuclear trophoblast infiltration within the uterus and its vessels. Rare villi may be present. Absence of cytotrophoblastic cell masses and the usual absence of syncytial cells differentiates the entity from choriocarcinoma. The process is largely composed of placental site cells (intermediate trophoblast, or X cells in our nomenclature) and blends with placental site nodules and plaques. Some of the

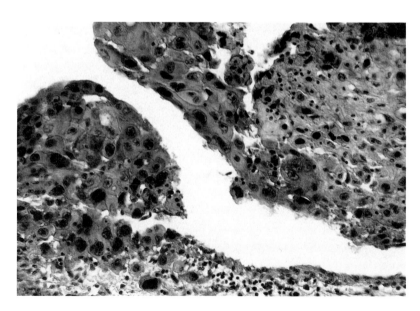

FIGURE 519. Trophoblastic pseudotumor (placental site trophoblastic tumor); same case as in Figure 518. H&E. ×160.

TABLE 24. Diagnostic differences between trophoblastic pseudotumor and other diseases.

Symptoms	Trophoblastic pseudotumor	Syncytial endometritis	Chorioadenoma destruens	Choriocarcinoma
Blood vessel invasion	+	−	−	+
Placental villi	−	−	+	−
Necrosis	±	±	+	+
Trophoblastic invasion	+	+	+	+
Syncytium/ cytotrophoblast	±	±	+/+	+/+
Hemorrhage	−	−	+	+

− = absent; + = present; ± = equivocal; +/+ = both present.

cells making up these lesions stain for human placental lactogen (hPL). Such a lesion is shown in Figures 518 and 519. We have found such a nodule 5 years after the last pregnancy when a patient had hysterectomy for cervical carcinoma.

Finkler and his colleagues (1988) treated seven patients with placental site trophoblastic tumors. They included a detailed review of this new entity. One of their apparent pseudotumors followed a CHM. The others occurred after abortion or premature delivery. All but one that followed an abortion pursued a benign course. Despite chemotherapy, this exceptional patient had metastatic disease in pelvic nodes. Although the authors did not provide any photomicrographs, they did describe an unprecedented high mitotic count. This point is particularly noteworthy because placental site cells (X cells) are not usually mitotic. Studies of major basic protein (MBP) levels from such patients would be highly informative.

An interesting study of this lesion was undertaken by Eckstein et al. (1985), who also reviewed the literature most competently. In their view, differentiation from choriocarcinoma should be easy because the lesion is a "well circumscribed yellowish mass in which hemorrhage and necrosis are less conspicuous than in choriocarcinoma." The histology is more like a placental site than like choriocarcinoma. The tumor in the aforementioned patient followed an apparently normal pregnancy but was eventually fatal with widespread metastases. It had a diploid DNA content, and biopsy samples were easily transplanted into nude mice. Unlike other lesions of this type, the tumor cells did not have a high mitotic rate. More recently, Fukunaga and Ushigome (1993a,b) reviewed the entire topic comprehensively and added three cases of placental site trophoblastic tumor to the literature. One of their patients died with widespread metastases. The patient had a term delivery and returned 9 months later with uterine, vaginal, bladder, and lung tumors, which resisted chemotherapy. Of the

three patients they reported, two recovered and all had diploid flow cytometric DNA values; all had pregnancies with female babies. Characteristically, many fewer mitoses were seen in these lesions than in true choriocarcinomas, and histochemically they showed significantly less hCG production and more hPL staining. As in eight other cases described, their fatal case had associated nephrotic syndrome, a complication not reported in choriocarcinoma. They estimated that perhaps 10% of placental site trophoblastic tumors behave in a malignant manner.

During the short time since the first description of the placental site trophoblastic tumor, some 80 cases have been reported. Perhaps it is presently overdiagnosed, considering that it is the rarest proliferative lesion of trophoblast; but it is also still somewhat difficult to define precisely, as it is not yet sufficiently differentiated morphologically from choriocarcinomas. Indeed, Fukunaga and Ushigome (1993a) believe that intermediate forms of these tumors exist. The case described by Hopkins et al. (1985) would thus perhaps still best be considered a choriocarcinoma following normal pregnancy, rather than a placental site tumor. Its histological composition most conformed to cytotrophoblast and syncytium, rather than to placental site giant cells. More precise methods to differentiate among these various lesions are desirable. Such efforts may be accomplished by the use of histochemistry, as performed by Wells and Bulmer (1988) and Fukunaga and Ushigome (1993a,b). These authors found in one such lesion the existence of a few tumor cells with hCG markers; more cells contained hPL antigen. Duncan and Mazur (1989) compared the ultrastructure of one such tumor (following normal pregnancy) with that of nine choriocarcinomas. The findings included an absence of cytotrophoblastic nests in the placental site tumor. The cellularity was composed primarily of intermediate trophoblast (X cells), with occasional interspersed syncytium. Surprisingly, the authors found by immunohistochemistry that some of the neoplastic X cells contained hPL as well as hCG, which is not usually the case.

Nagelberg and Rosen (1985) described other interesting biological features in such a patient. Their patient's tumor followed a normal pregnancy. The authors performed many endocrine studies because the tumor was accompanied by virilization due to testosterone production, possibly secondary to ovarian theca cell stimulation. It was also relatively resistant to chemotherapy. After an eventual hysterectomy, the pathologist found a solitary 2 cm mass of tumor cells. This report provided much insight into other endocrine parameters of this condition. A review of 20 cases of placental site nodules and plaques was undertaken by Young and colleagues (1990); and 40 cases were reviewed by Huetter and Gersell (1993). Most of the cells stained with antibodies to hPL and cytokeratin; all lesions were either incidental findings or followed a benign course. The prolonged production of hPL by the X cells of such a lesion was held to be responsible for the erythrocytosis in a patient reported by Brewer et al. (1992). After hysterectomy the symptoms disappeared; the lesion was a 6 cm hemorrhagic mass that infiltrated the myometrium but was primarily composed of X cells. There is now agreement that these nodules represent retained placental sites in which much hyalinization is found. Tsang et al. (1993) identified Mallory bodies in two cases, representing high-molecular-weight cytokeratins.

Yet another new tumor type was reported by Jauniaux and colleagues (1988). They called this lesion *chorangiocarcinoma*. It was described as a missing link, but these investigators still believed that "it is true malignant neoplasm or a voluminous chorangioma covered by extreme trophoblastic hyperplasia" (Hustin & Jauniaux, 1991). The unique lesion they described was a solitary chorioangioma with extensive trophoblastic hyperplasia at its borders. The authors concluded in that description that chorioangiomas are not hamartomas but true neoplasms.

Ultrastructure

Wynn and Davies (1964) studied the fine structure of trophoblastic neoplasms that were transplanted to hamster cheek pouches. They combined their morphological study with an endocrine assessment and were unable to demonstrate estrogenic activity. Except for excessive dilatation of syncytial cytoplasmic channels, the tumor resembled early human trophoblast. Larsen et al. (1967) made similar observations and showed that syncytial cells performed phagocytosis. Other studies were carried out directly on human choriocarcinomas that had not been transplanted (Inferrera et al., 1967;

Knoth et al., 1969a; Arai et al., 1976; Duncan & Mazur, 1989). The various investigators made the same observations. Several of the descriptions included cells that are truly intermediate between cytotrophoblast and syncytium (Figure 518), which was also shown in the choriocarcinomatous cell lines maintained in vitro by Knoth and colleagues (1969b).

ANTIGENIC STUDIES

Most choriocarcinomas have at least some paternal genome. Perhaps most (at least those derived from hydatidiform moles) have *only* paternal chromosomes. It is therefore possible that the tumor's antigenic determinants may engender immunological rejection. This assumption was central as an explanation for a frequently favorable prognosis. Elston (1969) described variably intense cellular reactions to the invading trophoblastic neoplasm and related it to outcome. Observations such as this one have led to the study of immune interactions of the tumors with the host and to the determination of HLA antigens in choriocarcinoma.

Mogensen and Kissmeyer-Nielsen (1968) studied HLA types in mothers, fathers and their children in conjunction with placenta-associated choriocarcinoma. Despite antigenic differences between father, and mother, most of the children were histocompatible with the mother. This compatibility, the authors suggested, made the tumors capable of growing in the uterus, rather than being rejected. Tomoda and his colleagues (1976) investigated HLA and ABO antigens in patients with gestational trophoblastic neoplasia and their husbands. ABO types had no correlation, but patients with choriocarcinoma were "frequently incompatible" at various HLA types. Nevertheless, patients with choriocarcinoma were more frequently histocompatible with their husbands than those having invasive moles. Rudolph and Thomas (1971) had found significantly different HLA antigens in the mother and child of a patient who developed choriocarcinoma. The authors thereby refuted the notion that the tumors develop because of a failure of trophoblast to be "rejected." Lawler et al. (1971) found that there was no increased histocompatibility between mothers and children in choriocarcinoma cases. There was a suggestion that major incompatibilities of HLA and ABO types protected the mother from disseminated disease. This aspect was further supported by findings of Mogensen and Kissmeyer-Nielsen (1971). Ivaskova and her colleagues (1969) found lymphocytotoxic antibodies against HLA antigens in 12 of 13 patients with choriocarcinoma or moles and speculated that these antigens may be important in tumor rejection. Differences in the population of the HLA_2 (MAC) antigen did not exist from controls in a French population of choriocarcinoma patients (Amiel & Lebovici, 1970). Ho et al. (1989) found that Whites did not share HLA antigens, whereas Chinese with choriocarcinomas did. Yamashita et al. (1984) performed direct tissue studies to ascertain the possible presence of histocompatibility antigens on choriocarcinoma cells. By this method, normal villi, hydatidiform moles, and two choriocarcinomas did not have any apparent class I and II antigens. Differences in responsiveness to class I and II antigens were concisely reviewed by Nepom (1989).

When ABO blood group antigens were studied in a Lebanese population, families with trophoblastic disease had a normal distribution, as did the controls (Iliya et al., 1969). Bagshawe et al. (1971) observed that blood group A women married to blood group O husbands have the highest risk of trophoblastic neoplasia; those married to blood group A husbands have the lowest risk. Blood group AB patients have tumors that metastasize widely and are least affected by chemotherapy. The investigators considered that these effects show immunological modulation of the tumor.

Because Rh(D) antigen is expressed on trophoblastic surfaces, Tomoda et al. (1981) suggested that hydatidiform moles [with Rh(D)] would be rejected by the Rh(d) host (see also Fischer et al., 1985), and that the difference in Rh antigens of Orientals could explain their high incidence of trophoblastic disease. Support for this idea has come from the early studies by Scott (1962, 1968).

It is not yet certain that biological trophoblast-specific antigen expression exists. Cheng and Johnson (1988) endeavored to produce antibodies to such possible antigens. When the antibodies were carefully absorbed, these authors found a low incidence (3.6%) of corresponding antibodies in serum samples of infertile women. These investigators suggested that the earlier results of Grimmer and colleagues (1988)—those that suggested a possible relation of these antibodies to lupus-like disorders—were erroneous. Srivannaboon (1971) found, in immunological studies with a trophoblast line, that choriocarcinoma contained an antigen that was not shared by normal trophoblast. The nature of this antigen was not identified.

There have also been attempts to treat gestational trophoblastic neoplasia with immunological methods. Doniach et al. (1958) immunized a patient with choriocarcinoma by injecting her husband's cells. Hackett and Beech (1961) injected concentrates of husband's leukocytes intradermally without inciting a reaction. They also employed Freund's adjuvant therapy and noted a gradual diminution in metastatic tumor nodules. Final resolution, however, occurred only after chemotherapy. The conclusion of these authors was that choriocarcinoma is not antigenic in the usual sense. Others have not agreed with this conclusion. Cinader et al. (1961) thought that their patient was successfully treated with leukocytes but were unable to rule out spontaneous remission. Although some spontaneous remissions of choriocarcinoma are well documented (Brewer et al., 1961), it is not a common event and certainly spontaneous remission cannot be reliably anticipated in clinical management. Ewing (1941), in fact, did not accept such lesions that regressed as being true choriocarcinomas.

The immunological tolerance of the husband's skin graft was explored in two patients with choriocarcinoma by Robinson et al. (1963); and Mathé et al. (1964) found variable skin graft survival in some patients with choriocarcinoma. There is no doubt that

some gestational trophoblastic neoplasia (GTN) elicits a cellular and immunological response and that it may be related to survival (see Ober, 1969). It is also the presumed explanation for the poorer response to chemotherapeutic agents of the testicular choriocarcinomas in men because they lack foreign antigens. Until the precise mechanism of graft rejection is understood and we know more about the tolerance afforded to normal placental trophoblast, it is useless to engage in further speculation. The reader is referred to the numerous papers from symposia that have dealt with this question (Edwards et al., 1975; Beer & Billingham, 1976; Wegmann & Gill, 1983; Gill et al., 1987).

EPIDEMIOLOGY

As with hydatidiform moles, the frequency of choriocarcinoma is irregularly distributed in different populations. It is also difficult to enumerate precisely because "malignant moles" are often included with choriocarcinoma. Nevertheless, there are major differences in prevalence. For instance, Ho et al. (1989) found the prevalence of GTN to be lowest in Whites (3 per 100,000 to 6 per 100,000) and highest in Chinese (68 per 100,000 to 202 per 100,000). They studied cellular antigens and found that Chinese had significant HLA antigen-sharing; Whites did not. This finding suggested to them that genetic and nongenetic factors are of etiological importance, and that it may also explain the generally better prognosis in Whites. Rolon and Lopez (1979) summarized much of the epidemiological aspects; their data and those of others are summarized in Table 25.

The higher incidence of choriocarcinoma in older women is apparent in most of these studies. Oettle (1961) made the point that despite the frequency of choriocarcinoma in Bantu women there is no increased frequency of hydatidiform moles in that population. They believed that the higher incidence of choriocarcinoma may result from higher ages at childbearing. In a study of Lebanese patients, Iliya et al. (1967) hypothesized that consanguinity is an important cause of choriocarcinoma. Parazzini et al. (1988a) adduced some data in favor of specific dietary deficiencies (e.g., vitamin A) in gestational trophoblastic neoplasia; "however, the limitation of available evidence still introduces serious uncertainties in the interpretation of these findings."

TABLE 25. Frequency of choriocarcinoma and chorioadenoma destruens among 100,000 live births.

Authors	Region	Choriocarcinoma	Chorioadenoma destruens
Hertig & Mansell (1956)	USA	43,000	
Wei & Cuyang (1963)	India	912	
Mills (1964)	England	70,000	
Tow (1965)	Singapore	5,000	
Acosta-Sison (1966)	Philippines	1,382–2,229	
Kolstad & Hognestad (1965)	Norway	20,000	
Aranda & Martinez (1969)	Puerto Rico	32,460	
Yen & MacMahon (1968)	Rhode Island	40,000	
Reddy & Rao (1969)	Taiwan	496	
Mogensen & Olsen (1972)	Denmark	49,000	126,000
Matalon et al. (1972)	Israel	15,000	
Baltazar (1976)	Philippines	5,747	
Rolon & Lopez (1979)	Paraguay	43,489	70,252

Modified from Rolon and Lopez (1979), with permission.

Endocrine Aspects

The most important endocrine consideration of chorio-carcinoma is its production of hCG or subunits thereof (see also Chapter 22). Follow-up of patients with CHM and choriocarcinomas is effectively done by assay of this hormone in serum (Delfs, 1959). Urine hCG values above 100,000 IU/24 hours (or serum levels of β-subunits measured by radioimmunoassay) strongly suggest the presence of a hydatidiform mole or malignant GTN. Conventionally, patients are monitored with weekly determination of hCG levels until none is detected for three consecutive weeks after the initial treatment of complete moles. In the usual case, hCG becomes undetectable within 8 to 173 days (Yuen et al., 1977). Chorionic gonadotropin is cleared by renal mechanisms, with a half-life of 35 hours (Midgley & Jaffe, 1968). Hammond et al. (1981) suggested that after the titers have disappeared hCG should be monitored for 1 year after evacuation of a mole. Even so, late recurrences have been reported, and they have frequently occurred despite adherence to this regimen (e.g., Kirk, 1965; Vaughn et al., 1980).

A possible improvement of monitoring cases with GTN is perhaps feasible with the determination of β-subunits of hCG in urine by radioimmunoassay (Wehmann et al., 1981). Through simultaneous measurements of serum and spinal fluid β-hCG levels, studies suggest that it may be possible to anticipate cerebral metastases (Soma et al., 1980).

Yazaki et al. (1980) compared isoelectric homogeneity of serum hCG in various types of normal and abnormal pregnancies. They found that normal gestations, CHM, and invasive moles had "normal" isoelectric peaks, whereas additional peaks were detected in sera of patients with choriocarcinoma. A variety of studies has shown that the hCG originates from the syncytial component of the choriocarcinoma. When Dawood (1975) measured progesterone levels in patients with chorio-carcinoma, he found that it correlated with hCG. He believed that the elevated progesterone levels resulted from its production by the hCG-stimulated ovaries, as many patients experience theca lutein cysts with this neoplasm (Kohorn, 1983), rather than the trophoblast. Lacking appropriate fetal adrenal precursors, estrogen production is sparse in choriocarcinoma patients, and its determination is not useful. It may be different in men with choriocarcinoma. They have excessive estrogen production and often suffer gynecomastia (Martin & Carden, 1963), presumably because of Leydig cell stimulation. Follow-up with hPL, MBP, and other trophoblastic proteins has either not been undertaken or has not been useful for therapeutic and management purposes.

Occasionally, choriocarcinoma is associated with excessive androgen production. These rare reports have been competently reviewed by Nagelberg and Rosen (1985). The origin of the androgens is still in dispute, although some in vitro work suggests a trophoblast origin. Searle et al. (1978) measured a placenta-specific β_1-glycoprotein in the serum of patients with GTN and found a moderate elevation in CHM and chorio-carcinoma patients—much less than that of hCG, however. They were not enthusiastic about the use of this marker in the management of patients. Nisbet et al. (1982) localized another placenta protein marker (PP5) to syncytium of placentas and its tumors. Serum levels, however, were not sufficiently elevated for its clinical use.

Ectopic Choriocarcinomas; Tumors in Men

Aside from the truly gestational choriocarcinoma, which most commonly follows a complete hydatidiform mole, choriocarcinoma has occasionally been reported in the fallopian tube, ovary, and other locations. These lesions may then be referred to as heterotopic chorioepithelioma (Nanke, 1959). Nanke, however, discovered such a tumor after hysterectomy performed for hydatidiform mole and it is most likely that the CHM was the tumor's antecedent of the cerebral, renal, and pulmonary metastases. The author opined that the tumor arose from deportation of benign trophoblast that subsequently dedifferentiated. He termed it chorioepitheliosis. As detailed in Chapter 22, such uncertainties can now be resolved when genetic markers are studied.

The primary choriocarcinoma in the lung of a patient without other lesions, reported by Tanimura et al. (1985), likely resulted from a prior therapeutic abortion. To support such a proposal, the authors examined the lungs of 10 patients dying after delivery or abortion and found pulmonary trophoblast in nine.

Tubal choriocarcinoma was reported by Madden (1950) following tubal abortion, as did most of the 48 other cases reviewed by the author. Other reports on tubal choriocarcinoma have come from Riggs et al. (1964) and Lurain et al. (1986). A comprehensive review was published by Ober and Maier (1981), who found 93 cases in the entire literature, deemed 58 to be acceptable, and added 18 of their own. These investigators indicated that small tumors are difficult to distinguish from ectopic pregnancy. They found two cases that still contained villi and thus should not be called chorio-carcinoma. Some patients were cured by simple hysterectomy, and others (94%) responded well to chemotherapy.

The fact that trophoblast is highly susceptible to methotrexate has led to many trials of the medical treatment of ectopic pregnancies with this agent (Ory et al., 1986; Carson et al., 1989). Five of six patients had no further need for therapy; one required subsequent salpingectomy. Barnes et al. (1982) reported the successful treatment of a placental choriocarcinoma, metastatic to the brain, that was later followed by a primary brain glioblastoma.

Some choriocarcinomas occur without known antecedent pregnancy (Acosta-Sison, 1957). Benjamin and Rorat (1978) reported ovarian choriocarcinomas as primary. Their patient developed the fatal ovarian (and hepatic) tumor apparently spontaneously. The uterine cavity contained only necrotic debris. The authors found six previous cases similar to theirs in the literature. Turner et al. (1964) reported on a successfully treated patient with an apparently primary ovarian choriocarcinoma. No antecedent or coincident pregnancy was found, although the authors called the tumor gestational. Cunanan et al. (1980) reported an ovarian choriocarcinoma that was associated with a normal uterine pregnancy delivered by hysterotomy several weeks after resection of the mass. The patient did well on chemotherapy; the infant and placenta were normal. This report included a review of 24 additional choriocarcinomas coexisting with pregnancy. In all, in 10 the tumor was found in the placenta, in 5 it was absent, and in the remaining 10 cases there was a lack of information. Axe et al. (1985) found six similar cases in their Registry of Ovarian Tumors. One of those patients died.

Manivel et al. (1987) reviewed the extensive literature of trophoblastic differentiation from germ cell tumors. This tumor is outside the scope of the present book. Suffice it to report that these investigators paid special attention to the presence of intermediate trophoblast in these germinal tumors. The cells were designated large mononuclear cells with a variety of immunological characteristics that had led Kurman et al. (1984) to call them intermediate trophoblast. Choriocarcinoma may differentiate from primary germ cell tumors of testis or mediastinum and from teratocarcinomas. Fine et al (1962) reviewed this topic adequately and reported a fatal case in which the tumor arose in the mediastinum and paid special attention to the endocrine aspects of the neoplasm.

Wenger et al. (1968) reported a mediastinal choriocarcinoma in a man. This tumor is unusual. The authors had seen only 17 choriocarcinomas in men at the Mayo Clinic. Chemotherapy is significantly less effective in men than for gestational trophoblastic neoplasms, which has been assumed to be due to the assistance of immunological "rejection" mechanisms in the gestational tumor. Soma et al. (1973), who studied the chromosomes of a man with gastric choriocarcinoma, identified fluorescent Y bodies in this hyperdiploid cell line. Fukunaga and Ushigome (1993a) found their eight tumors to be diploid and reviewed the evidence suggesting that chromosomes of these tumors are normal diploid. A primary choriocarcinoma without antecedent lesion was described in the lung of a 51-year-old man (Sullivan, 1989). A pulmonary choriocarcinoma was also reported in a 60-year-old woman (15 years after menopause). Because of her age, it is unlikely that it had derived from a preceding gestation (Pushchak & Farhi, 1987). Pushchak and Farhi speculated that it came from epithelial metaplasia, as she (and the patient of Sullivan) had been heavy smokers.

These cases must all be interpreted with caution, however, especially when one knows of the remarkable patient described by Dougherty et al. (1978): an 86-year-old woman with fatal pulmonary and cerebral metastases whose uterus had choriocarcinoma with degenerated villi. The inference was that the villi and trophoblast had existed since her last pregnancy, 34 years earlier. She had been amenorrheic after that pregnancy. This case is truly exceptional. Another remarkable case is that reported by Lathrop et al. (1978) of a choriocarcinoma that developed 14 years after tubal ligation.

THERAPY

Aside from the attempts at immunotherapy discussed previously, surgical and chemotherapy are used for the treatment of choriocarcinoma and its precursors. Initially, only surgical excision, perhaps prophylactic hysterectomy, was available for eradication of residual trophoblast after evacuation of hydatidiform moles. The survival rate after hysterectomy was only 31.9% with uncomplicated choriocarcinoma; when metastases were present it was 19.2% (Brewer et al., 1963). Some patients with metastases had spontaneous regression, a surprising observation then.

Much more rapid progress was made after the discovery that the folic acid antagonist methotrexate produced beneficial results (Li et al., 1956). The historical developments that followed were succinctly recalled by Hertz (1972) and Li (1972); in a larger thesis, Hertz (1978) provided a complete overview. So effective is methotrexate against proliferating trophoblast that it was even used for therapeutic abortion (Thiersch, 1952), and it is now occasionally employed for treatment of ectopic pregnancies (Ory et al., 1986). Others have employed this agent to cause the involution of residual trophoblast in abdominal implantations (St. Clair et al., 1969; Rahman et al., 1982). This method of therapy has improved patient survival remarkably (Brewer et al., 1964; Lewis et al., 1966; Goldstein, 1972). Many contributions have been published since these early studies and are aptly summarized in books by Goldstein and Berkowitz (1982) and Szulman and Buchsbaum (1987). Individual reports have established that immunological interactions occur when metastatic disease is treated chemotherapeutically in "incompatible" situations (Gallmeier et al., 1970). Even the feared cerebral metastases have a 50% remission rate when treated vigorously with chemotherapy and radiation (Weed & Hammond, 1980).

Despite these excellent results from methotrexate, actinomycin D, and other newer agents, there remains the problem of early diagnosis. This point is important. Delays and repeat chemotherapeutic treatment after a symptom-free interval often result in resistant metastases. Parazzini et al. (1988b) found that patients over age 40, those with AB blood group, and those with a history of complete mole had an especially poor outlook. Surwit et al. (1984) provided suggestions for aggressive therapy in other categories of "poor-prognosis GTN." Interestingly, students of this disease still disagree as to whether patients with hydatidiform moles should receive prophylactic chemotherapy in an effort to prevent the occurrence of choriocarcinoma. Bagshawe et al. (1969) believed it to be contraindicated. It is the experience of some physicians, however, that such a prophylactic regimen is not only safe but useful (Homesley et al., 1988). These considerations require a correct, precise diagnosis. We believe that patients with triploid, partial moles should be exempted from this consideration of prophylactic chemotherapy because no true choriocarcinoma follows such lesions. A most readable review of the progress made in the therapy of this tumor comes from the pen of Walter Jones (1990) who paid special tribute to Kenneth Bagshawe as having initiated a new age in the therapy of GTN.

It has often been asked if the multiple chemotherapeutic agents that are used to treat this neoplasm have an adverse effect on ovarian follicles. Several prospective studies have now affirmed that subsequent normal pregnancy is possible (Patterson, 1956; van Thiel et al., 1970; Walden & Bagshawe, 1976). Despite experimental evidence that these alkylating agents damage rodent ova, there is no reported increase in congenital anomalies and chromosomal anomalies of future offspring. Finally, occasional life-threatening hemorrhage may occur during the evolution of choriocarcinoma; Pearl and Braga (1992) were able to treat two such patients by embolization.

CHORIOCARCINOMA IN ANIMALS

Although there have been no reports of hydatidiform moles in animals, spontaneous choriocarcinoma has been observed a few times in several species. Lindsey et al. (1969) reported the first spontaneous choriocarcinoma in a rhesus monkey. The primary lesion was in the uterus and there were widespread pulmonary metastases. Pregnancy had been confirmed by rectal palpation, no known abortion had taken place and the tumor was unequivocally a choriocarcinoma by histological study. Madarame et al. (1989) found a localized hemorrhagic tumor in the uterus of a DDD mouse at age 601 days. Histologically, the pathology was clearly choriocarcinoma with appropriate immunochemical and electron microscopic characteristics. Experimental choriocarcinoma has often been produced in rats (Stein-Werblowsky, 1960; Shintani et al., 1966; Miyamoto, 1971), the nine-banded armadillo (Marin-Padilla & Benirschke, 1963), and the rabbit (Kushima et al., 1967).

Choriocarcinoma in Cell Lines and Genetics

It has long been possible to transplant trophoblastic neoplasms into the cheek pouches of Syrian hamsters (Galton et al., 1963). The transplanted tumor grows to a large size. This experimental system has been useful to determine susceptibility to chemotherapeutic agents and to study tumor biology and its cytogenetics. Immunological rejection processes could also be studied with this model. Apparently, the cheek pouch is an immunologically privileged site, and metastases do not occur in Syrian hamsters unless the neoplasm is transplanted to other sites (Ehrman & Gliserman, 1964). Chromosome numbers of such transplanted tumors are hyperdiploid ($2n \approx 80$) and increase with time. This finding coincides with the DNA studies of trophoblastic tumors by Makino et al. (1963) and Goldfarb et al. (1971). The latter investigators found mostly hyperdiploid (often tetraploid) values for choriocarcinomas, chorioadenoma destruens, and some moles, including values obtained for cytotrophoblastic cells (see also Atkin, 1965). Park (1957), who studied the Barr body content of the tumors, found that the tumor was equally aggressive whether it came from a male or a female pregnancy. With cytogenetic studies some choriocarcinomas have been shown to have chromosomal polymorphisms and heterozygosity, and many are aneuploid (Wake et al., 1981; Sheppard et al., 1985). The few other decisive modern chromosome and DNA studies that have been carried out on choriocarcinoma are referred to in Chapter 22 on molar pregnancies. Transplantation of choriocarcinoma into rhesus monkey brain was also successful, but not all implantations into the lung yielded tumor growth (Lewis et al., 1968). This finding suggested that immunological factors are involved in the rejection of such neoplasms. Carr (1979) found that when mouse trophoblast was transplanted into the lungs of mice it was accepted only by neonatal mice; adults failed to support trophoblast growth. Carr reviewed the well known deportation of chinchilla trophoblast to the lung during a normal gestation. Kato et al. (1982) made the interesting observation that when tissues from 21 hydatidiform moles and 10 invasive moles (chorioadenoma destruens) were transplanted into nude mice or immunosuppressed hamsters they were not accepted. Only seven of nine cases of choriocarcinoma could be successfully transplanted. Kato et al. therefore concluded that choriocarcinoma is a true neoplasm, but moles are not. Izhar et al. (1986) observed the development of trophoblast from human teratocarcinoma cell lines.

References

Acosta-Sison, H.: Apparent metastatic chorioepithelioma without demonstrable primary chorionic malignancy in the uterus: report of 3 cases; a new possible explanation of its occurrence. Obstet. Gynecol. 10:165–168, 1957.

Acosta-Sison, H.: The relative frequency of various anatomic sites as the point of first metastasis in 32 cases of chorionepithelioma. Am. J. Obstet. Gynecol. 75:1149–1152, 1958.

Acosta-Sison, H.: Choriocarcinoma from July 4, 1963 to June 30, 1965. Philippine J. Surg. 21:41–42, 1966.

Amiel, J.-L., and Lebovici, S.: Choriocarcinoma and the HL-A$_2$ antigen (MAC). Rev. Eur. Etud. Clin. Biol. 15: 191–192, 1970.

Arai, K., Soma, H., and Hokano, M.: Ultrastructure of trophoblastic tumor cells. J. Clin. Electron Microsc. 9:5–6, 1976.

Aranda, J.M., and Martinez, I.: Incidence of choriocarcinoma in Puerto Rico: a 15-year study. Cancer 23:506–507, 1969.

Arkwright, P.D., Rademacher, T.W., Dwek, R.A., and Redman, C.W.G.: Pre-eclampsia is associated with an increase in trophoblast glycogen content and glycogen synthase activity, similar to that found in hydatidiform moles. J. Clin. Invest. 91:2744–2753, 1993.

Atkin, N.B.: Sex chromosome studies on trophoblast. In, The Early Conceptus, Normal and Abnormal. pp. 130–134. University Court of the University of St. Andrews, Scotland, 1965.

Axe, S.R., Klein, V.R., and Woodruff, J.D.: Choriocarcinoma of the ovary. Obstet. Gynecol. 66:111–114, 1985.

Bagshawe, K.D.: Hydatidiform mole and chorioncarcinoma. B.M.J. 1:1509–1510, 1964.

Bagshawe, K.D.: Choriocarcinoma. The Clinical Biology of the Trophoblast and Its Tumors. Williams & Wilkins, Baltimore, 1969.

Bagshawe, K.D.: Pulmonary hypertension in gestational chorio-carcinoma: a West London syndrome? Lancet 2:223, 1988.

Bagshawe, K.D., and Noble, M.I.M.: Cardio-respiratory aspects of trophoblastic tumors. Q. J. Med. 35:39–54, 1966.

Bagshawe, K.D., Golding, P.R., and Orr, A.H.: Choriocarcinoma after hydatidiform mole: studies related to effectiveness of follow-up practice after hydatidiform mole. B.M.J. 2:733–737, 1969.

Bagshawe, K.D., Rawlins, G., Pike, M.C., and Lawler, S.D.: AB0 blood-groups in trophoblastic neoplasia. Lancet 1: 553–557, 1971.

Baltazar, J.C.: Epidemiological features of choriocarcinoma. Bull. W.H.O. 54:523–532, 1976.

Bardawil, W.A., and Toy, B.L.: The natural history of choriocarcinoma: problems of immunity and spontaneous regression. Ann. N.Y. Acad. Sci. 80:197–261, 1959.

Barnes, A.E., Liwnicz, B.H., Schellhaus, H.F., Altshuler, G., Aron, B.S., and Lippert, W.A.: Successful treatment of placental choriocarcinoma metastatic to brain followed by primary brain glioblastoma. Gynecol. Oncol. 13:108–114, 1982.

Beer, A.E., and Billingham, R.E.: The Immunobiology of Mammalian Reproduction. Prentice-Hall, Englewood Cliffs, NJ, 1976.

Benjamin, F., and Rorat, E.: Primary gestational choriocarcinoma of the ovary. Am. J. Obstet. Gynecol. 131:343–345, 1978.

Benson, P.F., Goldsmith, L.L.G., and Rankin, G.L.S.: Massive foetal haemorrhage into maternal circulation as a complication of choriocarcinoma. B.M.J. 1:841–842, 1962.

Blackburn, G.K.: Massive fetomaternal hemorrhage due to choriocarcinoma of the uterus. J. Pediatr. 89:680–681, 1976.

Brewer, C.A., Adelson, M.D., and Elder, R.C.: Erythrocytosis associated with a placental-site trophoblastic tumor. Obstet. Gynecol. 79:846–849, 1992.

Brewer, J.I., and Gerbie, A.B.: Early development of choriocarcinoma. Am. J. Obstet. Gynecol. 94:692–705, 1966.

Brewer, J.I., and Mazur, M.T.: Gestational choriocarcinoma: its origin in the placenta during seemingly normal pregnancy. Am. J. Surg. Pathol. 5:267–277, 1981.

Brewer, J.I., Rinehart, J.J., and Dunbar, R.W.: Choriocarcinoma. Am. J. Obstet. Gynecol. 81:574–583, 1961.

Brewer, J.I., Smith, R.T., and Pratt, G.B.: Choriocarcinoma: absolute 5 year survival rates of 122 patients treated by hysterectomy. Am. J. Obstet. Gynecol. 85:841–843, 1963.

Brewer, J.I., Gerbie, A.B., Dolkart, R.E., Skom, J.H., Nagle, R.G., and Torok, E.E.: Chemotherapy in trophoblastic diseases. Am. J. Obstet. Gynecol. 90:566–578, 1964.

Buckell, E.W.C., and Owen, T.K.: Chorionepithelioma in mother and infant. 61:329–330, 1954.

Carlson, J.A., Day, T.G., Kuhns, J.G., Howell, R.S., and Masterson, B.J.: Endoarterial pulmonary metastasis of malignant trophoblast associated with a term intrauterine pregnancy. Gynecol. Oncol. 17:241–248, 1984.

Carr, D.H.: Trophoblast growth in the lungs of mice. Obstet. Gynecol. 54:461–466, 1979.

Carson, S.A., Stovall, T., Umstot, E., Andersen, R., Ling, F., and Buster, J.E.: Rising human chorionic somatomammotropin predicts ectopic pregnancy rupture following methotrexate chemotherapy. Fertil. Steril. 51:593–597, 1989.

Chandra, S.A., Gilbert, E.F., Viseskul, C., Strother, C.M., Haning, R.V., and Javid, M.J.: Neonatal intracranial choriocarcinoma. Arch. Pathol. Lab. Med. 114:1079–1082, 1990.

Cheng, H.-M., and Johnson, P.M.: Specificity of trophoblast-reactive antibodies in human pregnancy. Arch. Pathol. Lab. Med. 112:1081, 1988.

Cinader, B., Hayley, M.A., Rider, W.D., and Warwick, O.H.: Immunotherapy of a patient with choriocarcinoma. Can. Med. Assoc. J. 84:306–309, 1961.

Cunanan, R.G., Lippes, J., and Tancinco, P.A.: Choriocarcinoma of the ovary with coexisting normal pregnancy. Obstet. Gynecol. 55:669–672, 1980.

Daamen, C.B.F., and Bloem, G.W.D.: Chorioepithelioma in mother and child. Ned. Tijdschr. Geneeskd. 105:651–656, 1961; J. Obstet. Gynaecol. Br. Commonw. 68:144–149, 1961.

Dawood, M.Y.: Serum progesterone and serum human chorionic gonadotropin in gestational and nongestational choriocarcinoma. Am. J. Obstet. Gynecol. 123:762–765, 1975.

Delfs, E.: Chorionic gonadotrophin determinations in patients with hydatidiform mole and choriocarcinoma. Ann. N.Y. Acad. Sci. 80:125–142, 1959.

Deligdisch, L., Driscoll, S.G., and Goldstein, D.P.: Gestational trophoblastic neoplasms: morphologic correlates of therapeutic response. Am. J. Obstet. Gynecol. 130:801–806, 1978.

Doniach, I., Crookston, J.H., and Cope, T.I.: Attempted treatment of a patient with choriocarcinoma by immunization with her husband's cells. J. Obstet. Gynaecol. Br. Emp. 65:553–556, 1958.

Dougherty, C.M., Cunningham, C., and Mickal, A.: Chorio-carcinoma with metastasis in a postmenopausal woman. Am. J. Obstet. Gynecol. 132:700–701, 1978.

Driscoll, S.G.: Choriocarcinoma: an "incidental finding" within a term placenta. Obstet. Gynecol. 21:96–101, 1963.

Driscoll, S.G.: Choriocarcinoma following delivery. Lab. Med. 48:21A, 1983.

Duleba, A.J., Miller, D., Taylor, G., and Effer, S.: Expectant management of choriocarcinoma limited to placenta. Gynecol. Oncol. 44:277–280, 1992.

Duncan, D.A., and Mazur, M.T.: Trophoblastic tumors: ultrastructural comparison of choriocarcinoma and placental-site trophoblastic tumor. Hum. Pathol. 20:370–381, 1989.

Dyke, P.C., and Fink, L.M.: Latent choriocarcinoma. Cancer 20:150–154, 1967.

Eckstein, R.P., Russell, P., Friedlaender, M., Tattersall, M.H.N., and Bradfield, A.: Metastasizing placental site trophoblastic tumor: a case study. Hum. Pathol. 16:632–636, 1985.

Edwards, R.G., Howe, C.W.S., and Johnson, M.H., eds.: Immunobiology of Trophoblast. Cambridge University Press, Cambridge, 1975.

Ehrman, R.L., and Gliserman, L.E.: Choriocarcinoma: growth patterns in hamster tissues. Nature 202:404–406, 1964.

Elston, C.W.: Cellular reaction to choriocarcinoma. J. Pathol. 97:261–268, 1969.

Evans, K.T., and Hendrickse, P. de V.: Pulmonary changes in malignant trophoblastic disease. Br. J. Radiol. 38:161–171, 1965.

Ewing, J.: Chorioma. Surg. Gynecol. Obstet. 10:366–392, 1910.

Ewing, J.R.: Neoplastic Diseases. 4th Ed. Saunders, Philadelphia, 1941.

Fahrner, R.J., McQueeney, A.J., Mosely, J.M., and Petersen, R.W.: Trophoblastic pulmonary thrombosis with cor pulmonale: report of a case due to malignant hydatidiform mole of five years' duration. J.A.M.A. 170:1898–1901, 1959.

Faul, P., Kelehan, P., and Dervan, P.: Interphase cytogenetic study of exaggerated placental site trophoblast using a biotin-labelled peroxidase method [abstract 503]. Mod. Pathol. 7:88A, 1994.

Feldman, K.: Choriocarcinoma with neonatal anemia. N. Engl. J. Med. 296:880, 1977.

Fine, G., Smith, R.W., and Pachter, M.R.: Primary extra-genital choriocarcinoma in the male subject: case report and review of the literature. Am. J. Med. 32:776–794, 1962.

Finkler, N.J., Berkowitz, R.S., Driscoll, S.G., Goldstein, D.P., and Bernstein, M.R.: Clinical experience with placental site trophoblastic tumors at the New England Trophoblastic Disease Center. Obstet. Gynecol. 71:854–857, 1988.

Fischer, H.E., Lichtiger, B., and Cox, I.: Expression of $Rh_0(D)$ antigen in choriocarcinoma of the uterus in an $Rh_0(D)$-negative patient: report of a case. Hum. Pathol. 16:1165–1167, 1985.

Fox, H., and Laurini, R.N.: Intraplacental choriocarcinoma: report of two cases. J. Clin. Pathol. 41:1085–1088, 1988.

Fukunaga, M., and Ushigome, S.: Malignant trophoblastic tumors: Immunohistochemical and flow cytometric comparison of choriocarcinoma and placental site trophoblastic tumors. Hum. Pathol. 24:1098–1106, 1993a.

Fukunaga, M., and Ushigome, S.: Metastasizing placental site trophoblastic tumor: an immunohistochemical and flow cytometric study of two cases. Am. J. Surg. Pathol. 17:1003–1010, 1993b.

Gallmeier, W.M., Bertrams, J., Kuwert, E., and Schmidt, C.G.: Regression des Chorionepithelioms: Zytostatikawirkung und/oder Immunreaktion? Dtsch. Med. Wochenschr. 95:1810–1815, 1970.

Galton, M., Goldman, P.B., and Holt, S.F.: Karyotypic and morphologic characterization of a serially transplanted human choriocarcinoma. J. Natl. Cancer Inst. 31:1019–1035, 1963.

Gill, T.J., Wegmann, G., and Nisbet-Brown, E.: Immuno-regulation and Fetal Survival. Oxford University Press, New York, 1987.

Goldfarb, S., Richart, R.M., and Okagaki, T.: A cytophotometric study of nuclear DNA content of cyto- and syncytiotrophoblast in trophoblastic disease. Cancer 27:83–92, 1971.

Goldstein, D.P.: The chemotherapy of gestational trophoblastic disease: principles of clinical management. J.A.M.A. 220:209–213, 1972.

Goldstein, D.P., and Berkowitz, R.S., eds.: Trophoblastic Neoplasms. Clinical Principles of Diagnosis and Management. Saunders, Philadelphia, 1982.

Greene, J.B., and McCue, S.A.: Choriocarcinoma with cerebral metastases coexistent with a first pregnancy. Am. J. Obstet. Gynecol. 131:253–254, 1978.

Grimmer, D., Landas, S., and Kemp, J.D.: IgM antitrophoblast antibodies in a patient with a pregnancy-associated lupuslike disorder, vasculitis, and recurrent intrauterine fetal demise. Arch. Pathol. Lab. Med. 112:191–193, 1988.

Hackett, E., and Beech, M.: Immunologic treatment of a case of choriocarcinoma. B.M.J. 2:1123–1126, 1961.

Hammond, C.B., Weed, J.C., Barnard, D.E., and Tyrey, L.: Gestational trophoblastic neoplasia. CA 31:322–332, 1981.

Heifetz, S.A., and Czaja, J.: In situ choriocarcinoma arising in partial hydatidiform mole: Implications for the risk of persistent trophoblastic disease. Pediatr. Pathol. 12:601–611, 1992.

Heller, E.L., and Householder, J.M.: Clinicopathologic conference. Am J. Clin. Pathol. 22:883–889, 1952.

Hertig, A.T., and Mansell, H.: Tumors of the female sex organs. Part I. Hydatidiform mole and choriocarcinoma. In, Atlas of Tumor Pathology. Sect. IX, Fasc. 33. Armed Forces of Pathology, Washington, DC, 1956.

Hertz, R.: Quantitative monitoring of chemotherapy of endocrine Tumors by hormone assay. J.A.M.A. 222:1163, 1972.

Hertz, R.: Choriocarcinoma and Related Gestational Trophoblastic Tumors in Women. Raven Press, New York, 1978.

Ho, H.-N., Gill, T.J., Klionsky, B., Ouyang, P.-C., Hsieh, C.-Y., and Kunschner, A.: Differences between white and Chinese populations in human leukocyte antigen sharing and gestational trophoblastic tumors. Am. J. Obstet. Gynecol. 161:942–948, 1989.

Homesley, H.D., Blessing, J.A., Rettenmaier, M., Capizzi, R.L., Major, F.J., and Twiggs, L.B.: Weekly intramuscular methotrexate for nonmetastatic gestational trophoblastic disease. Obstet. Gynecol. 72:413–418, 1988.

Hopkins, M., Nunez, C., Murphy, J.R., and Wentz, W.B.: Malignant placental site trophoblastic tumor. Obstet. Gynecol. 66:95S–100S, 1985.

Huber, H.: Das Chorionepitheliom. Arch. Gynecol. 207: 187–201, 1969.

Huetter, P.C., and Gersell, D.J.: Placental site nodule: an analysis of 40 cases [abstract 422]. Mod. Pathol. 4:74A, 1993.

Hustin, J., and Jauniaux, E.: Markedly elevated maternal serum alpha-fetoprotein associated with a normal fetus and choriocarcinoma of the placenta. Obstet. Gynecol. 77:329–330, 1991.

Hutchison, J.R., Peterson, E.P., and Zimmermann, E.A.: Coexisting metastatic choriocarcinoma and normal pregnancy: therapy during gestation with maternal remission and fetal survival. Obstet. Gynecol. 31:331–336, 1968.

Van Bogaert, L.J., and Staquet, J.P.: Chorionepitheliosis: a rare benign trophoblastic disease. Acta Obstet. Gynecol. Scand. 56:69–73, 1977.

Iliya, F.A., Khuri, F.P., and Khuri, S.F.: Multisystem blood group study in trophoblastic disease. Lebanese Med.J. 22: 707–711, 1969.

Iliya, F.A., Khuri, F.P., and Khuri, S.F.: Multisystem blood group study in trophoblastic disease. Lebanese Med. J. 22:707–711, 1969.

Inferrera, C., Pulle, C., Rigano, A., and Palmara, D.: Aspetti ultrastrutturali e citochimici del coriocarcinoma uterino. Arch. Ostet. Ginecol. 72:707–744, 1967.

Ivaskova, E., Jakoubkova, J., Zavadil, M., Schneid, v., Koldovasky, P., and Ivanyi, P.: HL-A antigens and choriocarcinoma. Transplant. Proc. 1:80–81, 1969.

Izhar, M., Siebert, P.D., Oshima, R.G., DeWolf, W.C., and Fukuda, M.N.: Trophoblastic differentiation of human teratocarcinoma cell line HT-H[1]. Dev. Biol. 116:510–518, 1986.

Jarrett, D.D., and Pratt-Thomas, H.R.: Metastatic choriocarcinoma appearing as a unilateral renal mass. Arch. Pathol. Lab. Med. 108:356–357, 1984.

Jauniaux, E., Zucker, M., Meuris, S., Verherst, A., Wilkin, P., and Hustin, J.: Chorangiocarcinoma: an unusual tumour of the placenta; the missing link? Placenta 9:607–613, 1988.

Jones, W.B.: Gestational trophoblastic disease: what have we learned in the past decade? Am. J. Obstet. Gynecol. 162: 1286–1295, 1990.

Kato, M., Tanaka, K., and Takeuchi, S.: The nature of trophoblastic disease initiated by transplantation into immunosuppressed animals. Am. J. Obstet. Gynecol. 142: 497–505, 1982.

Kirk, J.A.: Persistence of abnormal trophoblast. Am. J. Obstet. Gynecol. 92:667–669, 1965.

Knoth, M., Hesseldahl, H., and Larsen, J.F..: Ultrastructure of human choriocarcinoma. Acta Obstet. Gynecol. 48:100–118, 1969a.

Knoth, M., Pattillo, R.A., Garancis, J.C., Gey, G.O., Ruckert, A.C.F., and Mattingly, R.F.: Ultrastructure and hormone synthesis of choriocarcinoma. Am. J. Pathol. 54: 479–488, 1969b.

Kohorn, E.I.: Theca lutein ovarian cyst may be pathognomonic for trophoblastic neoplasia. Obstet. Gynecol. 62: 80S–81S, 1983.

Kolstad, P., and Hognestad, J.: Trophoblastic tumours in Norway. Acta Obstet. Gynecol. Scand. 44:80–88, 1965.

Kruseman, A.C.N., van Lent, M., Blom, A.H., and Lauw, G.P.: Choriocarcinoma in mother and child, identified by immunoenzyme histochemistry. Am. J. Clin. Pathol. 67: 279–283, 1977.

Kurman, R.J., Scully, R.E., and Norris, N.J.: Trophoblastic pseudotumor of the uterus: an exaggerated form of "syncytial endometritis" simulating a malignant tumor. Cancer 38:1214–1226, 1976.

Kurman, R.J., Main, C.S., and Chen, H.-C.: Intermediate trophoblast: a distinctive form of trophoblast with specific morphological, biochemical and functional features. Placenta 5:349–370, 1984.

Kushima, K., Noda, K., and Makita, M.: Experimental production of chorionic tumor in rabbits. Tohoku J. Exp. Med. 91:209–214, 1967.

Larsen, J.F., Ehrman, R.L., and Bierring, F.: Electron microscopy of human choriocarcinoma transplanted into hamster liver. Am. J. Obstet. Gynecol. 99:1109–1124, 1967

Lathrop, J.C., Wachtel, T.J., and Meissner, G.F.: Uterine choriocarcinoma fourteen years following bilateral tubal ligation. Obstet. Gynecol. 51:477–482, 1978.

Lawler, S.D., Klouda, P.T., and Bagshawe, K.D.: HL-A system in trophoblastic neoplasia. Lancet 2:834–837, 1971.

Lewis, J., Gore, H., Hertig, A.T., and Goss, D.A.: Treatment of trophoblastic disease. Am. J. Obstet. Gynecol. 86:710–722, 1966.

Lewis, J.L., Brown, W.E., Hertz, R., Davis, R.C., and Johnson, R.H.: Heterotransplantation of human choriocarcinoma in monkeys. Cancer Res. 28:2032–2038, 1968.

Li, M.C.: Chemotherapeutic and immunological aspects of choriocarcinoma. J.A.M.A. 222:1163–1164, 1972.

Li, M.C., Hertz, R., and Spencer, D.B.: Effect of methotrexate therapy upon choriocarcinoma and chorioadenoma. Proc. Soc. Exp. Biol. Med. 93:361–366, 1956.

Lindsey, J.R., Wharton, L.R., Woodruff, J.D., and Baker, H.J.: Intrauterine choriocarcinoma in a rhesus monkey. Pathol. Vet. 6:378–384, 1969.

Lurain, J.R., Sand, P.K., and Brewer, J.I.: Choriocarcinoma associated with ectopic pregnancy. Obstet. Gynecol. 68: 286–287, 1986.

Madarame, H., Sakural, H., and Konno, S.: Choriocarcinoma in a DDD mouse: a case report with immunohistochemical and ultrastructural studies. Lab. Anim. Sci. 39:255–258, 1989.

Madden, S.: Chorionepithelioma of the fallopian tube. J. Obstet. Gynaecol. Br. Emp. 57:68–70, 1950.

Makino, S., Sasaki, M.S., and Fukushima, T.: Preliminary notes on the chromosomes of human chorionic lesions. Proc. Jpn. Acad. 39:54–58, 1963.

Manivel, J.C., Niehans, G., Wick, M.R., and Dehner, L.P.: Intermediate trophoblast in germ cell neoplasms. Am. J. Surg. Pathol. 11:693–701, 1987.

Marchand, F.J.: Über die sogenannten "decidualen" Geschwülste im Anschluss an normale Geburt, Abort, Blasenmole und Extrauterinschwangerschaft. Monatsschr. Geburtshilfe Gynäkol. 1:419–438, 513–560, 1895.

Marin-Padilla, M., and Benirschke, K.: Thalidomide induced alterations in the blastocyst and placenta of the armdillo, Dasypus novemcinctus mexicanus, including a choriocarcinoma. Am. J. Pathol. 43:999–1016, 1963.

Marquez-Monter, H., and Velasco, A.F.: Patologia de los tumores trofoblasticos. Bol. Asoc. Mex. Patol. 5:11–16, 1967.

Martin, B.R., Orr, J.W., and Austin, J.M.: Cervical choriocarcinoma associated with an intrauterine contraceptive device: a case report. Am. J. Obstet. Gynecol. 147:343–344, 1983.

Martin, F.I.R., and Carden, A.B.G.: Gynaecomastia in chorion-epithelioma: oestrogen levels and probable pathogenesis. Acta Endocrinol. (Copenh.) 43:203–212, 1963.

Matalon, M., Paz, B., Modan, M., and Modan, B.: Malignant trophoblastic disorders: epidemiologic aspects and relationship to hydatidiform mole. Am. J. Obstet. Gynecol. 112:101–106, 1972.

Mathé, G., Dausset, J., Hervet, E., Amiel, J.L., Colombani, J., and Brule, G.: Immunological studies in patients with placental choriocarcinoma. J. Natl. Cancer Inst. 33:193–208, 1964.

Mercer, R.D., Lammert, A.C., Anderson, R., and Hazard, J.B.: Choriocarcinoma in mother and infant. J.A.M.A. 166:482–483, 1958.

Midgley, A.R., and Jaffe, R.B.: Regulation of human gonadotropins. II. Disappearance of human chorionic gonadotropin following delivery. J. Clin. Endocrinol. 28:1712–1718, 1968.

Miller, J.M., Surwit, E.A., and Hammond, C.B.; Choriocarcinoma following term pregnancy. Obstet. Gynecol. 53:207–212, 1979.

Mills, W.: Chorion-carcinoma in the midlands. Clin. Radiol. 15:260–262, 1964.

Miyamoto, M.: Experimental induction of choriocarcinoma in rats. Gann 62:55–56, 1971.

Mogensen, B., and Kissmeyer-Nielsen, F.: Histocompatibility antigens on the HL-A locus in generalised gestational choriocarcinoma: a family study. Lancet 1:721–724, 1968.

Mogensen, B., and Kissmeyer-Nielsen, F.: Current data on HL-A and AB0 typing in gestational choriocarcinoma and invasive mole. Transplant. Proc. 3:1267–1269, 1971.

Mogensen, B., and Olsen, S.: Gestational choriocarcinoma in Denmark 1940–1969: a reappraisal based on modern histologic criteria. Acta Obstet. Gynecol. Scand. 51:63–69, 1972.

Nagelberg, S.B., and Rosen, S.W.: Clinical and laboratory investigation of a virilized woman with placental-site trophoblastic tumor. Obstet. Gynecol. 65:527–534, 1985.

Nanke, E.: Über primär heterotopes (ektopisches) Chorionepitheliom und Chorionepitheliosis. Geburtshilfe Frauenheilkd. 19:523–531, 1959.

Nepom, G.T.: The effects of variations in human immune-response genes. N. Engl. J. Med. 321:751–752, 1989.

Nickels, J., Risberg, B., and Melander, S.: Trophoblastic pseudotumour of the uterus. Acta Pathol. Microbiol. Scand. A 86:14–16, 1978.

Nisbet, A.D., Brehmer, R.D., Horne, C.H.W., Brooker, D., Twiggs, L.B., and Okagaki, T.: Placental protein 5 in gestational trophoblastic disease: localization and circulating levels. Am. J. Obstet. Gynecol. 144:396–401, 1982.

Ober, W.B.: Gestational choriocarcinoma: immunological aspects, diagnosis and treatment. Excerpta Medica Int. Congr. Ser. 203:304–315, 1969.

Ober, W.B., and Fass, R.O.: The early history of choriocarcinoma. J. Hist. Med. Allied Sci. 16:492–73, 1961.

Ober, W.B., and Maier, R.C.: Gestational choriocarcinoma of the fallopian tube. Diagn. Gynecol. Obstet. 3:213–231, 1981.

Ober, W.B., Edgcomb, J.H., and Price, E.B.: The pathology of choriocarcinoma. Ann. N.Y. Acad. Sci. 172:299–426, 1971.

Oettle, A.G.: Malignant neoplasms of the uterus in the white, "coloured," Indian and Bantu races of the Union of South Africa. Acta Uni. Int. Contra Canc. 17:915–933, 1961.

Ollendorff, D.A., Goldberg, J.M., Abu-Jawdeh, G.M., and Lurain, J.R.: Markedly elevated maternal serum alpha-fetoprotein associated with a normal fetus and choriocarcinoma of the placenta. Obstet. Gynecol. 76:494–497, 1990.

Olive, D.L., Lurain, J.R., and Brewer, J.I.: Choriocarcinoma associated with term gestation. Am. J. Obstet. Gynecol. 148:711–716, 1984.

Ory, S.J., Villanueva, A.L., Sand, P.K., and Tamura, R.K.: Conservative treatment of ectopic pregnancy with methotrexate. Am. J. Obstet. Gynecol. 154:1299–1306, 1986.

Parazzini, F., La Vecchia, C., Mangili, G., Caminiti, C., Negri, E., Cecchetti, G., and Fasoli, M.: Dietary factors and risk of trophoblastic disease. Am. J. Obstet. Gynecol. 158:93–100, 1988a.

Parazzini, F., Mangili, G., Belloni, C., La Vecchia, C., Liati, P., and Marabini, R.: The problem of identification of prognostic factors for persistent trophoblastic disease. Gynecol. Oncol. 30:57–62, 1988b.

Park, W.W.: The occurrence of sex chromatin in chorionepitheliomas and hydatidiform moles. J. Pathol. Bacteriol. 74:197–206, 1957.

Park, W.W.: Choriocarcinoma: A Study of Its Pathology. Davis, Philadelphia, 1971.

Patterson, W.B.: Normal pregnancy after recovery from metastatic choriocarcinoma. Am. J. Obstet. Gynecol. 72:183–187, 1956.

Pearl, M.L., and Braga, C.A.: Percutaneous transcatheter embolization for control of life-threatening pelvic hemorrhage from gestational trophoblastic disease. Obstet. Gynecol. 80:571–574, 1992.

Pierce, G.B., and Midgley, A.R.: The origin and function of human syncytiotrophoblastic giant cells. Am. J. Pathol. 43:153–173, 1963.

Pushchak, M.J., and Farhi, D.C.: Primary choriocarcinoma of the lung. Arch. Pathol. Lab. Med. 111:477–479, 1987.

Rahman, M.S., Al-Suleiman, S.A., Rahman, J., and Al-Sibai, M.H.: Advanced abdominal pregnancy: observations in 10 cases Obstet. Gynecol. 59:366–372, 1982.

Rauter, B.: Zum Problem des Chorionepithelioms. Wien. Klin. Wochenschr. 80:634–636, 1968.

Reddy, D.B., and Rao, N.: Trophoblastic tumors. II. Choriocarcinoma: a review of 50 cases. Indian J. Med. 23:532–537, 1969.

Riggs, J.A., Wainer, A.S., Hahn, G.A., and Farell, D.M.: Extrauterine tubal choriocarcinoma. Am. J. Obstet. Gynecol. 88:637–641, 1964.

Robinson, E., Shulman, J., Ben-Hur, N., Zuckerman, H., and Neuman, Z.: Immunological studies and behaviour of husband and foreign homografts in patients with chorionepithelioma. Lancet 1:300–302, 1963.

Rolon, P.A., and Lopez, B.H.de: Malignant trophoblastic disease in Paraguay. J. Reprod. Med. 23:94–96, 1979.

Rosenheim, N.B., Wijnen, H., and Woodruff, J.D.: Clinical importance of the diagnosis of trophoblastic pseudotumors. Am. J. Obstet. Gynecol. 136:635–638, 1980.

Rudolph, R.H., and Thomas, E.D.: HL-A antigens and choriocarcinoma. Lancet 2:408–409, 1971.

Santamaria, M., Benirschke, K., Carpenter, P.M., Baldwin, V.J., and Pritchard, J.A.: Transplacental hemorrhage associated with placental neoplasms. Pediatr. Pathol. 7:601–615, 1987.

Schopper, W., and Pliess, G.: Über Chorionepitheliosis: ein Beitrag zur Genese, Diagnostik und Bedeutung ektopischer chorionepithelialer Wucherungen. Virchows Arch. 317:347–384, 1949.

Scott, J.S.: Choriocarcinoma. Am. J. Obstet. Gynecol. 83:185–193, 1962.

Scott, J.S.: Histocompatibility antigens in choriocarcinoma. Lancet 1:865–866, 1968.

Scully, R.E., and Young, R.H.: Trophoblastic pseudotumor: a reappraisal. Am. J. Surg. Pathol. 5:75–76, 1981.

Searle, F., Leake, B.A., Bagshawe, K.D., and Dent, J.: Serum-SP$_1$-pregnancy-specific-β-glycoprotein in choriocarcinoma and other neoplastic disease. Lancet 1:579–581, 1978.

Seckl, M.J., Rustin, G.J.S., Newlands, E.S., Gwyther, S.J., and Bomanji, J.: Pulmonary embolism, pulmonary hypertension, and choriocarcinoma. Lancet 338:1313–1315, 1991.

Sheppard, D.M., Fisher, R.A., and Lawler, S.D.: Karyotypic analysis and chromosome polymorphisms in four choriocarcinoma cell lines. Cancer Genet. Cytogenet. 16:251–258, 1985.

Shintani, S., Glass, L.E., and Page, E.W.: Studies of induced malignant tumors of placental and uterine origin in the rat. I. Survival of placental tissue following fetectomy. II. Induced tumors and their pathogenesis with special reference to choriocarcinoma. III. Identification of experimentally induced choriocarcinoma by detection of placental hormone. Am. J. Obstet. Gynecol. 95:542–549, 550–558, 559–563, 1966.

Silverberg S.G., and Kurman, R.J.: Tumors of the uterine corpus and gestational trophoblastic disease. In, Atlas of Tumor Pathology, Third Series, Fascicle 3. AFIP, Washington, DC, 1992.

Soma, H., Kiyokawa, T., Akaeda, T., Miyashita, T., and Matayoshi, K.: The chromosomes of a human choriocarcinoma cell line in vitro with special reference to the presence of Y chromosome. Acta Obstet. Gynaecol. Jpn. 20:239–242, 1973.

Soma, H., Takayama, M., Tokoro, K., Kikuchi, T., Kikuchi, K., and Saegusa, H.: Radioimmunoassay of hCG as an early diagnosis of cerebral metastases in choriocarcinoma patients. Acta Obstet. Gynecol. Scand. 59:445–448, 1980.

Soper, J.T., Mutch, D.G., Chin, N., Clarke-Pearson, D.L., and Hammond, C.B.: Renal metastases of gestational trophoblastic disease: a report of eight cases. Obstet. Gynecol. 72:796–798, 1988.

Spiegel, J.A.: Endoarterial choriocarcinoma of the lung: report of a case and review of the literature. Obstet. Gynecol. 24:740–748, 1964.

Srivannaboon, S.: Antigenicity of human choriocarcinoma. Int. J. Fertil. 16:36–41, 1971.

St. Clair, J.T., Wheeler, D.A., and Fish, S.A.: Methotrexate in abdominal pregnancy J.A.M.A. 208:529–531, 1969.

Stein-Werblowsky, T.: Induction of a chorin-epitheliomatous tumour in the rat. Nature 186:980, 1960.

Sullivan, L.G.: Primary choriocarcinoma of the lung in a man. Arch. Pathol. Lab. Med. 113:82–83, 1989.

Surwit, E.A., Alberts, D.S., Christian, C.D., and Graham, V.E.: Poor-prognosis gestational trophoblastic disease: an update. Obstet. Gynecol. 64:21–26, 1984.

Suzuki, T., Goto, S., Nawa, A., Kurauchi, O., Saito, M., and Tomoda, Y.: Identification of the pregnancy responsible for gestational trophoblastic disease by DNA analysis. Obstet. Gynecol. 82:629–634, 1993.

Szulman, A.E., and Buchsbaum, H.J., eds.: Gestational Trophoblastic Disease. Springer-Verlag, New York, 1987.

Tanimura, A., Natsuyama, H., Kawano, M., Tanimura, Y., Tanaka, T., and Kitazono, M.: Primary choriocarcinoma of the lung. Hum. Pathol. 16:1281–1284, 1985.

Teacher, J.H.: On chorionepithelioma and the occurrence of chorionepitheliomatous and hydatidiform mole-like structures in teratomata: a pathological and clinical study. J. Obstet. Gynaecol. Br. Emp. 4:1–64, 145–199, 1903.

Thiersch, J.B.: Therapeutic abortions with a folic acid antagonist, 4-aminopteroylglutamic acid (4-amino P.G.A.) administered by the oral route. Am. J. Obstet. Gynecol. 63:1298–1304, 1952.

Tomoda, Y., Fuma, M., Saiki, N., Ishizuka, N., and Akaza, T.: Immunologic studies in patients with trophoblastic neoplasia. Am. J. Obstet. Gynecol. 126:661–667, 1976.

Tomoda, Y., Kaseki, S., Goto, S., Nishi, H., Hara, T., and Naruki, M.: Rh-D factor in trophoblastic tumors: a possible cause of the high incidence in Asia. Am. J. Obstet. Gynecol. 139:742–743, 1981.

Tow, S.H.: Choriocarcinoma: a review of current concepts based on the Singapore experience. Singapore Med. J. 6:117–126, 1965.

Tsang, W.Y.W., Chum, N.P.Y., Tang, S.K., Tse, C.C.H., and Chan, J.K.C.: Mallory's bodies in placental site nodule. Arch. Pathol. Lab. Med. 117:547–550, 1993.

Turner, H.B., Douglas, W.M., and Gladding, T.C.: Chorio-carcinoma of the ovary. Obstet. Gynecol. 24:918–920, 1964.

Van Bogaert. L.-J., and Staquet, J.-P.: Chorionepitheliosis: a rare benign trophoblastic disease. Acta Obstet. Gynecol. Scand. 56:69–73, 1977.

Van Thiel, D.H., Ross, G.T., and Lipsett, M.B.: Pregnancies after chemotherapy of trophoblastic neoplasms. Science 169:1326–1327, 1970.

Vaughn, T.C., Surwit, E.A., and Hammond, C.B.: Late recurrences of gestational trophoblastic neoplasia. Am. J. Obstet. Gynecol. 138:73–76, 1980.

Veinot, J.P., Ford, S.E., and Price, R.G.: Subacute cor pulmonale due to tumor embolization. Arch. Pathol. Lab. Med. 116:131–134, 1992.

Wake, N., Tanaka, K., Chapman, V., Matsui, S., and Sandberg, A.A.: Chromosomes and cellular origin of choriocarcinoma. Cancer Res. 41:3137–3143, 1981.

Walden, P.A.M., and Bagshawe, K.D.: Reproductive per-formance of women successfully treated for gestational trophoblastic tumors. Am. J. Obstet. Gynecol. 125:1108–1114, 1976.

Weed, J.C., and Hammond, C.B.: Cerebral metastatic choriocarcinoma: intensive therapy and prognosis. Obstet. Gynecol. 55:89–94, 1980.

Wegmann, T.G., and Gill, T.J.: Immunology of Reproduc-tion. Oxford University Press, New York, 1983.

Wehmann, R.E., Ayala, A.R., Birken, S., Canfield, R.E., and Nisula, B.C.: Improved monitoring of gestational trophoblastic neoplasia using a highly sensitive assay for urinary human chorionic gonado tropin. Am. J. Obstet. Gynecol. 140:753–757, 1981.

Wei, P.Y., and Cuyang, P.C.: Trophoblastic disease in Taiwan: a review of 157 cases in a 10 year period. Am. J. Obstet. Gynecol. 85:844–849, 1963.

Wells, M., and Bulmer, J.N.: The human placental bed: histology, immunohistochemistry and pathology. Histo-pathology 13:483–498, 1988.

Wenger, M.E., Dines, D.E., Ahmann, D.L., and Good, C.A.: Primary mediastinal choriocarcinoma. Mayo Clin. Proc. 43:570–575, 1968.

Witzleben, C.L., and Bruninga, G.: Infantile choriocarcin-oma: a characteristic syndrome. J. Pediatr. 73:374–378, 1968.

Wolf, H.K., and Michalopoulos, G.K.: Proliferating cell nuclear antigen in human placenta and trophoblastic disease. Pediatr. Pathol. 12:147–154, 1992.

Wynn, R.M., and Davies, J.: Ultrastructure of transplanted choriocarcinoma and its endocrine implications. Am. J. Obstet. Gynecol. 88:618–633, 1964.

Yamashita, K., Nakamura, T., and Shimizu, T.: Absence of major histocompatibility complex antigens in choriocarcin-oma. Am. J. Obstet. Gynecol. 150:896–897, 1984.

Yazaki, K., Yazaki, C., Wakabayashi, K., and Igarashi, M.: Isoelectric heterogeneity of human chorionic gonadotropin: presence of choriocarcinoma specific components. Am. J. Obstet. Gynecol. 138:189–194, 1980.

Yen, S., and MacMahon, B.: Epidemiologic features of trophoblastic disease. Am. J. Obstet. Gynecol. 101:126–132, 1968.

Young, R.H., Kurman, R.J., and Scully, R.E.: Placental site nodules and plaques: a clinicopathologic analysis of 20 cases. Am. J. Surg. Pathol. 14:1001–1009, 1990.

Yuen, B.H., Cannon, W., Benedet, J.L., and Boyes, D.A.: Plasma β-subunit human chorionic gonadotropin assay in molar pregnancy and choriocarcinoma. Am. J. Obstet. Gynecol. 127:711–712, 1977.

24
Benign Tumors

Angiomas

With rare exceptions, vascular tumors are the only benign tumors of the placenta. Tumors designated chorioangiomas, chorangiomas, fibroangiomyxomas, fibromas, and the many other names that have been applied in the past are essentially similar, relatively common neoplasms of the placenta. Two large reviews have been published that bring together most of the literature. Fox (1967), who also reviewed the often confused nomenclature, indicated that Clarke described the first such tumor in 1798. Since then, the review by Siddall (1924) encompassed 130 cases, that by Marchetti (1939) comprised 209 cases, and Fox traced another 127 cases. Fox accounted for 344 published cases and gave incidence figures of 1 per 9,000 to 1 per 50,000 placentas. When careful study of placentas is undertaken, the real prevalence may be as high as 1 per 100 pregnancies, according to some authors, although in our experience this number is excessive. Wallenburg (1971) provided 13 new cases and summarized publications between 1939 and 1970. His reported incidence in consecutively collected placentas was 1 per 117. These authors provided an extensive literature documentation that would be redundant to repeat. Soma et al. (1991) found that the tumor existed in 0.2% of placentas in Japanese women but was more common (2.5–7.6%) in the high altitude population of Nepal.

The typical chorioangioma is composed of fetal blood vessels that are usually supported by only scant connective tissue. The tumors often bulge on the fetal surface of the placenta (Figure 520). When they are embedded in the villous tissue, they are located closer to the fetal surface (Figure 521). The vessels that comprise this tumor may be capillary or sinusoidal (Figure 522). Frequently, the stromal component is abundant, and the lesion resembles a fibroma (Figure 523). When Wharton's jelly-like material participates in the formation of the tumor, the appearance is that of a myxomatous neoplasm. The latter is particularly frequent when a chorioangioma arises near the base of the umbilical cord (Figures 265, 266). In such cases, a mucicarmine stain reveals the presence of mucus (Dunn, 1959). The tumor is invariably covered by trophoblast; one may envisage it as the proliferation of fetal capillaries of a villus whose surface thus expands (Figures 524, 525). The tumors often have degenerative changes, calcification, infarcts, and thromboses, which may leave hemosiderin behind (Dunn, 1959). At times, thrombosis and infarction are clinically manifest with cessation of maternal symptomatology, such as the frequent hydramnios that is associated with these lesions. Chazotte et al. (1990) observed such a lesion sonographically in a fetus who also had meconium peritonitis; when the chorangioma shrank, there was some improvement of the hydramnios. The 5 cm chorangioma in the 620 g placenta had focal infarcts. Hsieh and Soong (1992) challenged this report and represented a larger lesion with hydrops. It would now be possible to laser-fulgurate the vessels that supply symptomatic chorioangiomas and thus treat the hydrops fetalis at its root cause.

Chorioangiomas may be small and multiple (Figure 526); alternatively, they may constitute large masses that displace villous tissue and bulge on the fetal surface. They are fleshy, dark, often congested, and invariably benign. Previous authors, impressed with mitoses and the great cellularity of some tumors, suggested that occasional chorioangiomas represent sarcomas. Metastases and true invasion, however, have never been seen. Cary (1914) considered his case of "sarcoma" to be well authenticated, but he did not provide photographs. Moreover, mother and infant did not suffer any known deleterious consequences from the 6.5 × 4.0 × 3.0 cm, focally calcified tumor.

The tumors labeled hemangioendothelioblastomas by Williams (1921) were apparently benign. Variability of the histological appearance, often within the same

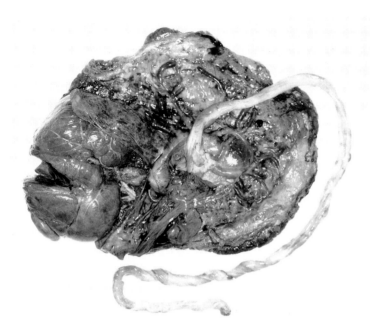

tumor, has confused many authors. Capillary, cavernous, endotheliomatous, fibrosing, and fibromatous tumors have been included in the nomenclature suggested by Schulz-Hetzel (1978). We believe that such precision is unwarranted because the clinical outcome is almost always the same, and it depends more on the size of the mass(es) than on the composition of the tumor(s). One may regard these tumors as hemangiomas or as hamartomas. The latter designation, however, probably is unwarranted as other placental elements (e.g., trophoblast) never participate in their composition. This would be expected if the designation ham-

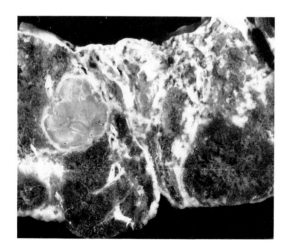

FIGURE 521. Partially infarcted 1 cm chorioangioma underneath the chorionic surface of an otherwise normal, mature placenta. It had a golden-yellow appearance and could easily have been mistaken for an infarct.

artoma were to apply, a point amply discussed by Marchetti (1939). This point was also examined in some detail by Barry et al. (1951) in a discussion of angiomas of cord and placenta. They ruled out that the lesions represent hamartomas and supported a neoplastic etiology.

It is theoretically possible to differentiate between a neoplasm or malformation-like tumor (hamartoma) with some precision. Linder and Gartler (1965) found that when they investigated leiomyomas of the uterus using glucose-6-phosphate dehydrogenase (G-6-PD) variants as markers in the frequently (15%) heterozygous black population, a single-cell origin was the rule for these neoplasms. The same was found to be true for most other tumors. "Congenital" tumors such as neurofibromas, on the other hand, had multiple cell derivation. They represent a malformation or hamartoma-like type of lesion. A study of chorioangiomas using this simple technique could be decisive in differentiating hamartoma from "true" neoplasm.

The relation of chorioangioma to hydramnios has been known at least since Siddall's extensive review in 1924. He observed that hydramnios was particularly associated with large tumors, but that the prognosis for the gravida was otherwise excellent. Marchetti (1939), who gathered 209 cases and added eight of his own, drew attention to the much commoner location of chorioangiomas near the fetal surface. He suggested their subdivision into three types and debated whether it represented a true tumor (he thought not) or a malformation, perhaps a hamartoma. The association with hydramnios was of particular interest to McInroy and Kelsey (1954). They saw a pregnancy from whose

FIGURE 522. Multiple chorioangiomas in a mature placenta, some of capillary type and others of more cavernous type. H&E. ×50.

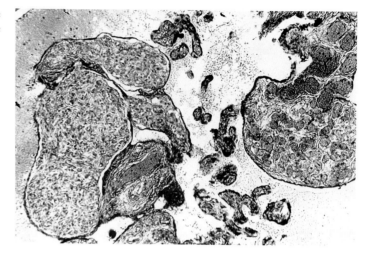

FIGURE 523. Chorioangioma with primarily fibromatous appearance. It measured 2.5 cm and occurred in a 29 weeks' gestation placenta. The cellularity of this lesion suggests that such tumors may represent sarcomas. H&E. ×170.

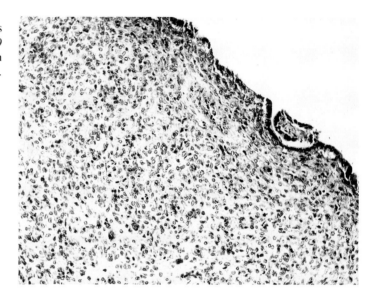

FIGURE 524. Chorioangioma that was associated with fetal transplacental exsanguination. The congested capillaries of the tumor are evident. The convexity of the tumor is covered by syncytiotrophoblast. H&E. ×160.

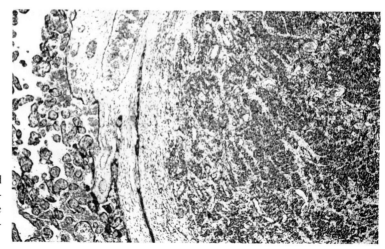

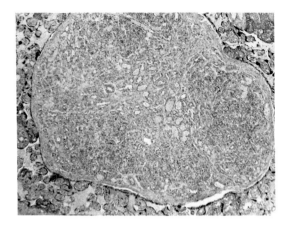

FIGURE 525. This chorioangioma displays the feature of overgrown capillaries in an enlarged villus covered by syncytium. H&E. ×40.

amnionic cavity 3,400 ml of amnionic fluid was withdrawn. The placental tumor weighed 454 g, measured 10.5 cm in greatest dimension, and had its own vascular pedicle. They suggested that the tumor represented "deadspace" and was therefore responsible for fluid exudation. Such a large tumor, associated with a stillborn fetus who had cardiomegaly, is shown in Figure 527. In an extensive consideration of this tumor, Kühnel (1933) opined that the tumor would have to cause venous obstruction before it could cause hydramnios.

Klaften (1929), who observed a patient with 6,000 ml of hydramnios and a 1,700 g stillbirth, found a fist-sized tumor bulging on the fetal surface of the placenta. He

discounted previous opinions that hydramnios was caused by the enlargement of amnionic surface from the bulging tumor mass. Rather, he believed that the tumor caused increased vascular resistance with transudation ensuing. A different mechanism for fetal hydrops was suggested by the case described in detail by Hirata et al. (1993). They discovered the 8.8 cm placental mass by Doppler and color flow mapping sonographically; and when hydrops developed, fetal blood sampling identified a hematocrit of only 17%. The hydrops improved after intrauterine transfusion. The anemia was attributed to microangiopathic hemolytic anemia, but a Kleihauer Betke test was not done on maternal blood. The latter might have shown transplacental bleeding, as has been observed in other cases.

Numerous large angiomas have been described. Lopez and Kristoffersen (1989) saw a patient with placenta previa at midgestation with sonographically recognized tumor. They suggested that placenta previa is one of several recognized complications with chorioangioma. The fetus was growth-retarded (899 g), and the placental tumor weighed 503 g. There are many reports of large chorioangiomas associated with hydramnios, hydrops fetalis, and fetal death. The placenta may be edematous and large in such cases. For instance, Knoth et al. (1976) found a 1,150 g placenta with multiple chorangiomas throughout the placenta, associated with a 3,250 g stillborn fetus. Other cases of fetal hydrops with large chorioangiomas were reported by Mandelbaum et al. (1969), Sweet et al. (1973), and Imakita et al. (1988).

The hearts of these newborns are often enlarged. The neonates may be severely anemic, and we believe that

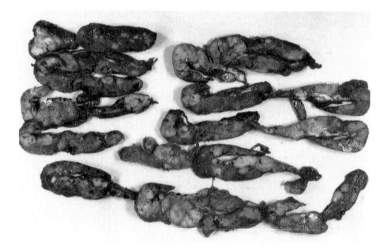

FIGURE 526. Chorioangiomatosis of the placenta. The nodular, pale lesions represent chorioangiomas, which comprise approximately 50% of the placenta. The lesions could easily have been mistaken for infarcts. The placenta weighed 430 g and was accompanied by a 3,200 g infant with cardiomegaly, anemia (hematocrit 40%), and thrombocytopenia at birth. Chromosomes were normal. (Courtesy Dr. P. Bromburger, Kaiser Hospital, San Diego.)

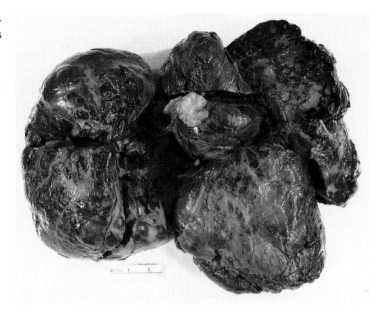

FIGURE 527. Exceptionally large (400 g) chorio-angioma shelled out from its placenta. The infant was stillborn and had cardiomegaly.

hydrops usually develops because of fetal heart failure. Similar observations are made when large fetal angiomas or arteriovenous fistulas cause hydrops (Cohen & Sinclair, 1963; Cooper & Bolande, 1965; Daniel & Cassady, 1968; Murray et al., 1969). Cardiomegaly alone was reported with the chorangioma described by Benson and Joseph (1961). That neoplasm measured 16 × 10 × 6 cm and weighed 542 g! High-output cardiac failure and hydramnios occurred with an 9 × 8 × 8 cm mass studied sonographically by Eldar-Geva et al. (1988).

Thrombocytopenia is also often observed in newborns whose placentas have chorioangiomas. It may be associated with heart failure and disseminated intravascular coagulation (Greene & Iams, 1984). Froehlich and Housler (1971) and Froehlich et al. (1971) described thrombocytopenia. The latter authors found the tumors to occur more frequently in white than in black mothers, more often with twins, and more often with malformed neonates. They mentioned an association with fetal angiomas, as did Leblanc and Carrier (1979). We have seen several neonates with hemangiomas whose placentas contained chorioangiomas, perhaps further supporting the notion that this tumor, similar to fetal angiomas, represents a congenital malformation, rather than a true neoplasm. Many authors have posed the same question. Drut et al. (1992) reported the presence of hemangioendotheliomas and multiple chorioangiomas in the Beckwith-Wiedemann syndrome and referred to a few case descriptions of similar combinations. The notion of hamartosis has also been inconclusively discussed. Demonstration of factor VIII within the neoplastic cells suggested to Majlessi and coauthors (1983) that the origin of the large and unusually cellular tumor

(327 g) they observed was endothelial. Sieracki et al. (1975), in a description of six cases, found one tumor with cells that resembled pericytes. Accordingly, they suggested the diagnosis of pericytoma. Hydropic bovine fetuses have been associated with chorioangiomas (Corcoran & Murphy, 1965), and Kirkbride et al. (1973) found an aborted calf with dermal, oral, and placental angiomas. Limaye and Tchabo (1989) observed maternal thrombocytopenia during the course of a pregnancy that was complicated by a 5 cm chorioangioma. They believed that the thrombocytopenia was the result of necrosis in the angioma.

Several authors have noted that chorioangiomas were associated with preeclampsia (e.g., Heggtveit et al., 1965). Stiller and Skafish (1986) found fetomaternal hemorrhage with a placenta that had eight chorioangiomas. Santamaria et al. (1987) saw fetal exsanguination result from such tumors. Perhaps the significantly increased fetal circulation caused by large tumors produces fetal growth retardation (Müller & Rieckert, 1967; Mahmood, 1977; King & Lovrien, 1978). In a series of seven chorioangiomas, Philippe et al. (1969) found four underdeveloped fetuses. Adducci (1975) reported fetal distress resulting from a large chorangioma. Aside from hydramnios, it is frequently reported that premature delivery and placenta previa are associated with chorioangiomas. Asadourian and Taylor (1968) described the occurrence of abruptio placentae with this placental tumor. Premature separation was also seen by Sulman and Sulman (1949), who additionally reported elevated maternal human chorionic gonadotropin (hCG) titers. Others have also found altered levels of pregnancy hormones with large chorioangiomas.

"Giant chorioangiomas" have been alluded to in several publications (e.g., Burrows et al., 1973: 570 g); the record is probably held by the 1,500 g (30 × 20 × 5 cm) tumor described by Arodi et al. (1985). It was associated with breech presentation, placenta previa, hydramnios, preeclampsia, and abruptio placentae. The 32 weeks' gestation fetus weighed 1,000 g and died from anemia and asphyxia.

Placental chorioangiomas present other challenging pathological features. Although placentomegaly, often with typical hydropic villi, is probably directly related to cardiac failure, anemia, and hypoproteinemia, there is no good explanation for an associated umbilical artery thrombosis as described by Sen (1970). Reiner and Fries (1965) found arteriovenous fistulas in their injection study of a chorioangioma; the neonate experienced rapidly disappearing cardiomegaly. Repetitive multiple chorioangiomas were noted by Battaglia and Woolever (1968), who speculated that sequestration of plasma proteins into the interstices of the lesion may have accounted for the associated hypoproteinemia and

edema of their case. Earn and Penner (1950) depicted a chorioangioma that was separate from the placenta; it was attached by a long vascular pedicle whose vein was diffusely calcified. The macerated fetus associated with this placenta was hydropic. Sonographic diagnosis has repeatedly been made of chorioangiomas and was well described by Dao et al. (1981), who found two large tumors (see also Hirata et al., 1993).

Because we had previously found a severely retarded fraternal twin that had a chromosomal error [46,XX t(2q−; 15q+)], with angiomatous masses in the placenta (Wurster et al., 1969) (Figure 528), we later studied a single chorangioma cytogenetically; it was normal (Kim et al., 1971). Ultrastructural studies done at the same time showed normal endothelial cells and capillaries. Subsequent electron microscopic studies of chorioangiomas were performed by Cash and Powell (1980); they revealed no major additional features. Soma et al. (1991) also studied the tumors electron microscopically and found them to be composed of angioblastic proliferation.

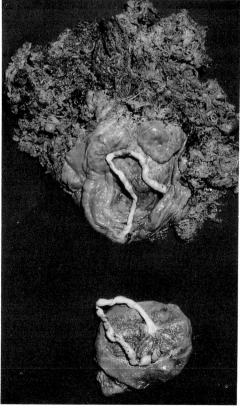
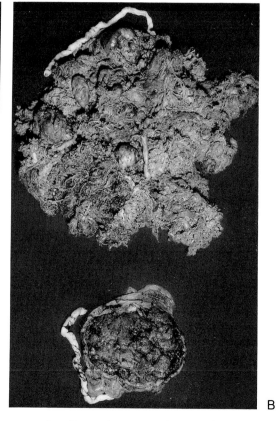

A

B

FIGURE 528. Placentas of dizygotic twins at term. The mother had had five pregnancies, was age 34, and suffered hydramnios at 36 weeks in this gestation. Twin A was a normal female infant (2,585 g) with a placenta that weighed 420 g. Twin B was male (1,642 g) with a placenta weighing 3,600 g; it was interpreted as a mole. Microscopically, there was primarily angiomatous change of the entire placenta, and the fetus had a translocation with duplication. (Reprinted with permission of Wurster, et al., Placental chorangiomata and mental deficiency in a child with 2/15 translocation. Cytogenetics 8:389–399, Karger, Basel, 1969.)

One publication suggested that a missing link might have been found between chorioangiomas and chorioarcinomas. Jauniaux et al. (1988) described a lesion they termed chorangiocarcinoma. The placenta of this 35 weeks' pregnancy contained a solitary small nodule fairly typical of a chorioangioma. Its surface, however, was covered by apparently proliferated trophoblastic epithelium. The mother and child did well; there was no other chemical or cytochemical evidence of chorioarcinoma. Electron microscopy was no more decisive in suggesting that it was a combination of the two disparate tumors.

OTHER BENIGN TUMORS

Some benign tumors of the placenta have been discussed in Chapters 12, 13, and 25. There are, for instance, rare teratomas (Castaldo et al., 1972; Fox, 1978), possibly representing twins. The partial hydatidiform moles, not representing true tumors, are covered in Chapters 21 and 22. Heterotopic tissues, such as adrenal gland, have occasionally occurred in the placenta. They were never neoplastic, but they have occasionally been associated with a growth-retarded infant (Cox & Chavrier, 1980). Fox (1978) had suggested that acceptable placental teratomas should reside on the fetal surface of the placenta.

Only one other report, that by Chen et al. (1986), presented a novel type of placental tumor. It was a presumed hepatocellular adenoma. The authors observed a small-for-gestational-age (1,781 g at 37 weeks) infant with a 530-g placenta that contained a 7.0 × 4.2 × 2.7 cm firm mass. The tumor was tan-white, sharply delimited, and composed of polyhedral cells that had the appearance of hepatocytes. There was no bile pigment, but the cells contained glycogen; and some of them reacted with antibodies to α-fetoprotein and α1-antitrypsin. Study by electron microscopy showed structures that strongly resembled bile canaliculi. The authors believed that the lesion was a "monodermal teratoma," although it was not on the placental surface. The fetus and mother had an entirely benign course.

Chorangiosis, Chorangiomatosis

The terminology for chorangiosis and chorioangiomatosis is poorly defined; indeed, Marchetti considered that this lesion was merely a diffuse ectasia of placental villous capillaries. One may possibly think of chorangiomatosis as representing multiple chorioangiomas, but chorangiosis is most certainly not a neoplastic condition. Because of its histological similarity to some aspects of chorioangioma, it may as well be discussed here, although it has a decidedly different pathogenesis. Meyenburg (1922) had considered this lesion as diffuse hemangiomatosis of the placenta, but it was Hörmann (1958) who coined the term chorioangiosis. Later authors suggested that it results from abnormal maturation of villi and hypoxia. In particular, the differentia-

tion from the congestion of diabetic mothers' placentas has caused confusion in the literature.

Caldwell et al. (1977) considered this lesion a "vascular anomaly of the placental villi with increased capillarity of their stroma." They saw a 3,100-g infant whose mother had received isoxsuprine over 5 months for vaginal bleeding and uterine contractions. The infant had thrombocytopenia and petechiae. Also present were hydramnios and a circumvallate placenta that weighed 1,770 g and measured 24.0 × 23.0 × 6.5 cm. It was unusually thick. The villi had hugely distended vessels that were numerically increased. As is true with chorioangiomas, the depressed platelet count was probably the result of sequestration in the placental capillaries.

It was not until Altshuler (1984) considered this entity in considerable detail that some clarity resulted about the nature of chorangiosis. He diagnosed the condition principally by low-power lens inspection of histological sections: "Chorangiosis was diagnosed when inspection with a ×10 objective, showed 10 villi, each with 10 or more vascular channels in 10 or more noninfarcted and nonischemic zones of at least three different placental areas." He graded chorangiosis from grade 1 to 3, depending on the profusion of vessels within villi. He found an overall incidence of 5.5% among 1,350 placentas and distinguished it clearly from congestion.

Chorangiosis is not common but has an ominous connotation (Benirschke, 1994a). Altshuler saw it associated with high frequency in stillbirths and many perinatal circumstances that suggest long-standing hypoxia. Thus it is more commonly observed in the placentas of babies who develop cerebral palsy. We find it often with cord problems of one kind or another (Benirschke, 1994b). The increase in capillary lumen cross sections seen in this lesion comes about, we believe, through endothelial proliferation. It thus takes time to develop. Perhaps it takes as long as weeks to develop full-blown marked chorangiosis. Its presence betrays a deleterious intrauterine environment for the fetus, and we see in its manifestation an attempt (teleologically speaking) of the placenta to enlarge its diffusional surface. It is thus not surprising to note that somewhat similar observations were made in placentas from high altitude when they were quantitatively compared with those of lower strata (Jackson et al., 1987; Reshetnikova et al., 1993; many others).

Placental villous congestion is particularly prominent with uncontrolled diabetes; and in my experience it may mask this lesion if one is not careful (Figure 529). With chorangiosis there is an obvious numerical increase of the vessels per villus; with congestion the vessels are merely distended. Chorangiosis correlates significantly with perinatal deaths (39%) (e.g., Keenan & Altshuler,

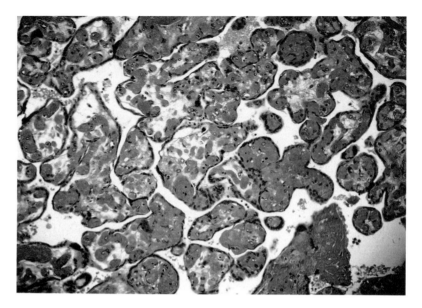

FIGURE 529. Severe villous congestion in a mature placenta from a trisomy 21 pregnancy. This picture is difficult to distinguish from that of chorangiosis. Quantitative measurements and vessel counts are necessary to make a clear distinction. H&E. ×160.

1975) and congenital anomalies (27%) and has thus been deemed to be an important signal for scrutiny, particularly in placentomegaly. Its final etiology, if a specific one really exists, remains to be elucidated.

References

Adducci, J.E.: Chorioangioma of the placenta: causing fetal distress. Minn. Med. 58:820–821, 1975.

Altshuler, G.: Chorangiosis: an important placental sign of neonatal morbidity and mortality. Arch. Pathol. Lab. Med. 108:71–74, 1984.

Arodi, J., Auslender, R., Atad, J., and Abramovici, H.: Case report: giant chorioangioma of the placenta. Acta Obstet. Gynecol. Scand. 64:91–92, 1985.

Asadourian, L.A., and Taylor, H.B.: Clinical significance of placental hemangiomas. Obstet. Gynecol. 31:551–555, 1968.

Barry, F.E., McCoy, C.P., and Callahan, W.P.: Hemangioma of the umbilical cord. Am. J. Obstet. Gynecol. 62:675–680, 1951.

Battaglia, F.C., and Woolever, C.A.: Fetal and neonatal complications associated with recurrent chorioangiomas. Pediatrics 41:62–66, 1968.

Benirschke, K.: Placenta pathology: questions to the perinatologist. J. Perinatol. (1994a).

Benirschke, K.: Obstetrically important lesions of the umbilical cord. J. Reprod. Med. 39:262–272, 1994b.

Benson, P.F., and Joseph, M.C.: Cardiomegaly in a newborn due to placental chorioangioma. B.M.J. 1:102–105, 1961.

Burrows, S., Gaines, J.L., and Hughes, F.J.: Giant chorioangioma. Am. J. Obstet. Gynecol. 115:579–580, 1973.

Caldwell, C., Purohit, D.M., Levkoff, A.H., Garvin, A.J., Williamson, H.O., and Horger III, E.O.: Chorangiosis of the placenta with persistent transitional circulation. Am. J. Obstet. Gynecol. 127:435–436, 1977.

Cary, W.H.: Report of a well-authenticated case of sarcoma of the placenta. Am. J. Obstet. 69:658–664, 1914.

Cash, J.B., and Powell, D.E.: Placental chorioangioma: presentation of a case with electron-microscopic and immunochemical studies. Am. J. Surg. Pathol. 4:87–92, 1980.

Castaldo, F., Guariglia, L., Lanzone, A., Marana, R., and Plotti, G.: Tumori non trofoblastici della placenta. I. Tumori primitivi. Recenti Prog. Med. 70:445–456, 1981.

Chazotte, C., Girz, B., Koenigsberg, M., and Cohen, W.R.: Spontaneous infarction of placental chorioangioma and associated regression of hydrops fetalis. Am. J. Obstet. Gynecol. 163:1180–1181, 1990.

Chen, K.T.K., Ma, C.K., and Kassel, S.H.: Hepatocellular adenoma of the placenta. Am. J. Surg. Pathol. 10:436–440, 1986.

Cohen, M.I., and Sinclair, J.C.: Neonatal death from congestive heart failure associated with large cutaneous cavernous hemangioma. Pediatrics 32:924–925, 1963.

Cooper, A.G., and Bolande, R.P.: Multiple hemangiomas in an infant with cardiac hypertrophy: postmortem angiographic demonstration of the arteriovenous fistulae. Pediatrics 35:27–35, 1965

Corcoran, C.J., and Murphy, E.C.: Rare bovine placental tumour—a case report. Vet. Rec. 77:1234–1235, 1965.

Cox, J.N., and Chavrier, F.: Heterotopic adrenocortical tissue within a placenta. Placenta 1:131–133, 1980.

Daniel, S.J., and Cassady, G.: Non-immunologic hydrops fetalis associated with a large hemangioendothelioma. Pediatrics 42:829–833, 1968.

Dao, A.H., Rogers, C.W., and Wong, S.W.: Chorioangioma of the placenta: report of 2 cases with ultrasound study in 1. Obstet. Gynecol. 57:46S–49S, 1981.

Drut, R., Drut, R.M., and Toulouse, J.C.: Hepatic hemangioendotheliomas, placental chorioangiomas, and dysmorphic kidneys in Beckwith-Wiedemann syndrome. Pediatr. Pathol. 12:197–203, 1992.

Dunn, R.I.S.: Haemangioma of the placenta (chorioangioma). J. Obstet. Gynaecol. Br. Emp. 66:51–57, 1959.

Earn, A.A., and Penner, D.W.: Five cases of chorioangioma. J. Obstet. Gynaecol. Br. Emp. 57:442–444, 1950.

Eldar-Geva, T., Hochner-Celnikier, D., Ariel, I., Ron, M., and Yagel, S.: Fetal high output cardiac failure and acute hydramnios caused by large placental chorioangioma: case report. Br. J. Obstet. Gynaecol. 95:1200–1203, 1988.

Fox, H.: Vascular tumors of the placenta. Obstet. Gynecol. Surv. 22:697–711, 1967.

Fox, H.: Pathology of the Placenta. Saunders, London, 1978.

Froehlich, L.A., and Housler, M.: Neonatal thrombocytopenia and chorangioma. J. Pediatr. 78:516–519, 1971.

Froehlich, L.A., Fujikura, T., and Fisher, P.: Chorioangiomas and their clinical implications. Obstet. Gynecol. 37:51–59, 1971.

Greene, E.E., and Iams, J.D.: Chorioangioma: a case presentation. Am. J. Obstet. Gynecol. 148:1146–1148, 1984.

Heggtveit, H.A., de Carvalho R., and Nuyens, A.J.: Chorioangioma and toxemia of pregnancy. Am. J. Obstet. Gynecol. 91:291–292, 1965.

Hirata, G.I., Masaki, D.I., O'Toole, M., Medearis, A.L., and Platt, L.D.: Color flow mapping and Doppler velocimetry in the diagnosis and management of a placental chorioangioma assocviated with nonimmune fetal hydrops. Obstet. Gynecol. 81:850–852, 1993.

Hörmann, G.: Zur Systematik einer Pathologie der menschlichen Plazenta. Arch. Gynecol. 191:297–344, 1958.

Hsieh, C.-C., and Soong, Y.-K.: Infarction of placental chorioangioma and associated regression of hydrops fetalis. Am. J. Obstet. Gynecol. 166:1306, 1992.

Imakita, M., Yutani, C., Ishibashi-Ueda, H., Murakami, M., and Chiba, Y.: A case of hydrops fetalis due to placental chorioangioma. Acta Pathol. Jpn. 38:941–945, 1988.

Jackson, M.R., Mayhew, T.M., and Haas, J.D.: Morphometric studies on villi in human term placentae and the effects of altitude, ethnic grouping and sex of newborn. Placenta 8:487–495, 1987.

Jauniaux, E., Zucker, M., Meuris, S., Verherst, A., Wilkin, P., and Hustin, J.: Chorangiocarcinoma: an unusual tumour of the placenta: the missing link? Placenta 9:607–613, 1988.

Keenan, W.J., and Altshuler, G.: Massive pulmonary hemorrhage in a neonate. J. Pediatr. 86:466–471, 1975.

Kim, C.K., Benirschke, K., and Connolly, K.S.: Chorangioma of the placenta: chromosomal and electron microscopic studies. Obstet. Gynecol. 37:372–376, 1971.

King, C.R., and Lovrien, E.W.: Chorioangioma of the placenta and intrauterine growth failure. J. Pediatr. 93:1027–1028, 1978.

Kirkbride, C.A., Bicknell, E.J., and Robl, M.G.: Hemangioma of a bovine fetus with a chorioangioma of the placenta. Vet. Pathol. 10:238–240, 1973.

Klaften, E.: Chorionhaemangioma placentae. Z. Geburtshilfe Gynäkol. 95:426–437, 1929.

Knoth, M., Rygaard, J., and Hesseldahl, H.: Chorioangioma with hydramnios and intra-uterine fetal death. Acta Obstet. Gynecol. Scand. 55:279–281, 1976.

Kühnel, P.: Placental chorangioma. Acta Obstet. Gynecol. Scand. 13:143–194, 1933.

Leblanc, A., and Carrier, C.: Chorio-angiome placentaire, angiomes cutanes et cholestase néonatale. Arch. Fr. Pediatr. 36:484–486, 1979.

Limaye, N.S., and Tchabo, J.-G.: Asymptomatic thrombocytopenia associated with chorioangioma of placenta. Am. J. Obstet. Gynecol. 161:76–77, 1989.

Linder, D., and Gartler, S.M.: Glucose-6-phosphate dehydrogenase mosaicism: utilization as a cell marker in the study of leiomyomas. Science 150:67–69, 1965.

Lopez, H.B.B., and Kristoffersen, S.E.: Chorioangioma of the placenta. Gynecol. Obstet. Invest. 28:108–110, 1989.

Mahmood, K.: Small chorioangiomas and small-for-gestational age baby. Am. J. Obstet. Gynecol. 127:440–442, 1977.

Majlessi, H.F., Wagner, K.M., and Brooks, J.J.: Atypical cellular chorangioma of the placenta. Int. J. Gynecol. Pathol. 1:403–408, 1983.

Mandelbaum, B., Ross, M., and Riddle, C.B.: Hemangioma of the placenta associated with fetal anemia and edema: report of a case. Obstet. Gynecol. 34:335–338, 1969.

Marchetti, A.A.: A consideration of certain types of benign tumors of the placenta. Surg. Gynecol. Obstet. 68:733–743, 1939.

McInroy, R.A., and Kelsey, H.A.: Chorio-angioma (haemangioma of placenta) associated with acute hydramnios. J. Pathol. Bacteriol. 68:519–523, 1954.

Meyenburg, H.V.: Über Hämangiomatosis diffusa placentae. Beitr. Pathol. Anat. Allg. Pathol. 70:510–512, 1922.

Müller, G., and Rieckert, H.: Beitrag zur Frage der Placentarinsuffizienz an Hand eines diffusen Chorangioms. Arch. Gynecol. 204:78–88, 1967.

Murray, D.E., Meyerowitz, B.R., and Hutter, J.J.: Congenital arteriovenous fistula causing congestive heart failure in the newborn. J.A.M.A. 209:770–771, 1969.

Philippe, E., Muller, G., Dehalleux, J.-M., Lefakis, P., and Gandar, R.: Le chorio-angiome et ses complications foetomaternelles. Rev. Fr. Gynecol. 64:335–341, 1969.

Reiner, L., and Fries, E.: Chorangioma associated with arteriovenous aneurysm. Am. J. Obstet. Gynecol. 93:58–64, 1965.

Reshetnikova, O.S., Burton, G.J., and Milovanov, A.P.: Hypoxia at altitude and villous vascularisation in the mature human placenta [abstract]. Placenta 14:A62, 1993.

Santamaria, M., Benirschke, K., Carpenter, P.M., Baldwin, V.J., and Pritchard, J.A.: Transplacental hemorrhage associated with placental neoplasms. Pediatr. Pathol. 7:601–615, 1987.

Schulz-Hetzel, I.: Über das Chorioangiom. Arch. Gynecol. 225:131–146, 1978.

Sen, D.K.: Placental hypertrophy associated with chorangioma. Am. J. Obstet. Gynecol. 107:652–654, 1970.

Siddall, R.S.: Chorioangiofibroma (chorioangioma). Am. J. Obstet. Gynecol. 8:430–456, 554–568, 1924.

Sieracki, J.C., Panke, T.W., Horvat, B.L., Perrin, E.V., and
Nanda, B.: Chorioangiomas. Obstet. Gynecol. 46:155–159,
1975.

Soma, H., Satoh, M., Higashi, S., Ogura, H., Horikiri, H.,
and Hata, T.: Ultrastructure of choriocarcinoma. J. Clin.
Electron Microsc. 24:5–6, 1991.

Stiller, A.G., and Skafish, P.R.: Placental chorangioma: a
rare cause of fetomaternal transfusion with maternal
hemolysis and fetal distress. Obstet. Gynecol. 67:296–298,
1986.

Sulman, F.G., and Sulman, E.: Increased gonadotrophin production in a case of detachment of placenta due to placental
haemangioma. J. Obstet. Gynaecol. Br. Emp. 56:1033–
1034, 1949.

Sweet, L., Reid, W.D., and Robertson, N.R.C.: Hydrops
fetalis in association with chorioangioma of the placenta.
J. Pediatr. 82:91–94, 1973.

Wallenburg, H.C.S.: Chorioangioma of the placenta: thirteen
new cases and a review of the literature from 1939–1970
with special reference to the clinical complications. Obstet.
Gynecol. Surv. 26:411–425, 1971.

Williams, J.T.: Angioma of the placenta: with pathological
report and microphotography by Dr. Frank B. Mallory.
Surg. Gynecol. Obstet. 32:523–526, 1921.

Wurster, D.H., Hoefnagel, D., Benirschke, K., and Allen,
F.H.: Placental chorangiomata and mental deficiency in
a child with 2/15 translocation; 46XX; t(2q−; 15q+).
Cytogenetics 8:389–399, 1969.

25
Multiple Pregnancy

In a remarkable paper that correlates prenatal events and discordance of twins with postnatal outcome, Price (1950) most emphasized the importance of "prenatal biases." He was much concerned with the influence of placentation on twin development, an aspect that had not often been considered in twin studies. Similar ideas have been echoed by Phillips (1993), who emphasized the influence of the proximity of twin placentas on their ability to support fetal growth. It was Galton (1875), however, cousin of Darwin and after whom the Galton Institute of Genetics in London is named, who was probably the first to suggest that twins, if properly studied, would yield information that might allow us to discriminate between the effects of heredity and those of the environment. It was his famous nature versus nurture concept. The extensive studies conducted by Friedrich Schatz at the same time suggested that prenatal influences among twins found reflection in the ultimate outcome of the twins. He was instrumental in clarifying that placental study is essential for this understanding. His extensive work is annotated in a bibliographic oddity (Schatz, 1900) that summarizes all of his papers and citations therein. His numerous contributions were partially translated for the book on twin placentation by Strong and Corney (1967). A concise review of the biological aspects of the human twinning process was published by Benirschke and Kim (1973), and a volume on twinning and twins by MacGillivray and his colleagues (1988) summarizes most relevant aspects of this interesting phenomenon of nature. Baldwin (1994) has produced a remarkable volume that contains all relevant aspects of placentation of multiple pregnancy, and it is well illustrated.

No doubt the complexity of human twinning cannot be understood without knowledge of the placentation of twins. Moreover, despite all the benefits reaped from animal studies, the placentation of most relevant species is often dissimilar from that of humans. Thus conclusions drawn from their multiple pregnancies must be interpreted with great care.

ZYGOSITY

There are "fraternal" (better named dizygotic, DZ) and "identical" (monozygotic, MZ) twins. With higher multiple births, these entities may be admixed. That such different classes of twins exist derives from several observations. Fraternal twins may be of different or like sex. A hypothesis is herein helpful: if all twins were DZ, one would expect a sex ratio similar to that for singletons (i.e. approximately 50% MF, 25% MM, and 25% FF). It is not the case. When large bodies of statistics of infants' sex at birth are studied, it is found that there is an excess of like-sex twins. This excess is presumed to result from the number of MZ (identical) twins. By subtracting the MZ twins from the total number of twins, an estimate is obtained for the distribution of MZ and DZ twins in a population—the so-called Weinberg rule (1901). [Hrubec and Robinette (1984) pointed out that the basis for this rule had previously been published by Bertillon (1874)]. Weinberg's "differential method" can be stated with the following formula:

$$\text{MZ twins} = \text{all twins} - \frac{\text{unlike-sex twins}}{2\,pq}$$

(p = frequency of male births; q = frequency of female births in a population).

Weinberg's formula should be taken as providing estimates, with considerable errors, if it is taken literally. It is particularly understandable when one considers the frequencies of different classes of twins as they exist at the time of conception, as there is much evidence that MZ twins have a higher prenatal death rate than do DZ twins. The Weinberg method cannot correct for losses of only one twin in a gestation—information that is also usually not recorded in birth statistics. It is therefore not surprising that the method has often been criticized (e.g., Renkonen, 1967; and reply by Cannings, 1969; James, 1971, 1983; Keith, 1974). Nevertheless, it is a unique and valuable tool for assessing the approximate frequency of DZ versus MZ twins in a population. Moreover, a prospective study that attempted to validate the method has found that the results agree well with findings from placentation and known zygosity of twins (Vlietinck et al., 1988). An interesting observation by James (1971) is that among DZ twins there is an excess of like-sex pairs. This observation is based on small samples of twins whose zygosity was ascertained by blood grouping. It has so far remained unexplained, but some additional data (James, 1977a,b) show an even more marked excess of females among monoamnionic, monochorionic (MoMo) twins and perhaps in acardiacs. More light has been shed on this phenomenon by the large study of Derom et al. (1988). These authors provided data from the Belgian prospective twin study that included zygosity diagnosis and placental assessment. Not only was the proportion of males reduced among MZ twins (irrespective of chorion status) but there was a marked reduction of male MoMo twins from what might be expected if this form of twinning occurred at random. The sex proportion of all MZ twins was 0.487 and that of MoMo 0.231; the DZ twins had a proportion of 0.518. Although no large data bodies are yet available, Derom et al., cited evidence that conjoined twins at term are more commonly female, whereas those of abortuses may be more often male. Of the two possibilities to explain this unexpected observation— higher frequency of late twinning in female conceptuses and higher abortion rate of male MoMo conceptuses—they favored the former. They referred to the suggestion made by Burn et al. (1986) that "unequal lyonization" of X chromosomes may be a cause of late twinning, and that it is unique to females. The apparent excess of female acardiacs is possibly further confirmation (James, 1977a,b).

Considerations of the MZ twinning rates come from Allen and Hrubec (1987), who proposed that a slight suggestion exists of a relation of the MZ twinning rate to maternal age, as is certain for DZ twins. These "constants" of DZ to MZ twin frequencies identified from various statistical considerations, however, are still considered to be arbitrary; and they appear to differ among various populations.

Other reasons for considering that a proportion of twins is "identical," or monozygotic, come from the numerous reports on genetic "identity" and the physical similarity exhibited by some twins. Twin research has traditionally involved ascertainment of zygosity by assessment of likeness. Dermatoglyphics (Newman, 1931a; Allen, 1968; Brismar, 1968; Herrlin et al., 1970; Reed et al., 1975), and blood grouping (Robertson, 1969; Selvin, 1970) are two of many parameters that have been employed. However, these methods have not always been decisive in assigning the zygosity for an individual set of twins, although their general reliability is high. For that reason, methods such as mixed leukocyte reaction (Jarvik et al., 1969), skin exchange graft survival (Stranc, 1966), and repeated blood group study (Osborne, 1958) have been advocated. Analysis of banded chromosomes, C bands and Q bands, has been used to ascertain monozygosity (Neurath et al., 1972; McCracken et al., 1978; Morton et al., 1981; Pedrosa et al., 1983). Until recently, this methodology has been the most reliable. These methods established mostly probabilities of twins' zygosity, and they were often somewhat imprecise. The mathematical aspects of phenotypic likeness studies have been treated by Meulepas et al. (1988). New methods have now been developed that are more decisive.

The new techniques for the direct comparison of DNA variants have much to be recommended as primary tools. They determine the restriction fragments lengths polymorphism (RFLP) of twins. These methods of comparing fragments of DNA are quick; they can be executed on placental tissue, blood, and other tissues; and they are decisive (Derom et al., 1985; Hill & Jeffreys, 1985). Importantly, the quantities of tissue needed for this study can be small when combined with the polymerase chain reaction (PCR). More recently, the use of microsatellites has proved useful and rapid in the definitive differential diagnosis of MZ versus DZ twins (Erdmann et al., 1993). Thus antenatal samples may readily be processed by this and related modern techniques for accurate determination of twin zygosity (Kovacs et al., 1988) and has been decisively used to identify the genetic relations between twins and

triplets (Motomura et al., 1987; Azuma et al., 1989). It is of further interest that this method can also be used to identify DNA patterns of macerated stillborn fetuses (Derom et al., 1989). Neuman and her colleagues (1990) have proved with RFLPs the dizygosity of tubal aborted twins and suggested that the alleged common monozygosity of ectopic twins is in error.

The least decisive method for the identification of the zygosity of twins—the likeness assessment—is also the most widely practiced method. It is the easiest method to execute, and it correctly asserts that physical characteristics are more alike in MZ twins than they are in DZ twins (e.g., tooth morphology: Lundström, 1963; skin color: Collins et al., 1966; cardiac findings: Preis & Srubarova, 1966; immunoglobulin levels: Sowards & Monif, 1972; cholesterol levels: Corey et al., 1975). A fairly reliable accuracy of zygosity diagnosis is said to be achieved with other simple tests, including the use of questionnaires (Cederlöf et al., 1961; Nichols & Bilbro, 1966). These oversimplifications have, however, also led to much misconception. Moreover, they have confused the neonatologist who cares for often markedly discordant twins during the neonatal period, who requires better guidelines for the care of neonatal twins than are generally available to clinicians.

It is now certain that MZ twins are frequently discordant in terms of development; some of this discordance can be secondary to unique placental vascular relations between twins (Schatz, 1886; Verschuer, 1927; Price, 1950); others have their cause in abnormal placentation. Discordance for congenital anomalies is higher in MZ twins than in DZ twins, a feature that has been critically analyzed by Boklage (1987a). Triplets share this feature, according to Suslak et al. (1987). Melnick and Myrianthopoulos (1979) found that the twofold increase of anomalies in MZ twins cannot be validly ascribed to the monochorionic placental status that is so prevalent in MZ twins. An exception, of course, are acardiacs and the destructive results from prenatal disseminated intravascular coagulation (DIC), which depend in their origin on the monochorionic status of the twin placenta. These authors suggested as a possible explanation that the impetus for MZ twinning may be similar to that which is the cause of the developmental anomalies. The relative frequency of anomalies in MZ twins (6–9%, with 80% discordance) has important implications with respect to prenatal diagnosis of early embryos (Jarmulowicz, 1989). It has been suggested that with the new methodology of PCR of DNA amplification, single blastomeres might be sexed and genetically defined in the future. It is unknown at this time if such loss of blastomeres could result in anomalies, or if the discordant anomalies of MZ twins are perhaps caused by the unequal splitting of the morula. These questions are important for future research.

Twin studies, as advocated by Galton (1875), endeavor to discern between genetic and environmental influences on fetal development. To be successful, they require accurate zygosity determination of the probands. Walker (1957) stated this requirement emphatically. Moreover, it has been found that if the linkage of genetic traits is not taken into consideration in the zygosity assignment, the probability of monozygosity is overestimated (Sorensen & Fenger, 1974). Kempthorne and Osborne (1961) and Allen and Hrubec (1979) have developed models to undertake such analyses. Allen (1965) has proposed excellent guidelines for the design of twin studies that should be consulted.

Placenta in the Study of Zygosity

To derive any benefit from placental studies for twin research, it is mandatory that the umbilical cords be labeled in the order they are delivered for identification of the infants. It is best done by placing one or more ties or clamps around the placental cut ends of the cords. Examination of twin placentas (and those of higher multiple births) may then contribute to the determination of zygosity and an understanding of abnormal events. It is also mandatory that a placental record be made. The latter is needed for an understanding of discordant development of twins and for our understanding of many other pathological features that twins present. The proposition that all monochorionic placentas belong to MZ twins (but that not all MZ twins have monochorial placentas) was first clearly stated in the seminal contribution of Curtius (1930). He then called for a detailed reexamination of the understanding of placentation in humans. In general, this proposition has been amply confirmed, for instance in the recent placental study of 182 like-sexed live-born twins by Ramos-Arroyo et al. (1988).

In principle, there are two types of twin placentation: monochorionic and dichorionic. With higher multiple births the types may be admixed, or one or the other types may be present. Monochorionic placentas, we believe, always come from MZ (identical) twins. The reason for this assumption is that no verified monochorial human placenta has been associated with twins of unlike sex. Furthermore, when genetic markers are studied in monochorionic twins, they are always identical (Corney et al., 1968); the rare exceptions are discussed below. Dichorionic placentas, however, may be associated with both DZ and MZ twins; most are associated with DZ twins. A decisive study of this topic is that of Cameron (1968), who examined the placentas of 668 twin pairs and determined their zygosity with studies of blood groups and placental enzymes. From the fetal sex and the structure of the placental membranes alone, the zygosity could be ascribed accurately in 55%. Genotyping was necessary in the remaining 45%. His analysis gave the following results.

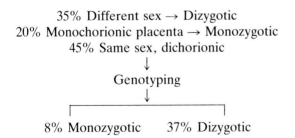

35% Different sex → Dizygotic
20% Monochorionic placenta → Monozygotic
45% Same sex, dichorionic
↓
Genotyping
↓

8% Monozygotic   37% Dizygotic

Of his 668 pairs, 80% had diamnionic, dichorionic (DiDi) placentas; and of these pairs, 90% were DZ. There were 20% monochorionic and therefore monozygotic twins. With the improved methodology of modern sonographic equipment, it is often possible to make the diagnosis of chorionic status before birth.

D'Alton and Dudley (1989) made the correct diagnosis in 68 of 69 prospectively studied cases using ultrasonography and counting the layers of the dividing membranes. Winn et al. (1989) suggested sonographic criteria for assessing the width of the dividing membranes. At amniocentesis done for genetic reasons, the thickness of this dividing membrane was measured in 32 patients. The cutoff point was a width of 2 mm. An accuracy of 82% was said to be achieved by this means. This method may be helpful in the future management of twin gestations. Finberg (1992) found that the "twin peak sign" was diagnostic of dichorionic twinning. He showed that a triangular projection of membranes can be seen above the placental surface in dichorionic twins or triplets.

Monochorionic twin placentas virtually always present as single disks. It is most unusual for monochorionic twin placentas to possess separate placental masses; and often they are then connected with small bridges. Nevertheless, Altshuler and Hyde (1993) have described such an exceptional case in which two completely separate disks were connected by a thin bridge. Underneath the chorion of this bridge was atrophied villous tissue. Rare observations of two disks in monochorionic twins have been made in conjoined twins (see below). Monochorionic twin placentas fall into two categories: (1) the monoamnionic monochorionic (MoMo) twin placentas in which the twins are in the same sac; and (2) the diamnionic, monochorionic (DiMo) placenta. The MoMo placenta is the least common. It is also associated with the highest perinatal mortality of twins. The higher mortality and complication rate for monozygotic twins has been critically examined by Kovacs et al. (1989). Multiple births not only have higher perinatal mortality, they also have greater morbidity. Because of the inordinate contribution to adverse outcomes, Powers and Kiely (1994) provided U.S.-based population figures that suggested "to lower the rates of adverse outcomes in twin pregnancies should become a major public health priority."

Dichorionic (DiDi) twin placentas may be fused into one mass (DiDi fused), or they may be separated (DiDi separate) organs (Benirschke, 1958). From a practical consideration of the analysis of the placentation of individual twins, it is important to first examine these membrane relations. It is most reliably done by making a cross section of the dividing membranes (i.e., the partition between the two sacs). By excising and rolling a square of these dividing membranes, the two types can then be differentiated (Figure 530). As an alternative method, one may take for histological study a section from the site where the membranes insert on the placental surface, a T section, as seen in Figure 531. This method has been particularly well illustrated by Allen and Turner (1971). Either of these methods for

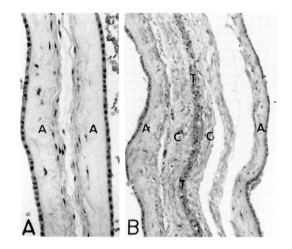

FIGURE 530. (A) Diamnionic monochorionic dividing membranes of identical (MZ) twins. There is always a space between the two amnions. The amnion consists of epithelial cells and connective tissue. (B) Diamnionic dichorionic dividing membranes. The right amnion is dislodged from the underlying chorion, a frequent artifact. The central trophoblastic remnants have fused. A = amnion; C = chorion; T = trophoblast. H&E. ×100.

this diagnosis can lead to improved outcome of these problematical gestations.

The other important point to be made is that monochorionic twin placentas usually have blood vessel connections between the fetal circulations; these connections are not present in dichorionic twin placentas. These anastomoses are discussed in greater detail later in the chapter. Note also that not all authorities have concurred with the ease of distinction between DiMo and DiDi placentas just elaborated. Thus the famous gemellologist Newman (1931b) believed that one could easily mistake a DiMo for a fused DiDi placenta. It is certainly not the case in experienced hands, but it points to the desirability of examining histological sections for affirmation. Moreover, it must be recognized that blood group studies in twins have the problem that fetal blood is commonly admixed because of the frequent blood vessel anastomoses. It then follows that if DZ twins were associated with a monochorionic placenta in which anastomoses existed their different blood antigens would permanently mingle. Only a highly sophisticated analysis of their blood groups would ascertain the presence of blood chimerism.

obtaining sections preserves a permanent record. For the experienced placentologist, it is just as effective to make the diagnosis of DiMo versus DiDi twin placentation by macroscopic inspection.

The dividing membranes of DiMo placentas are usually translucent (Figure 532). They are thin and not opaque, and there are no blood vessel remnants within them. When one separates the two amnions and comes to their insertion on the placental surface, one may continue to strip the amnions of a DiMo placenta away from the chorionic plate (Figure 533). Bleisch (1964) emphasized this point effectively. DiDi membrane partitions are considerably more opaque (Figure 534). They have remnants of villi and vessels in their four layers; and when by separating the two layers of each placental component one comes to the chorionic plate, further dissection is impossible (Figure 535). If one attempts to further cleave them, the surface of the placenta is disrupted.

As already stated, the advancements in sonographic equipment have made it possible to distinguish the thickness of the dividing membranes long before birth (Barss et al., 1985; Mahony et al., 1985; Hertzberg et al., 1987; Finberg, 1992). This diagnostic modality is particularly helpful in the diagnosis of MoMo twins who are at risk of cord entanglement. Belfort and his colleagues (1993) demonstrated by color flow Doppler sonography such cord entanglement in three sets of MoMo twins. They identified obstruction of flow in the umbilical vein by this means and made the point that

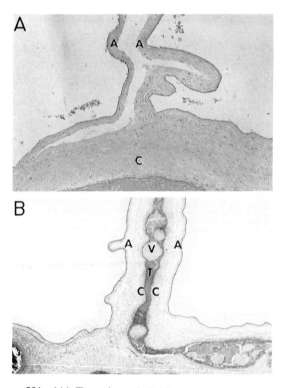

FIGURE 531. (A) T section of dividing membranes of monochorionic diamnionic twins. Note the contiguity of the chorion over the surface of the placenta at bottom and the separation of amnions. (B) T section of diamnionic dichorionic twin placenta. Note the atrophic villi and trophoblastic remnants between the two chorionic membranes. A = amnion; C = chorion; T = trophoblast; V = atrophic villi. H&E. ×40.

FIGURE 532. Diamnionic monochorionic twin placenta. The dividing membranes are held up to disclose their transparency. (See Figure 534 for contrast with DiDi placenta.)

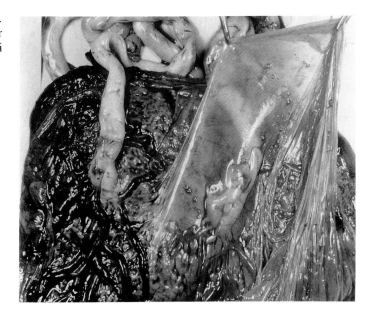

In this connection it is important to mention that Mortimer (1987) has challenged the concept that monochorionic placentas are diagnostic of MZ twins on the basis of blood studies. Cord blood grouping studies were conducted on 12 sets of monochorionic twins for 16 red blood cell antigens. In three sets there were discrepancies between the antigens despite the presence of artery-to-artery and vein-to-vein anastomoses. These discrepancies always involved single and minor blood groups. How such antigenic difference can come about is difficult to understand, as the anastomoses should have guaranteed complete mixing, as is the case in the few blood chimeras to be considered later. In our view, this study is incomplete evidence for Mortimer's proposition that 25% of the monochorionic twins studied were dizygotic. If it were so, there should be many more boy/girl twins found with monochorionic placentas, and it is not the case. Only two, perhaps three, such examples can be cited; and they were not well studied. The use of the DNA methods (with DNA

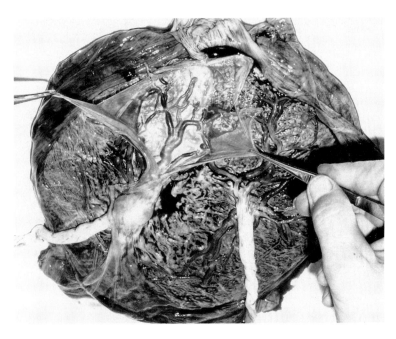

FIGURE 533. Diamnionic monochorionic twin placenta. The dividing membranes are being separated; at their base they are easily peeled off the chorionic surface. The vascular communications between the two fetal vascular beds are thus disclosed.

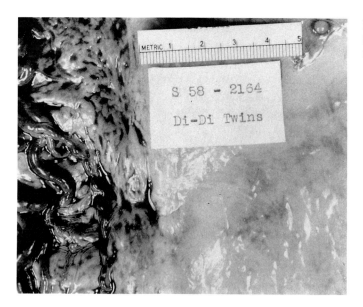

FIGURE 534. Dividing membranes of diamnionic dichorionic twins are characteristically opaque. They are only rarely translucent.

obtained from solid tissues!) discussed earlier will dispel any doubt in the future if twins with such apparent discrepancies come to light.

After it was recognized that monochorionic placentation is useful for identification of at least two-thirds of MZ twins, several larger series of twin placentas were published. They are summarized in Table 26. Note that marked differences exist in the distribution of the different twin groups in these reports. Thus the frequency of monochorial (MZ) twins is much lower in Nigeria, where the incidence of twinning is especially high, owing to the high frequency of DZ twins in the Yoruba tribe. Knox and Morley (1960) found western Nigerian Yoruba twin frequency to be as high as

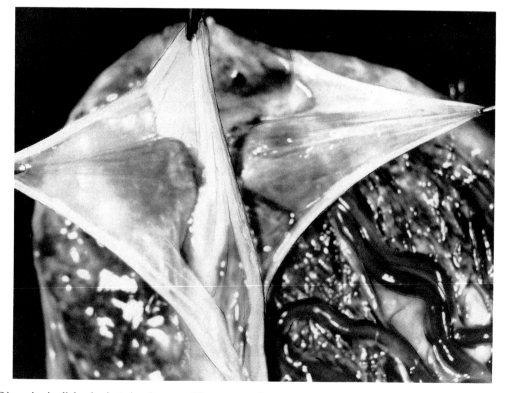

FIGURE 535. Diamnionic dichorionic twin placenta. The two amnions are being peeled off the central two chorionic leaves. The latter cannot be completely stripped off the placental mass without disrupting it.

TABLE 26. Distribution of placental types in twins.

Source	DiDi (%)	DiMo (%)	MoMo (% or ?)
Szendi (1938)	66	34	0
Vermelin & Ribon (1949)	45 (like sex) 32 (unlike sex)	23	
Benirschke (1961)	68.5	30	1.5
Potter (1963)	76	21	3.0?
Cameron (1968)	80	20	
Corney et al. (1968)	41 (like sex) 37 (unlike sex)	21.8	
Fujikura & Froehlich (1971)	73	24	2.4
Nylander (1970)	76 (Aberdeen) 92 (Yoruba-Nigeria)	19 5	5.0? 3.0?
Derom et al. (1988)	72	27	0.9
Barss (1988)	74.2	24.2	1.7

5.3%, with 91% being DZ. The converse is true of some Oriental populations. Sekiya and Hafez (1977) determined the type of placentation in 84 sets of Japanese twins. They found that 40 were dichorionic [26 fused (30.6%), 14 separate (16.75%)]; 41 were DiMo (48.8%), and 3 were MoMo (3.6%) (Figure 536).

The placental relations of DiMo and DiDi twins are easiest to identify in young pregnancies (Figure 537). The youngest implantation sites of DiDi twins (10–12 days) have been illustrated by Meyer and Meyer (1981). They featured tiny blastocysts that had implanted far away from one another in the uterine fundus. Finally, it may here be mentioned that Ohel et al. (1987) suggested that as seen by ultrasonographic "grading" methods the placentas of twins exhibit advanced maturation compared to age-matched singleton placentas.

Causes and Incidence of Multiple Births

A fundamental difference exists in the respective etiologies of DZ and MZ twins. DZ twins (and many higher multiples) are the result of polyovulation. It may be hereditary; it is age-related; and it can be induced by the administration of gonadotropins and other hormones. The strongest evidence that hormones (gonadotropins) are responsible for multiple ovulation comes from their therapeutic use in infertility patients. Intentional induction of multiple ovulation with gonadotropins is regularly employed in the livestock industry (e.g., Chupin et al., 1976) and is well studied in laboratory animals.

Milham (1964) therefore hypothesized that spontaneous DZ twinning in humans may be explained by a maternal increase in pituitary gonadotropin production. He based this idea on the increase in pituitary size with advancing age, the larger pituitaries possessed by Blacks, and the increase in size of the hypophysis after repeated pregnancies. These features correlate with an increase in DZ twinning rates. Numerous studies have since been undertaken to verify this hypothesis. In humans there is now good evidence that the recruitment of follicles for ovulation is controlled by follicle-stimulating hormone (FSH) (Vermesh & Kletzky, 1987). Marshall (1970) reviewed the findings following ovulation induction by gonadotropic hormones and clomiphene. The administration of clomiphene led to a 6% incidence of twins, and gonadotropin administration was followed by a 5% to 50% incidence of twins. These variable frequencies were found to be dose-related. Nylander (1973) determined that Nigerian women of the Yoruba tribe, known to have high rates of DZ twins, had elevated levels of FSH and luteinizing hormone (LH) compared to Whites. Soma et al. (1975),

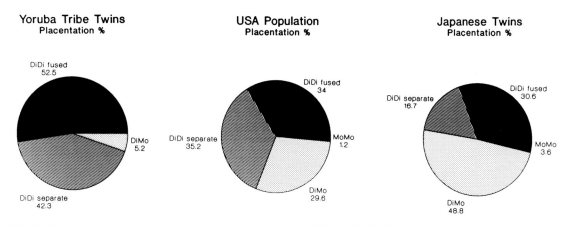

FIGURE 536. Twin placentation in three racial populations. The figures for the Yoruba (left) are from MacGillivray et al. (1975); those for the U.S. population come from Benirschke and Driscoll (1967); those for the Japanese population come from Sekiya and Hafez (1977).

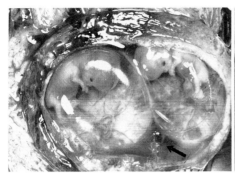
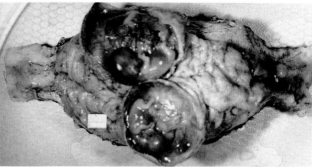

FIGURE 537. (Left) Uterus with diamnionic monochorionic (identical, or MZ) twins at 8 weeks' gestation. Note the two delicate amnions enclosed in a single chorion. Two yolk sacs are present at the arrow. (Right) Uterus with diamnionic dichorionic twin implantation. The uterus has been opened laterally, and the cervical halves are seen at either side. The two separate placenta membranes are easily seen. If these placentas expand, they will certainly collide and fuse.

noting the low frequency of DZ twins in Japanese when compared to other populations, measured the FSH and LH levels in 10 Japanese women. They found significantly lower values for both hormones than are present in Nigerian women. The values were also lower than those reported for the American populations (Figure 538). Because these two sets of data came from women near the time of expected ovulation, the validity of the results was questioned and the thesis then reexamined.

Presumably, recruitment of follicles for the next ovulation takes place around the time of menstruation. For that reason, Martin et al. (1984a,b) undertook a study of various hormonal levels in women during the first 4 days of their menstrual cycles. They compared women who had had at least one set of DZ twins with those who had had no twins. They also found that FSH and LH (less so) were elevated in twin-bearing mothers. Estradiol was also elevated. Spellacy et al. (1982) attempted to ascertain if the pituitaries of twin-bearing women were more responsive to the injection of gona-

dotropin-releasing hormone (GnRH). It proved not to be the case. It must be cautioned, however, that Spellacy's studies were undertaken during the luteal phase of the cycle and may thus not reflect the natural effect on FSH production needed for follicle recruitment.

The aforementioned hormone studies supported the notion that the genesis of DZ twins is indeed the result of excess production of FSH. Milham (1964) had suggested that the higher gonadotropin production he assumed to be the basis for DZ twinning is a racial characteristic of the hypophysis. This idea was challenged by Eriksson (1964), who pointed out that in some countries the DZ twinning rate has recently declined and that it could not be explained by an assumed lowering of the age of pregnant women and by differences in racial composition. His point was that DZ twinning is a "genetic trait." We believe that the gene responsible for higher FSH levels must now be considered to be the principal agent in familial twinning. The hormonal assays from many sources all point in this direction. Whether the effect of increased FSH production is the sequela of more pituitary cells or more GnRH production, or is also due to greater follicle sensitivity, needs to be studied. A further study supports the genetic nature of the multiple ovulation event. When women who had born DZ twins were followed sonographically it was found that they had considerably more ovulatory activity than controls (Martin et al., 1991).

In addition to inducing twin gestations, hormonal induction of ovulation is often followed by the birth of triplets and higher multiples. Schenker et al. (1981) reviewed this topic in detail, including the complications that arise from such pregnancies. They also made recommendations as to the prevention and management of multiple births.

Although it is true that multiple births are generally multizygotic, it has long been noted that among such

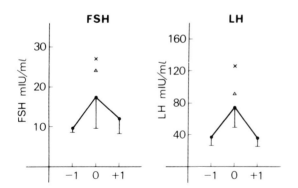

FIGURE 538. FSH and LH levels in women at around the time of ovulation. X = peak value in Yoruba tribe women of Africa; △ = peak value in U.S. Whites; solid line = Japanese women (n = 10). (Reprinted with permission from the American College of Obstetricians and Gynecologists (Obstetrics and Gynecology, Soma, et al., 1975, 46:311–312)).

multiple offspring there is often an admixture of DZ and MZ infants. For instance, Atlay and Pennington (1971) reported on quadruplets born after pituitary gonadotropin stimulation; two of the infants were monoamnionic and thus MZ twins. Whether the incidence of twinning rises following the discontinuation of chemical contraception ("the pill") is controversial. Rice-Wray et al. (1971) found no such increase in their study of 516 women, whereas Rothman (1977) and Bracken (1979) found that twinning was about doubled when pregnancy occurred within 1 to 2 months after cessation of oral contraception. The increase was found to be due to DZ twins in both of these studies. Bracken inferred that it results from pituitary response to oral contraceptives. Interesting discussion followed Bracken's paper (Bracken, 1979; Honoré, 1979; James et al., 1979) and suggested that after oral contraception pituitary gonadotropin release may in fact lead to DZ twinning. Whether it is also responsible for an increase in embryonic aneuploidy (particularly the occurrence of triploidy as has also been suggested) awaits further study. It has been hinted that currently a general rise in MZ twinning rates is occurring, and that it is perhaps related to the use of oral contraceptives (Bressers et al., 1987). Possible other environmental agents, however, could not be excluded by these investigators.

As had been noted by Weinberg (1909), twinning may be familial. Weinberg asserted that DZ twinning is inherited; however, it is not so for MZ twinning. Of course, such a genetic effect can be manifested only by a woman with the genetic background for twinning, not by the father of twins. He may pass on this gene to his offspring, but only double ovulation in women can *prove* the existence of the gene. It is thus sex-limited. The finding by Bulmer (1960) that increased twinning among relatives of fathers of twins is due to under-reporting of singletons does not seem to alter the inheritance of presumably higher FSH levels. These aspects are further elaborated by White and Wyshak (1964).

In our opinion, familial and racial predisposition to DZ twinning results from enhanced production of FSH. The racial relation to DZ twinning is most impressively shown by comparing the frequency in Nigerian women from the Yoruba tribe with Oriental women (Nylander & Corney, 1969; Nylander, 1971a). Nylander et al. observed that monochorial twins were rare in Nigerian women of the Yoruba tribe, and that zygosity determinations indicated a vast preponderance of DZ twins. The frequency of MZ twins was the same as that found in Whites (4.5 per 1,000). In the north of Nigeria, the twinning rate was 21 per 1,000, in the midregion 31 per 1,000, and in the western and eastern sections 45 per 1,000. These data contrast with reports from Japan, where the overall twinning rate is 6.1 per 1,000, with a

1.65:1.00 ratio of MZ/DZ twins (Inouye, 1957). Similar rates have been reported from Taiwan (Wei & Lin, 1967). In Europe there tends to be a "progressive decrease in the frequency of twins from north to south" (Eriksson, 1962).

The known higher frequency of DZ twins in older mothers may also be due to their enhanced FSH secretion. There is a steady rise in DZ twinning to the maternal age of 35; and after that age there is a sharp decline in DZ twinning. Although longitudinal studies of FSH secretion have not been reported for individual women, some data exist to indicate that FSH levels rise steadily with maternal age (Albert et al., 1956). This finding supports the notion that the increased DZ twinning frequency observed with advanced maternal age is due to enhanced FSH excretion by older women's pituitaries, but it does not prove it. The FSH levels are, of course, much higher still in postmenopausal women. Longitudinal studies are needed.

The interesting question has been raised as to whether the higher gonadotropin secretion of individuals with the genetic trait to produce twins is also manifest in men. For sheep and other domestic animal species, some evidence exists that in individual races there are differences in the frequency of DZ twinning (Land et al., 1973). It has also been suggested that the testicular weights from such animals is greater in males that carry the gene for twinning (Land, 1973; Islam et al., 1976). To study this further, Short (1984) has reported ethnic variations of testicular size in humans and found that Orientals have smaller testes than Europeans. There are no data yet from Yoruba men, but racially different testosterone levels have been reported by Ross et al. (1986). They tend to support the same principle and are viewed as being in support of the marked differences in prostatic cancer (Gittes, 1991). These and related aspects were considered in some detail in Diamond's stimulating editorial (1986). The differences of placentation in three well studied racial groups were depicted in Figure 536, which displays graphically how meaningfully different the placentas of twins are constructed when their zygosity is so variable.

The cause of MZ twinning is not fully understood. Whereas dizygotic twins (and multiples) derive from the fertilization of more than one ovum, monozygotic twins must originate from the spontaneous separation of blastomeres. Although this process occurs in all animals species with approximately the same frequency as that observed in humans, there are two species in which this polyembryony occurs with regularity: the two *Dasypus* species of armadillo: *Dasypus novemcinctus* (nine-banded armadillo) and *Dasypus septemcinctus al. hybridus* (seven-banded armadillos; mulita) (Fernandez, 1909; Newman & Patterson, 1910; Hamlett, 1933). The precise understanding of the mechanism of their polyembryony eludes us. Hamlett (1933) was critical of the statements made by Newman, who had inferred that it was the delayed implantation of armadillos that leads to impoverished nutrition and deficient oxygenation of the blastocyst, and it was thus the cause of polyembryony. Other species with delayed implantation do not share this phenomenon of polyembryony. Hamlett advocated that segregation of blastomeres is determined by genetic factors.

The nine-banded armadillo, ranging from Texas to Uruguay, always has identical quadruplets; the mulita may produce 7 to 12 male or female identical offspring. Although the mulita is much smaller, the two species are closely related and possess, for instance, identical chromosomes. The mulita is a common animal in Uruguay and Argentina; it has a single blastocyst (and corpus luteum) in a pregnancy that is also characterized by delayed implantation. Immediately after implantation the embryonic mass separates into multiple offspring. Whether it is by fission or budding was a hotly contended point of the discussions between Newman and Hamlett. In contrast to the monozygotic twinning in other mammals, the production of multiple births of these two armadillo species is so well regulated that anomalies such as conjoined twins, acardiacs, and most other abnormal events occurring in human MZ twins have not been observed (Hamlett, 1933). We deduced that one reason for these discrepancies may be that in these species the splitting of blastomeres is a precisely timed event. Also, placental anastomoses do not occur in armadillos (Anderson & Benirschke, 1963), possibly because of the different timing of their placentation. Perhaps it is the reason for their relative freedom from placental problems.

Other mammals that have rates of MZ twinning approximately similar to that in humans have no precisely timed monozygotic twinning period. In them and in humans, the splitting of the embryonic mass appears to occur at random during the early embryonic period. It has been observed that MZ twins commonly occur after surgical transfer of single bovine blastocysts into pseudopregnant cattle recipients (Moyaert et al., 1982; Kraay et al., 1983). Paulson et al. (1988) reported that triplets were born after the transfer of two previously frozen human embryos. Massip et al. (1983) observed cinematographically the atypical hatching of a cow blastocyst in vitro and suggested that it may be the mechanism by which dichorionic MZ twins take their origin. They observed partial protrusion of blastomeres from a zona; and after the "hatching" was complete, the two cell masses were connected only by a diminutive bridge. That hatched blastocysts are capable of twinning was demonstrated by surgical division of sheep embryos (Willadsen, 1979) as well as in mice (Tsunoda & McLaren, 1983), horses (Allen & Pashen, 1984), goats (Tsunoda et al., 1985), pigs (Nagashima et al., 1989), and other animals.

It is necessary to recognize that there are many temporal differences in the development of the inner cell mass and the setting aside of the trophectoderm in animals. Thus when different species are compared, it is difficult to draw good precise analogies to human development, especially placental growth. Thus the mouse segregates embryo from trophectoderm at the fourth cleavage stage (about 12–16 cells). The peripheral cells develop tight junctions and form the future placenta (Ziomek & Johnson, 1982), an event taking place much later in the sheep and cow. In humans, similar to the mouse, the event occurs at about the fifth division of cells. In 1% of cultured mouse embryos, spontaneous separation of blastomeres into MZ twins takes place, analogous to what would be expected of the process that leads to conjoined twins (Hsu & Gonda, 1980). Runner (1984) observed two inner cell masses in a mouse blastocyst at the stage of proamnion cavitation, which suggested to him late division of the embryonic mass and development of mirror imagery, which is also more commonly seen in MZ human twins. Experimental fission of quail embryos has also produced conjoined twins (Lutz & Lutz-Ostertag, 1963). The production of MZ twins in sea urchins was demonstrated by the isolation of first-cleavage blastomeres (Driesch, 1891). These embryos were rarely normal. Marcus (1979) showed that by shaking fertilized sea urchin eggs to remove their envelope and with subsequent exposure to hypertonic water he was able to promote separation of blastomeres. Many of these MZ twins were also underdeveloped. It is particularly interesting to note that there were many intertwin morphological differences. Ludwig (1927) had commented on the irregular division of hereditary material in MZ twins but did not believe that blastomeres were capable of separating. He thought twinning to be a late event and also expected that MZ twins would often be different.

When pregnant mice were exposed to low doses of vincristine on days 7 and 8, unexpectedly many MZ twins developed, some being monoamnionic (Kaufman & O'Shea, 1978). Kaufman and O'Shea cited the few other reports of conjoined twins produced by experimental teratogens. Perhaps best known are the experiments of Witschi (1934), in which he produced twins in the frog by fertilizing eggs that were 3 to 5 days' overripe. Witschi observed the development of several blastopores and gastrulation. Other sporadic observations of MZ animal twins have been cited by Corner (1955). He reviewed the few available specimens of early human MZ twin embryos, which are not dissimilar from those observed in experimental animals. Corner also cited the interesting observation of frequent admixture of MZ and DZ twins, to which we previously alluded.

The results of statistical surveys suggest that multiple ovulation due to hormonal stimulation is not the sole cause of enhanced multiple gestations. Derom et al. (1987) observed that MZ twinning (1.2%) is significantly higher than would be expected from random births (0.45%). Boklage (1987a) has in fact gone so far as to ascribe the causes of MZ twinning to factors that differ little from those that induce DZ twins. When all evidence is taken together, it must be said that spontaneous MZ twinning is still a poorly understood phenomenon. Boklage (1981) takes exception with the notion of embryonic "splitting" as the etiology of MZ twinning. He pointed out that the high embryonic mortality that occurred in the early experimental studies makes splitting an unlikely cause of MZ twins. There is no doubt any longer, however, that splitting can take place in mammals and it can definitely be done experimentally. Boklage also stated that none of the many experimental chimeras that have been produced in mice experimentally had resulted in MZ twins. This point in itself, however, is insufficient proof against splitting, it seems to us. Few mice eventuate in MZ twins in the first place, and not many offspring of experimental chimeras have been sufficiently studied to identify their possible monozygotic derivation. The arguments on this topic are not unlike the "splitting versus budding" controversy of the past and are well expressed as a "skirmish in semantics" by Hamlett (1933).

To explain MZ twinning, Boklage conceived that forces responsible for organizing a field, or gradient, in early embryos may be the reason for the MZ twinning event. He opined that a "weakness in the enforcement of that directive might allow a second such organizing center to induce a second developmental scheme." He was particularly concerned with understanding neural symmetry and with mirroring in twins.

In our opinion, the armadillo is the best animal from which to gain a better understanding of this puzzling yet frequent event of embryonic duplication. It is to be regretted that armadillos are difficult to breed in captivity, and so it is difficult to accumulate the relevant observations.

Other than for the pregnancy outcome, there is no good evidence that heredity in some way controls the MZ twinning event (other than in armadillos). Its incidence is nearly the same throughout the world. MZ twinning is not significantly influenced by maternal age or the environment. It appears to be a sporadic event. Because of the nature of the fetal placental membrane relation in human MZ twins, one assumes that MZ twinning can occur at any time during the first 2 weeks of development. It then appears to be randomly distributed.

For lack of a better term and better insight into the etiology of MZ twinning, we have referred to the cause as the twinning impetus. We make further inference that this impetus affects the developing embryos at random and that because of this randomness of the timing the different placental membrane relations shown in Figure 539 come about. We believe this impetus to be effective from days 1 to 14 of embryonic development. Our hypothesis further assumes that it is impossible for the impetus to split an already formed embryonic cavity such as the yolk sac, chorionic cavity, or amnion. The

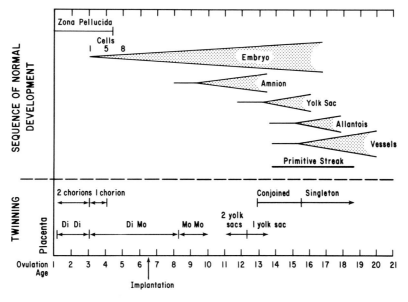

FIGURE 539. Interpretation of early events in the MZ twinning event. The earliest observed embryonic events are depicted in the upper portion. The bottom portion suggests that certain placental structures result if twinning occurs at certain times. Note that the DiDi/DiMo frequencies correspond roughly to the observed 1:3 ratio. It is also assumed that with later development (after day 8) MZ twinning becomes ever more difficult because of the enlarging embryonic/placental masses. Once the primitive streak is formed, conjoined twins may develop at first. Soon, however, the presumed twinning "impetus" is ineffective.

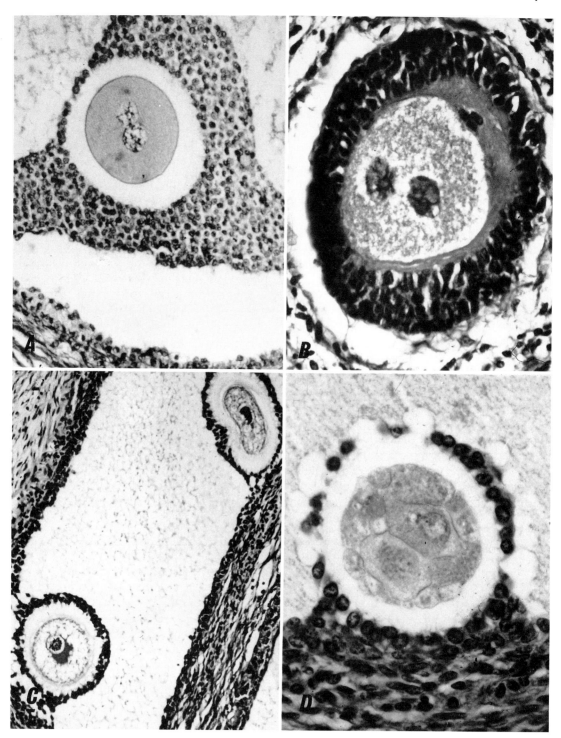

FIGURE 540. Four graafian follicles with abnormal ova whose future potential cannot be anticipated. (A, B) Binucleate ova in graafian follicles. (C) Binovular follicle. (D) Segmenting ovum within graafian follicle. H&E. A ×100; B ×160; C ×80; D ×100.

monozygotic twinning process, then, is a biological continuum during this early period.

The phenomenon was discussed by Gould (1982) in an entertaining thesis on the not so trivial question as to whether conjoined twins are one or two persons. Finally, an interesting result, with experimentally derived MZ mouse twins, has been reported by Gärtner and Baunack (1981). They produced MZ twins at the eight-cell stage and compared their growth with DZ twins in the same strain of mice. Despite the fact that they worked with an isogenic strain, the DZ twins differed more from each other in a variety of characteristics than did the MZ twins. The cause of this unexpected finding is not yet understood.

THIRD TYPE OF TWIN

The possibility of the existence of a third type of twin is occasionally considered in discussions of the twinning events. It proposes that MZ twins do not consist solely of identical twins, but that nonidentical twins, arising from a single ovulation event, make up part of the spectrum. It may amount to some 1% of twins who would usually be classed as DZ twins because of some dissimilarities of their genotypes. This concept envisages that polar body fertilization may occur. Thus the twins would then come from a single maternal, but two paternal, genomes. They would be intermediate in their genetic configuration between MZ and DZ twins. Such a possibility is supported by the occasional finding of polar bodies with a size similar to that of the normal oocyte. This event especially occurs in some bat species. Furthermore, there are some theoretical considerations detailed by Mijsberg (1957) that suggest the existence of third twins. In fact, the fertilization and further development of polar bodies has been observed. Dixon (1927) has described human polar bodies in mitosis, synchronous with the oocyte mitosis. It is also noteworthy that in humans and in a variety of animals binucleated ova are observed. They may produce such twins or even result in the development of chimeras. Binucleated eggs have been described repeatedly in the ovaries of a variety of animals, in women (Kennedy & Donahue, 1969) (Figure 540), and in children. Manivel et al. (1988) found binucleated oocytes in 19% and binovular follicles in 52% of their pediatric autopsy material. The fertilization of such abnormal ova has been observed by Zeilmaker and colleagues (1983).

The occurrence of "third twins" would explain the occasional finding of a single corpus luteum associated with fertilizations that were diagnosed to be DZ twins. The concept has been considered in some detail by Elston and Boklage (1978). Later, Boklage (1987b) suggested the term tertiary oocyte, rather than polar body fertilization, and critiqued the acceptance of the Weinberg formula in assigning zygosity, in particular for discordant twins. He also favored the notion that overripe ova may be responsible for some of these abnormal fertilization products. It must be cautioned, however, that mere inspection of ovaries (at operation) is insufficient evidence for the presence of a solitary corpus luteum. A second corpus luteum may be present and found buried underneath another, as is shown in Figure 541. The macroscopic inspection of the ovary in this case would have been misleading. Further complicating the resolution of the question is that two normal ova may reside in a single antrum (Figure 540). Such a Graafian follicle would result in a single corpus luteum and yet possibly produce

fraternal twins. Finally, it can be said that a possible instance of polar body twins, one an acardiac fetus with triploid chromosome constitution and the other diploid, has been studied in detail by Bieber et al. (1981). This subject is discussed in greater detail in the section on acardiac twins.

Twinning Incidence

The incidence of multiple pregnancy has been the topic of numerous investigations. This aspect was particularly well covered by Bulmer (1970) in his classical book on twinning in humans. It has also been the topic of several discussions, published in the third issue of the *Acta Geneticae Medicae et Gemellologiae* (Vol. 36, 1987). The rate for dizygotic twinning in various populations has been summarized by Diamond (1986) whose data are shown below.

Ethnic Group and locality	DZ twinning rate (per 1,000 births)
Asians	
Japanese	
Hawaii	2.2
Japan	2.3
Chinese	
Formosa	1.4
Hawaii	2.1
Malaya	2.8
Singapore	4.1
Hong Kong	6.8
Malays	
Hawaii	2.2
Manila	2.7
Malaya	5.2
Hawaiians	
Hawaii	3.9
Koreans	
Korea	5.1
Korea	5.8
Korea	7.9
Indians	
Bombay	6.8
Bangalore	7.3
Calcutta	8.1
Caucasians	
Europeans	
Spain	5.9
France	7.1
Switzerland	8.1
Holland	8.1
West Germany	8.2
Norway	8.3
Sweden	8.6
Britain	8.9

continued

Ethnic Group and locality	DZ twinning rate (per 1,000 births)
African Blacks	
Bantu	
Johannesburg	16.0
Leopoldville	19.0
Yoruba	
Ibadan	40.0
Ilesha	49.0

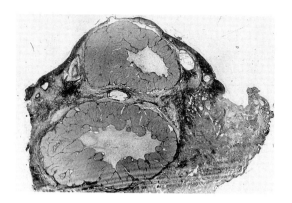

FIGURE 541. Cross section of an ovary at 8 weeks' gestation with two corpora lutea of pregnancy. One is hidden from external view because of its position, so only one would have been recognized by inspection. This specimen is from the diamnionic monochorionic (hence assumed to be MZ) twin gestation shown in Figure 537. H&E. ×4.

These data impressively show that DZ twinning has a profound racial variation. In contrast, the MZ twinning rate "is nearly constant at about three and a half per thousand in all races" (Bulmer, 1970). Eriksson (1962) has drawn attention to the decline of twinning rates from north to south in Europe, which is due to variations of DZ twinning rates. The twinning rates and outcomes for a large U.S. population have been analyzed by Myrianthopoulos (1970a,b). He reviewed the data of the US multicenter Collaborative Study, which analyzed 56,249 pregnancies with known outcome. It contained 615 twins (1 per 91.5 births). The differences in the ethnic background of that U.S. population and its relation to multiple pregnancy can be seen in the following data from his report.

Group	Twins (no.)	Population (no.)	DZ twins (no./births)
Whits	259	25,991	1/100.3
Blacks	331	26,080	1/78.8
Puerto Ricans	25	4,178	1/167.1

The zygosity of 508 of these twins was examined as well as possible, but a large number of twins remained unclassified. The results were as follows.

$$MZ = 29.6\%$$
$$DZ = 51.4\%$$
$$? \, Z = 19.0\%$$

The profound influence of maternal age is well documented in these reports. The incidence of DZ twinning rises until at 35 years maternal age there is an abrupt fall in the incidence. A greater frequency of twins in the U.S. black population had also been noted in the large database summarized by Guttmacher (1953). He reported on the frequency of triplets and higher multiple births at a time that preceded the use of fertility drugs. Over a 22-year period, viable twin births

occurred in 1 per 92.4 (Whites) and 1 per 73.8 (Blacks); triplets occurred in 1 per 9,828 (Whites) and 1 per 5,631 (Blacks).

The occurrence of higher multiple births, such as triplets and quadruplets, has commonly been estimated by the Hellin-Zeleny hypothesis: If twins occur with $1/n$, triplets occur with $(1/n)^2$ and quadruplets with $(1/n)^3$. This method is merely an approximation and is subject to maternal age, medical therapy, race, and other factors.

Multiple pregnancies showed a progressive decline from 1938 to 1949; more recent declines in the twinning rate have been studied by a number of investigators. Akesson et al. (1970) showed that the incidence of twinning in Sweden fell from 1.4% in 1871 to 1.1% in 1960. This change was due to fluctuations in the number of DZ twins born. Changes in maternal age were considered but not deemed to be the cause of this decline. Reports from the United States, Canada, Australia, and other countries have been similar (Elwood, 1973; James, 1973). The decrease in twin births in Holland was believed to be secondary to a decrease in maternal age at conception (Hoogendoorn, 1973). James (1975) suggested that the decline may relate to exogenous agents or that it is secondary to voluntary birth control. That the latter effect may have some significance is borne out by the apparent cessation of the DZ twinning decline in Canada (Elwood, 1983) and Hungary (Métneki & Czeizel, 1983); but James (1983) was not convinced. Allen (1987) provided data to show that there was no decline in U.S. twin births from 1964 to 1983.

The incidence of DZ twinning has been shown to have a seasonal relation. Timonen and Carpen (1968), who observed this phenomenon in the Finnish population, deduced that it results from the continuous light stimulation, which induces enhanced gonadotropin release. The peak of twin births occurred during early spring and summer. Elwood (1978) found the peak for a Canadian population to be in October, whereas Edwards (1938) had reported two peaks for conceptions (February and August) in a British population. The effect was more pronounced with twins than with singletons. Harlap et al. (1985) raised the possibility that an increase in DZ twins results from the development of overripe ova.

SUPERFETATION AND SUPERFECUNDATION

Twins may have different fathers through the process known as **superfecundation** (two ova are fertilized by spermatozoa from different fathers). That the concept is valid was proved by finding HLA antigen differences in the twins studied by Terasaki et al. (1978). In the accompanying editorial, Ryan (1978) referred to other cases and to its occurrence in test-tube babies. Another report, with one white and one black twin, was forthcoming from Harris (1982). This report is most remarkable because the fertilizations apparently occurred 1 week apart. Verma et al. (1992) proved superfecundation by two fathers with cytogenetic markers but were refused DNA fingerprinting. Harris (1982) also referred to a case of *superfetation* with twins of apparently different gestational ages (34 and 37 weeks). Rhine and Nance (1976) described the pedigree of a relevant family. They suggested that superfetation was the basis for the repeated dissimilarities of twins. They assumed it to be inherited as a dominant trait and expressed through a putative placental inability to suppress new ovulation after conception.

Vascular Anatomy of Twin Placentas

One of the most important observations to be made in the study of twin placentas is the accurate determination of the nature of fetal surface blood vessels. Their relation to one another is perhaps the single most important determinant for the outcome of many twin pregnancies. These aspects were first clearly demonstrated by Friedrich Schatz, whose numerous contributions have been summarized in English by Strong and Corney (1967). Price (1950) considered the various vascular anastomoses of monochorionic twin placentas to be the most important determinants for the frequently discordant development of MZ twins. This notion dates back more than a hundred years, and many observers since have reached similar conclusions.

The demonstration of anastomoses is relatively simple. Once learned, injection studies are rarely necessary. However, they aid in delineating the patterns for the novice and should be performed routinely. A simple method for the detection of anastomoses has been described by Coen and Sutherland (1970). They used milk for injection because it is so readily available and demonstrative, but other liquids are equally useful. For the purposes of injection it is best to cut the umbilical cords near their placental surface, so as to reduce vascular resistance. One should also have stripped the amnion from the chorionic surface, which exposes the fetal surface vessels well (Figure 542). The general examination of the placenta should have been com-

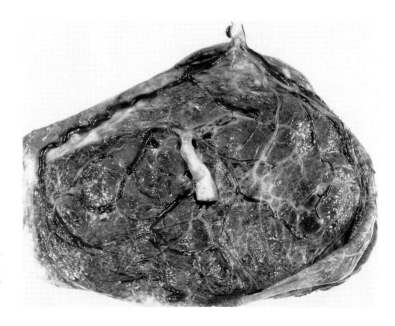

FIGURE 542. Diamnionic monochorionic twin placenta (26 weeks' gestation) with velamentous insertion of one cord. This twin had a much smaller portion of placental tissue and died.

pleted, of course, but it may be necessary to take samples for histological study only after the injection has been done. For optimal results, several tools are desirable and are depicted in Figure 543. It must be admitted, however, that a simple syringe and water are usually adequate. One must inspect the surface of the placenta carefully, follow major vessels to their ends, and determine, visually at first, which vessels are likely to have communications between the fetal circulations. In the normal placenta the fetal arteries terminate in the periphery, dip into the villous tissue, and emerge nearby as veins, which then course toward the umbilical cord. The arteries are recognized as those vessels that cross over veins, particularly those of a larger caliber. A 1:1 relation is usually found in the final vascular ramifications: one artery to one vein.

When no returning vein can be identified to accompany a peripheral arterial branch in a twin placenta, an artery-to-vein (A-V) communication may exist. This area then becomes important for the exploration of a deep anastomosis. These A-V anastomoses perfuse a common (or shared) cotyledon and form the basis for the transfusion syndrome, discussed below. They are common and constitute the "third circulation" of twin placentas. Most frequent are artery-to-artery anastomoses (A-A shunts); vein-to-vein (V-V) communications are the least frequent types of anastomoses, findings already made by Schatz in 1875 and more extensively in 1886. He believed that A-A anastomoses are more common because of the higher blood pressure existing in arteries; therefore V-V anastomoses are rare, and they were thought to obliterate more commonly before birth.

To document the presence of a direct A-A or V-V anastomosis, it is often sufficient to stroke blood back and forth through a major shunt. If one wishes to demonstrate it conclusively, injection of milk, colored water, or similar solution is feasible. To do so, one inserts a needle near the point of presumed anastomosis and then gently injects the liquid, which usually readily passes to the other side of the twin placenta (Figures 544, 545). The injection of as little as 5 to 10 ml of fluid is usually sufficient. Note that it may help to have a needle with a bead and to tie it into the vessels to allow more pressure to be exerted during injection. It is also important to recognize that one should not attempt to inject the entire placental bed from the vessels near the cord insertion. This measure requires so much volume of injection fluid that pressures are generally insufficient to demonstrate finer anastomoses (Figure 546). Moreover, twin placentas are often damaged during delivery and they leak when injected from the umbilical cord. This frequent disruption can make adequate demonstration of anastomoses difficult.

Identification of A-V shunts is usually the most difficult. It is best to inspect the surface carefully to identify possible areas of A-V shunts and then inject them successively. It is immaterial here whether one fills them from the arterial or the venous end. When the fluid is injected slowly, one sees an area of placenta distend and increase in thickness. After a short while, the fluid emerges from the other side, and it can then be traced to a larger vessel where its nature (artery or vein) can be ascertained. The delineation, direction, and number of these shunts is especially important if one wishes to understand the transfusion syndrome.

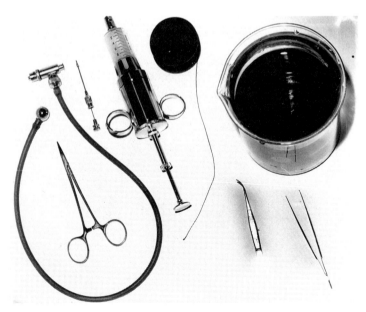

FIGURE 543. Ideal set of tools in inject twin placentas: syringe with beaded needle, string to tie needle in place, colored liquid (e.g., milk), clamps, forceps.

FIGURE 544. Injection of DiDi twin placenta. A potential anastomotic area has been isolated, the amnion is stripped, and a needle is inserted and tied in place.

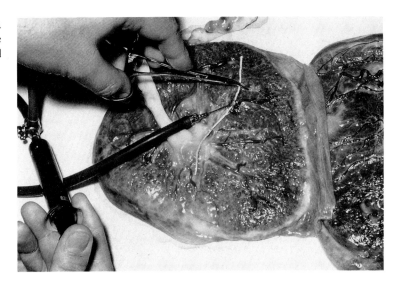

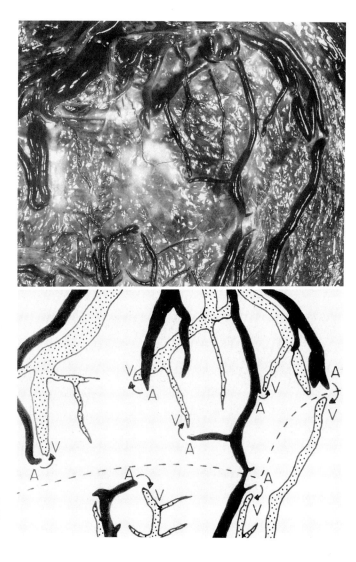

FIGURE 545. Vascular equator of a DiMo twin placenta to show A-A and A-V anastomoses, as well as the normal cotyledonary supply. The diagram is self-explanatory.

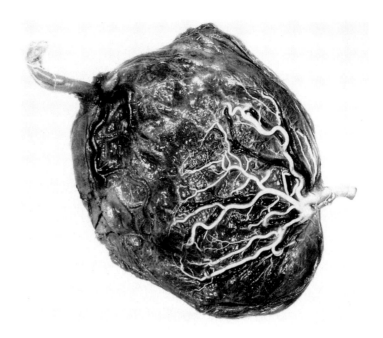

Figure 546. DiMo twin placenta with amnion stripped off; the right side has been injected with barium sulfate through one umbilical artery. There are no anastomoses. Both cords have a marginal insertion; arteries cross over veins. This method failed to disclose two small A-V shunts (bottom) because of the lack of sufficient pressure exerted when the entire tree is filled. (Courtesy Dr. S. Romney, New York.)

Finally, it is recommended that a drawing of the entire vascular relation is made for the record at the end of the procedure. Figures 547 and 548 show various types of anastomoses in two monochorionic twin placentas at their "vascular equators."

If one wishes to make injections of the placental vasculature with plastics for later corrosion, special procedures are necessary. The placenta must be intact. It must first be washed out with warm dextran to open all vessels and to remove the fetal blood. Saline has been found to be less satisfactory (Robertson & Neer, 1983). After the specimen has been flushed, one can then achieve gradual filling with plastics solutions in different colors and with ever increasing strength (see Torretta &

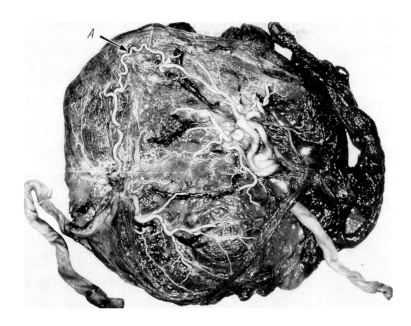

Figure 547. DiMo twin placenta with single large A-A anastomosis (A) at top left. It has been injected with barium. Finer A-V districts have not been filled.

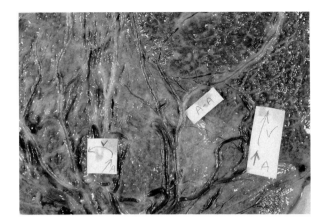

FIGURE 548. DiMo twin placenta, vascular equator. The amnions have been removed, and the various types of anastomosis are delineated on pieces of paper.

Cobellis, 1966). A diamnionic monochorionic twin placenta, thus prepared, is shown in Figure 550. Only exhaustive examination of such a specimen allows one to identify the possible presence of shared cotyledons. By and large, these preparations are more beautiful than they are useful. Only experienced observers (Hyrtl, 1870) profit from their preparation.

One might suspect that the proximity of cord insertions in twin placentas may influence the frequency and type of anastomoses, but that has not been our experience. Although it is true that in placentas with cords next to each other, as depicted for instance in Figures 549, 555, and 566, large communications often exist whose injection is scarcely needed, they cannot be assumed a priori. Many MoMo placentas have no communications, irrespective of their cords' proximity. This point was well made in the study by Wenner (1956). He

was surprised to find no anastomoses in the placental vascular ramifications of a thoracopagus. The demonstration of anastomoses is most difficult when one fetus has died before birth. It is thus often impossible to demonstrate vascular connections in DiMo placentas with a fetus papyraceus and also when the placenta has been fixed in formalin beforehand.

Despite numerous injection attempts, we have never seen anastomoses between blood vessels of dichorionic twin placentas. That they may exist in rare cases is not doubted. The finding of rare blood chimeras (see below) and occasional reports of such connections by competent observers (Figure 551) (Cameron, 1968:) make them a reality of great interest. In contrast, anastomoses occur frequently in the DZ twins of other species, such as marmosets and cattle. This aspect is discussed further below.

The observed frequency of intertwin blood vessel anastomoses in human MZ twins is difficult to assess because of the differences in techniques employed for their demonstration. We previously reported the following relations of anastomoses in 60 injected monochorionic twin placenta (Benirschke & Driscoll, 1967).

		Infant survival
Type of anastomosis	Total found	No.
A-A (one or more)	17	12
A-A + A-V	17	14
A-A + V-V	5	3
V-V	3	2
A-V	7	3
A-V + V-A	2	1
None	9	6

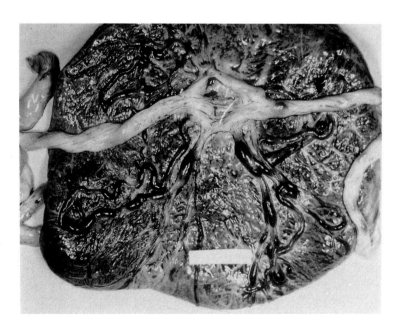

FIGURE 549. MoMo twin placenta with amnion removed. The cords insert next to each other, adjacent to major anastomoses.

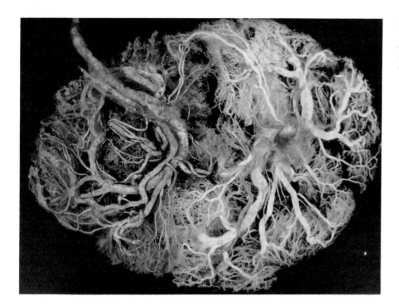

FIGURE 550. DiMo twin placenta that has been injected with colored plastics and then made into a corrosion cast. Many small anastomoses can be seen. Their nature is difficult to delineate.

Similar findings have been published by others. Robertson and Neer (1983) reported on 278 twin placentas (of 23,810 births; incidence 1/86; 7 triplets). They used dextran and heparin for injection, cannulated the vessels, and injected 100 ml over 30 minutes. The vessels were then infused with warmed solutions of dyes in colloid suspension. India ink did not work well. Nineteen placentas were damaged and excluded; 97 placentas were separate masses. Of 162 successfully injected fused placentas, 96 (59%) were DiDi; the remainder were monochorionic. Of 56 monochorionic twin placentas studied, all but one had demonstrable anastomoses. The one placenta without anastomoses had an infarcted area that had produced a separation between the two halves. There may have been a communication in the past, as obliteration of such anasto-

moses is not uncommon. In one dichorionic placenta, the injection material exchanged between the two sides through a tiny villous district. The longterm outcome of these twins is not known, as is true for Cameron's cases (Figure 551). These twins had identical blood groups, even though the pair was of different sex. As we indicated above, identical blood groups should be expected when vascular shunts exist in the placenta of twins. Four cases of the typical transfusion syndrome were found in the study by Robertson and Neer.

The topic of DZ twins having a monochorionic placenta and vascular intertwin anastomoses is somewhat controversial. Scipiades and Burg (1930) first described anastomoses in two boy/girl twin placentas. Lassen (1931) and Tüscher (1936) each added a rare case of MZ dichorial twins with fine anastomoses. It must be

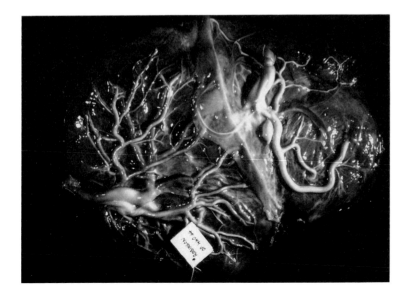

FIGURE 551. DiDi twin placenta with minute anastomosis coursing over the dividing membranes. The associated like-sex twins were MZ. (Reprinted with permission from Cameron: The Birmingham Twin Survey (Figure 5). Proc. R. Soc. Med. 61:229–234, 1968).

emphasized, however, that some of these cases are not well supported by pictorial or other conclusive evidence. Even Lassen (1931), who performed stereoradiography on a placenta, was not absolutely certain of the connections he demonstrated. The technique of stereoradiography is not satisfactory, as the findings in seven placentas from DZ twins with anastomoses have shown (Pérez et al., 1947). Szendi (1938) admitted this lack clearly in his discussion of the stereoscopic analysis in 4 of 20 dichorial placentas with putative anastomoses. Bleisch (1964) found arterial anastomoses in all 18 monochorionic, but in none of 42 dichorionic, twin placentas. He also succinctly explained why one should not accept the diagnosis of MoMo placentation in the boy/girl twin placenta reported by Pickering (1946). Wenner (1956) reemphasized Schatz' point of the rarity of V-V anastomoses. He found only three such cases among the perhaps 100 placentas that were studied. He suggested that this type of connection may have lethal consequences because "one fetus aspirates blood through these anastomoses from the other," a point to which we return later. In a later study, Bleisch (1965) found that all of his 75 monochorionic twin placentas had anastomoses. In all but one case the anastomoses were grossly identifiable, and the sizes of anastomoses were partially related to the distance of the cord insertions. He was unable to identify any specific reasons for the directions of flow, but death of one twin was associated with thrombosis. Only one V-V anastomosis was found, and Bleisch hypothesized first that the possibility exists for large blood shifts through large anastomoses, particularly given different intrauterine pressures. No connections were found between the circulations of dichorionic twins.

Twin placentas have other vascular peculiarities. Bhargava et al. (1971) made a detailed study of the vessels in the chorionic plate of 166 placentas from twins and triplets. They found many more placentas with arterial and venous tortuosities, "arteriovenous dissociations," and reversal of arteriovenous relations when they compared twin placentas with 167 singleton placentas. Their conclusion was that these vascular abnormalities are determined "mainly under the influence of the functional demands of the corresponding foetus." Identification of these anomalies may enhance our understanding of prenatal development.

The frequency of abnormal insertion of the umbilical cords in multiple gestation is particularly important, as was demonstrated in Table 17 (see Chapter 13). Kobak and Cohen (1939) described the incidence of velamentous insertion of one cord as being nine times higher in twins (routinely in triplets, according to De Lee, as quoted by these authors) than the 1% or so found in singleton placentas. Similar results were reported by Englert et al. (1987), when they observed abnormal

placental shapes and cord insertions in multiple pregnancies after in vitro fertilization. Eberle et al. (1993), who investigated the placental pathology of weight-discordant twins, found that discordant placental lesions were correlated more with dichorionic than monochorionic twins rather than this discordance being correlated with placental weight. Abnormal cord insertions are of concern to the perinatologist because of the possibly more frequent presence of vasa previa in twins. Kobak and Cohen (1939) described the stillbirth of a twin following vaginal bleeding that had resulted from disrupted vasa previa. Two similar cases of DiMo placentas and vasa previa were described by Whitehouse and Kohler (1960). Three of their six reported infants died from exsanguination. When this problem is anticipated, Kleihauer stains of the vaginal blood disclose the presence of fetal blood. We have seen several similar cases. In one, the fetal blood loss was recognized, and immediate neonatal transfusion with 100 ml of maternal blood saved the infant. A similar case has been described by Duenhoelter (1989). In another case we saw, vasa previa were present in the dividing membranes of DiDi twins. They ruptured, and fatal exsanguination occurred within 3 minutes of the second sac's rupture (Figures 552–554). Because there are often large anastomoses between DiMo twins, rapid exsanguination of the second twin may occur when vasa previa are ruptured in the first twin. It can also occur through an untied umbilical cord after delivery of the first twin. This potential exsanguination of a second twin is allegedly the reason for routine clamping of the placental end of the umbilical cord lest an undiagnosed twin bleed from the cut end of the first-born. Velamentous

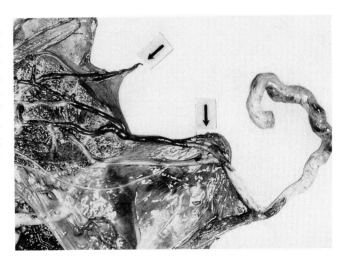

FIGURE 552. DiDi twin placenta with velamentous insertion of the cord from twin B. He exsanguinated within 3 minutes after rupture of the second sac. There was disruption of the velamentous vessels (arrows).

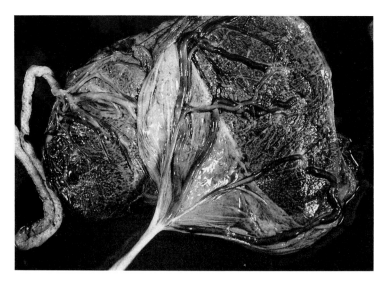

FIGURE 553. DiDi fused twin placenta with large vessels of twin A coursing over the dividing membranes. Twin A has a single umbilical artery. These twins delivered at 34 weeks' gestation. The superficial chorionic veins of twin B (right) were nearly completely thrombosed. The infants survived.

vessels of twins may thrombose before birth, or they may atrophy. Rarely are they of vitelline origin and then of no importance (Figure 555). Antoine et al. (1982) grossly underestimated the reported frequency of vasa previa in twin placentas, when they cited only eight cases. They described a case in which sinusoidal fetal heart rate patterns initiated appropriate fetal studies (e.g., amnioscopy and examination of the blood). Despite these efforts, both DiMo twins exsanguinated.

RamosArroyo et al. (1988) have also found that abnormal cord insertion was higher in twin gestations. Velamentous or marginal cords were found in 27.4% of monochorionic placentas, compared with 13.8% in dichorionic organs. They considered it evidence in favor of trophotropism (see Chapter 8). Conversely, Gavriil et al. (1993), who studied the placentas of in vitro fertilization, interpreted the more frequently eccentric insertion in twins as resulting from "oblique orientation

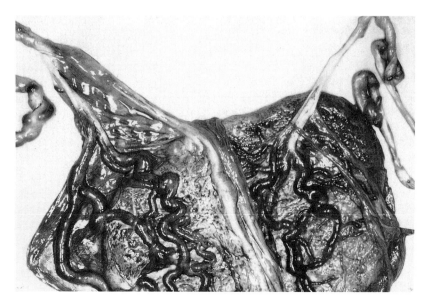

FIGURE 554. DiDi fused twin placenta with velamentous cord insertion of the left cord. Its fetal vessels are markedly dilated and course over the membranes at left. Note that the major vessels of these twins do not approach the dividing membranes.

of the blastocyst at the nidation" but provided no further explanation why it should happen. The excess frequency of velamentous cords in DiMo twin placentas has significant correlation with the transfusion syndrome. Fries et al. (1993) found that one-third of DiMo twin placentas had such abnormal cord insertions and that 64% were involved with transfusion syndrome cases and delivered significantly earlier. They thus sought an etiological role for this abnormal insertion. It may also be considered that velamentous insertion is so common in this syndrome because normal placental development failed to take place. We believe this situation possible because of the constant slight drainage of blood that occurs from the placenta with the velamentous cord into the other twin. Therefore this placenta with reduced pressure may not have grown as avidly and centrifugally as it should have. The primacy of the vascular component in villous capillary development was addressed by Giles et al. (1993). These authors studied sonographically abnormal umbilical artery waveforms (systolic/diastolic ratios) in twins and correlated them with villous vasculature. They found that microvascular disease of villi (reduction) correlates with growth retardation and abnormal S/Ds.

There is a wide spectrum of vascular relations in twin placentas. How do they come about, and what is so different in other species? In marmosets the assuredly DZ twins always have placental anastomoses; in artiodactyla (especially *Bos* but also *Sus*, *Ovis*, and others) DZ twins often have fused placentas, and blood tra-

verses from one fetus to the other. In marmosets it leads invariably to blood chimerism; but other than an occasional fetus papyraceus, the anastomoses cause no complications. With artiodactyla, however, in addition to the blood chimerism, the female twin becomes a freemartin when she is connected to a male's placental circulation. This result is not the case in humans, where dichorionic twins rarely have anastomoses, but where they have clearly occurred because of blood chimerism. Heterosexual blood chimerism is rare, and it is not associated with sterility (i.e., freemartinism in women).

The reason for the differences must be found in the early embryological development of the embryo and placenta. In marmosets, fusion of chorions occurs very early (Benirschke & Layton, 1969), but in human DZ twins no such fusion of chorionic circulations occurs. Here the placentas may become intimately fused, but they do not develop interplacental vascular anastomoses. Indeed, despite numerous suggestions to the contrary, villi do not fuse in the human placenta, however closely they may become approximated. When sections of India-ink-injected, intimately fused dichorionic twin placentas are prepared, one observes that the villi may intermingle, but they do not connect with one another. No blood vessels traverse from the villi of one fraternal twin to those of the co-twin.

To understand the vascular commonality of monochorionic twin placentas, it is easiest with a review of their early embryology (Figure 539). We suggest with the diagram in Figure 539 that, in human placental

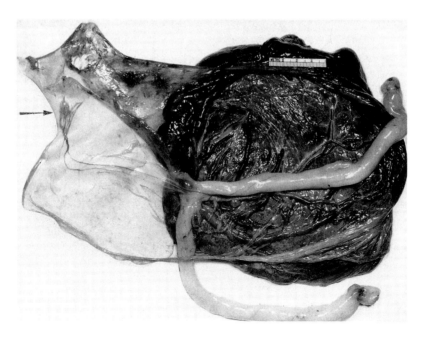

FIGURE 555. Immature DiMo twin placenta whose translucency of the dividing membranes is apparent. The cords seem to arise at the same spot but are nevertheless in separate amnionic compartments. Note the remains of a single yolk sac (arrow), from where omphalomesenteric vessels course toward the cords.

development, the single chorionic sac has long since formed when vessels develop from the yolk sac or in situ, at about the 13th day. One must envisage that these primitive vascular precursors sprout all over the inner surface of the primitive chorionic membrane; when the fetal heart gradually begins to pump, these fine vascular precursors start to fill with blood. The vessels undoubtedly link with one another at this early time. The type of anastomosis that ultimately develops is probably a matter of chance. Whether the vessels become arteries or veins is determined by the direction of blood flow and its pressure. Some of the anastomoses are kept open and others atrophy, depending on the velocity of flow. It may also be presumed that MZ twins often derive from embryonic splits with unequal cell numbers; it is therefore possible that one heart beats sooner or stronger, and that it influences the direction of flow in the anastomoses.

Monoamnionic Monochorionic Twin Placenta

The MoMo twin placenta is the least common type. It occurs in approximately one or two of 100 sets of twins in the U.S. population but has a nearly 50% perinatal mortality. Barss (1988) found that fetal demise occurred mostly before 24 weeks, when enough room for fetal motions and entanglement was still available in utero; Carr et al. (1990) found that after 30 weeks no further death occurred. Similarly Tessen and Zlatnik (1991), who reviewed 21 sets of MoMo twins, found that fetal death did not occur after 32 weeks. Double survival used to be so uncommon that many papers were published with the title, "MoMo twins with double survival." The classical paper on MoMo twins is that by Quigley (1935), who believed the condition to occur only once in 60,000 pregnancies. Quigley found only one case report during the preceding 12 years. Altogether perhaps 110 cases had been reported at the time of his review. More recent papers give an incidence of 1:10,000 to 1:16,000 pregnancies. Quigley found double survival in only 15.6% and an overall fetal mortality of 68%.

Most commonly, fetal death is due to entangling of umbilical cords because of fetal movements. This knotting of cords is unpredictable and is often found in young pregnancies, with abortion ensuing. It can now be visualized sonographically before birth, and management of such cases is changing. Thus Belfort et al. (1993) identified not only cord entanglement but also venous obstruction by color Doppler flow study. This diagnosis led to successful interruption of an otherwise endangered pregnancy. Tabsh (1990a) suggested that the diagnosis of monoamnionic twin placentation is easily made at amniocentesis by injection of indigo carmine, but the sonographic demonstration by Belfort and his colleagues (1993) indicated that this new method is superior to previous studies. They found cord entanglement and venous obstruction with Doppler flow studies that led to better management of their three pregnancies. Other complications occur in MoMo pregnancies, such as prenatal coagulation, exsanguination through placental anastomoses, or bleeding from one twin into the other through anastomoses, and congenital malformations.

One hopes, as died Belfort et al. (1993), that through prenatal diagnosis (Dunnihoo & Harris, 1966; Sutter et al., 1986) the chances of MoMo twin survival can be improved. Rodis et al. (1987) managed three sets of twins successfully despite their severely knotted cords; they also made suggestions for management. These authors identified one of these twins as having the typical transfusion syndrome. Driscoll (personal communication, 1970) has also seen the transfusion syndrome in MoMo twins. To find the transfusion syndrome in MoMo twins is otherwise uncommon (Wharton et al., 1968).

Table 27 presents a summary of the relevant literature on MoMo twin survival. Of 169 sets of MoMo twins, only 202 infants (60%) survived. The causes of death were predominantly cord entanglement with stillbirth (Figures 556, 563) or neonatal death, prematurity, and congenital anomalies. The aim of prenatal surveillance is to prevent the knots or entanglements of the cords to become fatal. It is not known when knots first form, but because it requires considerable fetal mobility to produce knots they are occasionally found already early in pregnancy, when more fluid exists (e.g., Figure 556). On the other hand, it must be noted that term neonatal MoMo twins can have extensive knotting without compromise of the umbilical circulation. One presumes that space limitations in the uterine cavity prevent the formation of new knots with advancing gestation, which may also be the reason why such knotting is uncommon in triplets. Only knots already present from an earlier gestation may have the potential to compromise the fetus.

Lee et al. (1988) endeavored to ascertain the best mode of pregnancy management when MoMo placentation is diagnosed sonographically. They surveyed perinatologists and ascertained 59 pregnancies with an overall perinatal mortality of 34.8%. A much higher mortality incidence was found when the diagnosis was made before 25 weeks' gestation than later. Although entangling of cords was an important cause of late death, there was an astonishing frequency of transfusion syndrome fatalities during earlier gestation. Frequent nonstress tests were recommended as the principal strategy for supervising these gestations.

TABLE 27. Reports of monoamnionic twin pregnancies (incomplete).

Source	Year	Sets of MoMo twins (no.)	Survivors (no.)	Remarks
Quigley	1935	1	1	Review of 109 cases
Litt & Strauss	1935	1	0	Knots, one anencephalic
Parks & Epstein	1940	1	2	Knot, no anastomoses
Coulton et al.	1947	2	4	No entangling
Wilson	1955	5	4	Anencephaly, CHD, knots, tangles, anastomoses, fold
Whitehouse	1955	1	1	1 Papyraceus, knots, anastomoses
Craig	1957	1	2	Entangling; 166 cases cited
Librach & Terrin	1957	3	6	One knotted
Walters & Whitehead	1957	2	2	Both knotted
Sinykin	1958	1	3	First triplets, entangling
Pickhardt & Breen	1958	1	2	No knots; anastomoses
Semmens	1958	1	0	1) Anemia, RDS. 2) CHD. No knots
Green et al.	1960	1	2	Knot, entangling
Zuckerman & Brzezinski	1960	2	1	2 Sets macerated, knots; other knots; 1 lived, 1 macerated
Tafeen et al.	1960	3	4	2 Knotted
Raphael	1961	5	5	2 Anomalies; 4 knot/entangling
Wensinger & Daly	1962	3	5	3 Knots/entangling
Timmons & de Alvarez	1963	4	4	3 Knots; 1 CNS damage; 1 fold
Goplerud	1964	1	2	No knots/entangling
Benirschke & Driscoll	1967	3	3	Knots
Dunnihoo & Harris	1966	1	2	No knots
Simonsen	1966	2	2	1 Knots
Wharton et al.	1968	18	24	1 CHD, 1 palsy, anastomoses
Larson et al.	1969a	1	0	Forked cord
Larson et al.	1969b	1	1	Both anomalies; no knots
Moestrup	1970	2	2	1 SUA (third case); no knots
Israelstam	1973	1	0	Knotting
Chapman	1974	3	2	Knotting
Mauer et al.	1974	1	1	Both discordant anomalies
Averback &	1977	1	1	No knots
Wigglesworth	1980	1	1	Macerated, entangling
Litschgi & Stucki	1981	1	2	Cord of twin. 2 around neck of twin. 1, cut during delivery, both velamentous, IUD
McLeod & McCoy	1982	1	2	Entangling
Colburn & Pasquale	1982	1	1	Torsion & thrombi of cord
Colgan & Luk	1984	1	1	SUA, severe anomalies; knots
Berry et al.	1986	23	13	4 Anomalies; knots/entangling
Lumme & Saarikoski	1986	1	2	Knots
Sutter et al.	1987	3	6	3 Knotted
Rodis et al.	1988	5	9	Knots in 1; transfusion syndrome; anomaly; twinning in 1/87 pregnancies, after 20 weeks
Barss	1988	59	77	Review of prenatally diagnosed MoMo twins
Lee et al.	1991	21	28	Controlled study; no deaths after 32 weeks
Tessen & Zlatnik	1990	2	4	Method for diagnosis in utero
Tabsh				
Total		192 (384 twins) 100%	234 Survivors (60%) 150 Dead (40%)	

RDS = respiratory distress syndrome. IUD = intrauterine death. CHD = congenital heart disease. CNS = central nervous system.

The proximity of cord insertion is apparently not the principal determinant of knotting. We have seen extensive knotting in cords that were inserted at opposite margins of the placenta and no knots in some placentas whose cords arose next to one another (Figure 549). When a cord is obstructed for long periods, it may become thin (Figure 557), a condition described in several papers (Table 27). One complication of MoMo twinning is that the accoucheur may inadvertently cut the wrong umbilical cord during delivery. Donald (1964) described such a case, and a similar set of MoMo twins was observed by McLeod and McCoy (1981). When the first twin could not be delivered because the cord was extensively entwined about the infant's neck, the cord

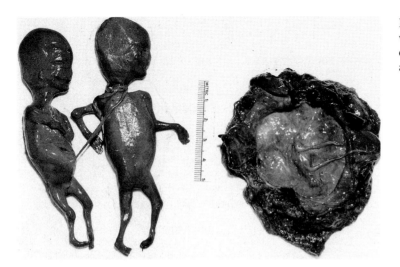

FIGURE 556. Macerated monoamnionic twins (12 weeks) with extensive knotting and entangling of cords. Fetal movements must have been extensive at an early embryonic age.

was severed. Only after the fetus was fully extracted was it realized that a mistake had been made. After rapid delivery of the second twin, both twins survived.

The placental surface of MoMo twin placentas usually has a continuous sheet of amnion without folds between the cord insertions. There have, however, been four observations of the existence of folds. Timmons and de Alvarez (1963), in a report of four cases of MoMo twins, found "a short fold of what was thought to be membrane . . . present in the midportion of the fetal surface but [it] did not extend between the origins of the umbilical cords." Another plica ("fringe") was described in one of the five MoMo twins reported by Wilson (1955). It inserted between the two cords of a set of MoMo macerated twins born with a surviving DZ triplet. A similar case has been described by Wolf (1920), and another is shown in Figures 558 and 559. One of these twins died during the neonatal period with the Klippel-Feil anomaly. The cords arose from a single point and had six vessels that merged into three (arrow

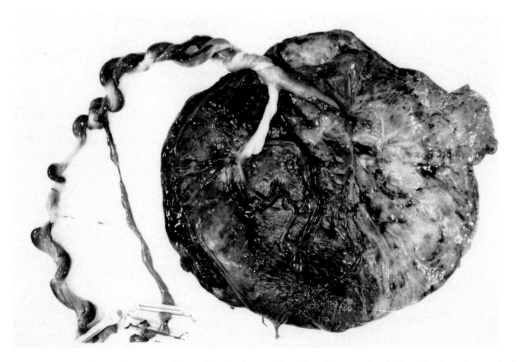

FIGURE 557. MoMo twins at 38 weeks' gestation with fetal death of one at 23 weeks (20 cm CR, 400 g macerated). Survivor is alive and well. Note the entangling and knotting of cords, the thin cord of the dead twin, and the extensive infarction of the right placental half. Anastomoses cannot be demonstrated this late after fetal death.

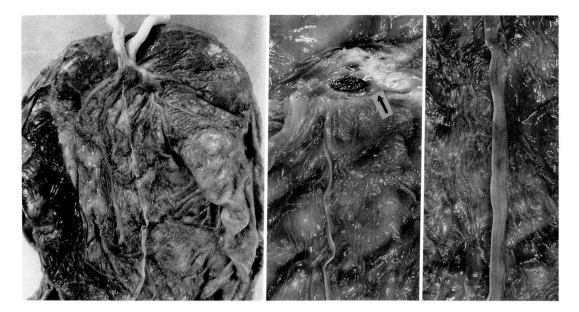

FIGURE 558. MoMo twin placenta; one twin had Klippel-Feil syndrome. The two cords arise from the same spot, where vessels merge (arrow). Thin plica, composed of two amnions, extends from the cord insertion to the margin. It is presumably the remains of an early attempt at formation of two amnionic cavities, interrupted by the twinning event.

in Figure 558) at their base. A thin, falciform plica extended from the cords to the margin of the placenta. The tip of this plica, which consisted of two fused amnions, showed degenerative changes and scarring (Figure 559). It is possible that disruption of two former amnionic cavities had occurred. It is also possible that the twinning took place just about at the time (7 days) the amnion is first set aside, thus preventing the forma-

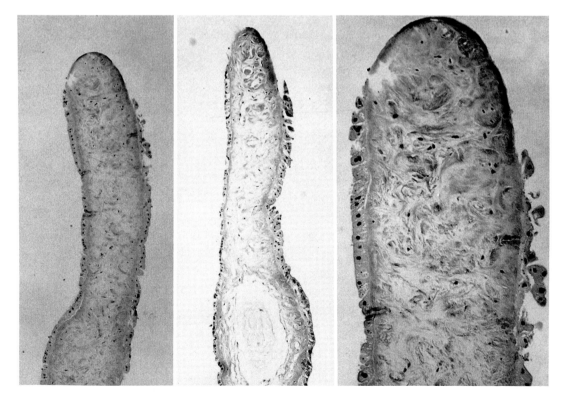

FIGURE 559. Sections through the tip of the plica shown in Figure 558. Note the degeneration of amnionic epithelium and the scarring of underlying connective tissue. H&E. ×260.

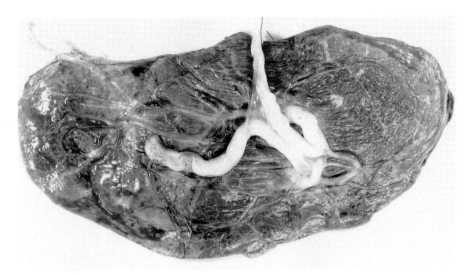

FIGURE 560. MoMo twin placenta at term with extensive interfetal vascular anastomoses. The nearly commonly arising cords are bound within an amnionic fold. This stage presumably arises shortly after the placenta shown in Figures 558 and 559.

tion of two complete amnionic sacs. It is difficult to conceive that an apparently single cavity could form from the spontaneous breakdown of the dividing membranes in a DiDi placenta, although it was assumed by Pickering (1946) in his description of boy/girl twins with a MoMo placenta. Nylander and Osunkoya (1970) also described "heterosexual twins with monochorionic placenta." They depicted a ridge with DiDi configuration present in one part and a DiMo relation in another portion of the placenta. Another unexplained case of monochorial placenta with fraternal twins was recorded by Verschuer (1925). He relied on the placental diagnosis of an assistant, and the dizygosity was based only on some physical differences (e.g., hair color). Gilbert and his colleagues (1991) not only identified several new cases of twins with rupture of dividing membrane occurring in utero ("pseudomonoamniotic" according to Megory et al., 1990), they also highlighted the morbidity that may ensue, such as entangling of extremities in bands and entangling of cords. Diamnionic placentas can be transformed into MoMo organs by amniocentesis and funipuncture (Magyar et al., 1991) and spontaneously, perhaps by fetal activity.

Tracing the history of MoMo twinning one step further, one may postulate that the placenta of Figure 560 was determined shortly after that which yielded the plica. Here the two cords, arising nearly one from the other, are bound together by a delicate amnionic membrane.

Anastomoses of fetal blood vessels seem to occur less commonly in MoMo placentas than in DiMo twin placentas. The proximity of the cord insertion again is not the sole determinant. Of greater importance, perhaps, is the possibility that when large communica-

tions exist the cell and blood traffic between the two fetuses may have the greatest influence on their wellbeing. The example depicted in Figure 561 features the placenta of a macerated MoMo twin and a co-twin who expired soon after birth (Benirschke, 1961). This case aroused much interest subsequently. The initially sur-

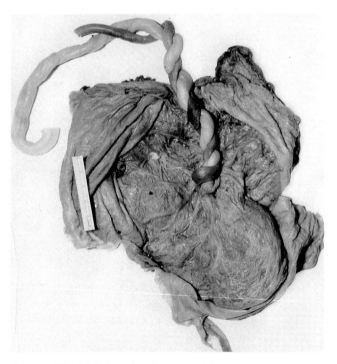

FIGURE 561. MoMo twin placenta with one macerated fetus (dark cord). The survivor, who had disseminated intravascular coagulation, died at age 62 hours (see Figure 562). (From Benirschke, 1961, with permission.)

viving infant died within 62 hours. Bilateral renal corti-cal necrosis, cerebral liquefaction, and other degenera-tive changes, including thrombi and focal mineralization (Figure 562), were present. These findings are descrip-tive of the sequelae of disseminated intravascular coagulation (DIC). We then postulated that thrombo-plastin from the macerating twin had entered the survivor's bloodstream via interplacental anastomoses prior to birth and had thus initiated DIC. There have been several other reports of neonatal deaths with findings of DIC (Table 28). During the past few years we have been consulted on many similar cases, where the medicolegal question arose as to possible preventive cesarean section after the death of one twin. Many of the descriptions in the literature are similar to the case shown here, but conclusive proof of prenatal DIC with definitive coagulation studies has been difficult to obtain. In a case of macerated MoMo twin with a term live-born co-twin, Bulla et al. (1987) found neonatal platelet counts of 67,000/mm^3 that later rose to 300,000/ mm^3. The infant died on day 10 with bilateral renal, splenic, and central nervous system (CNS) necroses. Patten et al. (1989b), who examined five co-twins with one fetus having died prenatally and who used the term twin embolization syndrome (TES), identified "active consumptive thrombocytopenia" in one of their cases with renal and CNS defects. Microcephaly and various other CNS abnormalities, in addition to in-testinal, peritoneal, and renal destructive lesions, were the focus of their observations. They urged prenatal sonographic studies of such pregnancies. As to the evidence of consumptive coagulopathy, diligent study of some other cases ruled out their existence when fetal demise of one twin had occurred (Hanna & Hill, 1984).

This complex issue is of great importance. Many investigators have tried to answer the many questions that arise from these observations. Litschgi and Stucki (1980) reviewed their twin material and found that in 13 cases of 191 twin pregnancies (6.8%; 0.07% of all births) a macerated fetus was delivered with a live twin. They found one MoMo, seven DiMo, and five DiDi cases and suggested that immediate delivery is not advisable when one twin has died. In view of the dis-tribution of deaths in relation to ultimate delivery, they recommended that all such pregnancies be terminated by 39 weeks. This aspect is discussed further in the section on fetus papyraceus. This pathological feature is not limited to MoMo placentation but affects all monochorial twins. Because the probability of thrombo-plastin infusion from a dead twin is highly unlikely, alternative explanations have been sought. They are completely summarized in a large paper by Liu et al. (1992) and are further discussed later in the chapter. Specifically, they suggest that acute hypotensive events occur in the surviving twin immediately after one twin dies because of the common placental vasculature. Jou

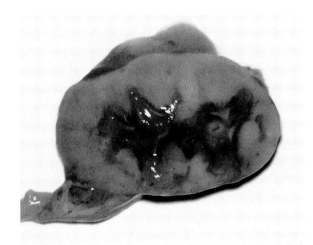

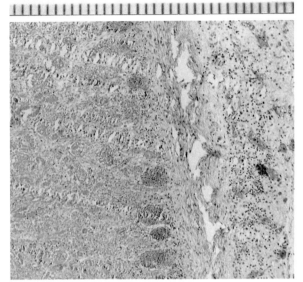

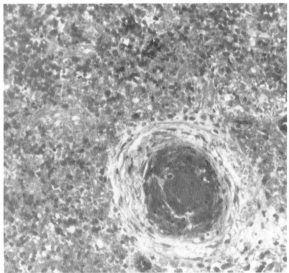

FIGURE 562. Organs of a premature neonate whose placenta is shown in Figure 561. Bilateral renal cortical necrosis and widespread thrombosis were present when this infant died at 62 hours. (Top) The kidney had diffuse, yellow, cortical infarction. (Center) Microscopic appearance of renal cortical necrosis. (Bottom) Splenic thrombus.

TABLE 28. Summary of twins with prenatal damage perhaps due to vascular transport of coagulation products or acute blood loss.

Source		Placenta	Remarks
Benirschke	1961	MoMo	Macerated twin; survivor with renal cortical necrosis, porencephaly; presumed DIC (Figures 561 and 562).
Figure 563	1959	MoMo	Macerated twin, thrombi in umbilical vessels; survivor died with extensive cerebral palsy.
Figures 567/568	1986	MoMo	32 Weeks; stillborn 1,800 g, survivor 2,400 g died with hydrops (? due to cord tangles); AA, A-V anastomoses, arthrogryposis, CNS atrophy.
Figure 569	1986	DiMo	Fetus papyraceus, velamentous cord; survivor has porencephaly; mother had DIC after delivery. Transfusion syndrome.
Timmons & de Alvarez	1963	MoMo	Case 4 had cerebral palsy from "embarrassed circulation."
Rosenquist	1963	DiMo	Adrenal, pulmonary, renal calcifications in donor of transfusion syndrome.
Moore et al.	1969	DiMo	(1) Singleton with velamentous cord and DIC. (2) Monochorionic, macerated; survivor developed DIC and died; blood studies were normal. (3) DiMo, one macerated stillborn, other had anemia and bilateral renal cortical necrosis but survived.
Dimmick et al.	1971	DiMo	Velamentous cord. CNS and renal necroses; unable to identify anastomoses; secondary to cord insertion?
Thomas	1974	Tri? Di	Male had IVH and coagulation disorder; one female macerated, one with mild coagulation disorder.
Durkin et al.	1976		Review of 8 cases; monochoriomics at highest risk.
Mannino et al.	1977	DiMo	Fetus papyraceus with aplasia cutis in survivor; review.
Melnick	1977	?	Macerated twin; CNS damage in survivor who died with CNS necrosis. Review of Collaborative Study and risk assessment.
Yoshioka et al.	1979	?, MZ	Three sets of twins had porencephaly and a macerated stillborn; thrombosis of cerebral artery. Authors considered emboli as cause.
Jung et al.	1984	?	Review of hydranencephaly and porencephaly; 11% had twins, most were macerated.
Barth & Harten	1985	DiMo	Term with macerated twin (death at 13–16 weeks); gastroschisis, CNS damage.
Nakayama et al.	1986	DiMo	Macerated fetuses with infarcts of CNS, kidney, spleen, liver. Reviewed 14 twins, only monochorionic twins had poor prognosis.
Hughes & Miskin	1986	DiMo?	Fetal death at 20 weeks, following which prenatally diagnosed CNS cysts, microcephaly, and renal dysplasia developed.
Yoshida & Soma	1986	DiMo	Review; macerated with cerebral palsy in survivor. Skin defects in male; macerated female co-twin.
Szymonowicz et al.	1986	? DiMo	Six cases with survivors having CNS deficits; other infarcts; review of total literature (53 cases).
Bulla et al.	1987	MoMo	Renal and CNS necroses; other was a macerated fetus. A-A and V-V anastomoses.
Leidig et al.	1988	?	Two of four cases with prenatal IVH were twins.
Jones	1988	?	Hydranencephaly; 30 cm fetus papyraceus.
Patten et al.	1989	DiMo	5 Cases with various brain, kidney, and intestinal defects.
Fisher & Siongco	1989	DiMo	Massive porencephaly; renal splenic infarcts.
Cherouny et al.	1989	MoMo	20 cases; one MoMo twin developed brain cysts, prenatal evaluation was reassuring.
Anderson et al.	1990	DiMo	Four cases, second trimester fetal deaths, CNS lesions, GI lesion in 2.
Larroche et al.	1990	DiMo	15 Monochorionic twins, vascular "instability."
Fusi et al.	1991	DiMo	CNS and renal necroses, no coagulation defect, transfusion.
Margono et al.	1992	DiMo	Foot necrosis before birth.
Liu et al.	1992	DiDi/DiMo/MoMo	38 Twins, 3 triplets. Damage in 19 offspring (72% monochorionics).

et al. (1993) observed sonographically the reversal of blood flow in the umbilical cord after fetal death of one twin. That such an event may occur is also evident from the detailed postmortem description of the original Siamese twins Chang and Eng Bunker (Kormann, 1869). After the death of Chang, Eng complained of chest tightness and expired within 2 hours. Large anastomoses were present in their xiphoid connections at autopsy through which exsanguination of Eng presumably occurred. An important case report has been published by Sherer et al. (1993) that shows the rapid development of the cerebral consequences of such fetal demise. They followed a twin transfusion set of twins with fetal death of one at 23 weeks, followed by spontaneous resolution of hydrops. They were able to demonstrate sonographically that echogenic changes had become prominent in the brain of the survivor within 48 hours. The authors considered these changes to be hemorrhages that eventuated into a severely microcephalic anomaly. Death of one MZ twin was observed at 27 weeks by Lander et al. (1993). Doppler sonographic observations within 24 hours after the death showed "remarkable variability in flow velocity waveforms in the umbilical artery of the surviving fetus. Changes from reversed to normal end-diastolic flow velocities were recorded within 6 minutes."

These suggestions are simplistic hemodynamic explanations for a complex dynamic state that exists in utero of ill-defined vascular communications. Because hemodynamic results of these anastomoses have been largely inaccessible to us until the event of Doppler flow studies, relatively little hard information is available at this time, and it is common to oversimplify from our incomplete knowledge. That the situation is much more complex in utero is to be inferred from the case report of Grafe (1993). She described DiMo liveborn premature twins, both with antenatal white matter necrosis; they died subsequently. Aside from a velamentous insertion of twin A's umbilical cord, there were artery-to-artery and vein-to-vein anastomoses. We assume that irregular flow back and forth through these anastomoses was responsible for the cerebral destructions.

At this point, it is important to understand the possible fates of placental tissue when one twin dies. If there are large interfetal vascular communications, the placental half of the dead fetus may continue to be perfused by the survivor. On the other hand, if the anastomoses are small, the dead fetus's placenta gradually atrophies and eventually appears infarcted. It is much the same as what happened when experimental fetal removal was practiced in rhesus monkeys. There is gradual atrophy of placenta, with much deposition of intervillous fibrin.

The problem of maternal DIC with a dead fetus is often discussed under the heading dead-fetus syndrome (Strauss et al., 1978). Although it has been described in some cases where one twin had died in utero (Skelly et al., 1982; Romero et al., 1984), in other patients it did not develop (Wittmann et al., 1986; Cherouny et al., 1989). The reason for the differences is not clear. This complex aspect is not treated further in this text.

To explain some cases of prenatal damage observed in twins after the death of the co-twin, it has also been postulated that thrombi in the fetal circulation embolize via the interfetal anastomoses, from the dead twin to the living twin. Although it is true that thrombi from fetal vascular occlusions can embolize to the fetus (Wolf et al., 1985), the lesions usually seen in the survivors of pregnancies with a macerated co-twin are not typical of those caused by emboli. Yoshioka et al. (1979) postulated that the CNS damage of the twins they examined, which had macerated co-twins, resulted from occlusion of large vessels. They believed that emboli from macerated co-twins were the most reasonable explanation for the damage. They cited a case described by Clark and Linell (1954) to support this hypothesis. The erythroblastotic stillborn described by Clark and Linell, whose mother had been treated with cortisone, had an occlusion of the internal carotid artery and cerebral vessels. The authors suggested that because the thrombus did not resemble loose clot it probably originated from an embolus; and they opined that it represented embolized placental tissue. This assumption cannot be the case, for there were no villous remains in the clot. Admittedly, it contained erythroblasts, but degenerating placental tissue never embolizes to the fetus. Clots could embolize from venous vessels, which have occasionally been shown to be thrombosed. Such an event is shown in the fetal vessels of Figure 563.

Massive plethora in a macerating twin masqueraded as the recipient of the twin transfusion syndrome in several cases. The transfusion syndrome could be ruled out, however, because the twins were of the same size, they had similar-sized hearts, and there were large placental anastomoses. We presumed that the plethoric twin had recently received large quantities of blood from the survivor via large vascular communications in the placenta. This acute transplacental fetus-to-fetus bleeding, with resulting plethora of one twin, was first mentioned by Lehndorff (1961) and was also described by Cameron (1968). Lehndorff correctly hypothesized that marked shifts may occur through large anastomoses during, or even before, delivery. Later, Bleisch (1965)

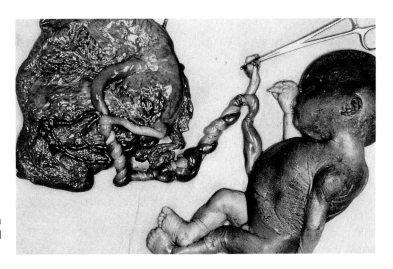

FIGURE 563. Macerated stillborn MoMo twin with extensive knotting of cords. The surviving infant died 3 months later with extensive brain necroses.

had the same thoughts. This phenomenon is different from the transfusion syndrome, which constitutes a specific entity and is discussed below.

All these cases have assumed great importance because cerebral palsy is common in twins (Durkin et al., 1976; Scheller & Nelson, 1992). Eastman et al. (1962) estimated it to be five times more common than in controls and assigned as the chief cause the prematurity of twins and an unfavorable intrauterine environment. This higher incidence of cerebral palsy (and of mental deficiency) affects primarily monozygotic twins (Berg & Kirman, 1960; Russell, 1961). Furthermore, a characteristic type of skin defect that is secondary to prenatal dermal necrosis (aplasia cutis) is also primarily associated with DiMo placentation and fetus papyraceus (Mannino et al., 1977). It is thus challenging to better understand what causes these prenatal insults. Moreover, as stated, there has been much litigation in cases of twins with cerebral palsy. In these legal suits it is commonly assumed that the obstetrician must be at fault when brain damage occurs in one of twins because had a quick cesarean section been done this damage would not have occurred—or so it is stated. It must be pointed out in this context that Bejar et al. (1990) have shown that porencephaly may already be present at birth, and that it correlates best with one of two circumstances: (1) fetal infection (chorioamnionitis, funisitis); or (2) MZ twins having placental vascular anastomoses. Leviton and Paneth (1990) reviewed the possible causes of CNS white matter necrosis. They concluded, as did Larroche et al. (1990), that circulatory phenomena were important aspects in the causation of cerebral palsy. Fusi and colleagues (1991) found no coagulation disorder but observed "acute twin-twin transfusion" as the cause of brain damage. They were emphatic that intervention would have to take place before fetal death occurred if CNS sequelae were to be prevented. Norman (1980, 1982) made somewhat similar observations on prenatal brain necrosis in DiMo twins.

For all these reasons it is of importance that we delineate more precisely the pathogenesis that leads to this prenatal CNS damage, so it may be anticipated and prevented if possible. Hurst and Abbitt (1989) observed that encephalomalacia and intraventricular CNS hemorrhage developed prenatally in a set of twins with the classical transfusion syndrome. In the case described by Hughes and Miskin (1986), bleeding complicated a known twin pregnancy at 20 weeks, and subsequently one twin became macerated. In the survivor, brain cyst development could be followed sonographically after 30 weeks and was found in the newborn after cesarean section at 37 weeks. Interestingly, the kidneys of this microcephalic, porencephalic infant had cystic changes, which we assume stemmed from former focal areas of necrosis. Nakayama et al. (1986) studied 14 live-born twins with macerated cotwins. Among the three with neonatal death, CNS, renal, splenic, and liver necroses were found. Relevant contributions have been forthcoming (Dudley & D'Alton, 1986; Liu et al., 1992), but a consensus as to the best management of monoamnionic twin pregnancies has not yet emerged (Hagay et al., 1985). Melnick (1977) estimated that some 3% of near-term monozygotic twins have a dead co-twin. Furthermore, one-third of the survivors, or possibly 1% of MZ twin births, have severe brain defects as a consequence of putative DIC (Jones, 1988).

These considerations are especially important in view of the evolving practice of intentional fetal elimination when discordant anomalies of twins are found, when too many fetuses are conceived, during the therapy of the prenatally diagnosed transfusion syndrome, and for prenatally diagnosed genetic disorders (Åberg et al., 1978). In these situations, it must be recognized that there are possible consequences for the second twin when one is eliminated (Wittmann et al., 1986).

The possibility of DIC developing in the remaining living twin after one had died led Cox et al. (1987) to sample the fetal vasculature of 19 twins. This evolving technique of fetal blood sampling promises much insight into the prenatal vascular relations among twins. It is for these complex reasons that we have summarized relevant case information in twin pregnancies with fetal death in one twin (Table 28). Other large tables may be found in Liu et al. (1992) where all relevant literature is also discussed. As is seen below, there is a good possibility that the survivor in cases of prenatal twin death experiences significant acute blood loss through superficial, large interplacental anastomoses. One can envisage that when one twin dies the other bleeds into this vascular bed, now devoid of counterpressure. Indeed, paradoxical plethora has been seen in discordant twins, in which the smaller (earlier dead) twin is plethoric.

In order to accumulate relevant prenatal information of such occurrences, Toubas et al. (1981) studied the fetal response to acute hemorrhage (15%) in the lamb. The arterial blood pressure, pH, and heart rate of the fetus fell significantly, and the cardiac output decreased. The blood flow in the fetus (kidneys, gastrointestinal tract, and lungs) and to the placenta were markedly reduced. Toubas et al. did not report any structural changes of these organs due to the hemorrhage. It is necessary that in future cases of prenatal death of one MZ twin we accumulate information on neonatal hematological parameters. Measurements of hematocrit, deformed red blood cells (schistocytes), split fibrin degradation products, platelet changes, and nucleated red blood cells can provide some of the information needed for better understanding this entity.

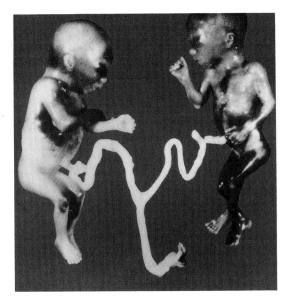

FIGURE 564. Forked umbilical cord of MoMo twin abortuses at 17 weeks' gestation. The smaller twin (right) had a single umbilical artery but no other anomalies. (Courtesy Dr. Marilyn Jones, San Diego.)

MoMo twins presumably arise at approximately days 8 to 10 of fertilization age and are next to last in the spectrum of the MZ twinning events (Coulton et al., 1947). This type of placenta is nearly always found with conjoined twins, only one exception having been reported (Weston et al., 1990). Monoamnionic twins may have a single or a forked umbilical cord (Figure 564) or two separate cords. Forked cords are occasionally found also in completely separate MoMo twins (Figure 564). In other MoMo twins, the cords originate close to each other on the placental surface, as in the cephalopagous conjoined twins whose placenta is shown in Figure 565. Forked cords have been described by Larson et al. (1969a) in a set of macerated abortuses. MoMo twins often have extensive vascular anastomoses between the fetal circulations, particularly when the cords are in close apposition (Figures 566–568). The impact that the cord position may have on the outcome of the surviving MoMo twin (after fetal death of one) is further documented in Table 28. When velamentous insertion of one cord complicates placentation in such cases, growth retardation and fetal death are especially common (Figure 569). Monoamnionic twins, as other MZ twins, may have remarkably different development, as was true of the case described by Larson et al. (1969a). Discordant anomalies are particularly common. Observations on MoMo twins have led to a better understanding of some types of congenital anomaly. Thus the occurrence of renal agenesis in one of MoMo twins (unilateral agenesis in the other, who survived) was not associated with the Potter syndrome, as expected. Rather, the adequate production of amnionic fluid by the more normal twin prevented this phenotype, indicating that it relates purely to the volume of amnionic fluid present (Mauer et al., 1974). The anomalous twin also had normal respiratory function. It died of uremia at 12 days of age. Similar observations were later made of MoMo twins, where one had sirenomelia.

Monoamnionic placentation has also been observed in MZ triplets. Sinykin (1958) described the triple survival of MoMo triplets whose placenta is shown in Figure 570. We have observed a monoamnionic triplet placenta of stillborns. The pregnancy was terminated with prostaglandins at 27 weeks, when fetal death had become evident. One was a tiny acardiac fetus, one was

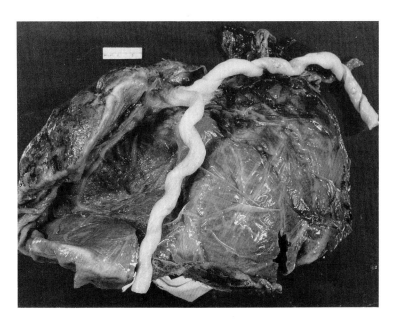

FIGURE 565. Forked umbilical cord of MoMo cephalopagous conjoined twins. (Courtesy Dr. S. Romanski, Los Angeles.)

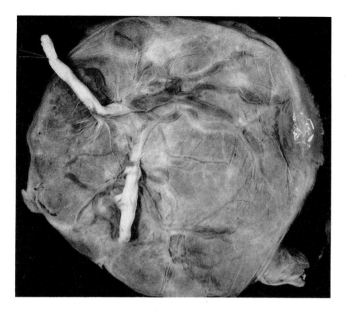

FIGURE 566. Term MoMo twin placenta. Note the extensive vascular anastomoses on the fetal surface.

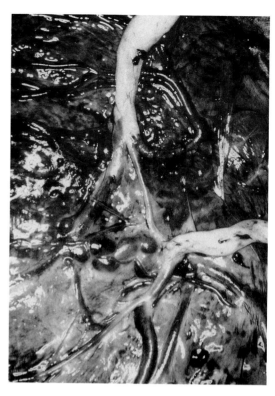

FIGURE 568. Large anastomoses are seen between cord vessels of the MoMo twin placenta shown in Figure 567.

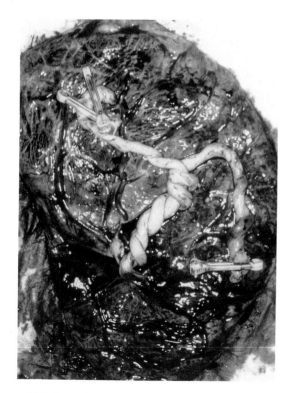

FIGURE 567. MoMo twin placenta with entangling of umbilical cords. Twin B (top left) died from nonimmune hydrops. At autopsy no cause was found for the hydrops. It was assumed to be the result of interference with venous return from the placenta. Figure 568 shows the large anastomoses after the cords have been untangled.

anencephalic, and the third was a normal macerated fetus (Figure 571). The long-standing nature of thrombotic events in such twins is evident from the frequent calcifications found in their placental vessels (Figure 572).

It would be expected that MoMo twins, who are probably determined between days 8 to 10 of development (Figure 539), may differ in the number of yolk sacs they possess. Figure 573 shows two early gestations of MoMo twins with an only partially divided yolk sac. It is considered to be the product of splitting on day 11 if the developmental table shown is correct. In another set of stillborn MoMo twins (with a dichorial triplet) we have seen two yolk sacs; that placenta also had two velamentous cords and presumably had its embryological origin prior to the placenta with partially divided yolk sac.

Diamnionic Monochorionic Twin Placenta

The DiMo twin placenta is the commonest form of placentation of identical, or monozygotic, twins. Each twin is enclosed in its own amnionic sac, and the "dividing membranes" are composed of two amnions only (Figures 530–533). As can be seen in the pho-

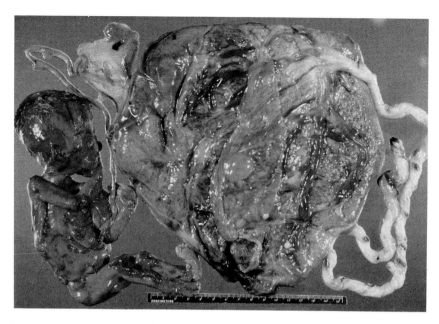

FIGURE 569. DiMo twin placenta with macerated fetus papyraceus at left, having velamentous insertion of its cord. The surviving fetus had porencephaly and was presumed to be the recipient in a transfusion syndrome.

tomicrographs, the amnion possesses epithelium and connective tissue. The presence of a layer of connective tissue has, regrettably, been mistaken as being diagnostic of chorion, the reason for being so didactic about the identification of these dividing membranes. These amnionic membranes can be moved freely over the chorionic surface. Because they often do so move before birth, it is not unusual to find the dividing membranes at a place that does not correspond with the "vascular equator" of the two twins' placental halves (Figure 574). DiMo placentas usually have two yolk sacs, and virtually all of them have vascular anastomoses, as was delineated earlier in the chapter. The cord insertion is, as in all twin placentas, more often marginal or velamentous than that of singletons. Single umbilical artery (SUA) is commoner in one or both of these twins (Thomas, 1961). Because the amnion does not have its own blood vessels, the dividing membranes

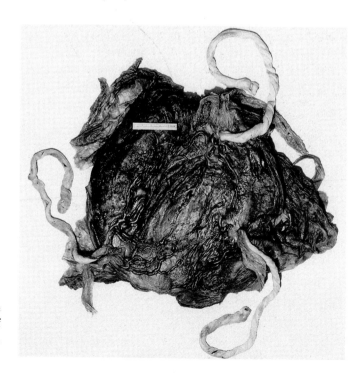

FIGURE 570. MoMo triplet placenta at term. There were anastomoses among all circulations and no entangling of cords. The triplets survived. (Courtesy Dr. M.B. Sinykin, San Antonio.)

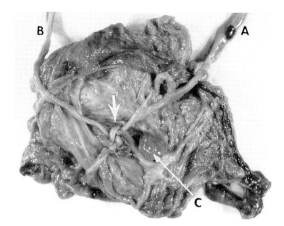

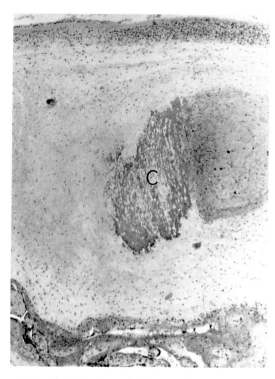

FIGURE 571. Monoamnionic triplets, all of whom were macerated. Labor was induced at 27 weeks. Triplet A was structurally normal; B was anencephalic; C was a diminutive acardiac fetus. Note the extensive knotting (large arrow).

FIGURE 572. Calcification of the vascular wall and an old thrombus in the placental surface vessel of one of MoMo twins that was macerated.

must survive on the nutrients and oxygen contained within the amnionic fluid. This notion is supported by the finding of amnion necrosis in cases of fetal death or amnion nodosum when one of the twins is oligohydramneic (Figure 575). In such cases, only the amnionic epithelium degenerates. The underlying connective tissue is generally intact. In cases of prenatal infection the inflammation is also lacking in these dividing membranes, and meconium pigmentation is sparse when it is found elsewhere in the amnionic cavity.

The lack of intersac transfer of solutes is illustrated by the results from injection of hypertonic saline when abortion is intended. Kovacs et al. (1972) injected 200 ml of a 20% NaCl solution into one sac after having removed 380 ml of amnionic fluid at 22 weeks. Cardiac activity stopped within 2 hours in one twin, and labor commenced 20 hours later. The DiMo twins weighed 300 g each; the injected fetus was macerated, but the

other was alive at delivery. Only the amnion of the injected side was necrotic. Hoch et al. (1972) made similar observations in a dichorionic twin pregnancy, but in this placentation it is more expected that solute transfer does not occur between the two sacs. Finally, a most unusual DiMo twin placenta, sent to us in consultation, is illustrated in Figure 576. This placenta shows one amnionic sac literally contained within the other; the twins differed appreciably in size.

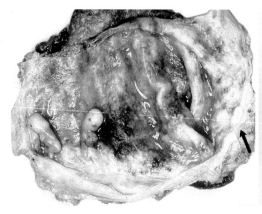

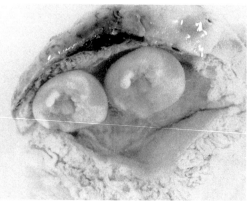

FIGURE 573. Monoamnionic twin abortuses, structurally normal (left). Note the partially duplicated, bean-shaped yolk sac (arrow). Therapeutic abortion of DiMo twins was done at 33 days' gestation (right).

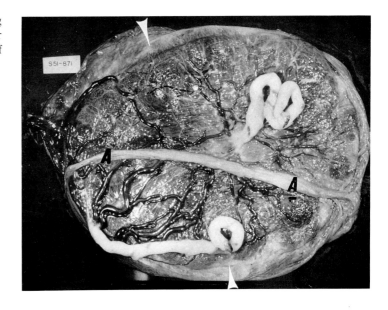

FIGURE 574. DiMo twin placenta with apposing amnions (A, A) meeting at angles to the vascular equator (arrowheads). Note the marginal insertion of the cord at left.

Diamnionic Dichorionic Twin Placenta

The DiDi twin placenta may be composed of separate disks, or the two placental portions may be intimately fused. It is the most common type of twin placentation and shares with others an increased frequency of marginal and velamentous insertion of umbilical cords. The fused placentas present the appearance seen in Figure 577. When the fetal vessels are injected, there is no exchange of fluid between the two fetuses. This finding is also borne out by a sharp line that divides the placentas, easily seen when one twin has died before

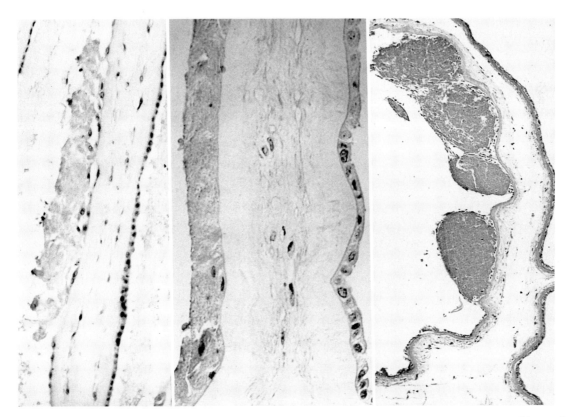

FIGURE 575. Degenerative features of the left amnion of dividing membranes in cases of DiMo placentas with one fetus dead (center, right) and amnion nodosum (left).

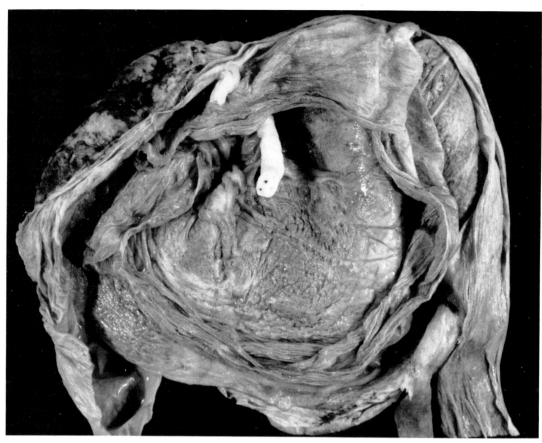

FIGURE 576. DiMo twin placenta (550 g) of MZ twins. One amnionic sac is enclosed by the other. The outer sac contained a smaller fetus with velamentous insertion of the cord. (Courtesy Drs. Anderson and Weinraub, Martin Luther King Hospital, Los Angeles.)

birth (Figure 578). A frequent and unusual feature of DiDi twin placentas is the phenomenon of irregular chorionic fusion, a feature well shown in Figure 579. In such placentas the membranes do not meet over the areas perfused by the individual fetuses; in fact, the placentas may be separated, and a portion of one may be covered by the membranes of the other. This phenomenon is best explained by assuming that the

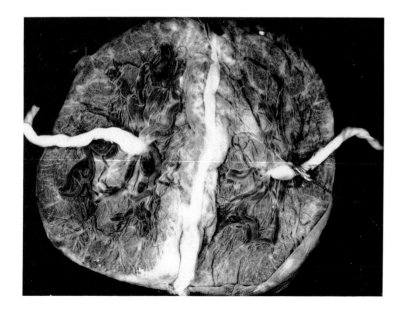

FIGURE 577. DiDi twin placenta, intimately fused. Left cord has SUA; right cord is being injected without transfer of fluids.

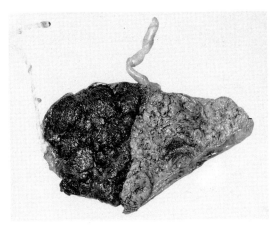

FIGURE 578. DiDi fused twin placenta, maternal surface. Twin at left is Rh-negative and living; twin at right is Rh-positive and macerated. There were two corpora lutea at delivery. Note the clear dividing line between the two placentas.

intraamnionic fluid pressure of one cavity gradually expands its sac, pushing the other away (Figure 580). It is not unlike the process of lifting the marginal chorion in cases of circumvallate placentation. It has no influence on the wellbeing of the fetuses, and no vascular fusion takes place in the areas of overlap.

When the fetal outcome of fused DiDi twin placentas is compared with that of separated DiDi placentas, Buzzard et al. (1983) found that there is a greater difference in birth weights with fused placentas. The inference is that placental proximity has a prenatal influence on fetal development, perhaps because of competition for space during placental expansion.

Vanishing Twin Phenomenon

It is not uncommon that one twin dies long before birth. If the pregnancy continues undisturbed, this fetus may disappear. It may become flattened (fetus compressus, fetus papyraceus); or when it is large, it may macerate and lose much of its fluid and become misshapen. Although fetus papyraceus has long been known, the phenomenon of a "vanishing twin" is a recent addition to our nomenclature. The term should be reserved for multiple pregnancies that are identified sonographically during the first 15 weeks of pregnancy and that have as their outcome a single fetus.

The seminal report on the vanishing twin was that of Levi (1976), who studied 6,690 early pregnancies sonographically. Of 118 patients identified to have twins, only 86 sets of twins were delivered. When the diagnosis of twins was made prior to 10 weeks, the rate of disappearance was 71%. When the diagnosis was made between 10 and 15 weeks, the disappearance rate was 62%. When twins were first diagnosed after 15 weeks, none disappeared. Similar figures of twin resorption (70%) were reported by Robinson and Caines (1977).

The vanishing twin is thus a feature of early pregnancy; its diagnosis is made by the ultrasonographic finding of two echogenic rings denoting the presence of two sacs. Although the existence of vanishing twins is not doubted, the possibility of error in the diagnosis of twin gestations was mentioned by Levi. It was described in greater detail by Landy et al. (1982), who reviewed the literature and made a letter-inquiry of colleagues. It is possible that a yolk sac or amnionic sac that is still separate from the chorion or other features of early

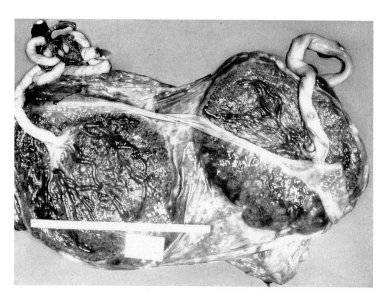

FIGURE 579. DiDi twin placenta with irregular chorionic fusion. The chorion laeve of the left placenta overlaps one-third of the placenta at right. There is no vascular fusion.

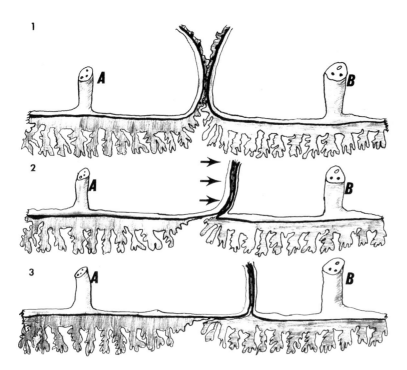

FIGURE 580. Presumed mechanism that leads to irregular chorionic fusion, as in Figure 579.

embryonic life are occasionally mistaken for twin cavities (e.g., Green & Hobbins, 1988). Moreover, only rare reports of placental examination have accompanied these studies. Even more rarely have empty sacs or old hemorrhage been identified. An exception is the report by Jauniaux and his colleagues (1988). They reported the placental findings of 10 such cases, five of which came from in vitro fertilization; five were spontaneous. First trimester bleeding was the only clinical evidence of this occurrence. In five cases, the vanished twins were identified as "well delineated plaques of perivillous fibrin deposition, associated in one case with embryonic remnants." There are other reports of frequent early vaginal bleeding episodes in these patients. Those events may represent the spontaneous abortions of twins. If the reported cases are applicable to the general population, the excessively high frequency of calculated twin gestations is surprising.

The term vanishing twin was perhaps first used by Jeanty et al. (1981). It is now an established entity in obstetrics, and more careful study of the placenta is needed to secure its place. When such a twin is found sonographically or only a remnant of a second sac is identified, every attempt should be made to obtain some karyotype information from the chorionic sac at birth. The results from such studies may eventually indicate whether these vanishing twins are chromosomally abnormal. Additionally, RLFP study should define zygosity readily.

Such fetuses would perhaps have been aborted were it not for a normal twin in the same uterus. Gruenwald

(1970) described three such specimens, two of which, however, are best considered to be fetus papyracei. One specimen consisted of a local thickening in the membranes that, when sectioned, disclosed ribs and other fetal tissues. We have seen several placentas with vanished twins enclosed in the membranes, but their presence had not been detected sonographically. Figures 581 to 584 show what their appearance may be. In all of these specimens, clear evidence of a second sac existed. In two of these cases and in several others observed, tiny embryos could be identified. Those embryos had surely died before 8 weeks' gestation. The fact that they were still recognizable suggests that when a vanished twin cannot be detected in the term placenta the diagnosis must have been either erroneous or an empty sac of a blighted ovum had been present and aborted. It is surprising in the embryos shown here how long an embryonic structure can coexist with a normally developing twin. A similar early, vanished embryo was first shown by Bergman et al. (1961) in their description of a blighted fetus. The tiny embryo, also present in the membranes, was essentially similar to the one shown in Figure 582. The empty sac feature was further discussed in the prospective study of 1,000 pregnancies by Landy et al. (1986). They calculated a minimum twinning incidence from this material as 3.29%, if not 5.39%. This figure is much higher than the currently estimated twinning frequency of the general population. These authors suggested that vanishing twins may be the source of rhesus sensitization. In view of the small quantities of blood potentially present to stimulate the

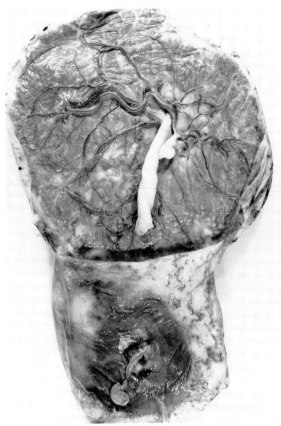 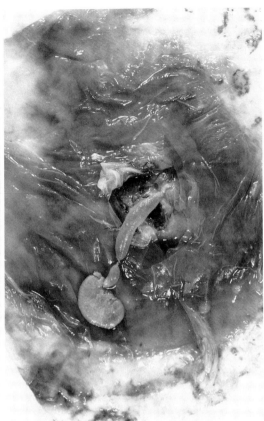

FIGURE 581. DiDi separated twin placenta at term. The patient presented with alleged abruptio. A normal term twin was delivered; a second placenta with a tiny (2 cm) embryo was found in the membranes. When its sac was opened (right), a yellow embryo of the opposite sex was attached to a swollen umbilical cord.

mother, this proposal seems to be an unduly pessimistic concern. Sulak and Dodson (1986) have presented evidence for two vanished triplets by demonstrating an empty chorionic sac. When the placental sac of the surviving singleton was studied, it was found to be filled with debris. Kapur et al. (1991) found an empty cavity of a former twin associated with a sirenomelic co-twin whose pregnancy was terminated at 18 weeks. Triplets had been diagnosed sonographically 4 weeks after conception by in vitro fertilization. It is more difficult to be certain that such structures as are shown in Figure 585 are the remains of vanished embryos, in this case a triplet, although we prefer to believe this view over ascribing these rests to be teratomas. In their study of 189 sonographically studied twin pregnancies, Yoshida and Soma (1986) found that 21 twins died. Nine qualified for the term vanishing twin. The association with prenatal bleeding was also emphasized by these observers.

In the differential diagnosis, it must be cautioned that retromembranous hemorrhages may occur after amniocentesis, and they can also occur spontaneously (i.e., without our knowing the cause). Such hemor-rhages must not be mistaken for vanished twins. The typical sonographic appearance of a small vanishing twin with normal co-twin at 14 weeks is shown in Figure 586.

The presence of vanished twins or fetus papyraceus has posed other difficult clinical problems. It has thus been reported that the maternal α-fetoprotein (AFP) may be significantly elevated in pregnancies complicated by a vanishing twin (Lange et al., 1979). The finding of high AFP levels has led to therapeutic abortion, the vanished twin not having been diagnosed (Winsor et al., 1987). There may also be an elevation of the amnionic fluid acetylcholinesterase levels. In the case described by Cruikshank and Granados (1988), this elevation was blamed on coexisting aplasia cutis.

Fetus Papyraceus

A fetus papyraceus forms when one of twins or higher multiple pregnancies dies during gestation and becomes compressed as pregnancy continues. There is no clear distinction between the vanishing twin and a fetus com-

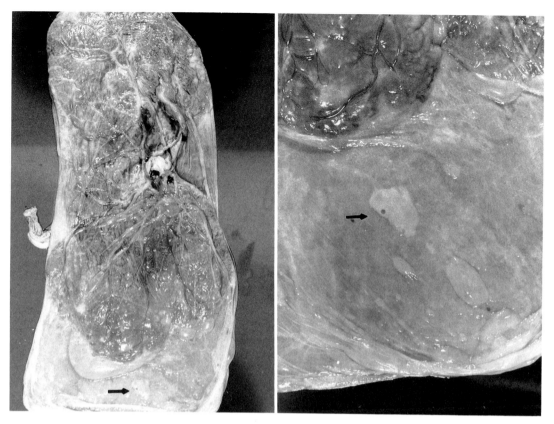

FIGURE 582. Term placenta with a separate embryo in the membranes (arrows). This embryo is similar to that shown by Bergman et al. (1961). The ocular pigment is readily seen. No placental remains were apparent.

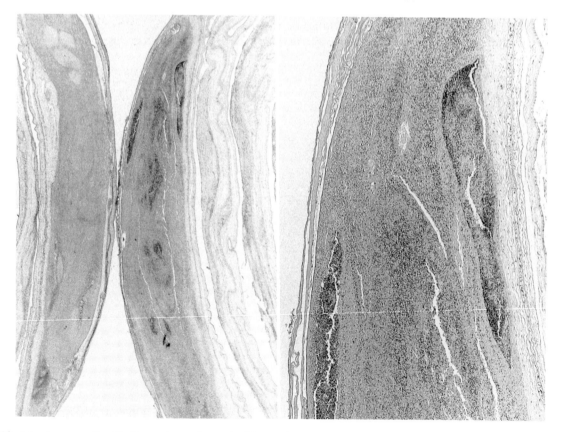

FIGURE 583. Membrane roll with the embryo shown in Figure 582. Macerated embryonic structures are visible. H&E. Left ×16; right ×60.

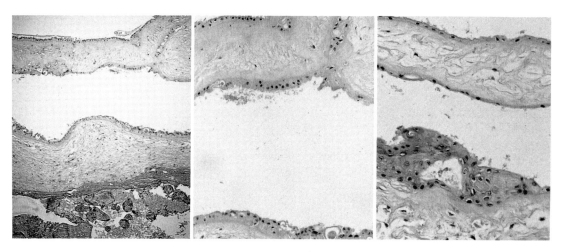

FIGURE 584. Mature placenta with vanished twin. A sub-amnionic sac containing debris is the remnant of a DiMo placenta. Note the squamous metaplasia (right), vacuolation (center), and amnion nodosum-like degeneration (left top). H&E. Left ×16; center ×40; right ×60.

pressus or papyraccus. Although such fetuses exist fairly frequently, they are often overlooked. They may be so compressed that small ones are found only with careful inspection of the placenta (Figure 587). We recommend that radiographs be obtained when such areas of thickened membranes are found and that the area be dissected carefully. The case shown in Figures 588 to 591 is a typical circumstance (Jackson & Benirschke, 1989). Sonographically, a typical fetus compressus was demonstrated (Figure 588); at delivery it was a separate mass of fibrin compressed in the membranes of the normal twin's placenta (Figure 589). Careful peeling of the DiDi membranes revealed the fetus compressus with umbilical cord (Figure 590), whose skeleton was normal by radiography (Figure 591). The fetus compressus of Figure 592, on the other hand, was enclosed in a separate amnion. It was acardiac with SUA and had six toes.

Several of these compressed fetuses had living co-twins with skin defects (Figure 593). Some have well defined, infarcted placentas (Figures 578, 593). In others, one can demonstrate that twisting of the umbilical cord at its fetal insertion is the presumed cause of demise. The cause of death, however, is not always

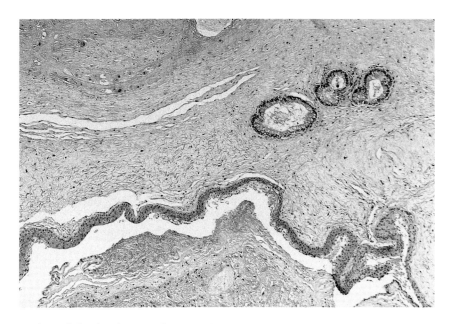

FIGURE 585. Remnant of a triplet in the membranes of a term DiMo twin placenta. Note the inclusion of columnar, mucus-producing epithelium and a cyst with squamous lining in the chorion. H&E. ×60.

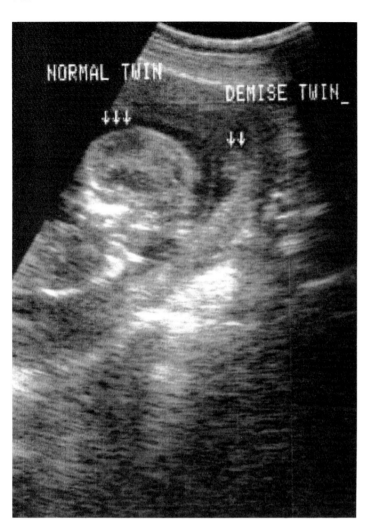

FIGURE 586. Sonogram at 14 weeks with one normal twin and one dead (vanishing) twin. The latter still has a separate cavity and measures 1.7 cm. (Courtesy Dr. J.D. Stephens, San Jose.)

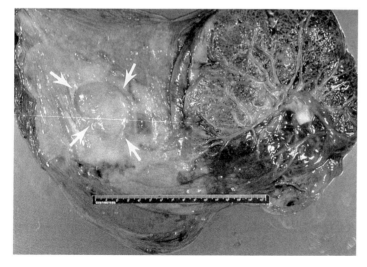

FIGURE 587. Diminutive fetus papyraceus in the membranes of a normal twin's placenta (arrows). Its dichorionic placenta was a flattened mass of fibrin.

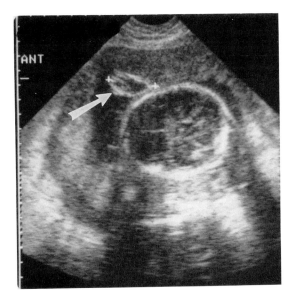

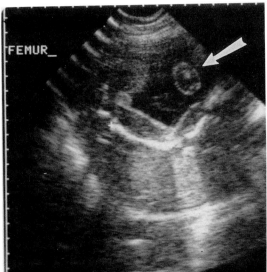

discerned. Thus when the donor dies, as in the transfusion syndrome, its placenta may be so atrophied or infarcted that the causative vascular anastomoses can no longer be verified. Chromosome preparations of the macerated twin may not be feasible, because of the advanced state of maceration. Cytogenetic examination may be possible, however, from the samples of the chorionic membranes, as would be RFLP study, which should be attempted. At least once, such a study of the DNA of a fetus papyraceus showed it to have a dizygotic relation to the living twin (Lemke et al., 1993). Acardiac fetuses are readily distinguished radiologically and by dissection from the normal, usual fetus papyraceus. A careful study of these vanished twins is doubtlessly worth the effort.

When maceration is advanced, the fetus may appear to be a lithopedion (Figure 594). This feature is more commonly found when a fetus is retained for months beyond the expected gestation; it need not be a twin (e.g., El-Sherbini, 1963). The formation of a lithopedion is particularly commonly described in retained fetuses of primates (e.g., Mueller-Heubach & Battelli, 1981; Swindle et al., 1981). Miller and Dillon (1989), who cited relevant literature on the frequency of lithopedion, estimated that perhaps 400 cases had been described. They presented the case of a 94-year-old woman with lithopedion that had been present for probably 61 years without doing harm. One of the most

FIGURE 588. Sonogram of a twin pregnancy with fetus papyraceus. The skull is seen at the arrows; the normal twin's skull is next to it (top). The femurs are at the bottom. (Courtesy Dr. G.R. Leopold, San Diego.)

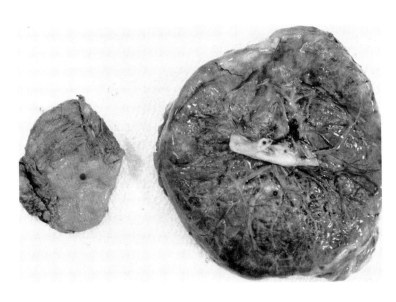

FIGURE 589. Specimen in Figure 588 is shown at term. The fetus papyraceus was in a separate mass (at left).

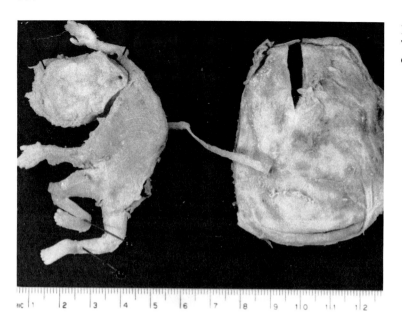

FIGURE 590. Same case as in Figures 588 and 589. The dissected fetus is attached to a short umbilical cord.

unusual placentas of a presumed former twin in our collection is depicted in Figure 595. It is the placenta of a normal infant at term, with marginal insertion of the cord. In the center of the larger placental mass was what appeared to have been the site of insertion of another cord, with fetal vessels radiating to it. No twin was found.

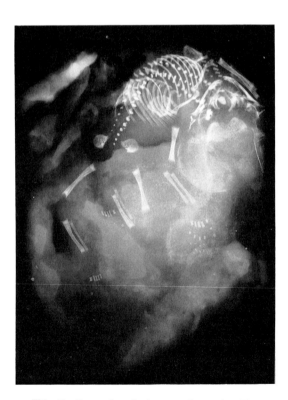

FIGURE 591. Radiograph of the specimen in Figure 590, showing a normal skeleton.

On occasion, a large fetus papyraceus presents with dystocia at delivery (Leppert et al., 1979). A fetus papyraceus may be one of triplets (Roos et al., 1957; Benelli, 1962) (Figure 571), and we have been advised of two of triplets found to be fetus papyracei at term (Shih, personal communication, 1986; see also Esposito, 1963). They may be of monochorionic or dichorionic gestations; congenital anomalies other than acardia have been occasionally identified on dissection. The co-twin of a fetus papyraceus may also have anomalies, such as microcephaly, absent ear (Roos et al., 1957), gastroschisis (Weiss et al., 1976), ileal atresia (Saier et al., 1975), or pulmonic stenosis (Baker & Doering, 1982; review by Szymonowicz et al., 1986). In a discussion of a case of ileal atresia, Sander (1983) drew attention to the possible cause of these anomalies. He suggested that they may have a prenatal thrombotic etiology, analogous to the phenomenon of DIC discussed above. Whether the scalp lesions in co-twins of fetus papyracei, also seen occasionally, are analogous to the aplasia cutis described by Mannino et al. (1977) is not clear. Demmel (1975), who reviewed all types of neonatal skin defect, does not mention the occurrence of macerated co-twins with these cases. The placenta was probably not examined in his somewhat older case population. A case similar to that of Mannino et al. (1977) was presented by McCrossin and Roberton (1989). Although their case was complicated by toxoplasmosis, the extensive skin defects of this neonate were essentially similar to those of Mannino et al. They were also in the process of healing at birth, and as early as 18 weeks' gestation a macerated, much smaller twin was demonstrated sonographically. Lemke and colleagues (1993) described extensive aplasia cutis in a twin asso-

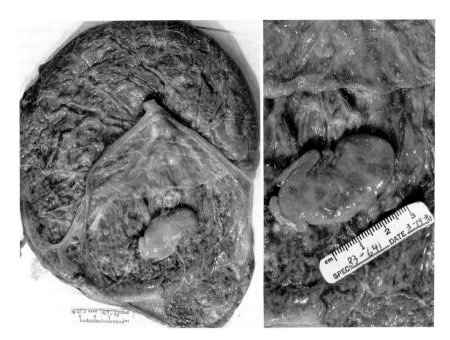

FIGURE 592. Fetus papyraceus in a separate amnion (DiMo placenta). It had SUA and six toes. It was shown to be acardiac upon dissection.

ciated with a dizygotic fetus papyraceus; regrettably, the placenta was not studied.

Innumerable reports of fetus papyracei have been published in the literature. The bulk of these cases from the older literature may be found in the comprehensive review by Kindred (1944) and publications of the material from the clinics of Litschgi and Stucki (1980), Yoshida and Soma (1986), and Johnson et al. (1986).

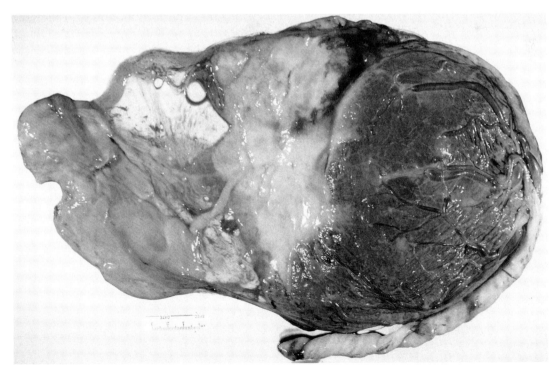

FIGURE 593. Typical fetus papyraceus with cord visibly attached to the infarcted twin placenta (DiMo). The surviving twin had scalp defects.

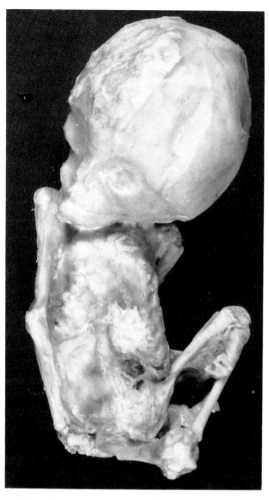

Figure 594. Fetus papyraceus with the appearance of a lithopedion.

Kindred reviewed 150 cases that had been published up to 1944. Of the 141 cases with adequate information given, 66% were dichorionic twins and three cases were MoMo twins. Mills (1949) was critical of many of Kindred's concepts. He reported three sets of monochorial twins, one of which was macerated. He wanted to separate mummified from compressed fetuses when many authors make such distinction. In my opinion, that question is moot. Litschgi and Stucki (1980) observed five dichorial and eight monochorial (one MoMo) twins. They suggested that when a macerated twin is recognized delivery should occur by the 39th week. That this advice is not uniformly accepted was mentioned earlier in the chapter.

For unknown reasons, death of the other twin may follow when a fetus papyraceus is present (Camiel, 1967; Yoshida & Soma, 1986). Forman (1956), who described a case with dichorionic placenta, stated that fetus papyraceus was first mentioned by Pliny (70 AD). Johnson et al. (1986) attempted to ascertain the incidence of fetus papyracei in 34,677 deliveries from their hospital. A total of 515 twins were observed, of which 27 (5%) had a single intrauterine fetal death; 16 of 25 liveborn co-twins survived (64%). The placenta was monochorial in 70%. One survivor had multiple infarcts, another had a gangrenous leg at birth, and several had thrombi. Puckett (1988) discussed the management of pregnancies when a second trimester twin dies, and Chescheir and Seeds (1988b) observed the spontaneous disappearance of hypofibrinogenemia following in utero death of a twin. They suggested that prophylactic heparin therapy is not warranted when one twin dies. Enbom (1985), who reported two cases of

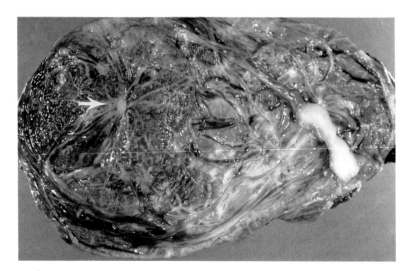

Figure 595. Term placenta with near-marginal insertion of the cord. At the arrow is a structure that has the appearance of a second cord, with fetal vessels radiating toward it. No twin was found.

antenatal death of one of DiMo twins, was also fearful of this complication with thrombosis and reviewed the literature. The survivors did not show sequelae of DIC. Foot necrosis and thrombosis of placental vessels were recorded in the survivor after fetal death of one twin by Margono et al. (1992). Bass et al. (1986) observed persistently elevated amnionic fluid AFP and acetylcholinesterase levels after the death of one twin, findings supported by Streit et al. (1989).

Carlson and Towers (1989) also found that of the 17 multiple gestations with fetal death of one twin they studied there was significant risk to the survivor. Their review suggested that fetal death of one twin occurs as often as in 2.6% of multiple gestations and three times more often in monochorionic than dichorionic twins. This occurrence is the reason Cox et al. (1987) have used fetal blood sampling for the surveillance of such surviving twins.

Szymoniwicz et al. (1986) reported six cases of a monozygotic twin surviving with CNS defects after the death of a co-twin 1 to 11 weeks before delivery. They also reviewed the 16 reports in the literature (with a total of 53 such cases) and concluded that delivery should be seriously considered when one twin dies in utero. In their survey of these cases, 72% had CNS defects, 19% had gastrointestinal (including liver and spleen) defects, 15% had renal lesions, and 8% had pulmonary lesions. Anderson et al. (1990) found not only CNS necrosis but also bowel injury in two of four cases with prenatal demise of a monochorionic twin. Szymoniwicz et al. described placental thrombi in some of their cases and continuing hematuria that lasted 2 weeks in such a survivor, suggesting a continuing process that was initiated before birth. Their vascular disruption hypothesis suggested infusion of thromboplastins, but they gave no account of the placental vascular anastomoses of their cases. The most recent report by Liu et al. (1992) of 41 cases with one prenatal death gave similar findings and suggested that exsanguination is the primary cause of injury to the survivor.

Transfusion Syndrome

The transfusion syndrome is considered to be a specific entity in twins, caused by the unidirectional, prenatal transfusion of blood through A-V anastomoses in the monochorionic twin placenta. One twin is the donor, and the other the recipient. The syndrome was first clearly delineated by Schatz (1882, 1886), when he observed a set of monochorial twins with gross discordance in size and development. One was edematous and urinated many times before dying at 12 hours of age; the other was a hypotrophic twin who never urinated and who had an empty bladder at death (53

hours). The atrophic twin had decubiti of the knees and ankles, much like the aplasia cutis described by Mannino et al. (1977). Schatz (1882) had already suggested that the fetal vessels were anastomotic through a "third circulation," which he was subsequently able to demonstrate clearly by injection of the DiMo placenta. He hypothesized also that the anastomoses were the cause of the fetus papyracei. In fact, he had described the "stuck twin" from clinical observations alone. This third circulation was then clearly perceived as proceeding from one of the donor's superficial (terminal) arteries into a shared cotyledon, from where it drained into the venous circulation of the recipient (Figure 596). This anastomosis is a capillary one. It is not always easy to demonstrate unless injections are made with thin liquids of selected areas in the placenta.

Because A-V anastomoses may be multiple and of varying size, and they may also proceed in opposite directions, the syndrome is variable in its consequences. This point has been elegantly shown with Doppler ultrasonographic studies of pregnancies complicated with this syndrome (Pretorius et al., 1988b). Pretorius et al. found it easy to demonstrate greater placental vascular resistance in one fetus, findings that were also shown in the therapeutic intervention in this syndrome by De Lia and Cruikshank (1989). Pretorius et al. (1988b) were unable to predict from their studies which was the donor and were also unable to anticipate the outcome. They confirmed that "the transfusion syndrome is an extremely complex dynamic physiologic state." De Lia and Cruikshank (1989) found markedly greater vascular resistance in the donor; Bromley et al. (1992) suggested from their experience with 12 sets that when clinical manifestations were clear-cut at 20 weeks the prognosis with conservative therapy was poorer than when the syndrome was diagnosed later in gestation.

Clinically, the transfusion syndrome is typically first recognized by acute hydramnios that develops around midgestation. Many other authors have made crucial observations since Schatz' description (e.g., Wurzbach & Bunkin, 1949). When sonograms or radiographs are obtained after the hydramnios appears, the twins are often recognized for the first time. Their sizes may already be significantly different (Schneider et al., 1985; Brown et al., 1989). In these cases, the placenta is almost always later found to be monochorial. The occurrence of acute hydramnios is considered to forewarn of a somber prognosis (Weir et al., 1979), and one twin may show edema, best recognized sonographically in the scalp (Wittmann et al., 1981). We have learned of a remarkable case of DiMo twins with severe hydramnios. At 20 weeks' gestation, the amount of amnionic fluid was 5,000 ml (withdrawn), with another estimated 2,000 ml unaspirated (K.L. Staisch, personal communication, 1976).

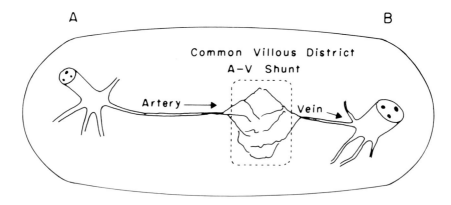

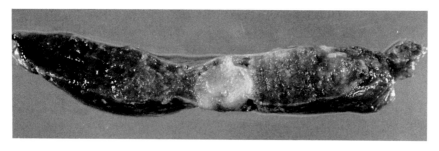

FIGURE 596. (A) Principal vasculature associated with the transfusion syndrome of MZ twins. (B) The shared cotyledon here was injected with water; it appears blanched. Note that the right half of this placenta is paler than the recipient's left half.

Not all authors agree with the concept that anastomoses may be the cause of the hydramnios in twin pregnancies (Krauer, 1964). Perhaps the first to voice his opposition to Schatz' notion of excessive urination of the "recipient twin" was Forssell (1912). He incorrectly interpreted that the placentas had "endarteritis" in their main stem vessels, and that the cause of the hydramnios was a degenerative amnionic epithelial change. These changes are clearly secondary. There is so much variation in the clinical expression of the transfusion syndrome that care must be exercised before making the diagnosis on clinical grounds alone (Wenstrom et al., 1992). Magnetic resonance imaging (MRI) has been usefully employed for the differential diagnosis (Brown & Weinreb, 1988). Not all hydramnios with twins, particularly chronic hydramnios, is due to the transfusion syndrome (Dorros, 1976). Accurate sonographic differentiation of the dividing membranes should therefore be attempted (Mahony et al., 1985; Townsend et al., 1988; D'Alton & Dudley, 1989). When acute hydramnios is found in a twin pregnancy, the second twin often has little or no amnionic fluid (oligohydramnios). This twin may move much less than the recipient, so the term "stuck twin" has been applied to this feature (Hashimoto et al., 1986; Brown et al., 1989; Patten et al., 1989a; Mahony et al., 1990).

To better explain the mechanism of hydramnios in this syndrome, Nageotte et al. (1989) proposed involvement of the atrial natriuretic peptide (atriopeptin) in the pathogenesis. They found markedly elevated atriopeptide levels in the recipient and lower levels in the donor of this syndrome (2,251 pg/ml versus 43 pg/ml; and 134 pg/ml versus 79 pg/ml). They suggested that the hormone is released because of the recipient's hypervolemia, and that its elevated levels may be responsible for the renal effects.

This prenatal unidirectional exchange of blood results in deprivation of nutrients to one twin and excessive development of the other. The twins may be remarkably discordant, as seen in the classical example shown in Figures 597 and 601. One twin was dehydrated and anemic and possessed organs that were significantly less developed than expected for the stage of development. The recipient was plethoric and had greatly enlarged organs. The discrepancy was particularly striking in the heart, but other organs were similarly affected. The A-V anastomosis responsible for this development is seen in Figures 598 and 599. The degree of discordance is variable. It probably depends on the number, size, and direction of the placental A-V communications. In general, when a simultaneous large (usually A-A) anastomosis coexists, the syndrome is prevented, and

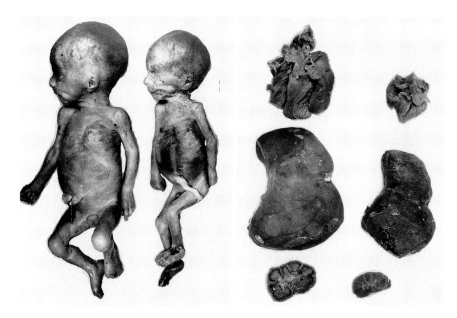

FIGURE 597. Twins with the typical transfusion syndrome. MZ twins were delivered at 27 weeks after two amniocenteses (4,000 ml and 3,000 ml) had partially relieved the hydramnios. (Left) The recipient weighed 540 g, exhibited edema, had a heart weight of 12.5 g, and the liver and one kidney were less severely hypertrophied. (Right) Donor weighed 410 g, and the heart weighed 2.7 g.

the twins reach greater gestational maturity. In its absence, the hydramnios leads to premature labor or to rupture of the membranes, with delivery before the 30th week of gestation. Alternatively, one twin may die and become a fetus papyraceus (Figure 600). In that case, the hydramnios ceases and the pregnancy may reach term. The same is true when the anastomoses are obliterated by laser (De Lia et al., 1990, 1993).

The development of intracranial hemorrhage has been witnessed in the recipient to have already occurred

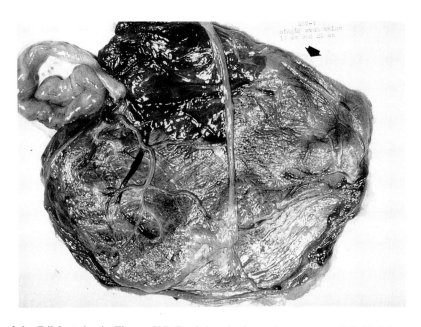

FIGURE 598. Placenta of the DiMo twins in Figure 597. Recipient had an edematous cord (left). The cord of the donor (right) is torn and was marginal. Note the area of "common villous district" (arrow) (see also Figure 599).

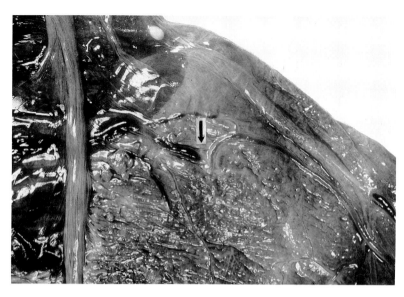

FIGURE 599. Common villous district of the case in Figures 597 and 598 is shown at the arrow. An artery from the donor (at right) dips into the placental tissue and emerges as a congested vein, coursing to the recipient (at left). The oval body at top is the remains of the yolk sac (single); there is also slight amnion nodosum in this cavity of the donor, who had oligohydramnios.

in utero, and periventricular encephalomalacia in the donor of this syndrome may also take place (Hurst & Abbitt, 1989). Other pathophysiological consequences of the syndrome have occasionally been recorded when prompt neonatal studies were undertaken. The set of DiMo twins with the transfusion syndrome whose data are shown next were delivered at 27 weeks' gestation and they were studied unusually well. The mother had preeclampsia, hydramnios, and placenta previa, and she had required a cesarean section. Both twins developed hyaline membrane disease and intraventricular hemorrhage. Their data were made available to us by colleagues from Minnesota. The results are so impressive they are shown here.

Some other cases in which clinical values are given are listed as follows (weight in grams, hemoglobin in grams per deciliter, hematocrit in percent).

Parameter	Donor twin	Recipient twin
Age at death (hours)	25	28
Birth weight (g)	732	1,100
Head circumference (cm)	23.5	26
Initial hemoglobin (g/dl)	3.2	22.4
Initial hematocrit (%)	12	70.5
Blood pressure (mm Hg)	20	50
Liver at autopsy (g)	42.4	32.2
Pancreas (g)	1.5	2.1
Kidneys, two (g)	7.7	13.8
Adrenal glands, two (g)	3.9	3.1

Source	Donor	Recipient
Klingberg et al. (1955)		
Weight	1,770	2,690
Hemoglobin	3.7	25.2
Hematocrit		87
Sacks (1959)		
Weight	1,431	2,084
Hemoglobin	5.5	24
Weight	1,424	1,843
Hemoglobin	18	30
Hematocrit	58	75
Weight	2,041	2,523
Hemoglobin	12.8	33
Hematocrit	93	
Weight	1,021	1,162
Hemoglobin	15	27
Hematocrit	41	80
Kresky (1964)		
Weight	1,900	2,600
Hemoglobin	11.3	22.1
Hematocrit	42	77
Bolens et al. (1968)		
Weight	2,410	2,510
Hemoglobin	25.9	13
Hematocrit	90	47

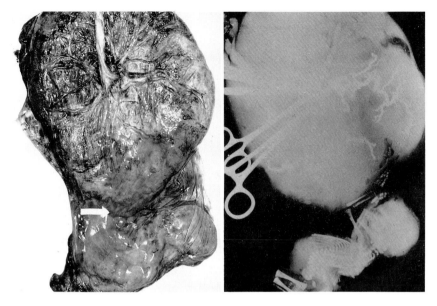

FIGURE 600. DiMo twin placenta with fetus papyraceus. Severe hydramnios at 20 weeks abated spontaneously. One twin died at that time. The pregnancy then normalized, and a normal twin was delivered at term with this fetus compressus. Its placental portion was completely infarcted.

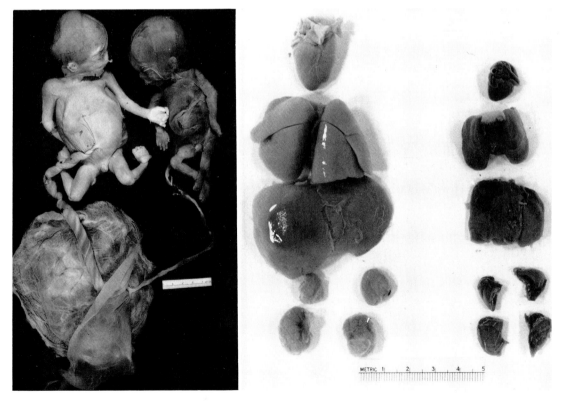

FIGURE 601. Macerated DiMo twins with the transfusion syndrome at 28 weeks' gestation. The donor (B) is plethoric, and the recipient (A) is edematous and pale. (A) Recipient: 285 g; 15 cm CR length; heart 3 g; lungs 10 g; liver 17.5 g; kidneys 1.5 g. (B) Donor: 189 g; 13 cm CR length; heart 0.7 g; lungs 3 g; liver 4 g; kidneys 1 g. The plethora of twin B is thought to be due to this twin's earlier death, with exsanguination of twin A into twin B.

Many other reports of blood values at birth have been published, with wide variations as seen in the tables above. At times the hematocrits reached astounding values. In a case referred to us, the plethoric newborn had necrosis of one leg due to arterial thrombosis. The other extremities infarcted shortly thereafter (J. Pritchard, personal communication). Some of the reports contain expressive color photographs of the twins (Becker & Glass, 1963). There is no correlation between the infants' size, the length of gestation, and the degree of plethora observed at birth. Moreover, the plethoric twin may be the smaller of the two, as seen in Figure 601. This discrepancy can be explained only when the anastomoses are carefully delineated and the circumstances of birth are known. This topic was especially well discussed in the case reports by Donnenfeld et al. (1989) and Bendon and Siddiqi (1989). An equally striking case is shown in Figures 602 and 603. The DiMo twins were both stillborn, but histological preservation was better in the anemic twin, and it is assumed that it died last. The weights of such twins (Figures 602–604) are important and are given next.

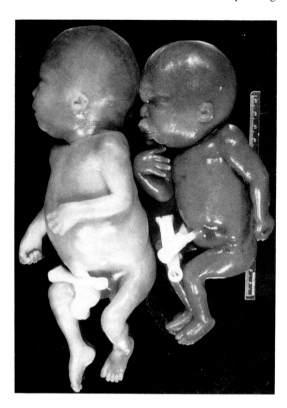

FIGURE 602. DiMo twins, the smaller being severely plethoric. The smaller size of the twin at right is due to the velamentous insertion of the umbilical cord.

Organs	Anemic twin	Plethoric twin
Body (g)	550	410
CR length (cm)	20	17.5
Heart (g)	11.3	3
Lung (g)	11.9	5
Spleen (g)	1	0.5
Liver (g)	37.2	8.3
Adrenals (g)	2.3	1.4
Kidneys (g)	4.9	2
Thymus (g)	0.9	0.2
Brain (g)	70	40

The smaller twin was growth-retarded because of its velamentous insertion of the cord. This case does *not* represent twin transfusion syndrome. The plethora was caused by reverse flow from the now-anemic twin, occurring through the large A-A anastomosis (demonstrated with milk injection) because of his longer survival. Another case of discordant twins we autopsied showed the donor to be plethoric. He was sonographically recorded as having died first; the anemic recipient died later from listeriosis. Autopsy confirmed the transfusion syndrome from the marked discordance of cardiac size (Benirschke, 1992). Other cases of prenatal demise and transfusion to the dead twin from the survivor were summarized in a later contribution (Benirschke, 1993).

Several authors have addressed similar unusual findings. Lehndorff (1961), who also reviewed the relevant literature, assumed that in most cases the

transfusion takes place during the terminal periods of delivery, when pressure changes occur because of uterine contractions. Klebe and Ingomar (1972) also believed that much of the transfer occurs during labor. With variable cord clamping practices, it may occur

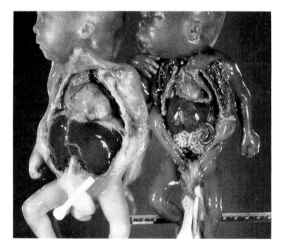

FIGURE 603. Same twins as in Figure 602. Note the smaller heart in the smaller, plethoric twin (right). See text.

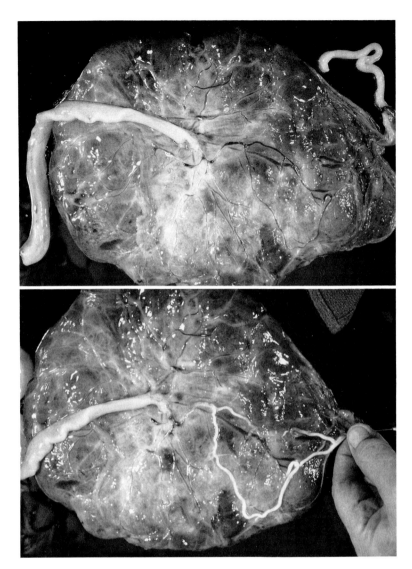

FIGURE 604. Placenta of twins in Figures 602 and 603. One large A-A anastomosis exists. The larger twin, who died last, must have exsanguinated into the plethoric twin through this anastomosis. This situation is *not* the transfusion syndrome.

immediately after birth. We have seen a pertinent case in this regard. Twins with significant birth weights, near term, had hematocrits of 32% and 63%, respectively. The smaller twin was plethoric and had no problems; the larger twin was anemic and required transfusion. The smaller twin had velamentous insertion of his umbilical cord, with much old retromembranous hemorrhage behind the cord insertion. Injection of the DiMo placenta showed that two large A-A anastomoses existed, in addition to A-V shunts. The villous blood content appeared similar, but the smaller twin's placental portion was much smaller. Our interpretation is that the growth-retarded twin (because of the velamentous cord insertion) was eventually unable to withstand the pressure column exerted from the larger twin that took place through the A-A anastomoses; he

thus became plethoric, perhaps during the terminal stages of labor. No cardiac hypertrophy was found in the larger twin, there was no hydramnios, and the fact that this pregnancy went to term suggested that it was not the classical twin transfusion syndrome. Features of long-term circulatory aberrations include cardiac hypertrophy, thromboses, and the presence of nucleated red blood cells. These findings bespeak the prolonged prenatal problem of adjustment to different circulatory phenomena.

The youngest specimens we observed to have signs of well established circulatory imbalance were a set of DiMo twin abortuses of about 10 to 12 weeks' gestation (Figure 605). Although those twins were still similar in size, their hearts were already grossly discordant. In another specimen of stillborn twins at 15 weeks, the

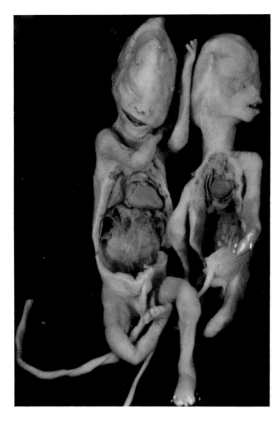

FIGURE 605. DiMo twin abortuses with the transfusion syndrome at about 11 weeks' gestation. The twins weighed 31 and 20 g, had 8 and 7 cm CR length, and had heart weights of 440 and 193 mg, respectively. This picture is the earliest evidence of the transfusion syndrome, with marked cardiac enlargement but relatively few bodily differences as yet.

plethora of the recipient was evident and the cardiac hypertrophy already well expressed (2.28 g versus 0.67 g). Despite this marked discrepancy, the bodies were virtually identical in their sizes and weights. The differences of fetal size commence later in gestation, usually after 25 weeks. Aherne et al. (1968) and Arts and Lohman (1971) reported that the anastomoses in typical transfusion syndrome twins are usually trans-villous and do not involve the larger surface vessels. It must be reemphasized that the mere plethora of one twin and anemia of the other do not necessarily signify the existence of the transfusion syndrome. To make the diagnosis of the transfusion syndrome it is important that the twins be of different size; and as minimal criteria they should have different heart sizes as well. It is clearly possible that large A-A or V-V anastomoses allow rapid transfer of blood when pressure relations change during parturition, and that the anastomoses can result in anemia or polycythemia, but differences in blood values alone do not justify the term transfusion syndrome. Indeed, there is much argument as to what clinical parameters to use when designating a set of twins as

having the transfusion syndrome. In some opinions, it is a hemoglobin difference of more than 5 g/dl; others also wish to include a coincident weight difference of more than 20%. These aspects were discussed by Danskin and Neilson (1989), who studied 178 consecutive twin pregnancies with a variety of parameters. They concluded that generally acceptable guidelines are not yet available, as dichorionic twins with such differences were found in their series who clearly did not have the syndrome.

Quantitative placental studies on the transfusion syndrome have rarely been undertaken. Sala and Matheus (1989) have addressed this issue with a relevant case. They found that the plethoric recipient had thinned trophoblastic villous covering and that the villous vessels were markedly distended. In contrast, the anemic "donor" had thick trophoblast and frequently "empty" villous capillaries. They also undertook stereological study of the villous architecture and provided quantitative data of differences in villous development. Their case is unusual in several ways. For instance, the hydramnios that one might have expected was apparently not present in this pregnancy; it was presumably absent because the pregnancy came to near term. That is distinctly unusual for the untreated transfusion syndrome. Although there was the expected marked difference in neonatal sizes (2,470 g versus 1,920 g), hemoglobin levels (29.3 g/dl versus 10.0 g/dl), and hematocrit values (75% versus 24%), the placenta had an A-A anastomosis. The smaller twin had velamentous insertion of the cord. The fact that there was an A-A anastomosis and that the pregnancy was carried to 36 weeks' gestation makes this observation unusual, and the data may not fit the usual cases of the immature gestation with the typical syndrome.

The frequency of the transfusion syndrome is difficult to estimate, but observations suggest that it is more common than is usually cited (Shah & Chaffin, 1989). Bebbington and Wittmann (1989) found 25 cases in their series of 595 multiple pregnancies (i.e., approximately 4% of twin gestations), which perhaps involves 5% to 10% of twins with monochorial placentas. Reviews of the syndrome are to be found in papers by Kloosterman (1963), de Marco (1964), Rausen et al. (1965), and Corney and Aherne (1965) and in more recent textbooks, but agreement of precise criteria is not easily obtained among the many points of view (Bruner & Rosemond, 1993). Single cases from different countries make other literature available: Littlewood (1963), van der Kolk (1964), Verger et al. (1963), Tojo et al. (1971), Koranyi and Kovacs (1975), Tuncer (1970), Sekiya and Hafez (1977), and others too numerous to cite. When the condition is diagnosed before 28 weeks' gestation, the overall survival rate was found to be only 21% (Gonsoulin et al., 1990a,b). Hydrops correlated with poor survival in this study, but decompression by amniocentesis was not beneficial in the outcome. The condition has also been described in one of triplets and higher multiple births, as for instance in the triplets described by Sekiya et al. (1973).

Aside from differences in weights and blood values, the transfusion syndrome has many other consequences. For instance, hyperbilirubinemia is often seen in the recipient (Conway, 1964), and Reisner et al. (1965) found symptomatic hypoglycemia in the donor to be a frequent neonatal complication. They speculated that it may be an etiological factor for "mental subnormality" in the twin's future. Falkner (1965) challenged this idea on the basis that the investigators had inadequate data. Reduced placental perfusion in the territory of the donor was held to be responsible for the marked differences seen during placental examination of these twins (Aherne et al., 1968). They suggested that the small placental volume may also have consequences related to reduced nutrient retrieval from the placenta, which they deduced would lead to fetal malnutrition. Conversely, one may speculate that the presumably lower blood pressure of the donor circulation prevents a normal placental expansion and that it may relate to the high incidence of velamentous cord insertion. The constant loss of blood proteins into the recipient twin through the A-V shunt may be another important factor for poor fetal growth. Abraham (1967) has shown dramatic differences in the villous structure of the two twins' placental villi. He suggested that the term parabiotic circulation, as used for experimental animal studies (Linke & Kuni, 1969) and sometimes applied to this syndrome, is not an appropriate designation. The term was popular at a time when immunological phenomena were first studied in depth, but it should no longer be used for twins. Abraham (1967) showed the lack of uniform concordance of hemoglobins with birth weights of 53 pairs in an interesting way.

Twin	No. with low hemoglobin	No. with high hemoglobin
Big	6	24
Small	19	4

The remarkable anemia of one twin's placental portion and polycythemia of the other's placenta was has been studied by Michaels (1967) and Aherne et al. (1968). Not only are the macroscopic features striking in their color difference but the histological structure of villi can differ substantially as well (Figures 606, 607).

The discordant organ development in twins with the transfusion syndrome has been variously studied by several authors. Thomas (1962) found not only hyper-trophy of cardiac muscle fibers in the plethoric twin but also that hyperplastic changes existed. Naeye (1964a,b, 1965; Naeye & Letts, 1964) undertook the most comprehensive organ analyses. Within this framework he was much concerned with hypoglycemia. By quantitative studies of tissue components, he found that the donor had significantly reduced, and the recipient significantly increased, cytoplasmic material. Differences of nuclear size and composition were less striking. He likened the findings to malnutrition in the donor and was particularly concerned with the reduction of brain weight. Studies of fetal growth parameters in various categories of twins (grouped according to placental type) confirm the essential findings of Naeye (Pridjian et al., 1991). DiMo twins were found to "have a high degree of brain-sparing growth restriction in the smaller twin and cardiac hyperplasia in the larger twin, most likely caused by hemodynamic inequalities."

Winner (1963) asserted that the different development was perhaps due to unequal genetic contribution from unequal splitting of the twins. That opinion does not bear in mind the complex nature of the syndrome. It is an ill-founded criticism. Naeye correctly retorted (1963), for example, that the presumed erythropoietin production by the donor would be equally distributed between the twins, and that the already plethoric twin would be stimulated to even greater hematopoiesis by infusion of blood from the anemic co-twin. Schwartz et al. (1984) described subcutaneous erythropoiesis in the donor twin, akin to the familiar blueberry muffin spots of newborns with cytomegalovirus and rubella virus infection.

Marx (1956) described the glomerular hyperplasia of the recipient twin's kidney in a report of a hydropic triplet with the transfusion syndrome. He conjectured that the increased perfusion of the kidney, under higher pressure, was responsible for this enhancement of glomerular development. He deduced, as did Schatz, that this situation led to the increased urination and hydramnios. The urine output (Kirshon, 1989) and pathophysiology of the syndrome were further elaborated on by Achiron et al. (1987), but the direct cause of this glomerular hyperplasia remains an unsolved question. Studies in patients with polycythemia (Corrin, 1961) have shown that it is not the cause. Glomerular hyperplasia has been observed in patients with tetralogy of Fallot (Bauer & Rosenberg, 1960) and cor pulmonale (Ellis, 1961). In these situations, hypoxia was thought to be the most important etiological factor. In addition to changes in glomerular structure, Naeye and Blanc (1972) found dilatation of renal tubules. They deduced that excessive urination was the cause of the hydramnios. That the recipient urinates excessively had already been decisively demonstrated by Schatz (1882). In the

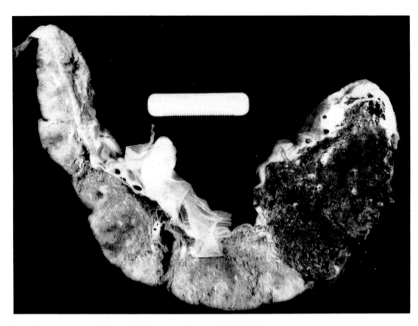

FIGURE 606. DiMo twin placenta at 34 weeks' gestation. Recipient had congestive heart failure (2,160 g, hyperbilirubinemia, blood pressure 70 mmHg). Its placental portion (right) is plethoric and thicker. The donor (anemic, thin portion of placenta at left) weighed 940 g and died neonatally. (Courtesy Dr. S. Kassel, Fresno.)

interesting discussion that followed that paper, Schatz expressed the opinion that the donor may have some amnionic fluid remaining because of sweating. Shah and Chaffin (1989) found a 55% overall mortality due to this syndrome. An interesting observation was reported by Popek et al. (1990). They found three monochorionic twins with prenatal calcification of the pulmonary artery in the absence of valvular anomalies. Two twins were "pump" twins of an acardiac and the other the "recipient" of the transfusion syndrome. The authors

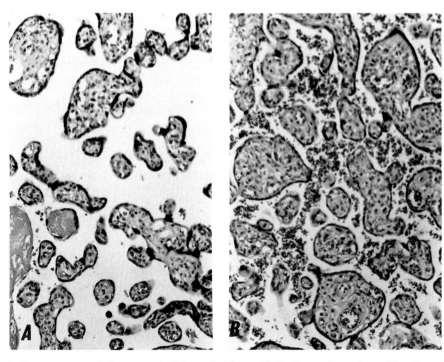

FIGURE 607. Histological appearance of the two twins' (seen in Figure 606) placental portions. The donor's placenta (right) is much more immature in appearance than the villi of the recipient (left), which are smaller. H&E. ×160.

speculated that this complication was due to increased cardiac output prenatally.

We have twice attempted to recreate the transfusion syndrome in sheep pregnant with fraternal twins (Resnik & Benirschke, unpublished). Having inserted intravascular catheters, we transferred daily 10 ml blood from the female to the male twin over 17 days. Our findings included (male/female): 3,600/3,375 g; hearts 24.5/23.5 g; livers 96.5/86.0 g; spleens 10.5/5.2 g; kidneys 27/22 g; cotyledon 440/370 g. The second experiment, done closer to term, gave similar results. Thus one can simulate the transfusion syndrome experimentally and perhaps better understand the adaptations that occur subsequent to the twin transfusion. Wilson (1979) studied the postnatal growth of dissimilar twins and concluded that "monozygotic twins become progressively more concordant with age ... while dizygotic twins became less concordant."

It was earlier stated that the recognition of twin-related hydramnios during early pregnancy has a bad outcome unless one twin dies. The transfusion then stops, and often the survivor is delivered near term and is normal (Figure 600). At the other end of the spectrum, various management schemes have been proposed for the twins *after* their birth; for example Shorland (1971) sought to correct the anemia, hypoglycemia, polycythemia, and hyperbilirubinemia. *Before* birth, incisive treatment is more difficult. The thoughtful review by Blickstein (1990) puts the various diagnostic modalities and treatment regimes into an unbiased perspective. Temporizing for a month by repeated amniocentesis and withdrawal of fluid is sometimes feasible for a while (Figures 597–599) but not for long (Feingold et al., 1986; Vetter & Schneider, 1988; Lange et al., 1989; Elliott, 1992; Reisner et al., 1993). There is a large body of literature on this topic, and the results are not uniform. Presumably they depend on the nature of the anastomoses and on the timing of the onset of hydramnios. Some authors advocate this modality of therapy strongly (Mahony et al., 1990; Urig et al., 1990; Saunders et al., 1992), whereas Gonsoulin et al. (1990a) showed in a careful study that the 21% overall survival rate was not improved by amniocentesis when the syndrome is diagnosed before 28 weeks. Pinette et al. (1993) also believed to have shown that early aggressive amniocentesis is an effective therapy. Bromley and colleagues (1992) found only a 25% survival rate when the diagnosis was made before 20 weeks, with a higher rate when the diagnosis was made later and conservative therapy instituted. Grischke and colleagues (1990) were similarly skeptical, and one wonders why the therapy is still being used at all. Bebbington and Wittmann (1989) found that gestational outcome depends mostly on age at delivery and that amniocentesis may be beneficial. For a pregnancy in

which hydrops and hydramnios had developed, De Lia et al. (1985a) treated the mother with digoxin at 27 weeks. They observed reversal of fetal cardiac failure in the recipient twin. The fetuses survived after cesarean section, which was done at 34 weeks. These authors estimated that 2,200 fetuses succumb annually in the United States from this syndrome alone. Jones et al. (1993) failed to arrest the syndrome in three pregnancies by administering indomethacin.

Wittmann et al. (1986) chose to sacrifice the donor of a severe transfusion syndrome case at 25 weeks' gestation. They inserted a needle into the heart under sonographic guidance. After the fetus died, the hydramnios disappeared and the pregnancy stabilized. No obvious maternal coagulopathy developed, and the healthy 2,890 g survivor was born at 37 weeks. The fetus papyraceus weighed 180 g. The placenta was DiMo. Subsequently, Baldwin and Wittmann (1990) summarized their favorable experience with this procedure in three cases of the transfusion syndrome. Weiner (1987) had earlier reported a similar experience. In the days that preceded sonography, we had unsuccessfully attempted a similar procedure (Benirschke & Driscoll, 1967). Another failure was reported by Chescheir and Seeds (1988a). They filled the pleural space of the donor with fluid until there was cessation of cardiac activity. This maneuver normalized the urine output of the survivor, but the hydramnios did not abate. Infection terminated the pregnancy prematurely.

Under ideal circumstances, it may become possible in the future to obliterate the interfetal vascular connections, which should then lead to complete normalization of the pregnancy. Schatz (1886) had early proposed that some vessels may thrombose and thus compromise blood exchange. De Lia et al. (1985b, 1989) have begun experimentation with the obliteration of selected fetal surface vessels by laser treatment in experimental animals. They were successful with this procedure in sheep and rhesus monkey and then successfully treated three patients with the transfusion syndrome (De Lia & Cruikshank, 1989). Delivery occurred several months after the vascular obliteration; and marked improvement of urination by the donor, with expansion of its amnionic sac, occurred immediately. The placentas showed the scarred cotyledons supplied by the coagulated vessels. Such therapy will probably be tried in many cases of the transfusion syndrome in the future, and one hopes that normative data of blood pressures, hemoglobin levels, and so on can be gathered for better understanding the physiology of this syndrome. De Lia et al. (1990) have since published more details of their experience, now comprising more than 20 cases, including a set of triplets. In one operated case, the authors pursued the vessels across a tear made in the dividing membranes. This disruption of dividing membranes may not be without hazard. As indicated earlier, amnionic bands may form or the MoMo twins resulting may entangle cords. The prenatal therapy by laser obliteration of vessels has since been practiced successfully by other teams (Natori et al., 1992; Ville et al., 1992) and was summarized by De Lia et al. (1993).

An unexplained finding in the transfusion syndrome is the recognition that the recipient has much higher levels of proteins, but that of immunoglobulin G (IgG) level was much out of line (Bryan & Slavin, 1974).

This chapter is not the place to review in detail the ultimate outcome of twin pregnancies. One aspect, nevertheless, is noteworthy. Because monozygosity eliminates genetic effects, the transfusion syndrome has served as a model to analyze aspects of the etiology of mental retardation. Several investigators have found that the smaller of MZ twins has a slightly lower IQ than the larger twin (Kaelber & Pugh, 1969; Hohenauer, 1971; Babson & Phillips, 1973). The larger the twins' size difference was at birth, the greater were the effects. Record et al. (1970) did not confirm these results using the data from the Birmingham Twin Study; they pointed out that the differences are *postnatal* in origin, rather than due to monozygosity and placentation. Likewise, Fujikura and Froehlich (1974) and Buckler and Robinson (1974) studied the postnatal equilibration of MZ twins who had been born with marked natal differences. They found only "negligible differences in . . . intelligence and educational attainment." The complexity of the problem is exemplified by reanalyses of the various data published by Munsinger (1977) and his critic Kamin (1978). The former believed that prenatal influences can be shown to have this deleterious effect; the latter did not. Both affirmed that future studies of this vexing question must include placental data. The criticism of former studies is echoed by O'Brien and Hay (1987) in an incisive analysis. These authors found differences when male co-twin development was compared with that of female co-twins. They also studied the effect of placentation on handedness.

Acardiac Twins

Acardiac twins are the most severely malformed fetuses that one can imagine. They range from small, teratoma-like masses to large fetuses with a great variety of anomalies. The absence of a heart is not obligatory to the diagnosis of this entity, as a severely malformed heart has occasionally been present. Schatz has called these twins hemicardia or hemiacardius, but Frutiger (1969) pointed out that this term is incorrect. He proposed the term pseudoacardius for those cases in which remnants of cardiac structures are found. A wide variety of names have been applied to this spectrum of acardiacs.

A veritable taxonomy was created, as in Schwalbe's and Schatz' writings. The most comprehensive treatise that encompasses all these attributes is the seminal book of Schatz (1898), who made the major contributions to our understanding of acardiacs. A total of 88 cases from Japan were summarized by Sato et al. (1984), and we have reviewed 49 acardiac pregnancies (Moore et al., 1990).

A human acardiac is one of MZ twins or higher multiple births whose development is severely disturbed and who usually has no cardiac remnants. There is good evidence that acardiacs are more common in higher multiple births than in twins (James, 1977a). That an acardiac can develop at all is due to the presence of two anastomoses in the monochorial placenta. An A-A anastomosis brings blood from an usually normal co-twin to the monster; and a V-V anastomosis returns the blood. The normal twin provides the cardiac flow to the monster but in a reversed fashion. The reversal of blood flow has been proved to exist with the use of Doppler sonography (Pretorius et al., 1988a). Schatz observed that the frequent presence of omphaloceles in acardiacs is an important obstruction to venous return and believed to play an etiological role. Later studies have not borne out this finding, as many acardiacs lack an omphalocele. Schatz believed that this kind of obstruction could be the cause of many such anomalous infants. We believe that the presence of the two types of placental anastomosis is the fundamental cause of the acardiac dysmorphism. Dichorionic (and DZ) human twins cannot develop into acardiacs, as they lack these communications in the placenta. No blood would be circulated through fetal vessels if a spontaneous acardia were to exist, and such an embryo would vanish. The fact, however, that such placental communications do exist among many fraternal (DZ) twins of some other species was recognized by Schatz, who discussed the acardiacs found in ruminants and carnivores.

The spectrum of acardiacs one can observe is illustrated in Figures 608 to 612. One of these fetuses had the appearance of a teratoma turned inside-out, another had remnants of a face and arms, and the third is unusual in that it had an exceptionally long umbilical cord. Despite the absence of any cerebral structures, the last-mentioned acardiac was sonographically witnessed to move actively. Also well shown in this fetus was the plethora, frequently observed in acardiacs. We believe it represents stagnation of blood, transfused by the pale, normal co-twin. The increased resistance to perfusion has been demonstrated by prenatal Doppler velocimetry (Sherer et al., 1989). The fetal mobility of an acardiac may be so great on occasion that they die because of cord entanglement (Figure 611). In all of the twins shown, the placenta was MoMo. Many others, though, have been described with a DiMo placenta. In

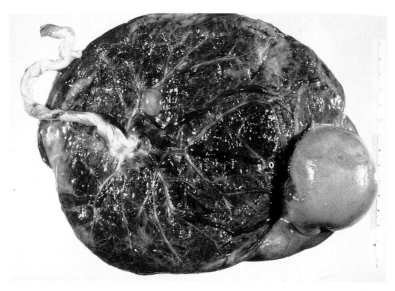

FIGURE 608. Acardiac twin, having the appearance of a teratoma. The normal twin weighed 2,910 g. The acardiac (holoacardius amorphus) twin weighed 40 g, had a diminutive cord, and was in a MoMo placenta with large anastomoses. (Courtesy the late Dr. N.J. Eastman, Baltimore.)

such cases, there is usually amnion nodosum of the acardiac's cavity because of its deficient or absent urine production. Sonographic examination of such cases then discovers a "stuck twin." Among the 30 acardiac twin pregnancies we studied and that had enough information, DiMo placentation was found in 22 cases and MoMo in 8 cases (Moore et al., 1990).

Dissection of the fetuses shows many gradations, ranging from a total absence of most organs to well differentiated structures of others, including gonads. Only liver tissue has never been observed by us, although we have been able to study numerous specimens. Schatz has written of the same experience. A female sex preponderance of acardiacs has been noted by James (1977a). For the study of acardiacs, it is usually best to obtain a radiograph of the specimen before dissection, as it gives some idea of the complexity of the abnormality, enables better classification, and delineates if a skull is present (Dicker et al., 1983; Bhatnagar et al., 1986).

Most acardiac fetuses have only a single umbilical artery (SUA). The absence of one umbilical artery, though, cannot be held responsible for the development of the anomaly, as it is not invariable. In contrast to Schatz' ideas, an omphalocele has been absent in at least one-half of the cases we have seen. One of the few hemiacardiacs we dissected possessed a two-chambered heart (Benirschke, 1970a). This heart and that of another hemiacardiac exhibited endocardial fibrosis. The first twin shown here also had a fairly well formed head with a brain and a bilateral cleft palate. One of monochorionic quintuplets with five amnions was an acardiac fetus (Hamblen et al., 1937) (Figure 612), and we described triplets with one acardiac in the previous edition of this book; and many other triplets, one being an acardiac are recorded in the literature. They may be MZ triplets (Ross, 1951; Landy et al., 1988) or multizygotic (Stoeckel, 1945; Wylin, 1971; Kirkland, 1982). The acardiacs described by Amatuzio and Gorlin (1981) were conjoined and associated with a MoMo triplet in heart failure.

The most remarkable specimen is that described by Fujikura and Wellings (1964) and shown in Figure 613. This malformed specimen was attached to the chorionic surface 1.5 cm from the insertion of the umbilical cord of a larger fetus. This more normal twin had amelia of the right arm, phocomelia of the right leg, hydrocephaly, and myelomeningocele; his right umbilical artery was absent. The acardiac was described as a teratoma-like mass. We have previously expressed our reservation about chorionic teratomas and prefer to think of this specimen as an acardiac that lacked the development of a defined umbilical cord. The presence of a cord is usually a prerequisite for the diagnosis of "acardiac fetus" (e.g., Joseph & Vogt, 1973), although the length of umbilical cords of acardiacs varies from 0 cm as in Figure 608 (see also Frutiger, 1969) to 53 cm as in Figure 610. The lack of organization, as emphasized by Fox and Butler-Manuel (1964) in a similar case, is not a strong argument that these masses are teratomas. Such disorganization occurs often in small holoacardii amorphi with good umbilical cords. Holoacardii amorphi are not true neoplasms (teratomas); they are part of the wide spectrum of acardiac twinning.

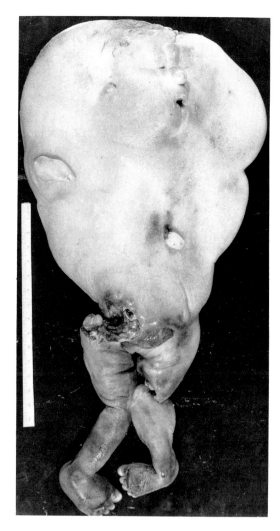

bability of a gross underestimate. More than 600 cases have been reported, and there are probably hundreds that go unpublished. Our own series now exceeds 50 cases, and many of these cases will remain undescribed.

Acardiacs often develop hydrops, and the pregnancy is thus frequently complicated by hydramnios. Hydropic acardiacs may then become much larger than the normal co-twin. The hydropic acardiac twin described by Pavlica (1967) was such a case. It weighed 2,150 g, whereas the co-twin was only 850 g. It was further remarkable that its umbilical cord forked from that of the normal co-twin. Markavy and Scanlon (1978) have described additional hydropic acardiacs with hydramnios and considered that this problem may result from hypoproteinemia. They also observed thrombosis of one umbilical artery in one of these acardiac fetuses.

Because the hydramnios may be severe and the large acardiac may present problems with dystocia (Loughead & Halbert, 1969), Platt et al. (1983) proposed that a ligature be placed around its umbilical cord through an amnioscope. Simpson et al. (1983) were successful

FIGURE 609. Well formed 1,210 g male acardiac fetus delivered at 28 weeks. Co-twin died neonatally and had aortic hypoplasia. The acardiac twin had a skull, remnants of brain, a small spinal cord, and many other organ remnants. (Courtesy Dr. J.D. Wilkes, New York.)

Kreyberg (1958) reported a similar case and had the same opinion. The differential diagnosis (acardiac or teratoma) was further considered by Stephens et al. (1989), who reviewed 96 cases and presented an additional bovine acardiac fetus. It was their opinion that the presence or absence of an umbilical cord was insufficient evidence for diagnosis, and they relied more heavily on the finding of an axial skeleton.

The incidence of acardiac pregnancies is difficult to ascertain, as most are not reported. Gillim and Hendricks (1953) estimated the incidence to be 1 per 34,600 births, or approximately 1 in 100 MZ twin pregnancies. This finding agrees with that derived by Napolitani and Schreiber (1960). Bhatnagar et al. (1986) based their estimate of 1 per 48,000 births on data from a variety of studies. They admitted the pro-

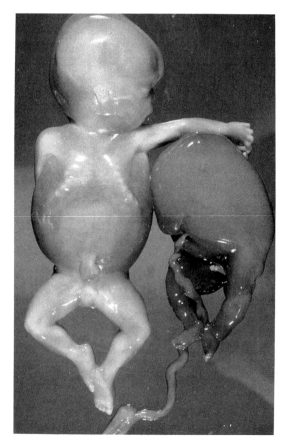

FIGURE 610. Exsanguinated premature MoMo plethoric acardiac twin fetus. This specimen is unusual because of the long umbilical cord. The fetus had been seen to move at sonography; it had no brain but a normal spinal cord.

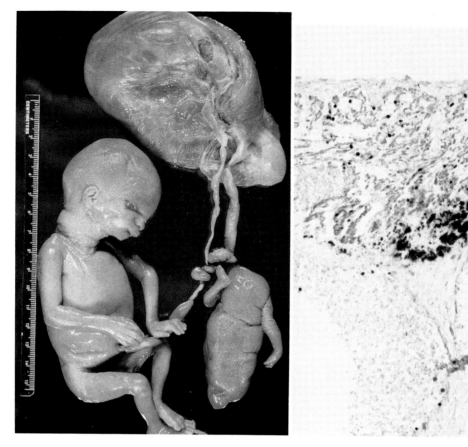

FIGURE 611. Macerated MoMo twins, one an acardiac (150 and 20 g, respectively). The twins died because of entangling of cords. Note the SUA of the cord and large A-A and V-V anastomoses. The acardiac twin had a remnant of heart with calcification in the remaining muscle fibers. H&E. ×160. (Courtesy Dr. S. Kassel, Fresno.)

in treating a pregnancy with a hydropic acardiac by digitalization.

The mechanism of hydramnios and congestive heart failure is complex. It is likely related to the size of the acardiac fetus, but suggestions in the literature allude to a correlation with the presence of renal tissue in the acardiac (Moore et al., 1990). Prospective studies, with ascertainment of urination by the acardiac, are needed.

Another way of treating an acardiac pregnancy is by selective removal of the anomalous twin, which has been successfully accomplished by Robie et al. (1989). These authors removed a sonographically identified acardiac fetus at 22.5 weeks' gestation that weighed 710 g. A normal twin was subsequently delivered at 33 weeks' gestation. Ash and colleagues (1990) successfully managed such a pregnancy with indomethacin. It led to marked reduction of amnionic fluid volume so a normal fetus (and a 785 g acardiac) were delivered at 34 weeks. Porreco et al. (1991) occluded the umbilical artery of an acardiac fetus in utero with a metal coil. It stopped reversed flow and led to normal delivery at 39 weeks. McCurdy et al. (1993) endoscopically attempted

to ligate the umbilical cord of an acardiac fetus at 18 weeks. Both twins died. More recently, however, Quintero et al. (1994) succeeded with ligating the umbilical cord near midgestation through a fetoscopic approach and salvaged the normal twin. The acardiac twin weighed 31 g at birth. Selective removal of an acardiac fetus was undertaken at 23 weeks after her death in utero by Ginsberg et al. (1992), with the normal twin proceeding normally to 39 weeks. Interestingly, the two cords branched one from another at their marginal insertion on the placenta; and both fetuses as well as normal members of the family had a chromosomal inversion [46,XX,inv (10)(p12q25)]. Wenstrom (1993) thought that elective removal of this acardiac was unnecessary.

Chitkara et al. (1989) reported on selective termination of 17 anomalous twins, 14 of which were aneuploid, but not acardiac fetuses. They emphasized the need for operator skill in this procedure and had much better success later in their series. Intracardiac injection of potassium chloride was the most effective means to accomplish the feticide. Neither the mothers nor the

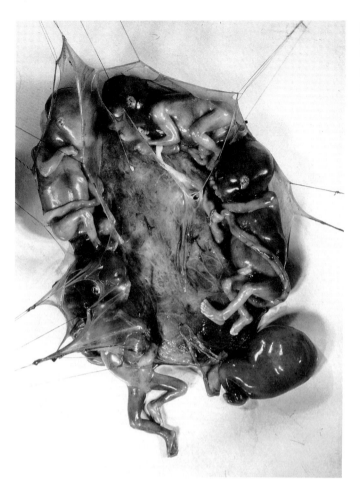

FIGURE 612. Acardiac quintuplet in monochorial placenta with five amnionic sacs (bottom right). Note its plethora. Three yolk sacs were identified. (Reprinted with permission of Hamblen, et al., J.A.M.A. 109:10–12, Copyright 1937, American Medical Association.)

surviving twins suffered DIC. Other cases were reviewed by Donnenfeld and his colleagues (1989). They attempted to ascertain the presence of intertwin anastomoses by prenatal angiography because of hydrocephaly in one twin. Complications led to fetal death and exsanguination of the normal twin into the abnormal fetus. Large A-A anastomoses were found in the monochorionic placenta.

Another acardiac fetus with forked cord (funiculopagus) has been described by Averback and Wigglesworth (1978). They also reviewed the literature of this uncommon event. Their acardius was in a separate amnionic sac and was rather well developed. The umbilical arteries, derived from the umbilical cords that had joined close to the placental surface, fused and provided a completely common circulation. It is interesting that this circulation could occur at all because of the presence of umbilical cord furcation, and in a DiMo placenta. When we ascertained the frequency of SUA in acardiacs, we found that SUA occurred 16 times in 29 cases; 13 had normal cords. Of 27 normal co-twins, 4 had SUA, and 23 were normal (Moore et al., 1990).

Not only are the acardiac twins malformed, but many of the co-twins have also congenital anomalies. Schinzel et al. (1979) suggested that about 10% of the co-twins are malformed. It is important to note that, with one possible exception, the sex of human acardiacs has been the same as that of the co-twin, providing it was accurately ascertained by, at least, a sex chromatin study (Benirschke, 1959), morphological identification of gonads (Kappelman, 1944), or cytogenetic analysis. Only Buxbaum and Wachsman (1938) described an aberrant case—that of a female twin with an apparently male acardiac co-twin. The sex of the latter was assessed by finding "a structure that closely resembled a penis." That this finding is insufficient evidence for its male gender has been demonstrated to us. We saw an acardiac with a sonographically identified penile structure that was subsequently delivered with a normal female co-twin. On dissection, this penile structure was an enlarged clitoris and normal ovaries were present. The reason for the clitoral enlargement remained obscure.

The most controversial aspect of acardiacs is their pathogenesis and etiology. Frutiger (1969), who de-

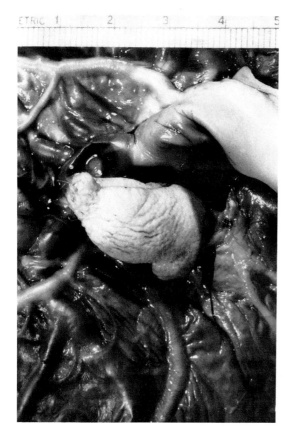

FIGURE 613. Diminutive acardiac twin that was likened to a teratoma. It is 1.5 cm from the cord insertion of a malformed twin with SUA. Large vessels led to the mass. (Courtesy Dr. T. Fujikura, Portland.)

scribed five acardiac cases, believed that the absence of the heart was secondary to the fetus suffering a deficient oxygen and nutrient supply, a suggestion that had previously been made popular by Loeschke (1948). He had the idea that the acardiac twin suffered malnutrition and hypoxia because it developed in the decidua capsularis, which, however, is clearly often not the case. Alderman (1973) challenged this notion and proposed a "primary failure of organ development." Köhn (1953) and Dahm (1955) also favored primary developmental problems. They suggested that "pathologic division" of the embryo and perhaps extraneous factors were responsible for acardiac development. They entertained the possibility of heritable causes. Gruenwald (1942) described a young, partially duplicated human embryo that might well have become an acardiac twin. He considered the two principal and opposing theories: (1) primary maldevelopment and (2) vascular reversal leading to suppression of cardiac development. His statement, that "an anomaly, anatomical or functional, intraembryonic or extraembryonic, may turn one twin into an acardius if its circulation becomes dependent on

that of the other embryo," probably best reflects our current thinking about the nature of these monsters. Lachman et al. (1980) have also presented reasonable theories of etiology in their discussion of a relevant case.

That vascular reversal nourishes the acardiac is without question. Much of the failure of organ systems to develop at all, or to do so in a diminutive fashion, is due to a deficient circulation. The circulating blood is not only deoxygenated but also arrives at a reduced pressure. The fact that the lower limbs of acardiacs are usually better formed than the arms has been considered to result from preferential perfusion of the legs as they are closest to incoming reversed arterial flow. The fact that the central nervous tissue is often reasonably well developed contradicts some notions that unimpaired neural development guarantees limb development, an area that has been summarized by Boulgakow (1926).

An important etiological consideration for the development of acardiacs is that these anomalies may occur in one of dizygotic twins of certain animals. Some species, in contrast to human twins, share anastomoses between fraternal twins. This situation is best known from the freemartin condition of cattle (Lillie, 1917). Here the male twin is responsible for atrophy of the female genitalia of the co-twin, with which he is vascularly connected, the basis of freemartinism. These connections also lead to permanent blood chimerism. Similar anastomoses are regularly present in the twins of marmosets and tamarins (Benirschke et al., 1962). In these species, however, sexual disturbances do not occur. Schatz (1898) had remarked that there are many ruminant acardiacs. Occasionally, they are found in carnivores but not in horses. Figure 614 shows a bovine acardiac monster, and such a twin from a goat is seen in Figure 615. Table 29 summarizes some of the literature of animal acardiacs. They are a crucial component when considering the genesis of these anomalies. One may speculate that these fraternal twins were originally normal but that, because of happenstance chorionic anastomoses, they became anomalous by virtue of circulatory reversal. This speculation is supported by the hypothesis of original normality, first enunciated by Claudius (1859) and later by Ahlfeld (1879). Schwalbe (1907) sided with Schatz in that he assumed a primary inequality of the twins, and that secondary alterations (macrocardia, microcardia, SUA, omphalocele) determine its ultimate outcome.

Evidence for a primary anomaly of at least some acardiacs has been gathered from cytogenetic studies. In several acardiac monsters, investigators have found abnormal karyotypes that were different from those of the co-twin. Other acardiacs have had normal chromosomal complements identical with those of the

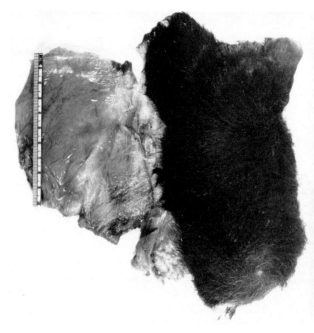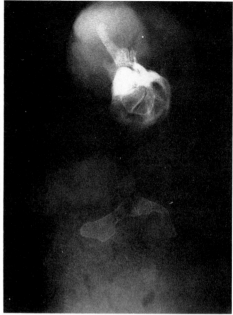

FIGURE 614. Bovine acardiac monster attached to remnants of membranes. This 600 g elongated structure had a semblance of pelvis (bottom right) and even more ossified cranial struc- tures (top right). Karyotype was 60,XX (From Benirschke, 1970b, with permission.)

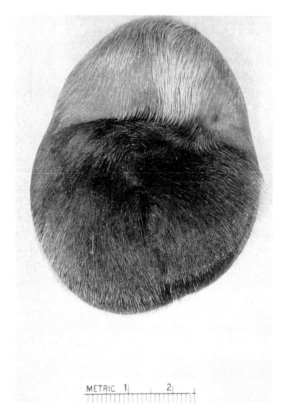

FIGURE 615. Amorphus globosus from the quadruplet pregnancy of a goat (♂♂♀), weighing 20 g. It had a short cord with two vessels and a small amount of cartilage and muscle amid fat.

normal co-twin, as in the example shown in Figure 616. These challenging findings are summarized in Table 30. One must caution, however, that only those studies in which the chromosome analysis was undertaken from the solid tissues of the acardiac specimens can be considered valid. The lymphocyte populations would be admixed a priori, and thus their karyotypic analysis is not helpful. Moreover, it is known that the lymphocyte contribution of the acardiac, who also usually lacks a thymus, may be minimal (Nigro, 1977). Finally it is of interest that at least two "normal" co-twins of acardiacs have had an abnormal chromosomal constitution (Table 30). Thus the cytogenetic picture is complex and does not lend itself to a resolution of which event is primary in the etiology of acardiacs. Acardiac twins may be observed at young gestations and then already have all the characteristic stigmata (Figure 617). We have concluded that whatever happens to their anatomical development it is an early process. Our own concept is that the reversal of circulations is the cause of the anomaly.

The characteristic vascular arrangement pertaining to most acardiacs is illustrated in Figure 618. It mirrors many descriptions of former authors. In these days of acronyms, the term TRAP (twin reversed arterial perfusion) has been applied to this "syndrome" (Allen et al., 1983). In this paper of Allen et al., which presents 14 acardiac cases, the spectrum of anomalies is well delineated. They described an additional specimen with

TABLE 29. Karyotypic studies in acardiac animals.

Source	Year	Species	Sex	Remarks
Sutton	1899	Cattle		Anidian monster
Simonds & Gowen	1925	Cattle		13 Amorphi
		Sheep/goat		3 Cases
		Bird		1 Cases; extensive literature
Cole & Craft	1945	Sheep	Female	
Roberts	1956	Horse		
		Cattle		
Dunn et al.	1967	Cattle	Female	60,XX; 61,XX (??mosaic)
			Male co-twin	60,XY
Neal & Wilcox	1967	Cattle		2 Amorphous twins, 1 heifer
Dennis & Leipold	1968	Sheep		1 Holoacardius acephalus
Herzog & Rieck	1969	Cattle	Female	60,XX misinterpreted
Benirschke	1970b	Cattle	Female	60,XX, normal co-twin
Dunn & Roberts	1972	Sheep	Male	54,XY (co-twin); 54,XY/53,XY
Crossman & Dickens	1974	Horse		Mass (500 g)
Höfliger	1974	Horse		Review
		Cattle		Acormus (head only)
Hein et al.	1985	Monkey	Female	DiMo; A-A anastomosis

TABLE 30. Karyotypic studies of human acardiac fetuses.

Source	Year	Donor	Acardiac	Placenta	Remarks
Richart & Benirschke	1963	ND	46,XY (F)	DiMo	
Rashad & Kerr	1966	46,XY (F)	46,XY (L)	DiMo	
		47,XY (F)	Extra C element		
Turpin et al.	1967	46,XX (F)	46,XX (F)	MoMo	
		47,XX (L)	Extra minute element		
Scott & Ferguson-Smith	1973	46,XY (L,F)	46,XY (L)	DiMo	
		46,XY (L)	Failed	DiMo	
Machin	1974	46,XX (F)	46,XX (F)	?	Triplets, 46,XX
Benirschke & Harper	1977	ND	46,XY (F)	MoMo	See Figure 617
Rehder et al.	1978	47,XXY (F)	47,XXY (F)	?	
Kaplan & Benirschke	1979	46,XX (F,L)	46,XX (F)	DiMo	
		46,XX (F,L)	46,XX (F)	DiMo	
Deacon et al.	1980	45,X (F)	46,XX (F,L)	?	
Bieber et al.	1981	46,XY (L)	69,XXX (F)	DiMo	Genetic studies indicated acardiac to derive from polar body
Gewolb et al.	1983	46,XY (?)	46,XY (?)	DiMo	Authors stated DiDi but depicted DiMo
Allen et al.	1983	46,XX (?)	45,XX t(4;21)del(4p)		Nature of chromosome study unknown;
Shapiro et al.	1986	46,XX (?)	46,XX	DiMo	
		47,XX + 11 (F)	?		
Buehler et al.	1986	47,XXY (?)	92,XXXXYY (?)	?	Review of the 16 previous acardiacs with karyotype
Bhatnagar etc.	1986	47,XX, tri 18	ND	?Mo	
Moore et al.	1987	47,XXY (L)	47,XXY (L)	DiMo	
		47,XXY (L)	92,XXXXYY (F,L)	DiMo	
Landy et al.	1988	45,X/46,XX(A)	46,XX (A,L,F)	TriMo	Triplets; mosaic fetus was normal female
Wolf et al.	1990	46,XX	46,X, i(Xp)	DiMo	Hydropic 3,720 g
Ginsberg et al.	1992	46,XX inv10	46,XX, inv10	MoMo	Normal members with same inversion
Benirschke	1992	46,XX	46,XX		Two normal acardiacs
Bolaji et al.	1992	46,XX	46,XX + 4n, +6n	TriMo	Triplets, well formed acardiac, hyperdiploid cells from "lymphoid aggregate" of acardiac

A = amnionic fluid cells; F = fibroblasts; L = lymphocytes; ND = not done.

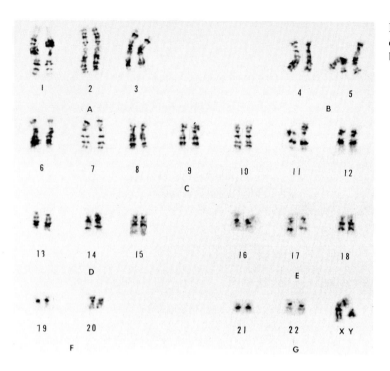

FIGURE 616. Normal male karyotype from the skin of the acardiac twin shown in Figure 609. Giemsa banding.

chromosomal error. We have recently karyotyped two new acardiacs and their co-twins and found both to have normal chromosome complements in solid tissues.

Conjoined Twins

Incompletely separated twins (conjoined, Siamese, x-pagi, double monsters) presumably take their origin after day 13 of embryogenesis. Because it has been most seriously questioned whether conjoined twins are one person or two, the reader is directed to the searching review of this topic by Gould (1982). Gould concluded that this question is not answerable, and perhaps it may even be an erroneous inquiry. The MZ twinning process is a continuum; sharp divisions do not exist, as is often the case with biological phenomena. Even more problematical is making clear decisions as to the classification of whole-body chimerae, as we see below. Moreover, the precise nature of the formation of conjoined twins is uncertain. Opposing views suggest incomplete splitting (unlikely) and partial fusion (more probable) of embryonic precursors. The reader is referred to the searching review of more than 500 cases by Weston (1992), who clearly has the largest experience with this topic.

Most fused twins are joined at the chest (thoracopagus), but all sorts of unions have been described (Harper et al., 1980). Numerous triplets have included conjoined twins (Koontz et al., 1985; Seo et al., 1985). With triplets, the placentas may be monochorionic

(Tan et al., 1971b), with the conjoints living in their separate amnionic cavity, or they may be dichorionic (Vestergaard, 1972). We have recently observed term thoracoomphalopagous girls with a monochorionic (diamnionic) normal female co-twin. The umbilical cord

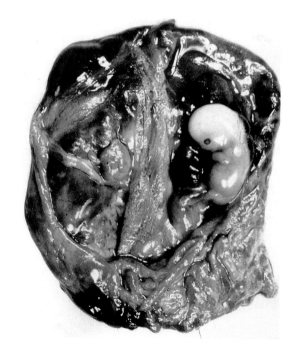

FIGURE 617. DiMo twin abortus at approximately 9 weeks' gestation. At left is a degenerating acardiac fetus. Note that it has a large amnionic cavity.

FIGURE 618. Usual vascular relations (anastomoses) between an acardiac twin and its co-twin.

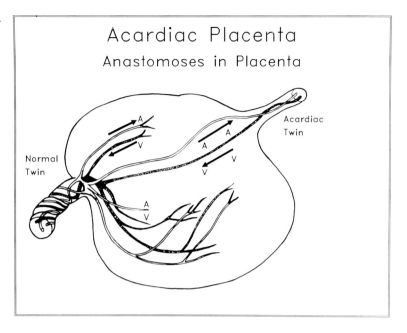

to the conjoined triplets was split (two arms with an artery and vein each) at the placental surface, which then joined to produce a cord with two arteries and two veins. Another of these rare diamnionic twin placentas with omphalopagous conjoined twins has been described by Weston and colleagues (1990). The typical placenta of conjoined twins, however, is a monoamnionic, monochorionic one. The former speculations that fusion of fraternal twins may be a mechanism of conjoint twinning is no longer tenable. For instance, chromosome studies of the twins have always been identical (Kreutner et al., 1963; Kim et al., 1971). In one case the twins and their mother had a pericentric inversion of one chromosome 9 (Delprado & Baird, 1984). Surprisingly, approximately 70% of conjoined twins are female (James, 1980). Burn et al. (1986) used this fact to support their hypothesis that "unequal lyonization" is associated with MoMo twinning. Incompletely separated twins have been described in a wide variety of species, for example, the rat (Levinsky, 1973; Mutinelli et al., 1992), swine (Selby et al., 1973), turtle (Szabuniewicz & McCrady, 1967; Lewis et al., 1992), and cetacea (Kawamura, 1969; Kawamura & Kashita, 1971). We have seen several California kingsnakes, calves, kittens, and other animals with double heads. Even in plants this event occurs with some frequency (Ahmad et al., 1977) (Figure 619) and is referred to as fasciation. It is remarkable and not yet fully understood why MZ bird twins have all been female. Conjoined chicken twins, described by Munro (1965), shared a single yolk sac.

Conjoined twins occur in approximately 1 of 50,000 births (Schmidt et al., 1981), or in 1 of 600 twins. The

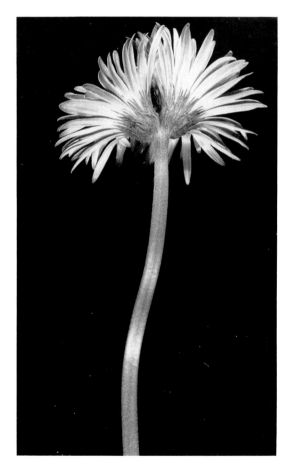

FIGURE 619. Conjoined "twin" Transvaal daisy (*Gerbera jamesonii*). The stem is fused; the flowers, with their identical number of petals (55/55), are separate.

figures vary substantially among surveys (Tan et al., 1971a; Bankole et al., 1972; Harper et al., 1980; Castilla et al., 1988); they are reported to be much higher in the Japanese population (Miyabara et al., 1973). Reports have also indicated that this anomaly occurs more commonly in Nigeria, and Bhettay et al. (1975) suggested a much higher rate to exist in South Africa. This statement, however, has been criticized by Hanson (1975). Difficulty of ascertainment was further discussed by Viljoen et al. (1983) in a large series of conjoined twins from southern Africa; contrary to earlier reports, these authors found no skewing in favor of the black population. Milham (1966) analyzed 22 sets and suggested local clustering of this anomaly, a suggestion supported by Viljoen et al. (1983).

The etiology of conjoined twinning remains unknown. Sporadic reports have suggested that it is due to exposure to teratogens (e.g., griseofulvin) (Rosa et al., 1987), and that its prevalence may include seasonal fluctuation. The relation of conjoined twinning to griseofulvin intake was disputed by the large data collected by Knudsen (1987), however. Ingalls (1969), who applied heat and hypoxia to zebra fish, was able to observe eight conjoined fish among 5,000 specimens; he described an "epidemic" in trout. Ferm (1969, 1978) found four conjoined hamsters whose mothers were subjected to teratogens. When Kao et al. (1986) injected solutions of lithium chloride into a blastomere of 32-cell-stage *Xenopus* eggs, a second head developed. Wan et al. (1982) observed conjoined twins in 0.4% of Swiss-Webster mice and in 0.06% of triplets. Treatment with vincristine or other manipulations did not increase the yield.

Whether these data are relevant to the human condition has not been decided. It is known, however, that conjoined twins frequently have other congenital anomalies, including cleft palate, anencephaly, and particularly congenital heart disease (Noonan, 1978; Marin-Padilla et al., 1981; Seo et al., 1985). Newman (1931a) noted marked differences in the development of various structures.

Keeler (1929) suggested that mirror imagery existed in 77% of conjoined twins, compared with 22% in monozygotic, separate twins. It must be cautioned, though, that situs inversus and mirroring are complex problems. Torgersen (1949) identified it to occur in 0.01% of a large population of Norwegians studied by mass radiography. Its incidence paralleled that of twinning, and he found that it was "not much higher" in MZ twins and was "rare" in DZ twins. (For further insight into situs inversus and related aspects, see Layton, 1976.) Hydramnios is said to occur in about one-half of conjoined twins (Wedberg et al., 1979). The frequency of various types of conjoined twins has been reported by Edmonds and Layde (1982), with

thoracoomphalopagus (28%) being the commonest form.

The placenta of conjoined twins is usually a single disk with MoMo membranes. The structure of the umbilical cords, however, varies widely, approximately 6% having two cords (Spencer, 1992). This fact much supports Spencer's view of fusion. The umbilical cord of Figure 620 was single and contained two arteries and a vein. It is similar to those described by Kreutner et al. (1963), de Leon (1974), and Itoh et al. (1974), who observed that the co-twins had a fused subdiaphragmatic aorta from where the umbilical arteries originated. Gilbert et al. (1972) and Tan et al. (1971b) described thoracopagi with one artery coming from one twin and the other from the second twin, who also received the single vein. The twins of Figure 621 had a single umbilical artery and a velamentous insertion of the umbilical cord. SUA was also found in four of seven conjoined twins reported by Miyabara et al. (1973). Kim et al. (1971) described thoracopagi with a single cord that possessed six vessels: four arteries and two veins. Mitrani (1968) saw one conjoined set of twins with six arteries and two veins. In the cases reported by Seo et al. (1985), two placentas had single cords with four arteries and one vein, one had three arteries and two veins, and three had normal cords with two arteries

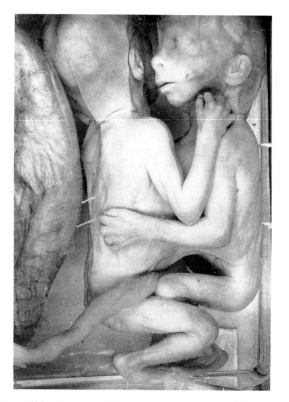

FIGURE 620. Thoracoabdominopagous twins with a monoamnionic placenta and a single umbilical cord.

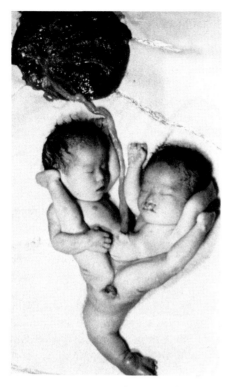

Fig	Clinical Data on "Conjoined Twins" at Katsushika Red Cross Maternity Hospital
Case:	T.S.(Born 2,Feb., 1972)
Gest.age:	40 wk
Mode of delivery:	C-section
Sex:	Both female
Birth weight.	4,465 g.
Apgar's score at one minute:	Both 2 (Died at 9 minutes after birth)
Type:	Diplopagus monster,dicephalus, tripus tetrabrachius
	Cleft lip and cleft palate and considerably smaller heart, 2 vaginas,1 anus,2 hearts,1 liver, & the sharing of the gastrointestinal tract
Placenta:	Size-22×17×2.6 cm weight-750 g
Umbilical cord:	Size 36×1.2 cm Single umbilical artery, Velamentous insertion of the cord

FIGURE 621. Conjoined twins (ischiopagi) with a MoMo placenta, a single velamentous umbilical cord, and SUA. They were delivered at 40 weeks' gestation. One had a cleft face and microcardia. There were two female genital tracts. (Courtesy Dr. S. Sekiya, Tokyo.)

and one vein. Two placentas, however, were separate disks; one of them had a fused cord. Delprado and Baird (1984) reported cephalothoracopagi with two cords. One was thick, ran in the membranes, and contained one artery and one vein; the smaller cord contained only one vessel. Another thoracopagous set of twins was reported by Freedman et al. (1962). These twins had two separate cords that inserted 1.5 cm apart and that fused 13 cm from the placental surface. The fused structure contained three arteries and two veins; the placenta was DiMo and contained a triplet of the same sex. Wiegenstein and Iozzo (1980) found two separated cords (11 cm apart) in a conjoined twin. The cords fused after having entangled in the placental portion and ran in a tented segment of amnion. A case with similarly fused, but separately originating, cords was described with a dicephalus, dibrachius pregnancy (Beischer & Fortune, 1968). In the thoracopagi examined by Marin-Padilla et al. (1981), the single cord split 9 cm before reaching the placental surface. One branch contained two arteries; the other cord had a velamentous insertion and contained the single vein. An interesting set of vessels was found in the umbilical cord of a thoracopagus studied by Chaurasia (1975). The smaller twin had a rudimentary heart, a large left and diminutive right umbilical artery, and no vein; the larger twin had a single large artery and vein. Reversal of circulation in the smaller twin was considered.

There is great variety in the spectrum of cord vasculature and structure, and no clear relations emerge as to the associated type of conjoined twin. One might expect that embryonic splitting at slightly different times produces different fusion anomalies and different cord structures and insertions. Future correlations may uncover these as yet unknown parameters. It is especially noteworthy that not all MoMo placentas of conjoined twins with two umbilical cords have vascular anastomoses on the placental surface. Finally, there exist anomalous fetuses with diminutive parasitic "twins" presenting as inclusions or appendages. They represent transitions to the next topic. Four such cases were described in some detail by Drut and his colleagues (1992). Because they have no relation to placental pathology they are not discussed further.

Sacrococcygeal Teratoma, Epignathus

Sacrococcygeal teratoma and epignathus are, in our opinion, malformed twins that represent a part of the spectrum of the monozygotic twinning continuum. Some may take exception to this concept. Nevertheless, findings of perfectly formed extremities, digits, and other structures favor this view. They are occasionally combined with more disorganized tumors (Cousins et al., 1980; Tokunaga et al., 1986). Schwalbe (1907) and Willis (1958) extensively discussed this aspect with illustrative material that also supports this notion. Exelby (1972) reviewed the origin and therapy of these tumors and found them to be much commoner in females (4F:1M); they also indicated that there is frequently a strong family history of twinning. In one parturient whose infant had a large sacrococcygeal teratoma, an ovarian teratoma was found simultaneously (Rayburn & Barr, 1982). These authors emphasized that recent genetic study had shown that these neoplasms have different genetic backgrounds.

There are also frequent concurrent anomalies in children with these tumors. Most of the neoplasms are benign, which is different from the rare teratomas of other sites, in which prenatal metastases have been reported (Semchyshyn et al., 1982). At times, however, an apparently benign sacrococcygeal teratoma eventuates in a malignancy. Lack et al. (1993) found an eventually fatal adenocarcinoma in a man 40 years after a sacrococcygeal teratoma had been incompletely removed at age 2 months. An alternate etiological point of view is that sacrococcygeal tumors and epignathi derive from misplaced germ cells. In a study of obstetrical complications with sacral tumors, Spitzer (1932) commented on the female sex preponderance and noted that the tumors are often complicated by hydramnios during pregnancy. That point has been reiterated in more recent publications of the prenatal diagnoses of

these lesions (Horger & McCarter, 1979; Hallgrimsson, 1981).

Placentomegaly has often been described to be a complication of sacrococcygeal teratomas (Cousins et al., 1980; Gergely et al., 1980; Kohga et al., 1980; Feige et al., 1982). The same is true of the placenta in epignathi (Kaplan et al., 1980; Chervenak et al., 1985), and yet other teratomas may be associated with hydramnios and fetal hydrops (Rosenfeld et al., 1979; Banfield et al., 1980; Semchyshyn et al., 1982; Mostoufi-Zadeh et al., 1985). The placental enlargement may be striking, and it is then usually exceptionally pale. There is severe edema of villi, which often appear to be excessively cellular, contain numerous Hofbauer cells, and are severely congested (Figure 622). One often finds numerous nucleated red blood cells in the fetal placental vessels. Ultrastructural examination of such specimens was first undertaken by Arai et al. (1977; see also Soma et al., 1979). It showed marked alterations of the syncytium, with distension of the transport vesicles (Figure 623), and unusually dense mitochondria. We believe that placental enlargement is the result of high output failure of the fetus and that it is similar to that found with large chorangiomas. This concept finds confirmation in the frequent fetal cardiac enlargement that is present. In effect, the teratoma acts as an arteriovenous fistula. The concept is further supported by the experience of Langer et al. (1989). They resected one of the tumors at 24 weeks and returned the fetus to the uterus (of three cases described). Hydrops improved, and Doppler study showed a decrease in cardiac output. Nakayama et al. (1991) made similar observa-

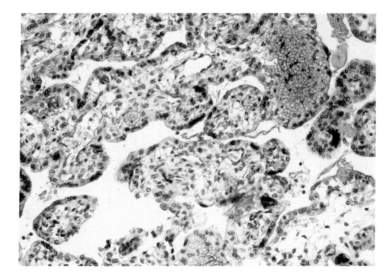

FIGURE 622. Villi of immature placenta in a patient with a large sacrococcygeal teratoma. Placenta weighed 880 g at 31 weeks. The neonate died with extensive cerebral necroses. The villi are irregular and patchily edematous, and they have distended fetal capillaries. There is focal hemorrhage, and numerous nucleated red blood cells are present. The cytotrophoblast is more prominent than expected at this age. H&E. ×160.

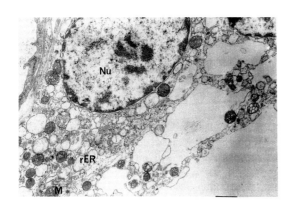

FIGURE 623. Ultrastructural view of villi in a sacrococcygeal teratoma, showing hugely distended syncytial transport vesicles. Data: 28 weeks' gestation; hydramnios; elevated hCG levels (9,830,400 IU/L), 680 g placenta. Nu = nucleus; rER = rough endoplasmic reticulum. ×5,600. (Courtesy Dr. H. Soma, Tokyo.)

tions when they resected the tumor in a newborn. Feige et al. (1982) unreasonably claimed that the placentomegaly represents an attempt by the placenta to compensate for the increased needs of the fetal tumor. Whenever karyotypic analysis has been done, the chromosomes of the tumors have been normal and identical to those of the host (Kaplan et al., 1979; Cousins et al., 1980).

CONGENITAL ANOMALIES

Twins have congenital anomalies more often than do singletons. Hendricks (1966) evaluated the outcome of 438 multiple pregnancies and found that their perinatal mortality rate is not only "startlingly high" (14%) but also that anomalies occurred with a frequency of 10.6% (approximately three times that of singletons). In a review of anomalies of Swedish twins, Källén (1986) noted that some anomalies (posthemorrhagic hydrocephalus, patent ductus) are undoubtedly an effect of the prematurity of many twins. Other anomalies, notably those referred to as the VACTERL association [vertebral abnormalities, anal atresia, cardiac abnormalities tracheoesophageal, fistula, renal agenesis and dysplasia, and limb defects, a variant of the VATER (vertebral, anal, tracheoesophageal, renal) association] and anencephaly, were overrepresented in twins. James (1976) found that anencephaly occurs in DZ twins with the same frequency as in singletons, but that its incidence is increased in one or both of MZ twins.

Schinzel et al. (1979) studied the structural defects of MZ twins in greater detail. They considered that some of these anomalies are related to the MZ twinning process per se. This concept is certainly true for the acardiacs, the conjoined twins, and probably also for those defects that arise as the result of vascular anastomoses (e.g., porencephaly, intestinal occlusions). When twin abortuses were studied, it was found that the incidence of twinning, particularly MZ twinning, is much higher than expected (1 in 35 abortions). The rate of associated anomalies was not significantly different from the rate in the total population (Livingston & Poland, 1980).

Livingston and Poland (1980) found that 35 of 53 pairs were monochorionic MZ, 2 were opposite sex (DZ), and 16 were same sex, dichorionic. Uchida et al. (1983) found 7 of 15 to be opposite sex.

A striking increase in twinning was found in infants with sirenomelia (symmelia). Usually, only one of the twins had that anomaly. Only rarely have both of MZ twins been concordantly affected by anomalies in general and symmelia in particular (Roberge, 1963). Davies et al. (1971) gathered 327 cases of sirenomelia from the literature and found that there is a 100-fold increase of this anomaly in MZ twins when compared with singletons. We have previously discussed that the hypoplasia of sirenomelics' lungs, the Potter syndrome features, and amnion nodosum are prevented by the presence of the normal amnionic environment, guaranteed by a normal co-twin. This idea is beautifully demonstrated in the case described by Kohler (1972).

Discordance for major anomalies in MZ twins seems to be the unexplained rule rather than the exception. It has been the topic of numerous publications (e.g., Fogel et al., 1965). Imaizumi (1989a) found that concordance of congenital hydrocephalus in Japan was only 15% for all twins (21% in like-sex twins), but that the corresponding figures from the literature were 4.6% and 7.8%, respectively. They also saw two sets of anencephaly and hydrocephaly in two sets of like-sex twins. Hernandez-Johnstone and Benirschke (1976) cited much of the relevant literature. This concept, however, has been considered to be a "tautology" (Boklage, 1987b). Boklage suggested that most surveys of anomalies in twins employ the Weinberg formula for the assignments of zygosity. We cannot agree with this statement. In numerous studies, the chorionic status was the method that decided the presence of MZ twins. Boklage was critical of the concept that MZ twinning and anomalies are related processes; he favored the interpretation that because such features as nonright-handedness and familial twinning are overrepresented in these anomalous twins the relation between MZ twinning and anomalies does not hold. His concept was that many such twins derive from "polar body" fertilization, which he considered to be tertiary oocytes. That twinning and cardiovascular anomalies may have common origins was detailed in a large study by Berg et al. (1989).

In some case, major disruptions of fetal structures can be explained by amnionic bands or adhesions of fetus to large sheets of amnion (Khudr & Benirschke, 1972; Donnenfeld et al., 1985). Boulot and colleagues (1990) proposed that the anencephaly-like anomaly they observed may have resulted from injury at "embryonic reduction." It is of parenthetical interest to point out that the presence of placental anastomoses in DiMo twins, one being anencephalic, has served to better understand the regulation of fetal adrenal development (Kohler & MacDonald, 1972).

In most of these anomalies, there is no evidence of a genetic component. It is perhaps even more surprising to learn that anomalies with a strong genetic etiology (e.g., cleft lip and cleft palate) are frequently discordant in MZ twins. Metrakos et al. (1958) reviewed 108 twin pairs and found the concordance in MZ twins to be 31%; in DZ twins it was 6.3%. These authors and others proved monozygosity for some pairs by means of exchange skin grafts. Discordance of facial clefts is unusually common in MZ twins. Their evidence and that from many other studies clearly indicates a familial disposition of cleft lip/palate. Studies of twins for other defects (e.g., club foot, dislocated hip) have led to the concept of causation by "polygenic genetic predisposition interacting with additional unknown intrauterine environmental triggers" (Carter, 1968). This concept of a quasicontinuous variation or a threshold character with anomalies of multifactorial etiology (Fraser, 1970) is currently the best way to interpret these seemingly contradictory findings. It remains to be elucidated as to what the prenatal factors are that place the affected twin beyond the critical threshold. It could be adverse placentation (e.g., velamentous insertion of cord or SUA), as we have championed; or it could be one of many other, as yet undetermined, factors. It may relate to unequal splitting. Too little is known of the placental conformation of most such twins to allow us to come to any definite conclusion. More data must be collected on the precise placentation of twins with discordance for defects.

Cytogenetics and "Heterokaryotypic MZ Twins"

Twins may have the same chromosomal errors as singletons. Rohmer et al. (1971) described a set of DZ twins with Down syndrome and collected 200 cases of trisomy 21 in the twin literature. One of these twins was a pure trisomic; the other had a small, subsequently diminishing population of trisomic cells; it had a normal phenotype. They speculated that blood chimerism might exist but were unable to verify it; the DiDi placenta contained no anastomoses. Most commonly MZ twins are concordant for a particular aneuploidy (e.g., 48,XXXY, in Simpson et al., 1974). Mosaicism has been observed on occasion, as in the MZ twins with trisomy 21 described by Shapiro and Farnsworth (1972).

A number of unusual, so-called heterokaryotypic twins have been reported. They were monozygotic by various criteria, but their chromosome number differed. The list of these heterokaryotypic MZ twins reported has become so large that it is impractical to summarize all the reports here. A complete review may be found in the contribution by Dallapiccola et al. (1985). They described a heterokaryotypic triplet and summarized, in table form, the 25 cases reported prior to their publication. The commonest variant is chromosomal discordance associated with the Turner syndrome. The 45,X genotype is prone to abort during early gestation. Of the relatively few survivors, most had mosaicism for cells composed of 45,X and 46,XX (or XY) genotypes. Mosaicism results from the simultaneous occurrence of twinning and somatic nondisjunction of chromosomes. If the Y chromosome of a 46,XY embryo is lost by nondisjunction during early development, male and female (45,X) MZ twins may be the outcome. This formerly inexplicable situation (MZ twins of different sex) has in fact been recorded in several instances to result from this event, as for instance Gonsoulin et al. (1990a). The 45,X MZ twin of their report was additionally hydropic. Investigators have more often documented MZ twins with various degrees and types of mosaicism, of X, XX, and XXX, or Y chromosomes. There is a wide spectrum. Kurosawa et al. (1992) have reported a set of MZ twins who were mosaic for two populations of cells—45,X and 47,XYY—in lymphocytes and fibroblasts. One twin had a greater proportion of male-determining cells and had a male phenotype; the other had a female phenotype. The fact that often both twins are mosaic may betray the influence of monochorionic placentation with anastomoses (when the mosaicism is confined to lymphocytes). Alternatively, when the fibroblasts of only one twin are mosaic or have a different complement from the karyotype of the co-twin, it suggests the loss of one chromosome in one twin after splitting has occurred. Most of the placentas associated with this phenomenon have been DiMo, but an occasional twin has had a MoMo placenta. Precise studies of placenta and of lymphocyte, fibroblast, and chorionic karyotypes will enhance our knowledge as to the timing of this unusual event.

Prenatal diagnosis of such errors was once difficult because the intentional sampling of individual amnionic cavities was impractical. Young et al. (1974) introduced a feasible method to sample the individual cavities for the surveillance of Rh-sensitized pregnancies. It has now been reported successfully accomplished for 79%, 94%, and 98% of cases, respectively (Librach et al., 1984; Taylor et al., 1984; Tabsh et al., 1985). This methodology has not only allowed precise diagnosis but has led to fetal transfusions, now practiced routinely (Bowman, 1985; Pijpers et al., 1988). An alternative method for aspirating the two cavities was advocated by Jeanty et al. (1990). These authors were nearly uniformly successful, but the possibility of destroying the dividing membranes exists with this technique. Selective feticide can then be undertaken when fetal trisomy is diagnosed by any of these techniques (Kerenyi & Chitkara, 1981; Chitkara et al., 1989; see also Donnenfeld et al., 1989). Pijpers et al. (1988) studied 83 pregnancies and obtained karyotypes of both twins in 77 cases (93%). They found elevated AFP levels (in both sacs) in two cases that were due to renal abnormalities. This finding suggested to them that AFP diffuses through the membranous partition. Unfortunately, the types of placenta present in these cases were not recorded. Franke and Estel (1978) had previously found that AFP permeates the membranes.

Chimerism, Mosaicism

It is not uncommon in cytogenetic studies to identify cell lines with different chromosome numbers or different complements. It has most recently become a problem in amniocentesis and placental cell cultures. The latter aspects are considered in the chapter on abortions; here it is essential to make the differential diagnosis of mosaicism and chimerism. Whole-body chimerism may develop when, during the early stages of development, dizygotic twin embryos fuse to form a single individual. The resulting genetic chimera, a whole-body chimera is an individual composed of two populations of cells whose origin are two genetically completely different fertilization products. In addition to this mechanism, the possibility exists that two spermatozoa fertilize an ovum and a polar body, and that these structures then make up a single embryo. This second explanation is the mechanism that is favored by most investigators for the production of chimeras. Chimeras differ from mosaics and should be clearly distinguished.

Mosaics are individuals composed of different cell lines but derived from a single embryonic precursor. Because of "lyonization," all females are mosaics. Not only may mosaics have different cell lines with different chromosome numbers but because of mutations they may also have lines of cells with different phenotypic expression. An individual with cancer, for instance, could be a mosaic; one line of cells would be the normal body constituents, and the other would be those cells that form the neoplasm. It is convenient and important to distinguish two pathogenetically different types of chimeras: (1) blood chimeras (also called twin chimeras by Tippett, 1984); and (2) whole-body chimeras (dispermic chimeras).

Blood chimeras have long been known to occur in cattle. In bovine fetuses the placentas often fuse, the fetal blood vessels join, and blood is exchanged between the embryonic twins. Because embryonic blood is largely like bone marrow, there is seeding of the other twin's marrow space with genotypically different hematopoietic elements and lymphocytes. It results in life-long admixture because these cells are not rejected by the immunologically impotent embryo. The foreign cells are subsequently regarded as "self." When male and female bovine fetuses are thus joined, it is easy to identify clones of male lymphocytes in the female and vice versa. This phenomenon is restricted to motile hematopoietic system cells. The fixed tissue cells do not participate.

The fact that chimerism first was recognized in cattle results from the masculinization of the female twin in heterosexual bovine co-twins. The female becomes a freemartin (Lillie, 1917), an animal that has external masculinization, an absent uterus, atrophied ovaries, and female genotype. The degree of masculinization does not depend on the percentage of chimeric male hemopoietic cells (Herzog, 1969). Complex chimerism may be detected when triplets or quadruplets are thus admixed (Basrur et al., 1970). Although long known, the virilization of female artiodactyl twins has not yet been satisfactorily explained. Lillie (1917) and most subsequent investigators have presumed that it was the result of embryonic hormone action secreted by the male gonads. Such an obvious hypothesis proved facile when it was discovered that marmoset monkeys of South America not only always have DZ twins but that they regularly have fused placentas and are all blood chimeric. Although 50% are XX/XY chimeric, the females are not sterilized in analogy to the freemartin effect (Benirschke, 1971; Gengozian, 1971). Currently, no rational explanation exists for this discrepancy among species. Freemartinism occurs in other artiodactyla, in birds, and in a few other species. We used to believe that some primitive germ cells might also travel through embryonic intertwin anastomoses to take up residence in the opposite-sex host; findings by Gengozian et al. (1980), however, have made it unlikely. In addition, many investigations have addressed issues of immunological tolerance in chimerism (Porter & Gengozian, 1969; Tippett, 1984).

In contrast to marmosets and cattle, anastomoses between DZ twin placentas of humans are rare indeed. One dichorionic twin placenta with an anastomosis has been described by Cameron (1968) and is depicted in Figure 551. Genetic study of the twins, however, showed them to be MZ. More recently, Lage et al. (1989) presented a dichorionic twin placenta with anastomoses that was accompanied by a mild form of the transfusion syndrome. The hematocrits of the twins were 43% and 59%, respectively. Altshuler and his colleagues (personal communication, 1993) saw a similar case at autopsy. These cases are exceptional. In addition to these two observations it must be recorded that spontaneous blood chimeras have been observed in occasional human fraternal twins. They have had no sexual abnormalities and are like marmosets in that respect. When their fixed tissue has been studied, it was not found to be admixed. The chimeras must, therefore, have received the foreign clone of blood cells either through placental anastomoses or, less likely, transplacentally. Kadowaki et al. (1965) reported the transfer of maternal lymphocytes to the fetus. They described a phenotypically normal male with XY/XX blood chimerism and apparent graft-versus-host rejection disease. Such transplacental exchange of lymphocytes, however, must be uncommon (Olding, 1972). Only on rare occasions have prospective studies shown minor transplacental lymphocyte chimerism. This transplacental traffic of cells is discussed in a separate chapter; it may affect singletons as well as twins.

The occurrence of blood chimerism in human DZ twins was first demonstrated by Dunsford et al. (1953). Since then, perhaps 32 cases have been described (Tippett, 1984). They are usually detected when blood group tests have peculiar results that then necessitate full genetic investigation; it usually happens long after birth. The associated placenta of such a chimera has been fully studied only in the case of Nylander and Osunkoya (1970). Hartemann et al. (1963) suggested that placental study of twin placentas would more often identify anastomoses among fraternal twins. It has not been our experience, despite the fact that we have tried on many occasions to verify anastomoses among DiDi twins by use of dye injections. Anastomoses that become apparent by radiographic examination of injected twin placentas and those discovered by corrosion casts prepared after a plastics injection (Scipiades & Burg, 1930; Pérez et al., 1947) give unreliable results. Crookston et al. (1970) described the unusual and complex immunological breakdown of tolerance that rarely occurs in such twins.

Whole-Body Chimerism

With whole-body chimeras, the entire body consists of cells with two or more genetic lineages that are derived from separate fertilization products. Most common among them is probably the fertilization of an ovum and a polar body by two spermatozoa, with the maternal contribution being similar. Such individuals represent, genetically speaking, fraternal twins fused into one body. They are not necessarily clinically manifest and may be fertile, even when XX and XY lineages coexist. Most are discovered when the two populations of cells have different sex chromosomes (XX/XY), which frequently results in gonadal abnormalities, most common among which is true hermaphroditism. The diagnosis was initially made by amniocentesis in a detailed report by Lawce (1985). The male neonate was entirely normal and had an overall 48/98 XX/XY cell admixture. Remarkably, the ratio was 40/8 in placental membranes but 1/39 in placental tissue. Other cytogenetic errors with multiple karyotypes are also known (Moreno & Sánchez, 1971). Whole-body chimeras may also be discovered during routine blood grouping tests. Still others may be found because of unusual phenotypic features, such as heterochromia (eyes of different color). Some such cases may even possess "striping" of skin, or they may have abnormal patches of the skin, resulting from the irregular distribution of melanocyte precursors that are derived from different genotypes (Zuelzer et al., 1964; Corey et al., 1967). This skin coloration is particularly obvious in the rare male tricolored (tortoiseshell) cats because the colors black and orange are allelic on the X chromosome in felines. Tricolored cats must all be female, or else they have chimerism (rarely are they endowed with 39,XXY chromosomes) as the basis for their abnormal coloration (Centerwall & Benirschke, 1975). It is thus important to clearly distinguish between mosaicism and chimerism, something not often duly considered in the literature. The placentas of these individuals never seem to have been examined, but then there is no reason to believe that they would be unusual.

The question of how spontaneous whole-body chimerism originates is unanswered. It is readily achieved experimentally by fusing morulae of experimental animals after their zonae pellucidae have been removed (Tarkowski, 1961). How it happens in vivo is speculative. The finding of diploid/triploid chimeras (e.g., Berghe & Verresen, 1970) was taken as evidence that fertilization of a large polar body (common in mice) produced such abnormal individuals (dispermic chimeras). Other proposed mechanisms, such as secondary nondisjunction of whole haploid sets (Jenkins et al., 1971), are much less likely. De la Chapelle et al. (1974) have suggested, as did other investigators, that early fusion of two embryos may be the way that whole-body chimeras are produced spontaneously, much as in the experimental model. This idea has subsequently been disputed because of the paucity of markers available. These concepts and the wide complexity of chimerism and hermaphroditism are topics of the review by Tippett (1984).

Triplets and Higher Multiple Births

The frequency of spontaneously conceived higher multiple births is customarily estimated with the help of Hellin's rule, discussed above. Because of ovulation induction with hormones, many higher multiple births have occurred; nonatuplets hold the record. For this reason it is presently difficult to ascertain the real and spontaneous occurrence of higher multiple births in any population. Many excessive numbers are reported only in the newspapers, and they are usually artificially induced. The patient who aborted the nonatuplets during the 12th week of pregnancy was not further described. Octuplets, born prematurely to a Mexican woman who had taken contraceptives until 8 months earlier, all died from complications of prematurity (Anonymous, 1967). The frequency of higher multiple births has increased enormously in recent years because of the practice of assisted reproduction. Thus Collins and Bleyl (1990) were able to summarize results of 71 quadruplet pregnancies. They advocated delivery by the 34th week of pregnancy because of the growth deficit occurring thereafter. Elliott and Radin (1992) reviewed their own 10 cases of quadruplet pregnancy and made specific management recommendations. They had no bad outcomes, even though the gestations terminated at about 32.5 weeks. Kiely et al. (1992) surveyed the trends of higher-order multiple births from 1972 to 1989. There had occurred a 113% increase among Whites and 22% increase among Black mothers, with a 50% reduction in perinatal mortality.

When Allen (1960) applied the Weinberg formula to higher multiple offspring, he observed for triplets that the proportion of MZ/DZ/TZ (TZ = trizygotic) was 1:3:2.0 among American Blacks, and or 1:2:1.0

among Whites; quadruplet Whites were 2:6:5:4. In Japan, with different rates of multiple births, the ratios for triplets were more like 2.5:1.0:1.0, reflecting the lower DZ twinning rate of this genetically different population (Imaizumi & Inouye, 1980). The high DZ rate of Nigerians is reflected in their distribution of zygosity in triplets, approximately 1:4:6 (Nylander, 1971b). The frequent admixture of monozygotic and dizygotic twins in plural births is well reflected in their placentation. They may all be monochorionic, or they have mono-, di-, and trichorionic placentation. Nylander and Corney (1971) found in the Yoruba population of triplets, 1 monochorionic, 10 dichorionic, and 29 trichorionic specimens. Similar data for other large populations cannot be found. Most reports are of single gestations or are from small series, such as those collected by Nylander and Corney (1971). Boyd and Hamilton (1970) had the following placentation in their eight cases of triplet pregnancy: four monochorionic, three dichorionic, and one trichorionic—different from that in African women and reflecting the different causes of twinning in the populations studied. Not all dichorionic triplets are polyzygotic. Thus the dichorionic triplets described by Komai and Fukuoka (1931) were shown to be monozygotic.

Triplets and higher plural births are not only smaller than expected for their gestational age (McKeown & Record, 1952), they also commonly deliver much earlier than twins or singletons. The perinatal mortality of 59 triplet pregnancies was 23% in the study of Itzkowic (1979). This investigator emphasized that cervical incompetence was not a significant factor in their premature deliveries. Others (Gabos, 1972) reported that cervical failure may require surgical intervention in these higher multiple gestations. O'Sullivan (1968) even advocated it routinely in multiple pregnancies with hydramnios. Michlewitz et al. (1981) found a perinatal mortality of 13% past 20 weeks and 7% when 15 triplet pregnancies past 28 weeks were studied. A large experience of the outcome of assisted reproduction from Norfolk (Seoud et al., 1992) found that there was the expected progressive increase of perinatal complications and prematurity with higher-order births.

Lipitz and his colleagues (1989) have shown that the outcome of triplet pregnancies has improved in recent years. They studied 78 triplet pregnancies between 1975 and 1988, with 88% occurring after ovulation induction. Their finding was that elective cerclage neither improved fetal loss nor enhanced the length of gestation. Of the infants they were able to follow, 10.5% had severe neurological handicaps. Some triplets have been delivered with long time intervals. Simpson et al. (1984) had the first infant born at 23 weeks' gestation (neonatal death with 505 g weight, congenital infection), and 99 days later (with Shirodkar stitch, antibiotics, and

isoxsuprine) a cesarean section was done at 37 weeks. One triplet was macerated, and the other lived (2,580 g); the placenta was a fused TriTri organ. Cardwell et al. (1988) described the survival of one triplet, with the first being born at 23 weeks (hyaline membrane disease); the second was born 4 days later and died with hyaline membrane disease. The third triplet delivered 16 days after the first and survived. Chorioamnionitis complicated this pregnancy as it does in many plural pregnancies. A pregnancy with one triplet aborting during the 16th week of pregnancy and the other triplets surviving to delivery at 35 weeks was reported by Banchi (1984). The aborted triplet had a separate chorionic sac; the survivors had a DiMo placenta. A remarkable case of triplets in a uterus didelphys was described by Mashiach et al. (1981). The clomiphene-induced pregnancy resulted in triplets: two in one horn and one in the other. One was found dead at 22 weeks; at 27 weeks, uterine contractions expelled a macerated triplet from the right horn, but cesarean section was done to deliver its co-twin who later died. The left horn did not go into labor. At 37 weeks, a normal triplet was delivered by cesarean section. Gonen et al. (1990a) reported on five triplet gestations with fetal death of one or two fetuses. Four of these fetuses were monochorionic, and delivery took place 30 (±26) days after the diagnosis of fetal death.

The various types of triplet placentations are shown in Figures 624 to 629. In addition to these three variants, the placentas of DiDi triplets may be separate. It is relatively uncommon, however, as the uterine surface area available for the implantation of multiple placentas is not large enough for them to remain separate. The liveborn monozygotic triplets whose placenta is shown in Figure 624 were monoamnionic and monochorionic (Sinykin, 1958). Triplet pregnancy does not always prevent entangling of cords when they are monoamnionic, as in the case shown in Figure 629, although entangling is less common than for twins. In this case, one anencephalic and a tiny acardiac fetus were associated with a normal triplet. All were aborted because of cord entanglements. Kohler and MacDonald (1972) reported triplets, one of whom was anencephalic and who had a normal DiMo co-twin. There was a normal separate chorionic triplet. The DiMo twins of the TriDi placenta shown in Figure 625 had suffered the typical transfusion syndrome, with A being the runted donor and B the recipient who died neonatally. All were female, with C representing a separate zygote, as established by blood grouping. Another TriDi set of triplets is seen in Figure 628. It has long been known that such admixture of MZ and DZ multiple births is more common than would be expected by chance. The reason is not clear. In addition to these examples, we have seen a DiMo triplet pregnancy abort with two mono-

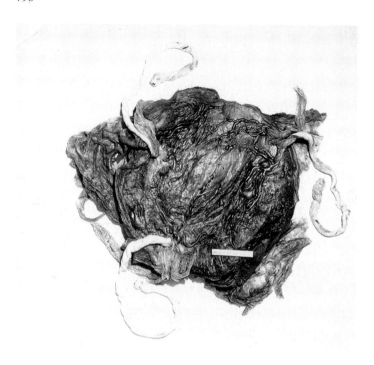

FIGURE 624. MoMo triplet term placenta without entangling of cords but anastomoses among all circulations. The triplets survived. (From Sinykin, 1958, with permission.)

amnionic pygopagous twins, a term DiMo triplet placenta with one set of thoracopagi, and a TriTri triplet pregnancy with two fetus papyracei, the other fetus coming to term and being normal. The prenatal death of the two fetuses may therein have been due to their velamentous cord insertions. A triplet pregnancy produced by in vitro fertilization is reported in Chapter 7. Five ova had been transferred; three implanted, and one became a placenta percreta that had to be removed from its interstitial implantation during the second month of pregnancy. The two remaining fetuses were delivered by cesarean section near term, one having amnionic bands. We have

witnessed yet another triplet placenta percreta. Thus plural pregnancies can present multiple problems with many anomalies of placentation alone.

It has often been asked how triplets or quintuplets (e.g., the famous Dionne quintuplets) can be MZ, as one might expect even numbers to result. Uneven numbers of monozygotic multiples may be explained by assuming that, on occasion, one embryo may not have survived or that "one division may set back development of the daughter products so that secondary division can occur at the same stage or even an earlier stage than did the primary division . . . or . . . three or

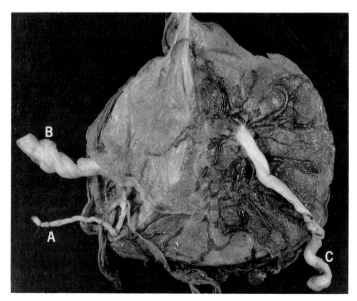

FIGURE 625. Triamnionic dichorionic triplets, all female. A is the donor of the transfusion syndrome, and B is the recipient in a DiMo placenta. C has a separate amnion and chorion, as well as blood groups different from those of the twins. (Blood groups courtesy Dr. F.H. Allen, New York.)

FIGURE 626. Triamnionic monochorionic triplet placenta at term. Many large anastomoses are present.

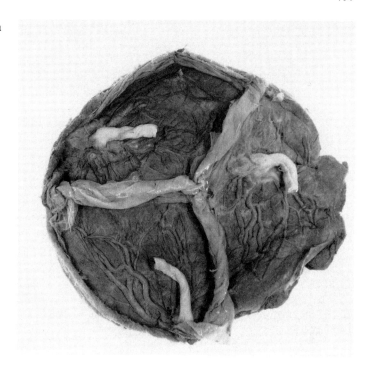

more embryonic centers might arise simultaneously instead of two" (Allen, 1960). Allen presented a graphic demonstration of the genesis of multiple embryos, assuming binary divisions as the principal modus operandi.

Quadruplets and quintuplets have also become more common in recent years. Whereas in the past most had not been induced by hormone administration, such treatment is clearly now a factor. We have met a diabetic patient who had three sets of fraternal triplets and then a set of fraternal twins, and her uterus finally had to be removed when it ruptured with a quadruplet pregnancy. Sinclair (1940) depicted the QuaTri placenta of a set of surviving quadruplets. A similar placenta from

three-egg quadruplets was described by Ryan and Wislocki (1954). Hamilton et al. (1959) reported the quadrichorial placenta depicted in Figure 630. They found in the 16 cases of the English literature that "every possible combination of ovulation had occurred except for double monozygous, often stated never to appear." Diddle and Burford (1935), however, described just such a case in stillborns. Atlay and Pennington (1971) observed a quadruplet pregnancy after ovulation induction with pituitary gonadotropins. It was composed of a set of monoamnionic twins, the others all having their separate amnion, and they were of different sex. The 30 weeks' gestation quadruplets had a good outcome. In this contribution, Atlay and Pennington provided much

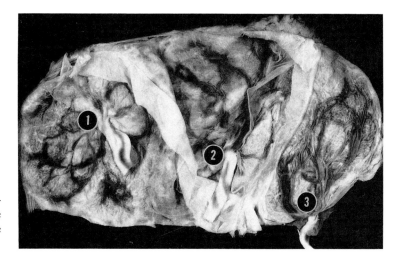

FIGURE 627. Triamnionic trichorionic term placenta. There are no anastomoses and, despite intimate fusion, no blood chimerism. Note the velamentous cord insertion of no. 3.

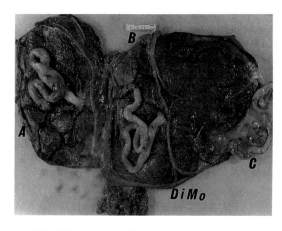

FIGURE 628. Triamnionic dichorionic triplet placenta at 36 weeks' gestation, all male. The diamnionic set of twins are at right with a single A-V anastomosis from C to B. All survived. The slightly separated dichorionic placenta of triplet A (at left) has an area of circummargination at the top, where the membranes of the right triplets pushed its membranes away.

hormonal data that may be helpful in the surveillance of plural pregnancies. McFee et al. (1974) reported on two sets of quadruplets, among which only one of the eight premature newborns succumbed. The authors gave detailed and helpful instructions as to preparations needed by staff and family for the anticipated delivery of plural births. Williams (1926) described the quadruplet pregnancy of a 38-year-old woman whose offspring all died. The placenta was TriTri and fused. He also reported on the fact that 24% of the 280 sets of twins observed at the Johns Hopkins Hospital were

monochorionic; of four triplets, three were TriDi, and one was TriTri. We have seen several quadruplet placentas with four chorions and one with four amnions and three chorions (Figure 631). Imaizumi (1989b) reported on 16 sets of quintuplets from Japan. Three sets were liveborn, eight were stillborn, and five were live- and stillborn, with 51 of 80 offspring being stillborn. The mean weight of 40 quintuplets was 1,048 g.

Nichols (1954) published a list of 17 quintuplet births in the United States and two in Canada, as well as five sextuplets in the United States. An editorial (Anonymous, 1968) estimated spontaneous quintuplets to occur as rarely as 1 in 8 million to 1 in 54 million births. The combined weights for four surviving sets were 10.61, 14.08, 12.11, and 23.52 pounds. We have seen surviving quintichorial quintuplets, conceived after clomiphene citrate (Clomid) induction and delivered at 31 weeks. Their combined weight was 8,200 g (1,420–1,820 g). Three of the umbilical cords had marginal insertions. As can be imagined, such enormous uterine distension gives rise to maternal dyspnea, hydramnios (?), excessive weight gain, preeclampsia, edema, varices, and cardiac failure. In another editorial (Anonymous, 1963a), 50 sets of quintuplets were listed as having been reported in the entire medical literature. It is interesting to note that several of the well described quintuplet placentas were diagnostic of MZ quintuplets, as were the Dionne quintuplets. The fact that one of the latter gave birth to a set of male twins is presumably a random occurrence.

A monozygotic quintuplet placenta was superbly studied by Gibbs et al. (1960); it is depicted in Figure 632. This placenta had a single chorion and five am-

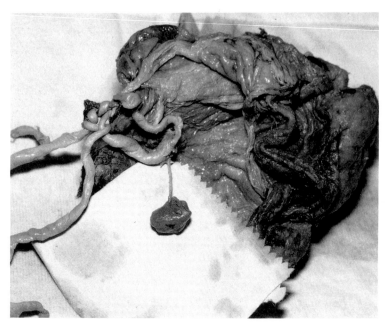

FIGURE 629. MoMo triplet placenta from a spontaneous abortion. Note the entangling of all umbilical cords. One was a normal fetus and one an anencephalic; the small fetus, placed separately on the piece of paper, was acardiac.

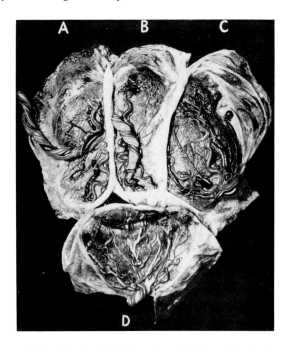

FIGURE 630. Quadruplet placenta with four chorionic sacs. All fetuses survived. (Reprinted with permission of Hamilton, et al. Another case of quadruplets. J. Obstet. Gynaecol Br. Emp. 66:409–412. Blackwell Scientific Publishing, Ltd., 1959.)

nions. There were many vascular anastomoses on the chorionic surface; several cords inserted marginally, and that of no. 5 had a single umbilical artery. All these extremely immature infants succumbed from hyaline membrane disease. The placenta was redescribed by Neubecker et al. (1962). Quintuplets reported by Berbos et al. (1964) were QuiQua (quintamnionic; quadrichorial); a quintuplet pregnancy induced with gonadotropins and studied by Aubert (1960) resulted in three male and two female infants, with QuiQua placenta, and the successful quintuplet pregnancy reported by Liggins and Ibbertson (1966) had five chorionic sacs (QuiQui). Bender and Brandt (1974) studied a quintuplet placenta by morphometry. It was induced by hormones and had QuiQui membranes. These authors drew attention to the "irregular chorionic fusion" of the dividing membranes, discussed earlier and depicted in Figures 579 and 580. G. Altshuler (personal communication, 1975) also observed a QuiQui placenta that, when injected with milk, exhibited no anastomoses. Finally, the monochorionic quintuplets (QuiMo) with one acardiac fetus reported by Hamblen et al. (1937) are shown in Figure 612.

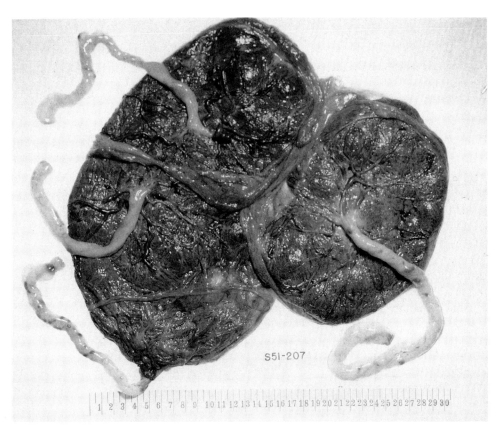

FIGURE 631. Quadruplet placenta (QuaTri), with DiMo monozygotic twins at bottom left, one having marginal insertion of the umbilical cord (35 weeks, 920 g).

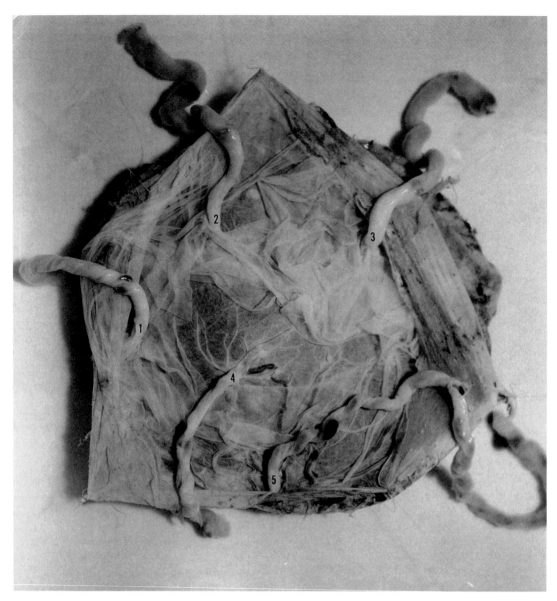

Figure 632. Monochorionic (quint-amnionic) quintuplet placenta, immature. All infants died from hyaline membrane disease; no. 5 had SUA. Large anastomoses are present.

(Reprinted with permission from The American College of Obstetricians and Gynecologists (Obstetrics and Gynecology, Gibbs, 1960, 16:464–468).)

No sextuplet placentas have been described as far as we can ascertain from the literature, and few sextuplets have been reported to have occurred. Figure 633 shows such a specimen from a patient treated with fertility drugs that was provided by Dr. M.A. Fletcher from a delivery in Washington, DC in 1983. It was a fused placenta with six amnions and six chorions. It also contained a fetus papyraceus, estimated to have died at 20 weeks' gestation. That fetus had a normal skeleton, but its cord had velamentous insertion, and this insertion was the presumed reason for his demise. Three other fetuses had marginal cord insertion. Two cords had a left, and three a right, spiral; that of the fetus

papyraceus was not spiraled at all. One specimen of a septuplet pregnancy, induced by gonadotropins and prematurely delivered (Turksoy et al., 1967), was depicted by Boyd and Hamilton (1970). The sacs each had their own chorion and amnion; one was separated, and the others were fused. The cords were mostly marginal and one had SUA.

Because plural gestations generally have poor outcomes, their early diagnosis and "selective reduction" of some cases is currently being advocated. By ultrasonography, Campbell and Dewhurst (1970) diagnosed hormone-induced quintuplets as early as at 19 weeks' gestation. The pregnancy went to 31 weeks. Labor

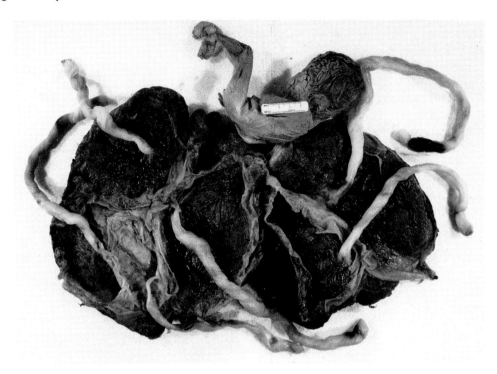

FIGURE 633. Sextuplet placenta with six chorionic sacs and a male fetus papyraceus. (Courtesy Dr. M.A. Fletcher, Washington, DC.)

ensued, and the healthy quintuplets were delivered by cesarean section. Kanhai et al. (1986) punctured the hearts of three quintuplets at 10 weeks' gestation (one was repeated at 11 weeks). The mother subsequently delivered full-term healthy twin girls. The placenta had only one 2.5-cm embryonic rest.

Another hormone-induced quintuplet pregnancy was managed by Farquharson et al. (1988). At 9 weeks two embryos had intracardiac injection of hypertonic saline. Five days later the procedure was repeated with another embryo. The maternal serum hCG levels declined substantially, and at 37 weeks heterosexual twins were delivered vaginally. Their placenta was DiDi. In the membranes, a plaque of atrophied villi and a cavity (but no fetuses) were found.

Evans and colleagues (1988) presented four such cases of therapeutic intervention. They also discussed the legal and other implications that attend this novel therapy. Their first case had nine gestational sacs at 7 weeks. Three fetuses were "needled" at 8 weeks and three additional ones at 9 weeks. The patient delivered two healthy male infants at 35 weeks. Their second case was a hormone-induced quadruplet pregnancy with elimination of two sacs by cardiac puncture at 10 weeks. Two healthy infants delivered at 36 weeks. In the third case in vitro fertilization led to implantation of four embryos; two embryos were eliminated at 10 weeks. One remaining fetus was then found to have Potter

syndrome. The other died in utero. In their fourth case, four fetuses had been induced with hormones, and two were eliminated at 11 weeks. The remaining twins were aborted because of cervical incompetence. They delivered, despite cerclage, at 19 weeks; the placentas were not described by these authors. They emphasized ethical issues and the need for regulated hormone induction of pregnancy for infertile patients, an aspect that was further elaborated on in a discussion by Weiner (1988). It might be mentioned parenthetically that there has been much discussion as to whether cerclage is indicated for multiple pregnancy because of the frequently observed cervical dilatation. Michaels et al. (1991) recommend that it not be used routinely; they used ultrasonographic criteria to select those patients who might benefit from this operation. Their results suggest that some patients' twin pregnancy is lengthened when cerclage is done. Berkowitz et al. (1988) reported their experience with selective embryocide in 12 multifetal pregnancies (2 × 6; 1 × 5; 5 × 4; 4 × 3). They reduced the number to two fetuses in 11 pregnancies and to three fetuses in one pregnancy. The surgery was undertaken between 9 and 13 weeks. Seven healthy twins were born. One produced a healthy singleton, and four had only fetal deaths. Later these authors reported on 200 multifetal reductions (Berkowitz et al., 1993). Boulot et al. (1993) concluded that the reduction reduces the incidence of preterm labor but does not prevent it. The difficulty and rationale for the procedure were highlighted in an editorial by Hobbins (1988). One such problem is the development of unforeseen complications in the survivor. Mahone et al. (1993) had such an experience. They described a twin transfusion syndrome at 23 weeks' gestation where the selective feticide of the hydropic recipient was followed quickly by hydrops in the remaining donor. They speculated that perhaps one mechanism of cardiac failure in the donor was the additional blood loss into the plethoric donor. Their photograph of the twins supports this notion. It also suggests to us that the best therapy for this ominous syndrome is interruption of the anastomosing vessels, as is practiced by De Lia (see below).

Since these early reports on embryo reduction there have been numerous reports that should be consulted. Thus Wapner et al. (1990) reviewed 46 cases with 80 fetuses remaining; 94% of them survived. Lynch et al. (1990) discussed 28 triplet, 47 quadruplet, 4 quintuplet, 4 sextuplet, 1 septuplet, and 1 nonatuplet pregnancies with reductions, usually to twins. Their outcomes were excellent. Tabsh (1990b) reviewed 40 cases, and Melgar et al. (1991) suggested that their results from the reduction of quadruplets indicated marked improvement in outcome, whereas that for triplets remains controversial. The intentional delivery of a 710 g acardiac fetus at 22 weeks' gestation by Robie et al. (1989) is also relevant in this regard. It was followed by delivery of a normal girl. The case is of special interest because the acardiac had a penile structure, yet possessed ovaries. She also had a normal female karyotype, and the co-twin was a normal girl. Itskovitz et al. (1989) and Gonen et al. (1990b,c) elected to use a transvaginal ultrasound approach for selective embryo reduction. The latter authors used intrathoracic potassium chloride injection and had one case of chorioamnionitis following the procedure. They considered the procedure to be not without significant risk. Tabsh (1993) reported the results of 131 transabdominal reductions done by one practitioner, with 103 deliveries ensuing. He had a 7% pregnancy loss rate from the intervention that occurred within 4 weeks and concluded that it is a safe procedure. Macones et al. (1993) showed that reducing triplets to twins markedly improves fetal survival.

Twins Associated with Abortion and Ectopic Pregnancy

Multiple pregnancies occur also as abortions and in ectopic gestations, but they are not often reported or perhaps are frequently overlooked. Many specimens from spontaneous abortions do not contain an embryo,

many are chromosomally abnormal, and many are fragmented when they are observed in the laboratory. Javert (1957) reviewed most of the relevant literature. He found citations of twin frequencies ranging from 6% to 20%. In his own material of 2,000 abortuses, he had an incidence of only 1.2%. Our own observations have yielded a still lower figure (0.3%) (Benirschke & Driscoll, 1967). There is general agreement, however, that monochorial twins are overrepresented in abortion material. Numerous MoMo twins, for instance, vanish during early development (Figures 571, 611); and still other twins succumb from the transfusion syndrome (Figure 605) or because they are acardiacs (Figure 617). It is impossible to give accurate figures. The great student of twinning, Guttmacher (1937), believed that twins were twice as common in abortions as in births (1 in 37 versus 1 in 86.5), and the investigations of Livingston and Poland (1980) and Uchida et al. (1983) pointed in the same direction.

It should be easier to identify ectopic twin gestations, as they are generally better preserved. Indeed, many such cases are on record (e.g., Starks, 1980). The exceptional case of a tubal triplet gestation was reported by Forbes and Natale (1968), who believed it to be only the fourth case published. It was TriMo, and only a single corpus luteum cyst was found. Fujii et al. (1981) described a unilateral tubal quadruplet pregnancy with QuaMo placenta and unequal development of the embryos. Twin ectopics have been seen more often. Considering the frequencies of ectopic pregnancy and twinning, it is surprising that Storch and Petrie (1976) found only 87 reported cases of ectopic twins. More astonishing still is the fact that most tubal ectopics are monochorionic. This finding is much out of proportion to the general distribution of twin placentation and the topic is discussed in detail by Neuman et al. (1990). They proved with RFLPs the dizygosity of tubal aborted twins and suggested that the alleged common monozygosity of ectopic twins may be in error. Arey (1923a,b) was the first to report that ectopic twins have a 15 times greater frequency of monochorionic placentation than do intrauterine gestations. He reported MoMo twins, quintuplets, three triplets, and one thoracopagus; and in an earlier publication (Arey, 1922) he suggested that these findings argued in favor of "chorionic fusion." The proof of this contention, the occurrence of monochorial heterosexual twins, has not been reported. Later, Arey considered the possibility of an environmental insult that produced MZ twins in this abnormal location. It is our opinion that most case reports are incomplete and too superficial, and so usually they do not allow a clear decision on this interesting point. Perhaps monochorial gestational sacs are larger ab initio and have more difficulty passing through the tube. Even less commonly described are twin ovarian ectopic pregnancies. Kalfayan and Gundersen (1980) reported a case of DiDi ovarian gestational sacs in a patient wearing an intrauterine device. They found three other reported cases.

"Heterotopic pregnancy is defined as a coexisting intrauterine and extrauterine pregnancy" (Goodno & Gentry, 1962). It is apparently more common than is usually assumed. Gamberdella and Marrs (1989), who described a much higher frequency in "assisted reproductive technology," considered heterotopic pregnancies to occur at a frequency of 1 per 30,000 pregnancies. It often involves an interstitial (cornual) and an intrauterine gestation. Sotrel et al. (1976) suggested that more than 600 cases had been reported in the literature. They identified a case that occurred after ovulation induction. These pregnancies are often complicated by placenta accreta/increta (Starks, 1980), and they are usually dichorionic. Because they were able to make the diagnosis early, Porreco et al. (1990) electively eliminated the ectopic fetus and allowed the intrauterine gestation to proceed to term. Laband et al. (1988), who reported four such cases, suggested that the incidence of this unusual, dangerous gestational complication may be greater than 1 per 30,000. Payne et al. (1971) have seen triplets in this situation after ovulation induction. A similar case is reported in Chapter 7 with interstitial placenta percreta, removed during the second month, with twins remaining in the uterus.

It is also surprising how many cases of twin gestation have been described in women with uterus didelphys and how frequently they have been delivered at different times. Laird et al. (1957) reported on a miscarriage from one side 6 months before the delivery of a normal twin from the other. Dawson and Ainslee (1958) saw premature twins delivering from a bicornuate uterus in short succession. Kennedy (1959) delivered an asphyxiated infant from one side, and 3 weeks later the other twin was born from the other uterus. Mingeot and Keirse (1971) delivered such twins within 9 hours of each other. Brown and Nelson (1967) reported that a patient with completely split genital tracts intentionally became pregnant on separate occasions in each uterus, with live infants resulting. A complex case was seen by Zervoudakis et al. (1976) in which curettage emptied an aborting pregnancy, but the patient remained pregnant in a blind uterine horn. Six weeks later the horn was surgically emptied when a chemical interruption failed. There were no apparent connections, although Loendersloot (1977) later suggested that a perforation may have been present from first curettage. Nhân and Huisjes (1983) induced the second uterine horn after delivery of a normal child from one horn. Finally, Ahram et al. (1984) delivered twins from both horns of a bicornuate uterus. They, as many before, had to initiate labor of the second horn before delivery could be effected. In most of these cases the placenta is not described. When it is discussed, the twins are usually considered to be binovular.

In a review of the obstetrical performance of 150 cases with uterine anomalies (with 325 pregnancies), Jones (1957) noted that twinning was not more common in these women. It may also be noted that delivery of twins at different times has been described in women with normal uteri. Thomsen (1978) reported a case where the first twin was delivered at 27 weeks and the second at 31 weeks. We have seen twins deliver 4 weeks apart, with the placenta of the first twin remaining in utero and becoming atrophied. The second twin survived. Previously, the maximum interval of 65 days was reported by Drucker et al. (1960), but Feichtinger et al. (1989) have described an even longer interval: The patient delivered one twin at 21 weeks' gestation, followed by tocolysis and cerclage. She delivered a healthy 1,750 g twin 12 weeks later; the placenta was dichorionic and had an infarcted portion. The survivor had a velamentous cord insertion. There was no inflammation. The most recent report on delayed delivery of second twins came from Vancouver (Wittmann et al., 1992). They observed four cases with delivery intervals ranging from 41 to 143 days, and then reviewed 21 cases from the literature. The overall salvage rate was 84%; careful management protocols are suggested by these authors.

Morbidity and Mortality

An abundant obstetrical literature discusses the causes for the excessive mortality of twins and the frequent obstetrical complications encountered during their delivery. Relatively rare and easy to understand is the phenomenon of "locked twins." Khunda (1972) discussed 37 such cases and estimated that it occurs with a frequency of 1 per 1,000 twin deliveries, and that it has a high stillbirth rate. Breech/vertex presentation of twins is the commonest factor; also common are primigravidity and large pelves. Cohen et al. (1965) had previously reported similar figures. In their experience, interlocking was present once in 817 twin deliveries and once in 87 breech/vertex presentations of twins. It is a particularly serious event when it occurs at or below the pelvic inlet, with death of twin A quickly ensuing. Amniotic sac dystocia has been described once, by Nickerson (1967). The membranes from twin 2 prolapsed in front of the first delivering twin. This abnormality was easily corrected, and delivery was accomplished.

Of the numerous maternal complications that attend multiple gestation, Seski and Miller (1963) listed in descending order: premature delivery, preeclampsia, hydramnios, placenta previa, abruptio placentae, cord prolapse, uterine inertia, and postpartum hemorrhage. Placental abnormalities often mirror these events. Hydramnios in twin pregnancies is most commonly due to the transfusion syndrome. Next most frequently, hydramnios results from fetal or placental anomalies. It has been debated as to whether preeclampsia is commoner with DZ twins than with MZ twins; that it is more frequent in twin gestations is not disputed. We have seen numerous dizygotic twin placentas in which only one placental half was affected with infarcts and decidual atherosis. It suggests that fetal and maternal interactions of respective genotypes are critical to the determination of pregnancy-induced hypertension (PIH, or preeclampsia). Campbell et al. (1977) studied this subject in great detail and reviewed the literature. They analyzed 343 twin pregnancies, with exact zygosity determination, and found that DZ and MZ twin pregnancies had the same incidence of mild and severe toxemia of pregnancy.

Perhaps the most debated topic in the management of twins is the manner in which the second twin is to be delivered and how rapidly it must be accomplished. Increased fetal mortality for the second twin has often been suggested but was also frequently not confirmed by studies in detail (Adam et al., 1991). In almost all respects (e.g., Apgar score, pH, weight) twin A is said to be favored (Young et al., 1985). The higher mortality of twin B was particularly evident in Spurway's (1962) report on the management of twin deliveries. Others have not found such dramatic differences, particularly when cases in which prenatal deaths (macerated stillborns, acardiacs) and infants weighing less than 1,500 g were excluded from such analyses (Thompson & Johnson, 1966; Rayburn et al., 1984; Adam et al., 1991). Nevertheless, the mortality of twins is much greater than that of singletons; and reports from the American, European, and African literature are summarized in the thoughtful review by Powers (1973). Those reports are shown in Table 31, as are more recent surveys. In general, the perinatal mortality of twins hovers around 10%, but the statistics are largely influenced by inclusion or exclusion of twins from early gestations and also depend on the date of study, as marked improvements have been achieved recently. Thus in a case-control study of Spellacy et al. (1990), the overall mortality of twins more than 500 g in weight now was 4.88% for twin A and 6.41% for twin B. As in this study, there is little doubt that prematurity, often the result of hydramnios, is the most important factor in determining outcome. Rouse et al. (1993) related fundal height measurement to preterm delivery. They decided that single measurement excessive fundal height does not predict premature labor. This hypothesis was to be expected, as excessive size alone cannot be the trigger for labor; rather, it is the rapid increase in uterine size

(as occurs with hydramnios from the transfusion syndrome) that has this effect. At times preterm labor is heavily influenced by the presence of the amnionic fluid infection syndrome (chorioamnionitis). Thus Naeye et al. (1978), who recorded a 13.8% twin perinatal mortality, found that infection was the cause of twin deaths in 2.3%, in contrast to 0.6% in singletons. The incidence was much higher (13.0% versus 1.8%) in Ethiopia. Premature rupture of membranes occurred more commonly in twins than singletons, but its outcome (latency to labor, infection) did not differ from singleton pregnancies (Mercer et al., 1993). These authors remarked on the paucity of abruptio occurring with multiple gestations. No significant differences between twins were found in the occurrence of the respiratory distress syndrome (Arnold et al., 1987) or cerebral hemorrhages (Pearlman & Batton, 1988). Most impressive, however, is the difference of perinatal mortality between monochorial and dichorial twins. Monochorionic twins have a significantly higher mortality, and that of monoamnionic twins is the highest (Benirschke, 1961; Cameron, 1968; Fujikura & Froehlich, 1971).

Early bed rest has been proposed to improve twin survival (Anonymous, 1963b). The cost of this measure is formidable (Powers & Miller, 1979), however, and careful appraisal with random trials has shown that it is inefficacious. In fact, with early admission and bed rest, the prematurity rate is increased. Robertson (1964b), who had earlier sought statistical improvement from early admission but did not find it, thought that random trials would be unethical. A study of the possible benefits was done by Rydhstrom (1988). Pregnancy outcome for 78 twin-bearing women who were prescribed prophylactic leave of absence from work to prevent preterm delivery was compared with that of a group of 78 twin-pregnant controls who did not take prophylactic leave. Gestational duration and birth weight did not differ between the two groups. The results indicated that prophylactic leave of absence from work did not improve the outcome of a twin pregnancy. Crowther et al. (1989) and MacLennan et al. (1990) also found that bed rest had no beneficial outcome in twin survivals. Indeed, "evidence is accumulating that rest may even increase premature labour" (Thornton & Rout, 1990; see also Andrews et al., 1991). Although cesarean section rates have increased from 3% (1963–1972) to 51% (1978–1984), Bell et al. (1986) were unable to show that even this modality of care improved the condition of twins at birth [see also Saunders et al. (1985) and Greig et al. (1992)]. Only attendance at prenatal twin care clinics seemed to have a beneficial effect on outcome (Ellings et al., 1993).

The excessive mortality of multiple offspring has been given as one reason for selective reduction during early pregnancy. Layzer (1988) noted that a 16% perinatal

TABLE 31. Perinatal motality of twins.

Source	Year	No. of twins	Toxemia (%)	Breech (%)	Mortality (%)
Powers	1973 (review)	794	33		18.8
Europe and Africa		2,012	25	18.4	12
		98	20.4	30	16
		944	24		11
		706	35.4	36.8	12.2
		510	24.4	32	18.8
		210	31		6
		992	32	20	14
		2,000	10.1	32.1	16.1
		412	26.2	24.5	10.9
		358	34		12.3
		3,152			9.5
Tow	1959	408			12.3
De Paepe	1959	108			8.8
Farrell	1964	1,000			16.1
Scholtes	1971	200			11.8
Bleker et al.	1979	1,655			14
Powers	1973 (review)	666	21.3	26.6	13.8
USA and Canada		270	16	30.5	28.6
		750	5	33	18.5
		504	21	28.3	15.6
		384	29.2		14
		1,000	28.2	21.2	9.8
		834			9.2
		384	27	31.3	14.1
		406	10.8	33	10.1
		17,168			9.9
		2,654	4.9	29.9	13.3
		986	37.5	24.4	9.9
		1,744	5	9.8	14.4
		2,798	14		11.8
		206	4.8	25	10.3
		1,046	16.5	31	10.8
		758			14
		1,054			13.4
		104			17.3
Ferguson	1964	3,238			9.3
Robertson	1964a	496	32		12.2
Myrianthopoulos	1970a	1,230			17.3
Ho & Wu	1975	177			10.7
Medearis et al.	1979	3,594			11.7
Keith et al.	1980	588			14.6
Hawrylyshyn et al.	1982	177			13.2
Laros & Dattel	1988	206			13.3
Fowler et al.	1991	41,554 White			4.71
		10,062 Black			7.93

mortality exists in triplets, and another 15% do not survive infancy. The figures for quadruplets and quintuplets are 21% and 22%, respectively; for sextuplets the respective figures are 41% and 50%. At the other end of this spectrum, large twins have also been recorded. Leonard (1957) has reviewed this topic and reported twins weighing 4,075 and 5,180 g (20.4 pounds together). They were, of course, dichorionic (male/female) and are the largest recorded in the literature.

Hormones in Twin Pregnancy

In efforts to predict twin pregnancies, various serological parameters have been studied for better surveillance. Halpin (1970) found excessively high hCG titers in a twin pregnancy, and Thiery et al. (1976) determined that hCG titers were 2.5 times higher in twins than in singletons. This increase was confirmed by studies of Jovanovic et al. (1977). Thiery et al. (1976) also reviewed the literature on the elevation of hCG levels during pregnancy and simultaneously studied the hPL levels. The latter were found to be 1.5 times higher than in singleton pregnancies. Other investigators have made similar observations (Gennser et al., 1975; Grennert et al., 1976a; Mägiste et al., 1976; Daw, 1977). In general, the values are 1 SD above those for singletons; and when one twin dies, a noticeable decrease has been recorded (Kenney et al., 1976). It has also been shown that following elective embryocide there is a marked fall in hCG levels, but that progesterone and estradiol levels remain stable (O'Keane et al., 1988). α-Fetoprotein was found to be elevated in seven of ten twin pregnancies reported by Ishiguro (1973), as was the level of cystylaminopeptidase (Einerh & Jacobsson, 1976). Because of the considerable scatter of hPL values during pregnancy, Dhont et al. (1976) suggested that simultaneous determination of hCG and hPL values gives more reliable results in the anticipation of twins (see reply by Grennert et al., 1976b).

References

Åberg, A., Mitelman, F., Cantz, M., and Gehler, J.: Cardiac puncture of fetus with Hurler's disease avoiding abortion of unaffected co-twin. Lancet 2:990–991, 1978.

Abraham, J.M.: Intrauterine feto-fetal transfusion syndrome: clinical observations and speculations on pathogenesis. Clin. Pediatr. 6:405–410, 1967.

Achiron, R., Rosen, N., and Zakut, H.: Pathophysiologic mechanism of hydramnios development in twin transfusion syndrome. J. Reprod. Med. 32:305–308, 1987.

Adam, C., Allen, A.C., and Baskett, T.F.: Twin delivery: Influence of the presentation and method of delivery on the second twin. Am. J. Obstet. Gynecol. 165:23–27, 1991.

Aherne, W., Strong, S.J., and Corney, G.: The structure of the placenta in the twin transfusion syndrome. Biol. Neonate 12:121–135, 1968.

Ahlfeld, F.: Beiträge zur Lehre von den Zwillingen. VI. Die Entstehung der Acardiaci. Arch. Gynäkol. 14:321–360, 1879.

Ahmad, Q.N., Britten, E.J., and Byth, D.E.: Haploid soybeans a rare occurrence in twin seedlings. J. Hered. 68:67, 1977.

Ahram. J.A., Toaff, M.E., Chandra, P., Laffey, P., and Chawla, H.S.: Successful outcome of a twin gestation in both horns of a bicornuate uterus. Am. J. Obstet. Gynecol. 150:323–324, 1984.

Akesson, H.O., Smith, G.F., and Thrybom, B.R.: Twinning and associated stillbirth in Sweden, 1871–1960. Hereditas 64:193–198, 1970.

Albert, A., Randall, R.V., Smith, R.A., and Johnson, C.E.: The urinary excretion of gonadotrophin as a function of age. In, Hormones and the Ageing Process. E.T. Engle and G. Pincus, eds., pp. 49–62. Academic Press, Orlando, FL, 1956.

Alderman, B.: Foetus acardius amorphus. Postgrad. Med. J. 49:102–105, 1973.

Allen, G.: A differential method for estimation of type frequencies in triplets and quadruplets. Am. J. Hum. Genet. 12:210–224, 1960.

Allen, G.: Twin research: problems and prospects. Prog. Med. Genet. 4:242–269, 1965.

Allen, G.: Diagnostic efficiency of fingerprint and blood group differences in a series of twins. Acta Genet. Med. Gemellol. 17:359–374, 1968.

Allen, G.: The non-decline in U.S. twin birth rates, 1964–1983. Acta Genet. Med. Gemellol. 36:313–323, 1987.

Allen, G., and Hrubec, Z.: Twin concordance: a more general model. Acta Genet. Med. Gemellol. 28:3–13, 1979.

Allen, G., and Hrubec, Z.: The monozygotic twinning rate: Is it really constant? Acta Genet. Med. Gemellol. 36:389–396, 1987.

Allen, M.I.v, Smith, D.W., and Shepard, T.H.: Twin reversed arterial perfusion (TRAP) sequence: a study of 14 twin pregnancies with acardius. Semin. Perinatol. 7:285–293, 1983.

Allen, M.S., and Turner, U.G.: Twin birth—identical or fraternal twins? Obstet. Gynecol. 37:538–542, 1971.

Allen, W.R., and Pashen, R.L.: Production of monozygotic (identical) horse twins by embryo micromanipulation. J. Reprod. Fertil. 71:607–613, 1984.

Altshuler, G., and Hyde, S.: Placental pathology case book: a bidiscoid, monochorionic placenta. J. Perinatol. 13:492–493, 1993.

Amatuzio, J.C., and Gorlin, R.J.: Conjoined acardiac monsters. Arch. Pathol. Lab. Med. 105:253–255, 1981.

Anderson, J.M., and Benirschke, K.: Fetal circulations in the placenta of Dasypus novemcinctus Linn. and their significance in tissue transplantation. Transplantation 1:306–310, 1963.

Anderson, R.L., Golbus, M.S., Curry, C.J.R., Callen, P.W., and Hastrup, W.H.: Central nervous system damage and other anomalies in surviving fetus following second trimester antenatal death of co-twin: report of four cases and literature review. Prenat. Diagn. 10:513–518, 1990.

Andrews, W.W., Leveno, K.J., Sherman, M.L., Mutz, J., Gilstrap, L.C., and Whalley, P.J.: Elective hospitalization in the management of twin pregnancies. Obstet. Gynecol. 77:826–831, 1991.

Anonymous: Quintuplet births. AMA News Nov. 25:3, 1963a.

Anonymous: Twin pregnancy. Lancet 2:79–80, 1963b.

Anonymous: Mexico City octuplets succumb within 13 hours. Med. World News, March 31, 1967.

Anonymous: Quintuplets. B.M.J. 1:534, 1968.

Antoine, C., Young, B.K., Silverman, F., Greco, M.A., and Alvarez, S.P.: Sinusoidal fetal heart rate pattern with vasa previa in twin pregnancy. J. Reprod. Med. 27:295–300, 1982.

Arai, K., Soma, H., and Hokano, M.: Ultrastructure of human placental villi in abortion, premature birth and stillbirth. J. Clin. Electron Microsc. 10:5–6, 1977.

Arey, L.B.: Chorionic fusion and augmented twinning in the human tube. Anat. Rec. 23:253–262, 1922.

Arey, L.B.: Tubal twins and tubal pregnancy. Surg. Gynecol. Obstet. 36:803–810, 1923a.

Arey, L.B.: Two embryologically important specimens of tubal twins. Surg. Gynecol. Obstet. 36:407–415, 1923b.

Arnold, C., McLean, F.H., Kramer, M.S., and Usher, R.H.: Respiratory distress syndrome in second-born versus first-born twins: a matched case-control analysis. N. Engl. J. Med. 317:1121–1125, 1987.

Arts, N.F.T., and Lohman, A.H.M: The vascular anatomy of monochorionic diamniotic twin placentas and the transfusion syndrome. Eur. J. Obstet. Gynecol. 3:85–93, 1971.

Ash, K., Harman, C.R., and Gritter, H.: TRAP sequence—successful outcome with indomethacin treatment. Obstet. Gynecol. 76:960–962, 1990.

Atlay, R.D., and Pennington, G.W.: The use of clomiphene citrate and pituitary gonadotropin in successive pregnancies: the Sheffield quadruplets. Am. J. Obstet. Gynecol. 109:402–407, 1971.

Aubert, L.: Développement aigu d'un kyste de l'ovaire et grossesse quintuple chez une femme ayant reçu successivement des gonadotrophines sériques et chorioniques. Ann. Endocrinol. (Paris) 21:176–182, 1960.

Averback, P., and Wigglesworth, F.W.: Monochorionic, monoamniotic, double-battledore placenta with stillbirth and postpartum cerebellar syndrome. Am. J. Obstet. Gynecol. 128:697–699, 1977.

Averback, P., and Wigglesworth, F.W.: Congenital absence of the heart: observation of human funiculopagous twinning with insertio funiculi furcata, fusion, forking, and interpositio velamentosa. Teratology 17:143–150, 1978.

Azuma, C., Kamiura, S., Nobunaga, T., Negoro, T., Saji, F., and Tanizawa, O.: Zygosity determination of multiple pregnancy by deoxyribonucleic acid fingerprints. Am. J. Obstet. Gynecol. 160:734–736, 1989.

Babson, S.G., and Phillips, D.S.: Growth and development of twins dissimilar in size at birth. N. Engl. J. Med. 289:937–940, 1973 (see also the editorial by J.B. Hardy, pp. 973–974).

Baker, V.V., and Doering, M.C.: Fetus papyraceus: an unreported congenital anomaly of the surviving infant. Am. J. Obstet. Gynecol. 143:234, 1982.

Baldwin, V.J.: Pathology of Multiple Pregnancy. Springer-Verlag, New York, 1994.

Baldwin, V.J., and Wittmann, B.K.: Pathology of intragestational intervention in twin-to-twin transfusion syndrome. Pediatr. Pathol. 10:79–93, 1990.

Banchi, M.T.: Triplet pregnancy with second trimester abortion and delivery of twins at 35 weeks' gestation. Obstet. Gynecol. 63:728–730, 1984.

Banfield, F., Dick, M., Behrendt, D.M., Rosenthal, A., Pescheria, A., and Scott, W.: Intracardial teratoma: a new and treatable cause of hydrops fetalis. Am. J. Dis. Child. 134:1174–1175, 1980.

Bankole, M.A., Oduntan, S.A., Oluwasanmi, J.O., Itayemi, S.O., and Khwaja, S.: The conjoined twins of Warri, Ibadan. Arch. Surg. 104:294–301, 1972.

Barss, V.A.: Monoamniotic twin pregnancy. In, Abstracts of the Society of Perinatal Obstetricians, Las Vegas, February 1988 [cited with the author's permission].

Barss, V.A., Benacerraf, B.R., and Frigoletto, F.D.: Ultrasonographic determination of chorion type in twin gestation. Obstet. Gynecol. 66:779–783, 1985.

Barth, P.G., and Harten, J.J. van der: Parabiotic twin syndrome with topical isocortical disruption and gastroschisis. Acta Neuropathol. (Basel) 67:345–349, 1985.

Basrur, P.K., Kosaka, S., and Kanagawa, H.: Blood cell chimerism and freemartinism in heterosexual bovine quadruplets. J. Hered. 61:15–18, 1970.

Bass, H.N., Oliver, J.B., Srinivasan, M., Petrucha, R., Ng, W., and Lee, J.O.S.: Persistently elevated AFP and AChE in amniotic fluid from a normal fetus following demise of its twin. Prenat. Diagn. 6:33–35, 1986.

Bauer, W.C., and Rosenberg, B.F.: Quantitative study of glomerular enlargement in children with tetralogy of Fallot: condition of glomerular enlargement without increase in renal mass. Am. J. Pathol. 37:695–772, 1960.

Bebbington, M.W., and Wittmann, B.K.: Fetal transfusion syndrome: antenatal factors predicting outcome. Am. J. Obstet. Gynecol. 160:913–915, 1989.

Becker, A.H., and Glass, H.: The twin-to-twin transfusion syndrome. Am. J. Dis. Child. 106:624–629, 1963.

Beischer, N.A., and Fortune, D.W.: Double monsters. Obstet. Gynecol. 32:158–170, 1968.

Bejar, R., Vigliocco, G., Gramajo, H., Solana, C., Benirschke, K., Berry, C., Coen, R., and Resnik, R.: Antenatal origin of neurologic damage in newborn infants. Part II. Multiple gestations. Am. J. Obstet. Gynecol. 162:1230–1236, 1990.

Belfort, M.A., Moise, K.J., Kirshon, B., and Saade, G.: The use of color flow Doppler ultrasonography to diagnose umbilical cord entanglement in monoamniotic twin gestation. Am. J. Obstet. Gynecol. 168:601–604, 1993.

Bell, D., Johansson, D., McLean, F.H., and Usher, R.H.: Birth asphyxia, trauma, and mortality in twins: has cesarean section improved outcome? Am. J. Obstet. Gynecol. 154:235–239, 1986.

Bender, H.G., and Brandt, G.: Morphologie und Morphometrie der Fünflings-Placenta. Arch. Gynecol. 216:61–72, 1974.

Bendon, R.W., and Siddiqi, T.: Clinical pathological conference: acute twin-to-twin in utero transfusion. Pediatr. Pathol. 9:591–598, 1989.

Benelli, A.: Gravidanza trigemina con trasformazione papiracea di un feto. Clin. Ostet. Gynecol. (Roma) 64:663–670, 1962.

Benirschke, K.: Placental membranes in twins. Obstet. Gynecol. Surv. 13:88–91, 1958.

Benirschke, K.: Nuclear sex of holoacardii amorphi. Obstet. Gynecol. 14:72–78, 1959.

Benirschke, K.: Twin placenta in perinatal mortality. N.Y. State J. Med. 61:1499–1508, 1961.

Benirschke, K.: Discordance for genetic defects in monozygous twins: a pathogenetic concept. Acta Facult. Med. Zagreb. Suppl. 1 18:15–24, 1970a.

Benirschke, K.: Spontaneous chimerism in mammals: a critical review. Curr. Top. Pathol. 51:1–61, 1970b.

Benirschke, K.: Chimerism, mosaicism and hybrids. In: Human Genetics, Proceedings Fourth International

Congress Human Genetics, Paris, pp. 212–231, Excerpta Medica, Amsterdam, 1971.

Benirschke, K.: The contribution of placental anastomoses to prenatal twin damage. Hum. Pathol. 23:1319–1320, 1992.

Benirschke, K.: Intrauterine death of a twin: mechanisms, implications for surviving twin, and placental pathology. Semin. Diagn. Pathol. 10:222–231, 1993.

Benirschke, K., and Driscoll, S.G.: The Pathology of the Human Placenta. Springer-Verlag, New York, 1967.

Benirschke, K., and Harper, V.D.R.: The acardiac anomaly. Teratology 15:311–316, 1977.

Benirschke, K., and Kim, C.K.: Multiple pregnancy. N. Engl. J. Med. 288:1276–1284, 1329–1336, 1973.

Benirschke, K., and Layton, W.: An early twin blastocyst of the golden lion marmoset, Leontocebus rosalia L. Folia Primatol. 10:131–138, 1969.

Benirschke, K., Anderson, J.M., and Brownhill, L.E.: Marrow chimerism in marmosets. Science 138:513–515, 1962.

Berbos, J.N., King, B.F., and Janusz, A.: Quintuple pregnancy: report of a case. J.A.M.A. 188:813–816, 1964.

Berg, J.M., and Kirman, B.H.: The mentally defective twin. B.M.J. 1:1911–1917, 1960.

Berg, K.A., Astemborski, J.A., Boughman, J.A., and Ferencz, C.: Congenital cardiovascular malformations in twins and triplets from a population-based study. Am. J. Dis. Child. 143:1461–1463, 1989.

Berghe, H.v.d., and Verresen, H.: Triploid-diploid mosaicism in the lymphocytes of a liveborn child with multiple malformations. Humangenetik 11:18–21, 1970.

Bergman, P., Lundin, P., and Malmstrom, T.: Twin pregnancy with early blighted fetus. Obstet. Gynecol. 18:348–351, 1961.

Berkowitz, R.L., Lynch, L., Chitkara, U., Wilkins, I.A., Mehalek, K.E., and Alvarez, E.: Selective reduction of multifetal pregnancies in the first trimester. N. Engl. J. Med. 318:1043–1047, 1988.

Berkowitz, R.L., Lynch, L., Lapinski, R., and Bergh, P.: First-trimester transabdominal multifetal pregnancy reduction: a report of two hundred completed cases. Am. J. Obstet. Gynecol. 169:17–21, 1993.

Berry, S.A., Johnson, D.E., and Thompson, T.R.: Agenesis of the penis, scrotal raphe, and anus in one of monoamniotic twins. Teratology 29:173–176, 1984.

Bertillon, M.: Des combinaisons de sexe dans les grossesses gémellaires (doubles ou triples), de leur cause et de leur caractère ethnique. Bull. Soc. Anthropol. 9:267–290, 1874.

Bhargava, I., Chakravarty, A., and Raja, P.T.K.: An anatomical study of the fetal blood vessels on the chorial surface of the human placenta. III. Multiple pregnancies. Acta Anat. (Basel) 80:465–479, 1971.

Bhatnagar, K.P., Sharma, S.C., and Bisker, J.: The holoacardius: a correlative computerized tomographic, radiologic, and ultrasonographic investigation of a new case with review of literature. Acta Genet. Med. Gemellol. 35: 77–89, 1986.

Bhettay, E., Nelson, M.M., and Beighton, P.: Epidemic of conjoined twins in Southern Africa? Lancet 2:741–743, 1975.

Bieber, F.R., Nance, W.E., Morton, C.C., Brown, J.A., Redwine, F.O., Jordan, R.L., and Mohanakumar, T.: Genetic studies of an acardiac monster: evidence of polar body twinning in man. Science 213:775–777, 1981.

Bleisch, V.R.: Diagnosis of monochorionic twin placentation. Am. J. Clin. Pathol. 42:277–284, 1964.

Bleisch, V.R.: Placental circulation of human twins. Am. J. Obstet. Gynecol. 91:862–869, 1965.

Bleker, O.P., Breur, W., and Huidekoper, B.L.: A study of birth weight, placental weight and mortality of twins as compared to singletons. Br. J. Obstet. Gynaecol. 86:111–118, 1979.

Blickstein, I.: The twin-twin transfusion syndrome: review. Obstet. Gynecol. 76:714–722, 1990.

Boklage, C.E.: On the timing of monozygotic twinning events. In, Twin Research 3. Part A: Twin Biology and Multiple Pregnancy. L. Gedda, P. Parisi, and W.E. Nance, eds., pp. 155–165. Liss, New York, 1981.

Boklage, G.E.: Race, zygosity, and mortality among twins: interaction of myth and method. Acta Genet. Med. Gemellol. 36:275–288, 1987a.

Boklage, C.E.: Twinning, nonrighthandedness, and fusion malformations: evidence for heritable causal elements held in common. Am. J. Med. Genet. 28:67–84, 1987b.

Bolaji, I.I., Mortimer, G., Meehan, F.P., England, S., and Greally, M.: Acardius in a triplet pregnancy: cytogenetic and morphological profile. Acta Genet. Med. Gemellol. 41:27–32, 1992 (Errata 41:365, 1992).

Bolens, M., Lacourt, G., and Mottu, T.H.E.: Un nouveau cas de transfusion interfoetale: surcharge ventriculaire droite et hypocoagulabilité chez la jumelle pléthorique; atteinte neurologique chez la jumelle anémique. Schweiz. Med. Wochenschr. 98:412–417, 1968.

Boulgakow, B.: Arrest of development of an embryo: a case of acephalus holoacardius showing arrest of development of all tissues in embryonic period. J. Anat. Physiol. 61:68–93, 1926.

Boulot, P., Hedon, B., Deschamps, F., Laffargue, F., Viala, J.L., Humeau, C., and Arnal, F.: Anencephaly-like malformation in surviving twin after embryonic reduction. Lancet 335:1155–1156, 1990.

Boulot, P., Hedon, B., Pelliccia, G., Lefort, G., Deschamps, F., Arnal, F., Humeau, C., Laffargue, F., and Viala, J.L.: Multifetal pregnancy reduction: a consecutive series of 61 cases. Br. J. Obstet. Gynaecol. 100:63–68, 1993.

Bowman, J.M.: Alloimmunization in twin pregnancies. Am. J. Obstet. Gynecol. 153:7–13, 1985.

Boyd, J.D., and Hamilton, W.J.: The Human Placenta. Heffer, Cambridge, 1970.

Bracken, M.J.: Oral contraception and twinning: an epidemiologic study. Am. J. Obstet. Gynecol. 133:432–434, 1979.

Bressers, W.M.A., Eriksson, A.W., Konstense, P.J., and Parisi, P.: Increasing trend in the monozygotic twinning rate. Acta Genet. Med. Gemellol. 36:397–408, 1987.

Brismar, B.: Dermatoglyphics of twins: a study based on a new systematics. Acta Genet. Med. Gemellol. 17:375–380, 1968.

Bromley, B., Frigoletto, F.D., Estroff, J.A., and Benacerraf, B.R.: The natural history of oligohydramnios/polyhydramnios sequence in monochorionic diamniotic twins. Ultrasound Obstet. Gynecol. 2:317–320, 1992.

Brown, C.E.L., and Weinreb, J.C.: Magnetic resonance imaging appearance of growth retardation in a twin pregnancy. Obstet. Gynecol. 71:987–988, 1988.

Brown, D.C., and Nelson, R.F.: Uterus didelphys and double vagina with delivery of a normal infant from each uterus. Can. Med. Assoc. J. 96:675–677, 1967.

Brown, D.L., Benson, C.B., Driscoll, S.G., and Doubilet, P.M.: Twin-twin transfusion syndrome: sonographic findings. Radiology 170:61–63, 1989.

Bruner, J.P., and Rosemond, R.L.: Twin-to-twin transfusion syndrome: a subset of the twin oligohydramnios-polyhydramnios sequence. Am. J. Obstet. Gynecol. 169:925–930, 1993.

Bryan, E., and Slavin, B.: Serum IgG levels in feto-fetal transfusion syndrome. Arch. Dis. Child. 49:908–910, 1974.

Buckler, J.M.H., and Robinson, A.: Matched development of a pair of monozygous twins of grossly different size at birth. Arch. Dis. Child. 49:472–76, 1974.

Buehler, B.A., McManus, B.M., and Mrocezek, E.C.: Acardiac monsters: clinical karyotypic and pathologic features [abstract]. Teratology 33:44C, 1986.

Bulla, M., von Lilien, T., Goecke, H., Roth, B., Ortmann, M., and Heising, J.: Renal and cerebral necrosis in survivor after in utero death of co-twin. Arch. Gynecol. 240:119–124, 1987.

Bulmer, M.G.: The familial incidence of twinning. Ann. Hum. Genet. 24:1–3, 1960.

Bulmer, M.G.: The Biology of Twinning in Man. Oxford University Press, London, 1970.

Burn, J., Povey, S., Boyd, Y., Munro, E.A., West, L., Harper, K., and Thomas, D.: Duchenne muscular dystrophy in one of monozygotic twin girls. J. Med. Genet. 23:494–500, 1986.

Buxbaum, H., and Wachsman, D.V.: A case of acephalus holoacardius. Am. J. Obstet. Gynecol. 36:1055–1057, 1938.

Buzzard, I.M., Uchida, I.A., Norton, J.A., and Christian, J.C.: Birth weight and placental proximity in like-sexed twins. Am. J. Hum. Genet. 35:318–323, 1983.

Cameron, A.H.: The Birmingham twin survey. Proc. R. Soc. Med. 61:229–234, 1968.

Camiel, M.R.: Fetus papyraceus with intrauterine sibling death. J.A.M.A. 202:247, 1967.

Campbell, D.M., MacGillivray, I., and Thompson, B.: Twin zygosity and pre-eclampsia. Lancet 2:97, 1977.

Campbell, S., and Dewhurst, C.J.: Quintuplet pregnancy diagnosed and assessed by ultrasonic compound scanning. Lancet 1:101–103, 1970.

Cannings, C.: A discussion of Weinberg's rule on the zygosity of twins. Ann. Hum. Genet. 32:403–405, 1969.

Cardwell, M.S., Caple, P., and Baker, L.C.: Triplet pregnancy on three separate days. Obstet. Gynecol. 71:448–449, 1988.

Carlson, N.J., and Towers, C.V.: Multiple gestation complicated by the death of one fetus. Obstet. Gynecol. 73:685–689, 1989.

Carr, S.R., Aronson, M.P., and Coustan, D.R.: Survival rates of monoamniotic twins do not decrease after 30 weeks' gestation. Am. J. Obstet. Gynecol. 163:719–722, 1990.

Carter, C.O.: Congenital defects. Proc. R. Soc. Med. 61:991–995, 1968.

Castilla, E.E., Lopez-Camelo, J.S., Orioli, I.M., Sanchez, O., and Paz, J.E.: The epidemiology of conjoined twins in Latin America. Acta Genet. Med. Gemellol. 37:111–118, 1988.

Cederlöf, R., Friberg, L., Jonsson, E., and Kaij, L.: Studies on similarity diagnosis in twins with the aid of mailed questionnaires. Acta Genet. (Basel) 11:338–362, 1961.

Centerwall, W.R., and Benirschke, K.: An animal model for the XXY Klinefelter syndrome in man: tortoiseshell and calico male cats. Am. J. Vet. Res. 36:1275–1280, 1975.

Chapman, K.: Monoamniotic twins. Lancet 2:1456, 1974.

Chaurasia, B.D.: Abnormal umbilical vessels and systemic circulatory reversal in thoracopagus twins. Acta Genet. Med. Gemellol. 24:261–268, 1975.

Cherouny, P.H., Hoskins, I.A., Johnson, T.R.B., and Niebyl, J.R.: Multiple pregnancy with late death of one fetus. Obstet. Gynecol. 74:318–320, 1989

Chervenak, F.A., Isaacson, G., Touloukian, R., Tortora, M., Berkowitz, R.L., and Hobbins, J.C.: Diagnosis and management of fetal teratomas. Obstet. Gynecol. 66:666–671, 1985.

Chescheir, N.C., and Seeds, J.W.: Polyhydramnios and oligohydramnios in twin gestations. Am. J. Obstet. Gynecol. 71:882–884, 1988a.

Chescheir, N.C., and Seeds, J.W.: Spontaneous resolution of hypofibrinogenemia associated with death of a twin in utero: a case report. Am. J. Obstet. Gynecol. 159:1183–1184, 1988b.

Chitkara, U., Berkowitz, R.L., Wilkins, I.A., Lynch, L., Mehalek, K.E., and Alvarez, M.: Selective second-trimester termination of the anomalous fetus in twin pregnancies. Obstet. Gynecol. 73:690–694, 1989.

Chupin, D., Huy, N.N., Azan, M., Mauléon, P., and Ortavant, R.: Induction hormonale de naissance gémellaires: principales conséquences sur les performances zootechniques. Ann. Zootech. 25:79–94, 1976.

Clark, M., and Linell, E.A.: Case report: prenatal occlusion of the internal carotid artery. J. Neurol. Neurosurg. Psychiatry 17:295–297, 1954.

Claudius, M.: Die Entwicklung der herzlosen Mißgeburten. Schwers, Kiel, 1859.

Coen, R.W., and Sutherland, J.M.: Placental vascular communications between twin fetuses. Am. J. Dis. Child. 120:332, 1970.

Cohen, M., Kohl, S.G., and Rosenthal, A.H.: Fetal interlocking complicating twin gestation. Am. J. Obstet. Gynecol. 91:407–412, 1965.

Colburn, D.W., and Pasquale, S.A.: Monoamniotic twin pregnancy. J. Reprod. Med. 27:165–168, 1982.

Cole, L.J., and Craft, W.A.: An ancephalic lamb monster in sheep. J. Hered. 36:29–32, 1945.

Colgan, T.J., and Luk, S.C.: Umbilical-cord torsion, thrombosis, and intrauterine death of a twin fetus. Arch. Pathol. Lab. Med. 106:101, 1982.

Collins, M.S., and Bleyl, J.A.: Seventy-one quadruplet pregnancies: Management and outcome. Am. J. Obstet. Gynecol. 162:1384–1392, 1990.

Collins, R.N., Lerner, A.B., and McGuire, J.S.: The relationship of skin color to zygosity in twins. J. Invest. Dermatol. 47:78–82, 1966.

Conway, C.F.: Transfusion syndrome in multiple pregnancy. Obstet. Gynecol. 23:745–751, 1964.

Corey, M.J., Miller, J.R., MacLean, R., and Chown, B.: A case of XX/XY mosaicism. Am. J. Hum. Genet. 19:378–387, 1967.

Corey, L.A., Harris, R.E., Kang, K.W., Christian, J.C., and Nance, W.E.: Variability of total cholesterol in monochorionic and dichorionic MZ twins. Am. J. Hum. Genet. 27:28A, 1975.

Corner, G.W.: The observed embryology of human single-ovum twins and other multiple births. Am. J. Obstet. Gynecol. 70:933–951, 1955.

Corney, G., and Aherne, W.: The placental transfusion syndrome in monozygous twins. Arch. Dis. Child. 40:264–270, 1965.

Corney, G., Robson, E.B., and Strong, S.J.: Twin zygosity and placentation. Ann. Hum. Genet. 32:89–96, 1968.

Corrin, B.: Glomerular size in polycythemia. J. Pathol. Bacteriol. 82:534–535, 1961.

Coulton, D., Hertig, A.T., and Long, W.N.: Monoamniotic twins. Am. J. Obstet. Gynecol. 54:119–123, 1947.

Cousins, L., Benirschke, K., Porreco, R., and Resnik, R.: Placentomegaly due to fetal congestive failure in a pregnancy with a sacrococcygeal teratoma. J. Reprod. Med. 25:142–144, 1980.

Cox, W.L., Forestier, F., Capella-Pavlovsky, M., and Daffos, F.: Fetal blood sampling in twin pregnancies: prenatal diagnosis and management of 19 cases. Fetal Ther. 2:101–108, 1987.

Craig, I.T.: Monoamniotic twins with double survival. Am. J. Obstet. Gynecol. 73:202–205, 1957.

Crookston, M.C., Tilley, C.A., and Crookston, J.H.: Human blood chimaera with seeming breakdown of immune tolerance. Lancet 2:1110–1112, 1970 (1:396, 1971).

Crossman, P.J., and Dickens, P.S.E.M.: Amorphus globosus in the mare. Vet. Rec. 95:22, 1974.

Crowther, C.A., Neilson, J.P., Verkuyl, D.A.A., Bannerman, C., and Ashurst, H.M.: Preterm labour in twin pregnancies: can it be prevented by hospital admission? Br. J. Obstet. Gynaecol. 96:850–853, 1989.

Cruikshank, S.H., and Granados, J.L.: Increased amniotic acetylcholinesterase activity with a fetus papyraceus and aplasia cutis congenita. Obstet. Gynecol. 71:997–999, 1988.

Curtius, F.: Nachgeburtsbefunde bei Zwillingen und Ähnlichkeitsdiagnose. Arch. Gynäkol. 140:361–366, 1930.

Dahm, K.: Über zwei Beobachtungen von Akardie und zur Frage ihrer Genese. Zentralbl. Allg. Pathol. Pathol. Anat. 93:41–50, 1955.

Dallapiccola, B., Stomeo, C., Ferranti, G., Di Lecci, A., and Purpura, M.: Discordant sex in one of three monozygotic triplets. J. Med. Genet. 22:6–11, 1985.

D'Alton, M.E., and Dudley, D.K.: The ultrasonographic prediction of chorionicity in twin gestation. Am. J. Obstet. Gynecol. 160:557–561, 1989.

Danskin, F.H., and Neilson, J.P.: Twin-to-twin transfusion syndrome: what are appropriate diagnostic criteria? Am. J. Obstet. Gynecol. 161:365–369, 1989.

Davies, J., Chazen, E., and Nance, W.E.: Symmelia in one of monozygotic twins. Teratology 4:367–378, 1971.

Daw, E.: Human placental lactogen and twin pregnancy. Lancet 2:299–300, 1977.

Dawson, W.M., and Ainslie, W.H.: Twin pregnancy in a uterus didelphys: a case report. J. Med. Soc. N.J. 55:649, 1958.

Deacon, J.S., Machin, G.A., Martin, J.M.E., Nicholson, S., Nwanko, D.C., and Wintemute, R.: Investigation of acephalus. Am. J. Med. Genet. 5:85–99, 1980.

De la Chapelle, A., Schröder, J., Rantanen, P., Thomasson, B., Niemi, M., Tilikainen, A., Sanger, R., and Robson, E.B.: Early fusion of two human embryos? Ann. Hum. Genet. 38:63–75, 1974.

De Leon, F.: Siamesische Zwillinge mit differenten Herzmißbildungen. Virchows Arch. [A] 362:51–57, 1974.

De Lia, J.E., and Cruikshank, D.P.: Fetoscopic laser occlusion of chorioangiopagus in severe twin transfusion syndrome [abstract]. Acta Genet. Med. Gemellol. 38:218, 1989

De Lia, J.E., Emery, M.G., Sheafor, S.A., and Jennison, T.A.: Twin transfusion syndrome: successful in utero treatment with digoxin. Int. J. Gynaecol. Obstet. 23:197–201, 1985a.

De Lia, J.E., Rogers, J.G., and Dixon, J.A.: Treatment of placental vasculature with a neodymium-yttrium-aluminum-garnet laser via fetoscopy. Am. J. Obstet. Gynecol. 151:1126–1127, 1985b.

De Lia, J.D., Cukierski, M.A., Lundergan, D.K., and Kochenour, N.K.: Neodymium:yttrium-aluminum-garnet laser occlusion of rhesus placental vasculature via fetoscopy. Am. J. Obstet. Gynecol. 160:485–489, 1989.

De Lia, J.E., Cruikshank, D.P., and Keye, W.R.: Fetoscopic neodymium:Yag laser occlusion of placental vessels in severe twin-twin transfusion syndrome. Obstet. Gynecol. 75:1046–1953, 1990.

De Lia, J.E., Kuhlmann, R.S., Cruikshank, D.P., and O'Bee, L.R.: Current topic: placental surgery: a new frontier. Placenta 14:477–485, 1993.

Delprado, W.J., and Baird, P.J.: Cephalothoracopagus syncephalus: a case report with previously unreported anatomical abnormalities and chromosomal analysis. Teratology 29:1–9, 1984.

De Marco, P.G.: Feto-fetal transfusions in monozygotic twins: review of the literature and report of two cases. Clin. Pediatr. 3:709–713, 1964.

Demmel, U.: Clinical aspects of congenital skin defects. Eur. J. Pediatr. 121:21–50, 1975.

Dennis, S.M., and Leipold, H.W.: Congenital cardiac defects in lambs. Am. J. Vet. Res. 29:2337–2340, 1968.

De Paepe, J.: Mortalité périnatale dans une série de grossesses gémellaires. Bull. Soc. R. Belge Gynecol. Obstet. 29:421–4433, 1959.

Derom, C., Bakker, E. Vlietninck, R., Derom, R., van den Berghe, H., Thiery, M., and Pearson, P.: Zygosity determination in newborn twins using DNA variants. J. Med. Genet. 22:279–282, 1985.

Derom, C., Vlietinck, R., Derom, R., van den Berghe, H., and Thiery, M.: Increased monozygotic twinning rate after ovulation induction. Lancet 1:1236–1238, 1987.

Derom, C., Vlietinck, R., Derom, R., van den Berghe, H., and Thiery, M.: Population-based study of sex proportion in monoamniotic twins. N. Engl. J. Med. 319:119–120, 1988.

Derom, C., Vlietninck, R. Derom, R., Thiery, M., and van den Berghe, H.: Genotyping macerated stillborn twin fetuses [abstract]. Acta Genet. Med. Gemellol. 38:148, 1989.

Dhont, M., Thiery, M., and Vandekerckhove, D.: Hormonal screening for detection of twin pregnancies. Lancet 2:861, 1976.

Diamond, J.M.: Variation in human testis size: ethnic differences. Nature 320:488–489, 1986.

Dicker, D., Peleg, D., Samuel, N., Feldberg, D., and Goldman, J.A.: Holoacardius: radiologic investigation. Early Hum. Devel. 9:59–65, 1983.

Diddle, A.W., and Burford, T.H.: Study of set of quadruplets. Anat. Rec. 61:281–293, 1935.

Dimmick, J.E., Hardwick, D.F., and Ho-Yuen, B.: A case of renal necrosis, and fibrosis in the immediate newborn period: association with the twin-to-twin transfusion syndrome. Am. J. Dis. Child. 122:345–347, 1971.

Dixon, A.F.: Human oocyte showing first polar body, and second polar body in metaphase. C. R. Assoc. Anat. 22:265–266, 1927.

Donald, J.G.: Unusual twin pregnancy. B.M.J. 2:1330, 1964.

Donnenfeld, A.E., Dunn, L.K., and Rose, N.C.: Discordant amniotic band sequence in monozygotic twins. Am. J. Med. Genet. 20:685–694, 1985.

Donnenfeld, A.E., Glazerman, L.R., Cutillo, D.M., Librizzi, R.J., and Weiner, S.: Fetal exsanguination following intrauterine angiographic assessment and selective termination of a hydrocephalic, monozygotic co-twin. Prenat. Diagn. 9:301–308, 1989.

Dorros, G.: The prenatal diagnosis of intrauterine growth retardation in one fetus of a twin gestation. Obstet. Gynecol. 48:46s–48s, 1976.

Driesch, H.: Entwicklungs-mechanische Studien. I. Der Werth der beiden ersten Furchungszellen in der Echinodermentwicklung: experimentelle Erzeugung von Theil-und Doppelbildungen. Z. Wiss. Zool. 53:160–184, 1891.

Drucker, P., Finkel, J., and Savel, L.E.: Sixty-five-day interval between the births of twins. Am. J. Obstet. Gynecol. 80:761–762, 1960.

Drut, R., Garcia, C., and Drut, R.M.: Poorly organized parasitic conjoined twins: report of four cases. Pediatr. Pathol. 12:691–700, 1992.

Dudley, D.K.L., and D'Alton, M.E.: Single fetal death in twin gestation. Semin. Perinatol. 10:65–72, 1986.

Duenhoelter, J.H.: Survival of twins after acute fetal hemorrhage from ruptured vasa previa. Obstet. Gynecol. 73:866–867, 1989.

Dunn, H.O., and Roberts, S.J.: Chromosome studies of an ovine acephalic-acardiac monster. Cornell Vet. 62:425–431, 1972.

Dunn, H.O., Lein, H., and Kenney, R.M.: The cytological sex of a bovine anidian (amorphous) twin monster. Cytogenetics 6:412–419, 1967.

Dunnihoo, D.R., and Harris, R.E.: The diagnosis of monoamniotic twinning by amniography. Am. J. Obstet. Gynecol. 96:894–895, 1966.

Dunsford, I., Bowley, C.C., Hutchison, A.M., Thompson, J.S., Sanger, R., and Race, R.R.: A human blood group chimera. B.M.J. 2:81, 1953.

Durkin, M.V., Kaveggia, E.G., Pendleton, E., Neuhaeser, G., and Opitz, J.M.: Analysis of etiologic factors in cerebral palsy with severe mental retardation. I. Analysis of gestational, parturitional and neonatal data. Eur. J. Pediatr. 123:67–81, 1976.

Eastman, N.J., Kohl, S.G., Maisel, J.E., and Kavaler, F.: The obstetrical background of 753 cases of cerebral palsy. Obstet. Gynecol. Surv. 17:459–500, 1962.

Eberle, A.M., Levesque, D., Vintzileos, A.M., Tsapanos, V., and Salafia, C.M.: Placental pathology in discordant twins. Am. J. Obstet. Gynecol. 169:931–935, 1993.

Edmonds, L.D., and Layde, P.M.: Conjoined twins in the United States. Teratology 25:301–308, 1982.

Edwards, J.: Season and rate of conception. Nature 142:357, 1938.

Einerh, Y., and Jacobsson, K.: Screening for early detection of twin pregnancies. Lancet 1:745, 1976.

Ellings, J.M., Newman, R.B., Hulsey, T.C., Bivins, H.A., and Keenan, A.: Reduction in very low birth weight deliveries and perinatal mortality in a specialized, multidisciplinary twin clinic. Obstet. Gynecol. 81:387–391, 1993.

Elliott, J.P.: Amniocentesis for twin-twin transfusion syndrome. Contemp. Ob/Gyn August: 30–42, 1992.

Elliott, J.P., and Radin, T.G.: Quadruplet pregnancy: contemporary management and outcome. Obstet. Gynecol. 80:421–424, 1992.

Ellis, P.A.: Renal enlargement in chronic cor pulmonale. J. Clin. Pathol. 14:552–556, 1961.

El-Sherbini, R.: Retention of an 8-month foetus in utero for two and a half years. J. Obstet. Gynaecol. Br. Commonw. 70:514–516, 1963.

Elston, R.C., and Boklage, C.E.: An examination of fundamental assumptions of the twin method. In, Twin Research: Psychology and Methodology, W.E. Nance, ed., pp. 189–199. Liss, New York, 1978.

Elwood, J.M.: Decline in dizygotic twinning. N. Engl. J. Med. 289:486, 1973.

Elwood, J.M.: Maternal and environmental factors affecting twin births in Canadian cities. Br. J. Obstet. Gynaecol. 85:351–358, 1978.

Elwood, J.M.: The end of the drop in twinning rates? Lancet 1:470, 1983.

Enbom, J.A.: Twin pregnancy with intrauterine death of one twin. Am. J. Obstet. Gynecol. 152:424–429, 1985.

Englert, Y., Imbert, M.C., van Rosendael, E., Belaisch, J., Segal, L., Feichtinger, W., Wilkin, P., Frydman, R., and Leroy, F.: Morphological anomalies in the placentae of IVF pregnancies: preliminary report of a multicentric study. Hum. Reprod. 2:155–157, 1987.

Erdmann, J., Nöthen, M.M., Stratmann, M., Fimmers, R., Franzek, E., and Propping, P.: The use of microsatellites in zygosity diagnosis of twins. Acta Genet. Med. Gemellol. 42:45–51, 1993.

Eriksson, A.: Variations in the human twinning rate. Acta Genet. (Basel) 12:242–250, 1962.

Eriksson, A.W.: Pituitary gonadotrophin and dizygotic twinning. Lancet 2:1298–1299, 1964.

Esposito, A.: Singolare caso di gravidanza trigemina con due feti mummeficati. Clin. Obstet. Gynecol. (Roma) 75:537–544, 1963.

Evans, M.I., Fletcher, J.C., Zador, I.E., Newton, B.W., Quigg, M.H., and Struyk, C.D.: Selective first-trimester termination in octuplet and quadruplet pregnancies: clinical and ethical issues. Obstet. Gynecol. 71:289–296, 1988.

Exelby, P.R.: Sacrococcygeal teratomas in children. CA 22:202–208, 1972.

Falkner, F.: The smaller of twins and hypoglycaemia. Lancet 1:869, 1965.

Farquharson, D.F., Wittmann, B.K., Hansmann, M., Yuen, B.H.Y., Baldwin, V.J., and Lindahl, S.: Management of quintuplet pregnancy by selective embryocide. Am. J. Obstet. Gynecol. 158:413–416, 1988.

Farrell, A.G.W.: Twin pregnancy: a study of 1,000 cases. S. Afr. J. Obstet. Gynaecol. 2:35–41, 1964.

Feichtinger, W., Breitenecker, G., and Fröhlich, H.: Prolongation of pregnancy and survival of twin B after loss of twin A at 21 weeks' gestation. Am. J. Obstet. Gynecol. 161:891–893, 1989.

Feige, A., Gille, J., v. Maillot, K., and Mulz, D.L.: Pränatale Diagnostik eines Steißbeinteratoms mit Hypertrophie der Plazenta. Geburtshilfe Frauenheilkd. 42:20–24, 1982.

Feingold, M., Cetrulo, C.L., Newton, E.R., Weiss, J., Shakr, C., and Shmoys, S.: Serial amniocenteses in the treatment of twin to twin transfusion complicated with acute hydramnios. Acta Genet. Med. Gemellol. 35:107–113, 1986.

Ferguson, W.F.: Perinatal mortality in multiple gestations: a review of perinatal deaths from 1609 multiple gestations. Obstet. Gynecol. 23:861–870, 1964.

Ferm, V.H.: Conjoined twinning in mammalian teratology. Arch. Environ. Health 19:353–357, 1969.

Ferm, V.H.: Cranio-dirachischisis totalis in cephalothoracopagus twins. Teratology 17:159–164, 1978.

Fernandez, M.: Beiträge zur Embryologie der Gürteltiere. I. Zur Keimblätterinversion und spezifischen Polyembryonie der Mulita (Tatusia hybrida Desm.) Morphol. Jahrb. 39:302–333, 1909.

Finberg, H.J.: The "twin peak" sign: reliable evidence of dichorionic twinning. J. Ultrasound Med. 11:571–577, 1992.

Fisher, J.E., and Siongco, A.: Case 3: complications from in utero death of a monozygous co-twin. Pediatr. Pathol. 9:765–771, 1989.

Fogel, B.J., Nitowsky, H.M., and Gruenwald, P.: Discordant abnormalities in monozygotic twins. Am. J. Obstet. Gynecol. 66:64–72, 1965.

Forbes, D.A., and Natale, A.: Unilateral tubal triplet pregnancy: report of a case. Obstet. Gynecol. 31:360–362, 1968.

Forman, R.C.: Twin pregnancy with one twin blighted. Am. J. Obstet. Gynecol. 72:1180–1181, 1956.

Forssell, O.H.: Zur Kenntnis des Amnionepithels in normalem und pathologischem Zustande. Arch. Gynäkol. 96:436–460, 1912.

Fowler, M.G., Kleinman, J.C., Kiely, J.L., and Kessel, S.S.: Am. J. Obstet. Gynecol. 165:L15–L22, 1991.

Fox, H., and Butler-Manuel, R.: A teratoma of the placenta. J. Pathol. Bacteriol. 88:137–140, 1964.

Franke, H., and Estel, C.: Untersuchungen über die Ultrastruktur und Permeabilität des Amnions unter besonderer Berücksichtigung mikrofilamentärer und mikrotubulärer Strukturen. Arch. Gynecol. 225:319–338, 1978.

Fraser, F.C.: The genetics of cleft lip and cleft palate. Am. J. Hum. Genet. 22:336–352, 1970.

Freedman, H.L., Tafeen, C.H., and Harris, H.: Conjoined thoracopagus twins: case report. Am. J. Obstet. Gynecol. 84:1904–1909, 1962.

Fries, M.H., Goldstein, R.B., Kilpatrick, S.J., Golbus, M.S., Callen, P.W., and Filly, R.A.: The role of velamentous cord insertion in the etiology of twin-twin transfusion syndrome. Obstet. Gynecol. 81:569–574, 1993.

Frutiger, P.: Zum Problem der Akardie. Acta Anat. (Basel) 74:505–531, 1969.

Fujii, S., Ban, C., Okamura, H., and Nishimura, T.: Unilateral tubal quadruplet pregnancy. Am. J. Obstet. Gynecol. 141:840–842, 1981.

Fujikura, T., and Froehlich, L.A.: Twin placentation and zygosity. Obstet. Gynecol. 37:34–43, 1971.

Fujikura, T., and Froehlich, L.A.: Mental and motor development in monozygotic co-twins with dissimilar birth weights. Pediatrics 53:884–889, 1974.

Fujikura, T., and Wellings, S.R.: A teratoma-like mass on the placenta of a malformed infant. Am. J. Obstet. Gynecol. 89:824–825, 1964.

Fusi, L., McParland, P., Fisk, N., Nicolini, U., and Wigglesworth, J.: Acute twin-twin transfusion: a possible mechanism for brain-damaged survivors after intrauterine death of a monochorionic twin. Obstet. Gynecol. 78:517–520, 1991.

Gabos, P.: Triplet pregnancy and cervical incompetence: a case report. Fertil. Steril. 23:940–942, 1972.

Galton, F.: The history of twins as a criterion of the relative powers of nature, and nurture. J. Br. Anthropol. Inst. 5:391–406, 1875.

Gamberdella, F.R., and Marrs, R.P.: Heterotopic pregnancy associated with assisted reproductive technology. Am. J. Obstet. Gynecol. 160:1520–1524, 1989.

Gärtner, K., and Baunack, E.: Is the similarity of monozygotic twins due to genetic factors alone? Nature 292:646–647, 1981.

Gavriil, P., Jauniaux, E., and Leroy, F.: Pathologic examination of placentas from singleton and twin pregnancies obtained after in vitro fertilization and embryo transfer. Pediatr. Pathol. 13:453–462, 1993.

Gengozian, N.: Male and female cell populations in the chimeric marmoset. In, Medical Primatology, pp. 926–938. Karger, New York, 1971.

Gengozian, N., Brewen, J.G., Preston, R.J., and Batson, J.S.: Presumptive evidence for the absence of functional germ cell chimerism in the marmoset. J. Med. Primatol. 9:9–27, 1980.

Gennser, G., Grennert, L., Kullander, S., Persson, P.H., and Wingerup, L.: Human placental lactogen in screening for multiple pregnancies. Lancet 1:274, 1975.

Gergely, R.Z., Eden, R., Schifrin, B.S., and Wade, M.E.: Antenatal diagnosis of congenital sacral teratoma. J. Reprod. Med. 24:229–231, 1980.

Gewolb, I.H., Freedman, R.M., Kleinman, C.S., and Hobbins, J.C.: Prenatal diagnosis of a human pseudoacardiac anomaly. Obstet. Gynecol. 61:657–662, 1983.

Gibbs, C.E., Boldt, J.W., Daly, J.W., and Morgan, H.C.: A quintuplet gestation. Obstet. Gynecol. 16:464–468, 1960.

Gilbert, E.F., Suzuki, H., Kimmel, D.L., Klingberg, W.G., and Lancaster, J.R.: A case of thoracopagus: conjoined twins. Teratology 6:197–200, 1972.

Gilbert, W.M., Davis, S.E., Kaplan, C., Pretorius, D., Merritt, T.A., and Benirschke, K.: Morbidity associated with prenatal disruption of the dividing membrane in twin gestations. Obstet. Gynecol. 78:623–630, 1991.

Giles, W., Trudinger, B., Cook, C., and Connelly, A.: Placental microvascular changes in twin pregnancies with abnormal umbilical artery waveforms. Obstet. Gynecol. 81:556–559, 1993.

Gillim, D.L., and Hendricks, C.H.: Holoacardius: review of the literature and case report. Obstet. Gynecol. 2:647–653, 1953.

Ginsberg, N.A., Applebaum, M., Rabin, S.A., Caffarelli, M.A., Kuuspalu, M., Daskal, J.L., Verlinsky, Y., Strom, C.M., and Barton, J.J.: Term birth after midtrimester hysterotomy and selective delivery of an acardiac twin. Am. J. Obstet. Gynecol. 167:33–37, 1992.

Gittes, R.F.: Carcinoma of the prostate. N. Engl. J. Med. 324:236–245, 1991.

Gonen, R., Heyman, E., Asztalos, E., and Milligan, J.E.: The outcome of triplet gestations complicated by fetal death. Obstet. Gynecol. 75:175–178, 1990a.

Gonen, R., Heyman, E., Asztalos, E., Ohlsson, A., Pitson, L.C., Shennan, A.T., and Milligan, J.E.: The outcome of triplet, quadruplet, and quintuplet pregnancies managed in a perinatal unit: obstetric, neonatal, and follow-up data. Am. J. Obstet. Gynecol. 162:454–459, 1990b.

Gonen, Y., Blankier, J., and Casper, R.F.: Transvaginal ultrasound in selective embryo reduction for multiple pregnancy. Obstet. Gynecol. 75:720–721, 1990c.

Gonsoulin, W., Copeland, K.L., Carpenter, R.J., Hughes, M.R., and Elder, F.B.: Fetal blood sampling demonstrating chimerism in monozygotic twins discordant for sex and tissue karyotype (46,XY and 45,X). Prenat. Diagn. 10:25–28, 1990a.

Gonsoulin, W., Moise, K.J., Kirshon, B., Cotton, D.B., Wheeler, J.M., and Carpenter, R.J.: Outcome of twin-twin transfusion diagnosed before 28 weeks of gestation. Obstet. Gynecol. 75:214–216, 1990b.

Goodno, J.A., and Gentry, W.: Coexistent interstitial and intra-uterine pregnancy: a case report. J.A.M.A. 179:295–296, 1962.

Goplerud, C.P.: Monoamniotic twins with double survival: report of a case. Obstet. Gynecol. 23:289–290, 1964.

Gould, S.J.: Living with connections: are Siamese twins one person or two? Natural Hist. 91:18–22, 1982.

Grafe, M.R.: Antenatal cerebral necrosis in monochorionic twins. Pediatr. Pathol. 13:15–19, 1993.

Green, J.J., and Hobbins, J.C.: Abdominal ultrasound examination of the first-trimester fetus. Am. J. Obstet. Gynecol. 159:165–175, 1988.

Green, Q.L., Jackson, J., and Miller, A.: Monoamniotic twins: report of a case with surviving normal infants. Am. J. Obstet. Gynecol. 79:1082–1084, 1960.

Greig, P.C., Veille, J.-C., Morgan, T., and Henderson, L.: The effect of presentation and mode of delivery on neonatal outcome in the second twin. Am. J. Obstet. Gynecol. 167:901–906, 1992.

Grennert, L., Persson, P.-H., Gennser, G., and Kullander, S.: Ultrasound and human-placental-lactogen screening for early detection of twin pregnancies. Lancet 1:4–6, 1976a.

Grennert, L., Persson, P.-H., Gennser, G., Kullander, S., and Thorell, J.: Hormonal screening for twin pregnancies. Lancet 2:1257–1258, 1976b.

Grischke, E.M., Boos, R., Schmidt W., and Bastert, G.: Twin pregnancies with fetofetal transfusion syndrome. Z. Geburtshilfe Perinatol. 194:17–21, 1990.

Gruenwald, P.: Early human twins with peculiar relations to each other and the chorion. Anat. Rec. 83:267–279, 1942.

Gruenwald, P.: Environmental influences on twins apparent at birth: a preliminary study. Biol. Neonate 15:79–93, 1970.

Guttmacher, A.F.: An analysis of 521 cases of twin pregnancy. I. Differences in single ovum and double ovum twinning. Am. J. Obstet. Gynecol. 34:76–84, 1937.

Guttmacher, A.F.: The incidence of multiple births in man and some of the other unipara. Obstet. Gynecol. 2:22–35, 1953.

Hagay, Z.J., Mazor, M., and Leiberman, J.R.: Multiple pregnancy complicated by a single intrauterine fetal death. Obstet. Gynecol. 66:837–838, 1985.

Hallgrimsson, J.T.: Sacro-coccygeal teratoma with acute hydramnios. Acta Obstet. Gynecol. Scand. 60:517–518, 1981.

Halpin, T.F.: Human chorionic gonadotropin titers in twin pregnancies. Am. J. Obstet. Gynecol. 106:317–318, 1970.

Hamblen, E.C., Baker, R.D., and Derieux, G.D.: Roentgenographic diagnosis and anatomic studies of a quintuple pregnancy. J.A.M.A. 109:10–12, 1937.

Hamilton, W.J., Brown, D., and Spiers, B.G.: Another case of quadruplets. J. Obstet. Gynaecol. Br. Emp. 66:409–412, 1959.

Hamlett, G.W.: Polyembryony in the armadillo: genetic or physiological? Q. Rev. Biol. 8:348–358, 1933.

Hanna, J.H., and Hill, J.M.: Single intrauterine fetal demise in multiple gestation. Obstet. Gynecol. 63:126–130, 1984.

Hanson, J.W.: Incidence of conjoined twinning. Lancet 2:1257, 1975.

Harlap, S., Shahar, S., and Baras, M.: Overripe ova and twinning. Am. J. Hum. Genet. 37:1206–1215, 1985.

Harper, R.G., Kenigsberg, K., Sia, C.G., Horn, D., Stern, D., and Bongiovi, V.: Xiphopagus conjoined twins: a 300-year review of the obstetric, morphopathologic, neonatal, and surgical parameters. Am. J. Obstet. Gynecol. 137:617–629, 1980.

Harris, D.W.: Letter to the editor. J. Reprod. Med. 27:39, 1982.

Hartemann, J., Peters, A., Dellestable, P., Duprez, A., and Touati, E.: Les transfusions foeto-foetales lors des grossesses biovulaires existent-elles? Gynecol. Obstet. (Paris) 62:663–668, 1963.

Hashimoto, B., Caallen, P.W., Filly, R.A., and Laros, R.K.: Ultrasound evaluation of polyhydramnios and twin pregnancy. Am. J. Obstet. Gynecol. 154:1069–1072, 1986.

Hawrylyshyn, P.A., Barkin, M., Bernstein, A., and Papsin, F.R.: Twin pregnancies—a continuing perinatal challenge. Obstet. Gynecol. 59:463–466, 1982.

Hein, P.R., van Groeninhen, J.C., and Puts, J.J.G.: A case of acardiac anomaly in the cynomolgus monkey (Macaca fascicularis): a complication of monozygotic monochorial twinning. J. Med. Primatol. 14:133–142, 1985.

Hendricks, C.H.: Twinning in relation to birth weight, mortality, and congenital anomalies. Obstet. Gynecol. 27: 47–53, 1966.

Hernandez-Johnstone, B., and Benirschke, K.: Monozygotic twins discordant for urinary tract anomalies and presenting as hydramnios. Obstet. Gynecol. 47:610–615, 1976.

Herrlin, K.-M., Hauge, M., and Eriksson, S.A.: Finger print patterns in an unselected series of triplets. Hum. Hered. 20:336–355, 1970.

Hertzberg, B.S., Kurtz, A.B., Choi, H.Y., Kaczmarczyl, J.M., Warren, W., Wapner, R.J., Needleman, R.J., Baltarowich, O.H., Pasto, M.E., Rifkin, M.D., Pennell, R.G., and Goldberg, B.B.: Significance of membrane thickness in the sonographic evaluation of twin gestations. A.J.R. 148:151–153, 1987.

Herzog, A.: Korrelieren die pathologisch-anatomischen Befunde an den Geschlechtsorganen von Rinderzwicken mit den quantitativen Relationen des Gonosomenchimärismus [XX/XY] in Blutzellen? Zuchthygiene 4:156–159, 1969.

Herzog, A., and Rieck, G.W.: Chromosomenanomalie bei einem Acardius (Amorphus globosus). Zuchthygiene 4:57–60, 1969.

Hill, A.V.S., and Jeffreys, A.J.: Use of minisatellite DNA probes for determination of twin zygosity at birth. Lancet 2:1394–1395, 1985.

Ho, S.K., and Wu, P.Y.K.: Perinatal factors and neonatal morbidity in twin pregnancy. Am. J. Obstet. Gynecol. 122: 979–987, 1975.

Hobbins, J.C.: Selective reduction-a perinatal necessity? N. Engl. J. Med. 318:1062–1063, 1988.

Hoch, Z., Peretz, B.A., Brandes, J.M., and Peretz, A.: Intraamniotic hypertonic saline treatment in a case of dizygotic twin pregnancy. Int. J. Gynaecol. Obstet. 10:156–160, 1972.

Höfliger, H.: Beitrag zur Kenntnis der Akardier. Schweiz. Arch. Tierheilk. 116:629–644, 1974 [extensive review].

Hohenauer, L.: Prenatal nutrition and subsequent development. Lancet 1:644–645, 1971.

Honoré, L.H.: Twinning in postpill spontaneous abortions. Am. J. Obstet. Gynecol. 135:700, 1979.

Hoogendoorn, D.: Daling van het aantal meerlinggeboorten. Ned. Tijdschr. Geneesk. 117:805–807, 1973.

Horger, E.O., and McCarter, L.M.: Prenatal diagnosis of sacrococcygeal teratoma. Am. J. Obstet. Gynecol. 134: 228–229, 1979.

Hrubec, Z., and Robinette, C.D.: The study of human twins in medical research. N. Engl. J. Med. 310:435–441, 1984.

Hsu, J., and Gonda, M.A.: Monozygotic twin formation in mouse embryos in vitro. Science 209:605–606, 1980.

Hughes, H.E., and Miskin, M.: Congenital microcephaly due to vascular disruption: in utero documentation. Pediatrics 78:85–87, 1986.

Hurst, R.W., and Abbitt, P.L.: Fetal intracranial hemorrhage and periventricular leukomalacia: complications of twin-twin transfusion syndrome. Am. J. Neurol. Res. 10:S62–S63, 1989.

Hyrtl, J.: Die Blutgefäße der Menschlichen Nachgeburt in normalen und abnormen Verhältnissen. Braumüller, Vienna, 1870.

Imaizumi, Y.: Concordance and discordance of congenital hydrocephalus in 107 twin pairs in Japan. Teratology 40: 1010–103, 1989a.

Imaizumi, Y.: Stillbirth rate and weight at birth of quintuplets in Japan. Acta Genet. Med. Gemellol. 38:65–69, 1989b.

Imaizumi, Y., and Inouye, E.: Analysis of multiple birth rates in Japan. III. Secular trend, maternal age effect and geographical variation in triplet rates. Jpn. J. Hum. Genet. 25:73–81, 1980.

Ingalls, T.H.: Conjoined twins in zebra fish. Arch. Environ. Health 19:344–352, 1969.

Inouye, E.: Frequency of multiple birth in three cities of Japan. Am. J. Hum. Genet. 9:317–320, 1957.

Ishiguro, T.: Alpha-fetoprotein in twin pregnancy. Lancet 2:1214, 1973.

Islam, A.B.M., Hill, W.G., and Land, R.B.: Ovulation rates in lines of mice selected for testis weight. Genet. Res. 27:23–32, 1976.

Israelstam, D.M.: Mono-amniotic twin pregnancy: a case report. S. Afr. Med. J. (Suppl. S. Afr. J. Obstet. Gynaecol.) 47:2026–2027, 1973.

Itoh, H., Kambe, S., Maeba, Y., and Hirai, T.: A case of duplicitas lateralis superior. Congen. Anom. (Japan) 14:1–11, 1974.

Itskovitz, J., Boldes, R., Thaler, I., Bronstein, M., Erlik, Y., and Brandes, J.M.: Transvaginal ultrasonography-guided aspiration of gestational sacs for selective abortion in multiple pregnancy. Am. J. Obstet. Gynecol. 160:215–217, 1989.

Itzkowic, D.: A survey of 59 triplet pregnancies. Br. J. Obstet. Gynaecol. 86:23–28, 1979.

Jackson, J., and Benirschke, K.: The recognition and significance of the vanishing twin. J. Am. Board Fam. Pract. 2:58–63, 1989.

James, W.H.: Excess of like sexed pairs of dizygotic twins. Nature 232:277–278, 1971.

James, W.H.: Decline in dizygotic twinning (cont.) N. Engl. J. Med. 289:1204–1205, 1973.

James, W.H.: The declines in dizygotic twinning rates and in birth rates. Ann. Hum. Biol. 2:81–84, 1975.

James, W.H.: Twinning and anencephaly. Ann. Hum. Biol. 3:401–409, 1976.

James, W.H.: A note on the epidemiology of acardiac monsters. Teratology 16:211–216, 1977a.

James, W.H.: The sex ratio of monoamniotic twin pairs. Ann. Hum. Biol. 4:143–153, 1977b.

James, W.H.: Sex ratio and placentation of twins. Ann. Hum. Biol. 7:273–276, 1980.

James, W.H.: Twinning rates. Lancet 1:934–935, 1983.

James, W.H.: Zygosity and Weinberg's rule. J. Reprod. Med. 13:197–199, 1984.

James, W.H., Bracken, M.B., and Honore, L.H.: Letters to the editor on: twinning rates and the "pill." Am. J. Obstet. Gynecol. 135:699–701, 1979.

Jarmulowicz, M.: Embryo biopsy. Lancet 1:547, 1989.

Jarvik, L.F., Falek, A., Schmidt, R., and Platt, M.: The mixed leukocyte reaction as a possible test of zygosity in twins. Hum. Hered. 19:668–673, 1969.

Jauniaux, E., Elkazen, N., Leroy, F., Wilkin, P., Rodesch, F., and Hustin, J.: Clinical and morphologic aspects of the vanishing twin phenomenon. Obstet. Gynecol. 72:577–581, 1988.

Javert, C.T.: Spontaneous and Habitual Abortion. Blakiston, New York, 1957.

Jeanty, P., Rodesch, F., Verhoogen, C., and Struyven, J.: The vanishing twin. Ultrasonics 2:25–31, 1981.

Jeanty, P., Shah, D., and Roussis, P.: Single-needle insertion in twin amniocentesis. J. Ultrasound Med. 9:511–517, 1990.

Jenkins, M.E., Eisen, J., and Seguin, F.: Congenital asymmetry and diploid-triploid mosaicism. Am. J. Dis. Child. 122:80–84, 1971.

Johnson, S., Barss, V., and Driscoll, S.: Incidence and impact of single intrauterine death in multiple gestation [abstract]. Lab. Invest. 54:29A, 1986.

Jones, K.L.: Smith's Recognizable Patterns of Human Malformation. 4th Ed. pp. 600–601. Saunders, Philadelphia, 1988.

Jones, J.M., Sbarra, A.J., Dilillo, L., Cetrulo, C.L., and D'Alton, M.E.: Indomethacin in severe twin-to-twin transfusion syndrome. Am. J. Perinatol. 10:24–26, 1993.

Jones, W.S.: Obstetric significance of female genital anomalies. Obstet. Gynecol. 10:113–127, 1957.

Joseph, T.J., and Vogt, P.J.: Placental teratomas. Obstet. Gynecol. 41:574–578, 1973.

Jou, H.-J., Ng, K.-Y., Teng, R.-J., and Hsieh, F.-J.: Doppler sonographic detection of reverse twin-twin transfusion after intrauterine death of the donor. J. Ultrasound Med. 5:307–309, 1993.

Jovanovic, L., Landesman, R., and Saxena, B.B.: Screening for twin pregnancy. Science 198:738, 1977.

Jung, J.H., Graham, J.M., Schultz, N., and Smith, D.W.: Congenital hydranencephaly/porencephaly due to vascular disruption in monozygotic twins. Pediatrics 73:467–469, 1984.

Kadowaki, J.-I., Thompson, R.I., Zuelzer, W.W., Woolley, P.V., Brough, A.J., and Gruber, D.: XX/XY lymphoid chimaerism in congenital immunological deficiency syndrome with thymic alymphoplasia. Lancet 2:1152–1156, 1965.

Kaelber, C.T., and Pugh, T.F.: Influence of intrauterine relations on the intelligence of twins. N. Engl. J. Med. 280:1030–1034, 1969; 281:332, 1969.

Kalfayan, B., and Gundersen, J.H.: Ovarian twin pregnancy. Obstet. Gynecol. 55:25S–27S, 1980.

Källén, B.: Congenital malformations in twins: a population study. Acta Genet. Med. Gemellol. 35:167–178, 1986.

Kamin, L.J.: Transfusion syndrome and the heritability of IQ. Ann. Hum. Genet. 42:161–171, 1978.

Kanhai, H.H.H., van Rijssel, E.J.C., Meerman, R.J., and Bennebroek Gravenhorst, J.: Selective termination in quintuplet pregnancy during first trimester. Lancet 1:1447, 1986.

Kao, K.R., Masui, Y., and Elinson, R.P.: Lithium-induced respecification of pattern in Xenopus laevis embryos. Nature 322:371–373, 1986.

Kaplan, C., and Benirschke, K.: The acardiac anomaly: new case reports and current status. Acta Genet. Med. Gemellol. 28:51–59, 1979.

Kaplan, C.G., Askin, F.B., and Benirschke, K.: Cytogenetics of extragonadal tumors. Teratology 19:261–266, 1979.

Kaplan, C., Perlmutter, S., and Molinoff, S.: Epignathus with placental hydrops. Arch. Pathol. Lab. Med. 104:374–375, 1980.

Kappelman, M.D.: Acardius amorphus. Am. J. Obstet. Gynecol. 47:412–416, 1944.

Kapur, R.P., Mahony, B.S., Nyberg, D.A., Resta, R.G., and Shephard, T.H.: Sirenomelia associated with a "vanishing twin." Teratology 43:103–108, 1991.

Kaufman, M.H., and O'Shea, K.S.: Induction of monozygotic twinning in the mouse. Nature 276:707–708, 1978.

Kawamura, A.: Siamese twins in the Sei whale Balaenoptera borealis Lesson. Nature 221:490–491, 1969.

Kawamura, A., and Kashita, K.: A rare double monster of dolphin, Stenella caeruleoalba. Sci. Rep. Whales Res. Inst. No.23:139–140, 1971.

Keeler, C.E.: On the amount of external mirror imagery in double monsters and identical twins. Proc. Natl. Acad. Sci. U.S.A. 15:839–842, 1929.

Keith, L.: Zygosity and Weinberg's rule. J. Reprod. Med. 13:195–197, 1974.

Keith, L., Ellis, R., Berger, G.S., Depp, R., Filstead, W., Hatcher, R., and Keith, D.M.: The Northwestern University multihospital twin study. I. A description of 588 twin pregnancies and associated pregnancy loss, 1971 to 1975. Am. J. Obstet. Gynecol. 138:781–789, 1980.

Kempthorne, O., and Osborne, R.H.: The interpretation of twin data. Am. J. Hum. Genet. 13:320–339, 1961.

Kennedy, J.F., and Donahue, R.P.: Binucleate human oocytes from large follicles. Lancet 1:754–755, 1969.

Kennedy, N.: Twin pregnancy in a double uterus. J.A.M.A. 169:2064, 1959.

Kenney, A., Hall, C.A., and McGrath, J.: H.P.L. and twins. Lancet 1:253–254, 1976.

Kerenyi, T.D., and Chitkara, U.: Selective birth in twin pregnancy with discordance for Down's syndrome. N. Engl. J. Med. 304:1525–1527, 1981.

Khudr, G., and Benirschke, K.: Discordant monozygous twins associated with amnion rupture: a case report. Obstet. Gynecol. 39:713–716, 1972.

Khunda, S.: Locked twins. Obstet. Gynecol. 39:453–459, 1972.

Kiely, J.L., Kleinman, J.C., and Kiely, M.: Triplets and higher-order multiple births: time trends and infant mortality. Am. J. Dis. Child. 146:862–868, 1992.

Kim, C.K., Barr, R.J., and Benirschke, K.: Cytogenetic studies of conjoined twins: a case report. Obstet. Gynecol. 38:877–881, 1971.

Kindred, J.E.: Twin pregnancies with one twin blighted. Am. J. Obstet. Gynecol. 48:642–682, 1944.

Kirkland, J.A.: An acardiac, acephalic monster in a triplet pregnancy. Aust. N.Z. J. Obstet. Gynaecol. 22:168–171, 1982.

Kirshon, B.: Fetal urine output in hydramnios. Obstet. Gynecol. 73:240–242, 1989.

Klebe, J.G., and Ingomar, C.J.: The fetoplacental circulation during parturition illustrated by the interfetal transfusion syndrome. Pediatrics 49:112–115, 1972.

Klingberg, W.G., Jones, B., Allen, W.M., and Dempsey, E.: Placental parabiotic circulation of single ovum human twins. Am. J. Dis. Child. 90:519–520, 1955.

Kloosterman, G.J.: The "third circulation" in identical twins. Ned. Tijdschr. Verlosk. 63:395–412, 1963.

Knox, G., and Morley, D.: Twinning in Yoruba women. J. Obstet. Gynaecol. Br. Emp. 67:981–984, 1960.

Knudsen, L.B.: No association between griseofulvin and conjoined twinning. Lancet 2:1097, 1987.

Kobak, A.J., and Cohen, M.R.: Velamentous insertion of cord with spontaneous rupture of vasa previa in twin pregnancy. Am. J. Obstet. Gynecol. 38:1063–1066, 1939.

Kohga, S., Nambu, T., Tanaka, K., Benirschke, K., Feldman, B.H., and Kishikawa, T.: Hypertrophy of the placenta and sacrococcygeal teratoma: report of two cases. Virchows Arch. A Histol. 386:223–229, 1980.

Kohler, H.G.: An unusual case of sirenomelia. Teratology 6:295–302, 1972.

Kohler, H.G., and MacDonald, H.N.: Discordant anencephaly in a set of triplets. Obstet. Gynecol. 40:607–611, 1972.

Köhn, K.: Beobachtungen zur Ätiologie der Acardier. Zentralbl. Allg. Pathol. Pathol. Anat. 90:209–218, 1953.

Komai, T., and Fukuoka, G.: A set of dichorionic identical triplets. J. Hered. 22:233–243, 1931.

Koontz, W.L., Layman, L., Adams, A., and Lavery, J.P.: Antenatal sonographic diagnosis of conjoined twins in a triplet pregnancy. Am. J. Obstet. Gynecol. 153:230–231, 1985.

Koranyi, G., and Kovacs, J.: Über das Zwillingstransfusionssyndrom. Acta Paediatr. Acad. Sci. Hung. 16:119–125, 1975.

Kormann, E.: Chang and Eng Bunker. Schmidts Jahrb. 143: 281, 1869.

Kovacs, B., Shahbahrami, B., Platt, L.D., and Comings, D.E.: Molecular genetic prenatal determination of twin zygosity. Obstet. Gynecol. 72:954–956, 1988.

Kovacs, B.W., Kirschbaum, T.H., and Paul, R.H.: Twin gestations. I. Antenatal care and complications. Obstet. Gynecol. 74:313–317, 1989.

Kovacs, L., Geallen, J., and Falkay, G.: Amniotic chloride concentrations in twin-pregnancy after intraamniotic injection of hypertonic saline. J. Obstet. Gynaecol. Br. Commonw. 79:54–59, 1972.

Kraay, G.J., Menard, D.P., and Bedoya, M.: Monozygous cattle twins as a result of transfer of a single embryo. Can. Vet. J. 24:281–283, 1983.

Krauer, F.: Das akute Hydramnion bei eineiigen Zwillingsschwangerschaften. Gynaecologia 158:395–399, 1964.

Kresky, B.: Transplacental transfusion syndrome. Clin. Pediatr. 3:600–603, 1964.

Kreutner, A.K., Levine, J., and Thiede, H.: A double truncus arteriosus in thoracopagus twins. N. Engl. J. Med. 268: 1388–1390, 1963.

Kreyberg, L.: A teratoma-like swelling in the umbilical cord possibly of acardius nature. J. Pathol. Bacteriol. 75:109–112, 1958.

Kurosawa, K., Kuromaru, R., Imaizumi, K., Nakamura, Y., Ishikawa, F., Ueda, K., and Kuroki, Y.: Monozygotic twins with discordant sex. Acta Genet. Med. Gemellol. 41:301–310, 1992.

Laband, S.J., Cherny, W.B., and Finberg, H.J.: Heterotopic pregnancy: report of four cases. Am. J. Obstet. Gynecol. 158:437–438, 1988.

Lachman, R., McNabb, M., Furmanski, M., and Karp, L.: The acardiac monster. Eur. J. Pediatr. 134:195–200, 1980.

Lack, E.E., Glaun, R.S., Hefter, L.G., Seneca, R.P., Steigman, C., and Athari, F.: Late occurrence of malignancy following resection of a histologically mature sacrococcygeal teratoma: report of a case and literature review. Arch. Pathol. Lab. Med. 117:724–728, 1993.

Lage, J.M., Vanmarter, L.J., and Mikhail, E.: Vascular anastomoses in fused, dichorionic twin placentas resulting in twin transfusion syndrome. Placenta 10:55–59, 1989.

Laird, E.G., Thomas, R.B., and Halabi, N.E.: Double pregnancy in a bicornuate uterus: a review of the literature with a case report. Del. Med. J. 29:78–83, 1957.

Land, R.B.: The expression of female sex-limited characters in the male. Nature 204:208–209, 1973.

Land, R.B., Pelletier, J., Thimonier, J., and Mauleon, P.: A quantitative study of genetic differences in the incidence of oestrus, ovulation and plasma luteinizing hormone concentration in the sheep. J. Endocrinol. 58:305–317, 1973.

Lander, M., Oosterhof, H., and Aarnoudse, J.G.: Death of one twin followed by extremely variable flow velocity waveforms in the surviving fetus. Gynecol. Obstet. Invest. 36: 127–128, 1993.

Landy, H.J., Keith, L., and Keith, D.: The vanishing twin. Acta Genet. Med. Gemellol. 31:179–194, 1982.

Landy, H.J., Weiner, S., Corson, S.L., Batzer, F.R., and Bolognese, R.J.: The "vanishing twin": ultrasonographic assessment of fetal disappearance in the first trimester. Am. J. Obstet. Gynecol. 155:14–19, 1986.

Landy, H.J., Larsen, J.W., Schoen, M., Larsen, M.E., Kent, S.G., and Weingold, A.B.: Acardiac fetus in a triplet pregnancy. Teratology 37:1–6, 1988.

Lange, A.P., Hebjorn, S., Moth, I., Fuglsand, E., Hasch, E., Bruun Petersen, G., and Norgaard-Pedersen, B.: Twin fetus papyraceus and alpha-fetoprotein: a clinical dilemma. Lancet 2:636, 1979.

Lange, I.R., Harman, C.R., Ash, K.M., Manning, F.A., and Menticoglou, S.: Twin with hydramnios: treating premature labor at source. Am. J. Obstet. Gynecol. 160:552–557, 1989.

Langer, J.C., Harrison, M.R., Schmidt, K.G., Silverman, N.H., Anderson, R.L., Goldberg, J.D., Filly, R.A., Crombleholme, T.M., Longaker, M.T., and Golbus, M.S.: Fetal hydrops and death from sacrococcygeal teratoma: rationale for fetal surgery. Am. J. Obstet. Gynecol. 160: 1145–1150, 1989.

Laros, R.K., and Dattel, B.J.: Management of twin pregnancy: the vaginal route is still safe. Am. J. Obstet. Gynecol. 158:1330–1338, 1988.

Larroche, J.Cl., Droullé, P., Delezoide, A.L., Narcy, F., and Nessmann, C.: Brain damage in monozygous twins. Biol. Neonate 57:261–278, 1990.

Larson, S.L., Kempers, R.D., and Titus, J.L.: Monoamniotic twins with a common umbilical cord. Am. J. Obstet. Gynecol. 105:635–636, 1969a.

Larson, S.L., Wilson, R.B., and Titus, J.L.: Monoamniotic hydrocephalic twins with survival: report of a case with cytogenetic study. Obstet. Gynecol. 34:419–421, 1969b.

Lassen, M.-T.: Nachgeburtsbefunde bei eineiigen Zwillingen und Ähnlichkeitsdiagnose. Arch. Gynäkol. 147:48–64, 1931.

Lawce, H.: Case report: prenatal chromosome findings in a case of XX/XY chimerism. Karyogram 11:93–94, 1985.

Layton, W.M.: Random determination of a developmental process: reversal of normal visceral asymmetry in the mouse. J. Hered. 67:336–338, 1976.

Layzer, R.B.: Selective reduction—a perinatal necessity? N. Engl. J. Med. 318:1062–1063, 1988.

Lee, C.Y., Madrazo, B., and Roberson, J.: Management of monoamniotic twins diagnosed by ultrasound. Personal communication, Flint, MI, 1988.

Lehndorff, H.: Intrauterines Bluten von einem Zwilling in den anderen. Neue Österr. Z. Kinderheilkd. 6:163–172, 1961.

Leidig, E., Dannecker, G., Pfeiffer, K.H., Salinas, R., and Pfeiffer, J.: Intrauterine development of posthaemorrhagic hydrocephalus. Eur. J. Pediatr. 147:26–29, 1988.

Lemke, R.P., Machin, G., Muttitt, S., Bamforth, F., Rao, S., and Welch, R.: A case of aplasia cutis congenita in dizygotic twins. J. Perinatol. 13:22–27, 1993.

Leonard, M.W.E.: Large twins: report of a case. Obstet. Gynecol. 9:219–220, 1957.

Leppert, P.C., Wartel, L., and Lowman, R.: Fetus papyraceus causing dystocia: inability to detect blighted twin antenatally. Obstet. Gynecol. 54:381–384, 1979.

Levi, S.: Ultrasonic assessment of the high rate of human multiple pregnancy in the first trimester. J. Clin. Ultrasound 4:3–5, 1976.

Levinsky, H.V.: A case of conjoined twins in the Sprague-Dawley rat. Lab. Anim. Sci. 23:903–904, 1973.

Leviton, A., and Paneth, N.: White matter damage in preterm newborns—an epidemiologic perspective. Early Hum. Dev. 24:1–22, 1990.

Lewis, S.H., Ryder, C., and Benirschke, K.: Omphalogopagus twins in Chelonia mydas. Herpetol. Rev. 23:69–70, 1992.

Librach, C.L., Doran, T.A., Benzie, R.J., and Jones, J.M.: Genetic amniocentesis in seventy twin pregnancies. Am. J. Obstet. Gynecol. 148:585–591, 1984.

Librach, S., and Terrin, A.J.: Monoamniotic twin pregnancy. Am. J. Obstet. Gynecol. 74:440–443, 1957.

Liggins, G.C., and Ibbertson, H.K.: A successful quintuplet pregnancy following treatment with human pituitary gonadotrophin. Lancet 1:114–117, 1966.

Lillie, F.R.: The free martin; a study of the action of sex hormones in the foetal life of cattle. J. Exp. Zool. 23: 371–452, 1917.

Linke, R.P., and Kuni, H.: Über unterschiedliche Blutfülle bei Parabiosepartnern: ein Beitrag zur Parabiosekrankheit. Z. Ges. Exp. Med. 149:233–250, 1969.

Lipitz, S., Reichman, B., Paret, G., Modan, M., Shalev, J., Serr, D.M., Mashiach, S., and Frenkel, Y.: The improving outcome of triplet pregnancies. Am. J. Obstet. Gynecol. 161:1279–1284, 1989.

Litschgi, M., and Stucki, D.: Verlauf von Zwillingsschangerschaften nach intrauterinem Fruchttod eines Föten. Z. Geburtshilfe Perinatol. 184:227–230, 1980.

Litt, S., and Strauss, H.A.: Monoamniotic twins, one normal, the other anencephalic; multiple true knots in the cords. Am. J. Obstet. Gynecol. 30:728–730, 1935.

Littlewood, J.M.: Polycythaemia, and anaemia in newborn monozygotic twin girls. B.M.J. 1:857–859, 1963.

Liu, S., Benirschke, K., Scioscia, A.L., and Mannino, F.L.: Intrauterine death in multiple gestation. Acta Genet. Med. Gemellol. 41:5–26, 1992.

Livingston, J.E., and Poland, B.J.: A study of spontaneously aborted twins. Teratology 21:139–148, 1980.

Loendersloot, E.W.: Twin pregnancy in double uterus. Am. J. Obstet. Gynecol. 127:682, 1977.

Loeschke, H.: Die Acardie, eine durch Anoxybiose und Nährstoffmangel verursachte Hemmungsbildung. Virchows Arch. Pathol. Anat. 315:499–533, 1948.

Loughead, J.R., and Halbert, D.R.: An acardiac amorphous twin presenting soft tissue dystocia. J. South. Med. Assoc. 62:1140–1142, 1969.

Ludwig, E.: Über die Verteilung der Erbmasse unter eineiige Zwillinge. Schweiz. Med. Wochenschr. 57:1041–1042, 1927.

Lumme, R.H., and Saarikoski, S.V.: Monoamniotic twin pregnancy. Acta Genet. Med. Gemellol. 35:99–105, 1986.

Lundström, A.: Tooth morphology as a basis for distinguishing monozygotic and dizygotic twins. Am. J. Hum. Genet. 15:34–43, 1963.

Lutz, H., and Lutz-Ostertag, Y.: Sur l'orientation des embryons jumeaux obtenus par fissuration parallèle à l'axe présumé du blastoderme non incubé de l'oef de Caille (Coturnix coturnix japonica). C. R. Proc. Acad. Sci. Paris 256:3752–3754, 1963.

Lynch, L., Berkowitz, R.L., Chitkara, U., and Alvarez, M.: First-trimester transabdominal multifetal pregnancy reduction: a report of 85 cases. Obstet. Gynecol. 75: 735–738, 1990.

MacGillivray, I., Nylander, P.P.S., and Corney, G.: Human Multiple Reproduction. Saunders, London, 1975.

MacGillivray, I., Campbell, D.M., and Thompson, B., eds.: Twinning and Twins. Wiley, Chichester, 1988.

Machin, G.A.: Malformations and chromosome anomalies in perinatal death. Ph.D. thesis, University of London, 1974 (quoted from Deacon et al., 1980).

MacLennan, A.H., Green, R.C., O'Shea, R., Brookes, C., and Morris, D.: Routine hospital admission in twin pregnancy between 26 and 30 weeks' gestation. Lancet 335: 267–269, 1990.

Macones, G.A., Schemmer, G., Pritts, E., Weiblatt, V., and Wapner, R.J.: Multifetal reduction of triplets to twins improves perinatal outcome. Am. J. Obstet. Gynecol. 169: 982–986, 1993.

Mägiste, M., v. Schenck, H., Sjöberg, N.-O., Thorell, J.I., and Åberg, A.: Screening for detecting twin pregnancy. Am. J. Obstet. Gynecol. 126:697–698, 1976.

Magyar, E., Weiner, E., Shalev, E., and Ohel, G.: Pseudo-amniotic twins with cord entanglement following genetic funipuncture. Obstet. Gynecol. 78:915–918, 1991.

Mahone, P.R., Sherer, D.M., Abramowicz, J.S., and Woods, J.R.: Twin-twin transfusion syndrome: rapid development of severe hydrops of the donor following selective feticide of the hydropic recipient. Am. J. Obstet. Gynecol. 169:166–168, 1993.

Mahony, B.S., Filly, R.A., and Callen, P.W.: Amnionicity and chorionicity in twin pregnancies: prediction using ultrasound. Radiology 155:205–209, 1985.

Mahony, B.S., Petty, C.N., Nyberg, D.A., Luthy, D.A., Hickok, D.E., and Hirsch, J.H.: The "stuck twin" phenomenon: ultrasonographic findings, pregnancy outcome, and management with serial amniocenteses. Am. J. Obstet. Gynecol. 163:1513–1522, 1990.

Manivel, J.C., Dehner, L.P., and Burke, B.: Ovarian tumor-like structures, biovular follicles, and binucleated oocytes in children: their frequency and possible pathologic significance. Pediatr. Pathol. 8:283–292, 1988.

Mannino, F.L., Jones, K.L., and Benirschke, K.: Congenital skin defects and fetus papyraceus. J. Pediatr. 91:559–564, 1977.

Marcus, N.H.: Developmental aberrations associated with twinning in laboratory-reared sea urchins. Dev. Biol. 70:274–277, 1979.

Margono, F., Feinkind, L., and Minkoff, H.L.: Foot necrosis in a surviving fetus associated with twin-twin transfusion syndrome and monochorionic placenta. Obstet. Gynecol. 79:867–869, 1992.

Marin-Padilla, M., Chin, A.J., and Marin-Padilla, T.M.: Cardiovascular abnormalities in thoracopagus twins. Teratology 23:101–113, 1981.

Markavy, K.L., and Scanlon, J.W.: Hydrops fetalis in a parabiotic, acardiac twin. Am. J. Dis. Child. 132:638–639, 1978.

Marshall, J.R.: Ovulation induction. Obstet. Gynecol. 35:963–970, 1970.

Martin, N.G., Beaini, J.L.E., Olsen, M.E., Bhatnagar, A.S., and Macourt, D.: Gonadotropin levels in mothers who have had two sets of DZ twins. Acta Genet. Med. Gemellol. 33:131–139, 1984a.

Martin, N.G., Olsen, M.E., Theile, H., Beaini, J.L.E., Handelsman, D., and Bhatnagar, A.S.: Pituitary-ovarian function in mothers who have had two sets of dizygotic twins. Fertil. Steril. 41:878–880, 1984b.

Martin, N.G., Shanley, S., Butt, K., Osborne, J., and O'Brien, G.: Excessive follicular recruitment and growth in mothers of spontaneous dizygotic twins. Acta Genet. Med. Gemellol. 40:291–301, 1991.

Marx, W.: Akutes Hydramnion bei Drillingsschwangerschaft mit hochgradigem Hydrops einer Frucht. Zentralbl. Gynakol. 78:101–109, 1956.

Mashiach, S., Ben-Rafael, Z., Dor, J., and Serr, D.M.: Triplet pregnancy in uterus didelphys with delivery interval of 72 days. Obstet. Gynecol. 58:519–520, 1981.

Massip, A., Zwalmen, P., and Mulnard, J.: Atypical hatching of a cow blastocyst leading to separation of complete twin half blastocysts. Vet. Rec. 112:301, 1983.

Mauer, S.M., Dorrin, R.S., and Vernier, R.L.: Unilateral and bilateral renal agenesis in monoamniotic twins. Am. J. Obstet. Gynecol. 84:236–238, 1974.

McCracken, A.A., Daly, P.A., Zolnick, M.R., and Clark, A.M.: Twins and Q-banded chromosome polymorphisms. Hum. Genet. 45:253–258, 1978.

McCrossin, D.B., and Roberton, N.R.C.: Congenital skin defects, twins and toxoplasmosis. J. R. Soc. Med. 82:108–109, 1989.

McCurdy, C.M., Childers, J.M., and Seeds, J.W.: Ligation of the umbilical cord of an acardiac-acephalus twin with an endoscopic intrauterine technique. Obstet. Gynecol. 82:708–711, 1993.

McFee, J.G., Lord, E.L., Jeffrey, R.L., O'Meara, O.P., Josepher, H.J., Butterfield, J., and Thompson, H.E.: Multiple gestations of high fetal number. Obstet. Gynecol. 44:99–106, 1974.

McKeown, T., and Record, R.G.: Observations on fetal growth in multiple pregnancy in man. J. Endocrinol. 8:386–401, 1952.

McLeod, F., and McCoy, D.R.: Monoamniotic twins with an unusual cord complication: case report. Br. J. Obstet. Gynaecol. 88:774–775, 1981.

Medearis, A.L., Jonas, H.S., Stockbauer, J.W., and Domke, H.R.: Perinatal deaths in twin pregnancy: a five-year analysis of statewide statistics in Missouri. Am. J. Obstet. Gynecol. 134:413–421, 1979.

Megory, E., Weiner, E., Shalev, E., and Ohel, G.: Pseudomonoamniotic twins with cord entanglement following genetic funipuncture. Obstet. Gynecol. 78:915–917, 1991.

Melgar, C.A., Rosenfeld, D.L., Rawlinson, K., and Greenberg, M.: Perinatal outcome after multifetal reduction to twins compared with nonreduced multiple gestations. Obstet. Gynecol. 78:763–767, 1991.

Melnick, M.: Brain damage in survivors after in-utero death of monozygous co-twin. Lancet 2:1287, 1977.

Melnick, M., and Myrianthopoulos, N.C.: The effects of chorion type on normal and abnormal developmental variation in monozygous twins. Am. J. Med. Genet. 4:147–156, 1979.

Mercer, B.M., Crocker, L.G., Pierce, F., and Sibai, B.M.: Clinical characteristics and outcome of twin gestation complicated by preterm premature rupture of the membranes. Am. J. Obstet. Gynecol. 168:1467–1473, 1993.

Métneki, J., and Czeizel, A.: Twinning rates. Lancet 1:935, 1983.

Metrakos, J.D., Metrakos, K., and Baxter, H.: Clefts of the lip and palate in twins: including a discordant pair whose monozygosity was confirmed by skin transplants. Plast. Reconstr. Surg. 23:109–122, 1958.

Meulepas, E., Vlietinck, R., and van den Berghe, H.: The probability of dizygosity of phenotypically concordant twins. Am. J. Hum. Genet. 43:817–826, 1988.

Meyer, W.R., and Meyer, W.W.: Report on a very young dizygotic human twin pregnancy. Arch. Gynecol. 231:51–56, 1981.

Michaels, L.: Unilateral ischemia of fused twin placenta: a manifestation of the twin transfusion syndrome? Can. Med. Assoc. J. 96:402–405, 1967.

Michaels, W.H., Schreiber, F.R., Padgett, R.J., Ager, J., and Pieper, D.: Ultrasound surveillance of the cervix in twin gestations: management of cervical incompetency. Obstet. Gynecol. 78:739–744, 1991.

Michlewitz, H., Kennedy, J., Kawada, C., and Kennison, R.: Triplet pregnancies. J. Reprod. Med. 26:243–246, 1981.

Mijsberg, W.A.: Genetic-statistical data on the presence of secondary oocytary twins among non-identical twins. Acta Genet. Statist. Med. 7:39–42, 1957.

Milham, S.: Pituitary gonadotrophin and dizygotic twinning. Lancet 2:566, 1964.

Milham, S.: Symmetrical conjoined twins: an analysis of the birth records of twenty-two sets. J. Pediatr. 69:643–647, 1966.

Miller, D.L., and Dillon, J.: An unusual abdominal mass in an elderly woman. N. Engl. J. Med. 321:1613–1614, 1989.

Mills, W.G.: Pathological changes in blighted twins. J. Obstet. Gynaecol. Br. Emp. 56:619–624, 1949.

Mingeot, R.A., and Keirse, M.J.: Twin pregnancy in a pseudodidelphys. Am. J. Obstet. Gynecol. 111:1121–1122, 1971.

Mitrani, A.: Conjoined thoracopagus twins. Harefuah 74: 95–97, 1968.

Miyabara, S., Okamoto, N., Akimoto, N., Satow, Y., and Nakagawa, S.: A study on dicephalic monsters, especially with regard to embryopathology. Hiroshima J. Med. Sci. 22:377–395, 1973.

Moestrup, J.K.: Monoamniotic twins: a case with vessel anomaly in one twin's umbilical cord. Acta Obstet. Gynecol. Scand. 49:85–87, 1970.

Moore, C.A., Buehler, B.A., McManus, B.M., Harmon, J.P., Mirkin, L.D., and Goldstein, D.J.: Brief clinical report: acephalus-acardia in twins with aneuploidy. Am. J. Med. Genet. Suppl. 3:139–143, 1987.

Moore, C.M., McAdams, A.J., and Sutherland, J.: Intrauterine disseminated intravascular coagulation: a syndrome of multiple pregnancy with a dead twin fetus. J. Pediatr. 74:523–528, 1969.

Moore, T.R., Gale, S.A., and Benirschke, K.: Perinatal outcome of forty-nine pregnancies complicated by acardiac twinning. Am. J. Obstet. Gynecol. 163:907–912, 1990.

Moreno, M.J., and Sanchez, O.: Mosaico cromosómico X0/XX/XY/XXY/, en un hermafrodita verdadero. Acta Cient. Venez. 22:14–18, 1971.

Mortimer, G.: Zygosity and placental structure in monochorionic twins. Acta Genet. Med. Gemellol. 36:417– 520, 1987.

Morton, C.C., Corey, L.A., Nance, W.E., and Brown, J.A.: Quinacrine mustard and nucleolar organizer region heteromorphisms in twins. Acta Genet. Med. Gemellol. 30:39–49, 1981.

Mostoufi-Zadeh, M., Weiss, L.M., and Driscoll, S.G.: Nonimmune hydrops fetalis: a challenge in perinatal pathology. Hum. Pathol. 16:785–789, 1985.

Motomura, K., Tateishi, H., Nishisho, I., Okazaki, M., Miki, T., Tonomura, A., Takai, S.-I., Mori, T., and Jeffreys,

A.J.: The zygosity determination of Japanese twins using a minisatellite core probe. Jpn. J. Hum. Genet. 32:9–14, 1987.

Moyaert, I., Bouters, R., and Bouquet, Y.: Birth of a monozygotic cattle twin following non surgical transfer of a single 7 day old embryo. Theriogenology 18:127–132, 1982.

Mueller-Heubach, E., and Battelli, A.F.: Prolonged in utero retention and mummification of a Macaca mulatta fetus. J. Med. Primatol. 10:265–268, 1981.

Munro, S.S.: Are monovular avian twins always female? J. Hered. 56:285–288, 1965.

Munsinger, H.: The identical-twin transfusion syndrome: a source of error in estimating IQ resemblance and heritability. Ann. Hum. Genet. 40:307–321, 1977.

Mutinelli, F., Nani, S., and Zampiron, S.: Conjoined twins (thoracopagus) in a Wistar rat (Rattus norvegicus). Lab. Anim. Sci. 42:612–613, 1992.

Myrianthopoulos, N.C.: An epidemiological survey of twins in a large, prospectively studied population. Am. J. Hum. Genet. 22:611–629, 1970a.

Myrianthopoulos, N.C.: A survey of twins in the population of a prospective collaborative study. Acta Genet. Med. Gemellol. 19:15–23, 1970b.

Naeye, R.: Parabiotic syndrome. N. Engl. J. Med. 269:1043, 1963.

Naeye, R.: Organ composition in newborn parabiotic twins with speculation regarding neonatal hypoglycemia. Pediatrics 34:415–418, 1964a.

Naeye, R.L.: The fetal and neonatal development of twins. Pediatrics 33:546–553, 1964b.

Naeye, R.: Organ abnormalities in a human parabiotic syndrome. Am. J. Pathol. 46:829–842, 1965.

Naeye, R.L., and Blanc, W.A.: Fetal renal structure and the genesis of amniotic fluid disorders. Am. J. Pathol. 67: 95–105, 1972.

Naeye, R.L., and Letts, H.W.: Body measurements of fetal and neonatal twins. Arch. Pathol. 77:393–396, 1964.

Naeye, R.L., Tafari, N., Judge, D., and Marboe, C.C.: Twins: causes of perinatal death in 12 United States cities and one African city. Am. J. Obstet. Gynecol. 131:267–272, 1978.

Nagashima, H., Kato, Y., and Ogawa, S.: Microsurgical bisection of porcine morulae and blastocysts to produce monozygotic twin pregnancy. Gamete Res. 23:1–10, 1989.

Nageotte, M.P., Hurwitz, S.R., Kaupke, C.J., Vaziri, N.D., and Pandian, M.R.: Atriopeptin in the twin transfusion syndrome. Obstet. Gynecol. 73:867–870, 1989.

Nakayama, A., Imai, S., and Takemura, T.: Intrauterine embolism syndrome: multiple infarction of co-twin caused by dead counterpart in utero [abstract]. Teratology 34:457, 1986.

Nakayama, D.K., Killian, A., Hill, L.M., Miller, J.P., Hannakan, C., Lloyd, D.A., and Rowe, M.I.: The newborn with hydrops and sacrococcygeal teratoma. J. Pediatr. Surg. 26:1435–1438, 1991.

Napolitani, F.D., and Schreiber, I.: The acardiac monster. Am. J. Obstet. Gynecol. 80:582–589, 1960.

Natori, M., Tanaka, M., Kohno, H., Ishimoto, H., Morisada, M., Kobayashi, T., and Nozawa, S.: A case of twin-twin transfusion syndrome treated with placental vessel occlusion using fetoscopic Nd:Yag laser system. Acta Obstet. Gynaecol. Jpn. 44:117–120, 1992.

Neal, F.C., and Wilcox, C.J.: Double acardius amorphus case in a brown Swiss cow. J. Dairy Sci. 50:236, 1967.

Neubecker, R.D., Blumberg, J.M., and Townsend, F.M.: A human monozygotic quintuplet placenta: report of a specimen. J. Obstet. Gynaecol. Br. Commonw. 69:137–139, 1962.

Neuman, W.L., Ponto, K., Farber, R.A., and Shangold, G.A.: DNA analysis of unilateral twin ectopic gestation. Obstet. Gynecol. 75: 479–483, 1990.

Neurath, P.W., Lin, P.-S., and Low, D.A.: Quantitative karyotyping: a model twin study. Cytogenetics 11:457–474, 1972.

Newman, H.H.: Differences between conjoined twins: in relation to a general theory of twinning. J. Hered. 22:201–215, 1931a.

Newman, H.H.: Palm-print patterns in twins: on the use of dermatoglyphics as an aid in the diagnosis of monozygotic and dizygotic twins. J. Hered. 22:41–49, 1931b.

Newman, H.H., and Patterson, J.T.: The development of the nine-banded armadillo from the primitive streak stage to birth; with especial reference to the question of specific polyembryony. J. Morphol. 21:359–424, 1910.

Nhân, V.Q., and Huisjes, H.J.: Double uterus with a pregnancy in each half. Obstet. Gynecol. 61:115–117, 1983.

Nichols, J.B.: Quintuplet and sextuplet births in the United States. Obstet. Gynecol. 3:124–125, 1954.

Nichols, R.C., and Bilbro, W.C.: The diagnosis of twin zygosity. Acta Genet. (Basel) 16:265–275, 1966.

Nickerson, C.W.: Amniotic sac dystocia in twins. Am. J. Obstet. Gynecol. 97:867–868, 1967.

Nigro, M.: Considérations immunologiques et endocrinologiques à propos d'un cas d'acardie. J. Gynecol. Obstet. Reprod. 6:963–970, 1977.

Noonan, J.A.: Twins, conjoined twins, and cardiac defects. Am. J. Dis. Child. 132:17–18, 1978.

Norman, M.G.: Bilateral encephaloclastic lesions in a 26 week gestation fetus: effect on neuroblast migration. J. Can. Sci. Neurol. 7:191–194, 1980.

Norman, M.G.: Mechanism of brain damage in twins. J. Can. Sci. Neurol. 9:339–344, 1982.

Nylander, P.P.S.: Placental forms and zygosity determination of twins in Ibadan, Western Nigeria: a study of 1475 twin maternities. Acta Genet. Med. Gemellol. 19:49–54, 1970.

Nylander, P.P.S.: Ethnic differences in twinning rates in Nigeria. J. Biosoc. Sci. 3:151–157, 1971a.

Nylander, P.P.S.: The incidence of triplets and higher multiple births in some rural and urban populations in Western Nigeria. Ann. Hum. Genet. 34:409–415, 1971b.

Nylander, P.P.S.: Serum levels of gonadotrophins in relation to multiple pregnancy in Nigeria. J. Obstet. Gynaecol. Br. Commonw. 80:651–653, 1973.

Nylander, P.P.S., and Corney, G.: Placentation and zygosity of twins in Ibadan, Nigeria. Ann. Hum. Genet. 33:31–40, 1969.

Nylander, P.P.S., and Corney, G.: Placentation and zygosity of triplets and higher multiple births in Ibadan, Nigeria. Ann. Hum. Genet. 34:417–426, 1971.

Nylander, P.P.S., and Osunkoya, B.O.: Unusual monochorionic placentation with heterosexual twins. Obstet. Gynecol. 36:621–625, 1970.

O'Brien, P.J., and Hay, D.A.: Birthweight differences, the transfusion syndrome, and the cognitive development of monozygotic twins. Acta Genet. Med. Gemellol. 36:181–196, 1987.

Ohel, G., Granat, M., Zeevi, D., Golan, A., Wexler, S., David, M.P., and Schenker, J.G.: Advanced ultrasonic placental maturation in twin pregnancies. Am. J. Obstet. Gynecol. 156:76–78, 1987.

O'Keane, J.A., Yuen, B.H., Farquharson, D.F., and Wittman, B.K.: Endocrine response to selective embryocide in a gonadotropin-induced quintuplet pregnancy. Am. J. Obstet. Gynecol. 155:364–367, 1988.

Olding, L.: The possibility of materno-foetal transfer of lymphocytes in man. Acta Paediatr. Scand. 61:73–75, 1972.

Osborne, R.H.: Serology in physical anthropology. Am. J. Phys. Anthropol. 16:187–195, 1958.

O'Sullivan, J.V.: Multiple pregnancy. Proc. R. Soc. Med. 61:235–236, 1968.

Parks, J., and Epstein, J.R.: Monoamniotic twin pregnancy with living infants. Am. J. Obstet. Gynecol. 39:140–142, 1940.

Patten, R.M., Mack, L.A., Harvey, D., Cyr, D.R., and Pretorius, D.H.: Disparity of amniotic fluid volume and fetal size: problem of the stuck twin—US studies. Radiology 172:153–157, 1989a.

Patten, R.M., Mack, L.A., Nyberg, D.A., and Filly, R.A.: Twin embolization syndrome: prenatal sonographic detection and significance. Radiology 173:685–689, 1989b.

Paulson, R.J., Lobo, R.A., Stein, A., Toker, R., Moegle, A., and Macaso, T.: Gestation of triplets after intrauterine implantation of two embryos. N. Engl. J. Med. 318:1339–1340, 1988.

Pavlica, F.: Über einen Fötus mit zahlreichen Entwicklungsanomalien. Padiatr. Padol. 3:27–33, 1967.

Payne, S., Dudge, J., and Bradbury, W.: Ectopic pregnancy concomitant with twin intrauterine pregnancy: a case report. Obstet. Gynecol. 38:905–906, 1971.

Pearlman, S.A., and Batton, D.G.: Effect of birth order on intraventricular hemorrhage in very low birth weight twins. Obstet. Gynecol. 71:358–360, 1988.

Pedrosa, M.P., Salzano, F.M., Mattevi, M.S., and Viegas, J.: Quantitative analysis of C-bands in chromosomes 1, 9, 16, and Y of twins. Acta Genet. Med. Gemellol. 32:257–260, 1983.

Pérez, M.L., Firpo, J.R., and Baldi, E.M.: Sobre las anastomosis circulatorias de las placentas dizigoticas. Obstet. Ginecol. Lat. 5:5–21, 1947.

Phillips, D.I.W.: Twin studies in medical research: can they tell us whether diseases are genetically determined? Lancet 341:1008–1009, 1993.

Pickering, G.H.: Monovular twins. B.M.J. 2:988, 1946.

Pickhardt, W.L., and Breen, J.L.: Monoamniotic twin pregnancy: report of a case. Obstet. Gynecol. 12:471–472, 1958.

Pijpers, L., Jahoda, M.G.J., Vosters, R.P.L., Niermeijer, M.F., and Sachs, E.S.: Genetic amniocentesis in twin pregnancies. Br. J. Obstet. Gynaecol. 95:323–326, 1988.

Pinette, M.G., Pan, Y.M.M., Pinette, S.G., and Stubblefield, P.G.: Treatment of twin-twin transfusion syndrome. Obstet. Gynecol. 82:841–846, 1993.

Platt, L.D., DeVore, G.R., Bieniarz, A., Benner, P., and Rao, R.: Antenatal diagnosis of acephalus acardia: a proposed management scheme. Am. J. Obstet. Gynecol. 146: 857–859, 1983.

Popek, E.J., Strain, J.D., Neumann, A., and Wilson, H.: In utero development of pulmonary artery calcification in monochorionic twins: report of three cases [abstract]. Mod. Pathol. 3(1):7P, 1990.

Porreco, R.P., Burke, M.S., and Parker, D.W.: Selective embryocide in the nonsurgical management of combined intrauterine-extrauterine pregnancy. Obstet. Gynecol. 75: 498–501, 1990.

Porreco, R.P., Barton, S.M., and Haverkamp, A.D.: Occlusion of umbilical artery in acardiac, acephalic twin. Lancet 337:326–327, 1991.

Porter, R.P., and Gengozian, N.: Immunological tolerance and rejection of skin allografts in the marmoset. Transplantation 8:653–665, 1969.

Potter, E.L.: Twin zygosity and placental form in relation to the outcome of pregnancy. Am. J. Obstet. Gynecol. 87: 566–577, 1963.

Powers, W.F.: Twin pregnancy: complications and treatment. Obstet. Gynecol. 42:795–808, 1973.

Powers, W.F., and Kiely, J.L.: The risks confronting twins: a national perspective. Am. J. Obstet. Gynecol. 170:456–461, 1994.

Powers, W.F., and Miller, T.C.: Bed rest in twin pregnancy: identification of a critical period and its cost implications. Am. J. Obstet. Gynecol. 134:23–29, 1979.

Preis, A., and Srubarova, M.: Cardiological findings in twins, with special references to their zygosity and peristasis. Acta Genet. Med. Gemellol. 15:190–198, 1966.

Pretorius, D.H., Leopold, G., Moore, T.R., Benirschke, K., and Sivo, J.J.: Acardiac twin: report of Doppler sonography. J. Ultrasound Med. 7:413–416, 1988a.

Pretorius, D.H., Manchester, D., Barkin, S., Parker, S., and Nelson, T.R.: Doppler ultrasound of twin transfusion syndrome. J. Ultrasound Med. 7:117–124, 1988b.

Price, B.: Primary biases in twin studies: review of prenatal and natal differences-producing factors in monozygotic pairs. Am. J. Hum. Genet. 2:293–352, 1950.

Pridjian, G., Nugent, C.E., and Barr, M.: Twin gestation: influence of placentation on fetal growth. Am. J. Obstet. Gynecol. 165:1394–1401, 1991.

Puckett, J.D.: Fetal death of second twin in second trimester. Am. J. Obstet. Gynecol. 159:740–741, 1988.

Quigley, J.K.: Mono-amniotic twin pregnancy: case record with review of literature. Am. J. Obstet. Gynecol. 29: 354–362, 1935.

Quintero, R.A., Reich, H., Puder, K.S., Bardicef, M., Evans, M.I., Cotton, D.B., and Romero, R.: Brief report: umbilical-cord ligation of an acardiac twin by fetoscopy at 19 weeks of gestation. N. Engl. J. Med. 330:469–471, 1994.

Ramos-Arroyo, M.A., Ulbright, T.M., and Christian, J.C.: Twin study: relationship between birth weight, zygosity, placentation, and pathologic placental changes. Acta Genet. Med. Gemellol. 37:229–238, 1988.

Raphael, S.I.: Monoamniotic twin pregnancy: a review of the literature and a report of 5 new cases. Am. J. Obstet. Gynecol. 81:323–330, 1961.

Rashad, M.N., and Kerr, M.G.: Observations on the so-called holoacardius amorphus. J. Anat. 100:425–426, 1966.

Rausen, A.R., Seki, M., and Strauss, L.: Twin transfusion syndrome: a review of 19 cases studied at one institution. J. Pediatr. 66:613–628, 1965.

Rayburn, W.F., and Barr, M.: Teratomas: concordance in mother and fetus. Am. J. Obstet. Gynecol. 144:110–112, 1982.

Rayburn, W.F., Lavin, J.P., Miodovnik, M., and Varner, M.W.: Multiple gestation: time interval between delivery of the first and second twins. Obstet. Gynecol. 63:502–506, 1984.

Record, R.G., McKeown, T., and Edwards, J.H.: An investigation of the difference on measured intelligence between twins and single births. Ann. Hum. Genet. 34:11–20, 1970.

Reed, T., Sprague, F.R., Kang, K.W., Nance, W.E., and Christian, J.C.: Genetic analysis of dermatoglyphic patterns in twins. Hum. Hered. 25:263–275, 1975.

Rehder, H., Geisler, M., Kleinbrecht, J., and Degenhardt, K.H.: Monozygotic twins with 47,XXY karyotype and discordant malformations. Teratology 17:5a, 1978.

Reisner, D.P., Mahony, B.S., Petty, C.N., Nyberg, D.A., Porter, T.F., Zingheim, R.W., Williams, M.A., and Luthy, D.A.: Stuck twin syndrome: outcome in thirty-seven consecutive cases. Am. J. Obstet. Gynecol. 169:991–995, 1993.

Reisner, S.H., Forbes, A.E., and Cornblath, M.: The smaller of twins and hypoglycaemia. Lancet 1:524–526, 1965.

Renkonen, K.O.: Is Weinberg's differential rule defective? Ann. Hum. Genet. 30:277–280, 1967.

Rhine, S.A., and Nance, W.E.: Familial twinning: a case for superfetation in man. Acta Genet. Med. Gemellol. 25: 66–69, 1976.

Rice-Wray, E., Cervantes, A., Gutierrez, J., and Marquez-Monter, H.: Pregnancy and progeny after hormonal contraceptives—genetic studies. J. Reprod. Med. 6:101–104, 1971.

Richart, R., and Benirschke, K.: Holoacardius amorphus: report of a case with chromosome analysis. Am. J. Obstet. Gynecol. 86:329–332, 1963.

Roberge, J.L.: Sympodia in identical twins: report of a case. J.A.M.A. 186:728–729, 1963.

Roberts, S.J.: Veterinary Obstetrics and Genital Diseases. Edwards Broths, Ann Arbor, 1956.

Robertson, E.G., and Neer, K.J.: Placental injection studies in twin gestation. Am. J. Obstet. Gynecol. 147:170–175, 1983.

Robertson, J.G.: Twin pregnancy: morbidity and fetal mortality. Obstet. Gynecol. 23:330–337, 1964a.

Robertson, J.G.: Twin pregnancy: influence of early admission on fetal survival. Obstet. Gynecol. 23:854–860, 1964b.

Robertson, J.G.: Blood grouping in twin pregnancy. Br. J. Obstet. Gynaecol. 76:154–156, 1969.

Robie, G.F., Payne, G.G., and Morgan, M.A.: Selective delivery of an acardiac, acephalic twin. N. Engl. J. Med. 320:512–513, 1989.

Robinson, H.P., and Caines, J.S.: Sonar evidence of early pregnancy failure in patients with twin conceptions. Br. J. Obstet. Gynaecol. 84:22–25, 1977.

Rodis, J.F., Vintzileos, A.M., Campbell, W.A., Deaton, J.L., Fumia, F., and Nochimson, J.: Antenatal diagnosis and management of monoamniotic twins. Am. J. Obstet. Gynecol. 157:1255–1257, 1987.

Rohmer, A., Ruch, J.-V., Schneegans, E., and Clavert, J.: Jumeaux dizygotes, l'un 47 XX 21+ et cliniquement mongolien, l'autre 46 XX/47 XX 21+ et cliniquement non mongolien. Pediatrie 26:209–213, 1971.

Romero, R., Duffy, T.P., Berkowitz, R.L., Chang, E., and Hobbins, J.C.: Prolongation of a preterm pregnancy complicated by death of a single twin in utero and disseminated intravascular coagulation: effects of treatment with heparin. N. Engl. J. Med. 310:772–774, 1984.

Roos, F.J., Roter, A.M., and Molina, F.A.: A case of triplets including anomalous twins and a fetus compressus. Am. J. Obstet. Gynecol. 73:1342–1345, 1957.

Rosa, F.W., Hernandez, C., and Carlo, W.A.: Griseofulvin teratology, including two thoracopagus conjoined twins. Lancet 1:171, 1987.

Rosenfeld, C.R., Coln, C.D., and Duenhoelter, J.H.: Fetal teratomas as a cause of polyhydramnios. Pediatrics 64:176–179, 1979.

Rosenquist, G.C.: Parabiotic syndrome. N. Engl. J. Med. 269:161–162, 1963.

Ross, J.R.W.: An acardius amorphus in a triplet pregnancy. J. Obstet. Gynaecol. Br. Emp. 58:835–838, 1951.

Ross, R.K., Bernstein, L., Judd, H., Hanisch, R., Pike, M., and Henderson, B.: Serum testosterone levels in healthy young black and white men. J. Natl. Cancer Inst. 76:45–48, 1986.

Rothman, K.J.: Fetal loss, twinning and birth weight after oral-contraceptive use. N. Engl. J. Med. 297:468–471, 1977.

Rouse, D.J., Skopec, G.S., and Zlatnik, F.J.: Fundal height as a predictor of preterm twin delivery. Obstet. Gynecol. 81:211–214, 1993.

Runner, M.N.: New evidence for monozygotic twins in the mouse: twinning initiated in the late blastocyst can account for mirror image asymmetries. Anat. Rec. 209:399–406, 1984.

Russell, E.M.: Cerebral palsied twins. Arch. Dis. Child. 36:328–336, 1961.

Ryan, K.J.: Paternity and pedigree, from superfecundation to "test-tube" babies. N. Engl. J. Med. 299:603, 1978.

Ryan, R.R., and Wislocki, G.B.: The birth of quadruplets, with an account of the placentas and fetal membranes. N. Engl. J. Med. 250:755–758, 1954.

Rydhstrom, H.: Twin pregnancy and the effects of prophylactic leave of absence on pregnancy duration and birth weight. Acta Obstet. Gynecol. Scand. 67:81–84, 1988.

Sacks, M.O.: Occurrence of anemia and polycythemia in phenotypically dissimilar single-ovum human twins. Pediatrics 24:604–608, 1959.

Saier, F., Burden, L., and Cavanagh, D.: Fetus papyraceus: an unusual case with congenital anomaly of the surviving fetus. Obstet. Gynecol. 45:217–220, 1975.

Sala, M.A., and Matheus, M.: Placental characteristics in twin transfusion syndrome. Arch. Gynecol. Obstet. 246:51–56, 1989.

Sander, C.H.: Fetus papyraceus. Am. J. Obstet. Gynecol. 145:895–896, 1983.

Sato, T., Kaneko, K., Konuma, S., Sato, I., and Tamada, T.: Acardiac anomalies: review of 88 cases in Japan. Asia Oceania J. Obstet. Gynaecol. 10:45–52, 1984.

Saunders, M.C., Dick, J.S., McPherson, K., and Chalmers, I.: The effect of hospital admission for bed rest on the duration of twin pregnancy: a randomized trial. Lancet 2:793–795, 1985.

Saunders, N.J., Snijders, R.J.M., and Nicolaides, K.H.: Therapeutic amniocentesis in twin-twin transfusion syndrome appearing in the second trimester of pregnancy. Am. J. Obstet. Gynecol. 166:820–824, 1992.

Schatz, F.: Zur Frage ber die Quelle des Fruchtwassers und über Embryones papyracei. Arch. Gynäkol. 7:336–338, 1875; 19:329, 1882.

Schatz, F.: Die Gefässverbindungen der Placentarkreisläufe eineiiger Zwillinge, ihre Entwicklung und ihre Folgen. Arch. Gynäkol. 27:1–72, 1886.

Schatz, F.: Die Acardii und ihre Verwandten. Hirschwald, Berlin, 1898.

Schatz, F.: Systematisches und alphabetisches Inhaltsverzeichniss von Friedrich Schatz: Placentakreisläufe eineiiger Zwillinge, ihre Entwicklung und ihre Folgen, in Band 19, 24, 27, 29, 30, 53, 55, 58, 60. Arch. Gynäkol. 60:559–584, 1900 [systematic index of Schatz's work on twins, with specific references to his citing various features of twin placentas, and authorities quoted].

Scheller, J.M., and Nelson, K.B.: Twinning and neurologic morbidity. Am. J. Dis. Child. 146:110–113, 1992.

Schenker, J.G., Yarkoni, S., and Granat, M.: Multiple pregnancies following induction of ovulation. Fertil. Steril. 35:105–123, 1981.

Schinzel, A.A.G.L., Smith, D.W., and Miller, J.R.: Monozygotic twinning and structural defects. J. Pediatr. 95:921–930, 1979.

Schmidt, W., Heberling, D., and Kubli, F.: Antepartum ultrasonographic diagnosis of conjoined twins in early pregnancy. Am. J. Obstet. Gynäkol. 139:961–963, 1981.

Schneider, K.T.M., Vetter, K., Huch, R., and Huch, A.: Acute polyhydramnios complicating twin pregnancies. Acta Genet. Med. Gemellol. 34:179–184, 1985.

Scholtes, G.: Zum Problem der Zwillingsschwangerschaft. Arch. Gynecol. 210:188–207, 1971.

Schwalbe, E.: Acardii und Verwandte. In, Die Missbildungen des Menschen und der Tiere. Vol. II. Die Doppelbildungen. Gustav Fischer, Jena, 1907.

Schwartz, J.L., Maniscalco, W.M., Lane, A.T., and Currao, W.J.: Twin transfusion syndrome causing cutaneous erythropoiesis. Pediatrics 74:527–529, 1984.

Scipiades, E., and Burg, E.: Über die Morphologie der menschlichen Plazenta mit besonderer Berücksichtigung auf unsere eigenen Studien. Arch. Gynäkol. 141:577–619, 1930.

Scott, J.M., and Ferguson-Smith, M.A.: Heterokaryotypic monozygotic twins and the acardiac monster. J. Obstet. Gynaecol. 80:52–59, 1973.

Sekiya, S., and Hafez, E.S.E.: Physiomorphology of twin transfusion syndrome: a study of 86 twin gestations. Obstet. Gynecol. 50:288–292, 1977.

Sekiya, S.-I., Akamatsu, H., Kaneko, K., and Takeishi, Y.: Report of a case: placental vascular communications between triplet fetuses; triplet transfusion syndrome. J. Jpn. Neonatol. Soc. (Nihon Shinseiji Gakkai Zasshi) 9:89–96, 1973.

Selby, L.A., Khalili, A., Stewart, R.W., Edmonds, L.D., and Marienfeld, C.J.: Pathology and epidemiology of conjoined twinning in swine. Teratology 8:1–10, 1973.

Selvin, S.: Twin zygosity diagnosis by blood group antigens. Hum. Hered. 20:540–548, 1970.

Semchyshyn, S., Mangurten, H., Benawra, R., Trujillo, Y., Fernandez, B., and McKeown, J.C.: Fetal tumor: antenatal diagnosis and its implications. J. Reprod. Med. 27:231–234, 1982.

Semmens, J.P.: Monoamniotic twin pregnancy: delivery of living premature twins after uterine rupture; a case report. Obstet. Gynecol. 12:75–77, 1958.

Seo, J.W., Shin, S.S., and Chi, J.G.: Cardiovascular system in conjoined twins: an analysis of 14 Korean cases. Teratology 32:151–161, 1985.

Seoud, M.A.-F., Toner, J.P., Kruithoff, C., and Muasher, S.J.: Outcome of twin, triplet, and quadruplet in vitro fertilization pregnancies: the Norfolk experience. Fertil. Steril. 57:825–834, 1992.

Seski, A.G., and Miller, L.A.: Plural pregnancies—the cause of plural problems. Obstet. Gynecol. 21:227–233, 1963.

Shah, D.M., and Chaffin, D.: Perinatal outcome in very preterm births with twin-twin transfusion syndrome. Am. J. Obstet. Gynecol. 161:1111–1113, 1989.

Shapiro, L.R., and Farnsworth, P.G.: Down's syndrome in twins. Clin. Genet. 2:364–370, 1972.

Shapiro, L.R., Wilmot, P.L., Duncan, P.A., Davidian, M.M., Fakhry, J., and Capone, A.J.: Holoacardius acephalus: cytogenetic abnormalities as the principle pathogenetic mechanism. Proc. Greenwood Genet. Center 5:128, 1986.

Sherer, D.M., Armstrong, B., Shah, Y.G., Metlay, L.A., and Woods, J.R.: Prenatal sonographic diagnosis, Doppler velocimetric umbilical cord studies, and subsequent management of an acardiac twin pregnancy. Obstet. Gynecol. 74:472–475, 1989.

Sherer, D.M., Abramowicz, J.S., Jaffe, R., Smith, S.A., Metlay, L.A., and Woods, J.R.: Twin-twin transfusion syndrome with abrupt onset of microcephaly in the surviving recipient following spontaneous death of the donor twin. Am. J. Obstet. Gynecol. 169:85–88, 1993.

Shorland, J.: Management of the twin transfusion syndrome. Clin. Pediatr. 10:160–163, 1971.

Short, R.V.: Testis size, ovulation rate and breast cancer. In, One Medicine. O.A. Ryder, and M.L. Byrd, eds., pp. 32–44. Springer-Verlag, New York, 1984.

Simonds, J.P., and Gowen, G.A.: Fetus amorphus. Surg. Gynecol. Obstet. 41:171–179, 1925.

Simonsen, M.: Monoamniotic twins. Acta Obstet. Gynecol. Scand. 45:43–52, 1966.

Simpson, C.W., Olatunbosun, O.A., and BaldwinLage, V.J.: Delayed interval delivery in triplet pregnancy: report of a single case and review of the literature. Obstet. Gynecol. 64:8S–11S, 1984.

Simpson, J.L., Morillo-Cucci, G., Horwith, M., Stiefel, F.H., Feldman, F., and German, J.: Abnormalities of human sex chromosomes. VI. Monozygotic twins with the complement 48,XXXY. Humangenetik 21:301–308, 1974.

Simpson, P.C., Trudinger, B.J., Walker, A., and Baird, P.J.: The intrauterine treatment of fetal cardiac failure in a twin pregnancy with an acardiac, acephalic monster. Am. J. Obstet. Gynecol. 147:842–844, 1983.

Sinclair, J.G.: The Badgett quadruplets. J. Hered. 31:163–164, 1940.

Sinykin, M.B.: Monoamniotic triplet pregnancy with triple survival. Obstet. Gynecol. 12:78–82, 1958.

Skelly, H., Marivate, M., Norman, R., Kenoyer, G., and Martin, R.: Consumptive coagulopathy following fetal death in a triplet pregnancy. Am. J. Obstet. Gynecol. 142:595–596, 1982.

Soma, H., Takayama, M., Kiyokawa, T., Akaeda, T., and Tokoro, K.: Serum gonadotropin levels in Japanese women. Obstet. Gynecol. 46:311–312, 1975.

Soma, H., Saito, T., Kikuchi, K., Arai, K., Takayama, M., Yoshida, K., and Terada, K.: Sacrococcygeal teratoma in a fetus and its placenta. Rinsho Fujinka Sanka (Clin. Gynecol. Obstet. Jpn.) 33:303–307, 1979.

Sorensen, S.A., and Fenger, K.: On the use of linked markers in the diagnosis of zygosity in twins. Hum. Hered. 24:529–539, 1974.

Sotrel, G., Rao, R., and Scommegna, A.: Heterotopic pregnancy following clomid treatment. J. Reprod. Med. 16:78–80, 1976.

Sowards, D.L., and Monif, R.G.: Serum immunoglobulin M levels between weeks 22 and 37 of gestation. Am. J. Obstet. Gynecol. 112:394–396, 1972.

Spellacy, W.N., Kalra, P.S., Buggie, J., and Birk, S.A.: Gonadotropin responses to graded GNRF injections in women with prior twin pregnancies. J. Reprod. Med. 27:435–438, 1982.

Spellacy, W.N., Handler, A., and Ferre, C.D.: A case-control study of 1253 twin pregnancies from 1982–1987 perinatal data base. Obstet. Gynecol. 75:168–171, 1990.

Spencer, R.: Conjoined twins: Theoretical embryological basis. Teratology 45:591–602, 1992.

Spitzer, W.: Zur geburtshilflichen Bedeutung der kongenitalen Sakraltumoren. Zentralbl. Gynäkol. 56:1403–1409, 1932.

Spurway, J.H.: The fate and management of the second twin. Am. J. Obstet. Gynecol. 83:1377–1388, 1962.

Starks, G.C.: Unilateral twin interstitial ectopic pregnancy: a case report. J. Reprod. Med. 25:79–82, 1980.

Stephens, T.D., Spall, R., Urfer, A.G., and Martin, R.: Fetus amorphus or placental teratoma? Teratology 40:1–10, 1989.

Stoeckel, W.: Lehrbuch der Geburtshilfe. p. 258. Gustav Fischer, Jena, 1945.

Storch, M.P., and Petrie, R.H.: Unilateral tubal twin gestation. Am. J. Obstet. Gynecol. 125:1148, 1976.

Stranc, M.F.: Skin homograft survival in a severely burned triplet: study of triplet zygotic type. Plast. Reconstr. Surg. 37:280–290, 1966.

Strauss, J.H., Ballard, J.O., and Chamlian, D.: Consumption coagulopathy associated with intrauterine fetal death: the role of heparin therapy. Int. J. Gynaecol. Obstet. 16:225–227, 1978.

Streit, J.A., Penick, G.D., Williamson, R.A., Weiner, C.P., and Benda, J.A.: Prolonged elevation of alphafetoprotein and detectable acetylcholinesterase after death of an anomalous twin. Prenat. Diagn. 9:1–6, 1989.

Strong, S.J., and Corney, G.: The Placenta in Twin Pregnancy. Pergamon, Oxford, 1967.

Sulak, L.E., and Dodson, M.G.: The vanishing twin: pathologic conformation of an ultrasonographic phenomenon. Obstet. Gynecol. 68:811–815, 1986.

Suslak, L., Mimms, G.M., and Desposito, F.: Monozygosity and holoprosencephaly: cleavage disorders of the "midline field." Am. J. Med. Genet. 28:99–102, 1987.

Sutter, J., Arab, H., and Manning, F.A.: Monoamniotic twins: antenatal diagnosis and management. Am. J. Obstet. Gynecol. 155:836–837, 1986.

Sutton, J.B.: An acardiac from a cow. Trans. Obstet. Soc. Lond. 41:97, 1899

Swindle, M.M., Adams, R.J., and Craft, C.F.: Intrauterine mummified fetus in a rhesus monkey (Macaca mulatta). J. Med. Primatol. 10:269–273, 1981.

Szabuniewicz, M., and McCrady, J.D.: A case of "Siamese" twins in the turtle (Pseudemys scripta elegans). Texas J. Sci. 19:232–233, 1967.

Szendi, B.: Über die Bedeutung der Struktur der Eihäute und des Gefässnetzes der Placenta auf Grund von 112 Zwillingsgeburten. Arch. Gynäkol. 167:108–129, 1938.

Szymonowicz, W., Preston, H., and Yu, Y.Y.H.: The surviving monozygotic twin. Arch. Dis. Child. 61:454–458, 1986.

Tabsh, K.: Genetic amniocentesis in multiple gestation: a new technique to diagnose monoamniotic twins. Obstet. Gynecol. 75:296–298, 1990a.

Tabsh, K.M.A.: Transabdominal multifetal pregnancy reduction: report of 40 cases. Obstet. Gynecol. 75:739–741, 1990b.

Tabsh, K.M.A.: A report of 131 cases of multifetal pregnancy reduction. Obstet. Gynecol. 82:57–60, 1993.

Tabsh, K.M.A., Crandall, B., Lebherz, T.B., and Howard, J.: Genetic amniocentesis in twin pregnancy. Obstet. Gynecol. 65:843–845, 1985.

Tafeen, C.H., Freedman, H.L., and Kahane, A.J.: Monoamniotic twins. Am. J. Obstet. Gynecol. 79:1078–1081, 1960.

Tan, K.L., Goon, S.M., Salmon, Y., and Wee, J.H.: Conjoined twins. Acta Obstet. Gynecol. Scand. 50:373–380, 1971a.

Tan, K.L., Tock, E.P.C., Dawood, M.Y., and Ratnam, S.S.: Conjoined twins in a triplet pregnancy. Am. J. Dis. Child. 122:455–458, 1971b.

Tarkowski, A.K.: Mouse chimaeras developed from fused eggs. Nature 190:875–860, 1961.

Taylor, M.B., Anderson, R.L., and Golbus, M.S.: One hundred twin pregnancies in a prenatal diagnosis program. Am. J. Med. Genet. 18:419–422, 1984.

Terasaki, P.I., Gjertson, D., Bernoco, D., Perdue, S., Mickey, M.R., and Bond, J.: Twins with two different fathers identified by HLA. N. Engl. J. Med. 299:590–592, 1978.

Tessen, J.A., and Zlatnik, F.J.: Monoamniotic twins: a retrospective controlled study. Obstet. Gynecol. 77:832–834, 1991.

Thiery, M., Dhont, M., and Vandekerckhove, D.: Serum hCG and hPL in twin pregnancies. Acta Obstet. Gynecol. Scand. 56:495–497, 1976.

Thomas, D.B.: Intrauterine intraventricular haemorrhage and disseminated intravascular coagulation in a triplet pregnancy. Aust. Paediatr. J. 10:25–27, 1974.

Thomas, J.: Untersuchungsergebnisse über die Aplasie einer Nabelarterie unter besonderer Berücksichtigung der Zwillingsschwangerschaft. Geburtshilfe Frauenheilkd. 21:984–992, 1961.

Thomas, J.: Morphologische Untersuchungen über das "große Herz" des Feten. Geburtshilfe Frauenheilkd. 22:1316–1323, 1962.

Thompson, J.P., and Johnson, C.E.: Survival and management of the second-born twin. Obstet. Gynecol. 27:827–832, 1966.

Thomsen, R.J.: Delayed interval delivery of a twin pregnancy. Obstet. Gynecol. 52:37s–40s, 1978.

Thornton, J.G., and Rout, D.J.: Hospital admission in twin pregnancy. Lancet 335:978, 1990.

Timmons, J.D., and de Alvarez, R.R.: Monoamniotic twin pregnancy. Am. J. Obstet. Gynecol. 86:875–881, 1963.

Timonen, S., and Carpen, E.: Multiple pregnancies and photoperiodicity. Ann. Chir. Gynaecol. Fenn. 57:135–139, 1968.

Tippett, P.: Human chimeras. In, Chimeras in Developmental Biology. N.L. Douarin, and A. McLaren, eds., pp. 165–178. Academic Press, Orlando, FL, 1984.

Tojo, R., Larripa, J., Iglesias, H., and Quiroga, E.: Sindrome de transfusion feto-fetal: a proposito de tres observaciones. Rev. Esp. Pediatr. 27:101–112, 1971.

Tokunaga, S., Ikeda, T., Matsuo, T., Maeda, H., Kurosaki, N., and Shimoda, H.: A case of sacral parasite. Congen. Anom. (Japan) 26:321–330, 1986.

Torgersen, J.: Genic factors in visceral asymmetry and in the development and pathologic changes of lungs, heart and abdominal organs. Arch. Pathol. 47:566–593, 1949.

Torretta, G., and Cobellis, G.: Aspetti vascolari della placenta monocoriale su calchi al neoprene. Arch. Ostet. Ginecol. 71:357–362, 1966.

Toubas, P.L., Silverman, N.H., Heyman, M.A., and Rudolph, A.M.: Cardiovascular effects of acute hemorrhage in fetal lambs. Am. J. Physiol. 240:H45–H48, 1981.

Tow, S.H.: Foetal wastage in twin pregnancy. J. Obstet. Gynaecol. Br. Emp. 66:444–451, 1959.

Townsend, R.R., Simpson, G.F., and Filly, R.A.: Membrane thickness in ultrasound prediction of chorionicity of twin gestations. J. Ultrasound Med. 7:327–332, 1988.

Tsunoda, Y., and McLaren, A.: Effect of various procedures on the viability of mouse embryos containing half the normal number of blastomeres. J. Reprod. Fertil. 69:315–322, 1983.

Tsunoda, Y., Tokunaga, T., Sugie, T., and Katsumata, M.: Production of monozygotic twins following the transfer of bisected embryos in the goat. Theriogenology 24:337–342, 1985.

Tuncer, M.: Placenta angiograms in the diagnosis of placental transfusion syndrome in twins. Hacettepe Bull. Med. Surg. 3:182–191, 1970.

Turksoy, R.N., Toy, B.L., Rogers, J., and Papageorge, W.: Birth of septuplets following human gonadotropin administration in Chiari-Frommel syndrome. Obstet. Gynecol. 30:692–697, 1967.

Turpin, R., Bocquet, L., and Grasset, J.: Étude d'un couple monozygote: fille normale—monstre acardiaque féminin: considérations anatomo-pathologiques et cytogénétiques. Ann. Genet. (Paris) 10:107–113, 1967.

Tüscher, H.: Zur Frage der Entscheidung über die Ein = oder Zeieiigkeit bei bichorischen biamniotischen Zwillingen mit Gefäßanastomosen in der Plazenta. Erbarzt 10:148–149, 1936.

Uchida, I.A., Freeman, V.C.P., Gedeon, M., and Goldmaker, J.: Twinning rate in spontaneous abortions. Am. J. Hum. Genet. 35:987–993, 1983.

Urig, M.A., Clewell, W.H., and Elliott J.P.: Twin-twin transfusion syndrome. Am. J. Obstet. Gynecol. 163:1522–1526, 1990.

van der Kolk, W.F.J.: De asymmetrische derde circulatie en haar gevolgen voor monozygote gemelli. Maandschr. Kindergenesk. 32:186–194, 1964.

Verger, P., Martin, C.L., and Cardinaud, M.-C.: Anémie-polygobulie des jumeaux univitellins et transfusion foeto-foetale. Pediatrie 18:533–541, 1963.

Verma, R.S., Luke, S., and Dhawan, P.: Twins with different fathers. Lancet 339:63–64, 1992.

Vermelin, H., and Ribon, M. (1949): Quoted from Corner, G.W. (1955).

Vermesh, M., and Kletzky, O.A.: Follicle-stimulating hormone is the main determinant of follicular recruitment and development in ovulation induction with human menopausal gonadotropin. Am. J. Obstet. Gynecol. 157:1397–1402, 1987.

Verschuer, O.v.: Ein Fall von Monochorie bei zweieiigen Zwillingen. Munch. Med. Wochenschr. 72:184, 1925.

Verschuer, O.v.: Die vererbungsbiologische Zwillingsforschung: Ihre biologischen Grundlagen: Studien an 102 eineiigen und 45 gleichgeschlechtlichen zweieiigen Zwillings- und 2 Drillingspaaren. Ergebn. Inn. Med. Kinderheilkd. 31:35–120, 1927.

Vestergaard, P.: Triplets pregnancy with a normal foetus and dicephalus dibrachius sirenomelus. Acta Obstet. Gynecol. Scand. 51:93–94, 1972.

Vetter, K., and Schneider, K.T.M.: Iatrogenous remission of twin transfusion syndrome. Am. J. Obstet. Gynecol. 158:221, 1988.

Viljoen, D.L., Nelson, M.M., and Beighton, P.: The epidemiology of conjoined twinning in southern Africa. Clin. Genet. 24:15–21, 1983.

Ville, Y., Hecher, K., Ogg, D., Warren, R., and Nicolaides, K.: Successful outcome after Nd:Yag laser separation of chorioangiopagus-twins under sonoendoscopic control. Ultrasound Obstet. Gynecol. 2:429–431, 1992.

Vlietinck, R., Derom, C., Derom, R., van der Berghe, H., and Thiery, M.: The validity of Weinberg's rule in the East Flanders prospective twin survey (EFPTS). Acta Genet. Med. Gemellol. 37:137–141, 1988.

Walker, N.F.: Determination of the zygosity of twins. Acta Genet. (Basel) 7:33–38, 1957.

Walters, D., and Whitehead, D.: Monoamniotic twin pregnancy. Am. J. Obstet. Gynecol. 73:1129–1131, 1957.

Wan, Y.-J., Wu, T.-C., and Damjanov, I.: Twinning and conjoined placentation in mice. J. Exp. Zool. 221:81–86, 1982.

Wapner, R.J., Davis, G.H., Johnson, A., Weinblatt, V.J., Fischer, R.L., Jackson, L.G., Chervenak, F.A., and McCullough, L.B.: Selective reduction of multifetal pregnancies. Lancet 335:90–93, 1990.

Wedberg, R., Kaplan, C., Leopold, G., Porreco, R., Resnik, R., and Benirschke, K.: Cephalothoracopagus (janiceps) twinning. Obstet. Gynecol. 54:390–396, 1979.

Wei, P.Y., and Lin, C.C.: Incidence of twin births among the Chinese in Taiwan. Am. J. Obstet. Gynecol. 98:881–884, 1967.

Weinberg, W.: Beiträge zur Physiologie und Pathologie der Mehrlingsgeburten beim Menschen. Pflüegers Arch. 88: 346–430, 1901.

Weinberg, W.: Die Anlage zur Mehrlingsgeburt beim Menschen und ihre Vererbung. Arch. Rass. Ges. Biol. 6:322–339, 470–482, 609–630, 1909.

Weiner, C.P.: Diagnosis and treatment of twin to twin transfusion in the mid-trimester of pregnancy. Fetal Ther. 2: 71–74, 1987.

Weiner, J.: Selective first-trimester termination in octuplet and quadruplet pregnancies: clinical and ethical issues. Obstet. Gynecol. 72:821, 1988.

Weir, P.E., Ratten, G.J., and Beischer, N.A.: Acute polyhydramnios—a complication of monozygous twin pregnancy. Br. J. Obstet. Gynaecol. 86:849–853, 1979.

Weiss, D.B., Aboulafia, Y., and Isachson, M.: Gastroschisis and fetus papyraceus in double ovum twins. Harefuah 91: 392–394, 1976.

Wenner, R.: Les examens vasculaires des placentas gemellaires et le diagnostic des jumeaux homozygotes. Bull. Soc. R. Belge Gynecol. Obstet. 26:773–783, 1956.

Wensinger, J.A., and Daly, R.F.: Monoamniotic twins. Am. J. Obstet. Gynecol. 83:1254–1256, 1962.

Wenstrom, K.D.: Midtrimester selective delivery of an acardiac twin [letter to editor]. Am. J. Obstet. Gynecol. 168:1647, 1993.

Wenstrom, K.D., Tessen, J.A., Zlatnik, F.J., and Sipes, S.L.: Frequency, distribution, and theoretical mechanisms of hematologic and weight discordance in monochorionic twins. Obstet. Gynecol. 80:257–261, 1992.

Weston, P.A., Ives, E.J., Honoré, R.L.H., Lees, G.M., Sinclair, D.B., and Schiff, D.: Monochorionic diamniotic minimally conjoined twins: a case report. Am. J. Med. Genet. 37:558–561, 1990.

Wharton, B., Edwards, J.H., and Cameron, A.H.: Mono-amniotic twins. J. Obstet. Gynaecol. Br. Commonw. 75: 158–163, 1968.

White, C., and Wyshak, G.: Inheritance in human dizygotic twinning. N. Engl. J. Med. 271:1003–1006, 1964.

Whitehouse, D.B.: Mono-amniotic twins with one blighted. J. Obstet. Gynaecol. Br. Emp. 62:610–611, 1955.

Whitehouse, D.B.B., and Kohler, H.G.: Vasa previa in twin pregnancy. J. Obstet. Gynaecol. Br. Emp. 67:281–283, 1960.

Wiegenstein, L., and Iozzo, R.V.: Unusual findings in a conjoined ("Siamese") twin placenta. Am. J. Obstet. Gynecol. 137:744–745, 1980.

Willadsen, S.M.: A method for culture of micromanipulated sheep embryos and its use to produce monozygotic twins. Nature 277:298–300, 1979.

Williams, J.W.: Note on placentation in quadruplet and triplet pregnancy. Bull. Johns Hopkins Hosp. 39:271–280, 1926.

Willis, R.: The Borderland of Embryology and Pathology. Butterworth, London, 1958.

Wilson, J.K.: Mono-amniotic multiple pregnancy: a report of five new cases. J. Obstet. Gynaecol. Br. Emp. 62:605–609, 1955.

Wilson, R.S.: Twin growth: initial deficit, recovery, and trends in concordance from birth to nine years. Ann. Hum. Biol. 6:205–220, 1979.

Winn, H.N., Gabrielli, S., Reece, E.A., Roberts, J.A., Salafia, C., and Hobbins, J.C.: Ultrasonographic criteria for the prenatal diagnosis of placental chorionicity in twin gestations. Am. J. Obstet. Gynecol. 161:1540–1542, 1989.

Winner, W.: Parabiotic syndrome. N. Engl. J. Med. 269:1043, 1963.

Winsor, E.J.T., Brown, B.S.J., Luther, E.R., Heifetz, S., and Welch, J.P.: Deceased co-twin as a cause of false positive amniotic fluid AFP and AChE. Prenat. Diagn. 7:485–489, 1987.

Witschi, E.: Appearance of accessory "organizers" in overripe eggs of the frog. Proc. Soc. Exp. Biol. Med. 31:419–420, 1934.

Wittmann, B.K., Baldwin, V.J., and Nichol, B.: Antenatal diagnosis of twin transfusion syndrome by ultrasound. Obstet. Gynecol. 58:123–127, 1981.

Wittmann, B.K., Farquharson, D.F., Thomas, W.D.S., Baldwin, V.J., and Wadsworth, L.D.: The role of feticide in the management of severe twin transfusion syndrome. Am. J. Obstet. Gynecol. 155:1023–1026, 1986.

Wittmann, B.K., Farquharson, D., Wong, G.P., Baldwin, V., Wadsworth, L.D., and Elit, L.: Delayed delivery of second twin: report of four cases and review of the literature. Obstet. Gynecol. 79:260–263, 1992.

Wolf, H., Macdonald, J., and Bradford, W.: Holoacardius anceps with abnormal karyotype and multicystic renal dysplasia with patent ductus arteriosus in a surviving co-twin [abstract]. Mod. Pathol. 3(1):10P, 1990.

Wolf, P.L., Jones, K.L., Longway, S.R., Benirschke, K., and Bloor, C.: Prenatal death from acute myocardial infarction and cardiac tamponade due to embolus from the placenta. Am. Heart J. 109:603–605, 1985.

Wolf, W.: Zwei neue Fälle monoamniotischer Zwillinge. Inaug. Diss. Leipzig, 1920 (quoted by Verschuer, O.v: Die vererbungsbiologische Zwillingsforschung. Ergebn. Inn. Med. Kinderheilkd. 31:35, 1927).

Wurzbach, F.A., and Bunkin, I.A.: Unilateral acute hydramnios in uniovular twin pregnancy. J. Obstet. Gynaecol. Br. Emp. 56:242–245, 1949.

Wylin, R.: Acardiac monster in a triplet pregnancy. J. Reprod. Med. 6:29–32, 1971.

Yoshida, K., and Soma, H.: Outcome of the surviving cotwin of a fetus papyraceus or of a dead baby. Acta Genet. Med. Gemellol. 35:91–98, 1986.

Yoshioka, H., Kadomoto, Y., Mino, M., Morikawa, Y., Kasabuchi, Y., and Kusunoki, T.: Multicystic encephalomalacia in liveborn twin with a stillborn macerated co-twin. J. Pediatr. 95:798–800, 1979.

Young, B.K., Suidan, J., Antoine, C., Silverman, F., Lustig, I., and Wasserman, J.: Differences in twins: the importance of birth order. Am. J. Obstet. Gynecol. 151:915–921, 1985.

Young, P.E., Carson, K.F., Prichard, L.L., and Jones, O.W.: A technique for obtaining precise chromosome and bilirubin studies on amniotic fluid in twin pregnancy. J. Reprod. Med. 13:163–166, 1974.

Zeilmaker, G.H., Alberda, A.T.H., and Gent, I.v.: Fertilization and cleavage of oocytes from binovular human ovarian follicle: a possible cause of dizygotic twinning and chimerism. Fertil. Steril. 40:841–843, 1983.

Zervoudakis, I.A., Lauersen, N.H., and Saary, Z.: Unusual twin pregnancy in a double uterus. Am. J. Obstet. Gynecol. 124:659–661, 1976.

Ziomek, C.A., and Johnson, M.H.: The roles of phenotype and position in guiding the fate of 16-cell mouse blastomeres. Dev. Biol. 91:440–447, 1982.

Zuckerman, H., and Brzezinski, A.: Monoamniotic twin pregnancy: report of two cases with review of the literature. Gynaecologia 150:290–298, 1960.

Zuelzer, W.W., Beattie, K.M., and Reisman, L.E.: Generalized unbalanced mosaicism attributable to dispermy and probable fertilization of a polar body. Am. J. Hum. Genet. 16:38–51, 1964.

26
Involution of Implantation Site and Retained Placenta

Involution of the Placental Site

Pathologists rarely obtain a postpartum uterus for a detailed study of the involutional changes that take place at the former site of implantation. Therefore involution of the normal placental site has been studied by only a few investigators. Normally, the postpartum lochia contain the decidual remnants, including perhaps the remains of the vasculature that had previously undergone the so-called physiological changes of pregnancy. Only when significant postpartum hemorrhage occurs and hysterectomy becomes necessary is the pathologist asked to seek the cause of the bleeding. He or she may then find remains of villi, incompletely thrombosed vessels, "placental polyps," and some degree of inflammatory reaction. These areas are difficult to study objectively because most pathologists have no experience with the normal, complex process of placental site involution. Williams (1931), in a classical paper, attempted to rectify this situation. His study should be read before any interpretation of such postpartum uteri is undertaken. It must also be recognized that in 85% of normal, delivered placentas the decidua basalis shows foci of polymorphonuclear leukocyte infiltration (Schneider, 1970). These cells are part of an apparently normal process of implantation and are not considered an expression of deciduitis or infection.

The placenta separates from the uterus in the decidua basalis, deep to Nitabuch's fibrin layer. This fibrin layer is usually present in the floor of the delivered placenta. Contrary to some opinions, it does not serve as the cleavage plane. Placental separation probably occurs largely because of the shearing action of the underlying myometrium against the noncontractile placenta. One may speculate that detachment might be easier when the placenta is more turgid and still filled with fetal blood, but it is apparently not the case. Walsh (1968) found that when the cord is clamped early and more

fetal blood remains in the placenta, postpartum hemorrhage is significantly more common than when this blood was allowed to drain into the fetus.

Immediately after delivery the uterine surface is covered with fibrin and blood clot; the contraction of the uterus clamps the vessels and stops bleeding. Ludwig (1971) and Ludwig and Metzger (1971) have made elegant electron microscopic observations of this area postpartum. In their scanning electron microscopic study, they speak of a "wallpapering" of the endometrial surface with a delicate meshwork of cross-linked fibrin that includes deformed erythrocytes. They had shown earlier that, with the first contraction after expulsion of the placenta, this fibrin is deposited and that it aids with hemostasis. There is pronounced furrowing of the inner surface of the uterus following delivery that is bridged by the "tapestry" of fibrin. Mukaida et al. (1975), who investigated this topic more recently, came to similar conclusions.

Friedländer (1870) found that most of the endometrium degenerates after birth and that regeneration takes place from the glands and stroma in the spongy layer of the endometrium; this process is largely completed by 4 weeks, at least in the area away from the implantation site. The endometrium of the implantation site itself is not reformed for several additional weeks after delivery. The controversy over what constitutes physiological changes after birth did not cease until Williams (1931) published his comprehensive study of normal uteri that had been removed up to 4 months after delivery. He showed that the detachment of the placental site proceeded with little inflammation or necrosis. The cessation of blood flow through the endometrial vessels was largely accomplished by contraction of the uterus itself. In the absence of contraction, as in cases following former overdistension (e.g., with multiple pregnancy, hydramnios), these vessels bleed extensively. This uterine atony presents a life-threatening situation that demands emergency attention.

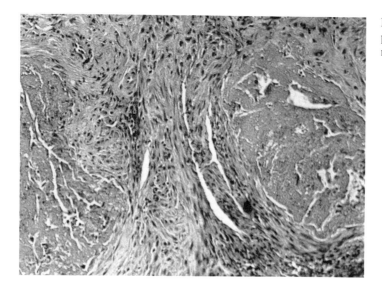

FIGURE 634. Poorly thrombosed uterine vessels of the placental site 2 weeks after delivery of a hydatidiform mole. H&E. ×160.

Normally, then, these vessels are clamped by uterine contraction; they thrombose subsequently (Figure 634), and the vascular placental site eventually becomes a mass of hyaline plaques (Figure 635). The vessels become "organized" by the ingrowth of fibrocytes and endothelium, and they are later recanalized. This process takes many weeks. One can then readily identify former implantation sites by the presence of these unusual hyalinized vessels and by the remains of some placental site giant cells. These residua of implantation have been demonstrated particularly impressively in several monkey species, in which they form macroscopically visible plaques (Bronson et al., 1972). Although the changes in monkeys are in general similar, they differ by involving usually both uterine sides, as their placenta is commonly bidiscoid. Moreover, they are much more massive and persist much longer than the approximately 7 weeks considered to be normal for women. Also, some calcification occurs in the hyaline areas of simian placental site involution, which is not often the case in humans.

The placental site is then "exfoliated," as Williams (1931) called it, rather than being absorbed into the myometrial tissue. At least the portions that are central to the myometrium are undermined. Williams (1931) considered that the decidual site is undermined by regrowth and by extension and downgrowth of endometrium that originates from remaining endometrial glands and stroma. He described it to be a "conservative" effort of nature to thus dispose of the thrombosed vessels. It must be borne in mind, however, that it applies only to the decidual portions of the placental site; the myometrial part has a much slower regressive curve.

The nature of the vascular changes that take place at the placental site postpartum was the topic of a study by

Maher (1959). He observed that the elastic membranes of placental site vessels lose their staining qualities for 25 to 30 days. After that the elastica is restored, but there is persistence of abnormalities in the pattern of the elastic membrane for a long time. Maher described striking involutional and regenerative changes of the placental site vessels and compared them with the much less prominent effect of pregnancy in those portions of

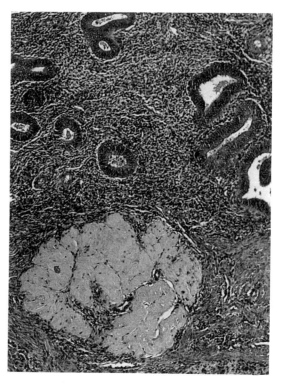

FIGURE 635. Agglomeration of hyaline masses from placental site vessels 6 weeks after normal delivery. H&E. ×64.

TABLE 32. Structural alterations in the postpartum placental site.

Time	Size (cm)	Slough	Glands	Decidua	Veins	Arteries
Term	9	Hemorrhage	Present	Viable	Hyaline	Fibrinoid
Days 1–3	7–8	Early necrosis	Prominent	Necrosis	Thrombosis	Obliterated
Days 3–5	6	With reaction	Atypia	Necrosis	Organization	Hyalinized
Days 5–8	4.5	Demarcated	Increased	Regression	Organization	Hyalinized
Weeks 4–20	2	Hemosiderin	Inactive	Absent	Recanalized	Remnants of hyaline

Reprinted with permission from Anderson and Davis placental site involution. Am J Obstet. Gynecol. 102:23–33, 1968.

the uterus and tube that are remote from the implantation site.

Anderson and Davis (1968) made the next major contribution to the study of placental site involution. They believed that vascular constriction and occlusion cause necrosis and sloughing of the former decidua basalis. They confirmed the findings of Sharman (1953), which were made from 626 postpartum biopsies and 11 uteri, removed 1 to 9 months after delivery. Anderson and Davis suggested that the absence of necrosis observed by Williams (1931) was due to his lack of appropriate material from days 4 to 7 postpartum. They corrected this deficiency and measured the placental site. Immediately after birth of the infant, the placental site was 18 cm; after the placenta detached it measured 9 cm (largely because of uterine contraction), and it was 4 mm in thickness. At 8 days postpartum, the placental site measured only 4.5 cm in diameter; and by 8 weeks it had shrunk to 2 cm. The latest time at which a normal placental site was visible macroscopically was 11 weeks after delivery. In contrast to Williams' (1931) opinion, a 6 mm deep area of necrosis of the placental site, extending onto the myometrium, was observed from 2 to 6 days. A mixed "granulocytic and mononuclear inflammatory infiltrate occurred in the slough and the viable endomyometrium." Anderson and Davis (1968) described the physiological adenomyosis that occurs in the superficial myometrium, particularly in the center of the former placental site, and they delineated the development of pleomorphic nucleated cells of the endometrial glands. In their experience, placental site giant cells persisted for several days, were confined to the superficial layers, and did not extend deep into the myometrium. Villi were found in four early specimens from apparently uncomplicated pregnancies. None of these elements normally persisted past 4 weeks. Vessels were described as thrombosed and showing "endophlebitis." Endothelial proliferation was a particularly prominent feature in the veins. Toward the end of the first week, the veins showed the beginning of organization of clots; arterial thrombosis was not a prominent feature. Because these normal changes are often misinterpreted, a summary of the features of sequential events is presented in Table 32.

Anderson and Davis (1968) were unable to resolve the nature of the placental site giant cells but favored a trophoblastic origin for these cellular elements. They stated emphatically that involution of the placental site does not lead to "fibrosis" of the uterus. They insisted that the term subinvolution must be understood within the framework of these normal involutional processes.

Sharman (1953) found that mitoses of the endometrium first occurred 8 days after delivery. By 16 days the endometrium was structurally intact again. He also observed an "appreciable number" of plasma cells to be present 6 weeks after birth in 50% of his cases (37% had plasma cells at 3 to 4 months postpartum). This result is surprising, as it implies infection in one-half of postpartum patients. It must be reiterated, however, that the inflammatory reaction of the normal placental site involutional process is usually sparse, and in most women it is confined to the first few days. Moreover, this infiltrate is made up of granulocytes and macrophages; plasma cells appear only late in this process.

Subinvolution

At times the uterus does not involute properly, and the clinical diagnosis of uterine subinvolution is entertained. What are the pathological equivalents of this condition? Khong and Khong (1993) are the most recent authors to have examined this phenomenon, with the evaluation of 169 specimens from "delayed postpartum hemorrhage" following a singleton delivery. They provided some reason why such studies should be divided into periods before and after 6 weeks postpartum, not an important issue for pathologists, we believe. Retained placental tissue was most common (45 cases), followed by "subinvolution" (i.e., widely patent uteroplacental arteries) in 30 patients. Endometritis ($n = 7$) was uncommon, and most other patients had essentially normal histological findings.

Normally the uterus shrinks rapidly, with dissolution of the myometrium. In 2 weeks its size reduces from about 1,000 g to nearly 100 g, and the endometrium and placental site are cast off. With subinvolution this regression is delayed; the uterus remains boggy and

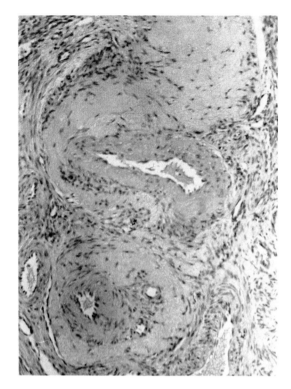

FIGURE 636. Myometrial remnants of a former placental site with hyalinization 2 years after normal delivery and death for unrelated reasons. H&E. ×160.

edematous and may actually be retroflexed and congested. Often there is bleeding and some remaining placental tissue ("placental polyp"), or an infection may cause uterine subinvolution. Thorsteinsson and Kempers (1970) studied the records of 148 patients with delayed postpartum bleeding (1%) and found that this

bleeding most commonly resulted from subinvolution of the placental site. Curettage was done in 94 patients, 78 of whom were found to harbor microscopic fragments of placental tissue; seven additional patients had grossly visible placental remains. Curettage cured most patients. It is interesting to note here also that most of the patients ($n = 135$) were said to have had normal placentas at delivery.

According to Stamm (1961), incompletely removed placentas have been the cause of litigation. He believed that evaluating the completeness of the placenta by injecting milk is inaccurate, and that it should not become a routine procedure. Tears in the placenta often occur, which makes it difficult to ascertain with certainty that removal was complete. Stamm suggested that manual exploration of the uterus is necessary when one is uncertain if a placenta has been removed completely.

Placental Polyps

Placental polyps were described in three patients by Hoberman and his colleagues (1963) who also reviewed the sparse English literature on this topic. Placental polyps are usually composed of remnants of villous tissue that have become encased in layered clot. At times one finds that the villi are directly attached to the myometrium; they are thus focal placentas accretas, but because of degenerative changes this diagnosis is often impossible to verify.

When these "polyps" are removed, the symptoms usually abate. If they are not removed, life-threatening bleeding may occur. This possibility was emphasized in the study of placental polyps undertaken by Dyer and

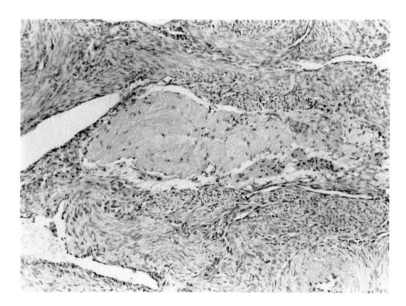

FIGURE 637. Finding similar to that in Figure 636 but deeper in the myometrium. H&E. ×160.

Bradburn (1971). They decried that this important complication of the puerperium is rarely mentioned in modern textbooks. Dyer and Bradburn described the immediate type polyp, which occurs during the first month after delivery, and the delayed type, where the tissue may be discovered months or even years later. They acknowledged that accretas may be part of the problem but believe that other, unrecognized factors play a role as well. Finally, they speculated that such retained fragments are the possible sites of future trophoblastic tumors. In our opinion, there is little evidence for the latter speculation, even though the placental site tumor has become a delineated entity (see Chapter 23). Philippe et al. (1968) claimed that deficient arterial occlusion at involution is a probable cause of postpartum hemorrhage. After studying and depicting the normal vascular occlusions, these authors showed hugely distended vessels with poorly organized thrombi, as well as increased hyaline masses, to be a cause of the bleeding that may take place later, when early postpartum hemorrhage has occurred. Philippe and his colleagues speculated that these vascular changes may result from inadequate hormonal effects on these vessels during the immediate postpartum period. They also suggested that therapy with 17 hydroxyprogesterone caproate may resolve the condition and that hysterectomy is not always indicated. Rutherford and Hertig (1945) demonstrated "placental polyps" in three postpartum patients who did not have placental remains and inflammation; they had hugely dilated, improperly occluded, placental site vessels. Perhaps this situation is "true" subinvolution, a process whose etiology is yet to be clarified. Most recently, late bleeding has been associated with the discovery of hyalinized masses ("placental site nodules"); when stained with antibodies to human placental lactogen (hPL), these masses were found to contain positively staining placental site giant cells (Young et al., 1988). The authors cautioned that they are benign remnants of placentation that must not be mistaken for tumor. Suffice it to say, retained placental villi are not always present in patients who experience postpartum hemorrhage. Incomplete occlusion of vessels alone may be the cause of subinvolution, as may idiopathic failure of trophoblastic placental site cells to involute.

In addition to these features of subinvolution, of course, there is postpartum endometritis, or "puerperal

→

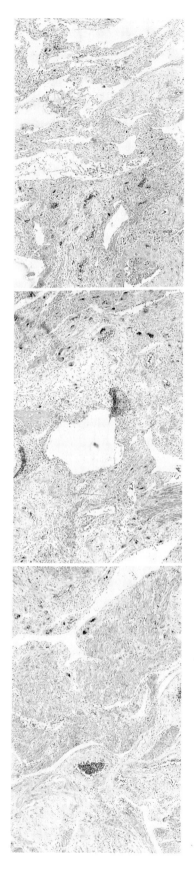

FIGURE 638. Composite of implantation site with endometrium above. This patient had retained placental tissue for 16 weeks (see Figure 639), and many of the placental site giant cells (dark) persist deep in the myometrium. No vascular thrombosis had occurred. H&E. ×16.

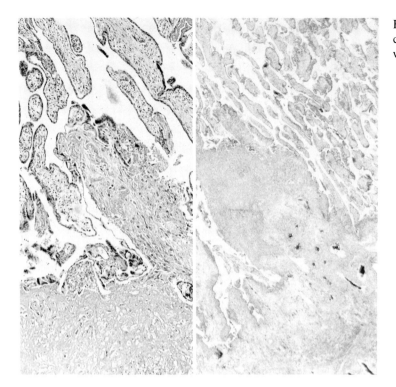

FIGURE 639. Live and necrotic villi forming the placental polyp of the uterus shown in Figure 638 at 16 weeks after delivery. H&E. ×64.

fever," an infection caused by a variety of microorganisms. Its prototype, however, is caused by group A streptococci. The histological features may be similar to those seen with other subinvolutional events, although additionally there are pronounced acute inflammation, infiltration with plasma cells, phlebothrombosis, and bacterial organisms. All are life-threatening processes that may also lead to pulmonary embolism. Various aspects of a placental polyp symptomatic 9 years after abortion of the last known pregnancy were reported by Lawrence et al. (1988). At the time of abortion the patient had undergone sterilization. The polyp was composed mostly of "necrotic and hyalinized villi, without identifiable trophoblast." A few syncytial cells exhibited human chorionic gonadotropin (hCG) immunohistochemically, and abundant X cells were present with the hPL reaction. Regrettably, the authors did not report on the status of the ovaries so as to rule out a possible recent pregnancy. They also reviewed the few case reports and case series from the literature, which included a placental polyp 21 years after pregnancy.

In our experience, the hyaline material of former placental sites may persist in the uterus for much longer than has been indicated in most of the literature cited here, much as the corpus albicans persists for years in the ovary. The myometrial remnants of former placental site vessels are shown in Figures 636 and 637, assuredly 2 years after the last pregnancy. Figure 638 shows the uterus of a patient with retained placental tissue who

died 16 weeks postpartum. Numerous trophoblastic cells can be seen throughout the myometrium of the placental site. Most, but not all, villi were completely necrotic in this patient (Figure 639).

Involution of a Remaining Placenta

Involution of remaining placenta is conveniently dealt with here because some of its features resemble the findings of retained placental tissue and placental polyps. When fetectomy is performed in monkeys between the 10th and 23rd weeks of pregnancy, it is alleged that the placenta is delivered on time (Van Wagenen & Newton, 1943). Lewis and Hertz (1966) found that most of their monkeys developed degenerated placentas when fetectomy was done between the 14th and 35th days of gestation. They had expected to find hydatid swelling, perhaps molar transformation; but it did not occur. In similar, larger experiments, Panigel and Myers (1972) also did not find hydatid changes following either fetectomy or ligation of the vessels that extend to the monkey's second placental disk (the bridging vessels). They observed that some villi remained structurally normal for several weeks, although their fetal capillaries and red blood cells soon disintegrated. The maintenance of some fine structural detail in these surviving villi is indeed remarkable. The villi become usually more compacted, rather than hydropic. Detaching a disk of the placenta and thereby interrupting the maternal perfusion in monkeys, however, led to placental infarction (Myers & Panigel, 1973). In many ways the villous changes found after prolonged retention of the placenta resemble those encountered following fetal demise (Fox, 1968). They are initiated by syncytial knotting, stromal fibrosis with loss of capillaries, and "fibrosis" of major stem vessels. Calcification and complete villous hyalinization are end-stages.

When investigation of the factors that initiate labor required reexamination of the role of fetectomy, specifically as it relates to the role played by the fetal adrenal and pituitary glands, Lanman et al. (1975) restudied the placental changes following fetectomy in the monkey. In the 13 animals these authors examined, fetectomy was performed between 65 and 143 days (term is 168 days). Nine of the placentas remained in situ beyond the expected date of delivery; two delivered near term; and two delivered prematurely. Histological study revealed empty vessels, stromal fibrosis of villi, hyalinization, and calcification 17 to 108 days after fetectomy. X cell hyperplasia was prominent in two placentas. The placental weights were similar to what was expected at the time of fetectomy. They were much smaller than expected for the gestational age of the placenta. Somewhat different results were obtained by Nathanielsz et al. (1992). These authors were unable to obtain the placentas for dissection but, because of the endocrine changes that occurred after fetectomy the authors decided that a functional fetal circulation in necessary for normal gestational control.

The anatomical results just reviewed are also the experience with retained placentas in women whose fetus has died or when only one fetus of twins survives. The placental tissue remains intact for a long time. It first loses its fetal vasculature and undergoes fibrosis, and much fibrin accumulates particularly in the intervillous space. The placenta eventually atrophies and comes to resemble an infarct. The result is not a true infarct, of course, because an infarct occurs only after interruption of the maternal intervillous circulation.

References

Anderson, W.R., and Davis, J.: Placental site involution. Am. J. Obstet. Gynecol. 102:23–33, 1968.

Bronson, R., Volk, T.L., and Ruebner, B.H.: Involution of placental site and corpus luteum in the monkey. Am. J. Obstet. Gynecol. 113:70–75, 1972.

Dyer, I., and Bradburn, D.M.: An inquiry into the etiology of placental polyps. Am. J. Obstet. Gynecol. 109:858–867, 1971.

Fox, H.: Morphological changes in the human placenta following fetal death. J. Obstet. Gynaecol. Br. Commonw. 75:839–843, 1968.

Friedländer, C.: Physiologisch-anatomische Untersuchungen über den Uterus. Simmel, Leipzig, 1870.

Hoberman, L.K., Hawkinson, J.A., and Beecham, C.T.: Placental polyp: report of 3 cases. Obstet. Gynecol. 22: 25–29, 1963.

Khong, T.Y., and Khong, T.K.: Delayed postpartum hemorrhage: a morphologic study of causes and their relation to other pregnancy disorders. Obstet. Gynecol. 82:17–22, 1993.

Lanman, J.T., Mitsudo, S.M., Brinson, A.O., and Thau, R.B.: Fetectomy in monkeys (Macaca mulatta); retention of the placenta past term. Biol. Reprod. 12:522–525, 1975.

Lawrence, W.D., Qureshi, F., and Bonakdar, M.I.: "Placental polyp": light microscopic and immunohistochemical observations. Hum. Pathol. 19:1467–1470, 1988.

Lewis, J., and Hertz, R.: Effects of early embryectomy and hormonal therapy on the fate of the placenta in pregnant rhesus monkeys. Proc. Soc. Exp. Biol. Med. 123:805–809, 1966.

Ludwig, H.: Surface structure of the human term placenta and of the uterine wall post partum in the screen scan electron microscope. Am. J. Obstet. Gynecol. 111:328–344, 1971.

Ludwig, H., and Metzger, H.: Das uterine Placentarbett post partum im Rasterelektronenmikroskop, zugleich ein Beitrag der extravasalen Fibrinbildung. Arch. Gynecol. 210:251–266, 1971.

Maher, J.A.: Morphologic and histochemical changes in postpartum uterine blood vessels. Arch. Pathol. 67:175–180, 1959.

Mukaida, T., Yoshida, K., and Soma, H.: A surface ultrastructural study of the placental separation site. J. Clin. Electron Microsc. 8:5–6, 1975.

Myers, R.E., and Panigel, M.: Experimental placental detachment in the rhesus monkey: changes in villous ultrastructure. J. Med. Primatol. 2:170–189, 1973.

Nathanielsz, P.W., Figueroa, J.P., and Honnebier, M.B.O.M.: In the rhesus monkey placental retention after fetectomy at 121 to 130 days' gestation outlasts the normal duration of pregnancy. Am. J. Obstet. Gynecol. 166:1529–1535, 1992.

Panigel, M., and Myers, R.E.: Histological and ultrastructural changes in rhesus monkey placenta following interruption of fetal placental circulation by fetectomy or interplacental umbilical vessel ligation. Acta Anat. (Basel) 81:481–506, 1972.

Philippe, E., Ritter, J., Renaud, R., Dellenbach, P., Fonck-Cussac, Y., and Gandar, R.: Les métrorrhagies tardives du post-partum par anomalie d'involution des artères utéro-placentaires. Rev. Fr. Gynecol. 63:255–262, 1968.

Rutherford, R.N., and Hertig, A.T.: Noninvolution of the placental site. Am. J. Obstet. Gynecol. 49:378–384, 1945.

Schneider, L.: Über Vorkommen und Bedeutung leukocytärer Infiltrate im Ablösungsbereich der spontan geborenen Placenta. Arch. Gynecol. 208:247–254, 1970.

Sharman, A.: Post-partum regeneration of the human endometrium. J. Anat. 87:1–10, 1953.

Stamm, H.: Alte und neue Probleme bei Plazentarpolypen. Gynaecologia 151:252–260, 1961.

Thorsteinsson, V.T., and Kempers, R.D.: Delayed postpartum bleeding. Am. J. Obstet. Gynecol. 107:565–571, 1970.

Van Wagenen, G., and Newton, W.H.: Pregnancy in the monkey after removal of the fetus. Surg. Gynecol. Obstet. 77:539–549, 1943.

Walsh, S.Z.: Maternal effects of early and late clamping of the umbilical cord. Lancet 1:996–997, 1968.

Williams, J.W.: Regeneration of the uterine mucosa after delivery, with especial reference to the placental site. Am. J. Obstet. Gynecol. 22:664–696, 793–796, 1931.

Young, R.H., Kurman, R.J., and Scully, R.E.: Placental site nodule. Mod. Pathol. 1:107A, 1988.

27
Legal Considerations

There continues to be a significant number of litigations against hospitals and obstetricians in which the placenta becomes an important participant in advising the disputing parties on prenatal circumstances. This litigation is initiated most often on behalf of children with cerebral palsy and occasionally with malformations, stillbirth, or other less than optimal or expected outcome (Rosenblatt & Hurst, 1989; Richards & Thomasson, 1992). Record-keeping of the clinical circumstances and a professional placental study prove to be of utmost importance in many cases. Weinstein (1988), who wrote a concise review on the topic, asserted that such litigation is principally the result of the following.

1. Society's belief that all wrongs must have a reason and that the wrongs must be put right
2. Pervasive lottery mentality
3. Inability of many individuals to accept responsibility for themselves or their actions
4. Increasing incidence of true medical negligence.

Many physicians who have become involved in this legal process in one way or another have witnessed that Weinstein's third point is now common reality. Physicians frequently take care of pregnant patients who continue the use of alcohol and tobacco during pregnancy despite many personal or public warnings against it. Other pregnant patients abuse themselves with cocaine, crack, and other agents and thus endanger their fetus simultaneously. This aspect of modern society was discussed in an incisive paper on wrongful births by Fleischer (1987). Unfortunately, these facts are rarely taken into serious consideration when malpractice claims are litigated, or they are casually dismissed as likely not being contributory. Other physicians argue that the fourth of the above statements is incorrect; they believe that there has been no true increase of medical malpractice—only the lawsuits that claim it to be true have increased. Sandmire (1989) provided

cogent evidence for this view. No doubt there has been an increase in the overall incidence of cerebral palsy as a result of the increasingly smaller babies for whom care is provided (Anonymous, 1989; Kuban & Leviton, 1994). Conversely, older causes of cerebral palsy-like condition, such as kernicterus, have all but disappeared, and fewer term babies now suffer this fate. However, the oversimplified allegations of intrapartum hypoxia and its blanket relation to neonatal pH or Apgar score and the ultimate infant performance are often incorrectly assessed, and assumption of negligence or guilt on the part of a perinatologist is frequently not justified. The understanding of how cerebral palsy develops is still imperfect, as reviewed by Nelson and Leviton (1991) and Kuban and Leviton (1994). Cases such as those described by Lopez-Zeno et al. (1990) should always be remembered before hasty conclusions are drawn. These authors observed the survival of a normal child delivered by cesarean section 22 minutes after maternal cardiac arrest had occurred, which was 45 minutes after the fatal shooting of the mother. Follow-up failed to show neurological damage; the placenta was not described. The complete anoxia incurred by this fetus is much longer and certainly more severe than is the case for many alleged cerebral palsy hypoxia cases. Thus careful evaluation is indicated. In a careful review, Perkins (1987) examined this complex field. It should be required reading before drawing unwarranted conclusions. It is especially noteworthy that Perkins concluded that "the number of infants injured before labor is highly underestimated," and that "of infants injured during labor is highly overestimated." The placental record can help materially in sorting out these discrepancies.

"The examination of the placenta may be viewed as a diary of the pregnancy," Gillan (1992) has aptly stated, and the placenta has therefore become an increasingly important organ in adjudicating medicolegal allegations. Regrettably, this aspect was not considered in the last review on cerebral palsy (Kuban & Leviton, 1994). Altshuler and Herman (1989) reviewed specific areas that need to be addressed by pathologists, and they considered some of the epidemiological principles in a thoughtful review of this medicolegal topic. Of particular interest is their capsular review of relevant pathological features of the placenta and the possible correlations of lesions with fetal hypoxic states. They were correct in reiterating that the placenta "is an objective diary, related to the outcome of pregnancy." More recently, Altshuler (1993a,b) has produced two incisive reviews of the principal lesions of the placenta that may be of paramount importance in reflecting a prenatal onset of hypoxic insults. The reviews suggested that the presence of nucleated red blood cells at term, chronic villitis, meconium damage, excessive fibrin deposits, chorioamnionitis, chorangiosis, and placental dysmaturity are the most important aspects to be considered in this context. The papers also provide a triage for placental study. Furthermore, an important meeting of pathologists, perinatologists, and the legal profession resulted in a volume that attempts to address the complexity of the medicolegal aspects of placental pathology (Travers & Schmidt, 1991).

The pathologist is often consulted to render specific advice on pathological findings and on other perinatal aspects of pregnancies with poor outcomes. This consultation prominently includes considerations of findings made at placental examinations. All too often, however, the placental material available is insufficient for an expert opinion. Recommendations are here made how to collect placentas for such possible need in the future. Altshuler and Herman (1989) suggested that one should briefly record findings from placental examination of *all* deliveries because cerebral palsy may occur with entirely normal deliveries. We agree with this view but find it to be an impractical task for most hospitals. In order to have placental material available for possible future study, they also suggested that formalin-fixed samples be embedded in paraffin and archived as uncut specimens. In our view, the value accruing to the child and pediatrician from an examination of the placenta at the time of delivery supersedes the storage of unexamined material. It is particularly regrettable, as happens occasionally, that erroneous testimony is given in best faith because the consultant has not properly evaluated all the facts of a given case. He or she may have reviewed only the slides without knowing the gross findings of the placenta, for instance, and based his or her opinions solely on those histological findings that were available, whereas detailed study of perinatal circumstances might have provided a more educated judgment. Of course, pathologists should not be put into the position of making judgments on monitor strips

and the like. They must, however, have a general idea of the entirety of the complex cases before the placental examination can be meaningfully interpreted. Even more unfortunate is testimony by "experts" who have little experience in placental pathology. Likewise, pathologists must be mindful not to render expert opinions on areas that are outside their field of competence, for instance regarding the findings of heart rate monitoring.

Litigations have had an impact on the practice of perinatal medicine without having much improved our knowledge of the cause(s) of cerebral palsy. Because the placental study often provides significant insight into prenatal life, however, it has become apparent to many health care providers that, when caring for problematical neonates or when difficulties during labor and delivery are encountered, the placenta should be examined professionally. The notion that it is imperative to examine the placenta, if only to establish the cause of the perinatal death, is not new. For instance, during efforts to understand the causes of fetal demise Davies and Arroyo (1985) were able to ascertain the cause of perinatal death by autopsy alone in 47.6%. For the purpose of ascribing a cause of death, however, placental study was necessary in an additional 34.0% of their material. We have reviewed our material of perinatal autopsies from 2 years and found that the true cause of perinatal death could not be established in 15.6% of the cases (Figure 640). Thrombosis of vessels, maternal floor infarct, villitis, and abruptio placentae are major reasons in singletons why the placenta must be studied. Driscoll (1965) found it also to be true for 16% of her case material; Salafia and Vintzileos (1990) were equally emphatic about the need to examine all placentas.

If the *cause* of perinatal mortality is strongly corroborated by placental findings, the same is likely to be true of possible perinatal fetal or neonatal damage, making the examination of this organ all the more mandatory. In order to have the placentas of neonates with developing problems available for study, suggestions were made in Chapter 2 how best to store placentas. This triage of the selection and other related aspects of placental study were well detailed in tabular form by Altshuler (1993a,b). Aside from the aspect of placental storage, to facilitate examination of the placenta in cases of possible neonatal difficulties it is our opinion that *all* placentas of twins, premature infants, and deliveries in which meconium staining or other obvious perinatal problems are apparent should be studied by the pathologist. It is imperative that these findings then become an entry in the patient's record. This practice is not only desirable for adjudicating many legal cases in which placental pathology can be helpful,

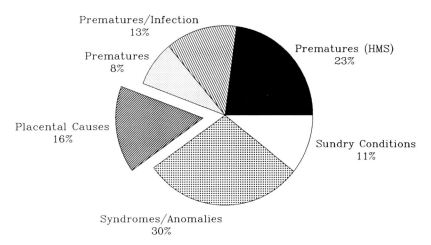

FIGURE 640. Perinatal autopsy findings in 122 consecutive cases (University of California, San Diego, 1981–1982). Placental examination was necessary in 19 (16%) to provide the cause of death. In many others, especially the premature infants and anomalies, there were abnormal placental findings, such as inflammation and single umbilical artery, but they were not the *cause* of death. HMS = hyaline membrane syndrome.

it may materially assist the obstetrician when counseling about future pregnancies and in the accumulation of data that may ultimately help our understanding of perinatal problems.

We have often wished in legal consults that a photograph of the placenta was available, particularly when confronted with the record of a poorly described or inadequately studied placenta. This desire has been made light of in litigations, but photography can be easily accomplished on delivery floors, where pictures of neonates are taken routinely. This step has also been advocated for regions where pathological support is inadequate (Ward, 1991). If photography is impractical, a drawing of salient findings (e.g., to indicate the insertion of the umbilical cord or the presence of twin vascular anastomoses) is often more helpful than a poor description of the gross features. Ideally, of course, all placentas would have an examination by a knowledgeable pathologist, but it is not likely to happen routinely. Those placentas that are studied, however, must be adequately sampled for histology. At least three sections of villous tissue plus one of cord and a membrane roll are optimal. When selecting the villous tissue, it is important that more than the obviously infarcted or pathological areas are sampled; infarcts all look the same microscopically. For an appreciation of the placental status (e.g., for the identification of Tenney-Parker changes in preeclampsia or chorangiosis and villitis) the more normal-appearing villous tissue is usually more informative than are sections of infarcts. In the membrane roll, the decidua capsularis must be included, as it is the best site for an analysis of maternal vessel pathology and for the appreciation of inflammatory processes. Formalin fixation of placentas before examination provides much less valuable information than examination of a fresh organ. The sooner the placenta is studied, the better are the results; however, storage in a refrigerator preserves the salient feature for many days. There is little autolysis when the placenta is refrigerated; it only loses some weight during storage by extrusion of villous water, particularly edematous organs. The pathologist must also become familiar with the artifacts produced by fixation, especially being cognizant of changes in weight after fixation (the weight increases).

As stated earlier, litigations have involved, most importantly, deliveries in which cerebral palsy became a problem in the future development of an infant. This development is, in general, much more common in prematurely born infants, in twins, and in infants born after prolonged pregnancies. The study of the causes of cerebral palsy is a difficult aspect of medicine, as no single etiology can possibly be assigned, despite the large prospective Collaborative Perinatal Study. Rosen and Dickinson (1992) estimated that 2.7 per 1,000 children age 5 to 7 years suffer a form of this illness. Nearly 36% have occurred in children with birth weights of less than 2,500 g, and they suggested that 70% had an antenatal onset. Interestingly, Rosen and Dickinson (1993) provided evidence that electronic fetal monitoring was unable to predict the development of cerebral palsy, even though this ability had been the original intent for this technology. Naeye and Peters (1987) examined the 7-year outcome of children from the aforementioned large Collaborative Perinatal Study of 56,000 pregnancies. Their overriding conclusion was that chronic, rather than acute, hypoxia has a greater influence on abnormal brain development (see comments by Harkavy, 1987, and those by Durant and Woodward, 1987). This study, as many others, well demonstrated how complex is the topic of the cause of cerebral palsy (see also Naeye et al., 1989; Naeye, 1992). The two reviews of Altshuler (1993a,b) cited many additional studies that should be consulted by the reader who wishes to obtain a rounded appreciation of this complex topic. At the same time, cerebral palsy also has obviously great social and medical importance; the disease often represents a major tragedy to the families involved, let alone the child. One of the most thoughtful reviews of this complexity was provided by Perkins (1987). Additional studies from Australia are summarized in the Collaborative Perinatal Study involving 608 children reported by Aylward et al. (1989). These authors also found only weak correlations to perinatal variables. Their instructive tables show impressively that many time-honored indicators of "asphyxia" have little or no bearing on the cerebral outcome of the neonate. Regrettably, items such as meconium staining and many more conditions of concern to us were not studied. Grant et al. (1989) have also concluded from their randomized study of the possible benefits of intrapartum monitoring that prevention of cerebral palsy is difficult. This study and others have been succinctly annotated in editorial comments (Anonymous, 1989; Freeman, 1990).

The findings collected during a competent placental examination, including histological examination, frequently identify abnormal prenatal circumstances that had not been recognized clinically. Thus they have often materially aided in advising the legal profession accurately. For the purpose of this chapter, we summarize salient points that have derived from our experience in this arena. More details on the conditions to be described may be found in the relevant sections of this book. It must be reemphasized that an interpretation of the placenta alone is often insufficient to arrive at a full appreciation of the complexity of individual cases. It is frequently necessary to know many facts in addition to the placental findings in order to render appropriate advice. For instance, one may need to know the identity of microrganisms in infectious cases. The social history may be of considerable importance; and an accurate estimation of the length of gestation, the complications known to have occurred during pregnancy, and so on must all be weighed in the context of the placental findings. These items provide valuable information with which one is in a better position to interpret subtle placental findings. Reviewed here are only some of the more common placental problems that we have encountered and observations we have made during the litigation process.

Twinning Problems

Placentas from twins provide the pathologist with the unique opportunity to compare different placental features with neonatal outcome. Thus the fetus accompanied by a velamentous insertion of the umbilical cord is usually more growth-retarded than one with a normal cord and is thus uniquely exposed also to the prenatal hazards of anomalous cord insertion. Multiple births not only have a much higher incidence of prematurity, they suffer a manifold increased frequency of cerebral palsy compared with singletons. Studies have suggested that some of these cerebral lesions have a prenatal onset because cystic areas of areas of former white matter necrosis are sometimes evident at birth (Bejar et al., 1990). Larroche (1986) described a case that also demonstrated these prenatal lesions; she found other cases of prenatal encephalopathies associated with trauma and other prenatal events. Central nervous system (CNS) damage of prenatal onset appears to be commoner in monozygotic monochorionic twins. It is therefore imperative that the membrane relation of *all* twins be firmly established at the time of delivery or during placental study if one wants to understand the origin of the lesions. This point is particularly important when one twin has died prenatally. Coagulative, destructive events in the survivor are then especially common; such events are usually confined to monochorionic twins. They generally have a prenatal onset, as sonographic studies have clearly shown (Patten et al., 1989), and commence soon after the death of one fetus (Liu et al., 1992; Benirschke, 1993).

As stated earlier, monochorionic twins not only have a higher rate of prematurity, they suffer perinatal mortality more frequently (Baldwin, 1994). The highest mortality attends monoamnionic twins. Monoamnionic monochorionic (MoMo) twins entangle their cords frequently, which causes restrictions to venous return from the placenta. This problem often kills one or both fetuses; in others one can infer venous return problems from existing thrombi. Vascular anastomoses between twins may allow rapid shifts of blood from one twin to the other, which may lead to acute anemia and hypotension in utero. Neonatal anemia in one of twins, where the other has died in utero, had been difficult to interpret prior to detailed placental studies. It goes without saying that the umbilical cords of twins must be labeled at delivery, so it becomes possible to assign specific placental lesions to individual infants. It is also necessary to identify and record the presence of a fetus papyraceus, as it may have greatly affected the development of the surviving twin through interplacental vascular anastomoses. Perhaps the cause of the death of one twin was sublethal to the other.

Furthermore, inflammatory processes have an important impact on fetal well-being, and they are frequently correlated with cerebral palsy. As was indicated in the consideration of infections, in twins chorioamnionitis more often affects twin A. When one has knowledge of the location of twins in utero, it may lead to a better appreciation of possible aspiration pneumonia and other fetal effects.

Twins have a high frequency of velamentous and marginal insertion of the umbilical cords, and these insertional abnormalities are at times correlated with single umbilical artery (SUA). The membranous vessels may have ruptured during delivery and have caused acute anemia; or they may be thrombosed, which often produces dire fetal sequelae. SUAs are also generally more common in twins, not only when the cords are marginally inserted. When twins are delivered by cesarean section, the twin located in the lower uterine segment may actually be delivered as the second twin. Therefore recording the distance of membrane rupture from the edge of the placenta aids in assigning the correct position of twins in utero when labeling of cords is inadequate. This point has particular relevance with respect to inflammation and to the possible rupture of velamentous vessels.

Twins with velamentous insertion of the umbilical cord are usually smaller than those with more normal cord position. Such discrepancy in size does not automatically affirm the diagnosis of the transfusion syndrome, as is all too readily done; that diagnosis requires the demonstration of the responsible arteri-ovenous (A-V) shunts in the monochorionic twin placenta. The transfusion syndrome is an important aspect of monozygotic twinning. It is largely responsible for the frequent occurrence of hydramnios in twin pregnancy that leads to the high frequency of premature delivery of monochorionic twins. Although anemia and plethora of the neonatal twins may be obvious, these findings alone do not accurately attest to the underlying cause, the presence of an A-V fistula in the placenta. Plethora can occur in one twin when, for instance, the first-born twin has been allowed to drain blood into the second while it is still in utero. A surviving twin also may partially and acutely exsanguinate into a stillborn twin while in utero with resulting acute hypotension. Knowledge of the time when clamping of the cords was done may be important when interpreting discordant hemoglobin values of twins. When one twin is small for gestational age, possibly because it had a velamentous insertion of the cord, large surface anastomoses may drain blood from the larger twin into the smaller member while still in situ, in apparent paradox to the transfusion syndrome. However, this situation is *not* the equivalent of the classical transfusion syndrome. For all these reasons it is important that the nature of interfetal placental blood vessel anastomoses be ascertained, possibly by injection of the placental vasculature. The findings are best recorded by making a drawing of these connections; they cannot otherwise be readily reconstructed.

Inflammation

As with the cause of some premature monochorionic twins, chorioamnionitis (membranitis) and funisitis are much overrepresented in children who develop cerebral palsy. These pathological changes are now clearly established as being the result of ascending infection. They cannot be explained by hypoxia occurring during labor or assigned to changes in amnionic pH, as had been previously suggested. Infections are not only much more common in premature deliveries, they are indeed probably a main reason for most premature births before 30 weeks' gestation (see Ornoy et al., 1976, for a consideration of its importance in stillbirths). Ascending infection also correlates with prenatal cystic changes in the brain. Studies have suggested that the hypoxia may be the result of vasoconstriction engendered by the release of prostaglandins, tumor necrosis factor, or other vasoactive agents that come either from the inflammatory exudate or from bacterial products suspended in the amnionic cavity.

Culturing the surface of the placenta is usually not as helpful for studying the cause of chorioamnionitis as is a meticulous histological study. The causative organisms of chorioamnionitis frequently do not grow readily in the laboratory, or they require special microbiological attention that is not always available. Moreover, the placenta is frequently contaminated by the birth process, making most routine cultures worthless, or the patient has received antibiotics before delivery. It may be more practical to obtain culture material from underneath the chorionic plate or to make touch preparations of the placental surface for the identification of organisms. Chorioamnionitis is an occasional cause of thrombosis in fetal surface vessels; it can be identified macroscopically by the appearance of white-yellow streaks on the surfaces of blood vessels. Altshuler and Herman (1989) referred to the mural thrombi as cushions, following De Sa's lead (1984) (Figure 641). They must be sampled for histological study.

When thrombi have developed in large fetal surface vessels, the distal fetal villous vascular bed degenerates, leading to defoliation of vascular endothelium, dispersion of blood, and disorganization of the vessels. It produces the appearance of hemorrhagic endovasculitis (HEV), which we consider not to be an inflammatory but a degenerative process. It is commonly found in the main stem placental vessels of stillborn infants, but this

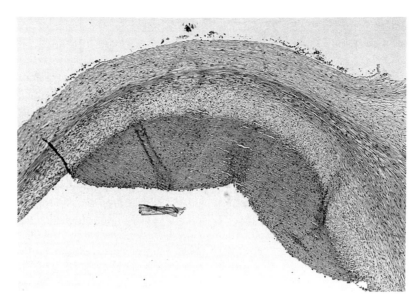

FIGURE 641. Mural thrombus in a placental surface vein ("cushion") of a child with unexplained cerebral palsy. Note that the vein wall is partially degenerated. The lesion was not recognized macroscopically or microscopically by the pathologist who signed out the case. H&E. ×160.

endothelial degeneration has then usually occurred *after* the fetus' death. Unfortunately, much inappropriate testimony has been given in the past, with this confusing entity of HEV supposedly indicating the existence of undiagnosed virus infections before birth. Perhaps the most informative finding for an understanding of HEV has come from finding the lesion confined to the placental bed of only the dead MZ twin of a diamnionic monochorionic (DiMo) twin placenta. The fact that the surviving twin's placental bed did not have HEV nearly invalidates the possible inference that HEV is a specific pathological finding of prenatal disease. In his study of placentas from stillborn fetuses, Genest (1992) depicted these changes and placed a time frame on their occurrence (see Chapter 13).

Villous tissue must be sampled for microscopy in all cases of a suspected virus infection. It must be admitted, however, that many virus infections are difficult to identify precisely by histopathological study alone. For instance, the immunodeficiency virus that is responsible for the acquired immunodeficiency syndrome (AIDS) leaves no characteristic alterations in the placenta. Hepatitis, Coxsackie virus infection, and other virus diseases cannot be reliably diagnosed histologically from placental material. Therefore these diseases cannot be ruled out by placental study alone. Cytomegalovirus (CMV) infection is perhaps the most common prenatal virus infection of relevance to cerebral palsy-type lesions. Significant damage to fetal brain and other organs occurs frequently, and the placenta may show characteristic alterations. These changes are often scattered in the placenta, sometimes affecting only a few

villi, and they may be difficult to find. Therefore several blocks of villous tissue should be prepared for histological study. It is probably best to obtain five blocks in order to optimally sample the suspect material. Of considerable importance are prenatal infections with herpes virus, as they may be responsible for porencephaly and neonatal death. It is commonly assumed that the infection is acquired only during the delivery process, and so cesarean section is often practiced when genital blisters exist. It is less well known that a number of cases have been described in which the infection was acquired *before* birth and where neonates had blisters from herpes simplex virus infection with positive cultures (see Chapter 20). These infants may progress to destructive encephalopathy; and when they come to autopsy, neither culture nor electron microscopy identifies the now vanished agent. For that reason, Schwartz and Caldwell (1991) proposed that in situ DNA hybridization studies be done on placental tissue for the correct diagnosis. Few absolutely specific placental changes of this virus infection exist, although Robb et al. (1986a,b) identified suggestive features. Premature infants delivered because of chorioamnionitis are often associated with decidual hemorrhage that clinically may give the appearance of an abruptio placentae. This hemorrhage, however, is usually due to bleeding from deciduitis at the placental margins and cannot be compared with the classical abruptio placentae seen with toxemia and trauma.

Villitis of unknown etiology (VUE) is a severe alteration of villi that includes infiltration with lymphocytes, macrophages, but only rarely plasma cells; it usually leads to destruction of villi. It may be indistinguishable from CMV-induced villitis. Considerable experience may be required to differentiate the two, and it is occasionally impossible without the use of CMV probes. VUE definitely reduces the area of placental exchange and is also often associated with fetal death and with growth retardation. The etiology of VUE is unknown at this time, but the dire significance of the entity cannot be in doubt. There are, however, also cases of villitis of unknown etiology that have no apparent effect on fetal development. VUE has a tendency to recur in future pregnancies. Evaluation of the significance of finding VUE in the placenta of a retarded child may be difficult, and it requires much experience with placental study.

Green Placenta

The presence of meconium at birth was a frequent reason for alleging that birth was delayed or inappropriately handled in the British examination of obstetrical malpractice claims (Capstick & Edwards, 1990). They doubted that preventive measures could avoid the alleged accidents and recommended that attention be paid to the immediate handling of incidents. Interestingly, meconium staining of the placental surface is not only a frequent finding in mature placentas, it is usually not associated with fetal distress or cerebral palsy. In our experience, meconium staining/discharge occurs in about 17% of births, most often after 40 weeks' gestation. Almost all are normal. One should bear in mind that when a meconium-stained placenta has been standing unrefrigerated for many hours some of the meconium pigment may actually travel slightly into the amnion and perhaps minimally discolor the chorion as well. Usually, however, it is then also associated with some autolysis of tissues and is thus recognizable as having been artifactually caused. Refrigeration minimizes this problem. Because of the nature of the hormonal control of the intestinal propulsion, meconium staining is more common in postmature organs and is rare in immature placentas. Some of the legal guidelines pertaining to meconium staining have been examined by Sepkowitz (1987). In his 8-year experience, 4.3% of newborns (1,368) were meconium-stained. His further data suggested that, because of legal negotiations, from 1982 to 1985 there was a marked increase in the reported incidence (14.4%) of meconium staining. Therapeutic measures such as laryngoscopy and oxygen administration to the neonate were increased as a consequence of these interventions, but they did not guarantee an overall improvement of the neonatal outcome. The author concluded that, "while the issuance of medical guidelines alone had little effect on the incidence and care of the meconium-stained newborn, the combination of the legal imperative with medical guidelines had a profound and corruptive effect."

Prolonged pregnancy is significantly correlated with meconium discharge, as are the complications from its aspiration and other hazards of prolonged pregnancy (Arias, 1987). The results of Arias' study suggested that "the increased incidence of complications in pregnancy prolonged beyond 40 weeks cannot be adequately predicted with antepartum electronic monitoring and ultrasound evaluation of fetal size, placental grade, and amniotic fluid volume." It is also noteworthy that not all meconium-stained placentas are accompanied by fetal meconium aspiration (Altshuler & Herman, 1989). Sunoo and his colleagues (1989) clearly identified that meconium discharge and aspiration may occur *before* labor and without evidence of fetal distress. They made a detailed study of 75 cases of meconium aspiration (among 14,527 deliveries) and identified four infants in whom the aspiration occurred during early labor and in whom it was accompanied by normal fetal heart tracings. Postmaturity in itself is also often a reason for litigation when it is associated with cerebral palsied offspring. Whether these events are truly related remains to be established. The oligohydramnios and meconium discharge that so often occur after 40 weeks' gestation are often considered to be signs of "placental insufficiency," a concept espoused by Vorherr (1975). We have not been impressed that good evidence for placental dysfunction has been identified, and Naeye (1978) agreed with this notion. Thus a definitive deleterious influence of postmaturity on placental growth and function has yet to be established.

When a placenta from a premature infant has a green surface, one must consider the possibility that this discoloration is not due to meconium but represents hemosiderin and related pigments. Hemosiderin deposits most frequently accompany the peripheral hemorrhages of circumvallate placentas, although retromembranous hematomas, thromboses, marginal hemorrhage, and fetal hemolysis can cause hemosiderin deposits on the placental surface owing to hemolysis. An iron stain of the placenta quickly reveals the nature of the pigment when doubt exists. Other discolorations, from brown to green, may be the result of other insults (e.g., infection with fusobacteria). The nature of those pigments is not always understood. Finally, it must be cautioned that the bilirubin pigment of meconium-laden macrophages may bleach when slides lie in sunlight.

Because meconium is gradually processed in macrophages, moving from the amnionic surface toward the chorion, a rough estimate of the minimum time elapsed between discharge and delivery may be available from microscopic examination of the placental surface; or when the amnion is stripped and the underlying chorion is examined and found to be green at gross examination, an approximate time frame is indicated by the depth of staining. It must be emphasized, however, that this evaluation is subject to a few errors that must be borne in mind when, as occurs frequently when giving testimony, one is asked about the probability for the meconium to have been discharged at such or such a time. In our estimation these parameters are not decisive when trying to understand cerebral palsy; rather, it may be the consequences of meconium discharge that are relevant. Furthermore, meconium may have been discharged days before delivery, and most of it may already have been transported away from the fetal surface when the placenta becomes available for study. It is also probable that repeated meconium discharge can occur in utero, which would be difficult to discern from placental examination. Thus a time estimate based on the only in vitro study of meconium transport may be misleading (Miller et al., 1985), although it is the best estimate we have at present. It is our opinion that the legal profession is overemphasizing the importance of meconium discharge without appreciating the complexity of this process and the complex etiology of spastic quadriplegia and other features of cerebral palsy. At the same time, when a damaged infant, even a stillborn, is under consideration and its birth had not been accompanied by meconium discharge, the question why this dead baby was *not* meconium-stained is never asked. Interestingly, most stillbirths we see have no meconium staining, even though ultimately anoxia was the cause of their death.

Meconium may be otherwise injurious to the fetal well-being, in part because of its effect on the umbilical circulation. It also causes severe degenerative changes in the vascular walls of the placenta and cord, as it does in the amnionic epithelium. Some evidence now exists to show that vasoconstriction is a consequence of meconium exposure rather than its cause (Altshuler & Hyde, 1989). Thus although meconium discharge has become the "red flag" in legal cases—in which it is usually suggested that the passage of meconium alone must be evidence of fetal distress—it is more likely that it is the meconium that damages the fetus by acting as a vasoconstrictive agent on the umbilical vein and superficial placental vessels. In so doing it perhaps reduces the venous return of oxygenated blood from the placenta; of course, there could also be constriction of arteries with reduced blood flow to the placenta. These avenues are now being explored experimentally; the courtroom, however, treats as given facts the association of meconium and cerebral palsy as being causally related, which is unjust in our opinion. Similar suggestions of umbilical cord vessel constriction by bacterial products in the amnionic sac infection syndrome have come from experimental studies by Hyde et al. (1989). Finally, we speculate that the real damage of the meconium aspiration syndrome of neonates may be a chemical injury to the alveolar epithelium, similar to its effect on amnion and cord vessels.

Vascular Abnormalities

Abnormalities of the umbilical cord and placental surface vessels are important findings during placental examinations. It has long become obvious that it is important to record the absence of one umbilical artery, as this frequent finding correlates well with a variety of fetal congenital anomalies and with growth retardation. It is particularly important also to look for thromboses in the fetal surface vessels of every placenta. Most surface vascular thrombi are evident macroscopically by the yellow-white streak that accompanies a chorionic vessel. Thrombi are more difficult to spot in the umbilical cord unless the cord is routinely sectioned in areas of discoloration that were not caused by clamping. Thromboses have many causes. They develop usually over a long period, although we have seen fresh, occlusive thrombi in cases of recent cord entanglement with stillbirth. The thrombi definitely point to significant prenatal fetal problems. We find thrombi most frequently associated with excessively long and heavily spiraled umbilical cords, in association with maternal lupus anticoagulant and with infections. Cytomegalovirus infection also has a propensity to affect the endothelium and to produce thrombi. Thrombosis of surface vessels may be a feature of diabetes complicating pregnancy, of toxoplasmosis, and of banal but severe chorioamnionitis, where one often finds mural thrombi and occasionally organized thrombi, the so-called cushions. We have reported that thrombi may embolize to the fetus and there they may cause infarcts. However, unless such an infant comes to autopsy, embolic sequelae are usually not evident.

Complete vascular obliteration, of course, leads to atrophy of the villous district subserved by the vessel. It is the frequent cause of avascular, apparently hyalinized villi, which may thus reduce the quantity of available "exchange membrane"; for this reason, chronic thrombosis correlates with growth retardation and hypoxia. Some fetal thrombi are found in association with maternal lupus anticoagulant, a condition that must be actively investigated, as it may produce few maternal symptoms. There are additionally many placentas with, at times, extensive thrombosis in which the etiology of the thrombi remains obscure. This is particularly true for the arterial thrombi. For the purpose of legal adjudication, it is important to recognize this point and to acknowledge that thrombosis is a long-standing event and that it can usually not be anticipated before birth. We have seen a child with cerebral palsy in which one umbilical artery was nearly completely occluded by an inflammatory thrombus. The pregnancy was not complicated in any way, and upon arrival at the hospital a cesarean section was performed immediately for fetal distress. Despite this knowledge the jury was led to believe that this tragedy could have been averted by better prenatal care.

Umbilical Cord

Aside from the cord accidents that occur with mono-amnionic twins, the cord displays lesions that often have a significant impact on fetal well-being. Green discoloration of the entire Wharton's jelly can be observed only macroscopically, as the relatively small number of cord macrophages in the umbilical cord does not stain prominently. The cord is also often discolored from hemolysis, especially when thrombi are present or when prenatal bleeding has occurred. At the site where the cord has been clamped, of course, hemorrhage is frequent, but it can be distinguished from spontaneous hemorrhage by the marks of the serrated clamps that are left embedded on the cord's surface. We have seen in a child with cerebral palsy that a true cord hematoma had histological features of an angioma, presumably secondary to its "organization." The mother had been traumatized during pregnancy. The surface of the cord may have tiny granular protuberances from candidal infection. The compression from knots or prolapsed cords may be seen. When it is present, there may be marked distension of blood vessels on one side but not the other, betraying the prenatal compromise of the circulation. Edematous cords occur in edematous and immature infants, whereas thin cords often accompany growth-retarded infants. Angiomas are rare, but when present they are of great significance. Usually the cord is spiraled. When the twists are especially numerous, the cord is also usually excessively long. That such excessive spiralling can lead to fetal death is not in doubt. Indeed, the remarkable twisting on the fetus' abdominal surface in some abortuses testifies to this lethal effect of twists. More problematical is the chronic effect that may ensue from excessive cord twists. They are often associated with fetal surface vessel (venous) thrombi, and reduced venous return (with oxygenated blood) from the placenta can be deduced. Future Doppler velocimetry and cordocentesis observations will have to clarify the hemodynamic aspects of cord twists.

Placental Villous Color

Aside from the meconium staining of the fetal surface, the color of the villous tissue is an important notation at placental delivery, especially in problematical cases.

The villous tissue is red because of its fetal hemoglobin content. Placentas of diabetic mothers are darker because of fetal plethora, and those of immature infants are lighter. Once a number of normal placentas has been examined with this fact in mind, the observer should be able to identify those placentas that are unusually light-colored. They may be from infants with hydrops, but more often they are associated with infants who had a fetomaternal hemorrhage. In that case, immediate Kleihauer stains on maternal blood are mandatory. This test is important so one may estimate the amount of fetal blood loss; it also provides information needed for the therapeutic transfusion that may have to be instituted.

In hydropic infants the cause of hydrops should be studied as well as possible. The protocol includes mandatory examination of the Rh status plus a search for nucleated red blood cells, parvovirus inclusions in red blood cell precursors, and the existence of other fetal infections (e.g., cytomegalovirus). There are many other causes of anemia and hydrops. For instance, cardiac arrhythmias often produce hydrops that the pathologist cannot detect at autopsy. These causes are detailed in Chapter 16. Here it is important to stress that the appreciation of an unusually light-colored placenta has relevance for legal purposes as well. Occasional hydropic infants are the result of high-output cardiac failure of the fetus that results from large placental chorioangiomas. They are readily apparent when the placenta is palpated and then sectioned. Neonatal anemia, of course, is obvious when a low hemoglobin value is found at neonatal examination. The adjustment of the fetal hematocrit may take some time after fetal blood loss, but we have only the most superficial knowledge of how quickly the hematocrit adjusts after fetal bleeding—information that would be useful for adjudicating the timing of fetal hemorrhage.

In patients with hepatitis and jaundice, the villous tissue may be a deep golden color, which is often difficult to visualize microscopically and is thus an important macroscopic descriptor. This discoloration also tends to bleach on the slides owing to office lighting alone.

The maternal surface may be yellow and firmer than normal in a condition known as *maternal floor infarction*. This condition is strongly correlated with diffuse fibrin deposition throughout the placenta and with fetal growth retardation. Some observers have suggested that increased fibrin deposition confirms the diagnosis of prolonged placental perfusion problems; however, the maternal floor infarction syndrome has an unknown etiology, although it is a frequent cause of stillbirth. Appropriate histological study verifies the existence of this condition. Such excessive fibrin deposits are frequently a repetitive event during subsequent pregnancies. Contrary to opinions expressed in the literature, this condition is not caused by fetal death.

Color changes on the maternal surface and behind the membranes may disclose an unrecognized *abruptio placentae*. Most cases of placental separation are clinically silent and can be observed only when the maternal surface is carefully scrutinized. A fresh retroplacental hematoma with indentation of the villous tissue is obvious. The clot may have dried (in contrast to the "currant jelly" clot of normal retroplacental blood), and it may be stringy and compacted. When placental separation is focal and occurred long before delivery, the clot may have largely disappeared, or it is replaced by a brown, filmy material. Still older clots leave a greenish (hemosiderin) residue.

Infarcts at the edge of the placenta are common; and when small, they are of little significance. Their age can be approximated from their initially red, then yellow, and eventually white color. Infarcts that are scattered throughout the placenta, however, signify maternal disease of some sort. This finding assumes particular importance in prematurely delivered infants, in whom infarcts are generally rare. Most commonly, the cause of such infarcts is preeclampsia, but the lesions due to lupus anticoagulant have a similar appearance; and when infarcts are found in the absence of signs of pregnancy toxemia, their cause requires further study. Moreover, for understanding the fetal impact of infarcts, it is probably beneficial that a percentage estimate of the amount of infarcted villous tissue be recorded. Altshuler suggested that most infarcts are not associated with fetal CNS changes (Altshuler & Herman, 1989).

Choriangiosis, on the other hand, is correlated with prolonged fetal oxygen deprivation. It is a highly abnormal condition that must be recognized as being associated with many perinatal problems. Although minor forms of choriangiosis are reasonably common, its value for our understanding fetal/placental/maternal relations has so far been underestimated. Altshuler (1984, 1993a,b) found choriangiosis in about 5% of neonates admitted to his intensive care unit—much more commonly than occurs in "routine" placentas. It is never found in normal cases. He made the point that choriangiosis is significantly different from congestion and that it probably relates to chronic low grade hypoxia. That suggestion is supported by the finding of choriangiosis in women gestating at high altitude. Choriangiosis if often seen with villitis of unknown etiology (VUE), and we find it peripheral to atrophying villi when old vascular thrombi have occluded the fetal vascular bed. There are other correlations to fetal death, diabetes, umbilical cord problems, and so on. The recognition of choriangiosis is an important feature of placental study. Whether "grading" the degree of choriangiosis as promoted by Altshuler (1984) is truly

helpful remains to be confirmed by new studies. Scheffen et al. (1990) provided beautiful evidence of the capillary adaptation in the guinea pig placenta following long-standing hypoxia. Although this system may differ from the histology of human adaptation processes, the underlying mechanism is the same and confirms the clinical findings. Other adaptations to low oxygen saturation were discussed in the context of preeclampsia in Chapter 19, including cytotrophoblast proliferation with syncytial excess, reduction of villous length, and the possible mediation of these processes through cytokines.

Other Types of Pathology

The fetal circulation of the placenta normally contains very few nucleated red blood cells (NRBCs). When they are found in sections of the placenta, the pathologist must seek an explanation for their presence. It may be obvious from hematological study that there is evidence of hemolytic disease or that transplacental bleeding or chronic infection exists, but often the cause of an excessive number of NRBCs in the fetal vessels is not immediately evident. Fox (1967) suggested that NRBCs are often found in the fetal circulation because of acute hypoxia. Presumably, the human fetus reacts to oxygen deficiency, as it does to anemia, by secreting NRBCs from the hepatic or bone marrow stores. How acutely this reaction occurs and whether it is a quantitative response to certain levels of oxygen deprivation is unknown. The finding of NRBCs in the fetal vessels merely signals to the pathologist that a careful review of the record is needed to explain this important observation that may otherwise be overlooked. As stated, how quickly such a response occurs is unknown, for which reason Shields et al. (1993) attempted to elucidate the blood replacement by experimental hemorrhage in ovine fetuses. Despite an initial increase in fetal erythropoietin (EPO) levels, a significant hemorrhage (40%) was not followed by a significant rise in the fetal reticulocyte count, nor were the former blood volume and hematocrit restored before birth. Thus the ovine model may not be appropriate to settle this important question. Older studies have suggested that sheep fetuses marshal some response; the current understanding of all of these aspects are discussed in admirable detail in Altshuler's review (1993a). It cites the study by Ruth et al. (1988), which determined the EPO levels at birth in preeclamptic pregnancies and those with severe asphyxia. EPO levels were elevated in most pregnancy-induced hypertension (PIH)-derived neonates, irrespective of CNS damage; the significant finding was the marked elevation of EPO levels in those infants who ultimately had CNS damage, but not others. We can relate two experiences from our files that help in understanding the time course in human fetuses to some extent: One patient was at term and had a major "gush of bright red blood" (later identified as fetal blood from disrupted velamentous vessels) upon insertion of an intrauterine pressure catheter. She was delivered by cesarean section 48 minutes later; the infant was pale, but the placenta otherwise entirely normal. The cord arterial pH was 7.05, hemoglobin 14.6 g/dl, hematocrit 44.8%, white blood cell count (WBC), 28,000/mm³, platelets 120,000/mm³ falling to 71,000/mm³. Three transfusions of packed red blood cells were given and the hemoglobin level was then only 10.3 g/dl and the hematocrit 29.9%. The first enumeration of NRBCs occurred 1.5 hours after delivery and showed 19 NRBCs/100 WBCs; 6 hours later it was 32 NRBCs/100 WBCs. Thus there was a continued hematological response after the delivery of the anemic child, and some degree of an initial NRBC response was detectable within an hour. This finding is contrary to the rapid decline of NRBCs postnatally when the hypoxic event has been more remote; under those circumstances most NRBCs have disappeared by the second day. Another case that is relevant came as a consultation: The mother had had a car accident with lap belt injury at 28 weeks' pregnancy. Approximately 12 hours later the fetus was born with a hematocrit of 25%. Kleihauer stains gave an estimated 40 to 50 ml fetal blood in the maternal circulation; 45 NRBCs/100 WBCs were found, and there was villous edema. It is entirely possible that acute blood loss as shown in these two cases initiates a stronger response than gradual hypoxia, which is consistent with Altshuler's (1993b) remark that "acute fetal blood loss and congenital septic hemolysis reduce the time it takes fetal hypoxia to cause fetal erythropoiesis and increased nucleated red blood cells." In another child, the 102 cm long umbilical cord had prolapsed and was hemorrhagic for one-half of its length. The neonate had 53 NRBCs/ 100 WBCs, but the placenta showed chorangiosis and mural thrombi in large vessels. The latter observations indicate long-standing fetal hypoxia, a more frequent finding in this complex situation that prevents adequate assessment of the temporal response of the fetal system. We do not know the complete answers to these questions at present and encourage colleagues to collect case material in order to gain a better understanding of the time course of the NRBC response. It should also be cautioned that fetal growth retardation is known to be associated with an increased number of NRBCs in their circulation (Nicolini et al., 1990). These authors deduced from the blood studies by cordocentesis that the only reasonable explanation for intrauterine growth retardation with the presence of NRBCs is long-standing hypoxia. Phelan et al. (1994) studied NRBCs in asphyxiated and normal neonates. They found that normal infants do not have NRBCs but that asphyxiated newborns have elevated counts. The most elevated NRBC counts were explicable only by assuming hypoxia to have occurred long before birth.

The pathologist is frequently asked to place a time frame for the lesion under discussion. He or she may be required to specify how quickly villi can become atrophic following thrombosis as well as the exact temporal evolution of thrombi. How long has a significant phlebitis been present, and is it correlated with the length of time from rupture of membranes? These and other probing questions are often difficult to adjudicate, and the answers (with respect to best medical judgment) may present problems for a conscientious witness. It requires experience, and it may be better to state the lack of our knowledge than to express unwarranted opinions that are contradicted in the courtroom or by other experts. This uncertainty is an indication for the pathologist to seek new information from appropriate cases in which clinical data corroborate a particular finding. It is the reason why the meticulous study of twin placentas can be so useful, as it often provides a "control," a fetus who has shared the same intrauterine environment as the case under litigation but who may be normal.

Another relevant feature found in the study of abnormal infants is villous "dysmaturity," the discrepancy of villous maturation with chronological age. It is not to say that this placenta is merely an immature one but, rather, that the placenta shows abnormalities, often irregularly distributed, such as an increase in fibrin, villous size and stromal cells, decreased syncytial knots, and frequently increased vascularity. Irregularly matured villi are frequent in placentas associated with a variety of chromosomal abnormalities, for instance. Similar villous changes are found with other placental disturbances, as shown in Figure 642, and they may be difficult to explain. In this case, they probably resulted from partial venous thrombosis of surface vessels (Figure 641) in a child whose outcome was cerebral palsy and who was involved in litigation. The ultimate "cause" of these lesions was not apparent, but it is clear that they were long-standing prenatal deviations from normal. Similar thromboses and degenerative changes may have taken place in the surviving fetus. We will never know. Tenney-Parker changes of villi (increased syncytial knotting) signify deficient uteroplacental blood flow of some duration, and focal villous edema may be associated with premature delivery and neonatal hypoxia. These notations are all microscopic findings that cannot be anticipated macroscopically. Their frequent presence with abnormal fetal outcomes signifies the importance of placental examination by a competent pathologist and knowledge of the spectrum of what is "normal."

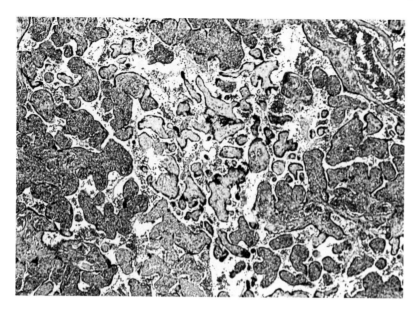

Figure 642. Irregular villous maturation and adjacent chorangiosis of the placenta in the cerebral palsy case shown in Figure 641. The vascularity of the central group of villi is apparent. It is presumed that this focal villous vascular loss is due to the same abnormality that was responsible for the mural thrombus. H&E. ×60.

It may be pertinent to review the presence of villous edema in this context. Edema of villi has been associated with poor fetal outcome and has also played a role in the litigation process. Naeye et al. (1983) noted that villous edema was frequent and severe in the immature placentas (more than 32 weeks) of pregnancy complications. It was believed to correlate with fetal hypoxia, and the authors postulated that the hypoxia was the result of compression of fetal villous capillaries by edema. We find villous edema exceedingly difficult to quantitate, especially when the placenta has been stored and has lost some of its fluid. Moreover, many mildly hydropic fetuses with marked villous edema have not had a hypoxic deficit due to compression of villous vessels, making us uneasy about using this criterion for our evaluation of abnormal placentas. No additional studies of this topic were published until the report by Shen-Schwarz et al. (1989). These investigators found villous edema in 13% of singleton placentas during the second half of pregnancy. In 11% of *term* placentas, edema was associated with fetal and neonatal deaths. They also detected edema more often in prematurely delivered placentas but were unable to relate villous edema to chorioamnionitis. Altshuler (1993a,b) was also uncertain that villous edema was a cause of fetal hypoxia, as resulting from compressing the villous capillaries. Further studies are needed to clarify the importance of villous edema as a correlate of fetal well-being and to delineate its precise pathogenesis.

References

Altshuler, G.: Chorangiosis: an important placental sign of neonatal morbidity and mortality. Arch. Pathol. Lab. Med. 108:71–74, 1984.

Altshuler, G.: A conceptual approach to placental pathology and pregnancy outcome. Semin. Diagn. Pathol. 10:204–221, 1993a.

Altshuler, G.: Some placental considerations related to neurodevelopmental and other disorders. J. Child Neurol. 8:78–94, 1993b.

Altshuler, G., and Herman, A.: The medicolegal imperative: placental pathology and epidemiology. In, Fetal and Neonatal Brain Injury: Mechanisms, Management and the Risk of Malpractice. D.K. Stevenson and P. Sunshine, eds., pp. 250–263. B.C. Decker, Toronto, 1989.

Altshuler, G., and Hyde, S.: Meconium induced vasoconstriction: a potential cause of cerebral and other fetal hypoperfusion and of poor pregnancy outcome. Child Neurol. 4:137–142, 1989.

Anonymous: Cerebral palsy, intrapartum care, and a shot in the foot. Lancet 2:1251–1252, 1989.

Arias, F.: Predictability of complications associated with prolongation of pregnancy. Obstet. Gynecol. 70:101–106, 1987.

Aylward, G.P., Verhulst, S.J., and Bell, S.: Correlation of asphyxia and other risk factors with outcome: a contemporary view. Dev. Med. Child Neurol. 31:329–340, 1989.

Baldwin, V.J.: Pathology of Multiple Pregnancy. Springer-Verlag, New York, 1994.

Bejar, R., Vigliocco, G., Gramajo, H., Solana, C., Benirschke, K., Berry, C., Coen, R., and Resnik, R.:

Antenatal origin of neurologic damage in newborn infants. Part II. Multiple gestations. Am. J. Obstet. Gynecol. 162: 1230–1236, 1990.

Benirschke, K.: Intrauterine death of a twin: Mechanisms, implications for surviving twin, and placental pathology. Semin. Diagn. Pathol. 10:222–231, 1993.

Capstick, J.B., and Edwards, P.J.: Trends in obstetric malpractice claims. Lancet 336:931–932, 1990.

Davies, B.R., and Arroyo, P.: The importance of primary diagnosis in perinatal death. Am. J. Obstet. Gynecol. 152:17–23, 1985.

De Sa, D.J.: Diseases of the umbilical cord. In, Pathology of the Placenta. E.V.D.K. Perrin, ed. Churchill Livingstone, New York, 1984.

Driscoll, S.G.: Pathology and the developing fetus. Pediatr. Clin. North Am. 12:493–514, 1965.

Durant, R.H., and Woodward, C.: Antenatal hypoxia and IQ values. Am. J. Dis. Child. 141:1150–1151, 1987.

Fleischer, L.D.: Wrongful births: when is there liability for prenatal injury? Am. J. Dis. Child. 141:1260–1265, 1987.

Fox, H.: The incidence and significance of nucleated erythrocytes in the foetal vessels of the mature human placenta. J. Obstet. Gynaecol. Br. Commonw. 74:40–43, 1967.

Freeman, R.: Intrapartum fetal monitoring—a disappointing story. N. Engl. J. Med. 322:624–626, 1990.

Genest, D.R.: Estimating the time of death in stillborn fetuses. II. Histologic evaluation of the placenta; a study of 71 stillborns. Obstet. Gynecol. 80:585–592, 1992.

Gillan, J.E.: Perinatal placental pathology. Curr. Opin. Obstet. Gynecol. 4:286–294, 1992.

Grant, A., O'Brien, N., Joy, M.-T., Hennessy, E., and MacDonald, D.: Cerebral palsy among children born during the Dublin randomized trial of intrapartum monitoring. Lancet 2:1233–1235, 1989.

Harkavy, K.L.: Antenatal hypoxia and IQ values. Am. J. Dis. Child. 141:1150, 1987.

Hyde, S., Smotherman, J., Moore, J.I., and Altshuler, G.: A model of bacterially induced umbilical vein spasm, relevant to fetal hypoperfusion. Obstet. Gynecol. 73:966–970, 1989.

Kuban, K.C.K., and Leviton, A.: Cerebral palsy. N. Engl. J. Med. 330:188–195, 1994.

Larroche, J.-C.: Fetal encephalopathies of circulatory origin. Biol. Neonate 50:61–74, 1986.

Liu, S., Benirschke, K., Scioscia, A.L., and Mannino, F.L.: Intrauterine death in multiple gestation. Acta Genet. Med. Gemellol. 41:5–26, 1992.

Lopez-Zeno, J.A., Carlo, W.A., O'Grady, J.P., and Fanaroff, A.A.: Infant survival following delayed postmortem cesarean delivery. Obstet. Gynecol. 76:991–992, 1990.

Miller, P.W., Coen, R.W., and Benirschke, K.: Dating the time interval from meconium passage to birth. Obstet. Gynecol. 66:459–462, 1985.

Naeye, R.L.: Causes of perinatal mortality excess in prolonged gestations. Am. J. Epidemiol. 108:429–433, 1978.

Naeye, R.L.: Disorders of the Placenta, Fetus, and Neonate. Diagnosis and Clinical Significance. Mosby Year Book, St. Louis, 1992.

Naeye, R.L., and Peters, E.C.: Antenatal hypoxia and low IQ values. Am. J. Dis. Child. 141:50–54, 1987.

Naeye, R., Maisels, M.J., Lorenz, R.P., and Botti, J.J.: The clinical significance of placental villous oedema. Pediatrics 71:588–594, 1983.

Naeye, R.L., Peters, E.C., Bartholomew, M., and Landis, R.: Origins of cerebral palsy. Am. J. Dis. Child. 143:1154–1161, 1989.

Nelson, K.B., and Leviton, A.: How much of neonatal encephalopathy is due to birth asphyxia? Am. J. Dis. Child. 145:1325–1331, 1991.

Nicolini, U., Nicolaides, P., Fisk, N.M., Vaughan, J.I., Fusi, L., Gleeson, R., and Rodeck, C.H.: Limited role of fetal blood sampling in prediction of outcome in intrauterine growth retardation. Lancet 336:768–772, 1990.

Ornoy, A., Crone, K., and Altshuler, G.: Pathological features of the placenta in fetal death. Arch. Pathol. Lab. Med. 100:367–371, 1976.

Patten, R.M., Mack, L.A., Nyberg, D.A., and Filly, R.A.: Twin embolization syndrome: prenatal sonographic detection and significance. Radiology 173:685–689, 1989.

Perkins, R.P.: Perspectives on perinatal brain damage. Obstet. Gynecol. 69:807–819, 1987.

Phelan, J.P., Ahn, N.O., Korst, L., and Martin, G.I.: Nucleated red blood cells: a marker for fetal asphyxia. Am. J. Obstet. Gynecol. 170: SPO abstracts 49, 286, 1993.

Richards, B.C., and Thomasson, G.: Closed liability claims analysis and the medical record. Obstet. Gynecol. 80: 313–316, 1992.

Robb, J.A., Benirschke, K., and Barmeyer, R.: Intrauterine latent herpes simplex virus infection. I. Spontaneous abortion. Hum. Pathol. 17:1196–1209, 1986a.

Robb, J.A., Benirschke, K., Mannino, F., and Voland, J.: Intrauterine latent herpes simplex virus infection. II. Latent neonatal infection. Hum. Pathol. 17:1210–1217, 1986b.

Rosen, M.G., and Dickinson, J.C.: The incidence of cerebral palsy. Am. J. Obstet. Gynecol. 167:417–423, 1992.

Rosen, M.G., and Dickinson, J.C.: The paradox of electronic fetal monitoring: more data may not enable us to predict or prevent infant neurologic morbidity. Am. J. Obstet. Gynecol. 168:745–751, 1993.

Rosenblatt, R.A., and Hurst, A.: An analysis of closed obstetric malpractice claims. Obstet. Gynecol. 74:710–714, 1989 (75:471–472, 1990).

Ruth, V., Autti-Rämö, I., Granström, M.-J., Korkman, M., and Raivio, K.O.: Prediction of perinatal brain damage by cord plasma vasopressin, erythropoietin, and hypoxanthine values. J. Pediatr. 113:880–885, 1988.

Salafia, C.M., and Vintzileos, A.M.: Why all placentas should be examined by a pathologist in 1990. Am. J. Obstet. Gynecol. 163:1282–1293, 1990.

Sandmire, H.F.: Malpractice—the syndrome of the 80s. Obstet. Gynecol. 73:145–146, 1989.

Scheffen, I., Kaufmann, P., Philippens, L., Leiser, R., Geisen, C., and Mottaghy, K.: Alterations of the fetal capillary bed in the guinea pig placenta following long-term hypoxia. In, Oxygen Transport to Tissue XII. J. Piiper et al., eds. Plenum, New York, 1990.

Schwartz, D.A., and Caldwell, E.: Herpes simplex virus infection of the placenta: the role of molecular pathology in the diagnosis of viral infection of placenta-associated tissues. Arch. Pathol. Lab. Med. 115:1141–1144, 1991.

Sepkowitz, S.: Influence of the legal imperative and medical guidelines on the incidence and management of the meconium-stained newborn. Am. J. Dis. Child. 141:1124–1127, 1987.

Shen-Schwarz, S., Ruchelli, E., and Brown, D.: Villous oedema of the placenta: a clinicopathological study. Placenta 10:297–307, 1989.

Shields, L.E., Widness, J.A., and Brace, R.A.: Restoration of fetal red blood cells and plasma proteins after a moderately severe hemorrhage in the ovine fetus. Am. J. Obstet. Gynecol. 169:1472–1478, 1993.

Sunoo, C., Kosasa, T.S., and Hale, R.W.: Meconium aspiration syndrome without evidence of fetal distress in early labor before elective cesarean delivery. Obstet. Gynecol. 73:707–709, 1989.

Travers, H., and Schmidt, W.A.: College of American Pathologists Conference XIX on the Examination of the Placenta. Arch. Pathol. Lab. Med. 115:660–731, 1991 [composite of many articles by numerous authors].

Vorherr, H.: Placental insufficiency and postmaturity. Eur. J. Obstet. Gynecol. Reprod. Biol. 5:109–122, 1975.

Ward, C.J.: Analysis of 500 obstetric and gynecologic malpractice claims: causes and prevention. Am. J. Obstet. Gynecol. 165:298–306, 1991.

Weinstein, L: Malpractice—the syndrome of the 80s. Obstet. Gynecol. 72:130–135, 1988.

28
Glossary

This glossary is intended to trace the roots of the often confusing terms used in placental pathology and perinatal development. The accents are placed for pronunciation.

Gk. = Greek; L. = Latin; Fr. = French; OE = Old English; ME = Middle English.

Abrúptio (placéntae): detachment of placenta [L. *abrumpere* = to break away]

Acárdius: malformed twin without heart, invariably one of monozygotic twins [Gk. *a* = without, not + *kardia* = heart]

Adventítia: outer layer of vessel wall [L. *advenire* = to add]

Allántoïs (allantóic): designation of one type of placenta, because of its roots in other mammals; thin membrane between amnion and chorion [Gk. *allantos* = sausage]

Ámnion: thin membrane surrounding the fetus; lamb's caul [Gk. *amnos* = lamb] (*Note*: Because we use chorionic and not choriotic, it is here preferred to speak of amnionic, rather than amniotic, Hyrtl, 1880, explored the various terminology used to describe placental structures. He concluded that amnios and amnion were both correct. It was first used by Galen, referring to skin. The reference to lamb comes from Vesalius.)

Androgénesis: development of male gender [Gk. *andros* = man + *gennan* = produce]

Anídian monster: a hideous fetus with peculiar features; a form of acardiac twin [Gk. *an* = not + *idios* = peculiar + L. *monstrum*]

Artiodáctyla: order of mammals, the even-hoofed animals (e.g., cow, deer) [Gk. *artios* = even + *daktylos* = toe]

Báttledore (placenta): marginal insertion of cord [OE = flat, wooden paddle used in the game of battledore to hit the shuttlecock]

Blástocyst: early germinative vesicle [Gk. *blaste* = germ + *kystis* = vesicle]

Bosselátion: surface granulation of placenta [Fr. *bosseler* = to ornament with bosses; from *bosse* = knob]

Capillary: hair-fine blood vessel [L. *capilla* = hair]

Céllular: belonging to the cell [*L. cellula* = small cabin, cell]

Extracellular: outside the cell

Intercellular: between cells

Intracellular: within cells

Transcellular: across cells

Chiméra (chímerism): the composite of several genotypes [Gk. *chimaira* = a monstrous beast; in Greek mythology a monster made of the head of a lion, body of a goat, and tail of a dragon]

Chirálity: the quality of being chiral [Gk. *chiro* = the hand; a three-dimensional form, as a molecule, that cannot be superimposed on its mirror image]

Chorioangiópagus parasíticus: a fetus, connected by blood vessels to another fetus [Gk. *chorion* = "little gut" = outer membranes around embryo + *angeios* = vessel + *pagos* = something set or fixed; *para* = next to + *sitos* = food]

Chórion: outer membrane around embryo [Gk. *chorion* = little gue]. (According to Hyrtl, 1880, the term was also used by Galen as the outer shell of the membranes.)

   C. frondósum: the placenta proper [L. *frondosus* = richly covered with leaves, as in tree]

   C. laéve: the membranous portion of the chorionic sac [L. *levis* = smooth, without villi]

Chorionepithelióma: malignant tumor of trophoblast = chorioepithelioma or choriocarcinoma [Gk. *chorion* = "little gut" (outer membrane enclosing an embryo) + *epi* = on + *thele* = nipple + *oma* = turmor]

Circumvállate (placenta): an abnormal form of placenta with circumferential, old hemorrhages [L. *circum* + *vallare* = to wall around]

Cirsoid: aneurysmal dilatation of vessel [Gk. *kirsos* = enlarged vein]

Cotylédon: originally name for the single spots of placental tissue in the ruminants; lobe of the human placenta [Gk. *kotyle* = cup]

Cytotrophoblast: cellular type of the trophoblast [Gk. *kytos* = cell + *trephein* = to nourish + *blaste* = germ]

Decídua: the endometrium at end of the luteal phase [L. *decidere* = fall, die]

   D. basalis: basal portion of placenta [Gk. *basis* = base]

   D. capsuláris: outer portion of membranes [L. *capsula* = little box]

D. parietális: endometrium of pregnancy, covering wall portion of uterus [L. *paries* = wall; *parietalis* = pertaining to wall]

D. véra: uterine decidua, contrasting it to pseudodecidua, outside of uterus, as in endometriosis [L. *verus* = true]

Désmosome: intercellular junction [Gk. *desmos* = ligament + *soma* = body]

Dizygótic: twins of two ova, "fraternal twins" [Gk. *dis* = twice, two + *zygon* = yoke]

Eclámpsia: coma and convulsive seizure during pregnancy [Gk. *eklampsis* = shining forth; or *ek* = out + *lampein* = to shine]

Émbryoblast: embryo-forming cells of the blastocyst [Gk. *embryon* = unborn child + *blaste* = germ]

Endométrium: innermost layer of the uterus [Gk. *endon* = inside + *metra* = uterus]

Endoplásmic reticulum: a net-like, membrane-lined cell organelle (Gk, *endon* = inside + *plasma* = juice; L. *reticulum* = small net]

Endothélium: innermost layer of blood vessels [Gk. *endon* = inside + *thele* = mamilla]

Epígnathus: tumorous mass in mouth, affixed to jaw, and possibly a twin [Gk. *epi* = upon, at, over + *gnathos* = jaw]

Epithelium: superficial cellular layer [Gk. *epi* = upon + *thele* = mamilla]

Fétus papyráceus: paper-like, macerated, compressed ("compressus") fetus [L. *papyrus* = plant from which paper is made]

Fíbrin: blood clot product [L. *fibra* = fiber]

Fíbrinoid: a substance similar to but not identical with fibrin [Gk. *-eides* = looking like]

Fíbroblast: connective tissue cell [Gk. *blaste* = germ]

Freemártin: the female of fraternal cattle twins, sterilized in utero by the male co-twin with whose placental vessels she is joined (The term presumably comes from the St. Martin's feast in England, when these animals were consumed.)

Funiculópagous (twins): twins joined at umbilical cord [L. *funis* = rope, cord + Gk. *pagos* = fixed]

Fúnis (funículus): umbilical cord (L. *funis* = rope, cord]

Funisítis: inflammation of umbilical cord [L. *funis* = rope]

Fúrcate (cord) ("insértio funículi furcáta"): forked insertion of the little rope [L. *furca* = fork]

Glycocálix: superficial layer of polysaccharides, covering the cell surface [Gk. *glycos* = sweet + *kalyx* = goblet]

Granulomatósis infantiséptica: neonatal disseminated listeriosis [L. *granulum* = little grain + Gk. *oma* = tumor]

Gynogénesis: female development [Gk. *gyne* = woman + *gennan* = produce]

Hemiacárdius: acardiac monster in which remnants of heart may be found [L. *hemi* = a half]

Holoacárdius: completely heartless monster (twin) [Gk. *Holos* = whole]

Hydatídiform (mole): severely hydropic placenta with bulbous, villous enlargement [Gk. *hydatis* = watery vesicle + L. *forma* = shape; L. *mola* = false conception]

Hydrámnios: excessive amount of amnionic fluid [Gk. *hydor* = water (*hydros* = sweat; some early authors believed that amnionic fluid was fetal sweat) + *amnion* = lamb's caul]

Implantátion: establishing of intimate fetomaternal contact in the uterus [L. *implantare* = to embed]

Intervíllous: between the placental villi (i.e., in the maternal blood space) [L. *inter* = between]

Intravíllous: within a villus [L. *intra* = in]

Lacúna: [L. = hole, gap]

Lithopédion: stone-like fetus [Gk. *lithos* = stone + *paidion* = child]

Lóchia (pl.): uterine discharges after birth [Gk. *lochia*]

Mácrophage: phagocytotic and paracrine cell type [Gk. *macros* = large + *phagein* = to eat]

Mágma reticuláre: jelly-like fluid in original embryonic sac [Gk. *magma* = suspension of finely divided material in small amount of water + L. *reticulum* = little net (network)]

Mármoset: family of small South American primates that always produce fraternal twins [Old, Fr. *marmouset* = grotesque figure]

Mecónium: fetal intestinal content [Gk. *mekonion* = poppy juice]

Mésenchyme: undifferentiated connective tissue [Gk. *mesos* = in the middle of + *chein* = to pour (something poured in between)]

Mésoderm: the middle germ layer [Gk. *derma* = skin]

Mésothelium: connective tissue-derived epithelial layer [Gk. *thele* = mamilla]

Microvíllus: finger-like extension of the cell surface.

Mitochóndrion: rod-shaped cell organelle [Gk. *mitos* = thread + *chondros* = grain]

Mole (hydatidiform, Breus'): vesicular mass of placenta [L. *mola* = false conception]

Monozygótic: single-egg-derived twins ("identical twins") [Gk. *monos* = single + *zygotos* = yoked]

Nódus spúrius vasculósus (gelatínus): false knot in umbilical cord of vascular genesis [L. *nodus* = knot + *spurius* = not genuine + *gelatina* = gelatin]

Núchal (cord): umbilical cord entwined around neck [L. *nucha* = nape of the neck]

Óctoploid: having eight sets of chromosomes [Gk. *okto* = eight + *ploos* = fold + *eidos* = form]

Oligohydrámnios: too little, or no, amnionic fluid [Gk. *oligos* = little + *hydor* = water (*hydros* = sweat) + *amnion* = lamb caul]

Ómphalo- (mesentéric): umbilicus [Gk. *omphalos* = navel]

Páraplacénta: those parts of the chorionic sac, not belonging to the placenta (e.g., membranes) [Gk. *para* = beside]

Périvillous: around the placental villi [Gk. *peri* = around]

Placénta: [L. flat cake](According to Hyrtl, 1880, this term, with an originally Greek root, was introduced in 1559 by Realdus Columbus. Others referred to it as secundines.)

P. accréta: unusually adherent placenta that fails to detach [L. *accrescere* = to grow together, adhere]

P. incréta: placenta that has grown into the myometrium [L. *increscere* = to grow into]

P. membranácea: thin placental membrane, the entire outside of which is covered with villi [L. *membrana* = from parchment, membrane]

P. percréta: placenta that has grown through the uterine wall [L. *percrebescrere* = to crowd everywhere]

P. prévia: placenta that is located in the lower uterus and is in the way before the fetus can be delivered [L. *praevius* = in front of, before, leading the way]

Plasmódium: multinucleate mass of protoplasm [Gk. *plasma* = a thing formed (juice) + *eidos* = to form]

Pólyploid: having many sets of chromosomes [Gk. *polys* = much, many + *ploos* = fold + *eidos* = form]

Pólypoid: protrusion of tissue, polyp [Gk. *polys* = many + *pous* = foot + *oid* = like]

Pyknósis: degenerative condensation of cells or nuclei [Gk. *pyknos* = dense]

Schístocytes: broken red blood cells in disseminated intravascular coagulation [Gk. *schistos* = split]

Secúndines: synonymous with afterbirth [L. *secundus* = following]

Sínusoid: enlarged capillary [L. *sinus* = bight + Gk. *eides* = looking like]

Siréniform (fétus): malformed infant with fused legs [Gk. *seiren* = mermaid]

Sirenomélia: malformed infant with fused legs [Gk. *seiren* = mermaid + *melos* = limb]

Stróma: connective tissue core of a organ [L. *stroma* = cushion]

Subchórial: under the chorionic plate [L. *sub* = below + Gk. *chorion* = leather, embryonic membrane]

Succentúriate (lobe): accessory lobe of placenta [L. *succenturiare* = to substitute]

Superfecundátion: fertilization of two or more ova at different times during the same menstrual period [L. *super* = beyond, excessively + *fecundus* = fertile]

Superfetátion: pregnancy on top of already existing pregnancy [L. *superfetare* = to bring forth while already pregnant; L. *fetus* = fruit, offspring]

Sympus: fetus with fused legs [Gk. *syn* = together + *pous* = foot (same as siren)]

Syncytiotrophoblast: syncytial type of trophoblast

Syncytium: multinuclear mass, derived from cell fusion [Gk. *syn* = together + *kytos* = cell]

Synéchia (pl. synéchiae): adhesion of parts, here in the uterus [Gk. *synecheia* = continuity]

Tessellátion: irregular surface of placenta [L. *tessella* = little square stone (from Gk. *tessares* = four)]

Tétraploid: having four sets of chromosomes [Gk. *tettares* = four + *ploos* = fold]

Thalassémias: hemoglobin disorders [from Gk. *thalassa* = the sea; generally referring to the Mediterranean]

Thixotrópic (thyxo-) gel: gel that liquefies when shaken, generally the extraembryonic fluid [Gk. *thixis* = touching + *trope* = turn]

Thoracopágus: twins, conjoined at chest [Gk. *thorax* = chest + *pagos* = fix]

Trabécula: small septum [L. small beam]

Tróphoblast: epithelium that covers the placenta [Gk. *trophe* = nourishment + *blastos* = germ]

Trophótropism: "wandering" of the placenta to the site of best nourishment [Gk. *trophe* = nourishment + *trope* = turn]

Urachus: connection of bladder to allantoic sac [Gk. *ourachos* ("that which has a tail") = cord that extends from bladder to navel]

Vas prévium (pl. Vása prévia): blood vessels within membranes that present before fetal parts during delivery [L. *vas* = vessel(s) that is (are) ahead ("previous") of fetal part]

Vas vasórum (vása vasórum): blood vessels that nourish the vessels [L. *vas* = vessel]

Velaméntous (cord insertion): membranous insertion of umbilical cord [L. *velamen* = veil + *velamentum* = cover]

Vérnix caseósa: sebum, hair, and other skin secretions from fetus [L. *vernix* = varnish + *caseus* = cheese]

Víllus (pl. vílli): ramifications of placenta with fetal vessels that are the "business end" of the placenta, covered with trophoblast [L. *villus* = tuft of hair]

Vitélline: belonging to the yolk sac [L. *vitellus* = yolk of an egg]

Bibilography

Haubrich, W.S.: Medical Meanings. A Glossary of Word Origins. Harcourt, Brace, Jovanovich, San Diego, 1984.

Hyrtl, J.: Onomatologia Anatomica. Braumüller, Vienna, 1880.

Thomas, C.L.: Taber's Cyclopedic Medical Dictionary. 15th Ed. Davis, Philadelphia, 1985.

Webster, D.: Webster's Unabridged Dictionary. Dorset & Baber, Cleveland, 1983.

Acknowledgment. We are grateful to Professor E.N. Genovese, San Diego State University, for his correcting the text.

Index